The Maud
Prescribin
in Psychia

Mersey Care NHS Trust
Service Governance Support Team

NHS

Mersey Care Knowledge and Library Service

Please return by date shown

30.05.17		

MCKLS, Mersey Care NHS Trust, Ashworth Library Indigo
Parkbourn Maghull Liverpool L31 1HW
. Tel: 0151 471 2431
E-mail: Ashworth.library@merseycare.nhs.uk

The Maudsley Prescribing Guidelines in Psychiatry

12th Edition

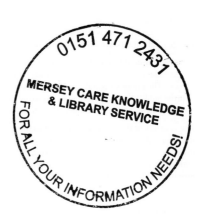

David Taylor

Director of Pharmacy and Pathology
South London and Maudsley NHS Foundation Trust
Professor of Psychopharmacology
King's College London, London, UK

Carol Paton

Chief Pharmacist
Oxleas NHS Foundation Trust
Joint Head of the Prescribing Observatory for Mental Health
Honorary Research Fellow, Imperial College London, London, UK

Shitij Kapur

Professor of Schizophrenia, Imaging and Therapeutics
Executive Dean and Head of Faculty, Institute of Psychiatry, Psychology and Neuroscience (IoPPN)
Deputy Vice Principal (Health Schools)
King's College London, London, UK

WILEY Blackwell

This edition first published 2015 © 2015 by David Taylor, Carol Paton and Shitij Kapur
Eleventh edition published 2012 © 2012 by David Taylor, Carol Paton and Shitij Kapur

Registered Office
John Wiley & Sons, Ltd, The Atrium, Southern Gate, Chichester, West Sussex, PO19 8SQ, UK

Editorial Offices
9600 Garsington Road, Oxford, OX4 2DQ, UK
The Atrium, Southern Gate, Chichester, West Sussex, PO19 8SQ, UK
111 River Street, Hoboken, NJ 07030-5774, USA

For details of our global editorial offices, for customer services and for information about how to apply for permission to reuse the copyright material in this book please see our website at www.wiley.com/wiley-blackwell

Library of Congress Cataloging-in-Publication Data

Taylor, David, 1946–, author.
  The Maudsley prescribing guidelines in psychiatry / David Taylor, Carol Paton, Shitij Kapur. – 12th edition.
    p. ; cm.
  Prescribing guidelines in psychiatry
  Includes bibliographical references and index.
  ISBN 978-1-118-75460-3 (pbk.)
  I. Paton, Carol, author.   II. Kapur, Shitij, author.   III. South London and Maudsley NHS Trust, issuing body.   IV. Title.   V. Title: Prescribing guidelines in psychiatry.
  [DNLM: 1. Mental Disorders–drug therapy–Great Britain.   2. Psychopharmacology–methods–Great Britain.   3. Psychotropic Drugs–administration & dosage–Great Britain.   4. Psychotropic Drugs–therapeutic use–Great Britain. WM 402]
  RC483
  616.89′18–dc23
                                    2014049389

A catalogue record for this book is available from the British Library.

Wiley also publishes its books in a variety of electronic formats. Some content that appears in print may not be available in electronic books.

Set in 10/12pt Sabon by SPi Publisher Services, Pondicherry, India
Printed and bound in Great Britain by TJ International Ltd.

1   2015

Contents

Preface

This 12th edition of *The Maudsley Prescribing Guidelines in Psychiatry* marks its 20th year in continuous production. Readers who have owned or used previous editions will find this edition no different in style from previous incarnations. This is deliberate – the feedback we receive suggests the organisation and structure are well liked. Each section of *The Guidelines* is a densely referenced but succinct review of the literature, set alongside some fairly broad recommendations for practice. Each of these sections has been updated and revised, and some new ones added (for example, interpreting clozapine plasma levels, post-mortem plasma levels, summary of depot pharmacokinetics). Much of the guidance provided in this edition has changed as a result of more recent research; some of it to a small extent, some of it to an extent amounting to a reversal of prior guidance (for example, on the use of fish oils in psychosis). These changes reflect the very nature of the scientific method – that hypotheses come and go as evidence mounts or is countered.

This edition of *The Guidelines* has a particularly international flavour. This is because the 11th edition sold more copies outside the UK than in it, and because there are, we think, at least ten translations of *The Guidelines* in existence. Although *The Guidelines* are still essentially our local guide to prescribing, we have made a special effort to widen, geographically speaking, its utility. This is most noticeable in the inclusion of drugs not licensed in the UK (e.g. ziprasidone, iloperidone, desvenlafaxine), but widely used in other countries. Readers should, therefore, not assume that every drug mentioned in *The Guidelines* is available in their own country. The reader should also be aware that no guideline could take account of every psychotropic drug used around the world, so omissions are inevitable.

As with previous editions, very special thanks are due to Maria O'Hagan who manages the writing and structuring of *The Guidelines*; an increasingly complex process given the size, complexity and heavily referenced nature of the current edition. Thanks are also due to the many expert contributors to *The Guidelines* who are listed overleaf, and to Adam Gilbert, our editor at Wiley.

David Taylor

Acknowledgements

We thank the following people for contributing their time and expertise to this 12th edition of *The Maudsley Prescribing Guidelines in Psychiatry.*

Adam Winstock
Adelaida Naumann-Sinden
Adrian Treloar
Allan Young
Andrea Danese
Anne Connolly
Argyris Stringaris
Ayesha Ali
Bimpe Idowu
Carmine Pariante
Celia Feetam
Cheryl Kipping
Daniel Harwood
Daniel Hayes
Dave Branford
David R. Coghill
Delia Bishara
Emily Finch
Eromona Whiskey
Faith Borgan
Fiona Gaughran
Flora Coker
Francis Keaney
Gay Sutherland
Georgina Boon
Gordana Milavic
Ifeoma Okonkwo
Irene Guerrini
James Bell

Jane Marshall
Jenny Bearn
Kalliopi Vallianatou
Katie Beck
Louise Howard
Marco Lyons
Marinos Kyriakopoulos
Maxine Patel
Michael Kelleher
Nada Zahreddine
Oliver Howes
Olubanke Olofinjana
Paul Gringras
Petrina Douglas-Hall
Rob McCutcheon
Robert Flanagan
Robert Howard
Robin Murray
Russell Foster
Sally Porter
Sarah Elliott
Seema Varma
Shubhra Mace
Siobhan Gee
Thomas Barnes
Tiago Marques
Tom Walker-Tilley
Tony Cleare
Vivienne Curtis

Notes on using *The Maudsley Prescribing Guidelines*

The main aim of *The Guidelines* is to provide clinicians with practical and useful advice on the prescribing of psychotropic agents in commonly encountered clinical situations. The advice contained in this handbook is based on a combination of literature review, clinical experience and expert contribution. We do not claim that this advice is necessarily 'correct' or that it deserves greater prominence than guidance provided by other professional bodies or special interest groups. We hope, however, to have provided guidance that helps to assure the safe, effective and economic use of medicines in psychiatry. We hope also to have made clear precisely the sources of information used to inform the guidance given.

Please note that many of the recommendations provided here go beyond the licensed or labelled indications of many drugs, both in the UK and elsewhere. Note also that, while we have endeavoured to make sure all quoted doses are correct, clinicians should always consult statutory texts before prescribing. Users of *The Guidelines* should also bear in mind that the contents of this handbook are based on information available to us in December 2014. Much of the advice contained here will become out-dated as more research is conducted and published.

No liability is accepted for any injury, loss or damage, however caused.

Notes on inclusion of drugs

The Guidelines are used in many other countries outside the UK. With this in mind, we have included in this edition those drugs in widespread use throughout the western world in December 2014. Thus, we have included, for example, ziprasidone and iloperidone, even though these drugs are not marketed in the UK at this time. Their inclusion gives *The Guidelines* relevance in those countries where ziprasidone and iloperidone are marketed, and may also be of benefit to UK readers, since many unlicensed drugs can be obtained through formal pharmaceutical importers. We have also tried to include information on drugs likely to be introduced into practice in the next two years. Many older drugs, or those not widely available (methotrimeprazine, pericyazine, maprotiline, zotepine, loxapine etc.), are either only briefly mentioned or not included on the basis that these drugs are not in widespread use at the time of writing.

List of abbreviations

AACAP	American Academy of Child and Adolescent Psychiatry	BPSD	behavioural and psychological symptoms of dementia
ACB	anticholinergic cognitive burden	BuChE	butyrylcholinesterase
ACE	angiotensin-converting enzyme	CAM	Confusion Assessment Method
ACh	acetylcholine	CAMS	Childhood Anxiety Multimodal Study
AChE	acetylcholinesterase		
ADAS-cog	Alzheimer's Disease Assessment Scale-cognitive subscale	CATIE	Clinical Antipsychotic Trials of Intervention Effectiveness
ADD	attention deficit disorder	CBT	cognitive behavioural therapy
ADH	alcohol dehydrogenase	CBZ	carbamazepine
ADHD	attention deficit hyperactivity disorder	CDRS	Children's Depression Rating Scale
		CES-D	Centre for Epidemiological Studies Depression scale
ADIS	Anxiety Disorders Interview Schedule		
ADL	activities of daily living	CGAS	Children's Global Assessment Scale
ALP	alkaline phosphatase	CGI	Clinical Global Impression scales
ALT	alanine transaminase/ aminotransferase	CIBIC-Plus	Clinician's Interview-Based Impression of Change
ANNSERS	Antipsychotic Non-Neurological Side-Effects Rating Scale	CIGH	clozapine-induced gastrointestinal hypomotility
APA	American Psychological Association	CIWA-Ar	Clinical Institute Withdrawal Assessment of Alcohol scale revised
ARB	angiotensin II receptor blocker		
ASD	autism spectrum disorders	CKD	chronic kidney disease
ASEX	Arizona Sexual Experience scale	CNS	central nervous system
AST	aspartate aminotransferase	COMT	catechol-O-methyltransferase
BAC	blood alcohol concentration	COPD	chronic obstructive pulmonary disease
BAD	bipolar affective disorder		
BAP	British Association for Psychopharmacology	COWS	Clinical Opiate Withdrawal Scale
		COX	cyclo-oxygenase
bd	*bis die* (twice a day)	CPP	child–parent psychotherapy
BDI	Beck Depression Inventory	CPSS	Child PTSD Symptom Scale
BDNF	brain-derived neurotrophic factor	CrCl	creatinine clearance
BED	binge eating disorder	CRP	C-reactive protein
BEN	benign ethnic neutropenia	CT	complementary therapy
BMI	body mass index	CUtLASS	Cost Utility of the Latest Antipsychotic Drugs in Schizophrenia Study
BP	blood pressure		
BPD	borderline personality disorder		

CVA	cerebrovascular accident	IM	intramuscular
CY-BOCS	Children's Yale-Brown Obsessive Compulsive Scale	IMHP	intramuscular high potency
		INR	international normalised ratio
CYP450	cytochrome P450	IR	immediate release
DAI	drug attitude inventory	IV	intravenous
DEXA	dual-energy X-ray absorptiometry	IVHP	intravenous high potency
DHEA	dehydroepiandrosterone	Kiddie-SADS	Kiddie-Schedule for Affective Disorders and Schizophrenia
DLB	dementia with Lewy bodies		
DMDD	disruptive mood dysregulation disorder	LAI	long-acting injection
		LDL	low-density lipoprotein
DVLA	Drivers and Vehicle Licensing Agency	LFT	liver function tests
EAD	early after depolarisation	MADRS	Montgomery-Asberg Depression Rating Scale
ECG	electrocardiogram		
ECT	electroconvulsive therapy	mane	morning
EEG	electroencephalogram	MAOI	monoamine oxidase inhibitor
eGFR	estimated glomerular filtration rate	MARS	Medication Adherence Rating Scale
EOSS	early-onset schizophrenia-spectrum		
EPA	eicosapentanoic acid	MASC	Multidimensional Anxiety Scale for Children
EPS	extrapyramidal side-effects		
ER	extended release	MCA	Mental Capacity Act
ERK	extracellular signal-regulated kinase	MCI	mild cognitive impairment
ES	effect size	MDRD	Modification of Diet in Renal Disease
ESR	erythrocyte sedimentation rate		
FBC	full blood count	MDT	multidisciplinary team
FDA	Food and Drug Administration (USA)	MHRA	Medicines and Healthcare Product and Regulatory Authority
FGA	first-generation antipsychotics		
FPG	fasting plasma glucose	MI	myocardial infarction
FTI	Fatal Toxicity Index	MMSE	Mini Mental State Examination
GABA	gamma-aminobutyric acid	MR	modified release
GASS	Glasgow Antipsychotic Side-effect Scale	MS	mood stabilisers
		MS	multiple sclerosis
GBL	gamma-butaryl-lactone	NAS	neonatal abstinence syndrome
G-CSF	granulocyte-colony stimulating factor	NICE	National Institute for Health and Clinical/Care Excellence
GFR	glomerular filtration rate		
GGT	gamma-glutamyl transferase	NMDA	N-methyl-D-aspartate
GHB	gamma-hydroxybutyrate	NMS	neuroleptic malignant syndrome
GI	gastrointestinal	NNH	number needed to harm
GM-CSF	granulocyte-macrophage colony-stimulating factor	NNT	number needed to treat
		nocte	at night
HADS	Hospital Anxiety and Depression Scale	NPI	neuropsychiatric inventory
		NRT	nicotine replacement therapy
HD	Huntington's disease	NSAID	non-steroidal anti-inflammatory drug
HDL	high-density lipoprotein		
HIV	human immune deficiency virus	NVC	neurovascular coupling
5-HMT	5-hydroxy-methyl-tolterodine	OCD	obsessive compulsive disorder
HPA	hypothalamic-pituitary-adrenal	od	*omni die* (once a day)
ICD	International Classification of Diseases	OD	overdose
		OGTT	oral glucose tolerance test
IG	intra-gastric	OOWS	Objective Opiate Withdrawal Scale
IJ	intra-jejunal	PA	pathologic aggression

PANDAS	Paediatric Autoimmune Neuropsychiatric Disorder Associated with Streptococcus	SAWS	Short Alcohol Withdrawal Scale
		SCARED	Screen for Child Anxiety and Related Emotional Disorders
PANSS	Positive and Negative Syndrome Scale	SGA	second-generation antipsychotics
		SIADH	syndrome of inappropriate antidiuretic hormone
PBA	pseudobulbar affect		
PDD	pervasive developmental disorders	SIB	severe impairment battery
PDD-NOS	pervasive developmental disorders-not otherwise specified	SJW	St John's wort
		SLE	systemic lupus erythematosus
P-gp	P-glycoprotein	SNRI	selective noradrenaline reuptake inhibitor
PHQ-9	Patient Health Questionnaire-9		
PICU	psychiatric intensive care unit	SOWS	Short Opiate Withdrawal Scale
PL	product licence	SPC	summary of product characteristics
PLC	pathological laughter and crying	SPECT	single photon emission computed tomography
PMR	post-mortem redistribution		
po	*per os* (by mouth)	SROM	slow release oral morphine
POMH-UK	Prescribing Observatory for Mental Health	SSRI	selective serotonin reuptake inhibitor
		STS	selegiline transdermal system
PPI	proton pump inhibitor	TADS	Treatment of Adolescents with Depression Study
prn	*pro re nata* (as required)		
PT	prothrombin time	TCA	tricyclic antidepressant
PTSD	post-traumatic stress disorder	TDM	therapeutic drug monitoring
qds	*quarter die sumendum* (four times a day)	tds	*ter die sumendum* (three times a day)
		TEAM	treatment of early age mania
RCADS	Revised Children's Anxiety and Depression Scale	TFT	thyroid function test
		TIA	transient ischaemic attack
RCT	randomised controlled trial	TMS	transcranial magnetic stimulation
RID	relative infant dose	TORDIA	Treatment of Resistant Depression in Adolescence
RLAI	risperidone long-acting injection		
ROMI	Rating of Medication Influences scale	TPR	temperature, pulse, respiration
		TS	Tourette's syndrome
RPG	random plasma glucose	TSH	thyroid stimulating hormone
RRBI	restricted repetitive behaviours and interests	U&E	urea and electrolytes
		UGT	UDP-glucuronosyl transferase
RT	rapid tranquillisation	VaD	vascular dementia
RTA	road traffic accident	VCFS	velo-cardio-facial syndrome
rTMS	repetitive transcranial magnetic stimulation	VNS	vagal nerve stimulation
		VTE	venous thromboembolism
RUPP	Research Units on Paediatric Psychopharmacology	WBC	white blood cell
		WCC	white cell count
SADQ	Severity of Alcohol Dependence Questionnaire	WHO	World Health Organisation
		YMRS	Young Mania Rating Scale

Plasma level monitoring of psychotropic drugs

Plasma drug concentration or plasma 'level' monitoring is a process surrounded by some confusion and misunderstanding. Drug level monitoring, when appropriately used, is of considerable help in optimising treatment and assuring adherence. However, in psychiatry, as in other areas of medicine, plasma level determinations are frequently undertaken without good cause and results acted upon inappropriately.[1] Conversely, in other instances, plasma levels are underused.

Before taking a blood sample for plasma level assay, make sure that the following criteria are satisfied.

- **Is there a clinically useful assay method available?** Only a minority of drugs have available assays. The assay must be clinically validated and results available within a clinically useful timescale. Check with your local laboratory.
- **Is the drug at 'steady state'?** Plasma levels are usually meaningful only when samples are taken after steady-state levels have been achieved. This takes 4–5 drug half-lives. A clear exception to this advice is suspected overdose; in such situations attainment of steady state is of no relevance.
- **Is the timing of the sample correct?** Sampling time is vitally important for many but not all drugs. If the recommended sampling time is, say, 12 hours post dose, then the sample should be taken 11–13 hours post dose if possible; 10–14 hours post dose, if absolutely necessary. For trough or 'pre-dose' samples, take the blood sample immediately before the next dose is due. Do not, under any circumstances, withhold the next dose for more than 1 or (possibly) 2 hours until a sample is taken. Withholding for longer than this will inevitably give a misleading result (it will give a lower result than that ever seen in the usual, regular dosing), and this may lead to an inappropriate dose increase. Sampling time is less critical with drugs with a long half-life (e.g. olanzapine) but, as an absolute minimum, prescribers should always record the time of sampling and time of last dose. This cannot be emphasised enough.

The Maudsley Prescribing Guidelines in Psychiatry, Twelfth Edition. David Taylor, Carol Paton and Shitij Kapur.
© 2015 David Taylor, Carol Paton and Shitij Kapur. Published 2015 by John Wiley & Sons, Ltd.

- If a sample is not taken within 1–2 hours of the required time, it has the potential to mislead rather than inform. The only exception to this is if toxicity is suspected – sampling at the time of suspected toxicity is obviously appropriate.
- **Will the level have any inherent meaning?** Is there a target range of plasma levels? If so, then plasma levels (from samples taken at the right time) will usefully guide dosing. If there is not an accepted target range, plasma levels can only indicate adherence or potential toxicity. However, if the sample is being used to check compliance, then bear in mind that a plasma level of zero indicates only that the drug has not been taken in the past several days. Plasma levels above zero may indicate erratic compliance, full compliance or even long-standing non-compliance disguised by recent taking of prescribed doses. Note also that target ranges have their limitations: patients may respond to lower levels than the quoted range and tolerate levels above the range; also, ranges quoted by different laboratories vary sometimes widely, often without explanation.
- **Is there a clear reason for plasma level determination?** Only the following reasons are valid:
  - to confirm compliance (but see above)
  - if toxicity is suspected
  - if drug interaction is suspected
  - if clinical response is difficult to assess directly (and where a target range of plasma levels has been established)
  - if the drug has a narrow therapeutic index and toxicity concerns are considerable.

Interpreting sample results

The basic rule for sample level interpretation is to act upon assay results only in conjunction with reliable clinical observation (*'treat the patient, not the level'*). For example, if a patient is responding adequately to a drug but has a plasma level below the accepted target range, then the dose should not normally be increased. If a patient has intolerable adverse effects but a plasma level within the target range, then a dose decrease may be appropriate.

Where a plasma level result is substantially different from previous results, a repeat sample is usually advised. Check dose, timing of dose and recent compliance but ensure, in particular, the correct timing of the sample. Many anomalous results are the consequence of changes in sample timing.

Table 1.1 shows the target ranges for some commonly prescribed psychotropic drugs.

Amisulpride

Amisulpride plasma levels are closely related to dose with insufficient variation to make routine plasma level monitoring prudent. Higher levels observed in women[17-19] and older age[17,19] seem to have little significant clinical implication for either therapeutic response or adverse effects. A (trough) threshold for clinical response has been suggested to be approximately 100 µg/L[20] and mean levels of 367 µg/L[19] have been noted in responders in individual studies. Adverse effects (notably extrapyramidal side-effects, EPS) have been observed at mean levels of 336 µg/L,[17] 377 µg/L[20] and 395 µg/L.[18] A plasma

Table 1.1 Interpreting plasma concentration sample results for psychotropic drugs

Drug	Target range	Sample timing	Time to steady state	Comments
Amisulpride	200–320 µg/L	Trough	3 days	See text
Aripiprazole	150–210 µg/L	Trough	15–16 days	See text
Carbamazepine[2,3]	>7 mg/L bipolar disorder	Trough	2 weeks	Carbamazepine induces its own metabolism. Time to steady state dependent on autoinduction
Clozapine	350–500 µg/L Upper limit of target range is ill-defined	Trough	2–3 days	See text
Lamotrigine[4–6]	Not established but suggest 2.5–15 mg/L	Trough	5 days Autoinduction is thought to occur, so time to steady state may be longer	Some debate over utility of lamotrigine levels, especially in bipolar disorder. Toxicity may be increased above 15 mg/L but normally well tolerated
Lithium[7–11]	0.6–1.0 mmol/L (0.4 mmol may be sufficient for some patients/indications; >1.0 mmol/L required for mania)	12 hours post-dose	5 days	Well-established target range, albeit derived from ancient data sources
Olanzapine	20–40 µg/L	12 hours	1 week 2 months depot	See text
Paliperidone[12]	20–60 µg/L (9-OH risperidone)	Trough	2–3 days oral 2 months depot	No obvious reason to suspect range should be any different from risperidone. Some practical confirmation. As with risperidone, plasma level monitoring is not recommended
Phenytoin[3]	10–20 mg/L	Trough	Variable	Follows zero-order kinetics. Free levels may be useful
Quetiapine	Around 50–100 µg/L?	Trough?	2–3 days oral	Target range not defined. Plasma level monitoring not recommended. See text
Risperidone	20–60 µg/L (active moiety – risperidone+9OH risperidone)	Trough	2–3 days oral 6–8 weeks depot	Plasma level monitoring is not recommended. See text
Tricyclics[13]	Nortriptyline 50–150 µg/L	Trough	2–3 days	Rarely used and of dubious benefit
	Amitriptyline 100–200 µg/L			Use electrocardiogram to assess toxicity
Valproate[2,3,14–16]	50–100 mg/L Epilepsy and bipolar	Trough	2–3 days	Some doubt over value of levels in epilepsy and in bipolar disorder. Some evidence that, in mania, levels up to 125 mg/L are tolerated and more effective than lower concentrations

level threshold of below 320 µg/L has been found to predict avoidance of EPS.[20] A review of the current literature[21] has suggested an approximate range of **200–320 µg/L** for optimal clinical response and avoidance of adverse effects.

In practice, only a minority of treated patients have 'therapeutic' plasma levels (probably because of poor adherence[22]) so plasma monitoring may be of some benefit. However, amisulpride plasma level monitoring is rarely undertaken and few laboratories offer amisulpride assays. The dose–response relationship is sufficiently robust (in trials, at least) to obviate the need for plasma sampling within the licensed dose range and adverse effects are well managed by dose adjustment alone. Plasma level monitoring is best reserved for those in whom clinical response is poor, adherence is questioned or in whom drug interactions or physical illness may make adverse effects more likely.

Aripiprazole

Plasma level monitoring of aripiprazole is rarely undertaken in practice. The dose–response relationship for aripiprazole is well established with a plateau in clinical response and D_2 dopamine occupancy seen in doses above approximately 10 mg/day.[23] Plasma levels of aripiprazole, its metabolite and the total moiety (parent plus metabolite) strongly relate linearly to dose, making it possible to predict, with some certainty, an approximate plasma level for a given dose.[24] Target plasma level ranges for optimal clinical response have been suggested as 146–254 µg/L[25] and 150–300 µg/L,[26] with adverse effects observed above 210 µg/L. Interindividual variation in aripiprazole plasma levels has been observed but not fully investigated, although gender appears to have little influence.[27,28] Age, metabolic enzyme genotype and interacting medications seem likely causes of variation[26–29] but there are too few reports regarding their clinical implication to recommend specific monitoring in respect to these factors. A putative range of between **150 µg/L and 210 µg/L**[24] has been suggested as a target for patients taking aripiprazole and these are broadly the concentrations seen in patients receiving depot aripiprazole at 300 mg and 400 mg monthly.[30] However, for reasons described here, plasma level monitoring is not advised in routine practice.

Clozapine

Clozapine plasma levels are broadly related to daily dose[31] but there is sufficient variation to make any precise prediction of plasma level impossible. Plasma levels are generally lower in younger patients, males[32] and smokers[33] and higher in Asians.[34] A series of algorithms has been developed for the approximate prediction of clozapine levels according to patient factors and these are strongly recommended.[35] Algorithms cannot, however, account for other influences on clozapine plasma levels such as changes in adherence, inflammation[36] and infection.[37,38]

The plasma level threshold for acute response to clozapine has been suggested to be 200 µg/L,[39] 350 µg/L,[40–42] 370 µg/L,[43] 420 µg/L,[44] 504 µg/L[45] and 550 µg/L.[46] Limited data suggest a level of at least 200 µg/L is required to prevent relapse.[47] Substantial variation in clozapine plasma level may also predict relapse.[48]

Despite these somewhat varied estimates of response threshold, plasma levels can be useful in optimising treatment. In those not responding to clozapine, dose should be adjusted to give plasma levels in the range 350–500 µg/L (a range reflecting a consensus of the above findings). Those not tolerating clozapine may benefit from a reduction to a dose giving plasma levels in this range. An upper limit to the clozapine target range has not been defined. Any upper limit must take into account two components: the level above which no therapeutic advantage is gained and the level at which toxicity/tolerability is unacceptable. Plasma levels do seem to predict electroencephalogram (EEG) changes[49,50] and seizures occur more frequently in patients with levels above 1000 µg/L[51] so levels should probably be kept well below this. Other non-neurological clozapine-related adverse effects also seem to be related to plasma level,[52] as might be expected. No 'therapeutic' upper limit has been defined although levels around 600–800 µg/L have been proposed.[53]

A further consideration is that placing an upper limit on the target range for clozapine levels may discourage potentially worthwhile dose increases within the licensed dose range. Before plasma levels were widely used, clozapine was fairly often given in doses up to 900 mg/day, with valproate being added when the dose reached 600 mg/day. It remains unclear whether using these high doses can benefit patients with plasma levels already above the accepted threshold. Nonetheless, it is prudent to use an anticonvulsant as prophylaxis against seizures and myoclonus when plasma levels are above 600 µg/L (a level based more on repeated recommendation than on a clear evidence-based threshold[53]) and certainly when levels approach 1000 µg/L.

Norclozapine is the major metabolite of clozapine. The ratio of clozapine to norclozapine averages 1.25 in populations[54] but may differ for individuals. In chronic dosing, the ratio should remain the same for a given patient. A decrease in ratio may suggest enzyme induction, while an increase suggests enzyme inhibition, a non-trough sample or recent missed doses. Note also that clozapine metabolism may become saturated at higher doses: the ratio of clozapine to norclozapine increases with increasing plasma levels, suggesting saturation.[55-57] The effect of fluvoxamine also suggests that metabolism via CYP1A2 to norclozapine can be overwhelmed.[58]

Olanzapine

Plasma levels of olanzapine are linearly related to daily dose[59] but there is substantial variation,[60] with higher levels seen in women,[45] non-smokers[61] and those on enzyme-inhibiting drugs.[61,62] With once-daily dosing, the threshold level for response in schizophrenia has been suggested to be 9.3 µg/L (trough sample),[63] 23.2 µg/L (12-hour post-dose sample)[45] and 23 µg/L at a mean of 13.5 hours post dose.[64] There is evidence to suggest that levels greater than around 40 µg/L (12-hour sampling) produce no further therapeutic benefit than lower levels.[65] Severe toxicity is uncommon but may be associated with levels above 100 µg/L, and death is occasionally seen at levels above 160 µg/L[66] (albeit when other drugs or physical factors are relevant). A target range for therapeutic use of 20–40 µg/L (12-hour post-dose sample) has been proposed[67] for schizophrenia; the range for mania is probably similar.[68]

Notably, significant weight gain seems most likely to occur in those with plasma levels above 20 µg/L.[69] Constipation, dry mouth and tachycardia also seem to be related to plasma level.[70]

In practice, the dose of olanzapine should be largely governed by response and tolerability. However, a survey of UK sample assay results suggested that around 20% of patients on 20 mg a day will have sub-therapeutic plasma levels and more than 40% have levels above 40 µg/L.[71] Plasma level determinations might then be useful for those suspected of non-adherence, those showing poor tolerability or those not responding to the maximum licensed dose. Where there is poor response and plasma levels are below 20 µg/L, dose may then be adjusted to give 12-hour plasma levels of 20–40 µg/L; where there is good response and poor tolerability, the dose should be tentatively reduced to give plasma levels below 40 µg/L.

Quetiapine (IR)

Dose of quetiapine is weakly related to trough plasma samples.[72] Mean levels reported within the dose range 150 mg/day to 800 mg/day range from 27 µg/L to 387 µg/L,[73–78] although the highest and lowest levels are not necessarily found at the lowest and highest doses. Age, gender and co-medication may contribute to the significant interindividual variance observed in therapeutic drug monitoring (TDM) studies, with female gender,[78,79] older age[77,78] and CYP3A4-inhibiting drugs[73,77,78] likely to increase quetiapine concentration. Reports of these effects are conflicting[79] and not sufficient to support the routine use of plasma level monitoring based on these factors alone. Despite the substantial variation in plasma levels at each dose, there is insufficient evidence to suggest a target therapeutic range to aim for (although a target range of 100–500 µg/L has been proposed[80]); thus plasma level monitoring is likely to have little value. Moreover, the metabolites of quetiapine have major therapeutic effects and their concentrations are only loosely associated with parent drug levels.[81]

Most current reports of quetiapine concentration associations are derived from analysis of trough samples. Because of the short half-life of quetiapine, trough levels tend to drop to within a relatively small range regardless of dose and previous peak level. Thus peak plasma levels may be more closely related to dose and clinical response[72] although monitoring of such is not currently justified in the absence of an established peak plasma target range.

Quetiapine has an established dose–response relationship, and appears to be well tolerated at doses well beyond the licensed dose range.[82] In practice, dose adjustment should be based on patient response and tolerability.

Risperidone

Risperidone plasma levels are rarely measured in the UK and very few laboratories have developed assay methods for its determination. In any case, plasma level monitoring is probably unproductive (dose–response is well described) except where compliance is in doubt and in such cases measurement of prolactin will give some idea of compliance.

The therapeutic range for risperidone is generally agreed to be **20–60 µg/L** of the active moiety (risperidone + 9-OH-risperidone)[83,84] although other ranges (25–150 µg/L and 25–80 µg/L) have been proposed.[85] Plasma levels of 20–60 µg/L are usually afforded by oral doses of between 3 mg and 6 mg a day.[83,86–88] Occupancy of striatal dopamine D_2 receptors has been shown to be around 65% (the minimum required for therapeutic effect) at plasma levels of approximately 20 µg/L.[84,89]

Risperidone long-acting injection (RLAI) (25 mg/2 weeks) appears to afford plasma levels averaging between 4.4 and 22.7 µg/L.[87] Dopamine D_2 occupancies at this dose have been variously estimated at between 25% and 71%.[84,90,91] There is considerable interindividual variation around these mean values with a substantial minority of patients with plasma levels above those shown. Nonetheless, these data do cast doubt on the efficacy of a dose of 25 mg/2 weeks although it is noteworthy that there is some evidence that long-acting antipsychotic preparations are effective despite apparently sub-therapeutic plasma levels and dopamine occupancies.[92] Perhaps more importantly, a report of assay results for patients receiving RLAI[93] found 50% of patients with levels below 20 µg/L and for 10% no risperidone/9-hydroxyrisperidone was detected. Thus therapeutic drug monitoring might be clinically helpful for those on RLAI but this rather defeats the object of a long-acting injection.

Limited data for paliperidone palmitate suggest that standard loading doses give plasma levels of 25–45 µg/L while at steady state, plasma levels ranged from 10–25 µg/L for 100 mg/month and 15–35 µg/L for 150 mg/month.[94]

References

1. Mann K et al. Appropriateness of therapeutic drug monitoring for antidepressants in routine psychiatric inpatient care. Ther Drug Monit 2006; 28:83–88.
2. Taylor D et al. Doses of carbamazepine and valproate in bipolar affective disorder. Psychiatr Bull 1997; 21:221–223.
3. Eadie MJ. Anticonvulsant drugs. Drugs 1984; 27:328–363.
4. Cohen AF et al. Lamotrigine, a new anticonvulsant: pharmacokinetics in normal humans. Clin Pharmacol Ther 1987; 42:535–541.
5. Kilpatrick ES et al. Concentration–effect and concentration–toxicity relations with lamotrigine: a prospective study. Epilepsia 1996; 37:534–538.
6. Johannessen SI et al. Therapeutic drug monitoring of the newer antiepileptic drugs. Ther Drug Monit 2003; 25:347–363.
7. Schou M. Forty years of lithium treatment. Arch Gen Psychiatry 1997; 54:9–13.
8. Anon. Using lithium safely. Drug Ther Bull 1999; 37:22–24.
9. Nicholson J et al. Monitoring patients on lithium –a good practice guideline. Psychiatr Bull 2002; 26:348–351.
10. National Institute for Health and Clinical Excellence. Bipolar disorder. The management of bipolar disorder in adults, children and adolescents, in primary and secondary care. Clinical Guideline 38, 2006. www.nice.org.uk
11. Severus WE et al. What is the optimal serum lithium level in the long-term treatment of bipolar disorder – a review? Bipolar Disord 2008; 10:231–237.
12. Nazirizadeh Y et al. Serum concentrations of paliperidone versus risperidone and clinical effects. Eur J Clin Pharmacol 2010; 66:797–803.
13. Taylor D et al. Plasma levels of tricyclics and related antidepressants: are they necessary or useful? Psychiatr Bull 1995; 19:548–550.
14. Perucca E. Pharmacological and therapeutic properties of valproate. CNS Drugs 2002; 16:695–714.
15. Allen MH et al. Linear relationship of valproate serum concentration to response and optimal serum levels for acute mania. Am J Psychiatry 2006; 163:272–275.
16. Bowden CL et al. Relation of serum valproate concentration to response in mania. Am J Psychiatry 1996; 153:765–770.
17. Muller MJ et al. Amisulpride doses and plasma levels in different age groups of patients with schizophrenia or schizoaffective disorder. J Psychopharmacol 2008; 23:278–286.
18. Muller MJ et al. Gender aspects in the clinical treatment of schizophrenic inpatients with amisulpride: a therapeutic drug monitoring study. Pharmacopsychiatry 2006; 39:41–46.
19. Bergemann N et al. Plasma amisulpride levels in schizophrenia or schizoaffective disorder. Eur Neuropsychopharmacol 2004; 14:245–250.
20. Muller MJ et al. Therapeutic drug monitoring for optimizing amisulpride therapy in patients with schizophrenia. J Psychiatr Res 2007; 41:673–679.
21. Sparshatt A et al. Amisulpride – dose, plasma concentration, occupancy and response: implications for therapeutic drug monitoring. Acta Psychiatr Scand 2009; 120:416–428.

22. Bowskill SV et al. Plasma amisulpride in relation to prescribed dose, clozapine augmentation, and other factors: data from a therapeutic drug monitoring service, 2002–2010. Hum Psychopharmacol 2012; 27:507–513.

23. Mace S et al. Aripiprazole: dose–response relationship in schizophrenia and schizoaffective disorder. CNS Drugs 2008; 23:773–780.

24. Sparshatt A et al. A systematic review of aripiprazole – dose, plasma concentration, receptor occupancy and response: implications for therapeutic drug monitoring. J Clin Psychiatry 2010; 17:1447–1456.

25. Kirschbaum KM et al. Therapeutic monitoring of aripiprazole by HPLC with column-switching and spectrophotometric detection. Clin Chem 2005; 51:1718–1721.

26. Kirschbaum KM et al. Serum levels of aripiprazole and dehydroaripiprazole, clinical response and side effects. World J Biol Psychiatry 2008; 9:212–218.

27. Molden E et al. Pharmacokinetic variability of aripiprazole and the active metabolite dehydroaripiprazole in psychiatric patients. Ther Drug Monit 2006; 28:744–749.

28. Bachmann CJ et al. Large variability of aripiprazole and dehydroaripiprazole serum concentrations in adolescent patients with schizophrenia. Ther Drug Monit 2008; 30:462–466.

29. Hendset M et al. Impact of the CYP2D6 genotype on steady–state serum concentrations of aripiprazole and dehydroaripiprazole. Eur J Clin Pharmacol 2007; 63:1147–1151.

30. Mallikaarjun S et al. Pharmacokinetics, tolerability and safety of aripiprazole once-monthly in adult schizophrenia: an open-label, parallel-arm, multiple-dose study. Schizophr Res 2013; 150:281–288.

31. Haring C et al. Influence of patient-related variables on clozapine plasma levels. Am J Psychiatry 1990; 147:1471–1475.

32. Haring C et al. Dose-related plasma levels of clozapine: influence of smoking behaviour, sex and age. Psychopharmacology 1989; 99 Suppl:S38–S40.

33. Taylor D. Pharmacokinetic interactions involving clozapine. Br J Psychiatry 1997; 171:109–112.

34. Ng CH et al. An inter-ethnic comparison study of clozapine dosage, clinical response and plasma levels. Int Clin Psychopharmacol 2005; 20:163–168.

35. Rostami-Hodjegan A et al. Influence of dose, cigarette smoking, age, sex, and metabolic activity on plasma clozapine concentrations: a predictive model and nomograms to aid clozapine dose adjustment and to assess compliance in individual patients. J Clin Psychopharmacol 2004; 24:70–78.

36. Haack MJ et al. Toxic rise of clozapine plasma concentrations in relation to inflammation. Eur Neuropsychopharmacol 2003; 13:381–385.

37. de Leon J et al. Serious respiratory infections can increase clozapine levels and contribute to side effects: a case report. Prog Neuropsychopharmacol Biol Psychiatry 2003; 27:1059–1063.

38. Espnes KA et al. A puzzling case of increased serum clozapine levels in a patient with inflammation and infection. Ther Drug Monit 2012; 34:489–492.

39. VanderZwaag C et al. Response of patients with treatment-refractory schizophrenia to clozapine within three serum level ranges. Am J Psychiatry 1996; 153:1579–1584.

40. Perry PJ et al. Clozapine and norclozapine plasma concentrations and clinical response of treatment refractory schizophrenic patients. Am J Psychiatry 1991; 148:231–235.

41. Miller DD. Effect of phenytoin on plasma clozapine concentrations in two patients. J Clin Psychiatry 1991; 52:23–25.

42. Spina E et al. Relationship between plasma concentrations of clozapine and norclozapine and therapeutic response in patients with schizophrenia resistant to conventional neuroleptics. Psychopharmacology 2000; 148:83–89.

43. Hasegawa M et al. Relationship between clinical efficacy and clozapine concentrations in plasma in schizophrenia: effect of smoking. J Clin Psychopharmacol 1993; 13:383–390.

44. Potkin SG et al. Plasma clozapine concentrations predict clinical response in treatment-resistant schizophrenia. J Clin Psychiatry 1994; 55 Suppl B:133–136.

45. Perry PJ. Therapeutic drug monitoring of antipsychotics. Psychopharmacol Bull 2001; 35:19–29.

46. Llorca PM et al. Effectiveness of clozapine in neuroleptic-resistant schizophrenia: clinical response and plasma concentrations. J Psychiatry Neurosci 2002; 27:30–37.

47. Xiang YQ et al. Serum concentrations of clozapine and norclozapine in the prediction of relapse of patients with schizophrenia. Schizophr Res 2006; 83:201–210.

48. Stieffenhofer V et al. Clozapine plasma level monitoring for prediction of rehospitalization schizophrenic outpatients. Pharmacopsychiatry 2011; 44:55–59.

49. Khan AY et al. Examining concentration-dependent toxicity of clozapine: role of therapeutic drug monitoring. J Psychiatr Pract 2005; 11:289–301.

50. Varma S et al. Clozapine-related EEG changes and seizures: dose and plasma-level relationships. Therapeut Adv Psychopharmacol 2011; 1:47–66.

51. Greenwood-Smith C et al. Serum clozapine levels: a review of their clinical utility. J Psychopharmacol 2003; 17:234–238.

52. Yusufi B et al. Prevalence and nature of side effects during clozapine maintenance treatment and the relationship with clozapine dose and plasma concentration. Int Clin Psychopharmacol 2007; 22:238–243.

53. Remington G et al. Clozapine and therapeutic drug monitoring: is there sufficient evidence for an upper threshold? Psychopharmacology (Berl) 2013; 225:505–518.

54. Couchman L et al. Plasma clozapine, norclozapine, and the clozapine:norclozapine ratio in relation to prescribed dose and other factors: data from a therapeutic drug monitoring service, 1993–2007. Ther Drug Monit 2010; 32:438–447.

55. Volpicelli SA et al. Determination of clozapine, norclozapine, and clozapine-N-oxide in serum by liquid chromatography. Clin Chem 1993; 39:1656–1659.

56. Guitton C et al. Clozapine and metabolite concentrations during treatment of patients with chronic schizophrenia. J Clin Pharmacol 1999; 39:721–728.

57. Palego L et al. Clozapine, norclozapine plasma levels, their sum and ratio in 50 psychotic patients: influence of patient-related variables. Prog Neuropsychopharmacol Biol Psychiatry 2002; 26:473–480.

58. Wang CY et al. The differential effects of steady-state fluvoxamine on the pharmacokinetics of olanzapine and clozapine in healthy volunteers. J Clin Pharmacol 2004; 44:785–792.

59. Bishara D et al. Olanzapine: a systematic review and meta-regression of the relationships between dose, plasma concentration, receptor occupancy, and response. J Clin Psychopharmacol 2013; 33:329–335.

60. Aravagiri M et al. Plasma level monitoring of olanzapine in patients with schizophrenia: determination by high-performance liquid chromatography with electrochemical detection. Ther Drug Monit 1997; 19:307–313.

61. Gex-Fabry M et al. Therapeutic drug monitoring of olanzapine: the combined effect of age, gender, smoking, and comedication. Ther Drug Monit 2003; 25:46–53.

62. Bergemann N et al. Olanzapine plasma concentration, average daily dose, and interaction with co-medication in schizophrenic patients. Pharmacopsychiatry 2004; 37:63–68.

63. Perry PJ et al. Olanzapine plasma concentrations and clinical response in acutely ill schizophrenic patients. J Clin Psychopharmacol 1997; 6:472–477.

64. Fellows L et al. Investigation of target plasma concentration–effect relationships for olanzapine in schizophrenia. Ther Drug Monit 2003; 25:682–689.

65. Mauri MC et al. Clinical outcome and olanzapine plasma levels in acute schizophrenia. Eur Psychiatry 2005; 20:55–60.

66. Rao ML et al. [Olanzapine: pharmacology, pharmacokinetics and therapeutic drug monitoring]. Fortschr Neurol Psychiatr 2001; 69:510–517.

67. Robertson MD et al. Olanzapine concentrations in clinical serum and postmortem blood specimens – when does therapeutic become toxic? J Forensic Sci 2000; 45:418–421.

68. Bech P et al. Olanzapine plasma level in relation to antimanic effect in the acute therapy of manic states. Nord J Psychiatry 2006; 60:181–182.

69. Perry PJ et al. The association of weight gain and olanzapine plasma concentrations. J Clin Psychopharmacol 2005; 25:250–254.

70. Kelly DL et al. Plasma concentrations of high-dose olanzapine in a double-blind crossover study. Hum Psychopharmacol 2006; 21:393–398.

71. Patel MX et al. Plasma olanzapine in relation to prescribed dose and other factors: data from a therapeutic drug monitoring service, 1999–2009. J Clin Psychopharmacol 2011; 31:411–417.

72. Sparshatt A et al. Relationship between daily dose, plasma concentrations, dopamine receptor occupancy, and clinical response to quetiapine: a review. J Clin Psychiatry 2011; 72:1108–1123.

73. Hasselstrom J et al. Quetiapine serum concentrations in psychiatric patients: the influence of comedication. Ther Drug Monit 2004; 26:486–491.

74. Winter HR et al. Steady-state pharmacokinetic, safety, and tolerability profiles of quetiapine, norquetiapine, and other quetiapine metabolites in pediatric and adult patients with psychotic disorders. J Child Adolesc Psychopharmacol 2008; 18:81–98.

75. Li KY et al. Multiple dose pharmacokinetics of quetiapine and some of its metabolites in Chinese suffering from schizophrenia. Acta Pharmacol Sin 2004; 25:390–394.

76. McConville BJ et al. Pharmacokinetics, tolerability, and clinical effectiveness of quetiapine fumarate: an open-label trial in adolescents with psychotic disorders. J Clin Psychiatry 2000; 61:252–260.

77. Castberg I et al. Quetiapine and drug interactions: evidence from a routine therapeutic drug monitoring service. J Clin Psychiatry 2007; 68:1540–1545.

78. Aichhorn W et al. Influence of age, gender, body weight and valproate comedication on quetiapine plasma concentrations. Int Clin Psychopharmacol 2006; 21:81–85.

79. Mauri MC et al. Two weeks' quetiapine treatment for schizophrenia, drug-induced psychosis and borderline personality disorder: a naturalistic study with drug plasma levels. Expert Opin Pharmacother 2007; 8:2207–2213.

80. Patteet L et al. Therapeutic drug monitoring of common antipsychotics. Ther Drug Monit 2012; 34:629–651.

81. Fisher DS et al. Plasma concentrations of quetiapine, N-desalkylquetiapine, o-desalkylquetiapine, 7-hydroxyquetiapine, and quetiapine sulfoxide in relation to quetiapine dose, formulation, and other factors. Ther Drug Monit 2012; 34:415–421.

82. Sparshatt A et al. Quetiapine: dose–response relationship in schizophrenia. CNS Drugs 2008; 22:49–68.

83. Olesen OV et al. Serum concentrations and side effects in psychiatric patients during risperidone therapy. Ther Drug Monit 1998; 20:380–384.

84. Remington G et al. A PET study evaluating dopamine D2 receptor occupancy for long-acting injectable risperidone. Am J Psychiatry 2006; 163:396–401.

85. Seto K et al. Risperidone in schizophrenia: is there a role for therapeutic drug monitoring? Ther Drug Monit 2011; 33:275–283.

86. Lane HY et al. Risperidone in acutely exacerbated schizophrenia: dosing strategies and plasma levels. J Clin Psychiatry 2000; 61:209–214.

87. Taylor D. Risperidone long-acting injection in practice – more questions than answers? Acta Psychiatr Scand 2006; 114:1–2.

88. Nyberg S et al. Suggested minimal effective dose of risperidone based on PET-measured D2 and 5-HT2A receptor occupancy in schizophrenic patients. Am J Psychiatry 1999; 156:869–875.

89. Uchida H et al. Predicting dopamine D receptor occupancy from plasma levels of antipsychotic drugs: a systematic review and pooled analysis. J Clin Psychopharmacol 2011; **31**:318–325.
90. Medori R et al. Plasma antipsychotic concentration and receptor occupancy, with special focus on risperidone long-acting injectable. Eur Neuropsychopharmacol 2006; **16**:233–240.
91. Gefvert O et al. Pharmacokinetics and D2 receptor occupancy of long-acting injectable risperidone (Risperdal Consta™) in patients with schizophrenia. Int J Neuropsychopharmacol 2005; **8**:27–36.
92. Nyberg S et al. D2 dopamine receptor occupancy during low-dose treatment with haloperidol decanoate. Am J Psychiatry 1995; **152**:173–178.
93. Bowskill SV et al. Risperidone and total 9-hydroxyrisperidone in relation to prescribed dose and other factors: data from a therapeutic drug monitoring service, 2002–2010. Ther Drug Monit 2012; **34**:349–355.
94. Pandina GJ et al. A randomized, placebo-controlled study to assess the efficacy and safety of 3 doses of paliperidone palmitate in adults with acutely exacerbated schizophrenia. J Clin Psychopharmacol 2010; **30**:235–244.

Acting on clozapine plasma concentration results

In most developed countries, clozapine plasma concentration monitoring is widely employed. Table 1.2 gives some general advice about actions that should be taken when clozapine levels fall within a certain range. The ranges shown are somewhat arbitrary and convenient – the concentration at which a particular patient might respond cannot be known without a trial of clozapine. Most adverse effects are linearly related to dose or plasma level. That is, there is no step-change in risk of seizures, for example, at a particular dose or plasma concentration.[1] As a consequence, Table 1.2 should be considered more an aid to decision making rather than a rigorous, unbending evidence-based instruction. Note also the effect of tolerance to adverse effects – many patients have a significant adverse effect burden before therapeutic levels are reached.[2]

Table 1.2 Clozapine plasma concentration monitoring*

Plasma concentration	Response status	Tolerability status	Suggest action
<350 µg/L	Poor	Poor	Increase dose very slowly to give level of 350 µg/L
	Poor	Good	Increase dose to give level of 350 µg/L
	Good	Poor	Maintain dose. Consider dose reduction if tolerability does not improve
	Good	Good	Continue to monitor. No action required
350–500 µg/L	Poor	Poor	Increase dose slowly, according to tolerability, to give level of >500 µg/L. Consider prophylactic anticonvulsant.[†] If no improvement, consider augmentation
	Poor	Good	Increase dose slowly, according to tolerability, to give level of >500 µg/L. Consider prophylactic anticonvulsant.[†] If no improvement, consider augmentation
	Good	Poor	Maintain dose to see if tolerability improves. Consider dose reduction to give plasma level of around 350 µg/L
	Good	Good	Continue to monitor. No action required
500–1000 µg/L	Poor	Poor	Consider use of prophylactic anticonvulsant.[†] Consider augmentation. Attempt dose reduction if augmentation successful
	Poor	Good	Consider use of prophylactic anticonvulsant.[†] Consider augmentation
	Good	Poor	Attempt slow dose reduction to give plasma level of 350–500 µg/L unless there is known non-response at lower level. If this is the case, maintain dose and consider adding anticonvulsant.[†] Optimise treatment of adverse effects
	Good	Good	Consider use of prophylactic anticonvulsant.[†] Maintain dose if good tolerability continues

(Continued)

Table 1.2 (*Continued*)

Plasma concentration	Response status	Tolerability status	Suggest action
>1000 µg/L	Poor	Poor	Add anticonvulsant. Attempt augmentation. Reduce dose to give level of <1000 µg/L. Consider abandoning clozapine treatment
	Poor	Good	Add anticonvulsant. Attempt augmentation. If augmentation successful, reduce dose to give level <1000 µg/L. If unsuccessful, consider abandoning clozapine treatment
	Good	Poor	Add anticonvulsant. Attempt dose reduction to give plasma level <1000 µg/L
	Good	Good	Add anticonvulsant. Monitor closely; attempt dose reduction only if tolerability declines

Notes:

Poor response   No response or unsatisfactory response to clozapine. Not sufficiently well to be discharged.

Good response   Obvious positive changes related to use of clozapine. Likely to be suitable for discharge to supported or unsupported care in the community.

Poor tolerability   Dose constrained by adverse effects such as tachycardia, sedation, hypersalivation, hypotension (see Chapter 2 for suggestions of treatment for adverse effects).

Good tolerability   Patient tolerates treatment well and there are no signs of serious toxicity.

Augmentation   Adding another antipsychotic or mood stabiliser (see Chapter 2).

In all situations, ensure adequate treatment for clozapine-induced constipation, which is dose related. Ensure regular bowel movements and record bowel function. Stimulant laxatives such as senna often required (see Chapter 2).

Seizures are dose- and plasma-level dependent. Suitable anticonvulsants are valproate, lamotrigine and, rarely, topiramate. Use lamotrigine if response poor; valproate if affective symptoms present (see Chapter 2).

*This table applies to results for patients on a stable clozapine dose with confirmed good adherence.

†Anticonvulsants should be used in patients whose plasma level exceeds 600 µg/L, unless electroencephalogram is normal.

References

1. Varma S et al. Clozapine-related EEG changes and seizures: dose and plasma-level relationships. Therapeut Adv Psychopharmacol 2011; 1:47–66.
2. Yusufi B et al. Prevalence and nature of side effects during clozapine maintenance treatment and the relationship with clozapine dose and plasma concentration. Int Clin Psychopharmacol 2007; 22:238–243.

Interpreting post-mortem blood concentrations

A great many drugs are subject to post-mortem concentration changes but, for obvious practical reasons, research into the mechanisms and extent of these effects is very limited. The best that can be said is that a drug *plasma* concentration measured during life may be very different from the (usually *whole blood*) concentration measured some time after death.

A number of processes are responsible for these changes in concentration. In life, active mechanisms serve to concentrate some drugs in certain organs or tissues. After death, passive diffusion occurs as cell membranes break down and this will mean that post-mortem blood samples will, for some drugs, show higher concentrations than were seen during life. (This is known as post-mortem redistribution (PMR) and has been described as a 'toxicological nightmare'[1] because of the number of different processes involved.) In addition, central blood vessels surrounding major organs often reveal much higher drug concentrations than relatively distant peripheral samples.[2] PMR and other processes are temperature- and time-dependent and so time since death and conditions of storage are important determinants of blood concentration changes.[3] Post-mortem redistribution tends to be greater with drugs with a large volume of distribution (i.e. those for which tissue concentrations in life vastly exceed blood concentrations), especially when given over a long period during life.

Other processes of importance[4] include the post-mortem synthesis of certain compounds. The body can generate γ-hydroxybutyrate and trauma may allow the introduction of yeasts that metabolise glucose to alcohol. Another phenomenon is the

Table 1.3 Factors affecting post-mortem blood concentrations

Factor	Examples	Consequences
Redistribution of drug from tissues to blood compartment	Most drugs with large volume of distribution, e.g. clozapine,[6,7] olanzapine,[8] methadone,[9] SSRIs, TCAs, mirtazapine[10]	Post-mortem levels up to 10x higher than in-life levels, sometimes higher
Uneven distribution of drugs in the blood compartment and in organs (i.e. site of blood collection affects concentration)	Most drugs,[11,12] e.g. clozapine, TCAs, SSRIs, benzodiazepines	Concentrations may vary several-fold according to site of collection at post-mortem, e.g. femoral blood versus heart blood
Decay of drugs in post-mortem tissue (usually by bacterial degradation)	Not widely studied but known to occur with olanzapine, risperidone[13] and some benzodiazepines	Post-mortem levels may be lower than in-life levels
Post-mortem metabolism/ degradation	Cocaine metabolised/degraded post-mortem. Many other drugs are unstable in post-mortem samples. Yeasts may produce ethanol following trauma[4]	Post-mortem levels may be lower (cocaine) or higher (alcohol) than in-life levels

SSRI, selective serotonin reuptake inhibitor; TCA, tricyclic antidepressant.

degradation of drugs by bacteria (e.g. clonazepam and nitrazepam). Also, the metabolism of some drugs (cocaine, for example) appears to continue after death (although this may be simple chemical instability of the parent compound).

Table 1.3 lists some of the factors relevant to drug concentration changes after death and the possible consequences of these processes. Generally speaking, an isolated post-mortem blood concentration cannot be sensibly interpreted. Even where in-life levels are available, experts agree that, for most drugs in most circumstances, interpretation of blood levels after death is near impossible: high concentrations should certainly not be taken, in the absence of other evidence, to indicate death by overdose. Expert advice should always be sought when considering the role of medication in a death.[5]

References

 1. Pounder DJ et al. Post-mortem drug redistribution – a toxicological nightmare. Forensic Sci Int 1990; **45**:253–263.
 2. Ferner RE. Post-mortem clinical pharmacology. Br J Clin Pharmacol 2008; **66**:430–443.
 3. Flanagan RJ et al. Analytical toxicology: guidelines for sample collection postmortem. Toxicol Rev 2005; **24**:63–71.
 4. Kennedy MC. Post-mortem drug concentrations. Intern Med J 2010; **40**:183–187.
 5. Flanagan RJ. Poisoning: fact or fiction? Med Leg J 2012; **80**:127–148.
 6. Flanagan RJ et al. Effect of post-mortem changes on peripheral and central whole blood and tissue clozapine and norclozapine concentrations in the domestic pig (Sus scrofa). Forensic Sci Int 2003; **132**:9–17.
 7. Flanagan RJ et al. Suspected clozapine poisoning in the UK/Eire, 1992–. Forensic Sci Int 2005; **155**:91–99.
 8. Saar E et al. The time-dependant post-mortem redistribution of antipsychotic drugs. Forensic Sci Int 2012; **222**:223–227.
 9. Caplehorn JR et al. Methadone dose and post-mortem blood concentration. Drug Alcohol Rev 2002; **21**:329–333.
10. Launiainen T et al. Drug concentrations in post-mortem femoral blood compared with therapeutic concentrations in plasma. Drug Test Anal 2014; **6**:308–316.
11. Rodda KE et al. The redistribution of selected psychiatric drugs in post-mortem cases. Forensic Sci Int 2006; **164**:235–239.
12. Han E et al. Evaluation of postmortem redistribution phenomena for commonly encountered drugs. Forensic Sci Int 2012; **219**:265–271.
13. Butzbach DM et al. Bacterial degradation of risperidone and paliperidone in decomposing blood. J Forensic Sci 2013; **58**:90–100.

Schizophrenia

This chapter covers the treatment of schizophrenia with antipsychotic drugs, the adverse effect profile of these drugs and how adverse effects can be managed. It also discusses the use of clozapine and other drugs in the treatment of refractory schizophrenia, the adverse effects of clozapine and the treatment of these effects.

ANTIPSYCHOTIC DRUGS

General introduction

Classification

Before the 1990s antipsychotics (or major tranquillisers as they were then known) were classified according to their chemistry. The first antipsychotic, chlorpromazine, was a phenothiazine compound – a tricyclic structure incorporating a nitrogen and a sulphur atom. Further phenothiazines were generated and marketed, as were chemically similar thioxanthenes such as flupentixol. Later, entirely different chemical structures were developed according to pharmacological paradigms. These included butyrophenones (haloperidol), diphenylbutylpiperidines (pimozide) and substituted benzamides (sulpiride).

Chemical classification remains useful but is made somewhat redundant by the large range of chemical entities now available and by the absence of clear structure–activity relationships for newer drugs. The chemistry of older drugs does relate to their propensity to cause movement disorder. Piperazine phenothiazines (e.g. fluphenazine), butyrophenones and thioxanthines are most likely to cause extrapyramidal side-effects (EPS), and piperidine phenothiazines (e.g. pipotiazine) and benzamides least likely. Aliphatic phenothiazines (e.g. chlorpromazine) and diphenybutylpiperidines are perhaps somewhere in between.

The Maudsley Prescribing Guidelines in Psychiatry, Twelfth Edition. David Taylor, Carol Paton and Shitij Kapur.
© 2015 David Taylor, Carol Paton and Shitij Kapur. Published 2015 by John Wiley & Sons, Ltd.

Relative propensity for EPS was originally the primary factor behind typical/atypical classification. Clozapine has long been known as an atypical antipsychotic on the basis of its inability to cause EPS and its failure in animal-based antipsychotic screening tests. Its re-marketing in 1990 signalled the beginning of a mass of introductions of other drugs claimed, with varying degrees of accuracy, also to be atypical. Of these, perhaps only clozapine and quetiapine are 'fully' atypical, seemingly having no propensity whatever for EPS. Others show dose-related effects, although therapeutic activity can usually be gained without EPS. This is perhaps the real distinction between typical and atypical drugs: the ease with which a dose can be chosen (within the licensed dosage range) which is effective but which does not cause EPS (compare haloperidol with olanzapine).

The typical/atypical dichotomy does not lend itself well to classification of antipsychotics in the middle ground of EPS propensity. Thioridazine was widely described as atypical in the 1980s but is a 'conventional' phenothiazine. Sulpiride was marketed as an atypical but is often classified as typical. Risperidone, at its maximum dose of 16 mg/day (10 mg in the US) is just about as 'typical' as a drug can be. Alongside these difficulties is the fact that there is nothing either pharmacologically or chemically which clearly binds these so-called atypicals together as a group, save a general, but not universal finding, of preference for D2 receptors outside the striatum. Nor are atypicals characterised by improved efficacy over older drugs (clozapine and one or two others excepted) or the absence of hyperprolactinaemia (which is probably worse with risperidone and amisulpride than with typical drugs).

In an attempt to get round some of these problems, typicals and atypicals were re-classified as first- or second-generation antipsychotics (FGA/SGA). All drugs introduced since 1990 are classified as SGAs (i.e. all atypicals) but the new nomenclature dispenses with any connotations regarding atypically, whatever that may mean. However, the FGA/SGA classification remains problematic because neither group is defined by anything other than time of introduction – hardly the most sophisticated pharmacological classification system. Perhaps more importantly, date of introduction is often wildly distant from date of first synthesis. Clozapine is one of the oldest antipsychotics (synthesised in 1959) while olanzapine is hardly in its first flush of youth having first been patented in 1971. These two drugs are of course SGAs; apparently the most modern of antipsychotics.

In this edition of *The Guidelines* we conserve the FGA/SGA distinction more because of convention than some scientific basis. Also we feel that most people know which drugs belong to each group – it thus serves as a useful shorthand. However, it is clearly more sensible to consider the properties of *individual* antipsychotics when choosing drugs to prescribe, or in discussions with patients and carers.

Choosing an antipsychotic

The NICE guideline for medicines adherence[1] recommends that patients should be as involved as possible in decisions about the choice of medicines that are prescribed for them, and that clinicians should be aware that illness beliefs, and beliefs about medicines, influence adherence. Consistent with this general advice that covers all of healthcare, the NICE guideline for schizophrenia emphasises the importance of patient choice rather than specifically recommending a class or individual antipsychotic as first line treatment.[2]

Antipsychotics are effective in both the acute and maintenance treatment of schizophrenia and other psychotic disorders. They differ in their pharmacology, kinetics, overall efficacy/effectiveness and tolerability, but perhaps more importantly, response and tolerability differs between patients. This variability of individual response means that there is no clear first line antipsychotic suitable for all.

Relative efficacy

Further to the publication of CATIE[3] and CUtLASS,[4] the World Psychiatric Association reviewed the evidence relating to the relative efficacy of 51 first-generation antipsychotics and 11 second-generation antipsychotics and concluded that, if differences in EPS could be minimised (by careful dosing) and anticholinergic use avoided, there is no convincing evidence to support any advantage for SGAs over FGAs.[5] As a class, SGAs may have a lower propensity for EPS and tardive dyskinesia[6] but this is somewhat offset by a higher propensity for metabolic side-effects. A recent meta-analysis of antipsychotics for first episode psychosis[7] found few differences between FGAs and SGAs as groups of drugs but minor advantages for olanzapine and amisulpride individually.

When individual non-clozapine SGAs are compared with each other, it would appear that olanzapine is more effective than aripiprazole, risperidone, quetiapine and ziprasidone, and that risperidone has the edge over quetiapine and ziprasidone.[8] FGA-controlled trials also suggest an advantage for olanzapine, risperidone and amisulpride over older drugs.[9,10] A recent network meta-analysis[11] broadly confirmed these findings, ranking amisulpride second behind clozapine and olanzapine third. These three drugs were the only ones to show clear efficacy advantages over haloperidol. The magnitude of these differences is small (but potentially substantial enough to be clinically important)[11] and must be weighed against the very different side-effect profiles associated with individual antipsychotics.

Both FGAs and SGAs are associated with a number of adverse effects. These include weight gain, dyslipidaemia, increases in plasma glucose/diabetes,[12,13] hyperprolactinaemia, hip fracture,[14] sexual dysfunction, EPS including neuroleptic malignant syndrome (NMS),[15] anticholinergic effects, venous thromboembolism (VTE),[16] sedation and postural hypotension. The exact profile is drug-specific (see individual sections on adverse effects), although comparative data are not robust[17] (see Leucht meta-analysis[11] for rankings of some adverse effect risks). Adverse effects are a common reason for treatment discontinuation[18] particularly when efficacy is poor.[11] Patients do not always spontaneously report side-effects however,[19] and psychiatrists' views of the prevalence and importance of adverse effects differs markedly from patient experience.[20] Systematic enquiry along with a physical examination and appropriate biochemical tests is the only way accurately to assess their presence and severity or perceived severity. Patient-completed checklists such as the Glasgow Antipsychotic Side-effect Scale (GASS)[21] can be a useful first step in this process. The clinician-completed Antipsychotic Non-Neurological Side-Effects Rating Scale (ANNSERS) facilitates more detailed assessment.[22]

Non-adherence to antipsychotic treatment is common and here the guaranteed medication delivery associated with depot preparations is potentially advantageous. In comparison with oral antipsychotics, there is a strong suggestion that depots are associated with a reduced risk of relapse and rehospitalisation.[23–25]

In patients whose symptoms have not responded adequately to sequential trials of two or more antipsychotic drugs, clozapine is the most effective treatment[26–28] and its use in these circumstances is recommended by NICE.[2] The biological basis for the superior efficacy of clozapine is uncertain.[29] Olanzapine should probably be one of the two drugs used before clozapine.[8,30]

References

1. National Institute for Health and Clinical Excellence. Medicines adherence: involving patients in decisions about prescribed medicines and supporting adherence. Clinical Guideline **CG76**, 2009. http://www.nice.org.uk/
2. National Institute for Health and Clinical Excellence. Schizophrenia: core interventions in the treatment and management of schizophrenia in adults in primary and secondary care (update). Clinical Guideline **82**, 2009. http://www.nice.org.uk/
3. Lieberman JA et al. Effectiveness of antipsychotic drugs in patients with chronic schizophrenia. N Engl J Med 2005; 353:1209–1223.
4. Jones PB et al. Randomized controlled trial of the effect on Quality of Life of second- vs first-generation antipsychotic drugs in schizophrenia: Cost Utility of the Latest Antipsychotic Drugs in Schizophrenia Study (CUtLASS 1). Arch Gen Psychiatry 2006; 63:1079–1087.
5. Tandon R et al. World Psychiatric Association Pharmacopsychiatry Section statement on comparative effectiveness of antipsychotics in the treatment of schizophrenia. Schizophr Res 2008; 100:20–38.
6. Tarsy D et al. Epidemiology of tardive dyskinesia before and during the era of modern antipsychotic drugs. Handb Clin Neurol 2011; 100:601–616.
7. Zhang JP et al. Efficacy and safety of individual second-generation vs. first-generation antipsychotics in first-episode psychosis: a systematic review and meta-analysis. Int J Neuropsychopharmacol 2013; 16:1205–1218.
8. Leucht S et al. A meta-analysis of head-to-head comparisons of second-generation antipsychotics in the treatment of schizophrenia. Am J Psychiatry 2009; 166:152–163.
9. Davis JM et al. A meta-analysis of the efficacy of second-generation antipsychotics. Arch Gen Psychiatry 2003; 60:553–564.
10. Leucht S et al. Second-generation versus first-generation antipsychotic drugs for schizophrenia: a meta-analysis. Lancet 2009; 373:31–41.
11. Leucht S et al. Comparative efficacy and tolerability of 15 antipsychotic drugs in schizophrenia: a multiple-treatments meta-analysis. Lancet 2013; 382:951–962.
12. Manu P et al. Prediabetes in patients treated with antipsychotic drugs. J Clin Psychiatry 2012; 73:460–466.
13. Rummel-Kluge C et al. Head-to-head comparisons of metabolic side effects of second generation antipsychotics in the treatment of schizophrenia: a systematic review and meta-analysis. Schizophr Res 2010; 123:225–233.
14. Sorensen HJ et al. Schizophrenia, antipsychotics and risk of hip fracture: a population-based analysis. Eur Neuropsychopharmacol 2013; 23:872–878.
15. Trollor JN et al. Comparison of neuroleptic malignant syndrome induced by first- and second-generation antipsychotics. Br J Psychiatry 2012; 201:52–56.
16. Masopust J et al. Risk of venous thromboembolism during treatment with antipsychotic agents. Psychiatry Clin Neurosci 2012; 66:541–552.
17. Pope A et al. Assessment of adverse effects in clinical studies of antipsychotic medication: survey of methods used. Br J Psychiatry 2010; 197:67–72.
18. Falkai P. Limitations of current therapies: why do patients switch therapies? Eur Neuropsychopharmacol 2008; 18 Suppl 3:S135–S139.
19. Yusufi B et al. Prevalence and nature of side effects during clozapine maintenance treatment and the relationship with clozapine dose and plasma concentration. Int Clin Psychopharmacol 2007; 22:238–243.
20. Day JC et al. A comparison of patients' and prescribers' beliefs about neuroleptic side-effects: prevalence, distress and causation. Acta Psychiatr Scand 1998; 97:93–97.
21. Waddell L et al. A new self-rating scale for detecting atypical and second-generation antipsychotic side effects. J Psychopharmacol 2008; 22:238–243.
22. Ohlsen RI et al. Interrater reliability of the Antipsychotic Non-Neurological Side-Effects Rating Scale measured in patients treated with clozapine. J Psychopharmacol 2008; 22:323–329.
23. Tiihonen J et al. Effectiveness of antipsychotic treatments in a nationwide cohort of patients in community care after first hospitalisation due to schizophrenia and schizoaffective disorder: observational follow-up study. BMJ 2006; 333:224.
24. Leucht C et al. Oral versus depot antipsychotic drugs for schizophrenia--a critical systematic review and meta-analysis of randomised long-term trials. Schizophr Res 2011; 127:83–92.
25. Leucht S et al. Antipsychotic drugs versus placebo for relapse prevention in schizophrenia: a systematic review and meta-analysis. Lancet 2012; 379:2063–2071.

26. Kane J et al. Clozapine for the treatment-resistant schizophrenic. A double-blind comparison with chlorpromazine. Arch Gen Psychiatry 1988; **45**:789–796.

27. McEvoy JP et al. Effectiveness of clozapine versus olanzapine, quetiapine, and risperidone in patients with chronic schizophrenia who did not respond to prior atypical antipsychotic treatment. Am J Psychiatry 2006; **163**:600–610.

28. Lewis SW et al. Randomized controlled trial of effect of prescription of clozapine versus other second-generation antipsychotic drugs in resistant schizophrenia. Schizophr Bull 2006; **32**:715–723.

29. Stone JM et al. Review: The biological basis of antipsychotic response in schizophrenia. J Psychopharmacol 2010; **24**:953–964.

30. Agid O et al. An algorithm-based approach to first-episode schizophrenia: response rates over 3 prospective antipsychotic trials with a retrospective data analysis. J Clin Psychiatry 2011; **72**:1439–1444.

General principles of prescribing

- There is evidence to suggest that some antipsychotics are more effective than others: clozapine is the treatment of choice for refractory illness, and olanzapine, amisulpride, and perhaps risperidone, are more effective than other SGAs and FGAs.[1,2] Antipsychotics differ markedly with respect to their side-effect profiles[2] and patients differ in the side-effects they are and are not willing to tolerate. It is therefore important that the **patient is involved in the choice of antipsychotic drug**.

- The **lowest possible dose** should be used. For each patient, the dose should be titrated to the lowest known to be effective (see section on 'Minimum effective doses' in this chapter); dose increases should then take place only after one or two weeks of assessment during which the patient shows poor or no response. With depot medication, where no loading dose is given, plasma levels rise substantially for 6–12 weeks after initiation, even without a change in dose. Dose increases during this time are therefore inappropriate and difficult to evaluate.

- There is no evidence that high doses of antipsychotics have any advantages over standard doses but high doses are clearly associated with a greater side-effect burden[3] (see section on 'High-dose antipsychotics: prescribing and monitoring' in this chapter). The vast majority of patients should receive a **standard dose**.

- For the large majority of patients, the use of a **single antipsychotic** (with or without additional mood stabiliser or sedatives) is recommended (see section on 'Combined antipsychotics' in this chapter). Apart from exceptional circumstances (e.g. clozapine augmentation) antipsychotic polypharmacy should be avoided because of the risk of an increased frequency and severity of adverse effects, particularly that associated with QT prolongation and sudden cardiac death.[4]

- **Combinations** of antipsychotics should only be used where response to a single antipsychotic (including clozapine) has been clearly demonstrated to be inadequate. In such cases, the effect of the combination against target symptoms and the side-effects should be carefully evaluated and documented. Where there is no clear benefit, treatment should revert to single antipsychotic therapy.

- In general, **antipsychotics should not be used as 'prn' sedatives**. Short courses of benzodiazepines or general sedatives (e.g. promethazine) are recommended.

- Responses to antipsychotic drug treatment should be **assessed by recognised rating scales** and be documented in patients' records.

- Those receiving antipsychotics should undergo **close monitoring of physical health** (including blood pressure, pulse, ECG, plasma glucose and plasma lipids) (see later sections in this chapter) and **regular assessment of adverse effects**. The latter may be facilitated by the use of rating scales: for example, GASS[5] can be completed by the patient and broadly captures the most common side-effects associated with antipsychotic drugs, while ANNSERS[6] is completed by the clinician and allows detailed assessment of non-neurological side-effects. Systematic inquiry reveals considerably more adverse effects than patients spontaneously report.[7]

References

1. Leucht S et al. Second-generation versus first-generation antipsychotic drugs for schizophrenia: a meta-analysis. Lancet 2009; 373:31–41.
2. Leucht S et al. Comparative efficacy and tolerability of 15 antipsychotic drugs in schizophrenia: a multiple-treatments meta-analysis. Lancet 2013; 382:951–962.
3. Royal College of Psychiatrists. Consensus statement on high-dose antipsychotic medication. Council Report CRXX, 2014.
4. Ray WA et al. Atypical antipsychotic drugs and the risk of sudden cardiac death. N Engl J Med 2009; 360:225–235.
5. Waddell L et al. A new self-rating scale for detecting atypical or second-generation antipsychotic side effects. J Psychopharmacol 2008; 22:238–243.
6. Ohlsen RI et al. Interrater reliability of the Antipsychotic Non-Neurological Side-Effects Rating Scale measured in patients treated with clozapine. J Psychopharmacol 2008; 22:323–329.
7. Yusufi B et al. Prevalence and nature of side effects during clozapine maintenance treatment and the relationship with clozapine dose and plasma concentration. Int Clin Psychopharmacol 2007; 22:238–243.

CHAPTER 2

Minimum effective doses

Table 2.1 suggests the minimum dose of antipsychotic likely to be effective in schizophrenia (first or multi-episode). At least some patients will respond to the dose suggested, although others may require higher doses. Given the variation in individual response, all doses should be considered approximate. Primary references are provided where available, but consensus opinion has also been used. Only oral treatment with commonly used drugs is covered.

Table 2.1 Antipsychotics: minimum effective dose/day

Drug	First episode	Multi-episode
FGAs		
Chlorpromazine	200 mg*	300 mg
Haloperidol[1–6]	2 mg	4 mg
Sulpiride[7]	400 mg*	800 mg
Trifluoperazine[8]	10 mg*	15 mg
SGAs		
Amisulpride[9–12]	400 mg*	Unclear ?400 mg
Aripiprazole[13–16]	10 mg	10 mg
Asenapine[17]	10 mg*	10 mg
Iloperidone[6,18]	4 mg*	8 mg
Lurasidone[19]	37 mg base/40 mg HCl	37 mg base/40 mg HCl
Olanzapine[5,6,20–22]	5 mg	7.5 mg
Quetiapine[23–28]	150 mg*	300 mg
Risperidone[4,29–31]	2 mg	3 mg
Sertindole[32]	Not appropriate	12 mg
Ziprasidone[6,33–35]	40 mg*	80 mg

*Estimate – too few data available.
FGA, first-generation antipsychotic; HCl, hydrochloride; SGA, second-generation antipsychotic.

References

1. Oosthuizen P et al. Determining the optimal dose of haloperidol in first-episode psychosis. J Psychopharmacol 2001; **15**:251–255.
2. McGorry PD. Recommended haloperidol and risperidone doses in first-episode psychosis. J Clin Psychiatry 1999; **60**:794–795.
3. Waraich PS et al. Haloperidol dose for the acute phase of schizophrenia. Cochrane Database Syst Rev 2002; CD001951.
4. Schooler N et al. Risperidone and haloperidol in first-episode psychosis: a long-term randomized trial. Am J Psychiatry 2005; **162**:947–953.
5. Keefe RS et al. Long-term neurocognitive effects of olanzapine or low-dose haloperidol in first-episode psychosis. Biol Psychiatry 2006; **59**:97–105.
6. Liu CC et al. Aripiprazole for drug-naive or antipsychotic-short-exposure subjects with ultra-high risk state and first-episode psychosis: an open-label study. J Clin Psychopharmacol 2013; 33:18–23.
7. Soares BG et al. Sulpiride for schizophrenia. Cochrane Database Syst Rev 2000; CD001162.

8. Armenteros JL et al. Antipsychotics in early onset Schizophrenia: Systematic review and meta-analysis. Eur Child Adolesc Psychiatry 2006; 15:141–148.

9. Mota NE et al. Amisulpride for schizophrenia. Cochrane Database Syst Rev 2002; CD001357.

10. Puech A et al. Amisulpride, and atypical antipsychotic, in the treatment of acute episodes of schizophrenia: a dose-ranging study vs. haloperidol. The Amisulpride Study Group. Acta Psychiatr Scand 1998; 98:65–72.

11. Moller HJ et al. Improvement of acute exacerbations of schizophrenia with amisulpride: a comparison with haloperidol. PROD-ASLP Study Group. Psychopharmacology 1997; 132:396–401.

12. Sparshatt A et al. Amisulpride - dose, plasma concentration, occupancy and response: implications for therapeutic drug monitoring. Acta Psychiatr Scand 2009; 120:416–428.

13. Taylor D. Aripiprazole: a review of its pharmacology and clinical utility. Int J Clin Pract 2003; 57:49–54.

14. Cutler AJ et al. The efficacy and safety of lower doses of aripiprazole for the treatment of patients with acute exacerbation of schizophrenia. CNS Spectr 2006; 11:691–702.

15. Mace S et al. Aripiprazole: dose-response relationship in schizophrenia and schizoaffective disorder. CNS Drugs 2008; 23:773–780.

16. Sparshatt A et al. A systematic review of aripiprazole – dose, plasma concentration, receptor occupancy and response: implications for therapeutic drug monitoring. J Clin Psychiatry 2010; 71:1447–1456.

17. Citrome L. Role of sublingual asenapine in treatment of schizophrenia. Neuropsychiatr Dis Treat 2011; 7:325–339.

18. Crabtree BL et al. Iloperidone for the management of adults with schizophrenia. Clin Ther 2011; 33:330–345.

19. Leucht S et al. Dose equivalents for second-generation antipsychotics: the minimum effective dose method. Schizophr Bull 2014; 40:314–326.

20. Sanger TM et al. Olanzapine versus haloperidol treatment in first-episode psychosis. Am J Psychiatry 1999; 156:79–87.

21. Kasper S. Risperidone and olanzapine: optimal dosing for efficacy and tolerability in patients with schizophrenia. Int Clin Psychopharmacol 1998; 13:253–262.

22. Bishara D et al. Olanzapine: a systematic review and meta-regression of the relationships between dose, plasma concentration, receptor occupancy, and response. J Clin Psychopharmacol 2013; 33:329–335.

23. Small JG et al. Quetiapine in patients with schizophrenia. A high- and low-dose double-blind comparison with placebo. Seroquel Study Group. Arch Gen Psychiatry 1997; 54:549–557.

24. Peuskens J et al. A comparison of quetiapine and chlorpromazine in the treatment of schizophrenia. Acta Psychiatr Scand 1997; 96:265–273.

25. Arvanitis LA et al. Multiple fixed doses of "Seroquel" (quetiapine) in patients with acute exacerbation of schizophrenia: a comparison with haloperidol and placebo. Biol Psychiatry 1997; 42:233–246.

26. Kopala LC et al. Treatment of a first episode of psychotic illness with quetiapine: an analysis of 2 year outcomes. Schizophr Res 2006; 81:29–39.

27. Sparshatt A et al. Quetiapine: dose-response relationship in schizophrenia. CNS Drugs 2008; 22:49–68.

28. Sparshatt A et al. Relationship between daily dose, plasma concentrations, dopamine receptor occupancy, and clinical response to quetiapine: a review. J Clin Psychiatry 2011; 72:1108–1123.

29. Lane HY et al. Risperidone in acutely exacerbated schizophrenia: dosing strategies and plasma levels. J Clin Psychiatry 2000; 61:209–214.

30. Williams R. Optimal dosing with risperidone: updated recommendations. J Clin Psychiatry 2001; 62:282–289.

31. Ezewuzie N et al. Establishing a dose-response relationship for oral risperidone in relapsed schizophrenia. J Psychopharmacol 2006; 20:86–90.

32. Lindstrom E et al. Sertindole: efficacy and safety in schizophrenia. Expert Opin Pharmacother 2006; 7:1825–1834.

33. Bagnall A et al. Ziprasidone for schizophrenia and severe mental illness. Cochrane Database Syst Rev 2000; CD001945.

34. Taylor D. Ziprasidone – an atypical antipsychotic. Pharm J 2001; 266:396401.

35. Joyce AT et al. Effect of initial ziprasidone dose on length of therapy in schizophrenia. Schizophr Res 2006; 83:285–292.

Further reading

Davis JM et al. Dose response and dose equivalence of antipsychotics. J Clin Psychopharmacol 2004; 24:192–208.

CHAPTER 2

Quick reference for licensed maximum doses

Table 2.2 lists the EU-licensed maximum doses of antipsychotics, according to the EMA labelling (as of December 2014).

Table 2.2 EU-licensed maximum doses of antipsychotics, according to the EMA labelling (December 2014)

Drug	Maximum dose
FGAs - oral	
Chlorpromazine	1000 mg/day
Flupentixol	18 mg/day
Haloperidol	20 mg/day
Levomepromazine	1000 mg/day
Pericyazine	300 mg/day
Perphenazine	24 mg/day
Pimozide	20 mg/day
Sulpiride	2400 mg/day
Trifluoperazine	None (suggest 30 mg/day)
Zuclopenthixol	150 mg/day
SGAs - oral	
Amisulpride	1200 mg/day
Aripiprazole	30 mg/day
Asenapine	20 mg (sublingual)
Clozapine	900 mg/day
Iloperidone*	24 mg/day
Lurasidone	148 mg base/160 mg HCl
Olanzapine	20 mg/day
Paliperidone	12 mg/day
Quetiapine	750 mg/day schizophrenia 800 mg/day bipolar affective disorder
Risperidone	16 mg/day
Sertindole	24 mg/day
Ziprasidone*	160 mg/day
Depots	
Aripiprazole depot	400 mg/month
Flupentixol depot	400 mg/week
Fluphenazine depot	50 mg/week
Haloperidol depot	300 mg every 4 weeks

Table 2.2 (*Continued*)

Drug	Maximum dose
Paliperidone depot	150 mg/month
Pipotiazine depot	200 mg every 4 weeks
Risperidone	50 mg every 2 weeks
Zuclopenthixol depot	600 mg/week

*US labelling.
FGA, first-generation antipsychotic; HCl, hydrochloride; SGA, second-generation antipsychotic.

CHAPTER 2

Equivalent doses

Antipsychotic drugs vary greatly in potency (which is not the same as efficacy) and this is usually expressed as differences in 'neuroleptic' or 'chlorpromazine' 'equivalents'. Knowledge of equivalent doses is useful when switching between FGAs with different potencies and similar pharmacological actions, but in the absence of individual dose–response relationships being known. Some of the estimates relating to neuroleptic equivalents are based on early dopamine binding studies and some on clinical experience or expert panel opinion. Licensed maximum doses for antipsychotic drugs bear little relationship to their 'neuroleptic equivalents' – these maxima represent wildly different neuroleptic equivalents.

Table 2.3 gives some approximate equivalent doses for FGAs.[1-3] The values should be seen as a rough guide when transferring from one conventional drug to another. An early review of progress is essential.

It is inappropriate to convert SGA doses into 'equivalents' since, unlike with FGAs, the dose–response relationship is usually well-defined for these drugs and because, with different pharmacological actions, switching between drugs may not be sensible. Dosage guidelines are discussed under each individual drug. A rough guide is given in Table 2.4 below.[3-6] Clozapine is not included because its action is clearly not equivalent to any other antipsychotic.

Table 2.3 First-generation antipsychotics – equivalent doses

Drug	Equivalent dose (consensus)	Range of values in literature
Chlorpromazine	100 mg/day	–
Flupentixol	3 mg/day	2–3 mg/day
Flupentixol depot	10 mg/week	10–20 mg/week
Fluphenazine	2 mg/day	1–5 mg/day
Fluphenazine depot	5 mg/week	1–12.5 mg/week
Haloperidol	2 mg/day	1.5–5 mg/day
Haloperidol depot	15 mg/week	5–25 mg/week
Perphenazine	10 mg/day	10 mg/day
Pimozide	2 mg/day	2 mg/day
Pipotiazine depot	10 mg/week	10–12.5 mg/week
Sulpiride	200 mg/day	200–300 mg/day
Trifluoperazine	5 mg/day	2.5–5 mg/day
Zuclopenthixol	25 mg/day	25–60 mg/day
Zuclopenthixol depot	100 mg/week	40–100 mg/week

Table 2.4 Second-generation antipsychotics – equivalent doses

Drug	Approximate equivalent dose (per day, unless stated)
Aripiprazole	10 mg
Asenapine	10 mg
Iloperidone	8 mg
Lurasidone	37 mg base/40 mg HCl
Olanzapine	7.5–10 mg
Paliperidone palmitate	75 mg/month
Quetiapine	300 mg
Risperidone oral	3 mg
Risperidone LAI	37.5 mg/2 weeks
Sertindole	12 mg
Ziprasidone	40 mg

Comparing potencies of FGAs with SGAs introduces yet more uncertainty in respect to dose equivalence. Very approximately, 100 mg chlorpromazine is equivalent to 1.5 mg risperidone.[3]

References

1. Foster P. Neuroleptic equivalence. Pharm J 1989; **243**:431–432.
2. Atkins M et al. Chlorpromazine equivalents: a consensus of opinion for both clinical and research implications. Psychiatr Bull 1997; **21**:224–226.
3. Patel MX et al. How to compare doses of different antipsychotics: a systematic review of methods. Schizophr Res 2013; **149**:141–148.
4. Woods SW. Chlorpromazine equivalent doses for the newer atypical antipsychotics. J Clin Psychiatry 2003; **64**:663–667.
5. Gardner DM et al. International consensus study of antipsychotic dosing. Am J Psychiatry 2010; **167**:686–693.
6. Leucht S et al. Dose equivalents for second-generation antipsychotics: the minimum effective dose method. Schizophr Bull 2014; **40**:314–326.

High-dose antipsychotics: prescribing and monitoring

'High dose' can result from the prescription of either:

- a single antipsychotic in a dose that is above the recommended maximum, or
- two or more antipsychotics that, when expressed as a percentage of their respective maximum recommended doses and added together, result in a cumulative dose of >100%.

Efficacy

There is no firm evidence that high doses of antipsychotics are any more effective than standard doses. This holds true for the use of antipsychotics in rapid tranquillisation, the management of acute psychotic episodes, chronic aggression and relapse prevention. In the UK, approximately one-quarter to one-third of hospitalised patients are prescribed high-dose antipsychotics, the vast majority through the cumulative effect of combinations.[1,2] The common practice of prescribing antipsychotic drugs on a prn basis makes a major contribution.[1] The national audit of schizophrenia conducted in the UK in 2013, reported on prescribing practice for over 5000 predominantly community-based patients; overall 10% were prescribed a high dose of antipsychotics.[3]

Reviews of the dose–response effects of a variety of antipsychotics have revealed very little evidence for increasing doses above accepted licensed ranges.[2,4,5] Effect appears to be optimal at low doses: 4 mg/day risperidone;[6] 300 mg/day quetiapine,[7] olanzapine 10 mg,[8,9] etc. Similarly, 100 mg two-weekly risperidone depot offers no benefits over 50 mg two-weekly,[10] and 320 mg/day ziprasidone[11] is no better than 160 mg/day. All currently available antipsychotics (with the possible exception of clozapine) exert their antipsychotic effect primarily through antagonism (or partial agonism) at post-synaptic dopamine receptors. There is increasing evidence that in some patients with schizophrenia, symptoms do not seen to be driven through dysfunction of dopamine pathways;[12,13] and so increasing dopamine blockade in such patients is clearly futile.

There are a small number of randomised controlled trials (RCTs) that examine the efficacy of high versus standard doses in patients with treatment-resistant schizophrenia.[14,15] Some demonstrated benefit[16] but the majority of these studies are old, the number of patients randomised is small, and study design is poor by current standards. Some studies used daily doses equivalent to more than 10 g chlorpromazine. In a study of patients with first-episode schizophrenia, increasing the dose of olanzapine to up to 30 mg/day and the dose of risperidone to up to 10 mg/day in non-responders to standard doses, yielded only a 4% absolute increase in overall response rate; switching to an alternative antipsychotic, including clozapine was considerably more successful.[17] One small (n = 12) open study of high dose quetiapine (up to 1400 mg/day) found modest benefits in a third of subjects[18] (other, larger studies of quetiapine have shown no benefit for higher doses[7,19,20]). A further small (n = 40) RCT of high dose olanzapine (up to 45 mg/day) versus clozapine, high dose olanzapine suggested similar efficacy to clozapine.[21] In all studies, the side-effect burden associated with high dose treatment was considerable.

Adverse effects

The majority of side-effects associated with antipsychotic treatment are dose-related. These include EPS, sedation, postural hypotension, anticholinergic effects, QTc prolongation and sudden cardiac death.[22,23] High-dose antipsychotic treatment clearly worsens adverse effect incidence and severity.[11,20,24,25] There is some evidence that dose reduction from very high (mean 2253 mg chlorpromazine equivalents per day) to high (mean 1315 mg chlorpromazine equivalents per day) dose leads to improvements in cognition and negative symptoms.[26]

Recommendations:

- The use of high dose antipsychotics should be an exceptional clinical practice and only ever employed when an adequate trial of standard treatments, including clozapine, have failed.
- Documentation of target symptoms, response and side-effects, ideally using validated rating scales, should be standard practice so that there is ongoing consideration of the risk benefit ratio for the patient. Close physical monitoring (including ECG) is essential.

Prescribing high-dose antipsychotics

Before using high doses, ensure that:

- sufficient time has been allowed for response
- at least two different antipsychotics have been tried sequentially (one FGA, and if possible, olanzapine)
- clozapine has failed or not been tolerated due to agranulocytosis or other serious adverse effect. Most other side-effects can be managed. A very small proportion of patients may also refuse clozapine outright
- compliance is not in doubt (use of blood tests, liquids/dispersible tablets, depot preparations, etc)
- adjunctive medications such as antidepressants or mood stabilisers are not indicated
- psychological approaches have failed or are not appropriate.

The decision to use high doses should:

- be made by a senior psychiatrist
- involve the multidisciplinary team
- be done, if possible, with patient's informed consent.

Process

- Rule out contraindications (ECG abnormalities, hepatic impairment).
- Consider and minimise any risks posed by concomitant medication (e.g. potential to cause QTc prolongation, electrolyte disturbance or pharmacokinetic interactions via CYP inhibition).
- Document the decision to prescribe high doses in the clinical notes along with a description of target symptoms. The use of an appropriate rating scale is advised.

CHAPTER 2

CHAPTER 2

- Adequate time for response should be allowed after each dosage increment before a further increase is made.

Monitoring

- Physical monitoring should be carried out as outlined in the section on 'Monitoring' in this chapter.
- All patients on high doses should have regular ECGs (base-line, when steady-state serum levels have been reached after each dosage increment, and then every 6 to 12 months). Additional biochemical/ECG monitoring is advised if drugs that are known to cause electrolyte disturbances or QTc prolongation are subsequently co-prescribed.
- Target symptoms should be assessed after 6 weeks and 3 months. If insufficient improvement in these symptoms has occurred, the dose should be decreased to the normal range.

References

1. Paton C et al. High-dose and combination antipsychotic prescribing in acute adult wards in the UK: the challenges posed by p.r.n. prescribing. Br J Psychiatry 2008; 192:435–439.
2. Royal College of Psychiatrists. Consensus statement on high-dose antipsychotic medication. College Report CR190 2014: in press.
3. Patel MX et al. Quality of prescribing for schizophrenia: evidence from a national audit in England and Wales. Eur Neuropsychopharmacol 2014; 24:499–509.
4. Davis JM et al. Dose response and dose equivalence of antipsychotics. J Clin Psychopharmacol 2004; 24:192–208.
5. Gardner DM et al. International consensus study of antipsychotic dosing. Am J Psychiatry 2010; 167:686–693.
6. Ezewuzie N et al. Establishing a dose-response relationship for oral risperidone in relapsed schizophrenia. J Psychopharmacol 2006; 20:86–90.
7. Sparshatt, A et al. Quetiapine: dose-response relationship in schizophrenia. CNS Drugs 2008; 22:49–68.
8. Kinon BJ et al. Standard and higher dose of olanzapine in patients with schizophrenia or schizoaffective disorder: a randomized, double-blind, fixed-dose study. J Clin Psychopharmacol 2008; 28:392–400.
9. Bishara D et al. Olanzapine: a systematic review and meta-regression of the relationships between dose, plasma concentration, receptor occupancy, and response. J Clin Psychopharmacol 2013; 33:329–335.
10. Meltzer HY et al. A six month randomized controlled trial of long acting injectable risperidone 50 and 100 mg in treatment resistant schizophrenia. Schizophr Res 2014; 154:14–22.
11. Goff DC et al. High-dose oral ziprasidone versus conventional dosing in schizophrenia patients with residual symptoms: the ZEBRAS study. J Clin Psychopharmacol 2013; 33:485–490.
12. Kapur S et al. Relationship between dopamine D2 occupancy, clinical response, and side effects: a double-blind PET study of first-episode schizophrenia. Am J Psychiatry 2000; 157:514–520.
13. Demjaha A et al. Dopamine synthesis capacity in patients with treatment-resistant schizophrenia. Am J Psychiatry 2012; 169:1203–1210
14. Hirsch SR et al. Clinical use of high-dose neuroleptics. Br J Psychiatry 1994; 164:94–96
15. Thompson C. The use of high-dose antipsychotic medication. Br J Psychiatry 1994; 164:448–458.
16. Aubree JC et al. High and very high dosage antipsychotics: a critical review. J Clin Psychiatry 1980; 41:341–350.
17. Agid O et al. An algorithm-based approach to first-episode schizophrenia: response rates over 3 prospective antipsychotic trials with a retrospective data analysis. J Clin Psychiatry 2011; 72:1439–1444.
18. Boggs DL et al. Quetiapine at high doses for the treatment of refractory schizophrenia. Schizophr Res 2008; 101:347–348.
19. Lindenmayer JP et al. A randomized, double-blind, parallel-group, fixed-dose, clinical trial of quetiapine at 600 versus 1200 mg/d for patients with treatment-resistant schizophrenia or schizoaffective disorder. J Clin Psychopharmacol 2011; 31:160–168.
20. Honer WG et al. A randomized, double-blind, placebo-controlled study of the safety and tolerability of high-dose quetiapine in patients with persistent symptoms of schizophrenia or schizoaffective disorder. J Clin Psychiatry 2012; 73:13–20.
21. Meltzer HY et al. A randomized, double-blind comparison of clozapine and high-dose olanzapine in treatment-resistant patients with schizophrenia. J Clin Psychiatry 2008; 69:274–285.
22. Ray WA et al. Atypical antipsychotic drugs and the risk of sudden cardiac death. N Engl J Med 2009; 360:225–235.
23. Weinmann S et al. Influence of antipsychotics on mortality in schizophrenia: systematic review. Schizophr Res 2009; 113:1–11.
24. Bollini P et al. Antipsychotic drugs: is more worse? A meta-analysis of the published randomized control trials. Psychol Med 1994; 24:307–316.
25. Baldessarini RJ et al. Significance of neuroleptic dose and plasma level in the pharmacological treatment of psychoses. Arch Gen Psychiatry 1988; 45:79–90.
26. Kawai N et al. High-dose of multiple antipsychotics and cognitive function in schizophrenia: the effect of dose-reduction. Prog Neuropsychopharmacol Biol Psychiatry 2006; 30:1009–1014.

Antipsychotic prophylaxis

First episode of psychosis

Antipsychotics provide effective protection against relapse, at least in the short to medium term. A meta-analysis of placebo-controlled trials found that 26% of first episode patients randomised to receive maintenance antipsychotic relapsed after 6–12 months compared with 61% randomised to receive placebo.[1] After 1–2 years of being well on antipsychotic medication, the risk of relapse remains high (figures of 10–15% per month have been quoted), but this area is less well researched.[2] Although the current consensus is that antipsychotics should be prescribed for 1–2 years after a first episode of schizophrenia,[3,4] Gitlan et al.[5] found that withdrawing antipsychotic treatment in line with this consensus led to a relapse rate of almost 80% after one year medication-free and 98% after 2 years. Other studies in first episode patients have found that discontinuing antipsychotics increases the risk of relapse 5-fold[6] and confirmed that only a small minority of patients who discontinue remain well 1–2 years later.[7-10] However, a 5-year follow-up of a 2-year RCT, during which patients received either maintenance antipsychotic treatment or had their antipsychotic dose reduced or discontinued completely, found that while there was a clear advantage for maintenance treatment with respect to reducing short-term relapse this advantage was lost in the medium-term. Further, the dose-reduction/discontinuation group were receiving lower doses of antipsychotic drugs at follow-up and had better functional outcomes.[11] There are numerous interpretations of these outcomes but the most that can be concluded at this stage is dose reduction is a possible option in first episode psychosis.

It should be noted that definitions of relapse usually focus on the severity of positive symptoms, and largely ignore cognitive and negative symptoms: positive symptoms are more likely to lead to hospitalisation while cognitive and negative symptoms (which respond less well, and in some circumstances may even be exacerbated by antipsychotic treatment) have a greater overall impact on quality of life.

With respect to antipsychotic choice: in the context of a RCT, clozapine did not offer any advantage over chlorpromazine in the medium term in first episode patients with non-refractory illness.[12] But in a large naturalistic study of patients with a first admission for schizophrenia, clozapine and olanzapine fared better with respect to preventing re-admission than other oral antipsychotics.[13] In this same study, the use of a long-acting antipsychotic injection (depot) seemed to offer advantages over oral antipsychotics despite confounding by indication (depots will have been prescribed to poor compliers, oral to good compliers).[13] Note that in this study first admission may not be the same as first episode.

In practice, a firm diagnosis of schizophrenia is rarely made after a first episode and the majority of prescribers and/or patients will have at least attempted to stop antipsychotic treatment within one year.[14] It is vital that patients, carers and key-workers are aware of the early signs of relapse and how to access help. Antipsychotics should not be considered the only intervention. Psychosocial and psychological interventions are clearly also important.[15]

CHAPTER 2

Multi-episode schizophrenia

The majority of those who have one episode of schizophrenia will go on to have further episodes. Patients with residual symptoms, a greater side-effect burden and a less positive attitude to treatment are at greater risk of relapse.[16] With each subsequent episode, the baseline level of functioning deteriorates[17] and the majority of this decline is seen in the first decade of illness. Suicide risk (10%) is also concentrated in the first decade of illness. Antipsychotic drugs, when taken regularly, protect against relapse in the short, medium and long term.[1,18] Those who receive targeted antipsychotics (i.e. only when symptoms re-emerge) seem to have a worse outcome than those who receive prophylactic antipsychotics[19,20] and the risk of tardive dyskinesia may also be higher. Similarly, low dose antipsychotics are less effective than standard doses.[21]

Table 2.5 summarises the known benefits and harms associated with maintenance antipsychotic treatment as reported in a meta-analysis by Leucht et al. (2012).[1]

Depot preparations may have an advantage over oral preparations in maintenance treatment, most likely because of guaranteed medication delivery. Meta-analyses of clinical trials have shown that the relative and absolute risks of relapse with depot maintenance treatment were 30% and 10% lower respectively, than with oral treatment.[1,23] Long-acting preparations of antipsychotics may thus be preferred by both prescribers and patients.

A recent meta-analysis concluded that the risk of relapse with newer antipsychotics is similar to that associated with older drugs.[1] (Note that lack of relapse is not the same as good functioning.[24]) The proportion of multi-episode patients who achieve remission is small and may differ between antipsychotic drugs. The CATIE study reported that only 12% of patients treated with olanzapine achieved remission for at least 6 months, compared with 8% treated with quetiapine and 6% with risperidone.[25] The advantage seen here for olanzapine is consistent with that seen in an acute efficacy multiple treatments meta-analysis.[26]

Table 2.5 Benefits and harms associated with maintenance antipsychotic treatment

Benefits				Harms			
Outcome	Antipsychotic	Placebo	NNT	Adverse effect	Antipsychotic	Placebo	NNH*
Relapse at 7–12 months	27%	64%	3	Movement disorder	16%	9%	17
Re-admission	10%	26%	5	Anticholinergic effects	24%	16%	11
Improvement in mental state	30%	12%	4	Sedation	13%	9%	20
Violent/aggressive behaviour	2%	12%	11	Weight gain	10%	6%	20

NNH, number treated for one patient to be harmed; NNT, number needed to treat for one patient to benefit.
*Likely to be a considerable underestimate as adverse effects are rarely systematically assessed in clinical trials.[22]

Patients with schizophrenia often receive a number of sequential antipsychotic drugs during the maintenance phase.[27] Such switching is a result of a combination of suboptimal efficacy and poor tolerability. In both CATIE[28] and SOHO,[29,30] the attrition rate from olanzapine was lower than the attrition rate from other antipsychotic drugs, suggesting that olanzapine may be more effective than other antipsychotic drugs (except clozapine). Note though that olanzapine is associated with a high propensity for metabolic side-effects. In the SOHO study, the relapse rate over a 3 year period was relatively constant, supporting the benefit for maintenance treatment.[31,32]

In summary:

- relapse rates in patients not receiving antipsychotics are extremely high
- antipsychotics significantly reduce relapse, re-admission and violence/aggression
- long-acting depot formulations provide the best protection against relapse.

Adherence to antipsychotic treatment

Amongst people with schizophrenia, non-adherence with antipsychotic treatment is high. Only 10 days after discharge from hospital up to 25% are partially or non-adherent, rising to 50% at 1 year and 75% at 2 years.[33] Not only does non-adherence increase the risk of relapse, it may also increase the severity of relapse and the duration of hospitalisation.[33] The risk of suicide attempts also increases four-fold.[33]

Dose for prophylaxis

Many patients probably receive higher doses than necessary (particularly of the older drugs) when acutely psychotic.[34,35] In the longer term a balance needs to be made between effectiveness and adverse-effects. Lower doses of the older drugs (8 mg haloperidol/day or equivalent) are, when compared with higher doses, associated with less severe side-effects,[36] better subjective state and better community adjustment.[37] Very low doses increase the risk of psychotic relapse.[34,38] There are no data to support the use of lower than standard doses of the newer drugs as prophylaxis. Doses that are acutely effective should generally be continued as prophylaxis[39,40] although an exception to this is prophylaxis after a first episode where careful dose reduction is supportable.

How and when to stop[41]

The decision to stop antipsychotic drugs requires a thorough risk–benefit analysis for each patient. Withdrawal of antipsychotic drugs after long-term treatment should be gradual and closely monitored. The relapse rate in the first 6 months after abrupt withdrawal is double that seen after gradual withdrawal (defined as slow taper down over at least 3 weeks for oral antipsychotics or abrupt stopping of depot preparations).[42] Abrupt withdrawal may also lead to discontinuation symptoms (e.g. headache, nausea, insomnia) in some patients.[43]

The following factors should be considered.[41]

- Is the patient symptom-free, and if so, for how long? Long-standing, non-distressing symptoms which have not previously been responsive to medication may be excluded.

- What is the severity of adverse-effects (EPS, tardive dyskinesia, sedation, obesity, etc.)?
- What was the previous pattern of illness? Consider the speed of onset, duration and severity of episodes and any danger posed to self and others.
- Has dosage reduction been attempted before, and, if so, what was the outcome?
- What are the patient's current social circumstances? Is it a period of relative stability, or are stressful life events anticipated?
- What is the social cost of relapse (e.g. is the patient the sole breadwinner for a family)?
- Is the patient/carer able to monitor symptoms, and, if so, will they seek help?

As with first-episode patients, patients, carers and key-workers should be aware of the early signs of relapse and how to access help. Be aware that targeted relapse treatment is much less effective than continuous prophylaxis.[9] Those with a history of aggressive behaviour or serious suicide attempts and those with residual psychotic symptoms should be considered for life-long treatment.

Key points that patients should know

- Antipsychotics do not 'cure' schizophrenia. They treat symptoms in the same way that insulin treats diabetes.
- Some antipsychotic drugs may be more effective than others.
- Many antipsychotic drugs are available. Different drugs suit different patients. Perceived adverse-effects should always be discussed, so that the best tolerated drug can be found.
- Long-term treatment is generally required to prevent relapses.
- Antipsychotics should never be stopped suddenly.
- Psychological and psychosocial interventions increase the chance of staying well.[15]

Alternative views

While it is clear that antipsychotics effectively reduce symptom severity and rates of relapse, a minority view is that antipsychotics might also sensitise patients to psychosis. Thus, relapse on withdrawal can be seen as a type of discontinuation reaction resulting from super-sensitivity of (probably) dopamine receptors. This phenomenon might explain better outcomes seen in first episode patients who receive lower doses of antipsychotics.

The concept of 'super-sensitivity psychosis' was much discussed decades ago[44,45] although one rarely sees mention of it now. It is also striking that dopamine antagonists used for non-psychiatric conditions can induce withdrawal psychosis.[46–48] Whilst these theories and observations do not alter recommendations made in this section, they do emphasise the need for using the lowest possible dose of antipsychotic in all patients.

References

1. Leucht S et al. Antipsychotic drugs versus placebo for relapse prevention in schizophrenia: a systematic review and meta-analysis. Lancet 2012; 379:2063–2071.
2. Nuechterlein KH et al. The early course of schizophrenia and long-term maintenance neuroleptic therapy. Arch Gen Psychiatry 1995; 52:203–205.
3. American Psychiatric Association. Guideline Watch (September 2009): Practice Guideline for the Treatment of Patients With Schizophrenia. 2009. http://www.psychiatryonline.com/content.aspx?aid=501001

4. Sheitman BB et al. The evaluation and treatment of first-episode psychosis. Schizophr Bull 1997; **23**:653–661.

5. Gitlin M et al. Clinical outcome following neuroleptic discontinuation in patients with remitted recent-onset schizophrenia. Am J Psychiatry 2001; **158**:1835–1842.

6. Robinson D et al. Predictors of relapse following response from a first episode of schizophrenia or schizoaffective disorder. Arch Gen Psychiatry 1999; **56**:241–247.

7. Wunderink L et al. Guided discontinuation versus maintenance treatment in remitted first-episode psychosis: relapse rates and functional outcome. J Clin Psychiatry 2007; **68**:654–661.

8. Chen EY et al. Maintenance treatment with quetiapine versus discontinuation after one year of treatment in patients with remitted first episode psychosis: randomised controlled trial. BMJ 2010; **341**:c4024.

9. Gaebel W et al. Relapse prevention in first-episode schizophrenia--maintenance vs intermittent drug treatment with prodrome-based early intervention: results of a randomized controlled trial within the German Research Network on Schizophrenia. J Clin Psychiatry 2011; **72**:205–218.

10. Caseiro O et al. Predicting relapse after a first episode of non-affective psychosis: a three-year follow-up study. J Psychiatr Res 2012; **46**:1099–1105.

11. Wunderink L et al. Recovery in remitted first-episode psychosis at 7 years of follow-up of an early dose reduction/discontinuation or maintenance treatment strategy: long-term follow-up of a 2-year randomized clinical trial. JAMA Psychiatry 2013; **70**:913–920.

12. Girgis RR et al. Clozapine v. chlorpromazine in treatment-naive, first-episode schizophrenia: 9-year outcomes of a randomised clinical trial. Br J Psychiatry 2011; **199**:281–288.

13. Tiihonen J et al. A nationwide cohort study of oral and depot antipsychotics after first hospitalization for schizophrenia. Am J Psychiatry 2011; **168**:603–609.

14. Johnson DAW et al. Professional attitudes in the UK towards neuroleptic maintenance therapy in schizophrenia. Psychiatr Bull 1997; **21**:394–397.

15. National Institute for Health and Clinical Excellence. Schizophrenia: core interventions in the treatment and management of schizophrenia in adults in primary and secondary care (update). Clinical Guideline **82**, 2009. http://www.nice.org.uk/

16. Schennach R et al. Predictors of relapse in the year after hospital discharge among patients with schizophrenia. Psychiatr Serv 2012; **63**:87–90.

17. Wyatt RJ. Neuroleptics and the natural course of schizophrenia. Schizophr Bull 1991; **17**:325–351.

18. Almerie MQ et al. Cessation of medication for people with schizophrenia already stable on chlorpromazine. Schizophr Bull 2008; **34**:13–14.

19. Jolley AG et al. Trial of brief intermittent neuroleptic prophylaxis for selected schizophrenic outpatients: clinical and social outcome at two years. Br Med J 1990; **301**:837–842.

20. Herz MI et al. Intermittent vs maintenance medication in schizophrenia. Two-year results. Arch Gen Psychiatry 1991; **48**:333–339.

21. Schooler NR et al. Relapse and rehospitalization during maintenance treatment of schizophrenia. The effects of dose reduction and family treatment. Arch Gen Psychiatry 1997; **54**:453–463.

22. Pope A et al. Assessment of adverse effects in clinical studies of antipsychotic medication: survey of methods used. Br J Psychiatry 2010; **197**:67–72.

23. Leucht C et al. Oral versus depot antipsychotic drugs for schizophrenia--a critical systematic review and meta-analysis of randomised long-term trials. Schizophr Res 2011; **127**:83–92.

24. Schooler NR. Relapse prevention and recovery in the treatment of schizophrenia. J Clin Psychiatry 2006; **67** Suppl 5:19–23.

25. Levine SZ et al. Extent of attaining and maintaining symptom remission by antipsychotic medication in the treatment of chronic schizophrenia: evidence from the CATIE study. Schizophr Res 2011; **133**:42–46.

26. Leucht S et al. Comparative efficacy and tolerability of 15 antipsychotic drugs in schizophrenia: a multiple-treatments meta-analysis. Lancet 2013; **382**:951–962.

27. Burns T et al. Maintenance antipsychotic medication patterns in outpatient schizophrenia patients: a naturalistic cohort study. Acta Psychiatr Scand 2006; **113**:126–134.

28. Lieberman JA et al. Effectiveness of antipsychotic drugs in patients with chronic schizophrenia. N Engl J Med 2005; **353**:1209–1223.

29. Haro JM et al. Three-year antipsychotic effectiveness in the outpatient care of schizophrenia: observational versus randomized studies results. Eur Neuropsychopharmacol 2007; **17**:235–244.

30. Haro JM et al. Antipsychotic type and correlates of antipsychotic treatment discontinuation in the outpatient treatment of schizophrenia. Eur Psychiatry 2006; **21**:41–47.

31. Ciudad A et al. The Schizophrenia Outpatient Health Outcomes (SOHO) study: 3-year results of antipsychotic treatment discontinuation and related clinical factors in Spain. Eur Psychiatry 2008; **23**:1–7.

32. Suarez D et al. Overview of the findings from the European SOHO study. Expert Rev Neurother 2008; **8**:873–880.

33. Leucht S et al. Epidemiology, clinical consequences, and psychosocial treatment of nonadherence in schizophrenia. J Clin Psychiatry 2006; **67** Suppl 5:3–8.

34. Baldessarini RJ et al. Significance of neuroleptic dose and plasma level in the pharmacological treatment of psychoses. Arch Gen Psychiatry 1988; **45**:79–90.

35. Harrington M et al. The results of a multi-centre audit of the prescribing of antipsychotic drugs for in-patients in the UK. Psychiatr Bull 2002; **26**:414–418.

36. Geddes J et al. Atypical antipsychotics in the treatment of schizophrenia: systematic overview and meta-regression analysis. Br Med J 2000; **321**:1371–1376.

37. Hogarty GE et al. Dose of fluphenazine, familial expressed emotion, and outcome in schizophrenia. Results of a two-year controlled study. Arch Gen Psychiatry 1988; **45**:797–805.

38. Marder SR et al. Low- and conventional-dose maintenance therapy with fluphenazine decanoate. Two-year outcome. Arch Gen Psychiatry 1987; **44**:518–521.

39. Rouillon F et al. Strategies of treatment with olanzapine in schizophrenic patients during stable phase: results of a pilot study. Eur Neuropsychopharmacol 2008; **18**:646–652.

40. Wang CY et al. Risperidone maintenance treatment in schizophrenia: a randomized, controlled trial. Am J Psychiatry 2010; **167**:676–685.

41. Wyatt RJ. Risks of withdrawing antipsychotic medications. Arch Gen Psychiatry 1995; **52**:205–208.

42. Viguera AC et al. Clinical risk following abrupt and gradual withdrawal of maintenance neuroleptic treatment. Arch Gen Psychiatry 1997; **54**:49–55.

43. Chouinard G et al. Withdrawal symptoms after long-term treatment with low-potency neuroleptics. J Clin Psychiatry 1984; **45**:500–502.

44. Chouinard G et al. Neuroleptic-induced supersensitivity psychosis: clinical and pharmacologic characteristics. Am J Psychiatry 1980; **137**:16–21.

45. Kirkpatrick B et al. The concept of supersensitivity psychosis. J Nerv Ment Dis 1992; **180**:265–270.

46. CHAFFIN DS. Phenothiazine-induced acute psychotic reaction: the "psychotoxicity" of a drug. Am J Psychiatry 1964; **121**:26–32.

47. Lu ML et al. Metoclopramide-induced supersensitivity psychosis. Ann Pharmacother 2002; **36**:1387–1390.

48. Roy-Desruisseaux J et al. Domperidone-induced tardive dyskinesia and withdrawal psychosis in an elderly woman with dementia. Ann Pharmacother 2011; **45**:e51.

CHAPTER 2

Combined antipsychotics

A recent systematic review of the efficacy of monotherapy with antipsychotic drugs concluded that the magnitude of the clinical improvement that is seen is generally modest.[1] It is therefore unsurprising that the main clinical rationale for prescribing combined antipsychotics is to improve residual psychotic symptoms[2,3] but there is no good objective evidence that combined antipsychotics (that do not include clozapine) offer any efficacy advantage over the use of a single antipsychotic. There are three negative RCTs of non-clozapine combinations[4] while the 'evidence base' supporting such combinations consists for the most part of small open studies and case series.[4,5] Placebo response and reporting bias (nobody reports the failure of polypharmacy) are clearly important factors in this flimsy evidence base. Two-thirds of patients established on combined antipsychotics can be successfully switched to monotherapy[6] while one-third fare poorly.

Some antipsychotic polypharmacy makes scientific sense. It has been shown that co-prescribed aripiprazole reduces weight in those given clozapine[7] and normalises prolactin in those on haloperidol[8] and risperidone long-acting injection (LAI)[9] (although not amisulpride[10]). Polypharmacy with aripiprazole in such circumstances may thus represent worthwhile, evidence-based practice, albeit in the absence of regulatory trials demonstrating safety. In many cases, however, using aripiprazole alone might be a more logical choice.

Evidence for harm is perhaps more compelling. There are a number of published reports of clinically significant side-effects such as an increased prevalence of EPS,[11] severe EPS,[12] increased metabolic side-effects,[13] sexual dysfunction,[14] increased risk of hip fracture,[15] paralytic ileus,[16] grand mal seizures,[17] prolonged QTc[18] and arrhythmias[3] associated with combined antipsychotics. Switching to monotherapy has been shown to lead to worthwhile improvements in cognitive functioning.[19] With respect to systematic studies, one that followed a cohort of patients with schizophrenia prospectively over a 10-year period found that receiving more than one antipsychotic concurrently was associated with substantially increased mortality[20] while there was no association between mortality and any measure of illness severity. These findings imply that it is the co-prescription of antipsychotics that increase mortality, rather than the more severe or refractory illness for which they are prescribed. Another study that followed-up 99 patients with schizophrenia over a 25 year period found that those who were prescribed three antipsychotics simultaneously were twice as likely to die as those who were prescribed only one.[21] A negative case-control and a database study[22,23] also exist. Combined antipsychotics have also been associated with longer hospital stay and more frequent adverse effects.[24] It follows that it should be standard practice to document the rationale for combined antipsychotics in individual cases in clinical records along with a clear account of any benefits and side-effects. Medico-legally, that would seem to be wise although in practice it is rarely done.[25]

Despite the adverse risk–benefit balance, prescriptions for combined antipsychotics are commonly seen,[26] are often long-term,[27] and the prevalence of such prescribing is not decreasing.[28] A UK quality improvement programme conducted through the Prescribing Observatory for Mental Health (POMH-UK) found that combined antipsychotics were prescribed for 43% of patients in acute adult wards in the UK at baseline and 39% at re-audit one year later.[29] In the majority of cases, the second antipsychotic was prescribed prn and the most common reason given for prescribing in this way was to manage behavioural disturbance.[29] National surveys have repeatedly shown that up to 50% of patients prescribed atypical antipsychotics receive a typical drug as well.[29–32] Anticholinergic medication is then often required.[31] Combined antipsychotics are associated with younger age, male gender, increased illness severity, acuity, complexity and chronicity, poorer functioning, inpatient status and a diagnosis of schizophrenia.[2,28,33,34] These associations largely reinforce the idea that polypharmacy is used where monotherapy proves inadequate.

The situation in the community is different. A recent, systematic, audit of 5000 community patients from nearly 60 different NHS Trusts in the UK shows that 60% of the patients received a single antipsychotic (FGA or SGA; oral or injectable) and a further 18% received clozapine, and 5% received no antipsychotics at a given time – suggesting that less than one in five received antipsychotic combinations. This highlights a clear difference between inpatient and outpatient practices – probably a reflection of patient selection, disease severity and prescribing cultures.[35]

Combining antipsychotic drugs is clearly an established custom and practice. A questionnaire survey of US psychiatrists found that, in patients who did not respond to a single antipsychotic, two-thirds of psychiatrists switched to another single antipsychotic, while a third added a second antipsychotic. Those who switched were more positive about outcomes than those who augmented.[36] A further questionnaire study conducted in Denmark revealed that almost two-thirds of psychiatrists would rather combine antipsychotics than prescribe clozapine.[37] One observational study found that patients who derived no benefit from antipsychotic monotherapy were more likely to be switched to an alternative antipsychotic, while those who partially responded were more likely to have a second antipsychotic added.[38] This may partly explain why some patients are prescribed combined antipsychotics early in a treatment episode[3,39] and the use of combined antipsychotics in a third of patients prior to initiating clozapine.[40] Combined antipsychotics are likely to involve depots/LAIs,[41] quetiapine[33] and FGAs,[29] perhaps due to the frequent use of the last of these as prn. Initiatives to reduce the prevalence of combined antipsychotic prescribing appear to have only modest effects.[6,29]

Overall, on the basis of lack of evidence for efficacy, and the potential for serious adverse effects such as QT prolongation (common to almost all antipsychotics), routine use of combined antipsychotics should be avoided. Note, however, that clozapine augmentation strategies often involve combining antipsychotics and this is perhaps the sole therapeutic area where such practice is supportable.[42–46] See section on 'Clozapine augmentation' in this chapter. While there is little evidence for starting polypharmacy, stopping it is not easy. As mentioned above, switching to monotherapy, even when done in a graded fashion, does entail a slightly higher risk of an exacerbation – although it is usually rewarded with lesser side-effects and the exacerbations can be successfully managed.[47]

Summary

- There is very little evidence supporting the efficacy of combining non-clozapine antipsychotics.
- Substantial evidence supports the potential for harm, and so the use of combined antipsychotics should generally be avoided.

- Combined antipsychotics are often prescribed and this practice is resistant to change.
- As a minimum requirement, all patients who are prescribed combined antipsychotics should have their side-effects systematically assessed (including ECG monitoring) and any beneficial effect on symptoms carefully documented.
- Some antipsychotic polypharmacy (e.g. combinations with aripiprazole) show clear benefits for tolerability but not efficacy.

References

1. Lepping P et al. Clinical relevance of findings in trials of antipsychotics: systematic review. Br J Psychiatry 2011; 198:341–345.
2. Correll CU et al. Antipsychotic polypharmacy: a comprehensive evaluation of relevant correlates of a long-standing clinical practice. Psychiatr Clin North Am 2012; 35:661–681.
3. Grech P et al. Long-term antipsychotic polypharmacy: how does it start, why does it continue? Ther Adv Psychopharmacol 2012; 2:5–11.
4. Tracy DK et al. Antipsychotic polypharmacy: still dirty, but hardly a secret. A systematic review and clinical guide. Curr Psychopharmacol 2013; 2:143–171.
5. Barnes TR et al. Antipsychotic polypharmacy in schizophrenia: benefits and risks. CNS Drugs 2011; 25:383–399.
6. Tani H et al. Interventions to reduce antipsychotic polypharmacy: a systematic review. Schizophr Res 2013; 143:215–220.
7. Fleischhacker WW et al. Effects of adjunctive treatment with aripiprazole on body weight and clinical efficacy in schizophrenia patients treated with clozapine: a randomized, double-blind, placebo-controlled trial. Int J Neuropsychopharmacol 2010; 13:1115–1125.
8. Shim JC et al. Adjunctive treatment with a dopamine partial agonist, aripiprazole, for antipsychotic-induced hyperprolactinemia: a placebo-controlled trial. Am J Psychiatry 2007; 164:1404–1410.
9. Trives MZ et al. Effect of the addition of aripiprazole on hyperprolactinemia associated with risperidone long-acting injection. J Clin Psychopharmacol 2013; 33:538–541.
10. Chen CK et al. Differential add-on effects of aripiprazole in resolving hyperprolactinemia induced by risperidone in comparison to benzamide antipsychotics. Prog Neuropsychopharmacol Biol Psychiatry 2010; 34:1495–1499.
11. Carnahan RM et al. Increased risk of extrapyramidal side-effect treatment associated with atypical antipsychotic polytherapy. Acta Psychiatr Scand 2006; 113:135–141.
12. Gomberg RF. Interaction between olanzapine and haloperidol. J Clin Psychopharmacol 1999; 19:272–273.
13. Suzuki T et al. Effectiveness of antipsychotic polypharmacy for patients with treatment refractory schizophrenia: an open-label trial of olanzapine plus risperidone for those who failed to respond to a sequential treatment with olanzapine, quetiapine and risperidone. Hum Psychopharmacol 2008; 23:455–463.
14. Hashimoto Y et al. Effects of antipsychotic polypharmacy on side-effects and concurrent use of medications in schizophrenic outpatients. Psychiatry Clin Neurosci 2012; 66:405–410.
15. Sorensen HJ et al. Schizophrenia, antipsychotics and risk of hip fracture: a population-based analysis. Eur Neuropsychopharmacol 2013; 23:872–878.
16. Dome P et al. Paralytic ileus associated with combined atypical antipsychotic therapy. Prog Neuropsychopharmacol Biol Psychiatry 2007; 31:557–560.
17. Hedges DW et al. New-onset seizure associated with quetiapine and olanzapine. Ann Pharmacother 2002; 36:437–439.
18. Beelen AP et al. Asymptomatic QTc prolongation associated with quetiapine fumarate overdose in a patient being treated with risperidone. Hum Exp Toxicol 2001; 20:215–219.
19. Hori H et al. Switching to antipsychotic monotherapy can improve attention and processing speed, and social activity in chronic schizophrenia patients. J Psychiatr Res 2013; 47:1843–1848.
20. Waddington JL et al. Mortality in schizophrenia. Antipsychotic polypharmacy and absence of adjunctive anticholinergics over the course of a 10-year prospective study. Br J Psychiatry 1998; 173:325–329.
21. Joukamaa M et al. Schizophrenia, neuroleptic medication and mortality. Br J Psychiatry 2006; 188:122–127.
22. Baandrup L et al. Antipsychotic polypharmacy and risk of death from natural causes in patients with schizophrenia: a population-based nested case-control study. J Clin Psychiatry 2010; 71:103–108.
23. Tiihonen J et al. Polypharmacy with antipsychotics, antidepressants, or benzodiazepines and mortality in schizophrenia. Arch Gen Psychiatry 2012; 69:476–483.
24. Centorrino F et al. Multiple versus single antipsychotic agents for hospitalized psychiatric patients: case-control study of risks versus benefits. Am J Psychiatry 2004; 161:700–706.
25. Taylor D et al. Co-prescribing of atypical and typical antipsychotics – prescribing sequence and documented outcome. Psychiatr Bull 2002; 26:170–172.
26. Harrington M et al. The results of a multi-centre audit of the prescribing of antipsychotic drugs for in-patients in the UK. Psychiatr Bull 2002; 26:414–418.
27. Procyshyn RM et al. Persistent antipsychotic polypharmacy and excessive dosing in the community psychiatric treatment setting: a review of medication profiles in 435 Canadian outpatients. J Clin Psychiatry 2010; 71:566–573.
28. Gallego JA et al. Prevalence and correlates of antipsychotic polypharmacy: a systematic review and meta-regression of global and regional trends from the 1970s to 2009. Schizophr Res 2012; 138:18–28.

29. Paton C et al. High-dose and combination antipsychotic prescribing in acute adult wards in the UK: the challenges posed by p.r.n. prescribing. Br J Psychiatry 2008; 192:435–439.

30. Taylor,D et al. A prescription survey of the use of atypical antipsychotics for hospital inpatients in the United Kingdom. Int J Psychiatry Clin Pract 2000; 4:41–46.

31. Paton C et al. Patterns of antipsychotic and anticholinergic prescribing for hospital inpatients. J Psychopharmacol 2003; 17:223–229.

32. De Hert M et al. Pharmacological treatment of hospitalised schizophrenic patients in Belgium. Int J Psychiatry Clin Pract 2006; 10:285–290.

33. Novick D et al. Antipsychotic monotherapy and polypharmacy in the treatment of outpatients with schizophrenia in the European Schizophrenia Outpatient Health Outcomes Study. J Nerv Ment Dis 2012; 200:637–643.

34. Baandrup L et al. Association of antipsychotic polypharmacy with health service cost: a register-based cost analysis. Eur J Health Econ 2012; 13:355–363.

35. Patel MX et al. Quality of prescribing for schizophrenia: evidence from a national audit in England and Wales. Eur Neuropsychopharmacol 2014; 24:499–509.

36. Kreyenbuhl J et al. Adding or switching antipsychotic medications in treatment-refractory schizophrenia. Psychiatr Serv 2007; 58:983–990.

37. Nielsen J et al. Psychiatrists' attitude towards and knowledge of clozapine treatment. J Psychopharmacol 2010; 24:965–971.

38. Ascher-Svanum H et al. Comparison of patients undergoing switching versus augmentation of antipsychotic medications during treatment for schizophrenia. Neuropsychiatr DisTreat 2012; 8:113–118.

39. Goren JL et al. Antipsychotic prescribing pathways, polypharmacy, and clozapine use in treatment of schizophrenia. Psychiatr Serv 2013; 64:527–533.

40. Howes OD et al. Adherence to treatment guidelines in clinical practice: study of antipsychotic treatment prior to clozapine initiation. Br J Psychiatry 2012; 201:481–485.

41. Aggarwal NK et al. Prevalence of concomitant oral antipsychotic drug use among patients treated with long-acting, intramuscular, antipsychotic medications. J Clin Psychopharmacol 2012; 32:323–328.

42. Shiloh R et al. Sulpiride augmentation in people with schizophrenia partially responsive to clozapine. A double-blind, placebo-controlled study. Br J Psychiatry 1997; 171:569–573.

43. Josiassen RC et al. Clozapine augmented with risperidone in the treatment of schizophrenia: a randomized, double-blind, placebo-controlled trial. Am J Psychiatry 2005; 162:130–136.

44. Paton C et al. Augmentation with a second antipsychotic in patients with schizophrenia who partially respond to clozapine: a meta-analysis. J Clin Psychopharmacol 2007; 27:198–204.

45. Barbui C et al. Does the addition of a second antipsychotic drug improve clozapine treatment? Schizophr Bull 2009; 35:458–468.

46. Taylor DM et al. Augmentation of clozapine with a second antipsychotic - a meta-analysis of randomized, placebo-controlled studies. Acta Psychiatr Scand 2009; 119:419–425.

47. Essock SM et al. Effectiveness of switching from antipsychotic polypharmacy to monotherapy. Am J Psychiatry 2011; 168:702–708.

Negative symptoms

The aetiology of negative symptoms is complex and it is important to determine the most likely cause in any individual case before embarking on a treatment regime. Negative symptoms can be either primary (transient or enduring) or secondary to positive symptoms (e.g. asociality secondary to paranoia), EPS (e.g. bradykinesia, lack of facial expression), depression (e.g. social withdrawal) or institutionalisation.[1] Secondary negative symptoms are obviously best dealt with by treating the relevant cause (EPS, depression, etc.).

The EUFEST (European First Episode Schizophrenia Trial) study found that 7% of first episode patients had persistent negative symptoms and that these were associated with a longer DUP (duration of untreated psychosis) and a deleterious effect on global functioning.[2] Negative symptoms are seen to a varying degree in up to three-quarters of people with established schizophrenia,[3] with up to 20% having persistent primary negative symptoms.[4] The findings of EUFEST related to global functioning have also been reported in those with established illness.[5]

The literature pertaining to the pharmacological treatment of negative symptoms largely consists of sub-analyses of acute efficacy studies, correlation analysis and path analyses.[6] Few studies specifically recruit patients with persistent negative symptoms.

In general:

- The earlier a psychotic illness is effectively treated, the less likely is the development of negative symptoms over time.[7,8] In first-episode patients, response of negative symptoms to antipsychotic treatment may be determined by $5HT_{1A}$ genotype.[9]
- Older antipsychotics have a modest effect against primary negative symptoms[10,11] but some can cause secondary negative symptoms (via EPS).
- Some SGAs have been shown to be statistically superior to FGAs in the treatment of negative symptoms,[12] in the context of overall treatment response in non-selected populations.[11,13] However the effect size is small[12] and unlikely to be clinically meaningful. Interestingly, in a recent meta-analysis, quetiapine (which has one of the best EPS profiles[14]) was the only SGA to fare worse than haloperidol in head-to-head studies that addressed efficacy against negative symptoms.[11]
- Data support the effectiveness of amisulpride in primary negative symptoms,[15,16] but not clear superiority over low dose haloperidol.[17] There are many, mostly small RCTs in the literature reporting equivalent efficacy for different SGAs, e.g. quetiapine and olanzapine;[18] ziprasidone and amisulpride,[19] asenapine and olanzapine (note that the discontinuation rate in this study was considerably higher with asenapine than with olanzapine).[20] A well-conducted study appeared to show superiority for olanzapine (only at 5 mg/day) over amisulpride.[21] A further small study shows superiority of olanzapine over haloperidol but the magnitude of the effect was modest.[22]
- Low serum folate[23] and glycine[24] concentrations have been found in patients with predominantly negative symptoms. Supplementation with folate and oral B12 has been demonstrated to lead to modest improvements in those with specific functional variants of folate-related genes.[25]

With respect to non-antipsychotic pharmacological interventions, several drugs that modulate glutamate pathways have been directly tested; there are negative RCTs of glycine,[26] d-serine,[27] modafinil,[28] and armodafinil[29] augmentation of antipsychotics, minocycline[30,31] and of LY2140023 monotherapy[32] (an agonist at mGlu 2/3 receptors) and a small preliminary positive RCT of pregnenolone.[33] With respect to decreasing glutamate transmission, there is a positive meta-analysis of lamotrigine augmentation of clozapine[34] and a positive[35] and negative[36] RCT of memantine (the negative study being much the larger of the two).

With respect to antidepressant augmentation of an antipsychotic for negative symptoms, a Cochrane review concluded that this may be an effective strategy for reducing affective flattening, alogia and avolition,[37] while a meta-analysis of selective serotonin reuptake inhibitor (SSRI) augmentation of an antipsychotic was less positive.[38] A more recent meta-analysis that included available data for all antidepressants was cautiously optimistic[39] but the authors noted that their findings were not definitive. A meta-analysis supports the efficacy of mirtazapine and mianserin (postulated to be related to their α_2-adrenergic antagonist effects).[25]

Meta-analyses support the efficacy of augmentation of an antipsychotic with *Ginkgo biloba*[40] and a COX-2 inhibitor (albeit with a small effect size)[41] while small RCTs have demonstrated some benefit for selegiline,[42,43] pramiprexole,[44] testosterone (applied topically),[45] ondansetron[46] and granisetron.[47] Data for repetitive transcranial magnetic stimulation are mixed.[48–50] A large (n=250) RCT in adults[51] and a smaller RCT in elderly patients[52] each found no benefit for donepezil and there is a further negative RCT of galantamine.[53]

Patients who misuse psychoactive substances experience fewer negative symptoms than patients who do not.[54] It is not clear if this cause or effect.

Recommendations

The following recommendations are derived from the British Association for Psychopharmacology (BAP) schizophrenia guideline.[55]

- Psychotic illness should be identified and treated as early as possible as this may offer some protection against the development of negative symptoms.
- For any given patient, the antipsychotic that gives the best balance between overall efficacy and adverse effects should be used.

Where negative symptoms persist beyond an acute episode of psychosis:

- Ensure EPS (specifically bradykinesia) and depression are detected and treated if present, and consider the contribution of the environment to negative symptoms (e.g. insitutionalisation, lack of stimulation).
- Consider augmentation of antipsychotic treatment with an antidepressant such as an SSRI, or mirtazapine ensuring that choice is based on minimising the potential for compounding side-effects through pharmacokinetic or pharmacodynamic drug interactions.
- If clozapine is prescribed, consider augmenting with lamotrigine or a suitable second antipsychotic.
- There are insufficient data to make recommendations about other pharmacological strategies, but pregnenolone, minocycline, selegiline, pramiprexole, *Ginkgo biloba*, testosterone and ondansetron may have potential.

References

1. Carpenter WT. The treatment of negative symptoms: pharmacological and methodological issues. Br J Psychiatry 1996; **168**:17–22.
2. Galderisi S et al. Persistent negative symptoms in first episode patients with schizophrenia: results from the European First Episode Schizophrenia Trial. Eur Neuropsychopharmacol 2013; **23**:196–204.
3. Selten JP et al. Distress attributed to negative symptoms in schizophrenia. Schizophr Bull 2000; **26**:737–744.
4. Bobes J et al. Prevalence of negative symptoms in outpatients with schizophrenia spectrum disorders treated with antipsychotics in routine clinical practice: findings from the CLAMORS study. J Clin Psychiatry 2010; **71**:280–286.
5. Rabinowitz J et al. Negative symptoms have greater impact on functioning than positive symptoms in schizophrenia: analysis of CATIE data. Schizophr Res 2012; **137**:147–150.
6. Buckley PF et al. Pharmacological treatment of negative symptoms of schizophrenia: therapeutic opportunity or cul-de-sac? Acta Psychiatr Scand 2007; **115**:93–100.
7. Waddington JL et al. Sequential cross-sectional and 10-year prospective study of severe negative symptoms in relation to duration of initially untreated psychosis in chronic schizophrenia. Psychol Med 1995; **25**:849–857.
8. Melle I et al. Prevention of negative symptom psychopathologies in first-episode schizophrenia: two-year effects of reducing the duration of untreated psychosis. Arch Gen Psychiatry 2008; **65**:634–640.
9. Reynolds GP et al. Effect of 5-HT1A receptor gene polymorphism on negative and depressive symptom response to antipsychotic treatment of drug-naive psychotic patients. Am J Psychiatry 2006; **163**:1826–1829.
10. Levine SZ et al. Delayed- and early-onset hypotheses of antipsychotic drug action in the negative symptoms of schizophrenia. Eur Neuropsychopharmacol 2012; **22**:812–817.
11. Darba J et al. Efficacy of second-generation-antipsychotics in the treatment of negative symptoms of schizophrenia: a meta-analysis of randomized clinical trials. Rev Psiquiatr Salud Ment 2011; **4**:126–143.
12. Leucht S et al. Second-generation versus first-generation antipsychotic drugs for schizophrenia: a meta-analysis. Lancet 2009; **373**:31–41.
13. Erhart SM et al. Treatment of schizophrenia negative symptoms: future prospects. Schizophr Bull 2006; **32**:234–237.
14. Leucht S et al. Comparative efficacy and tolerability of 15 antipsychotic drugs in schizophrenia: a multiple-treatments meta-analysis. Lancet 2013; **382**:951–962.
15. Boyer P et al. Treatment of negative symptoms in schizophrenia with amisulpride. Br J Psychiatry 1995; **166**:68–72.
16. Danion JM et al. Improvement of schizophrenic patients with primary negative symptoms treated with amisulpride. Amisulpride Study Group. Am J Psychiatry 1999; **156**:610–616.
17. Speller JC et al. One-year, low-dose neuroleptic study of in-patients with chronic schizophrenia characterised by persistent negative symptoms. Amisulpride v. haloperidol. Br J Psychiatry 1997; **171**:564–568.
18. Stauffer VL et al. Responses to antipsychotic therapy among patients with schizophrenia or schizoaffective disorder and either predominant or prominent negative symptoms. Schizophr Res 2012; **134**:195–201.
19. Olie JP et al. Ziprasidone and amisulpride effectively treat negative symptoms of schizophrenia: results of a 12-week, double-blind study. Int Clin Psychopharmacol 2006; **21**:143–151.
20. Buchanan RW et al. Asenapine versus olanzapine in people with persistent negative symptoms of schizophrenia. J Clin Psychopharmacol 2012; **32**:36–45.
21. Lecrubier Y et al. The treatment of negative symptoms and deficit states of chronic schizophrenia: olanzapine compared to amisulpride and placebo in a 6-month double-blind controlled clinical trial. Acta Psychiatr Scand 2006; **114**:319–327.
22. Lindenmayer JP et al. A randomized controlled trial of olanzapine versus haloperidol in the treatment of primary negative symptoms and neurocognitive deficits in schizophrenia. J Clin Psychiatry 2007; **68**:368–379.
23. Goff DC et al. Folate, homocysteine, and negative symptoms in schizophrenia. Am J Psychiatry 2004; **161**:1705–1708.
24. Sumiyoshi T et al. Prediction of the ability of clozapine to treat negative symptoms from plasma glycine and serine levels in schizophrenia. Int J Neuropsychopharmacol 2005; **8**:451–455.
25. Hecht EM et al. Alpha-2 receptor antagonist add-on therapy in the treatment of schizophrenia; a meta-analysis. Schizophr Res 2012; **134**:202–206.
26. Buchanan RW et al. The Cognitive and Negative Symptoms in Schizophrenia Trial (CONSIST): the efficacy of glutamatergic agents for negative symptoms and cognitive impairments. Am J Psychiatry 2007; **164**:1593–1602.
27. Weiser M et al. A multicenter, add-on randomized controlled trial of low-dose d-serine for negative and cognitive symptoms of schizophrenia. J Clin Psychiatry 2012; **73**:e728–e734.
28. Pierre JM et al. A randomized, double-blind, placebo-controlled trial of modafinil for negative symptoms in schizophrenia. J Clin Psychiatry 2007; **68**:705–710.
29. Kane JM et al. Adjunctive armodafinil for negative symptoms in adults with schizophrenia: a double-blind, placebo-controlled study. Schizophr Res 2012; **135**:116–122.
30. Levkovitz Y et al. A double-blind, randomized study of minocycline for the treatment of negative and cognitive symptoms in early-phase schizophrenia. J Clin Psychiatry 2010; **71**:138–149.
31. Chaudhry IB et al. Minocycline benefits negative symptoms in early schizophrenia: a randomised double-blind placebo-controlled clinical trial in patients on standard treatment. J Psychopharmacol 2012; **26**:1185–1193.
32. Patil ST et al. Activation of mGlu2/3 receptors as a new approach to treat schizophrenia: a randomized Phase 2 clinical trial. Nat Med 2007; **13**:1102–1107.
33. Marx CE et al. Proof-of-concept trial with the neurosteroid pregnenolone targeting cognitive and negative symptoms in schizophrenia. Neuropsychopharmacology 2009; **34**:1885–1903.

34. Tiihonen J et al. The efficacy of lamotrigine in clozapine-resistant schizophrenia: a systematic review and meta-analysis. Schizophr Res 2009; 109:10–14.

35. Rezaei F et al. Memantine add-on to risperidone for treatment of negative symptoms in patients with stable schizophrenia: randomized, double-blind, placebo-controlled study. J Clin Psychopharmacol 2013; 33:336–342.

36. Lieberman JA et al. A randomized, placebo-controlled study of memantine as adjunctive treatment in patients with schizophrenia. Neuropsychopharmacology 2009; 34:1322–1329.

37. Rummel C et al. Antidepressants for the negative symptoms of schizophrenia. Cochrane Database Syst Rev 2006; 3:CD005581.

38. Sepehry AA et al. Selective serotonin reuptake inhibitor (SSRI) add-on therapy for the negative symptoms of schizophrenia: a meta-analysis. J Clin Psychiatry 2007; 68:604–610.

39. Singh SP et al. Efficacy of antidepressants in treating the negative symptoms of chronic schizophrenia: meta-analysis. Br J Psychiatry 2010; 197:174–179.

40. Singh V et al. Review and meta-analysis of usage of ginkgo as an adjunct therapy in chronic schizophrenia. Int J Neuropsychopharmacol 2010; 13:257–271.

41. Sommer IE et al. Nonsteroidal anti-inflammatory drugs in schizophrenia: ready for practice or a good start? A meta-analysis. J Clin Psychiatry 2012; 73:414–419.

42. Singh V et al. Review and meta-analysis of usage of ginkgo as an adjunct therapy in chronic schizophrenia. Int J Neuropsychopharmacol 2010; 13:257–271.

43. Amiri A et al. Efficacy of selegiline add on therapy to risperidone in the treatment of the negative symptoms of schizophrenia: a double-blind randomized placebo-controlled study. Hum Psychopharmacol 2008; 23:79–86.

44. Kelleher JP et al. Pilot randomized, controlled trial of pramipexole to augment antipsychotic treatment. Eur Neuropsychopharmacol 2012; 22:415–418.

45. Ko YH et al. Short-term testosterone augmentation in male schizophrenics: a randomized, double-blind, placebo-controlled trial. J Clin Psychopharmacol 2008; 28:375–383.

46. Zhang ZJ et al. Beneficial effects of ondansetron as an adjunct to haloperidol for chronic, treatment-resistant schizophrenia: a double-blind, randomized, placebo-controlled study. Schizophr Res 2006; 88:102–110.

47. Khodaie-Ardakani MR et al. Granisetron as an add-on to risperidone for treatment of negative symptoms in patients with stable schizophrenia: randomized double-blind placebo-controlled study. J Psychiatr Res 2013; 47:472–478.

48. Novak T et al. The double-blind sham-controlled study of high-frequency rTMS (20Hz) for negative symptoms in schizophrenia: Negative results. Neuro Endocrinol Lett 2006; 27:209–213.

49. Mogg A et al. Repetitive transcranial magnetic stimulation for negative symptoms of schizophrenia: a randomized controlled pilot study. Schizophr Res 2007; 93:221–228.

50. Prikryl R et al. Treatment of negative symptoms of schizophrenia using repetitive transcranial magnetic stimulation in a double-blind, randomized controlled study. Schizophr Res 2007; 95:151–157.

51. Keefe RSE et al. Efficacy and safety of donepezil in patients with schizophrenia or schizoaffective disorder: significant placebo/practice effects in a 12-week, randomized, double-blind, placebo-controlled trial. Neuropsychopharmacology 2007; 33:1217–1228.

52. Mazeh D et al. Donepezil for negative signs in elderly patients with schizophrenia: an add-on, double-blind, crossover, placebo-controlled study. Int Psychogeriatr 2006; 18:429–436.

53. Conley RR et al. The effects of galantamine on psychopathology in chronic stable schizophrenia. Clin Neuropharmacol 2009; 32:69–74.

54. Potvin S et al. A meta-analysis of negative symptoms in dual diagnosis schizophrenia. Psychol Med 2006; 36:431–440.

55. Barnes TR. Evidence-based guidelines for the pharmacological treatment of schizophrenia: recommendations from the British Association for Psychopharmacology. J Psychopharmacol 2011; 25:567–620.

Monitoring

Table 2.6 summarises suggested monitoring for those receiving antipsychotics. More detail and background is provided in specific sections in this chapter.

Table 2.6 Monitoring of metabolic parameters for patients receiving antipsychotic drugs

Parameter/ test	Suggested frequency	Action to be taken if results outside reference range	Drugs with special precautions	Drugs for which monitoring is not required
Urea and electrolytes (including creatinine or estimated GFR)	Baseline and yearly as part of a routine physical health check	Investigate all abnormalities detected	Amisulpride and sulpiride renally excreted – consider reducing dose if GFR reduced	None
Full blood count (FBC)[1–6]	Baseline and yearly as part of a routine physical health check and to detect chronic bone marrow suppression (small risk associated with some antipsychotics)	Stop suspect drug if neutrophils fall below 1.5 × 10⁹/L Refer to specialist medical care if neutrophils below 0.5 × 10⁹/L Note high frequency of benign ethnic neutropenia in certain ethnic groups	Clozapine – FBC weekly for 18 weeks, then fortnightly up to one year, then monthly (schedule varies from country to country)	None
Blood lipids[7,8] (cholesterol; triglycerides) Fasting sample, if possible	Baseline, at 3 months then yearly to detect antipsychotic-induced changes, and generally monitor physical health	Offer lifestyle advice Consider changing antipsychotic and/or initiating statin therapy	Clozapine, olanzapine, quetiapine, phenothiazines – 3 monthly for first year, then yearly	Some antipsychotics (e.g. aripiprazole) not clearly associated with dyslipidaemia but prevalence is high in this patient group[9–11] so all patients should be monitored
Weight[7,8,11] (include waist size and BMI, if possible)	Baseline, frequently for 3 months then yearly to detect antipsychotic-induced changes, and generally monitor physical health	Offer lifestyle advice Consider changing antipsychotic and/or dietary/pharmacological intervention	Clozapine, olanzapine – 3 monthly for first year, then yearly	Aripiprazole, ziprasidone and lurasidone not clearly associated with weight gain but monitoring recommended nonetheless – obesity prevalence high in this patient group
Plasma glucose (fasting sample, if possible)	Baseline, at 4–6 months, then yearly to detect antipsychotic-induced changes, and generally monitor physical health	Offer lifestyle advice Obtain fasting sample or non-fasting and HbA1C Refer to GP or specialist	Clozapine, olanzapine, chlorpromazine – test at baseline, one month, then 4–6 monthly	Some antipsychotics not clearly associated with IFG but prevalence is high in this patient group[12,13] so all patients should be monitored

Continued

CHAPTER 2

Table 2.6 (*Continued*)

Parameter/ test	Suggested frequency	Action to be taken if results outside reference range	Drugs with special precautions	Drugs for which monitoring is not required
ECG	Baseline and after dose increases (ECG changes rare in practice[14]) on admission to hospital and before discharge if drug regimen changed If an antipsychotic associated with moderate-high risk of QTc prolongation is prescribed	Discuss with/refer to cardiologist if abnormality detected	Haloperidol, pimozide, sertindole – ECG mandatory Ziprasidone – ECG mandatory in some situations	Risk of sudden cardiac death increased with most antipsychotics[15] Ideally, all patients should be offered an ECG at least yearly
Blood pressure	Baseline; frequently during dose titration to detect antipsychotic-induced changes, and generally monitor physical health	If severe hypotension or hypertension (clozapine) observed, slow rate of titration Consider switching to another antipsychotic if symptomatic postural hypotension Treat hypertension in line with NICE guidelines	Clozapine, chlorpromazine and quetiapine most likely to be associated with postural hypotension	Amisulpride, aripiprazole, lurasidone, trifluoperazine, sulpiride
Prolactin	Baseline, then at 6 months, then yearly to detect antipsychotic-induced changes	Switch drugs if hyperprolactinaemia confirmed and symptomatic Consider tests of bone mineral density (e.g. DEXA scanning) for those with chronically raised prolactin.	Amisulpride, risperidone and paliperidone particularly associated with hyperprolactinaemia	Asenapine, aripiprazole, clozapine, lurasidone, quetiapine, olanzapine (<20 mg), ziprasidone usually do not elevate prolactin, but worth measuring if symptoms arise
Liver function tests (LFTs)[16–18]	Baseline, then yearly as part of a routine physical health check and to detect chronic antipsychotic-induced changes (rare)	Stop suspect drug if LFTs indicate hepatitis (transaminases × 3 normal) or functional damage (PT/albumin change)	Clozapine and chlorpromazine associated with hepatic failure	Amisulpride, sulpiride
Creatine phosphokinase (CPK)	Baseline, then if neuroleptic malignant syndrome (NMS) suspected	See section on 'Neuroleptic malignant syndrome'	NMS more likely with first-generation antipsychotics	None

Other tests:

Patients on clozapine may benefit from an **EEG**[19,20] as this may help determine the need for valproate (although interpretation is obviously complex). Those on quetiapine should have **thyroid** function tests yearly although the risk of abnormality is very small.[21,22]

BMI, body mass index; DEXA, dual-energy X-ray absorptiometry; ECG, electrocardiogram; EEG, electrocephalogram; GFR, glomerular filtration rate; IFG, impaired fasting glucose; PT, prothrombin time.

References

1. Burckart GJ et al. Neutropenia following acute chlorpromazine ingestion. Clin Toxicol 1981; **18**:797–801.
2. Grohmann R et al. Agranulocytosis and significant leucopenia with neuroleptic drugs: results from the AMUP program. Psychopharmacology 1989; **99** Suppl:S109–S112.
3. Esposito D et al. Risperidone-induced morning pseudoneutropenia. Am J Psychiatry 2005; **162**:397.
4. Montgomery J. Ziprasidone-related agranulocytosis following olanzapine-induced neutropenia. Gen Hosp Psychiatry 2006; **28**:83–85.
5. Cowan C et al. Leukopenia and neutropenia induced by quetiapine. Prog Neuropsychopharmacol Biol Psychiatry 2007; **31**:292–294.
6. Buchman N et al. Olanzapine-induced leukopenia with human leukocyte antigen profiling. Int Clin Psychopharmacol 2001; **16**:55–57.
7. Marder SR et al. Physical health monitoring of patients with schizophrenia. Am J Psychiatry 2004; **161**:1334–1349.
8. Fenton WS et al. Medication-induced weight gain and dyslipidemia in patients with schizophrenia. Am J Psychiatry 2006; **163**:1697–1704.
9. Weissman EM et al. Lipid monitoring in patients with schizophrenia prescribed second-generation antipsychotics. J Clin Psychiatry 2006; **67**:1323–1326.
10. Cohn TA et al. Metabolic monitoring for patients treated with antipsychotic medications. Can J Psychiatry 2006; **51**:492–501.
11. Paton C et al. Obesity, dyslipidaemias and smoking in an inpatient population treated with antipsychotic drugs. Acta Psychiatr Scand 2004; **110**:299–305.
12. Taylor D et al. Undiagnosed impaired fasting glucose and diabetes mellitus amongst inpatients receiving antipsychotic drugs. J Psychopharmacol 2005; **19**:182–186.
13. Citrome L et al. Incidence, prevalence, and surveillance for diabetes in New York State psychiatric hospitals, 1997-2004. Psychiatr Serv 2006; **57**:1132–1139.
14. Novotny T et al. Monitoring of QT interval in patients treated with psychotropic drugs. Int J Cardiol 2007; **117**:329–332.
15. Ray WA et al. Atypical antipsychotic drugs and the risk of sudden cardiac death. N Engl J Med 2009; **360**:225–235.
16. Hummer M et al. Hepatotoxicity of clozapine. J Clin Psychopharmacol 1997; **17**:314–317.
17. Erdogan A et al. Management of marked liver enzyme increase during clozapine treatment: a case report and review of the literature. Int J Psychiatry Med 2004; **34**:83–89.
18. Regal RE et al. Phenothiazine-induced cholestatic jaundice. Clin Pharm 1987; **6**:787–794.
19. Centorrino F et al. EEG abnormalities during treatment with typical and atypical antipsychotics. Am J Psychiatry 2002; **159**:109–115.
20. Gross A et al. Clozapine-induced QEEG changes correlate with clinical response in schizophrenic patients: a prospective, longitudinal study. Pharmacopsychiatry 2004; **37**:119–122.
21. Twaites BR et al. The safety of quetiapine: results of a post-marketing surveillance study on 1728 patients in England. J Psychopharmacol 2007; **21**:392–399.
22. Kelly DL et al. Thyroid function in treatment-resistant schizophrenia patients treated with quetiapine, risperidone, or fluphenazine. J Clin Psychiatry 2005; **66**:80–84.

Relative adverse effects – a rough guide

A rough guide to the relative adverse effects of antipsychotic drugs is shown in Table 2.7.

The table is made up of approximate estimates of relative incidence and/or severity, based on clinical experience, manufacturers' literature and published research. See individual sections for more precise information.

Other side-effects not mentioned in this table do occur. Please see dedicated sections on other side-effects included in this book for more information.

Table 2.7 Relative adverse effects of antipsychotic drugs

Drug	Sedation	Weight gain	Akathisia	Parkinsonism	Anti-cholinergic	Hypotension	Prolactin elevation
Amisulpride	–	+	+	+	–	–	+++
Aripiprazole	–	–	+	–	–	–	–
Asenapine	+	+	+	–	–	–	+
Benperidol	+	+	+	+++	+	+	+++
Chlorpromazine	+++	++	+	++	++	+++	+++
Clozapine	+++	+++	–	–	+++	+++	–
Flupentixol	+	++	++	++	++	+	+++
Fluphenazine	+	+	++	+++	++	+	+++
Haloperidol	+	+	+++	+++	+	+	++
Iloperidone	–	++	+	+	–	+	–
Loxapine	++	+	+	+++	+	++	+++
Lurasidone	+	–	+	+	–	–	+
Olanzapine	++	+++	+	–	+	+	+
Paliperidone	+	++	+	+	+	++	+++
Perphenazine	+	+	++	+++	+	+	+++
Pimozide	+	+	+	+	+	+	+++
Pipothiazine	++	++	+	++	++	++	+++
Promazine	+++	++	+	+	++	++	++
Quetiapine	++	++	–	–	+	++	–
Risperidone	+	++	+	+	+	++	+++
Sertindole	–	+	–	–	–	+++	–
Sulpiride	–	+	+	+	–	–	+++
Trifluoperazine	+	+	+	+++	+	+	+++
Ziprasidone	+	–	+	–	–	+	+
Zuclopenthixol	++	++	++	++	++	+	+++

dence/severity, ++ moderate, + low, – very low.

Treatment algorithms for schizophrenia

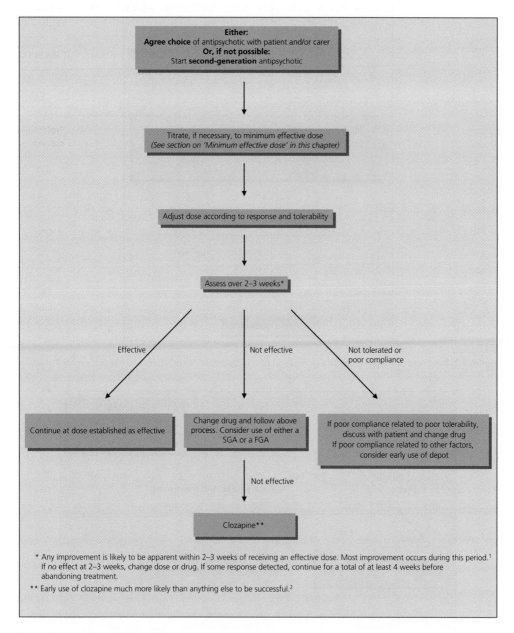

Either:
Agree choice of antipsychotic with patient and/or carer
Or, if not possible:
Start **second-generation** antipsychotic

Titrate, if necessary, to minimum effective dose
(*See section on 'Minimum effective dose' in this chapter*)

Adjust dose according to response and tolerability

Assess over 2–3 weeks*

Effective

Not effective

Not tolerated or
poor compliance

Continue at dose established as effective

Change drug and follow above
process. Consider use of either a
SGA or a FGA

If poor compliance related to poor tolerability,
discuss with patient and change drug
If poor compliance related to other factors,
consider early use of depot

Not effective

Clozapine**

* Any improvement is likely to be apparent within 2–3 weeks of receiving an effective dose. Most improvement occurs during this period.[1]
If *no* effect at 2–3 weeks, change dose or drug. If some response detected, continue for a total of at least 4 weeks before
abandoning treatment.
** Early use of clozapine much more likely than anything else to be successful.[2]

Figure 2.1 Treatment of first-episode schizophrenia.

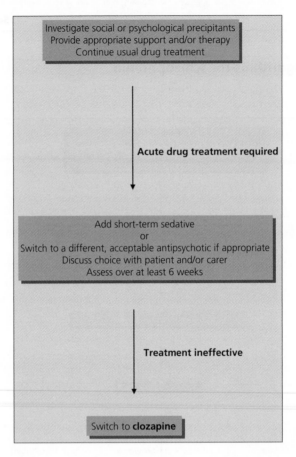

Figure 2.2 Treatment of relapse or acute exacerbation of schizophrenia (full adherence to medication confirmed).

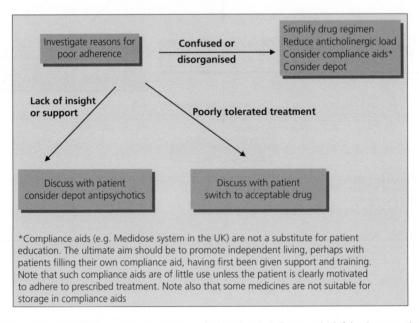

Figure 2.3 Treatment of relapse or acute exacerbation of schizophrenia (adherence doubtful or known to be poor).

Notes

- First-generation drugs may be slightly less efficacious than some SGAs.[3,4] FGAs should probably be reserved for second-line use because of the possibility of poorer outcome compared with FGAs and the higher risk of movement disorder, particularly tardive dyskinesia.[5,6]
- Choice is, however, based largely on comparative adverse effect profile and relative toxicity. Patients seem able to make informed choices based on these factors[7,8] although in practice they may only very rarely be involved in drug choice.[9]
- Where there is prior treatment failure (but not confirmed treatment refractoriness) olanzapine or risperidone may be better options than quetiapine.[10] Olanzapine, because of the wealth of evidence suggesting slight superiority over other antipsychotics, should always be tried before clozapine unless contraindicated.[11-14]
- Where there is confirmed treatment resistance (failure to respond to at least two antipsychotics) evidence supporting the use of clozapine (and only clozapine) is overwhelming.[15,16]

References

1. Agid O et al. The "delayed onset" of antipsychotic action--an idea whose time has come and gone. J Psychiatry Neurosci 2006; **31**:93–100.
2. Agid O et al. An algorithm-based approach to first-episode schizophrenia: response rates over 3 prospective antipsychotic trials with a retrospective data analysis. J Clin Psychiatry 2011; **72**:1439–1444.
3. Davis JM et al. A meta-analysis of the efficacy of second-generation antipsychotics. Arch Gen Psychiatry 2003; **60**:553–564.
4. Leucht S et al. Second-generation versus first-generation antipsychotic drugs for schizophrenia: a meta-analysis. Lancet 2009; **373**:31–41.
5. Schooler N et al. Risperidone and haloperidol in first-episode psychosis: a long-term randomized trial. Am J Psychiatry 2005; **162**:947–953.
6. Oosthuizen PP et al. Incidence of tardive dyskinesia in first-episode psychosis patients treated with low-dose haloperidol. J Clin Psychiatry 2003; **64**:1075–1080.
7. Whiskey E et al. Evaluation of an antipsychotic information sheet for patients. Int J Psychiatry Clin Pract 2005; **9**:264–270.
8. Stroup TS et al. Results of phase 3 of the CATIE schizophrenia trial. Schizophr Res 2009; **107**:1–12.
9. Olofinjana B et al. Antipsychotic drugs - information and choice: a patient survey. Psychiatr Bull 2005; **29**:369–371.
10. Stroup TS et al. Effectiveness of olanzapine, quetiapine, risperidone, and ziprasidone in patients with chronic schizophrenia following discontinuation of a previous atypical antipsychotic. Am J Psychiatry 2006; **163**:611–622.
11. Haro JM et al. Remission and relapse in the outpatient care of schizophrenia: three-year results from the Schizophrenia Outpatient Health Outcomes study. J Clin Psychopharmacol 2006; **26**:571–578.
12. Novick D et al. Recovery in the outpatient setting: 36-month results from the Schizophrenia Outpatients Health Outcomes (SOHO) study. Schizophr Res 2009; **108**:223–230.
13. Tiihonen J et al. Effectiveness of antipsychotic treatments in a nationwide cohort of patients in community care after first hospitalisation due to schizophrenia and schizoaffective disorder: observational follow-up study. BMJ 2006; **333**:224.
14. Leucht S et al. A meta-analysis of head-to-head comparisons of second-generation antipsychotics in the treatment of schizophrenia. Am J Psychiatry 2009; **166**:152–163.
15. McEvoy JP et al. Effectiveness of clozapine versus olanzapine, quetiapine, and risperidone in patients with chronic schizophrenia who did not respond to prior atypical antipsychotic treatment. Am J Psychiatry 2006; **163**:600–610.
16. Lewis SW et al. Randomized controlled trial of effect of prescription of clozapine versus other second-generation antipsychotic drugs in resistant schizophrenia. Schizophr Bull 2006; **32**:715–723.

CHAPTER 2

CHAPTER 2

First-generation antipsychotics – place in therapy

'Typical' and 'atypical' antipsychotics are not categorically differentiated. Typical (first-generation) drugs are those which can be expected to give rise to acute EPS, hyperprolactinaemia and, in the longer term, tardive dyskinesia. Atypicals (second-generation antipsychotics), by any sensible definition, might be expected not to be associated with these adverse effects. However, some atypicals show dose-related EPS, some induce hyperprolactinaemia (often to a greater extent than with FGAs) and all may eventually give rise to tardive dyskinesia. To complicate matters further, it has been suggested that the therapeutic and adverse effects of typical drugs can be separated by careful dosing[1] – thus making FGAs potentially 'atypical' (although there is much evidence to the contrary[2–4]).

Given these observations, it seems unwise and unhelpful to consider so-called typical and atypical drugs as distinct groups of drugs. The essential difference between the two groups is the size of the therapeutic index in relation to acute EPS; for instance haloperidol has an extremely narrow index (probably less than 0.5 mg/day); olanzapine a wide index (20–40 mg/day).

FGAs still play an important role in schizophrenia and offer a valid alternative to atypicals where atypicals are poorly tolerated or where typicals are preferred by patients themselves. Typicals may be less effective than some non-clozapine SGAs (amisulpride, olanzapine and risperidone may be more efficacious[5,6]). CATIE[7] and CUtLASS,[8] however, found few important differences between SGAs and FGAs (mainly sulpiride and perphenazine). The main drawbacks of FGAs are, of course, acute EPS, hyperprolactinaemia and tardive dyskinesia. Hyperprolactinaemia is probably unavoidable in practice and, even when not symptomatic, may grossly affect hypothalamic function.[9] It is also associated with sexual dysfunction,[10] but be aware that the autonomic effects of some atypicals may also cause sexual dysfunction.[11] In addition, some SGAs (risperidone, paliperidone, amisulpride) increase prolactin more than FGAs.[12]

Tardive dyskinesia probably occurs much more frequently with FGAs than SGAs[13–16] (notwithstanding difficulties in defining what is atypical), although there remains some uncertainty.[16–18] Careful observation of patients and the prescribing of the lowest effective dose are essential to help reduce the risk of this serious adverse event.[19,20] Even with these precautions, the risk of tardive dyskinesia with FGAs may be unacceptably high.[21]

A good example of the relative merits of SGAs and a carefully dosed FGA is the recent trial comparing paliperidone palmitate with haloperidol decanoate.[22] Paliperidone produced more weight gain and prolactin change, but haloperidol was associated with significantly more akathisia and parkinsonism and numerically more tardive dyskinesia. Actual efficacy was identical.

References

1. Oosthuizen P et al. Determining the optimal dose of haloperidol in first-episode psychosis. J Psychopharmacol 2001; 15:251–255.
2. Zimbroff DL et al. Controlled, dose-response study of sertindole and haloperidol in the treatment of schizophrenia. Sertindole Study Group. Am J Psychiatry 1997; 154:782–791.
3. Jeste DV et al. Incidence of tardive dyskinesia in early stages of low-dose treatment with typical neuroleptics in older patients. Am J Psychiatry 1999; 156:309–311.
4. Meltzer HY et al. The effect of neuroleptics on serum prolactin in schizophrenic patients. Arch Gen Psychiatry 1976; 33:279–286.
5. Davis JM et al. A meta-analysis of the efficacy of second-generation antipsychotics. Arch Gen Psychiatry 2003; 60:553–564.
6. Leucht S et al. Second-generation versus first-generation antipsychotic drugs for schizophrenia: a meta-analysis. Lancet 2009; 373:31–41.

7. Lieberman JA et al. Effectiveness of antipsychotic drugs in patients with chronic schizophrenia. N Engl J Med 2005; 353:1209–1223.

8. Jones PB et al. Randomized controlled trial of the effect on Quality of Life of second- vs first-generation antipsychotic drugs in schizophrenia: Cost Utility of the Latest Antipsychotic Drugs in Schizophrenia Study (CUtLASS 1). Arch Gen Psychiatry 2006; 63:1079–1087.

9. Smith S et al. The effects of antipsychotic-induced hyperprolactinaemia on the hypothalamic-pituitary-gonadal axis. J Clin Psychopharmacol 2002; 22:109–114.

10. Smith SM et al. Sexual dysfunction in patients taking conventional antipsychotic medication. Br J Psychiatry 2002; 181:49–55.

11. Aizenberg D et al. Comparison of sexual dysfunction in male schizophrenic patients maintained on treatment with classical antipsychotics versus clozapine. J Clin Psychiatry 2001; 62:541–544.

12. Leucht S et al. Comparative efficacy and tolerability of 15 antipsychotic drugs in schizophrenia: a multiple-treatments meta-analysis. Lancet 2013; 382:951–962.

13. Tollefson GD et al. Blind, controlled, long-term study of the comparative incidence of treatment-emergent tardive dyskinesia with olanzapine or haloperidol. Am J Psychiatry 1997; 154:1248–1254.

14. Beasley C et al. Randomised double-blind comparison of the incidence of tardive dyskinesia in patients with schizophrenia during long-term treatment with olanzapine or haloperidol. Br J Psychiatry 1999; 174:23–30.

15. Correll CU et al. Lower risk for tardive dyskinesia associated with second-generation antipsychotics: a systematic review of 1-year studies. Am J Psychiatry 2004; 161:414–425.

16. Novick D et al. Tolerability of outpatient antipsychotic treatment: 36-month results from the European Schizophrenia Outpatient Health Outcomes (SOHO) study. Eur Neuropsychopharmacol 2009; 19:542–550.

17. Halliday J et al. Nithsdale Schizophrenia Surveys 23: movement disorders. 20-year review. Br J Psychiatry 2002; 181:422–427.

18. Miller DD et al. Extrapyramidal side-effects of antipsychotics in a randomised trial. Br J Psychiatry 2008; 193:279–288.

19. Jeste DV et al. Tardive dyskinesia. Schizophr Bull 1993; 19:303–315.

20. Cavallaro R et al. Recognition, avoidance, and management of antipsychotic-induced tardive dyskinesia. CNS Drugs 1995; 4:278–293.

21. Oosthuizen P et al. A randomized, controlled comparison of the efficacy and tolerability of low and high doses of haloperidol in the treatment of first-episode psychosis. Int J Neuropsychopharmacol 2004; 7:125–131.

22. McEvoy JP et al. Effectiveness of paliperidone palmitate vs haloperidol decanoate for maintenance treatment of schizophrenia: a randomized clinical trial. JAMA 2014; 311:1978–1987.

CHAPTER 2

Omega-3 fatty acid (fish oils) in schizophrenia

Fish oils contain the omega-3 fatty acids, eicosapentanoic acid (EPA) and docosahexanoic acid (DHA) – also known as polyunsaturated fatty acids or PUFAs. These compounds are thought to be involved in maintaining neuronal membrane structure, in the modulation of membrane proteins and in the production of prostaglandins and leukotrienes.[1] High intake of PUFAs seems to protect against psychosis[2] and antipsychotic treatment may normalise PUFA deficits.[3] Animal models suggest a protective effect for PUFAs.[4] They have been suggested as treatments for a variety of psychiatric illnesses[5,6] but most research relates to their use in schizophrenia, where case reports,[7–9] case series[10] and prospective trials appear to suggest useful efficacy.[11–15]

A meta-analysis of these RCTs[16] concluded that EPA has 'no beneficial effect in established schizophrenia', although the estimate of effect size (0.242) approached statistical significance. Since then, a further RCT of 97 subjects in acute psychosis showed no advantage for EPA 2 g daily[17] and a relapse prevention study of EPA 2 g + DHA 1 g a day failed to demonstrate any value for PUFAs over placebo (relapse rate was 90% with PUFAs, 75% with placebo).[18]

On balance, evidence suggests that EPA (2–3 g daily) is unlikely to be a worthwhile option in schizophrenia when added to standard treatment. Set against doubts over efficacy are the observations that fish oils are relatively cheap, well tolerated (mild gastrointestinal symptoms may occur) and benefit physical health.[1,19–22] In addition, a study of 700 mg EPA + 480 mg DHA in adolescents and young adults at high risk of psychosis showed that such treatment greatly reduced emergence of psychotic symptoms compared with placebo[23] (although a recent review described this study as 'very low quality evidence'[24]).

PUFAs are no longer recommended for the treatment of residual symptoms of schizophrenia. If used, careful assessment of response is important and fish oils should be withdrawn if no effect is observed after 3 months' treatment, unless required for their beneficial metabolic effects. In younger people at risk of psychosis there seems to be no reason not to give PUFAs although supporting evidence remains weak.

Recommendations

- Patients at high risk of first-episode psychosis
  - Suggest **EPA 700 mg/day** (2 × Omacor or 6 × Maxepa capsules)
- Residual symptoms of multi-episode schizophrenia (added to antipsychotic)
  - Not recommended. If used, suggest dose of **EPA 2 g/day** (5 × Omacor or 10 × Maxepa capsules)

References

1. Fenton WS et al. Essential fatty acids, lipid membrane abnormalities, and the diagnosis and treatment of schizophrenia. Biol Psychiatry 2000; 47:8–21.

2. Hedelin M et al. Dietary intake of fish, omega-3, omega-6 polyunsaturated fatty acids and vitamin D and the prevalence of psychotic-like symptoms in a cohort of 33,000 women from the general population. BMC Psych 2010; 10:38.

3. Sethom MM et al. Polyunsaturated fatty acids deficits are associated with psychotic state and negative symptoms in patients with schizophrenia. Prostaglandins Leukot Essent Fatty Acids 2010; 83:131–136.

4. Zugno AI et al. Omega-3 prevents behavior response and brain oxidative damage in the ketamine model of schizophrenia. Neuroscience 2014; **259**:223–231.

5. Freeman MP. Omega-3 fatty acids in psychiatry: a review. Ann Clin Psychiatry 2000; **12**:159–165.

6. Ross BM et al. Omega-3 fatty acids as treatments for mental illness: which disorder and which fatty acid? Lipids Health Dis 2007; **6**:21–.

7. Richardson AJ et al. Red cell and plasma fatty acid changes accompanying symptom remission in a patient with schizophrenia treated with eicosapentaenoic acid. Eur Neuropsychopharmacol 2000; **10**:189–193.

8. Puri BK et al. Eicosapentaenoic acid treatment in schizophrenia associated with symptom remission, normalisation of blood fatty acids, reduced neuronal membrane phospholipid turnover and structural brain changes. Int J Clin Pract 2000; **54**:57–63.

9. Su KP et al. Omega-3 fatty acids as a psychotherapeutic agent for a pregnant schizophrenic patient. Eur Neuropsychopharmacol 2001; **11**:295–299.

10. Sivrioglu EY et al. The impact of omega-3 fatty acids, vitamins E and C supplementation on treatment outcome and side effects in schizophrenia patients treated with haloperidol: an open-label pilot study. Prog Neuropsychopharmacol Biol Psychiatry 2007; **31**:1493–1499.

11. Mellor JE et al. Schizophrenic symptoms and dietary intake of n-3 fatty acids. Schizophr Res 1995; **18**:85–86.

12. Peet M et al. Two double-blind placebo-controlled pilot studies of eicosapentaenoic acid in the treatment of schizophrenia. Schizophr Res 2001; **49**:243–251.

13. Fenton WS et al. A placebo-controlled trial of omega-3 fatty acid (ethyl eicosapentaenoic acid) supplementation for residual symptoms and cognitive impairment in schizophrenia. Am J Psychiatry 2001; **158**:2071–2074.

14. Emsley R et al. Randomized, placebo-controlled study of ethyl-eicosapentaenoic acid as supplemental treatment in schizophrenia. Am J Psychiatry 2002; **159**:1596–1598.

15. Berger GE et al. Ethyl-eicosapentaenoic acid in first-episode psychosis: a randomized, placebo-controlled trial. J Clin Psychiatry 2007; **68**:1867–1875.

16. Fusar-Poli P et al. Eicosapentaenoic acid interventions in schizophrenia: meta-analysis of randomized, placebo-controlled studies. J Clin Psychopharmacol 2012; **32**:179–185.

17. Bentsen H et al. A randomized placebo-controlled trial of an omega-3 fatty acid and vitamins E + C in schizophrenia. Transl Psychiatry 2013; **3**:e335.

18. Emsley R et al. A randomized, controlled trial of omega-3 fatty acids plus an antioxidant for relapse prevention after antipsychotic discontinuation in first-episode schizophrenia. Schizophr Res 2014.

19. Scorza FA et al. Omega-3 fatty acids and sudden cardiac death in schizophrenia: if not a friend, at least a great colleague. Schizophr Res 2007; **94**:375–376.

20. Caniato RN et al. Effect of omega-3 fatty acids on the lipid profile of patients taking clozapine. Aust N Z J Psychiatry 2006; **40**:691–697.

21. Emsley R et al. Safety of the omega-3 fatty acid, eicosapentaenoic acid (EPA) in psychiatric patients: results from a randomized, placebo-controlled trial. Psychiatry Res 2008; **161**:284–291.

22. Das UN. Essential fatty acids and their metabolites could function as endogenous HMG-CoA reductase and ACE enzyme inhibitors, anti-arrhythmic, anti-hypertensive, anti-atherosclerotic, anti-inflammatory, cytoprotective, and cardioprotective molecules. Lipids Health Dis 2008; **7**:37.

23. Amminger GP et al. Long-chain omega-3 fatty acids for indicated prevention of psychotic disorders: a randomized, placebo-controlled trial. Arch Gen Psychiatry 2010; **67**:146–154.

24. Stafford MR et al. Early interventions to prevent psychosis: systematic review and meta-analysis. BMJ 2013; **346**:f185.

CHAPTER 2

New and developing drugs to treat schizophrenia

Since the introduction of the 'atypical' antipsychotics nearly two decades ago, there have been no major new developments in the drug treatment of schizophrenia. The industry is following three different approaches:

- further refinement of dopamine-based antipsychotics with the aim of reducing side-effect burden
- development of non-dopamine antipsychotics
- development of add-on treatments that target specific aspects of schizophrenia (e.g. negative symptoms, cognitive symptoms, refractory symptoms, etc).

Further refined dopamine-related antipsychotics

Cariprazine

Cariprazine is a D_3-prefering D_3/D_2 partial agonist with limited activity at other receptor types.[1,2] The parent drug has a plasma half-life of several days and is metabolised by CYP3A4 to active compounds with even longer plasma half-lives.[3] Published data are very limited, but doses of 3–9 mg/day seem to be effective in schizophrenia and bipolar mania with minimal effects on metabolic parameters, prolactin or the ECG.[3] Currently (as of late 2014), cariprazine is being evaluated for regulatory approval and is not as yet available for routine clinical use.

Brexpiprazole

Brexpiprazole[4] is a D_2 partial agonist and $5HT_{2A}$ antagonist which also inhibits serotonin re-uptake and is chemically related to aripiprazole. It has been investigated as a treatment for attention deficit hyperactivity disorder (ADHD), adjunct in refractory unipolar depression and schizophrenia. Its main adverse effects are akathisia, weight gain and nasopharyngitis (all with placebo-corrected incidences of <5%). It appears to have no effect on the cardiac QT interval. Currently (as of late 2014), brexpiprazole is being evaluated for regulatory approval and is not as yet available for routine clinical use.

ITI-007

ITI-007 is a new compound being investigated by the drug company Intracellular Therapies – and while the drug was chosen because of its effects on intracellular signalling – it seems to achieve this effect via actions on dopamine and serotonin receptors. The compound has been evaluated in Phase I and Phase II trials in patients with schizophrenia and has shown promise in the treatment of positive and negative symptoms with limited side-effects.[5] The compound will need to be evaluated in Phase III trials to confirm efficacy and differential value. Those studies are currently being planned.

Inhaled loxapine

This represents a new form of delivery of antipsychotics for acute dosing. It uses the conventional antipsychotic loxapine, in a powder form and delivers it via a breath-actuated single-use inhaler at doses of 5 mg and 10 mg of loxapine equivalent. Pharmacokinetically, this delivers a peak concentration within 2–3 minutes and a clinically discernible effect within 10 minutes. In addition to side-effects related to loxapine, the delivery method leads to dysgeusia (distorted taste sense or bad taste) in a small number, and bronchospasm rarely. The method does require active patient participation, thus limiting use in acutely agitated situations. The drug is approved for use in the US and Europe but not widely marketed.

Non-dopamine approaches to antipsychotic effect

Phosphodiesterase 10A inhibitors

All antipsychotics block dopamine receptors. One effect of dopamine blockade is an alteration in intracellular cyclic adenosine monophosphate (AMP). Phosphodiesterase (PDE) enzyme systems regulate intracellular cyclic AMP, and since PDE 10A is expressed mainly in cells bearing dopamine receptors, it is possible to bypass the D2 receptors and achieve the same effect (in cells) via PDE 10A inhibitors.[6] A number of companies are exploring this strategy to treat schizophrenia. Pfizer has already evaluated PF-02545920 in Phase II trials, without success. Other companies (Amgen [AMG579], Lundbeck [AF111167], Omeros [OMS643762] Roche, Takeda, Forum, ICT) are developing different compounds for the same target.[7] None of these agents is available for clinical use as yet.

Add-on treatments for schizophrenia

Bitopertin and others – for negative symptoms

Bitopertin is a glycine re-uptake inhibitor which modulates glutamate and dopamine in the brain.[8] Similar agents Org 25935 (Organon) and AMG 747 (Amgen) were also being developed for the treatment for negative symptoms as an adjunct to regulate atypical antipsychotic treatment. Bitopertin is generally well tolerated and has minimal effects on the QT interval.[9] By inhibiting the glycine type 1 (GlyT1) transporter, bitopertin also inhibits haemoglobin synthesis and most patients show a dose-related reduction in plasma Hb, although reductions of >10% are uncommon.[10] While the Phase II trials showed evidence of an antipsychotic effect,[11] much larger Phase III trials have failed to replicate this effect.[12] Bitopertin is not currently available for clinical trials and it is unclear if any of these agents are being developed further.

Bitopertin and others – for refractory symptoms

Bitopertin is also being investigated as an add-on agent for patients for whom the conventional (dopamine-blocking) antipsychotics do not provide a sufficient clinical response on positive symptoms. Phase III studies have been initiated based on mechanistic reasoning, though the early results have not been encouraging.

Cholinergic approaches for cognitive symptoms

It is widely recognised that despite good control of psychosis, most patients suffer with cognitive symptoms which limit their functional potential. A number of pathways have been implicated but there is considerable interest in enhancing cholinergic transmission, especially via the nicotinic alpha-7 receptor.[13] Targacept's TC 5619 and Forum's EVP-6124, both of which are partial agonists at this receptor have been actively investigated at scale. After initially encouraging results[14] which were not replicated in subsequent larger trials, TC 5619 is not being further developed. After a positive Phase II study in which EVP-6124 was superior to placebo in both cognitive test improvement and functional symptoms improvement it is being evaluated for further Phase III trials. These agents are not available for clinical use.

References

1. Kiss B et al. Cariprazine (RGH-188), a dopamine D(3) receptor-preferring, D(3)/D(2) dopamine receptor antagonist-partial agonist antipsychotic candidate: in vitro and neurochemical profile. J Pharmacol Exp Ther 2010; 333:328–340.

2. Seneca N et al. Occupancy of dopamine D(2) and D(3) and serotonin 5-HT(1)A receptors by the novel antipsychotic drug candidate, cariprazine (RGH-188), in monkey brain measured using positron emission tomography. Psychopharmacology (Berl) 2011; 218:579–587.

3. Citrome L. Cariprazine: chemistry, pharmacodynamics, pharmacokinetics, and metabolism, clinical efficacy, safety, and tolerability. Expert Opin Drug Metab Toxicol 2013; 9:193–206.

4. Citrome L. A review of the pharmacology, efficacy and tolerability of recently approved and upcoming oral antipsychotics: an evidence-based medicine approach. CNS Drugs 2013; 27:879–911.

5. Intra-Cellular Therapies. Intra-Cellular Therapies Announces Positive Topline Phase II Clinical Results of ITI-007 for the Treatment of Schizophrenia. http://www.intracellulartherapies.com/press-room/press-releases/10-press-releases/38-dec-9-2013.html, 2013.

6. Siuciak JA. The role of phosphodiesterases in schizophrenia : therapeutic implications. CNS Drugs 2008; 22:983–993.

7. Schizophrenia Research Forum. Drugs in Trials. http://www.schizophreniaforum.org/res/drc/drug_tables.asp, 2014.

8. Alberati D et al. Glycine reuptake inhibitor RG1678: a pharmacologic characterization of an investigational agent for the treatment of schizophrenia. Neuropharmacology 2012; 62:1152–1161.

9. Hofmann, C et al. Evaluation of the effects of bitopertin (RG1678) on cardiac repolarization: a thorough corrected QT study in healthy male volunteers. Clin Ther 2012; 34:2061–2071.

10. Stark FS et al. Semi-physiologic Population PKPD Model Characterizing the Effect of Bitopertin (RG1678) Glycine Reuptake Inhibitor on Hemoglobin Turnover in Humans. PAGE 21 (2012) Abstr 2553. www.page-meeting.org/?abstract=2553: http://www.page-meeting.org/?abstract=2553, 2013.

11. Umbricht D et al. Effect of bitopertin, a glycine reuptake inhibitor, on negative symptoms of schizophrenia: a randomized, double-blind, proof-of-concept study. JAMA Psychiatry 2014; 71:637–646.

12. Goff DC. Bitopertin: the good news and bad news. JAMA Psychiatry 2014; 71:621–622.

13. Martin LF et al. Schizophrenia and the alpha7 nicotinic acetylcholine receptor. Int Rev Neurobiol 2007; 78:225–246.

14. Lieberman, JA et al. A Randomized Exploratory Trial of an Alpha-7 Nicotinic Receptor Agonist (TC-5619) for Cognitive Enhancement in Schizophrenia. Neuropsychopharmacology 2013; 38:968–975.

NICE guidelines for the treatment of schizophrenia[1]

The 2009 NICE guidelines[2] differed importantly from previous guidelines. There was no longer an imperative to prescribe an 'atypical' as first line treatment and it was recommended only that clozapine be 'offered' (rather than prescribed) after the prior failure of two antipsychotics. These semantic differences pointed respectively towards a disillusionment with SGAs and a recognition of the delay in prescribing clozapine in practice. Much emphasis was placed on involving patients and their carers in prescribing decisions. There is some evidence that this is rarely done[3] but that it can be done.[4] New NICE guidelines appeared in February 2014. Few changes were made to recommendations regarding drug treatment but psychological treatments are now more strongly promoted (perhaps reflecting the make-up of the NICE review panel).

NICE guidelines – a summary

- For people with newly diagnosed schizophrenia, offer oral antipsychotic medication. Provide information and discuss the benefits and side-effect profile of each drug with the service user. The choice of drug should be made by the service user and healthcare professional together, considering:
  - the relative potential of individual antipsychotic drugs to cause extrapyramidal side-effects (including akathisia), cardiovascular side-effects, metabolic side-effects (including weight gain), hormonal side-effects and other side-effects (including unpleasant subjective experiences)
  - the views of the carer where the service user agrees.
- Before starting antipsychotic medication, offer the person with schizophrenia an electrocardiogram (ECG) if:
  - specified in the summary of product characteristics (SPC)
  - a physical examination has identified specific cardiovascular risk (such as diagnosis of high blood pressure)
  - there is personal history of cardiovascular disease, or
  - the service user is being admitted as an inpatient.

- Treatment with antipsychotic medication should be considered an explicit individual therapeutic trial. Include the following:
  - record the indications and expected benefits and risks of oral antipsychotic medication, and the expected time for a change in symptoms and appearance of side-effects
  - at the start of treatment give a dose at the lower end of the licensed range and slowly titrate upwards within the dose range given in the British National Formulary (BNF) or SPC
  - justify and record reasons for dosages outside the range given in the BNF or SPC.

- Monitor and record the following regularly and systematically throughout treatment, but especially during titration:
  - efficacy, including changes in symptoms and behaviour
  - side-effects of treatment, taking into account overlap between certain side-effects and clinical features of schizophrenia, for example the overlap between akathisia and agitation or anxiety

- adherence
- physical health
- nutritional status, diet and physical activity
- record the rationale for continuing, changing or stopping medication, and the effects of such changes
- carry out a trial of the medication at optimum dosage for 4–6 weeks (although half of this period is probably sufficient if no effect at all is seen).

- Physical monitoring is to be the responsibility of the secondary care team for one year or until the patient is stable.
- Do not use a loading dose of antipsychotic medication (often referred to as 'rapid neuroleptisation'). (Note that this does not apply to loading doses of depot forms of olanzapine and paliperidone.)
- Do not routinely initiate regular combined antipsychotic medication, except for short periods (for example, when changing medication).
- If prescribing chlorpromazine, warn of its potential to cause skin photosensitivity. Advise using sunscreen if necessary.
- Consider offering depot/long-acting injectable antipsychotic medication to people with schizophrenia:
  - who would prefer such treatment after an acute episode
  - where avoiding covert non-adherence (either intentional or unintentional) to antipsychotic medication is a clinical priority within the treatment plan.

- Offer clozapine to people with schizophrenia whose illness has not responded adequately to treatment despite the sequential use of adequate doses of at least two different antipsychotic drugs alongside psychological therapies. At least one of the drugs should be a non-clozapine second-generation antipsychotic. (See Figure 2.2 – we recommend that one of the drugs should be olanzapine).
- For people with schizophrenia whose illness has not responded adequately to clozapine at an optimised dose, healthcare professionals should establish prior compliance with optimised antipsychotic treatment (including measuring drug levels) and engagement with psychological treatment before adding a second antipsychotic to augment treatment with clozapine. An adequate trial of such an augmentation may need to be up to 8–10 weeks (some data suggest 6 weeks may be enough[5]). Choose a drug that does not compound the common side-effects of clozapine.

References

1. National Institute for Health and Care Excellence. Psychosis and schizophrenia in adults: treatment and management. Clinical Guideline **178**, 2014. http://www.nice.org.uk/Guidance/CG178
2. National Institute for Health and Clinical Excellence. Schizophrenia: core interventions in the treatment and management of schizophrenia in adults in primary and secondary care (update). Clinical Guideline **82**, 2009. http://www.nice.org.uk/
3. Olofinjana B et al. Antipsychotic drugs - information and choice: a patient survey. Psychiatr Bull 2005; **29**:369–371.
4. Whiskey E et al. Evaluation of an antipsychotic information sheet for patients. Int J Psychiatry Clin Pract 2005; **9**:264–270.
5. Taylor D et al. Augmentation of clozapine with a second antipsychotic. A meta analysis. Acta Psychiatr Scand 2012; **125**:15–24.

Antipsychotic response – to increase the dose, to switch, to add or just wait – what is the right move?

For any clinician taking active care of patients with schizophrenia the single most common clinical dilemma is what to do when the current antipsychotic is not optimal for the patient. This may be for two broad reasons: firstly when the symptoms are well controlled but side-effects are problematic and, secondly, where there is inadequate response. Fortunately, given the diversity of antipsychotics available, it is usually possible to find an antipsychotic that has a side-effect profile that is acceptable to the patient. The more difficult question is when there is inadequate symptom response. If the patient has already had 'adequate' trials of two antipsychotics for 'sufficient' duration then clozapine should clearly be considered. However, the majority of the patients in the clinic are those who are either as yet not ready for clozapine or unwilling to choose that option. In those instances the clinician has four main choices: to increase the dose of the current medication; to switch to another antipsychotic; to add an adjunct medication or just to wait.

When to increase the dose?

While optimal doses of typical antipsychotics were always a matter of debate, the recommended doses of the newer atypical antipsychotics were generally based on careful and extensive clinical trials but even then the consensus on optimal doses has changed with time. For example, when risperidone was first launched it was suggested that optimal titration was from 2 mg to 4 mg to 6 mg or more for all patients, however, practising psychiatrists have tended towards lower doses.[1] On the other hand, when quetiapine was introduced, 300 mg was considered the optimal dose and the overall consensus now is towards higher doses,[2] although the evidence does not support this shift.[2,3] Nonetheless, most clinicians feel comfortable in navigating within the recommended clinical doses. The more critical question is what one should do if one has hit the upper limit of these dose ranges and the patient is tolerating the medication well with limited efficacy benefit.

Dose–response observations

Davis and Chen performed a systematic meta-analysis of the data available up to 2004 and concluded that the average dose that produces maximal benefit was 4 mg for risperidone, 16 mg of olanzapine, 120 mg of ziprasidone and 10–15 mg of aripiprazole (they could not determine such a dose for quetiapine using their method).[4] More recent trials have tried to compare 'high-dose' versus the standard dose. Kinon et al[5] studied the dose–response relationship of standard and higher doses of olanzapine in a randomized, double-blind, 8-week, fixed-dose study comparing olanzapine 10 mg, 20 mg and 40 mg and found no benefit of the higher doses (i.e. 40 mg was no better than even 10 mg) and found clear evidence for increasing side-effects (weight gain and prolactin) with dose. Similarly, the initial licensing studies of risperidone had compared the usual doses, 2–6 mg/day, to the higher doses, 8–16 mg/day, and had chosen the lower dose ranges as they found no additional benefit at higher doses, but, a clear signal for greater side-effects (extrapyramidal side-effects and prolactin). These more recent studies are in accord with older studies involving fixed-doses of haloperidol.[6] However, it is important to keep in mind that these doses are extracted from group evidence where patients are assigned to different doses, which is a different question from the clinical one where one considers increasing a dose only in those who have failed an initial dose. To our knowledge only one study has systematically addressed this question in its clinically relevant dimension. Kinon et al.[7] examined patients who failed to respond to the (then) standard dose of fluphenazine (20 mg) and tested three strategies: increasing dose to 80 mg, switching to haloperidol or watchful waiting (on the original dose). All three strategies were equivalent in terms of efficacy. Thus, it seems that at a group level (as opposed to an individual level) there is little evidence to support treatment beyond the recommended doses. This evidence from structured trials is corroborated by the practice norms – Hermes and Rosenheck examined the CATIE data to identify clinical factors that predicted the physician's decision to increase the dose and found that decisions for dose change (within the therapeutic ranges) were only weakly associated with clinical measures.[8]

Plasma level variations

However, group level evidence cannot completely determine individual decisions. There is significant inter-individual variation in plasma levels in patients treated with antipsychotics. One can often encounter a patient who, when at the higher end of the dose range (say 6 mg of risperidone or 20 mg of olanzapine) would have plasma levels that are well below the range expected for 2 mg risperidone or 10 mg of olanzapine respectively. In such patients, one can make a rational case for increasing the dose, provided the patient is informed and the side-effects are tolerable, to bring the plasma levels to the median optimal range for the particular medication. More details on plasma levels and their interpretation are provided in Chapter 1. However, one often encounters an unresponsive compliant patient, whose dose has reached the ceiling and plasma levels are also sufficient – what next?

Treatment choices

There are essentially three options here, clozapine, switch to another drug or add another (non-clozapine) drug. If the patient meets the criteria for clozapine it is undoubtedly the preferred option. Yet, in the most recent audit of community (not inpatient) practice in the UK, covering some 5000 patients in 60 different NHS Trusts, it was shown that nearly 40% of the patients who met criteria for treatment resistance did not receive clozapine; and of those who did the vast majority (85%) received their clozapine after a much longer wait after the failure of two antipsychotics that is advised in most guidelines.[9]

Nonetheless, there is a set of patients who do not like the idea of regular blood testing, the side-effect profile and the regular appointments required to receive clozapine. In these patients the choice is to switch to another medication or to add another antipsychotic. The data on switching are sparse. While almost every clinical trial in patients with chronic schizophrenia has entailed the patient switching from one antipsychotic to another - there are no rigorous studies of preferred switch combinations (e.g. if risperidone fails – what next? Olanzapine, quetiapine, aripiprazole or ziprasidone?). If one looks at only the switching trials which have been sponsored by the drug companies – it leads to a rather confusing picture, with the trials results being very closely linked to the sponsors' interest (see 'Why olanzapine beats risperidone, risperidone beats quetiapine, and quetiapine beats olanzapine: an exploratory analysis of head-to-head comparison studies of second-generation antipsychotics'.[10])

CATIE, a major US-based publicly funded comparative trial, examined patients who had failed their first atypical antipsychotic and were then randomly assigned to a different second one.[11] Patients who were switched to olanzapine and risperidone did better than those switched to quetiapine and ziprasidone. This greater effectiveness is supported by a recent meta-analysis that compared a number of atypicals to first-generation typical antipsychotics and concluded that, other than clozapine, only amisulpride, risperidone and olanzapine were superior to first-generation agents in efficacy;[12] and a meta-analysis comparing atypicals amongst themselves which suggests that olanzapine and risperidone (in that order) may be more effective than others.[13] This suggests that if a patient has not tried olanzapine or risperidone as yet, it would be a reasonable decision to switch to these drugs provided the side-effect balance is favourable. Between these two drugs, the data is somewhat limited. However, a number of controlled, but open label studies do show an asymmetrical advantage (i.e. switching to olanzapine being more effective, than risperidone) – providing some direction, albeit incomplete.[14,15]

What to choose for someone who fails olanzapine and risperidone (other than clozapine) is not yet clear. Should one switch (to, say, aripiprazole or ziprasidone or even an older typical agent) or should one add another antipsychotic. It should be borne in mind that after 'switching', adding another antipsychotic is probably the second most common clinical move as 39–43% of patients in routine care are on more than one antipsychotic.[16] Often a second antipsychotic is added to get an additional profile (e.g. sedation with quetiapine, or decrease prolactin with the addition of aripiprazole) – these matters are discussed elsewhere. We concern ourselves solely with the addition of an antipsychotic to another antipsychotic to increase efficacy. From a theoretical point of view since all antipsychotics block D_2 receptors (unlike antihypertensives, which use different mechanisms) there is limited rationale for addition. Studies of add-ons have often chosen combinations of convenience or based on clinical lore and perhaps the most systematic evidence is available for the addition of antipsychotics to clozapine[17] – perhaps supported by the rationale that since clozapine has low D_2 occupancy, increasing its D_2 occupancy may yield additional benefits.[18] A meta-analysis of all systematic antipsychotic add-on studies seem to suggest a modest benefit at best – the benefit being more likely when the patient is on clozapine, when a first-generation antipsychotic is added, and when both antipsychotics are used at effective doses.[19]

However, a move to polypharmacy should not be seen as a one-way street. While there is some evidence for augmentation with another antipsychotic, in general this ought to be avoided. Nonetheless, under some conditions of acute exacerbations or agitation the physician may find this to be the only practicable solution. Or quite often the physician may inherit the care of a patient on antipsychotic polypharmacy. Can this be safely reversed? Essock et al[20] provide evidence from a large trial (127 patients who were stable on antipsychotic polypharmacy). They examined the efficacy of returning these patients to their one major antipsychotic. Over a 12-month period this strategy was successful in about two-thirds of the patients. In the cases where the move to monotherapy resulted in a return of symptoms, the most common recourse was to go back to the original polypharmacy, and this was achieved without any significant worsening in this group. As an advantage the monotherapy group was exposed to less medication, had equivalent symptoms and even lost some weight.

When to just 'stay'? A review of the above evidence suggests that no one strategy – increasing the dose, switching or augmenting – is a clear winner in all situations. Increase the dose if plasma levels are low; switch if the patient has not tried olanzapine or risperidone; and if failing on clozapine – augmentation may help. Given the limited efficacy of these manoeuvres perhaps an equally important call by the treating doctor is when to just 'stay' with the current pharmacotherapy and focus on non-pharmacological means: engagement in case-management, targeted psychological treatments and vocational rehabilitation as means of enhancing patient well-being. While it may seem a passive option – staying may often do less harm that aimless switching.

Summary – when treatment fails

- If dose has been optimised, consider watchful waiting.
- Consider increasing antipsychotic dose according to tolerability and plasma levels.
- If this fails, consider switching to olanzapine or risperidone (if not already used).
- If this fails, use clozapine (supporting evidence very strong).
- If clozapine fails, use time-limited augmentation strategies (supporting evidence variable).

References

1. Ezewuzie N et al. Establishing a dose-response relationship for oral risperidone in relapsed schizophrenia. J Psychopharmacol 2006; 20:86–90.
2. Sparshatt A et al. Quetiapine: dose-response relationship in schizophrenia. CNS Drugs 2008; 22:49–68.
3. Honer WG et al. A randomized, double-blind, placebo-controlled study of the safety and tolerability of high-dose quetiapine in patients with persistent symptoms of schizophrenia or schizoaffective disorder. J Clin Psychiatry 2012; 73:13–20.
4. Davis JM et al. Dose response and dose equivalence of antipsychotics. J Clin Psychopharmacol 2004; 24:192–208.
5. Kinon BJ et al. Standard and higher dose of olanzapine in patients with schizophrenia or schizoaffective disorder: a randomized, double-blind, fixed-dose study. J Clin Psychopharmacol 2008; 28:392–400.
6. Van PT et al. A controlled dose comparison of haloperidol in newly admitted schizophrenic patients. Arch Gen Psychiatry 1990; 47:754–758.
7. Kinon BJ et al. Treatment of neuroleptic-resistant schizophrenic relapse. Psychopharmacol Bull 1993; 29:309–314.
8. Hermes E et al. Predictors of antipsychotic dose changes in the CATIE schizophrenia trial. Psychiatry Res 2012; 199:1–7.
9. Patel MX et al. Quality of prescribing for schizophrenia: evidence from a national audit in England and Wales. Eur Neuropsychopharmacol 2014; 24:499–509.
10. Heres S et al. Why olanzapine beats risperidone, risperidone beats quetiapine, and quetiapine beats olanzapine: an exploratory analysis of head-to-head comparison studies of second-generation antipsychotics. Am J Psychiatry 2006; 163:185–194.
11. Stroup TS et al. Effectiveness of olanzapine, quetiapine, risperidone, and ziprasidone in patients with chronic schizophrenia following discontinuation of a previous atypical antipsychotic. Am J Psychiatry 2006; 163:611–622.
12. Leucht S et al. Second-generation versus first-generation antipsychotic drugs for schizophrenia: a meta-analysis. Lancet 2009; 373:31–41.
13. Leucht S et al. A meta-analysis of head-to-head comparisons of second-generation antipsychotics in the treatment of schizophrenia. Am J Psychiatry 2009; 166:152–163.
14. Hong J et al. Clinical consequences of switching from olanzapine to risperidone and vice versa in outpatients with schizophrenia: 36-month results from the Worldwide Schizophrenia Outpatients Health Outcomes (W-SOHO) study. BMC Psychiatry 2012; 12:218.
15. Agid O et al. Antipsychotic response in first-episode schizophrenia: efficacy of high doses and switching. Eur Neuropsychopharmacol 2013; 23:1017–1022.
16. Paton C et al. High-dose and combination antipsychotic prescribing in acute adult wards in the UK: the challenges posed by p.r.n. prescribing. Br J Psychiatry 2008; 192:435–439.

17. Taylor DM et al. Augmentation of clozapine with a second antipsychotic – a meta-analysis of randomized, placebo-controlled studies. Acta Psychiatr Scand 2009; **119**:419–425.

18. Kapur S et al. Increased dopamine D2 receptor occupancy and elevated prolactin level associated with addition of haloperidol to clozapine. Am J Psychiatry 2001; **158**:311–314.

19. Correll CU et al. Antipsychotic combinations vs monotherapy in schizophrenia: a meta-analysis of randomized controlled trials. Schizophr Bull 2009; **35**:443–457.

20. Essock SM et al. Effectiveness of switching from antipsychotic polypharmacy to monotherapy. Am J Psychiatry 2011; **168**:702–708.

Antipsychotic long-acting injections

Antipsychotic long-acting injections (LAIs) are recommended where a patient has expressed preference for such a formulation because of its convenience or where avoidance of covert non-adherence is a clinical priority.[1,2] It is estimated that between one-quarter and one-third of people with schizophrenia are prescribed a LAI,[3] although this prevalence varies from country to country. Approximately half are also prescribed an oral antipsychotic drug, which often results in so-called high dose prescribing and seems counterintuitive.

Advice on prescribing LAIs

- **For FGAs, give a test dose.** Because they are long-acting, any adverse effects that result from injection are likely to be long-lived. For FGAs a test dose consisting of a small dose of active drug in a small volume of oil serves a dual purpose; it is a test of the patient's sensitivity to EPS and of any sensitivity to the base oil. For SGAs test doses are not required (less propensity to cause EPS and aqueous base not known to be allergenic).

- **Begin with the lowest therapeutic dose.** There are few data showing clear dose–response effects for LAIs. There is some information indicating that low doses (within the licensed range) are at least as effective as higher ones.[4-6] Low doses are likely to be better tolerated and are certainly less expensive.

- **Administer at the longest possible licensed interval.** All LAIs can be safely administered at their licensed dosing intervals, bearing in mind the maximum recommended single dose. There is no evidence whatsoever to suggest that shortening the dose interval improves efficacy although this fantasy persists. Moreover, injections are painful, so less frequent administration is desirable. The 'observation' that some patients deteriorate in the days before the next dose is due is not supported by fact. For some hours (or even days with some preparations) plasma levels of antipsychotics continue to fall, albeit slowly, after the next injection. Thus, patients are most at risk of deterioration immediately after a LAI and not before it. Moreover, in trials, relapse seems only to occur 3–6 months after withdrawing therapy; roughly the time required to clear steady-state LAI drug levels from the blood.

- **Adjust doses only after an adequate period of assessment.** Attainment of peak plasma levels, therapeutic effect and steady-state plasma levels are all delayed with LAIs. Doses may be *reduced* if adverse effects occur, but should only be increased after careful assessment over at least one month, and preferably longer. The use of adjunctive oral medication to assess dosage requirements of LAIs may be helpful, but is complicated by the slow emergence of antipsychotic effects. Note that at the start of therapy, plasma levels of antipsychotic released from a LAI increase over several weeks to months without increasing the given dose. (This is due to accumulation: steady state is only achieved after 6–8 weeks.) Dose increases during this time to steady-state plasma levels are thus illogical and impossible to evaluate properly. Monitoring and recording of efficacy, side-effects and impact on physical health during therapy is recommended

- **Depot preparations are not recommended for those who are antipsychotic-naïve.** Tolerance to some LAIs can be established by using the oral form of the same drug for two weeks before starting the LAI. Good examples here are haloperidol, aripiprazole and paliperidone (using oral risperidone).

Differences between LAIs

There are few differences between individual FGA LAIs. Pipotiazine may be associated with relatively less frequent EPS, and fluphenazine with relatively more EPS, but perhaps less weight gain.[7] Cochrane reviews have been completed for pipotiazine,[8] flupentixol,[9] zuclopenthixol,[10] haloperidol[11] and fluphenazine.[12] With the exception of zuclopenthixol (see below), these preparations are equally effective, both with respect to oral antipsychotics and each other. Standard doses are said to be as effective as high doses for flupentixol.[9]

Table 2.8 Antipsychotic LAIs: suggested doses and frequencies[2]

Drug	Trade Name	Licenced injection site	Test dose (mg)	Dose range (mg/week)	Dosing interval (weeks)	Comments
Aripiprazole	Abilify Maintena	Buttock	Not required**	300–400 mg monthly	Monthly	Does not increase prolactin
Flupentixol decanoate	Depixol	Buttock or thigh	20	50 mg every 4 weeks to 400 mg a week	2–4	Maximum licensed dose is very high relative to other LAIs
Fluphenazine decanoate	Modecate	Gluteal region	12.5	12.5 mg every 2 weeks to 100 mg every 2 weeks	2–5	High EPS
Haloperidol decanoate	Haldol	Gluteal region	25*	50–300 mg every 4 weeks	4	High EPS
Olanzapine pamoate	ZypAdhera	Gluteal	Not required**	150 mg every 4 weeks to 300 mg every 2 weeks	2–4	Note risk of post injection syndrome
Paliperidone palmitate	Xeplion	Deltoid or gluteal	Not required**	50–150 mg monthly	Monthly	Loading dose required at treatment initiation
Pipothiazine palmitate	Piportil	Gluteal region	25	50–200 mg every 4 weeks	4	? Lower incidence of EPS (unproven)
Risperidone microspheres	Risperidal Consta	Deltoid or gluteal	Not required**	25–50 mg every 2 weeks	2	Drug release delayed for 2–3 weeks
Zuclopenthixol decanoate	Clopixol	Buttock or thigh	100	200 mg every 3 weeks to 600 mg a week	2–4	? Slightly better efficacy than some FGAs

- The doses above are for adults. Check formal labelling for appropriate doses in the elderly.
- After a test dose, wait 4–10 days then titrate to maintenance dose according to response (see product information for individual drugs).
- Avoid using shorter dose intervals than those recommended except in exceptional circumstances (e.g. long interval necessitates high volume (>3–4 mL) injection). Maximum licensed single dose overrides longer intervals and lower volumes. For example, zuclopenthixol 500 mg every week is licensed whereas 1000 mg every 2 weeks is not (more than the licensed maximum of 600 mg is administered). Always check official manufacturer's information.

*Test dose not stated by manufacturer.
**Tolerability and response to the oral preparation should be established before administering the LAI. With respect to paliperidone LAI, oral risperidone can be used for this purpose.

Two differences that do exist between FGA LAIs are:

- zuclopenthixol may be more effective in preventing relapses than others, although this may be at the expense of an increased burden of side-effects[13,14]
- flupentixol decanoate can be given in very much higher 'neuroleptic equivalent' doses than the other LAI preparations and still remain 'within licensed dosing limits'. It is doubtful that this confers any real therapeutic advantage.

Aripiprazole, paliperidone, risperidone and olanzapine LAIs have a relatively lower propensity for EPS. Risperidone however increases prolactin, and because of its pharmacokinetic profile, dosage adjustment can be complex. Olanzapine can cause significant weight gain and is associated with inadvertent intravascular injection or post injection syndrome[15]. Unlike risperidone LAI, it is effective within a few days. Paliperidone is also rapidly released and effective within a few days, as is aripiprazole LAI.

Although the use of LAIs does not guarantee good treatment adherence, for those who continue with LAIs, there may be some adherence advantage over oral antipsychotics, which is indicated by a longer time to medication discontinuation.[16,17] There is also some evidence to suggest a better global outcome with LAIs as compared with oral antipsychotics with a reduced risk of rehospitalisation.[1,16] It has been argued that compliance with oral antipsychotics decreases over time and that relapse rates in patients prescribed depots decrease in comparison to oral antipsychotics only in the longer term.[18] That is, depots reveal advantages over oral treatment only after several years.

Table 2.8 summarises suggested doses and frequencies for administration of antipsychotic LAIs.

Intramuscular anticholinergics and LAIs

Antipsychotic LAIs do not produce acute movement disorders at the time of administration:[19] this may take hours to days. The administration of intramuscular procyclidine routinely with each dose is illogical, as the effects of the anticholinergic drug will have worn off before plasma antipsychotic levels peak.

References

1. National Institute for Health and Care Excellence. Psychosis and schizophrenia in adults: treatment and management. Clinical Guideline **178**, 2014. http://www.nice.org.uk/Guidance/CG178
2. Barnes TR. Evidence-based guidelines for the pharmacological treatment of schizophrenia: recommendations from the British Association for Psychopharmacology. J Psychopharmacol 2011; 25:567–620.
3. Barnes T. Antipsychotic long acting injections: prescribing practice in the UK. Br J Psychiatry 2009; 195:S37–S42.
4. Kane JM et al. A multidose study of haloperidol decanoate in the maintenance treatment of schizophrenia. Am J Psychiatry 2002; 159:554–560.
5. Taylor D. Establishing a dose-response relationship for haloperidol decanoate. Psychiatr Bull 2005; 29:104–107.
6. McEvoy JP et al. Effectiveness of paliperidone palmitate vs haloperidol decanoate for maintenance treatment of schizophrenia: a randomized clinical trial. JAMA 2014; 311:1978–1987.
7. Taylor D. Psychopharmacology and adverse effects of antipsychotic long acting injections. Br J Psychiatry 2009; 195:S13–S19.
8. Dinesh M et al. Depot pipotiazine palmitate and undecylenate for schizophrenia. Cochrane Database Syst Rev 2004; CD001720.
9. Mahapatra J et al. Flupenthixol decanoate (depot) for schizophrenia or other similar psychotic disorders. Cochrane Database Syst Rev 2014; 6: CD001470.
10. Coutinho E et al. Zuclopenthixol decanoate for schizophrenia and other serious mental illnesses. Cochrane Database Syst Rev 2000; CD001164.
11. Quraishi S et al. Depot haloperidol decanoate for schizophrenia. Cochrane Database Syst Rev 2000; CD001361.

12. David Aet al. Depot fluphenazine decanoate and enanthate for schizophrenia. Cochrane Database Syst Rev 2005; CD000307.

13. da Silva Freire Coutinho E et al. Zuclopenthixol decanoate for schizophrenia and other serious mental illnesses. Cochrane Database Syst Rev 2006; CD001164.

14. Shajahan P et al. Comparison of the effectiveness of depot antipsychotics in routine clinical practice. Psychiatrist 2010; 34:273–279.

15. Citrome L. Olanzapine pamoate: a stick in time? Int J Clin Pract 2009; 63:140–150.

16. Tiihonen J et al. A Nationwide Cohort Study of Oral and Depot Antipsychotics After First Hospitalization for Schizophrenia. Am J Psychiatry 2011; 168:603–609.

17. Leucht C et al. Oral versus depot antipsychotic drugs for schizophrenia--a critical systematic review and meta-analysis of randomised long-term trials. Schizophr Res 2011; 127:83–92.

18. Schooler NR. Relapse and rehospitalization: comparing oral and depot antipsychotics. J Clin Psychiatry 2003; 64 Suppl 16:14–17.

19. Kane JM et al. Guidelines for depot antipsychotic treatment in schizophrenia. European Neuropsychopharmacology Consensus Conference in Siena, Italy. Eur Neuropsychopharmacol 1998; 8:55–66.

Further reading

Patel MX et al. Antipsychotic long-acting (depot) injections for the treatment of schizophrenia. Br J Psychiatry 2009; 195 Suppl 52:S1–S67.

CHAPTER 2

Depot antipsychotics – pharmacokinetics

Table 2.9 summarises the pharmacokinetics of depot antipsychotics.

Table 2.9 Pharmacokinetics of depot antipsychotics

Drug	Trade name	Time to peak* (days)	Plasma half-life (days)	Time to steady state (weeks)[†]
Aripiprazole[1]	Abilify Maintena	7	30–46	~20
Flupentixol decanoate[2]	Depixol	7	8–17	~9
Fluphenazine decanoate[3–5]	Modecate	8–12[‡]	10	~8
Haloperidol decanoate[6,7]	Haldol	7	21	~14
Olanzapine pamoate[8,9]	ZypAdhera	2–3	30	~12
Paliperidone palmitate[10]	Xeplion	13	29–45	~20
Pipotiazine palmitate[11,12]	Piportil	7–14	15	~9
Risperidone microspheres[13,14]	Risperidal Consta	35	4	~8
Zuclopenthixol decanoate[2,11,15]	Clopixol	4–7	19	~12

*Time to peak is not the same as time to reach therapeutic plasma concentration but both are dependent on dose. For large (loading) doses, therapeutic activity is often seen before attaining peak levels. For low (test) doses, the initial peak level may be sub-therapeutic.

[†]Attainment of steady state (SS) follows logarithmic, not linear characteristics: around 90% of SS levels are achieved in three half-lives. Time to attain steady state is independent of dose and dosing frequency (that is, you can't hurry it up by giving more, more often). Loading doses can be used to produce prompt therapeutic plasma levels but time to SS remains the same.

[‡]Earlier estimates suggest peak concentrations after only a few hours.[15,16] It is likely that fluphenazine decanoate produces two peaks – one on the day of injection and a second slightly higher peak a week or so later.[6]

References

1. Mallikaarjun S et al. Pharmacokinetics, tolerability and safety of aripiprazole once-monthly in adult schizophrenia: an open-label, parallel-arm, multiple-dose study. Schizophr Res 2013; 150:281–288.
2. Jann MW et al. Clinical pharmacokinetics of the depot antipsychotics. Clin Pharmacokinet 1985; 10:315–333.
3. Simpson GM et al. Single-dose pharmacokinetics of fluphenazine after fluphenazine decanoate administration. J Clin Psychopharmacol 1990; 10:417–421.
4. Balant-Gorgia AE et al. Antipsychotic drugs. Clinical pharmacokinetics of potential candidates for plasma concentration monitoring. Clin Pharmacokinet 1987; 13:65–90.
5. Gitlin MJ et al. Persistence of fluphenazine in plasma after decanoate withdrawal. J Clin Psychopharmacol 1988; 8:53–56.
6. Wiles DH et al. Pharmacokinetics of haloperidol and fluphenazine decanoates in chronic schizophrenia. Psychopharmacology (Berl) 1990; 101:274–281.
7. Nayak RK et al. The bioavailability and pharmacokinetics of oral and depot intramuscular haloperidol in schizophrenic patients. J Clin Pharmacol 1987; 27:144–150.
8. Heres S et al. Pharmacokinetics of olanzapine long-acting injection: the clinical perspective. Int Clin Psychopharmacol 2014;.29:299–312.
9. Mitchell M et al. Single- and multiple-dose pharmacokinetic, safety, and tolerability profiles of olanzapine long-acting injection: an open-label, multicenter, nonrandomized study in patients with schizophrenia. Clin Ther 2013; 35:1890–1908.
10. Hoy SM et al. Intramuscular paliperidone palmitate. CNS Drugs 2010; 24:227–244.
11. Barnes TR et al. Long-term depot antipsychotics. A risk-benefit assessment. Drug Saf 1994; 10:464–479.
12. Ogden DA et al. Determination of pipothiazine in human plasma by reversed-phase high-performance liquid chromatography. J Pharm Biomed Anal 1989; 7:1273–1280.

13. Ereshefsky L et al. Pharmacokinetic profile and clinical efficacy of long-acting risperidone: potential benefits of combining an atypical antipsychotic and a new delivery system. Drugs R D 2005; **6**:129–137.

14. Eerdekens M et al. Pharmacokinetics and tolerability of long-acting risperidone in schizophrenia. Schizophr Res 2004; **70**:91–100.

15. Viala A et al. Comparative study of the pharmacokinetics of zuclopenthixol decanoate and fluphenazine decanoate. Psychopharmacology (Berl) 1988; **94**:293–297.

16. Soni SD et al. Plasma levels of fluphenazine decanoate. Effects of site of injection, massage and muscle activity. Br J Psychiatry 1988; **153**:382–384.

Management of patients on long-term depots

All patients receiving long-term treatment with antipsychotic medication should be seen by their responsible psychiatrist at least once a year (ideally more frequently) in order to review their progress and treatment. A systematic assessment of side-effects should constitute part of this review. For most people with multi-episode schizophrenia long-term, even lifelong, treatment is necessary. However with long-term depot treatment dose reduction might be considered in stable patients. There is some evidence to suggest that FGA depots are prescribed in excessive doses: haloperidol decanoate is optimally effective at 75 mg every 4 weeks;[1,2] other depots almost saturate dopamine receptors at low doses (e.g. flupentixol 40 mg per week[3]). There is no simple formula for deciding when or whether to reduce the dose of maintenance antipsychotic treatment; therefore, a risk–benefit analysis must be done for every patient. Many patients, it should be noted, are happy to receive depots.[4] When considering dose reduction, the following prompts may be helpful.

- Is the patient symptom-free and if so for how long? Long-standing, non-distressing symptoms which have not previously been responsive to medication may be excluded.
- What is the severity of the side-effects (EPS, tardive dyskinesia, obesity, etc.)?
- What is the previous pattern of illness? Consider the speed of onset, duration and severity of episodes and any danger posed to self or others.
- Has dosage reduction been attempted before? If so, what was the outcome?
- What are the patient's current social circumstances? Is it a period of relative stability, or are stressful life events anticipated?
- What is the social cost of relapse (e.g. is the patient the sole breadwinner for a family)?
- Is the patient able to monitor his/her own symptoms? If so, will he/she seek help?

If after consideration of the above, the decision is taken to reduce medication dose, the patient's family should be involved and a clear explanation given of what should be done if symptoms return/worsen. It would then be reasonable to proceed in the following manner.

- If it has not already been done, oral antipsychotic medication should be discontinued first.
- The interval between injections should be increased to up to 4 weeks before decreasing the dose given each time. Note: *not* with risperidone.
- The dose should be reduced by no more than one-third at any one time. Note: special considerations apply to risperidone.
- Decrements should, if possible, be made no more frequently than every 3 months, preferably every 6 months.
- Discontinuation should not be seen as the ultimate aim of the above process although it sometimes results. NICE[5] (2014) now suggest that intermittent treatment (symptom-triggered) is preferable to no treatment.

If the patient becomes symptomatic, this should be seen not as a failure, but rather as an important step in determining the minimum effective dose that the patient requires.

References

1. Taylor D. Establishing a dose-response relationship for haloperidol decanoate. Psychiatr Bull 2005; **29**:104–107.
2. McEvoy JP et al. Effectiveness of paliperidone palmitate vs haloperidol decanoate for maintenance treatment of schizophrenia: a randomized clinical trial. JAMA 2014; **311**:1978–1987.
3. Uchida H et al. Dose and dosing frequency of long-acting injectable antipsychotics: a systematic review of PET and SPECT data and clinical implications. J Clin Psychopharmacol 2014; Epub ahead of print: DOI: 10.1097/JCP.0000000000000065.
4. Heres S et al. The attitude of patients towards antipsychotic depot treatment. Int Clin Psychopharmacol 2007; **22**:275–282.
5. National Institute for Health and Care Excellence. Psychosis and schizophrenia in adults: treatment and management. Clinical Guideline **178**, 2014. http://www.nice.org.uk/Guidance/CG178

CHAPTER 2

Aripiprazole LAI

Aripiprazole lacks the prolactin-related and metabolic adverse effects of other SGA LAIs and so is a useful alternative to them. Placebo-controlled studies show a good acute and longer term effect[1] but aripiprazole LAI has not been compared with other depots. For most patients, a suitable dosing regimen is oral aripiprazole 10–20 mg/day for 14 days (to establish tolerability and response) then 400 mg aripiprazole LAI once monthly. Oral aripiprazole should be continued for 14 days after the first injection. In such a regimen, peak plasma levels are seen at 1–2 weeks after injection and the lowest trough at 4 weeks.[2] At steady state, peak plasma levels are up to 50% higher than the first dose peak and trough plasma levels only slightly below the first dose peak.[2] Dose adjustments should take this into account. A lower dose of 300 mg a month can be used in those not tolerating 400 mg. A dose of 200 mg a month may only be used for those patients receiving particular enzyme inhibiting drugs. The incidence of akathisia, insomnia, nausea and restlessness is similar to that seen with oral aripiprazole.[3,4]

There are no formal recommendations for switching to aripiprazole but we present recommendations based on our interpretation of available pharmacokinetic data in Table 2.10.

Table 2.10 Switching to aripiprazole LAI

Switching from	Aripiprazole LAI regimen
Oral antipsychotics	Cross taper antipsychotic with oral aripiprazole* over 2 weeks. Start LAI, continue aripiprazole oral for 2 weeks then stop
Depot antipsychotics (**not** risperidone LAI)	Start oral aripiprazole* on day last depot injection was due. Start aripiprazole LAI after 2 weeks then stop oral aripiprazole 2 weeks later
Risperidone LAI	Start oral aripiprazole* 5–6 weeks** after the last risperidone injection. Start aripiprazole LAI 2 weeks later; discontinue oral aripiprazole 2 weeks after that

*If prior response and tolerability to aripiprazole known, oral aripiprazole may not be required. Switch straight to aripiprazole LAI on the day oral would have started.
**This gap seems excessive, but the last injection of risperidone will provide therapeutic levels 4–6 weeks later; a post-dose peak at 5 weeks.

References

1. Shirley M et al. Aripiprazole (ABILIFY MAINTENA(R)): a review of its use as maintenance treatment for adult patients with schizophrenia. Drugs 2014; **74**:1097–1110.
2. Mallikaarjun S et al. Pharmacokinetics, tolerability and safety of aripiprazole once-monthly in adult schizophrenia: an open-label, parallel-arm, multiple-dose study. Schizophr Res 2013; **150**:281–288.
3. Kane JM et al. Aripiprazole intramuscular depot as maintenance treatment in patients with schizophrenia: a 52-week, multicenter, randomized, double-blind, placebo-controlled study. J Clin Psychiatry 2012; **73**:617–624.
4. Potkin SG et al. Safety and tolerability of once monthly aripiprazole treatment initiation in adults with schizophrenia stabilized on selected atypical oral antipsychotics other than aripiprazole. Curr Med Res Opin 2013; **29**:1241–1251.

Olanzapine LAI

Like all esters, olanzapine pamoate (embonate, in some countries) is very poorly water soluble. An aqueous suspension of olanzapine pamoate, when injected intramuscularly, affords both prompt and sustained release of olanzapine. Peak plasma levels are seen within one week of injection[1] and efficacy can be demonstrated after only 3 days.[2] Only gluteal injection is licensed; deltoid injection is less effective.[3] Olanzapine LAI is effective when given every 4 weeks, with 2-weekly administration only required when the highest dose is prescribed. It has not been compared with other long-acting injections. Loading doses are recommended in some dose regimens (Table 2.11). Formal labelling/SPC suggests that patients be given oral olanzapine to assess response and tolerability. This rarely happens in practice. Oral supplementation after the first depot injection is not necessary.

Switching

Direct switching to olanzapine LAI, ideally following an oral trial, is usually possible. So, when switching from another LAI (but not risperidone) olanzapine oral or LAI can be started on the day the last LAI was due. Likewise for switching from oral treatment – a direct switch is possible but prior antipsychotics are probably best reduced slowly after starting olanzapine (either oral or LAI). When switching from risperidone RLAI, olanzapine should be started, we suggest, 3–4 weeks after the last injection was due (e.g. 5–6 weeks after the last injection).

Post-injection syndrome

Post-injection syndrome occurs when olanzapine pamoate is inadvertently exposed to high blood volumes (probably via accidental intravasation). Olanzapine plasma levels may reach 600 µg/L and delirium and somnolence result.[4] The incidence of post-injection syndrome is less than 0.1% of injections; almost all reactions (86%) occur within 1 hour of injection.[5] In most countries, olanzapine LAI may only be given in healthcare facilities under supervision and patients need to be kept under observation for 3 hours after the injection is given.

Table 2.11 Olanzapine – dosing schedules

Oral olanzapine equivalent	Loading dose	Maintenance dose (given 8 weeks after the first dose)
10 mg/day	210 mg every 2 weeks 405 mg every 4 weeks	300 mg/4 weeks (or 150 mg every 2 weeks)
15 mg/day	300 mg every 2 weeks	405 mg/4 weeks (or 210 mg every 2 weeks)
20 mg/day	None – give 300 mg every 2 weeks	300 mg every 2 weeks

In the EU, the exact wording of the SPC[6] is as follows:

After each injection, patients should be observed in a healthcare facility by appropriately qualified personnel for at least 3 hours for signs and symptoms consistent with olanzapine overdose.

Immediately prior to leaving the healthcare facility, it should be confirmed that the patient is alert, oriented, and absent of any signs and symptoms of overdose. If an overdose is suspected, close medical supervision and monitoring should continue until examination indicates that signs and symptoms have resolved. The 3-hour observation period should be extended as clinically appropriate for patients who exhibit any signs or symptoms consistent with olanzapine overdose.

For the remainder of the day after injection, patients should be advised to be vigilant for signs and symptoms of overdose secondary to post-injection adverse reactions, be able to obtain assistance if needed, and should not drive or operate machinery.

This monitoring requirement has undoubtedly adversely affected the popularity of olanzapine LAI. No patient or medical factor has been identified which might predict post-injection syndrome[4] except that those experiencing the syndrome are more likely to have previously has an injection-site related adverse effect.[7]

References

1. Heres S et al. Pharmacokinetics of olanzapine long-acting injection: the clinical perspective. Int Clin Psychopharmacol 2014; **29**:299–312.
2. Lauriello J et al. An 8-week, double-blind, randomized, placebo-controlled study of olanzapine long-acting injection in acutely ill patients with schizophrenia. J Clin Psychiatry 2008; **69**:790–799.
3. Mitchell M et al. Single- and multiple-dose pharmacokinetic, safety, and tolerability profiles of olanzapine long-acting injection: an open-label, multicenter, nonrandomized study in patients with schizophrenia. Clin Ther 2013; **35**:1890–1908.
4. McDonnell DP et al. Post-injection delirium/sedation syndrome in patients with schizophrenia treated with olanzapine long-acting injection, II: investigations of mechanism. BMC Psych 2010; **10**:45.
5. Bushes CJ et al. Olanzapine long-acting injection: review of first experiences of post-injection delirium/sedation syndrome in routine clinical practice. 2013. Eli Lilly Personal Communication.
6. Eli Lilly and Company Limited, Eli Lilly and. Summary of Product Characteristics. ZYPADHERA 210 mg, 300 mg, and 405 mg, powder and solvent for prolonged release suspension for injection. 2014. http://www.medicines.org.uk/
7. Atkins S et al. A pooled analysis of injection site-related adverse events in patients with schizophrenia treated with olanzapine long-acting injection. BMC Psychiatry 2014; **14**:7.

Paliperidone palmitate LAI

Paliperidone was the third SGA to be developed as a LAI. It is the major active metabolite of risperidone: 9-hydroxyrisperidone. Following an intramuscular injection, active paliperidone plasma levels are seen within a few days, therefore co-administration of oral paliperidone or risperidone during initiation is not required.[1] Dosing consists of two initiation doses (deltoid) followed by monthly maintenance doses (deltoid or gluteal) – see Table 2.12. Following administration of a single IM dose to the deltoid muscle, on average 28% higher peak concentration is observed compared with IM injection to the gluteal muscle.[1] Thus, the two deltoid muscle injections on days 1 and 8 help to quickly attain therapeutic drug concentrations.

Paliperidone LAI has been compared with haloperidol depot given in a loading dose schedule matching that of paliperidone.[2] The two formulations were equally effective in preventing relapse but paliperidone increased prolactin to a greater extent and caused more weight gain. Haloperidol caused more akathisia, more acute movement disorder

Table 2.12 Paliperidone dose and administration information[1]

	Dose	Route
Initiation		
Day 1	150 mg IM (234 mg)*	Deltoid only
Day 8 (+/– 4 days)	100 mg IM (156 mg)*	Deltoid only
Maintenance		
Every month (+/– 7 days) thereafter	50–150 mg IM† (78–234 mg)*	Deltoid or gluteal

*Paliperidone palmitate dose can be expressed in terms of active moiety (50–150 mg) or weight of compound (78–234 mg).
†The maintenance dose is perhaps best judged by consideration of what might be a suitable dose of oral risperidone and then giving paliperidone palmitate in an equivalent dose (see below).
IM, intramuscular.

Table 2.13 Approximate dose equivalent[1,3]

Risperidone oral (mg/day) (bioavailability = 70%)[4]	Paliperidone oral (mg/day) (bioavailability = 28%)[5]	Risperidone LAI (Consta) (mg/2 weeks)	Paliperidone palmitate (mg/monthly)
2	4	25	50
3	6	37.5	75
4	9	50	100
6	12	–	150

Table 2.14 Switching to paliperidone palmitate

Switching from	Recommended method of switching	Comments
No treatment	Give the two initiation doses: 150 mg IM deltoid on day 1 and 100 mg IM deltoid on day 8 Maintenance dose starts 1 month later	In general the lowest most effective maintenance dose should be used The manufacturer recommends a dose of 75 mg monthly for the general adult population.[1] This is approximately equivalent to 3 mg/day oral risperidone (see Table 2.13). In practice the modal dose is 100 mg/month[6] Maintenance dose adjustments should be made monthly. However the full effect of the dose adjustment may not be apparent for several months[3]
Oral paliperidone/ risperidone	Give the two initiation doses followed by the maintenance dose (see Table 2.13 and prescribe equivalent dose)	Oral paliperidone/risperidone supplementation during initiation is not necessary
Oral antipsychotics	Reduce the dose of the oral antipsychotic over 1–2 weeks following the first injection of paliperidone. Give the two initiation doses followed by the maintenance dose	
Depot antipsychotic	For risperidone LAI, begin paliperidone 5–6 weeks after the last injection NB. No initiation doses are required	Doses of paliperidone palmitate IM may be difficult to predict. The manufacturer recommends a dose of 75 mg monthly for the general adult population. If switching from RLAI see Table 2.13 and prescribe equivalent dose Maintenance dose adjustments should be made monthly. However the full effect of the dose adjustment may not be apparent for several months[3]
Antipsychotic polypharmacy with depot	Start paliperidone (at the maintenance dose) when the next injection is due NB. No initiation doses are required Reduce the dose of the oral antipsychotic over 1–2 weeks following the first injection of paliperidone	Aim to treat the patient with paliperidone palmitate IM as the sole antipsychotic The maintenance dose should be governed as far as possible by the total dose of oral and injectable antipsychotic (see Table 2.13)

IM, intramuscular; RLAI, risperidone long-acting injection.

and there was a trend for a higher incidence of tardive dyskinesia. The average dose of haloperidol was around 75 mg a month; a dose rarely used in practice.

The second initiation dose may be given 4 days before or after day 8 (after the first initiation dose on day one).[3] Similarly the manufacturer recommends that patients may be given maintenance doses up to 7 days before or after the monthly time point.[3] This flexibility should help minimise the number of missed doses. There is a complex schedule of recommendations to be adhered to when doses are missed – please see SPC or formal labelling.

Some points to note:

- Paliperidone palmitate is an esterified form of paliperidone and utilises Elan Technologies' NanoCrystal® Technology; is formulated as an aqueous suspension engineered for sustained release.
- Paliperidone palmitate IM does not require cold storage.
- Paliperidone palmitate IM is available as pre-filled syringes and does not require reconstitution or suspension before administration.
- No oral supplementation is required on initiation for paliperidone palmitate.
- No test dose is required for paliperidone palmitate (but patients should (ideally) be currently stabilised on or have previously responded to oral paliperidone or risperidone).
- The median time to maximum plasma concentrations is 13 days.[1]

The approximate dose equivalents of different formulations of risperidone and paliperidone are shown in Table 2.13. Switching to paliperidone palmitate is shown in Table 2.14.

References

1. Janssen Pharmaceuticals. Highlights of Prescribing Information. INVEGA SUSTENNAR (paliperidone palmitate) extended-release injectable suspension, for intramuscular use. 2014. http://www.janssencns.com/sustenna-prescribing-information

2. McEvoy JP et al. Effectiveness of paliperidone palmitate vs haloperidol decanoate for maintenance treatment of schizophrenia: a randomized clinical trial. JAMA 2014; 311:1978–1987.

3. Janssen-Cilag Ltd. Summary of Product Characteristics. XEPLION 50 mg, 75 mg, 100 mg and 150 mg prolonged release suspension for injection. 2013. http://www.medicines.org.uk/

4. Janssen-Cilag Ltd, Janssen. Summary of Product Characteristics. Risperdal Tablets, Liquid and Quicklet. 2014. http://www.medicines.org.uk/

5. Janssen-Cilag Ltd. Summary of Product Characteristics. INVEGA 1.5 mg, 3 mg, 6 mg, 9 mg, 12 mg prolonged-release tablets. 2013. http://www.medicines.org.uk/

6. Attard A et al. Paliperidone palmitate long-acting injection–prospective year-long follow-up of use in clinical practice. Acta Psychiatr Scand 2014; 130:46–51.

Risperidone LAI

Risperidone was the first 'atypical' drug to be made available as a depot, or long-acting, injectable formulation. Doses of 25–50 mg every 2 weeks appear to be as effective as oral doses of 2–6 mg/day.[1] The long-acting injection also seems to be well tolerated – fewer than 10% of patients experienced EPS and fewer than 6% withdrew from a long-term trial because of adverse effects.[2] Oral risperidone increases prolactin,[3] as does RLAI[4] but levels appear to reduce somewhat following a switch from oral to injectable risperidone.[5-7] Rates of tardive dyskinesia are said to be low.[8] There are no direct comparisons with standard depots but switching from FGA depots in stable patients to risperidone LAI has been shown to be less successful than remaining on the FGA depot.[9]

Uncertainty remains over the dose–response relationship for RLAI. Studies randomising subjects to different fixed doses of RLAI show no differences in response according to dose.[10] One randomised, fixed-dose year-long study suggested better outcome for 50 mg every 2 weeks than with 25 mg, although no observed difference reached statistical significance.[11] Naturalistic studies indicate doses higher than 25 mg/2 weeks are frequently used.[12,13] One study suggested higher doses were associated with better outcome.[14,15]

Plasma levels afforded by 25 mg/2 weeks seem to be similar to, or even lower than, levels provided by 2 mg/day oral risperidone.[16,17] (One study found 9.5% of plasma samples from people apparently receiving risperidone LAI contained no risperidone or 9-hydroxyrisperidone[18]). Striatal dopamine D_2 occupancies are similarly low in people receiving 25 mg/2 weeks.[19,20] So, although fixed dose studies have not revealed clear advantages for doses above 25 mg/2 weeks other indicators cast doubt on the assumption that 25 mg/2 weeks will be adequate for all or even most patients. While this conundrum remains unresolved the need for careful dose titration becomes of great importance. This is perhaps most efficiently achieved by establishing the required dose of oral risperidone and converting this dose into the equivalent injection dose. Trials have clearly established that switching from 2 mg oral to 25 mg injection and 4 mg oral to 50 mg injection is usually successful[2,21,22] (switching from 4 mg/day to 25 mg/2 weeks increases the risk of relapse[23]). There remains a question over the equivalent dose for 6 mg oral: in theory, patients should be switched to 75 mg injection but this showed no advantage over lower doses in trials and is in any case above the licensed maximum dose. Paliperidone palmitate 150 mg a month is equivalent to oral risperidone 6 mg/day. In fact, for many reasons paliperidone palmitate (9-hydroxyrisperidone) may be preferred to risperidone injection: it acts acutely, can be given monthly, does not require cold storage and has a wider, more useful dose range (see section on 'Paliperidone palmitate intramuscular long-acting injection' in this chapter).

Risperidone long-acting injection differs importantly from other depots and the following points should be noted.

- Risperidone depot is not an esterified form of the parent drug. It contains risperidone coated in polymer to form microspheres. These microspheres have to be suspended in an aqueous base immediately before use.
- The injection must be stored in a fridge (consider the practicalities for community staff).

Table 2.15 Switching to risperidone long-acting injection (RLAI)

Switching from	Recommended method of switching	Comments
No treatment (new patient or recently non-compliant)	Start risperidone oral at 2 mg/day and titrate to effective dose. If tolerated, prescribe equivalent dose of RLAI Continue with oral risperidone for at least 3 weeks then taper over 1–2 weeks. Be prepared to continue oral risperidone for longer	Use oral risperidone before giving injection to assure good tolerability Those stabilised on 2 mg/day start on 25 mg/2 weeks Those on higher doses, start on 37.5 mg/2 weeks and be prepared to use 50 mg/2 weeks
Oral risperidone	Prescribe equivalent dose of RLAI	See above
Oral antipsychotics (not risperidone)	**Either:** Switch to oral risperidone and titrate to effective dose. If tolerated, prescribe equivalent dose of RLAI Continue with oral risperidone for at least 3 weeks then taper over 1–2 weeks. Be prepared to continue oral risperidone for longer **Or:** Give RLAI and then slowly discontinue oral antipsychotics after 3–4 weeks. Be prepared to continue oral antipsychotics for longer	Dose assessment is difficult in those switching from another antipsychotic. Broadly speaking, those on low oral doses should be switched to 25 mg/2 weeks. 'Low' in this context means towards the lower end of the licensed dose range or around the minimum dose known to be effective Those on higher oral doses should receive 37.5 mg or 50 mg every 2 weeks. The continued need for oral antipsychotics after 3–4 weeks may indicate that higher doses of RLAI are required
Depot antipsychotic	Give RLAI one week **before** the last depot injection is given	Dose of RLAI difficult to predict. For those on low doses (see above) start at 25 mg/2 weeks and then adjust as necessary Start RLAI at 37.5 mg/2 weeks in those previously maintained on doses in the middle or upper range of licensed doses. Be prepared to increase to 50 mg/2 weeks
Antipsychotic polypharmacy with depot	Give RLAI one week before the last depot injection is given Slowly taper oral antipsychotics 3–4 weeks later. Be prepared to continue oral antipsychotics for longer	Aim to treat patient with RLAI as the sole antipsychotic. As before, RLAI dose should be dictated, as far as is possible, by the total dose of oral and injectable antipsychotic

- It is available as doses of 25, 37.5 and 50 mg. The whole vial must be used (because of the nature of the suspension). This means that there is limited flexibility in dosing.
- A test dose is not required or sensible. (Testing tolerability with oral risperidone is desirable but not always practical.)
- It takes 3–4 weeks for the first injection to produce therapeutic plasma levels. Peak plasma levels are reached after 5 weeks. Patients must be maintained on a full dose of

their previous antipsychotic for at least 3 weeks after the administration of the first risperidone injection. Oral antipsychotic cover is sometimes required for longer (6–8 weeks). If the patient is not already receiving an oral antipsychotic, oral risperidone should be prescribed. (See Table 2.15 for advice on switching from depots.) **Patients who refuse oral treatment and are acutely ill should not be given RLAI because of the long delay in drug release.**

- Risperidone depot must be administered every 2 weeks. The Product Licence does not allow longer intervals between doses. There is little flexibility to negotiate with patients about the frequency of administration although monthly injections may be effective.[24]
- The most effective way of predicting response to RLAI is to establish dose and response with oral risperidone.
- Risperidone injection is not considered suitable for patients with treatment refractory schizophrenia although one study showed good effect with 50 mg and 100 mg two weekly.[25]

For guidance on switching to risperidone long-acting injection see Table 2.15.

References

1. Chue P et al. Comparative efficacy and safety of long-acting risperidone and risperidone oral tablets. Eur Neuropsychopharmacol 2005; 15:111–117.
2. Fleischhacker WW et al. Treatment of schizophrenia with long-acting injectable risperidone: a 12-month open-label trial of the first long-acting second-generation antipsychotic. J Clin Psychiatry 2003; 64:1250–1257.
3. Kleinberg DL et al. Prolactin levels and adverse events in patients treated with risperidone. J Clin Psychopharmacol 1999; 19:57–61.
4. Fu DJ et al. Paliperidone palmitate versus oral risperidone and risperidone long-acting injection in patients with recently diagnosed schizophrenia: a tolerability and efficacy comparison. Int Clin Psychopharmacol 2014; 29:45–55.
5. Bai YM et al. A comparative efficacy and safety study of long-acting risperidone injection and risperidone oral tablets among hospitalized patients: 12-week randomized, single-blind study. Pharmacopsychiatry 2006; 39:135–141.
6. Bai YM et al. Pharmacokinetics study for hyperprolactinemia among schizophrenics switched from risperidone to risperidone long-acting injection. J Clin Psychopharmacol 2007; 27:306–308.
7. Peng PW et al. The disparity of pharmacokinetics and prolactin study for risperidone long-acting injection. J Clin Psychopharmacol 2008; 28:726–727.
8. Gharabawi GM et al. An assessment of emergent tardive dyskinesia and existing dyskinesia in patients receiving long-acting, injectable risperidone: results from a long-term study. Schizophr Res 2005; 77:129–139.
9. Covell NH et al. Effectiveness of switching from long-acting injectable fluphenazine or haloperidol decanoate to long-acting injectable risperidone microspheres: an open-label, randomized controlled trial. J Clin Psychiatry 2012; 73:669–675.
10. Kane JM et al. Long-acting injectable risperidone: efficacy and safety of the first long-acting atypical antipsychotic. Am J Psychiatry 2003; 160:1125–1132.
11. Simpson GM et al. A 1-year double-blind study of 2 doses of long-acting risperidone in stable patients with schizophrenia or schizoaffective disorder. J Clin Psychiatry 2006; 67:1194–1203.
12. Turner M et al. Long-acting injectable risperidone: safety and efficacy in stable patients switched from conventional depot antipsychotics. Int Clin Psychopharmacol 2004; 19:241–249.
13. Taylor DM et al. Early clinical experience with risperidone long-acting injection: a prospective, 6-month follow-up of 100 patients. J Clin Psychiatry 2004; 65:1076–1083.
14. Taylor DM et al. Prospective 6-month follow-up of patients prescribed risperidone long-acting injection: factors predicting favourable outcome. Int J Neuropsychopharmacol 2006; 9:685–694.
15. Taylor DM et al. Risperidone long-acting injection: a prospective 3-year analysis of its use in clinical practice. J Clin Psychiatry 2009; 70:196–200.
16. Nesvag R et al. Serum concentrations of risperidone and 9-OH risperidone following intramuscular injection of long-acting risperidone compared with oral risperidone medication. Acta Psychiatr Scand 2006; 114:21–26.
17. Castberg I et al. Serum concentrations of risperidone and 9-hydroxyrisperidone after administration of the long-acting injectable form of risperidone: evidence from a routine therapeutic drug monitoring service. Ther Drug Monit 2005; 27:103–106.
18. Bowskill SV et al. Risperidone and total 9-hydroxyrisperidone in relation to prescribed dose and other factors: data from a therapeutic drug monitoring service, 2002–2010. Ther Drug Monit 2012; 34:349–355.
19. Gefvert O et al. Pharmacokinetics and D2 receptor occupancy of long-acting injectable risperidone (Risperdal Consta™) in patients with schizophrenia. Int J Neuropsychopharmacol 2005; 8:27–36.

20. Remington G et al. A PET study evaluating dopamine D2 receptor occupancy for long-acting injectable risperidone. Am J Psychiatry 2006; **163**:396–401.
21. Lasser RA et al. Clinical improvement in 336 stable chronically psychotic patients changed from oral to long-acting risperidone: a 12-month open trial. Int J Neuropsychopharmacol 2005; **8**:427–438.
22. Lauriello J et al. Long-acting risperidone vs. placebo in the treatment of hospital inpatients with schizophrenia. Schizophr Res 2005; **72**:249–258.
23. Bai YM et al. Equivalent switching dose from oral risperidone to risperidone long-acting injection: a 48-week randomized, prospective, single-blind pharmacokinetic study. J Clin Psychiatry 2007; **68**:1218–1225.
24. Uchida H et al. Monthly administration of long-acting injectable risperidone and striatal dopamine D2 receptor occupancy for the management of schizophrenia. J Clin Psychiatry 2008; **69**:1281–1286.
25. Meltzer HY et al. A six month randomized controlled trial of long acting injectable risperidone 50 and 100 mg in treatment resistant schizophrenia. Schizophr Res 2014; **154**:14–22.

ANTIPSYCHOTICS – ADVERSE EFFECTS

Extrapyramidal side-effects

Details of the extrapyramidal side-effects of antipsychotic drug treatment are shown in Table 2.16.

Table 2.16 Most common extrapyramidal side-effects

	Dystonia (uncontrolled muscular spasm)	Pseudo-parkinsonism (tremor, etc.)	Akathisia (restlessness)[1]	Tardive dyskinesia (abnormal movements)
Signs and symptoms[2]	Muscle spasm in any part of the body, e.g. ■ eyes rolling upwards (oculogyric crisis) ■ head and neck twisted to the side (torticollis) ■ the patient may be unable to swallow or speak clearly ■ in extreme cases, the back may arch or the jaw dislocate Acute dystonia can be both painful and very frightening	Symptoms include: ■ tremor and/or rigidity ■ bradykinesia (decreased facial expression, flat monotone voice, slow body movements, inability to initiate movement) ■ bradyphrenia (slowed thinking) ■ salivation Pseudo-parkinsonism can be mistaken for depression or the negative symptoms of schizophrenia	A subjectively unpleasant state of inner restlessness where there is a strong desire or compulsion to move, e.g. ■ foot stamping when seated ■ constantly crossing/uncrossing legs ■ rocking from foot to foot ■ constantly pacing up and down Akathisia can be mistaken for psychotic agitation and has been linked with suicidal ideation[3] and aggression towards others[4]	A wide variety of movements can occur such as: ■ lip smacking or chewing ■ tongue protrusion (fly catching) ■ choreiform hand movements (pill rolling or piano playing) ■ pelvic thrusting Severe orofacial movements can lead to difficulty speaking, eating or breathing. Movements are worse when under stress
Rating scales	No specific scale. Small component of general EPS scales	Simpson–Angus EPS Rating Scale[5]	Barnes Akathisia Scale[6]	Abnormal Involuntary Movement Scale[7] (AIMS)
Prevalence (with older drugs)	Approximately 10%,[8] but more common:[9] ■ in young males ■ in the neuroleptic-naive ■ with high potency drugs (e.g. haloperidol) Dystonic reactions are rare in the elderly	Approximately 20%,[10] but more common in: ■ elderly females ■ those with pre-existing neurological damage (head injury, stroke, etc.)	Approximately 25%,[11] less with SGAs; in decreasing order: aripiprazole, lurasidone, risperidone, olanzapine, quetiapine and clozapine[12]	5% of patients per year of antipsychotic exposure.[13] More common in: ■ elderly women ■ those with affective illness ■ those who have had acute EPS early in treatment Tardive dyskinesia may be associated with neurocognitive deficits[14]

Table 2.16 (Continued)

	Dystonia (uncontrolled muscular spasm)	Pseudo-parkinsonism (tremor, etc.)	Akathisia (restlessness)[1]	Tardive dyskinesia (abnormal movements)
Time taken to develop	Acute dystonia can occur within hours of starting antipsychotics (minutes if the IM or IV route is used) Tardive dystonia occurs after months to years of antipsychotic treatment	Days to weeks after antipsychotic drugs are started or the dose is increased	Acute akathisia occurs within hours to weeks of starting antipsychotics or increasing the dose. Tardive akathisia takes longer to develop and can persist after antipsychotics have been withdrawn	Months to years Approximately 50% of cases are reversible[13,14]
Treatment	Anticholinergic drugs given orally, IM or IV depending on the severity of symptoms:[9] ■ remember the patient may be unable to swallow ■ response to IV administration will be seen within 5 minutes ■ response to IM administration takes around 20 minutes ■ tardive dystonia may respond to ECT[15] ■ where symptoms do not respond to simpler measures including switching to an antipsychotic with a low propensity for EPS, botulinuim toxin may be effective[16] ■ rTMS may be helpful[17]	Several options are available depending on the clinical circumstances: ■ reduce the antipsychotic dose ■ change to an antipsychotic with lower propensity for pseudo-parkinsonism (see section on 'Relative adverse effects of antipsychotics' in this chapter) (as antipsychotic monotherapy) ■ prescribe an anticholinergic. The majority of patients do not require long-term anticholinergics. Use should be reviewed at least every 3 months. Do not prescribe at night (symptoms usually absent during sleep)	Several options are available depending on the clinical circumstances: ■ reduce the antipsychotic dose ■ change to an antipsychotic drug with lower propensity for akathisia (see section on 'Akathisia and relative adverse effects of antipsychotics') ■ a reduction in symptoms may be seen with:[18] propranolol 30–80 mg/day (evidence poor), clonazepam (low dose) 5HT$_2$ antagonists such as: cyproheptadine,[15] mirtazapine,[18] trazodone,[19,20] mianserin,[21] and cyproheptadine may help, as may diphenhydramine[22] All are unlicenced for this indication Anticholinergics are generally unhelpful[23]	Several options are available depending on the clinical circumstances: ■ stop anticholinergic if prescribed ■ reduce dose of antipsychotic ■ change to an antipsychotic with lower propensity for tardive dyskinesia;[24–27] note data are conflicting[28,29] ■ clozapine is the antipsychotic most likely to be associated with resolution of symptoms.[30] Quetiapine may also be useful in this regard[31] ■ tetrabenazine and Ginkgo biloba[32] have some efficacy as add on treatments. For other treatment options see the review by the American Academy of Neurology[33] and the section on 'Tardive dyskinesia' in this chapter

ECT, electroconvulsive therapy; EPS, extrapyramidal side-effects; IM, intramuscular; IV, intravenous; rTMS, repetitive transcranial magnetic stimulation.

CHAPTER 2

EPS are:

- dose-related
- most likely with high doses of high potency FGAs
- less common with other antipsychotics, particularly clozapine, olanzapine, quetiapine and aripiprazole,[34] but once present may be persistent.[35] Note that CUtLASS reported no difference in EPS between FGAs and SGAs[36] (although sulpiride was widely used in the FGA group). Vulnerability to EPS may be genetically determined.[37]

Beware that in never-medicated patients with first-episode schizophrenia, 1% have dystonia, 8% Parkinsonian symptoms and 11% akathisia.[38] Parkinsonian symptoms in such patients are associated with cognitive impairment.[39] In never-treated patients with established illness, 9% exhibit spontaneous dyskinesias and 17% Parkinsonian symptoms.[40] Patients who experience one type of EPS may be more vulnerable to developing others.[41] Substance misuse increases the risk of dystonia, akathisia and tardive dyskinesia.[42] Alcohol abuse is associated with akathisia.[43]

References

1. Barnes TRE. The Barnes akathisia scale – revisited. J Psychopharmacol 2003; 17:365–370.
2. Gervin M et al. Assessment of drug-related movement disorders in schizophrenia. Adv Psychiatr Treat 2000; 6:332–341.
3. Seemuller F et al. Akathisia and suicidal ideation in first-episode schizophrenia. J Clin Psychopharmacol 2012; 32:694–698.
4. Leong GB et al. Neuroleptic-induced akathisia and violence: a review. J Forensic Sci 2003; 48:187–189.
5. Simpson GM et al. A rating scale for extrapyramidal side effects. Acta Psychiatr Scand 1970; 212:11–19.
6. Barnes TRE. A rating scale for drug-induced akathisia. Br J Psychiatry 1989; 154:672–676.
7. Guy W. ECDEU Assessment Manual for Psychopharmacology. Washington, DC: US Department of Health, Education, and Welfare 1976:534–537.
8. Association AP. Practice guideline for the treatment of patients with schizophrenia. Am J Psychiatry 1997; 154 Suppl 4:1–63.
9. van Harten PN et al. Acute dystonia induced by drug treatment. Br Med J 1999; 319:623–626.
10. Bollini P et al. Antipsychotic drugs: is more worse? A meta-analysis of the published randomized control trials. Psychol Med 1994; 24:307–316.
11. Halstead SM et al. Akathisia: prevalence and associated dysphoria in an in-patient population with chronic schizophrenia. Br J Psychiatry 1994; 164:177–183.
12. Hirose S. The causes of underdiagnosing akathisia. Schizophr Bull 2003; 29:547–558.
13. Association AP. Tardive dyskinesia: a task force report of the American Psychiatric Association. Hosp Community Psychiatry 1993; 44:190.
14. Caroff SN et al. Treatment outcomes of patients with tardive dyskinesia and chronic schizophrenia. J Clin Psychiatry 2011; 72:295–303.
15. Miller CH et al. Managing antipsychotic-induced acute and chronic akathisia. Drug Saf 2000; 22:73–81.
16. Hennings JM et al. Successful treatment of tardive lingual dystonia with botulinum toxin: case report and review of the literature. Prog Neuropsychopharmacol Biol Psychiatry 2008; 32:1167–1171.
17. Jankovic J. Treatment of hyperkinetic movement disorders. Lancet Neurol 2009; 8:844–856.
18. Poyurovsky M et al. Efficacy of low-dose mirtazapine in neuroleptic-induced akathisia: a double-blind randomized placebo-controlled pilot study. J Clin Psychopharmacol 2003; 23:305–308.
19. Stryjer R et al. Treatment of neuroleptic-induced akathisia with the 5-HT2A antagonist trazodone. Clin Neuropharmacol 2003; 26:137–141.
20. Stryjer R et al. Trazodone for the treatment of neuroleptic-induced acute akathisia: a placebo-controlled, double-blind, crossover study. Clin Neuropharmacol 2010; 33:219–222.
21. Stryjer R et al. Mianserin for the rapid improvement of chronic akathisia in a schizophrenia patient. Eur Psychiatry 2004; 19:237–238.
22. Vinson DR. Diphenhydramine in the treatment of akathisia induced by prochlorperazine. J Emerg Med 2004; 26:265–270.
23. Rathbone J et al. Anticholinergics for neuroleptic-induced acute akathisia. The Cochrane database of systematic reviews 2006: CD003727.
24. Glazer WM. Expected incidence of tardive dyskinesia associated with atypical antipsychotics. J Clin Psychiatry 2000; 61 Suppl 4:21–26.
25. Kinon BJ et al. Olanzapine treatment for tardive dyskinesia in schizophrenia patients: a prospective clinical trial with patients randomized to blinded dose reduction periods. Prog Neuropsychopharmacol Biol Psychiatry 2004; 28:985–996.
26. Bai YM et al. Risperidone for severe tardive dyskinesia: a 12-week randomized, double-blind, placebo-controlled study. J Clin Psychiatry 2003; 64:1342–1348.

27. Tenback DE et al. Effects of antipsychotic treatment on tardive dyskinesia: a 6-month evaluation of patients from the European Schizophrenia Outpatient Health Outcomes (SOHO) Study. J Clin Psychiatry 2005; 66:1130–1133.

28. Woods SW et al. Incidence of tardive dyskinesia with atypical versus conventional antipsychotic medications: a prospective cohort study. J Clin Psychiatry 2010; 71:463–474.

29. Pena MS et al. Tardive dyskinesia and other movement disorders secondary to aripiprazole. Mov Disord 2011; 26:147–152.

30. Simpson GM. The treatment of tardive dyskinesia and tardive dystonia. J Clin Psychiatry 2000; 61 Suppl 4:39–44.

31. Peritogiannis V et al. Can atypical antipsychotics improve tardive dyskinesia associated with other atypical antipsychotics? Case report and brief review of the literature. J Psychopharmacol 2010; 24:1121–1125.

32. Zhang WF et al. Extract of ginkgo biloba treatment for tardive dyskinesia in schizophrenia: a randomized, double-blind, placebo-controlled trial. J Clin Psychiatry 2011; 72:615–21.

33. Bhidayasiri R et al. Evidence-based guideline: treatment of tardive syndromes: report of the Guideline Development Subcommittee of the American Academy of Neurology. Neurology 2013; 81:463–469.

34. Leucht S et al. Comparative efficacy and tolerability of 15 antipsychotic drugs in schizophrenia: a multiple-treatments meta-analysis. Lancet 2013; 382:951–962.

35. Tenback DE et al. Incidence and persistence of tardive dyskinesia and extrapyramidal symptoms in schizophrenia. J Psychopharmacol 2010; 24:1031–1035.

36. Peluso MJ et al. Extrapyramidal motor side-effects of first- and second-generation antipsychotic drugs. Br J Psychiatry 2012; 200:387–392.

37. Zivkovic M et al. The association study of polymorphisms in DAT, DRD2, and COMT genes and acute extrapyramidal adverse effects in male schizophrenic patients treated with haloperidol. J Clin Psychopharmacol 2013; 33:593–599.

38. Rybakowski JK et al. Extrapyramidal symptoms during treatment of first schizophrenia episode: Results from EUFEST. Eur Neuropsychopharmacol 2014; 24:1500–1505.

39. Cuesta MJ et al. Spontaneous Parkinsonism is associated with cognitive impairment in antipsychotic-naive patients with first-episode psychosis: a 6-month follow-up study. Schizophr Bull 2014; 40:1164–1173.

40. Pappa S et al. Spontaneous movement disorders in antipsychotic-naive patients with first-episode psychoses: a systematic review. Psychol Med 2009; 39:1065–1076.

41. Kim JH et al. Prevalence and characteristics of subjective akathisia, objective akathisia, and mixed akathisia in chronic schizophrenic subjects. Clin Neuropharmacol 2003; 26:312–316.

42. Potvin S et al. Substance abuse is associated with increased extrapyramidal symptoms in schizophrenia: a meta-analysis. Schizophr Res 2009; 113:181–188.

43. Hansen LK et al. Movement disorders in patients with schizophrenia and a history of substance abuse. Human psychopharmacol 2013; 28:192–197.

Further reading

Dayalu P et al. Antipsychotic-induced extrapyramidal symptoms and their management. Expert Opin Pharmacother 2008; 9:1451–1462.

El Sayeh HG et al. Non-neuroleptic catecholaminergic drugs for neuroleptic-induced tardive dyskinesia. Cochrane Database Syst Rev 2006; CD000458.

Akathisia

Akathisia is a common motor adverse effect of most antipsychotics although some SGAs are less likely to be associated with it. Akathisia is subjectively unpleasant and is fairly strongly linked to the emergence (often sudden) of suicidal ideation.[1,2] Figure 2.4 suggests a programme of treatment options for drug-induced akathisia.

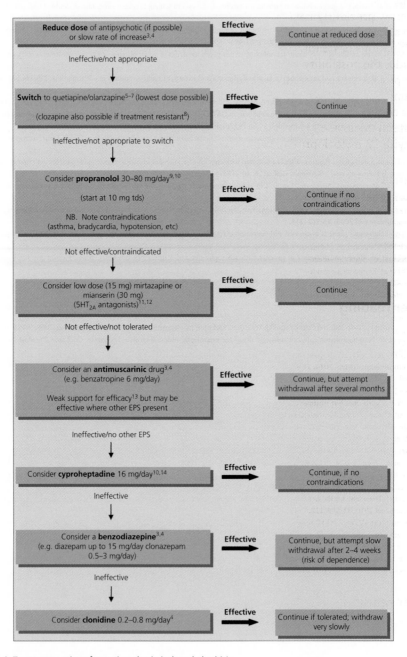

Figure 2.4 Treatment options for antipsychotic-induced akathisia.

Notes

- Akathisia is sometimes difficult to diagnose with certainty. A careful history of symptoms, medication and illicit substance use is essential.
- Evaluate efficacy of each treatment option over at least 1 month. Some effect may be seen after a few days but it may take much longer to become apparent in those with chronic akathisia.
- Withdraw previously ineffective akathisia treatments before starting the next option in the algorithm.
- Combinations of treatment may be used in refractory cases if carefully monitored.
- Consider the possibility of tardive akathisia in patients on long-term therapy.
- Other possible treatments for acute akathisia include vitamin B6,[15,16] pregabalin,[17] diphenhydramine,[18] trazodone[11,19] and zolmitriptan.[20,21] Always read the primary literature before considering any of the options.
- Parenteral midazolam (1.5 mg) has been successfully used to prevent akathisia associated with IV metoclopramide.[22]

CHAPTER 2

References

1. Seemuller F et al. Akathisia and suicidal ideation in first-episode schizophrenia. J Clin Psychopharmacol 2012; 32:694–698.
2. Seemuller F et al. The relationship of Akathisia with treatment emergent suicidality among patients with first-episode schizophrenia treated with haloperidol or risperidone. Pharmacopsychiatry 2012; 45:292–296.
3. Fleischhacker WW et al. The pharmacologic treatment of neuroleptic-induced akathisia. J Clin Psychopharmacol 1990; 10:12–21.
4. Sachdev P. The identification and management of drug-induced akathisia. CNS Drugs 1995; 4:28–46.
5. Kumar R et al. Akathisia and second-generation antipsychotic drugs. Curr Opin Psychiatry 2009; 22:293–299.
6. Miller DD et al. Extrapyramidal side-effects of antipsychotics in a randomised trial. Br J Psychiatry 2008; 193:279–288.
7. Rummel-Kluge C et al. Second-Generation Antipsychotic Drugs and Extrapyramidal Side Effects: A Systematic Review and Meta-analysis of Head-to-Head Comparisons. Schizophr Bull 2012; 38:167–177.
8. Kane JM et al. Akathisia: an updated review focusing on second-generation antipsychotics. J Clin Psychiatry 2009; 70:627–643.
9. Adler L et al. A controlled assessment of propranolol in the treatment of neuroleptic-induced akathisia. Br J Psychiatry 1986; 149:42–45.
10. Fischel T et al. Cyproheptadine versus propranolol for the treatment of acute neuroleptic-induced akathisia: a comparative double-blind study. J Clin Psychopharmacol 2001; 21:612–615.
11. Laoutidis ZG et al. 5-HT2A receptor antagonists for the treatment of neuroleptic-induced akathisia: a systematic review and meta-analysis. Int J Neuropsychopharmacol 2014; 17:823–832.
12. Poyurovsky M et al. Mirtazapine – a multifunctional drug: low dose for akathisia. CNS Spectr 2011; 16:63.
13. Rathbone J et al. Anticholinergics for neuroleptic-induced acute akathisia. Cochrane Database Syst Rev 2006; CD003727.
14. Weiss D et al. Cyproheptadine treatment in neuroleptic-induced akathisia. Br J Psychiatry 1995; 167:483–486.
15. Miodownik C et al. Vitamin B6 versus mianserin and placebo in acute neuroleptic-induced akathisia: a randomized, double-blind, controlled study. Clin Neuropharmacol 2006; 29:68–72.
16. Lerner V et al. Vitamin B6 treatment in acute neuroleptic-induced akathisia: a randomized, double-blind, placebo-controlled study. J Clin Psychiatry 2004; 65:1550–1554.
17. De BD et al. Reversal of aripiprazole-induced tardive akathisia by addition of pregabalin. J Neuropsychiatry Clin Neurosci 2013; 25:E9–10.
18. Friedman BW et al. A randomized trial of diphenhydramine as prophylaxis against metoclopramide-induced akathisia in nauseated emergency department patients. Ann Emerg Med 2009; 53:379–385.
19. Stryjer R et al. Trazodone for the treatment of neuroleptic-induced acute akathisia: a placebo-controlled, double-blind, crossover study. Clin Neuropharmacol 2010; 33:219–222.
20. Gross-Isseroff R et al. The 5-HT1D receptor agonist zolmitriptan for neuroleptic-induced akathisia: an open label preliminary study. Int Clin Psychopharmacol 2005; 20:23–25.
21. Avital A et al. Zolmitriptan compared to propranolol in the treatment of acute neuroleptic-induced akathisia: A comparative double-blind study. Eur Neuropsychopharmacol 2009; 19:476–482.
22. Erdur B et al. A trial of midazolam vs diphenhydramine in prophylaxis of metoclopramide-induced akathisia. Am J Emerg Med 2012; 30:84–91.

Further reading

Poyurovsky M. Acute antipsychotic-induced akathisia revisited. Br J Psychiatry 2010; 196:89–91.

Weight gain

Antipsychotics have long been recognised as weight-inducing agents. Suggested mechanisms include $5HT_{2C}$ antagonism, H_1 antagonism, hyperprolactinaemia and increased serum leptin (leading to leptin desensitisation).[1-4] There is no evidence that drugs exert any direct metabolic effect: weight gain seems to result from increased food intake and, in some cases, reduced energy expenditure.[5,6] Risk of weight gain appears to be related to clinical response[7] (although the association is too small to be clinically important[8]) and may also have a genetic basis.[9,10]

All available antipsychotics have been associated with weight gain, although mean weight gained varies substantially between drugs. With all drugs, some patients lose weight, some gain no weight and some gain a great deal of weight. Knowledge of the mean weight gained is often not useful in predicting how much weight an individual might gain. Assessment of relative risk for different drugs is based largely on short term studies. Table 2.17 suggests approximate relative risk of weight gain and the extent of mean weight gain.

See the following section for advice on treating drug-induced weight gain.

Table 2.17 Antipsychotic-induced weight gain[11-15]

Drug	Risk/extent of weight gain
Clozapine	**High**
Olanzapine	
Chlorpromazine	**Moderate**
Iloperidone	
Quetiapine	
Risperidone	
Paliperidone	
Amisulpride	**Low**
Asenapine	
Aripiprazole	
Haloperidol	
Lurasidone	
Sulpiride	
Trifluoperazine	
Ziprasidone	

References

1. Monteleone P et al. Pronounced early increase in circulating leptin predicts a lower weight gain during clozapine treatment. J Clin Psychopharmacol 2002; **22**:424–426.
2. Herran A et al. Effects of long-term treatment with antipsychotics on serum leptin levels. Br J Psychiatry 2001; **179**:59–62.
3. McIntyre RS et al. Mechanisms of antipsychotic-induced weight gain. J Clin Psychiatry 2001; **62 Suppl** 23:23–29.
4. Kroeze WK et al. H1-histamine receptor affinity predicts short-term weight gain for typical and atypical antipsychotic drugs. Neuropsychopharmacology 2003; **28**:519–526.
5. Virkkunen M et al. Decrease of energy expenditure causes weight increase in olanzapine treatment – a case study. Pharmacopsychiatry 2002; **35**:124–126.

6. Sharpe JK et al. Energy expenditure and physical activity in clozapine use: implications for weight management. Aust N Z J Psychiatry 2006; **40**:810–814.

7. Czobor P et al. Antipsychotic-induced weight gain and therapeutic response: a differential association. J Clin Psychopharmacol 2002; **22**:244–251.

8. Hermes E et al. The association between weight change and symptom reduction in the CATIE schizophrenia trial. Schizophr Res 2011; **128**:166–170.

9. Basile VS et al. Genetic dissection of atypical antipsychotic-induced weight gain: novel preliminary data on the pharmacogenetic puzzle. J Clin Psychiatry 2001; **62 Suppl** 23:45–66.

10. Reynolds GP et al. Polymorphism of the promoter region of the serotonin 5-HT(2C) receptor gene and clozapine-induced weight gain. Am J Psychiatry 2003; **160**:677–679.

11. Allison D et al. Antipsychotic-induced weight gain: A comprehensive research synthesis. Am J Psychiatry 1999; **156**:1686–1696.

12. Rummel-Kluge C et al. Head-to-head comparisons of metabolic side effects of second generation antipsychotics in the treatment of schizophrenia: a systematic review and meta-analysis. Schizophr Res 2010; **123**:225–233.

13. Leucht S et al. Comparative efficacy and tolerability of 15 antipsychotic drugs in schizophrenia: a multiple-treatments meta-analysis. Lancet 2013; **382**:951–962.

14. Cutler AJ et al. Long-term safety and tolerability of iloperidone: results from a 25-week, open-label extension trial. CNS Spectr 2013; **18**:43–54.

15. McEvoy JP et al. Effectiveness of paliperidone palmitate vs haloperidol decanoate for maintenance treatment of schizophrenia: a randomized clinical trial. JAMA 2014; **311**:1978–1987.

CHAPTER 2

Treatment of drug-induced weight gain

Weight gain is an important adverse effect of nearly all antipsychotics with obvious consequences for self-image, morbidity and mortality. Prevention and treatment are therefore matters of clinical urgency.

Monitoring

Patients starting antipsychotic treatment or changing drugs should, as an absolute minimum, be weighed and their weight clearly recorded. Estimates of body mass index and waist circumference should, ideally, also be made at baseline and later at least every 6 months.[1] Weekly monitoring of weight is recommended early in treatment, for the first 3 months at least. There is evidence that only a minority patients have anywhere near adequate monitoring of weight.[2] Clearly, monitoring of weight parameters is essential to assess the value of preventative and remedial measures.

Treatment and prevention

Most of the relevant literature in this area relates to attempts at reversing antipsychotic-related weight gain;[3] although there are now useful data suggesting that early interventions can prevent or mitigate weight gain.[4–6]

When weight gain occurs, initial options involve switching drugs or instituting behavioural programmes (or both). Switching always presents a risk of relapse and treatment discontinuation[7] but there is fairly strong support for switching to aripiprazole,[7–13] ziprasidone[14–16] or lurasidone[17,18] as a method for reversing weight gain. It is possible that switching to other drugs with a low propensity for weight gain is also beneficial.[19,20] Another option is to add aripiprazole to existing treatment – weight loss has been observed when aripiprazole was added to clozapine[21–23] and to olanzapine.[24] Stopping antipsychotic treatment altogether will reverse weight gain[25] but this course of action would not be sensible for the large majority of people with multi-episode schizophrenia. Note that, while some switching and augmentation strategies may minimise further weight gain or facilitate weight loss, the overall effect is generally modest; many patients continue to be overweight. Additional behavioural interventions are often required if BMI is to remain in/move towards the normal range.

A variety of behavioural methods have been proposed and evaluated with fairly good results.[26] Methods include calorie restriction,[27] low glycaemic index diet,[28] Weight Watchers[29] and diet/exercise programmes.[3,5,6,30–33] A meta-analysis of RCTs showed a robust effect for both prevention and intervention with these methods.[34] Pharmacological methods should be considered only where behavioural methods or switching have failed or where obesity presents clear, immediate physical risk to the patient. Some options are described in the table; metformin is now probably considered to be the drug of choice for the prevention and treatment of antipsychotic-induced weight gain. Table 2.18 lists drug treatment options for antipsychotic-induced weight gain (in alphabetical order).

Table 2.18 Drug treatment of antipsychotic-induced weight gain

Drug	Comments
Amantadine[35–38] (100–300 mg/day)	May attenuate olanzapine-related weight gain. Seems to be well tolerated. May (theoretically, at least) exacerbate psychosis. Weak evidence for benefit.[39] Not recommended.
Bupropion[40,41] (amfebutamone)	Seems to be effective in obesity when combined with calorie-restricted diets. Few data of its effects on drug-induced weight gain. Not recommended
Fluoxetine[42,43] (and other SSRIs)	Probably not effective.[39] Not recommended
H₂ antagonists[44–48] (e.g. nizatidine 300 mg bd, ranitidine 300 mg bd or famotidine 40 mg/day)	Some positive studies but most negative. Effect, if any, is small. Few data supporting a reversal of weight gain.
Metformin[49,50] (1.5–2.0 g/day)	Now a substantial database (in non-diabetic patients) supporting the use of metformin in both reducing and reversing weight gain caused by antipsychotics (mainly olanzapine). Beneficial effects on other metabolic parameters. Some negative studies, but clear and significant effect in meta-analyses.[39] Three more positive RCTs published since then.[51–53] Ideal for those with weight gain and diabetes or polycystic ovary syndrome. Note that metformin treatment increases the risk of vitamin B12 deficiency[54]
Melatonin[55] (3 mg at night)	One RCT showing attenuation of olanzapine-induced weight gain.
Methylcellulose (1500 mg ac)	Old-fashioned and rather unpalatable preparation. No data in drug-induced weight gain but once fairly widely used. Also acts as a laxative so may be suitable for clozapine-related weight gain
Orlistat[56–60] (120 mg tds ac/pc)	Reliable effect in obesity, especially when combined with calorie restriction. Few published data in drug-induced weight gain but widely used in practice with some success. When used without calorie restriction in psychiatric patients effects are very limited.[61,62] Failure to adhere to a low fat diet will result in fatty diarrhoea and possible malabsorbtion of orally administered medication. Good choice for clozapine-induced weight gain where it reduces both weight and the incidence of constipation[63]
Reboxetine[64,65] (4–8 mg daily)	Attenuates olanzapine-induced weight gain. Reverses some metabolic changes.[66] Effective when combined with betahistine[67]
Topiramate[68–78] (Up to 300 mg daily)	Reliably reduces weight even when drug-induced, but data are mainly observational. Problems may arise because of topiramate's propensity for causing sedation, confusion and cognitive impairment. May be antipsychotic[78,79]
Zonisamide[80] (150–600 mg/day)	Anticonvulsant drug with weight reducing properties. An RCT of 150 mg a day[81] showed significant weight reduction in people receiving SGAs

ac, *ante cibum* (before meals); bd, *bis in die* (twice a day); pc, *post cibum* (after meals); RCT, randomised controlled trial; SGA, second-generation antipsychotic; SSRI, selective serotonin reuptake inhibitor; tds, *ter die sumendum* (three times a day).

References

1. Marder SR et al. Physical health monitoring of patients with schizophrenia. Am J Psychiatry 2004; **161**:1334–1349.
2. Paton C et al. Obesity, dyslipidaemias and smoking in an inpatient population treated with antipsychotic drugs. Acta Psychiatr Scand 2004; **110**:299–305.
3. Kwon JS et al. Weight management program for treatment-emergent weight gain in olanzapine-treated patients with schizophrenia or schizoaffective disorder: A 12-week randomized controlled clinical trial. J Clin Psychiatry 2006; **67**:547–553.
4. Littrell KH et al. The effects of an educational intervention on antipsychotic-induced weight gain. J Nurs Scholarsh 2003; **35**:237–241.
5. Mauri M et al. Effects of an educational intervention on weight gain in patients treated with antipsychotics. J Clin Psychopharmacol 2006; **26**:462–466.
6. Alvarez-Jimenez M et al. Attenuation of antipsychotic-induced weight gain with early behavioral intervention in drug-naive first-episode psychosis patients: A randomized controlled trial. J Clin Psychiatry 2006; **67**:1253–1260.
7. Stroup TS et al. A randomized trial examining the effectiveness of switching from olanzapine, quetiapine, or risperidone to aripiprazole to reduce metabolic risk: Comparison of Antipsychotics for Metabolic Problems (CAMP). Am J Psychiatry 2011; **168**:947–956.
8. Casey DE et al. Switching patients to aripiprazole from other antipsychotic agents: a multicenter randomized study. Psychopharmacology (Berl) 2003; **166**:391–399.
9. De Hert M et al. A case series: evaluation of the metabolic safety of aripiprazole. Schizophr Bull 2007; **33**:823–830.
10. Lin SK et al. Reversal of antipsychotic-induced hyperprolactinemia, weight gain, and dyslipidemia by aripiprazole: A case report. J Clin Psychiatry 2006; **67**:1307.
11. Newcomer JW et al. A multicenter, randomized, double-blind study of the effects of aripiprazole in overweight subjects with schizophrenia or schizoaffective disorder switched from olanzapine. J Clin Psychiatry 2008; **69**:1046–1056.
12. Kim SH et al. Metabolic impact of switching antipsychotic therapy to aripiprazole after weight gain: a pilot study. J Clin Psychopharmacol 2007; **27**:365–368.
13. Mukundan A et al. Antipsychotic switching for people with schizophrenia who have neuroleptic-induced weight or metabolic problems. The Cochrane database of systematic reviews 2010: CD006629.
14. Weiden PJ et al. Improvement in indices of health status in outpatients with schizophrenia switched to ziprasidone. J Clin Psychopharmacol 2003; **23**:595–600.
15. Montes JM et al. Improvement in antipsychotic-related metabolic disturbances in patients with schizophrenia switched to ziprasidone. Prog Neuropsychopharmacol Biol Psychiatry 2007; **31**:383–388.
16. Karayal ON et al. Switching from quetiapine to ziprasidone: a sixteen-week, open-label, multicenter study evaluating the effectiveness and safety of ziprasidone in outpatient subjects with schizophrenia or schizoaffective disorder. J Psychiatr Pract 2011; **17**:100–109.
17. McEvoy JP et al. Effectiveness of lurasidone in patients with schizophrenia or schizoaffective disorder switched from other antipsychotics: a randomized, 6-week, open-label study. J Clin Psychiatry 2013; **74**:170–179.
18. Stahl SM et al. Effectiveness of lurasidone for patients with schizophrenia following 6 weeks of acute treatment with lurasidone, olanzapine, or placebo: a 6-month, open-label, extension study. J Clin Psychiatry 2013; **74**:507–515.
19. Gupta S et al. Weight decline in patients switching from olanzapine to quetiapine. Schizophr Res 2004; **70**:57–62.
20. Ried LD et al. Weight change after an atypical antipsychotic switch. Ann Pharmacother 2003; **37**:1381–1386.
21. Englisch S et al. Combined antipsychotic treatment involving clozapine and aripiprazole. Prog Neuropsychopharmacol Biol Psychiatry 2008; **32**:1386–1392.
22. Fleischhacker WW et al. Effects of adjunctive treatment with aripiprazole on body weight and clinical efficacy in schizophrenia patients treated with clozapine: a randomized, double-blind, placebo-controlled trial. Int J Neuropsychopharmacol 2010; **13**:1115–1125.
23. Schorr SG et al. A 12-month follow-up study of treating overweight schizophrenic patients with aripiprazole. Acta Psychiatr Scand 2008; **118**:246–250.
24. Henderson DC et al. Aripiprazole added to overweight and obese olanzapine-treated schizophrenia patients. J Clin Psychopharmacol 2009; **29**:165–169.
25. de Kuijper G et al. Effects of controlled discontinuation of long-term used antipsychotics on weight and metabolic parameters in individuals with intellectual disability. J Clin Psychopharmacol 2013; **33**:520–524.
26. Werneke U et al. Behavioural management of antipsychotic-induced weight gain: a review. Acta Psychiatr Scand 2003; **108**:252–259.
27. Cohen S et al. Weight gain with risperidone among patients with mental retardation: effect of calorie restriction. J Clin Psychiatry 2001; **62**:114–116.
28. Smith H et al. Low glycaemic index diet in patients prescribed clozapine: pilot study. Psychiatr Bull 2004; **28**:292–294.
29. Ball MP et al. A program for treating olanzapine-related weight gain. Psychiatr Serv 2001; **52**:967–969.
30. Pendlebury J et al. Evaluation of a behavioural weight management programme for patients with severe mental illness: 3 year results. Hum Psychopharmacol 2005; **20**:447–448.
31. Vreeland B et al. A program for managing weight gain associated with atypical antipsychotics. Psychiatr Serv 2003; **54**:1155–1157.
32. Ohlsen RI et al. A dedicated nurse-led service for antipsychotic-induced weight gain: An evaluation. Psychiatr Bull 2004; **28**:164–166.
33. Chen CK et al. Effects of a 10-week weight control program on obese patients with schizophrenia or schizoaffective disorder: a 12-month follow up. Psychiatry Clin Neurosci 2009; **63**:17–22.
34. Caemmerer J et al. Acute and maintenance effects of non-pharmacologic interventions for antipsychotic associated weight gain and metabolic abnormalities: a meta-analytic comparison of randomized controlled trials. Schizophr Res 2012; **140**:159–168.
35. Floris M et al. Effect of amantadine on weight gain during olanzapine treatment. Eur Neuropsychopharmacol 2001; **11**:181–182.

36. Gracious BL et al. Amantadine treatment of psychotropic-induced weight gain in children and adolescents: case series. J Child Adolesc Psychopharmacol 2002; **12**:249–257.

37. Bahk WM et al. Open label study of the effect of amantadine on weight gain induced by olanzapine. Psychiatry Clin Neurosci 2004; **58**:163–167.

38. Deberdt W et al. Amantadine for weight gain associated with olanzapine treatment. Eur Neuropsychopharmacol 2005; **15**:13–21.

39. Maayan L et al. Effectiveness of medications used to attenuate antipsychotic-related weight gain and metabolic abnormalities: a systematic review and meta-analysis. Neuropsychopharmacology 2010; **35**:1520–1530.

40. Gadde KM et al. Bupropion for weight loss: an investigation of efficacy and tolerability in overweight and obese women. Obes Res 2001; **9**:544–551.

41. Jain, AK et al. Bupropion SR vs. placebo for weight loss in obese patients with depressive symptoms. Obes Res 2002; **10**:1049–1056.

42. Poyurovsky M et al. Olanzapine-induced weight gain in patients with first-episode schizophrenia: a double-blind, placebo-controlled study of fluoxetine addition. Am J Psychiatry 2002; **159**:1058–1060.

43. Bustillo JR et al. Treatment of weight gain with fluoxetine in olanzapine-treated schizophrenic outpatients. Neuropsychopharmacology 2003; **28**:527–529.

44. Cavazzoni P et al. Nizatidine for prevention of weight gain with olanzapine: a double-blind placebo-controlled trial. Eur Neuropsychopharmacol 2003; **13**:81–85.

45. Pae CU et al. Effect of nizatidine on olanzapine-associated weight gain in schizophrenic patients in Korea: a pilot study. Hum Psychopharmaco 2003; **18**:453–456.

46. Poyurovsky M et al. The effect of famotidine addition on olanzapine-induced weight gain in first-episode schizophrenia patients: a double-blind placebo-controlled pilot study. Eur Neuropsychopharmacol 2004; **14**:332–336.

47. Atmaca M et al. Nizatidine for the treatment of patients with quetiapine-induced weight gain. Hum Psychopharmacol 2004; **19**:37–40.

48. Ranjbar F et al. The effect of ranitidine on olanzapine-induced weight gain. Biomed Res Int 2013; **2013**:639391

49. Praharaj SK et al. Metformin for olanzapine-induced weight gain: a systematic review and meta-analysis. Br J Clin Pharmacol 2011; **71**:377–382.

50. Ehret M et al. The effect of metformin on anthropometrics and insulin resistance in patients receiving atypical antipsychotic agents: a meta-analysis. J Clin Psychiatry 2010; **71**:1286–1292.

51. Wu RR et al. Metformin for treatment of antipsychotic-induced amenorrhea and weight gain in women with first-episode schizophrenia: a double-blind, randomized, placebo-controlled study. Am J Psychiatry 2012; **169**:813–821.

52. Jarskog LF et al. Metformin for weight loss and metabolic control in overweight outpatients with schizophrenia and schizoaffective disorder. Am J Psychiatry 2013; **170**:1032–1040.

53. Chen CH et al. Effects of adjunctive metformin on metabolic traits in nondiabetic clozapine-treated patients with schizophrenia and the effect of metformin discontinuation on body weight: a 24-week, randomized, double-blind, placebo-controlled study. J Clin Psychiatry 2013; **74**:e424–e430.

54. de Jager J et al. Long term treatment with metformin in patients with type 2 diabetes and risk of vitamin B-12 deficiency: randomised placebo controlled trial. BMJ 2010; **340**:c2181

55. Modabbernia A et al. Melatonin for prevention of metabolic side-effects of olanzapine in patients with first-episode schizophrenia: randomized double-blind placebo-controlled study. J Psychiatr Res 2014; **53**:133–140.

56. Sjostrom L et al. Randomised placebo-controlled trial of orlistat for weight loss and prevention of weight regain in obese patients. European Multicentre Orlistat Study Group. Lancet 1998; **352**:167–172.

57. Hilger E et al. The effect of orlistat on plasma levels of psychotropic drugs in patients with long-term psychopharmacotherapy. J Clin Psychopharmacol 2002; **22**:68–70.

58. Werneke U et al. Options for pharmacological management of obesity in patients treated with atypical antipsychotics. Int Clin Psychopharmacol 2002; **17**:145–160.

59. Pavlovic ZM. Orlistat in the treatment of clozapine-induced hyperglycemia and weight gain. Eur Psychiatry 2005; **20**:520

60. Carpenter LL et al. A case series describing orlistat use in patients on psychotropic medications. Med Health R I 2004; **87**:375–377.

61. Joffe G et al. Orlistat in clozapine- or olanzapine-treated patients with overweight or obesity: a 16-week randomized, double-blind, placebo-controlled trial. J Clin Psychiatry 2008; **69**:706–711.

62. Tchoukhine E et al. Orlistat in clozapine- or olanzapine-treated patients with overweight or obesity: a 16-week open-label extension phase and both phases of a randomized controlled trial. J Clin Psychiatry 2011; **72**:326–330.

63. Chukhin E et al. In a randomized placebo-controlled add-on study orlistat significantly reduced clozapine-induced constipation. Int Clin Psychopharmacol 2013; **28**:67–70.

64. Poyurovsky M et al. Attenuation of olanzapine-induced weight gain with reboxetine in patients with schizophrenia: a double-blind, placebo-controlled study. Am J Psychiatry 2003; **160**:297–302.

65. Poyurovsky M et al. Attenuating effect of reboxetine on appetite and weight gain in olanzapine-treated schizophrenia patients: a double-blind placebo-controlled study. Psychopharmacology (Berl) 2007; **192**:441–448.

66. Amrami-Weizman A et al. The effect of reboxetine co-administration with olanzapine on metabolic and endocrine profile in schizophrenia patients. Psychopharmacology (Berl) 2013; **230**:23–27.

67. Poyurovsky M et al. Reducing antipsychotic-induced weight gain in schizophrenia: a double-blind placebo-controlled study of reboxetine-betahistine combination. Psychopharmacology (Berl) 2013; **226**:615–622.

68. Binkley K et al. Sibutramine and panic attacks. Am J Psychiatry 2002; **159**:1793–1794.

69. Taflinski T et al. Sibutramine-associated psychotic episode. Am J Psychiatry 2000; **157**:2057–2058.

CHAPTER 2

70. Dursun SM et al. Clozapine weight gain, plus topiramate weight loss. Can J Psychiatry 2000; 45:198

71. Levy E et al. Topiramate produced weight loss following olanzapine-induced weight gain in schizophrenia. J Clin Psychiatry 2002; 63:1045

72. Van Ameringen M et al. Topiramate treatment for SSRI-induced weight gain in anxiety disorders. J Clin Psychiatry 2002; 63:981–984.

73. Appolinario JC et al. Topiramate use in obese patients with binge eating disorder: an open study. Can J Psychiatry 2002; 47:271–273.

74. Chengappa KN et al. Changes in body weight and body mass index among psychiatric patients receiving lithium, valproate, or topiramate: an open-label, nonrandomized chart review. Clin Ther 2002; 24:1576–1584.

75. Pavuluri MN et al. Topiramate plus risperidone for controlling weight gain and symptoms in preschool mania. J Child Adolesc Psychopharmacol 2002; 12:271–273.

76. Cates ME et al. Efficacy of add-on topiramate therapy in psychiatric patients with weight gain. Ann Pharmacother 2008; 42:505–510.

77. Egger C et al. Influence of topiramate on olanzapine-related weight gain in women: an 18-month follow-up observation. J Clin Psychopharmacol 2007; 27:475–478 .

78. Hahn MK et al. Topiramate augmentation in clozapine-treated patients with schizophrenia: clinical and metabolic effects. J Clin Psychopharmacol 2010; 30:706–710.

79. Afshar H et al. Topiramate add-on treatment in schizophrenia: a randomised, double-blind, placebo-controlled clinical trial. J Psychopharmacol 2009; 23:157–162.

80. Gadde KM et al. Zonisamide for weight loss in obese adults: a randomized controlled trial. JAMA 2003; 289:1820–1825.

81. Ghanizadeh A et al. The effect of zonisamide on antipsychotic-associated weight gain in patients with schizophrenia: a randomized, double-blind, placebo-controlled clinical trial. Schizophr Res 2013; 147:110–115.

Tardive dyskinesia

Tardive dyskinesia (TD) is now a somewhat less commonly encountered problem than in previous decades,[1] probably because of the introduction and widespread use of SGAs.[2–5] Treatment of established TD is often unsuccessful, so prevention, early detection and early treatment are essential. TD is associated with greater cognitive impairment,[6] more severe psychopathology[7] and higher mortality.[8]

There is fairly good evidence that SGAs are less likely to cause TD[9–13] although TD certainly does occur with these drugs albeit at quite different rates.[14–18] The observation that SGAs produce less TD than typical drugs is consistent with the long-held belief that early acute movement disorders and akathisia predict later TD.[19–21] Note, also, that TD can occur after minuscule doses of conventional drugs (and in the absence of portentous acute movement disorder[22]) and following the use of other dopamine antagonists such as metoclopramide.[23] It can also occur in never-medicated patients with both first-episode[24] and established[25] schizophrenia. FGA depot treatments may be particularly likely to bring about TD.[18] Risk of TD may be related to the extent of D_2 receptor occupancy (higher occupancy, higher risk).[26] It follows that the lower doses of FGAs that are now becoming routine in clinical practice may be associated with a lower risk of TD, perhaps approaching that seen with SGAs, but this has not yet been systematically explored.

Treatment – first steps

Most authorities recommend the withdrawal of any anticholinergic drugs and a reduction in the dose of antipsychotic as initial steps in those with early signs of TD[27,28] (dose reduction may initially worsen TD). Cochrane, however found little support for this approach[29] and the American Academy of Neurology does not recommend it.[30] It has now become common practice to withdraw the antipsychotic prescribed when TD was first observed and to substitute another drug. The use of clozapine[27] is probably best supported in this regard, but quetiapine, another weak striatal dopamine antagonist, is also effective.[31–37] Olanzapine and aripiprazole are also options.[38,39,39–42] There are a few supporting data for risperidone[40] but this might not be considered a logical choice in a patient with established TD, given that risperidone is more likely than clozapine, olanzapine and quetiapine to be associated with movement disorders in its own right. Again, the evidence for benefit in switching to particular SGAs is considered weak.[30]

Treatment – additional agents

Switching or withdrawing antipsychotics is not always effective or advisable and so additional agents are often used. Table 2.19 below describes the most frequently prescribed add-on drugs for TD, in order of preference.

Treatment – other possible options

The large number of proposed treatments for TD undoubtedly reflects the somewhat limited effectiveness of standard remedies. Table 2.20 lists some of these putative treatments in alphabetical order.

Table 2.19 Most frequently prescribed additional drugs for the treatment of tardive dyskinesia

Drug	Comments
Tetrabenazine[41,42]	Only licensed treatment for TD in UK. Has antipsychotic properties but reported to be depressogenic. Drowsiness, parkinsonism and akathisia also occur.[43,44] Dose is 25–200 mg/day. Reserpine (similar mode of action) also effective but rarely, if ever, used
Benzodiazepines[27,28]	Widely used and considered effective but Cochrane review suggests benzodiazepines are 'experimental'.[45] Intermittant use may be necessary to avoid tolerance to effects. Most used are clonazepam 1–4 mg/day and diazepam 6–25 mg/day. Better supporting evidence for clonazepam[30,44]
Vitamin E[46,47]	Numerous studies but efficacy remains to be conclusively established. Cochrane suggest there evidence only for slowing deterioration of TD.[48] Dose is in the range 400–600 IU/day
Ginkgo biloba[49]	One good RCT showing significant benefit over placebo. Well tolerated
Propranolol[50,51]	Open label studies only but formerly a widely used treatment. Dose is 40–120 mg/day. Beware contraindications (asthma, bradycardia, hypotension)

IU, international units; RCT, randomised controlled trial; TD, tardive dyskinesia.

Table 2.20 Less commonly prescribed additional drugs for the treatment of tardive dyskinesia

Drug	Comments
Amantadine[52,53]	Rarely used but apparently effective at 100–300 mg a day
Amino acids[54]	Use is supported by a small randomised, placebo-controlled trial. Low risk of toxicity
Botulinum toxin[55–58]	Case reports of success for localised dyskinesia. Probably now treatment of choice for disabling or distressing focal symptoms
Calcium antagonists[59]	A few published studies but not widely used. Cochrane is dismissive
Donepezil[60–62]	Supported by a single open study and case series. One negative RCT (n=12). Dose is 10 mg/day
Fish oils[63,64]	Very limited support for use of EPA at dose of 2 g/day
Fluvoxamine[65]	Three case reports. Dose is 100 mg/day. Beware interactions
Gabapentin[66]	Adds weight to theory that GABAergic mechansims improve TD. Dose is 900–1200 mg/day
Levetiracetam[67–70]	Three published case studies. One RCT. Dose up to 3000 mg/day
Melatonin[71]	Use is supported by a well-conducted trial. Usually well tolerated. Dose is 10 mg/day. Some evidence that melatonin receptor genotype determines risk of TD[72]
Naltrexone[73]	May be effective when added to benzodiazepines. Well tolerated. Dose is 200 mg/day
Ondansetron[74,75]	Limited evidence but low toxicity. Dose is up to 12 mg/day
Pyridoxine[76]	Supported by a well conducted trial. Dose is up to 400 mg/day
Quercetin[77]	Plant compound which is thought to be an antioxidant. No human studies in TD but widely used in other conditions
Sodium oxybate[78]	One case report. Dose was 8 g/day
Transcranial magnetic stimulation[79] (rTMS)	Single case report
Zolpidem[80]	Three case reports. Dose 10–30 mg a day

EPA, eicosapentanoic acid; GABA, gamma-aminobutyric acid; RCT, randomised controlled trial; TD, tardive dyskinesia.

References

1. Merrill RM et al. Tardive and spontaneous dyskinesia incidence in the general population. BMC Psychiatry 2013; **13**:152.

2. de Leon J. The effect of atypical versus typical antipsychotics on tardive dyskinesia : A naturalistic study. Eur Arch Psychiatry Clin Neurosci 2007; **257**:169–172.

3. Halliday J et al. Nithsdale Schizophrenia Surveys 23: movement disorders. 20-year review. Br J Psychiatry 2002; **181**:422–427.

4. Kane JM. Tardive dyskinesia circa 2006. Am J Psychiatry 2006; **163**:1316–1318.

5. Eberhard J et al. Tardive dyskinesia and antipsychotics: a 5-year longitudinal study of frequency, correlates and course. Int Clin Psychopharmacol 2006; **21**:35–42.

6. Wu JQ et al. Tardive dyskinesia is associated with greater cognitive impairment in schizophrenia. Prog Neuropsychopharmacol Biol Psychiatry 2013; **46**:71–77.

7. Ascher-Svanum H et al. Tardive dyskinesia and the 3-year course of schizophrenia: results from a large, prospective, naturalistic study. J Clin Psychiatry 2008; **69**:1580–1588.

8. Chong SA et al. Mortality rates among patients with schizophrenia and tardive dyskinesia. J Clin Psychopharmacol 2009; **29**:5–8.

9. Beasley C et al. Randomised double-blind comparison of the incidence of tardive dyskinesia in patients with schizophrenia during long-term treatment with olanzapine or haloperidol. Br J Psychiatry 1999; **174**:23–30.

10. Glazer WM. Expected incidence of tardive dyskinesia associated with atypical antipsychotics. J Clin Psychiatry 2000; **61 Suppl** 4:21–26.

11. Correll CU et al. Lower risk for tardive dyskinesia associated with second-generation antipsychotics: a systematic review of 1-year studies. Am J Psychiatry 2004; **161**:414–425.

12. Dolder CR et al. Incidence of tardive dyskinesia with typical versus atypical antipsychotics in very high risk patients. Biol Psychiatry 2003; **53**:1142–1145.

13. Correll CU et al. Tardive dyskinesia and new antipsychotics. Curr Opin Psychiatry 2008; **21**:151–156.

14. Gafoor R et al. Three case reports of emergent dyskinesia with clozapine. Eur Psychiatry 2003; **18**:260–261.

15. Keck ME et al. Ziprasidone-related tardive dyskinesia (Letter). Am J Psychiatry 2004; **161**:175–176.

16. Maytal G et al. Aripiprazole-related tardive dyskinesia. CNS Spectr 2006; **11**:435–439.

17. Fountoulakis KN et al. Amisulpride-induced tardive dyskinesia. Schizophr Res 2006; **88**:232–234.

18. Novick D et al. Incidence of extrapyramidal symptoms and tardive dyskinesia in schizophrenia: thirty-six-month results from the European schizophrenia outpatient health outcomes study. J Clin Psychopharmacol 2010; **30**:531–540.

19. Sachdev P. Early extrapyramidal side-effects as risk factors for later tardive dyskinesia: a prospective study. Aust N Z J Psychiatry 2004; **38**:445–449.

20. Miller DD et al. Clinical correlates of tardive dyskinesia in schizophrenia: baseline data from the CATIE schizophrenia trial. Schizophr Res 2005; **80**:33–43.

21. Tenback DE et al. Evidence that early extrapyramidal symptoms predict later tardive dyskinesia: a prospective analysis of 10,000 patients in the European Schizophrenia Outpatient Health Outcomes (SOHO) Study. Am J Psychiatry 2006; **163**:1438–1440.

22. Oosthuizen PP et al. Incidence of tardive dyskinesia in first-episode psychosis patients treated with low-dose haloperidol. J Clin Psychiatry 2003; **64**:1075–1080.

23. Kenney C et al. Metoclopramide, an increasingly recognized cause of tardive dyskinesia. J Clin Pharmacol 2008; **48**:379–384.

24. Puri BK et al. Spontaneous dyskinesia in first episode schizophrenia. J Neurol Neurosurg Psychiatry 1999; **66**:76–78.

25. McCreadie RG et al. Spontaneous dyskinesia and parkinsonism in never-medicated, chronically ill patients with schizophrenia: 18-month follow-up. Br J Psychiatry 2002; **181**:135–137.

26. Yoshida K et al. Tardive dyskinesia in relation to estimated dopamine D2 receptor occupancy in patients with schizophrenia: analysis of the CATIE data. Schizophr Res 2014; **153**:184–188.

27. Duncan D et al. Tardive dyskinesia: how is it prevented and treated? Psychiatric Bulletin 1997; **21**:422–425.

28. Simpson GM. The treatment of tardive dyskinesia and tardive dystonia. J Clin Psychiatry 2000; **61 Suppl** 4:39–44.

29. Soares-Weiser K et al. Neuroleptic reduction and/or cessation and neuroleptics as specific treatments for tardive dyskinesia. The Cochrane database of systematic reviews 2006: CD000459.

30. Bhidayasiri R et al. Evidence-based guideline: treatment of tardive syndromes: report of the Guideline Development Subcommittee of the American Academy of Neurology. Neurology 2013; **81**:463–469.

31. Vesely C et al. Remission of severe tardive dyskinesia in a schizophrenic patient treated with the atypical antipsychotic substance quetiapine. Int Clin Psychopharmacol 2000; **15**:57–60.

32. Alptekin K et al. Quetiapine-induced improvement of tardive dyskinesia in three patients with schizophrenia. Int Clin Psychopharmacol 2002; **17**:263–264.

33. Nelson MW et al. Adjunctive quetiapine decreases symptoms of tardive dyskinesia in a patient taking risperidone. Clin Neuropharmacol 2003; **26**:297–298.

34. Emsley R et al. A single-blind, randomized trial comparing quetiapine and haloperidol in the treatment of tardive dyskinesia. J Clin Psychiatry 2004; **65**:696–701.

35. Bressan RA et al. Atypical antipsychotic drugs and tardive dyskinesia: relevance of D2 receptor affinity. J Psychopharmacol 2004; **18**:124–127.

36. Sacchetti E et al. Quetiapine, clozapine, and olanzapine in the treatment of tardive dyskinesia induced by first-generation antipsychotics: a 124-week case report. Int Clin Psychopharmacol 2003; **18**:357–359.

37. Gourzis P et al. Quetiapine in the treatment of focal tardive dystonia induced by other atypical antipsychotics: a report of 2 cases. Clin Neuropharmacol 2005; **28**:195–196.

CHAPTER 2

38. Soutullo CA et al. Olanzapine in the treatment of tardive dyskinesia: a report of two cases. J Clin Psychopharmacol 1999; **19**:100–101.

39. Kinon BJ et al. Olanzapine treatment for tardive dyskinesia in schizophrenia patients: a prospective clinical trial with patients randomized to blinded dose reduction periods. Prog Neuropsychopharmacol Biol Psychiatry 2004; **28**:985–996.

40. Bai YM et al. Risperidone for severe tardive dyskinesia: a 12-week randomized, double-blind, placebo-controlled study. J Clin Psychiatry 2003; **64**:1342–1348.

41. Jankovic J et al. Long-term effects of tetrabenazine in hyperkinetic movement disorders. Neurology 1997; **48**:358–362.

42. Leung JG et al. Tetrabenazine for the treatment of tardive dyskinesia. Ann Pharmacother 2011; **45**:525–531.

43. Kenney C et al. Long-term tolerability of tetrabenazine in the treatment of hyperkinetic movement disorders. Mov Disord 2007; **22**:193–197.

44. Rana AQ et al. New and emerging treatments for symptomatic tardive dyskinesia. Drug Des Devel Ther 2013; **7**:1329–1340.

45. Bhoopathi PS et al. Benzodiazepines for neuroleptic-induced tardive dyskinesia. The Cochrane database of systematic reviews 2006; **3**: CD000205.

46. Adler LA et al. Vitamin E treatment for tardive dyskinesia. Arch Gen Psychiatry 1999; **56**:836–841.

47. Zhang XY et al. The effect of vitamin E treatment on tardive dyskinesia and blood superoxide dismutase: a double-blind placebo-controlled trial. J Clin Psychopharmacol 2004; **24**:83–86.

48. Soares-Weiser K et al. Vitamin E for neuroleptic-induced tardive dyskinesia. The Cochrane database of systematic reviews 2011: CD000209.

49. Zhang WF et al. Extract of Ginkgo biloba treatment for tardive dyskinesia in schizophrenia: a randomized, double-blind, placebo-controlled trial. J Clin Psychiatry 2011; **72**:615–621.

50. Perenyi A et al. Propranolol in the treatment of tardive dyskinesia. Biol Psychiatry 1983; **18**:391–394.

51. Pitts FN, Jr. Treatment of tardive dyskinesia with propranolol. J Clin Psychiatry 1982; **43**:304.

52. Angus S et al. A controlled trial of amantadine hydrochloride and neuroleptics in the treatment of tardive dyskinesia. J Clin Psychopharmacol 1997; **17**:88–91.

53. Pappa S et al. Effects of amantadine on tardive dyskinesia: a randomized, double-blind, placebo-controlled study. Clin Neuropharmacol 2010; **33**:271–275.

54. Richardson MA et al. Efficacy of the branched-chain amino acids in the treatment of tardive dyskinesia in men. Am J Psychiatry 2003; **160**:1117–1124.

55. Tarsy D et al. An open-label study of botulinum toxin A for treatment of tardive dystonia. Clin Neuropharmacol 1997; **20**:90–93.

56. Brashear A et al. Comparison of treatment of tardive dystonia and idiopathic cervical dystonia with botulinum toxin type A. Mov Disord 1998; **13**:158–161.

57. Hennings JM et al. Successful treatment of tardive lingual dystonia with botulinum toxin: case report and review of the literature. Prog Neuropsychopharmacol Biol Psychiatry 2008; **32**:1167–1171.

58. Beckmann YY et al. Treatment of intractable tardive lingual dyskinesia with botulinum toxin. J Clin Psychopharmacol 2011; **31**:250–251.

59. Essali A et al. Calcium channel blockers for neuroleptic-induced tardive dyskinesia. The Cochrane database of systematic reviews 2011: CD000206.

60. Caroff SN et al. Treatment of tardive dyskinesia with donepezil. J Clin Psychiatry 2001; **62**:128–129.

61. Bergman J et al. Beneficial effect of donepezil in the treatment of elderly patients with tardive movement disorders. J Clin Psychiatry 2005; **66**:107–110.

62. Ogunmefun A et al. Effect of donepezil on tardive dyskinesia. J Clin Psychopharmacol 2009; **29**:102–104.

63. Emsley R et al. The effects of eicosapentaenoic acid in tardive dyskinesia: a randomized, placebo-controlled trial. Schizophr Res 2006; **84**:112–120.

64. Vaddadi K et al. Tardive dyskinesia and essential fatty acids. Int Rev Psychiatry 2006; **18**:133–143.

65. Albayrak Y et al. Benefical effects of sigma-1 agonist fluvoxamine for tardive dyskinesia and tardive akathisia in patients with schizophrenia: report of three cases. Psychiatry Investig 2013; **10**:417–420.

66. Hardoy MC et al. Gabapentin in antipsychotic-induced tardive dyskinesia: results of 1-year follow-up. J Affect Disord 2003; **75**:125–130.

67. McGavin CL et al. Levetiracetam as a treatment for tardive dyskinesia: a case report. Neurology 2003; **61**:419.

68. Meco G et al. Levetiracetam in tardive dyskinesia. Clin Neuropharmacol 2006; **29**:265–268.

69. Woods SW et al. Effects of levetiracetam on tardive dyskinesia: a randomized, double-blind, placebo-controlled study. J Clin Psychiatry 2008; **69**:546–554.

70. Chen PH et al. Rapid improvement of neuroleptic-induced tardive dyskinesia with levetiracetam in an interictal psychotic patient. J Clin Psychopharmacol 2010; **30**:205–207.

71. Shamir E et al. Melatonin treatment for tardive dyskinesia: a double-blind, placebo-controlled, crossover study. Arch Gen Psychiatry 2001; **58**:1049–1052.

72. Lai IC et al. Analysis of genetic variations in the human melatonin receptor (MTNR1A, MTNR1B) genes and antipsychotics-induced tardive dyskinesia in schizophrenia. World J Biol Psychiatry 2011; **12**:143–148.

73. Wonodi I et al. Naltrexone treatment of tardive dyskinesia in patients with schizophrenia. J Clin Psychopharmacol 2004; **24**:441–445.

74. Sirota P et al. Use of the selective serotonin 3 receptor antagonist ondansetron in the treatment of neuroleptic-induced tardive dyskinesia. Am J Psychiatry 2000; **157**:287–289.

75. Naidu PS et al. Reversal of neuroleptic-induced orofacial dyskinesia by 5-HT3 receptor antagonists. Eur J Pharmacol 2001; **420**:113–117.

76. Lerner V et al. Vitamin B(6) in the treatment of tardive dyskinesia: a double-blind, placebo-controlled, crossover study. Am J Psychiatry 2001; **158**:1511–1514.

CHAPTER 2

77. Naidu PS et al. Reversal of haloperidol-induced orofacial dyskinesia by quercetin, a bioflavonoid. Psychopharmacology (Berl) 2003; **167**:418–423.

78. Berner JE. A case of sodium oxybate treatment of tardive dyskinesia and bipolar disorder. J Clin Psychiatry 2008; **69**:862.

79. Brambilla P et al. Transient improvement of tardive dyskinesia induced with rTMS. Neurology 2003; **61**:1155.

80. Waln O et al. Zolpidem improves tardive dyskinesia and akathisia. Mov Disord 2013; **28**:1748–1749.

Further reading

Aia PG et al. Tardive dyskinesia. Curr Treat Options Neurol 2011; **13**:231–241.

Paleacu D et al. Tetrabenazine treatment in movement disorders. Clin Neuropharmacol 2004; **27**: 230–233.

CHAPTER 2

Neuroleptic malignant syndrome

Neuroleptic malignant syndrome (NMS) is a rare, but potentially serious or even fatal, adverse effect of all antipsychotics. It is a syndrome essentially of muscular rigidity and sympathetic hyperactivity occurring as a result of dopaminergic antagonism in the context of psychological stressors and genetic predisposition.[1] Although widely seen as an acute, severe syndrome, NMS may, in many cases, have few signs and symptoms; 'full-blown' NMS may thus represent the extreme of a range of non-malignant related symptoms.[2] Certainly, asymptomatic rises in plasma creatine kinase (CK) are fairly common.[3]

The incidence and mortality rate of NMS are difficult to establish and probably vary as drug use changes and recognition of NMS increases. It has been estimated that fewer than 1% of all patients treated with conventional antipsychotics will experience NMS.[4] Incidence figures for SGA drugs are not available, but all have been reported to be associated with the syndrome,[5–12] even newer drugs like ziprasidone,[13,14] iloperidone,[15]

Table 2.21 Diagnosis and management of neuroleptic malignant syndrome

Signs and symptoms[1,4,16,17] (presentation varies considerably)[18]	Fever, diaphoresis, rigidity, confusion, fluctuating consciousness Fluctuating blood pressure, tachycardia Elevated creatine kinase, leukocytosis, altered liver function tests
Risk factors[16,17,19–23]	High potency typical drugs, recent or rapid dose increase, rapid dose reduction, abrupt withdrawal of anticholinergics, antipsychotic polypharmacy Psychosis, organic brain disease, alcoholism, Parkinson's disease, hyperthyroidism, psychomotor agitation, mental retardation Agitation, dehydration
Treatments[4,16,24–27]	**In the psychiatric unit:** Withdraw antipsychotics, monitor temperature, pulse, blood pressure. Consider benzodiazepines if not already prescribed – IM lorazepam has been used[28] **In the medical/A&E unit:** Rehydration, bromocriptine + dantrolene, sedation with benzodiazepines, artificial ventilation if required L-dopa, apomorphine, and carbamazepine have also been used, among many other drugs. Consider ECT for treatment of psychosis
Restarting antipsychotics[16,24,29]	Antipsychotic treatment will be required in most instances and re-challenge is associated with acceptable risk Stop antipsychotics for at least 5 days, preferably longer. Allow time for symptoms and signs of NMS to resolve completely Begin with very small dose and increase very slowly with close monitoring of temperature, pulse and blood pressure. Creatine kinase monitoring may be used, but is controversial.[17,30] Close monitoring of physical and biochemical parameters is effective in reducing progression to 'full-blown' NMS[31,32] Consider using an antipsychotic structurally unrelated to that previously associated with NMS, or a drug with low dopamine affinity (quetiapine or clozapine). Aripiprazole may also be considered[33] but it has a long plasma half-life and has been linked to an increased risk of NMS[22] Avoid depots (of any kind) and high potency conventional antipsychotics

A&E, accident and emergency; ECT, electroconvulsive therapy; IM, intramuscular; NMS, neuroleptic malignant syndrome.

aripiprazole,[34-37] paliperidone,[38] asenapine[39] and risperidone injection.[40] Mortality is probably lower with SGAs,[41-43] but symptoms are the same as those seen with FGAs[44] except that rigidity is less common.[42] NMS is also sometimes seen with other drugs such as antidepressants[45-48] and lithium.[49] Combinations of antipsychotics with SSRIs[50] or cholinesterase inhibitors[51,52] may increase the risk of NMS. NMS-type syndromes induced by SGA/SSRI combinations may share their symptoms and pathogenesis with serotonin syndrome.[53] The use of benzodiazepines has been linked to an important increase in the risk of NMS.[22,23]

The characteristics of NMS and its management are summarised in Table 2.21.

References

1. Gurrera RJ. Sympathoadrenal hyperactivity and the etiology of neuroleptic malignant syndrome. Am J Psychiatry 1999; **156**:169–180.

2. Bristow MF et al. How "malignant" is the neuroleptic malignant syndrome? BMJ 1993; **307**:1223–1224.

3. Meltzer HY et al. Marked elevations of serum creatine kinase activity associated with antipsychotic drug treatment. Neuropsychopharmacology 1996; **15**:395–405.

4. Guze BH et al. Current concepts. Neuroleptic malignant syndrome. N Engl J Med 1985; **313**:163–166.

5. Sing KJ et al. Neuroleptic malignant syndrome and quetiapine (Letter). Am J Psychiatry 2002; **159**:149–150.

6. Suh H et al. Neuroleptic malignant syndrome and low-dose olanzapine (Letter). Am J Psychiatry 2003; **160**:796.

7. Gallarda T et al. Neuroleptic malignant syndrome in an 72-year-old-man with Alzheimer's disease: A case report and review of the literature. Eur Neuropsychopharmacol 2000; **10 (Suppl** 3):357.

8. Stanley AK et al. Possible neuroleptic malignant syndrome with quetiapine. Br J Psychiatry 2000; **176**:497.

9. Sierra-Biddle D et al. Neuropletic malignant syndrome and olanzapine. J Clin Psychopharmacol 2000; **20**:704–705.

10. Hasan S et al. Novel antipsychotics and the neuroleptic malignant syndrome: a review and critique. Am J Psychiatry 1998; **155**:1113–1116.

11. Tsai JH et al. Zotepine-induced catatonia as a precursor in the progression to neuroleptic malignant syndrome. Pharmacotherapy 2005; **25**:1156–1159.

12. Gortney JS et al. Neuroleptic malignant syndrome secondary to quetiapine. Ann Pharmacother 2009; **43**:785–791.

13. Leibold J et al. Neuroleptic malignant syndrome associated with ziprasidone in an adolescent. Clin Ther 2004; **26**:1105–1108.

14. Borovicka MC et al. Ziprasidone- and lithium-induced neuroleptic malignant syndrome. Ann Pharmacother 2006; **40**:139–142.

15. Guanci N et al. Atypical neuroleptic malignant syndrome associated with iloperidone administration. Psychosomatics 2012; **53**:603–605.

16. Levenson JL. Neuroleptic malignant syndrome. Am J Psychiatry 1985; **142**:1137–1145.

17. Hermesh H et al. High serum creatinine kinase level: possible risk factor for neuroleptic malignant syndrome. J Clin Psychopharmacol 2002; **22**:252–256.

18. Picard LS et al. Atypical neuroleptic malignant syndrome: diagnostic controversies and considerations. Pharmacotherapy 2008; **28**:530–535.

19. Viejo LF et al. Risk factors in neuroleptic malignant syndrome. A case-control study. Acta Psychiatr Scand 2003; **107**:45–49.

20. Spivak B et al. Neuroleptic malignant syndrome during abrupt reduction of neuroleptic treatment. Acta Psychiatr Scand 1990; **81**:168–169.

21. Spivak B et al. Neuroleptic malignant syndrome associated with abrupt withdrawal of anticholinergic agents. Int Clin Psychopharmacol 1996; **11**:207–209.

22. Su YP et al. Retrospective chart review on exposure to psychotropic medications associated with neuroleptic malignant syndrome. Acta Psychiatr Scand 2014; **130**:52–60.

23. Nielsen RE et al. Neuroleptic malignant syndrome-an 11-year longitudinal case-control study. Can J Psychiatry 2012; **57**:512–518.

24. Olmsted TR. Neuroleptic malignant syndrome: guidelines for treatment and reinstitution of neuroleptics. South Med J 1988; **81**:888–891.

25. Shoop SA et al. Carbidopa/levodopa in the treatment of neuroleptic malignant syndrome (Letter). Ann Pharmacother 1997; **31**:119.

26. Terao T. Carbamazepine in the treatment of neuroleptic malignant syndrome (Letter). Biol Psychiatry 1999; **45**:381–382.

27. Lattanzi L et al. Subcutaneous apomorphine for neuroleptic malignant syndrome. Am J Psychiatry 2006; **163**:1450–1451.

28. Francis A et al. Is lorazepam a treatment for neuroleptic malignant syndrome? CNS Spectr 2000; **5**:54–57.

29. Wells AJ et al. Neuroleptic rechallenge after neuroleptic malignant syndrome: case report and literature review. Drug Intell Clin Pharm 1988; **22**:475–480.

30. Klein JP et al. Massive creatine kinase elevations with quetiapine: report of two cases. Pharmacopsychiatry 2006; **39**:39–40.

31. Shiloh R et al. Precautionary measures reduce risk of definite neuroleptic malignant syndrome in newly typical neuroleptic-treated schizophrenia inpatients. Int Clin Psychopharmacol 2003; **18**:147–149.

32. Hatch CD et al. Failed challenge with quetiapine after neuroleptic malignant syndrome with conventional antipsychotics. Pharmacotherapy 2001; **21**:1003–1006.

33. Trutia A et al. Neuroleptic rechallenge with aripiprazole in a patient with previously documented neuroleptic malignant syndrome. J Psychiatr Pract 2008; **14**:398–402.

34. Spalding S et al. Aripiprazole and atypical neuroleptic malignant syndrome. J Am Acad Child Adolesc Psychiatry 2004; **43**:1457–1458.

35. Chakraborty N et al. Aripiprazole and neuroleptic malignant syndrome. Int Clin Psychopharmacol 2004; **19**:351–353.

36. Rodriguez OP et al. A case report of neuroleptic malignant syndrome without fever in a patient given aripiprazole. J Okla State Med Assoc 2006; **99**:435–438.

37. Srephichit S et al. Neuroleptic malignant syndrome and aripiprazole in an antipsychotic-naive patient. J Clin Psychopharmacol 2006; **26**:94–95.

38. Duggal HS. Possible neuroleptic malignant syndrome associated with paliperidone. J Neuropsychiatry Clin Neurosci 2007; **19**:477–478.

39. Singh N et al. Neuroleptic malignant syndrome after exposure to asenapine: a case report. Prim Care Companion J Clin Psychiatry 2010; **12**:e1.

40. Mall GD et al. Catatonia and mild neuroleptic malignant syndrome after initiation of long-acting injectable risperidone: case report. J Clin Psychopharmacol 2008; **28**:572–573.

41. Ananth J et al. Neuroleptic malignant syndrome and atypical antipsychotic drugs. J Clin Psychiatry 2004; **65**:464–470.

42. Trollor JN et al. Comparison of neuroleptic malignant syndrome induced by first- and second-generation antipsychotics. Br J Psychiatry 2012; **201**:52–56.

43. Nakamura M et al. Mortality of neuroleptic malignant syndrome induced by typical and atypical antipsychotic drugs: a propensity-matched analysis from the Japanese Diagnosis Procedure Combination database. J Clin Psychiatry 2012; **73**:427–430.

44. Trollor JN et al. Neuroleptic malignant syndrome associated with atypical antipsychotic drugs. CNS Drugs 2009; **23**:477–492.

45. Kontaxakis VP et al. Neuroleptic malignant syndrome after addition of paroxetine to olanzapine. J Clin Psychopharmacol 2003; **23**:671–672.

46. Young C. A case of neuroleptic malignant syndrome and serotonin disturbance. J Clin Psychopharmacol 1997; **17**:65–66.

47. June R et al. Neuroleptic malignant syndrome associated with nortriptyline. Am J Emerg Med 1999; **17**:736–737.

48. Lu TC et al. Neuroleptic malignant syndrome after the use of venlafaxine in a patient with generalized anxiety disorder. J Formos Med Assoc 2006; **105**:90–93.

49. Gill J et al. Acute lithium intoxication and neuroleptic malignant syndrome. Pharmacotherapy 2003; **23**:811–815.

50. Stevens DL. Association between selective serotonin-reuptake inhibitors, second-generation antipsychotics, and neuroleptic malignant syndrome. Ann Pharmacother 2008; **42**:1290–1297.

51. Stevens DL et al. Olanzapine-associated neuroleptic malignant syndrome in a patient receiving concomitant rivastigmine therapy. Pharmacotherapy 2008; **28**:403–405.

52. Warwick TC et al. Neuroleptic malignant syndrome variant in a patient receiving donepezil and olanzapine. Nat Clin Pract Neurol 2008; **4**:170–174.

53. Odagaki Y. Atypical neuroleptic malignant syndrome or serotonin toxicity associated with atypical antipsychotics? Curr Drug Saf 2009; **4**:84–93.

Catatonia

Catatonia is a word usually used to describe a state of stupor occurring in the context of a psychotic illness. There are two problems with this. First, catatonic schizophrenia describes either immobile stupor or a state of chaotic physical and psychological agitation.[1] Second, stupor is seen in many other non-organic conditions such as depression, mania and conversion disorder.[2–6]

Catatonia is thus one type of stupor, a condition characterised by at least two of the following symptoms:

- marked psychomotor retardation sometimes with complete immobility
- mutism
- waxy flexibility (no resistance from a patient to an attempt to move a limb into the most awkward position and maintenance of its position)
- negativism (strong opposite direction movement responses to an attempt to move a patients limb) or automatic obedience
- peculiar voluntary movements, e.g. posturing, mannerisms, stereotyped movements and grimacing
- echolalia, echopraxia
- refusal to eat and/or drink.

If psychiatric stupor is left untreated, physical health complications are unavoidable and develop rapidly. Prompt treatment is crucial as it may prevent complications, which include dehydration, venous thrombosis, pulmonary embolism, pneumonia, and ultimately death.[7]

There are three psychiatric illnesses which can present with stupor. Amongst them, stupor is mostly seen in psychotic illness. As outlined above, catatonic schizophrenia presents not only with an immobile mute picture of stupor, but also with a catatonic excitement, when a patient experiences the opposite to stupor – a chaotic psychomotor agitation and pronouncedly increased volume of speech, most of which is incoherent. The second psychiatric cause of stupor is affective illness, where an immobile mute clinical picture can occur in both depressive and manic states.[2,4,8–11] The third cause is one of the most intriguing and rare psychiatric conditions – conversion disorder stupor, which sometimes is referred to as psychosomatic or hysterical catatonia.[12–15]

There are also developmental disorders such as autism, as well as neurodegenerative[16,17] and organic disorders which can present with a catatonia-like picture of a mute and immobile patient. These include a number of medical disorders such as:

- subarachnoid haemorrhages
- basal ganglia disorders
- non-convulsive status epilepticus
- locked-in and akinetic mutism states
- endocrine and metabolic disorders, e.g. Wilson's disease[18]
- Prader-Willi syndrome
- antiphospholidid syndrome[19]
- systemic lupus erythematosus (SLE)[20]

- infections
- dementia
- and drug withdrawal and toxic drug states can precipitate catatonic symptoms, e.g. after abrupt withdrawal of clozapine and withdrawal of zolpidem, temazepam and many non-psychotropics including the medicines used in oncology.

The treatment of stupor is dependent on its cause. Benzodiazepines are the drugs of choice for stupor occurring in the context of affective and conversion disorders.[8,9,21] It is postulated that benzodiazepines may act by increasing GABAergic transmission or reducing levels of brain-derived neurotropic factor.[22] There is most experience with lorazepam. Many patients will respond to standard doses (up to 4 mg per day), but repeated and higher doses (between 8 and 24 mg per day) may be needed.[23] One observational study of 9 years duration in patients with stupor of a mood disorder causality[8] – either major depressive episodes or bipolar I – reported an 83.3% response to intramuscular lorazepam 2 mg administered within first 2 hours of presentation, and a 100% response if 10 mg diazepam IV in 500 mL normal saline was added in cases of IM treatment failure. Where benzodiazepines are effective, their benefit is seen very quickly.

Catatonia in schizophrenia is somewhat less likely to respond to benzodiazepines, with a response in the range of 40–50%.[24] A double-blind, placebo-controlled, crossover trial with lorazepam up to 6 mg per day demonstrated no effect on catatonic symptoms in patients with chronic schizophrenia,[25] similar to the poor effect of lorazepam in a non-randomised trial.[26] A further complication of schizophrenia is that of differential diagnosis. Debate continues on the similarities and differences between catatonic stupor in psychosis and NMS.[27,28] Two terms have been coined – lethal catatonia and malignant catatonia[29] to describe stupor which is accompanied by autonomic instability or hyperthermia. This potentially fatal condition cannot be distinguished either clinically or by laboratory testing from NMS, leading to a suggestion that NMS is a variant form of malignant catatonia.[30] However, the absence of any prior administration of dopamine antagonist can help rule out NMS.

In stupor associated with schizophrenia, electroconvulsive therapy (ECT) and benzodiazepines remain first-choice treatments (Figure 2.5). The vast majority of current published evidence and evidence published over previous decades suggests that prompt ECT remains the most successful treatment.[26,31–45] As with benzodiazepines, response to ECT may be lower in patients with schizophrenia (or who have been treated with antipsychotics) than in patients with mood disorders.[46] In malignant catatonia, every effort should be made to maximise the effect of ECT by using liberal-stimulus dosing to induce well-generalised seizures.[47] Physical health needs should be also priorities and in-patient medical care obtained when necessary, especially for those showing autonomic imbalance and those whose dietary intake cannot be managed in psychiatric care.

The use of antipsychotics should be carefully considered (Table 2.22). Some authors recommend that antipsychotics should be avoided altogether in catatonic patients, although there are case reports of successful treatment with aripiprazole, risperidone, olanzapine, ziprasidone and clozapine.[48–53] There is probably most evidence supporting clozapine and olanzapine.

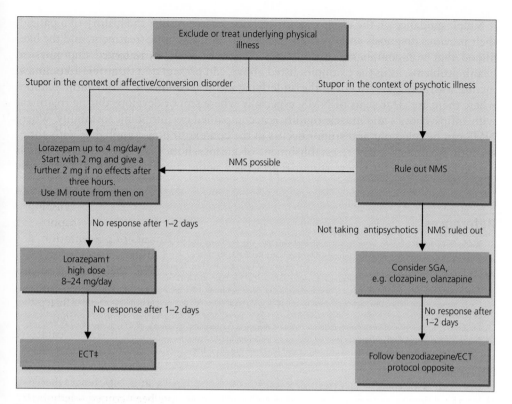

Figure 2.5 Algorithm for treating stupor[54]
*Lorazepam is absorbed sublingually and is tasteless. This route may be preferred in non co-operative patients or those who cannot swallow.
†Intravenous diazepam may be considered here.
‡Do not wait to give ECT if there is significant danger to life.

Table 2.22 Alternative treatments for catatonia/stupor. Listed in alphabetical order – no preference implied by order

Antipsychotics[48-53,55-58]

- aripiprazole
- clozapine
- olanzapine

- risperidone
- ziprasidone

Experimental treatments* [9,10,41,59-64]

- amantadine
- amitriptyline
- carbamazepine
- fluoxetine
- fluvoxamine
- lithium

- memantine
- methyphenidate
- mirtazapine
- tramadol
- valproate
- zolpidem

*Always read the primary literature before using anything in this section.

CHAPTER 2

Simple guidance on the usage of antipsychotics is to consider the history of a patient, their previous diagnosis and previous response to antipsychotic treatment, and the likelihood that non-compliance precipitated stupor. It needs to be noted that physical health problems, as in the examples listed above, can present as a catatonia-like clinical picture warranting treatment of the underlying medical condition. Avoid antipsychotics where there are clear signs of NMS, especially where stupor develops during treatment with antipsychotics and muscle rigidity is accompanied by autonomic instability. Where NMS can be ruled out and stupor occurs in the context of non-compliance with antipsychotic treatment, early re-establishment of antipsychotics is recommended. This is particularly important where stupor represents a withdrawal syndrome (as commonly seen with clozapine).

References

1. Walther S. Dysfunctions of the motor system in schizophrenia. Eur Arch Psychiatry Clin Neurosci 2013; **263 Suppl**1:S16.
2. Takacs R et al. Catatonia in Affective Disorders. Curr Psychiatry Rev 2013; **9**:101–105.
3. Fink M. Rediscovering catatonia: the biography of a treatable syndrome. Acta Psychiatr Scand Suppl 2013;**1–47**.
4. Campos Mangas.M.C. et al. P-167 - Catatonia in bipolar disorder. Eur Psychiatry 2012; **27 Suppl** 1:1.
5. Bartolommei N et al. Catatonia: a critical review and therapeutic recommendation. J Psychopathol 2012; **18**:234–246.
6. Lee J. Dissociative catatonia: Dissociative-catatonic reactions, clinical presentations and responses to benzodiazepines. Aust N Z J Psychiatry 2011; **45**:A42
7. Petrides G et al. Synergism of lorazepam and electroconvulsive therapy in the treatment of catatonia. Biol Psychiatry 1997; **42**:375–381.
8. Huang YC et al. Rapid relief of catatonia in mood disorder by lorazepam and diazepam. Biomed J 2013; **36**:35–39.
9. Vasudev K et al. What works for delirious catatonic mania? BMJ Case Rep 2010; **2010**.
10. Neuhut R et al. Resolution of catatonia after treatment with stimulant medication in a patient with bipolar disorder. Psychosomatics 2012; **53**:482–484.
11. Ghaffarinejad AR et al. Periodic catatonia. Challenging diagnosis for psychiatrists. Neurosciences (Riyadh) 2012; **17**:156–158.
12. Suzuki K et al. Hysteria presenting as a prodrome to catatonic stupor in a depressive patient resolved with electroconvulsive therapy. J ECT 2006; **22**:276.
13. Alwaki A et al. Catatonia: an elusive diagnosis. Neurology 2013; **80 Suppl** 1.
14. Dhadphale M. Eye gaze diagnostic sign in hysterical stupor. Lancet 1980; **2**:374–375.
15. Gomez J. Hysterical stupor and death. Br J Psychiatry 1980; **136**:105–106.
16. Mazzone L et al. Catatonia in patients with autism: prevalence and management. CNS Drugs 2014; **28**:205–215.
17. Dhossche DM, Wachtel LE. Catatonia in Psychiatric Illnesses. In: Fatemi SH, Clayton PJ, eds. The Medical Basis of Psychiatry. Totowa, NJ: Humana Press; 2008. pp. 471–486.
18. Shetageri VN et al. Case report: catatonia as a presenting symptom of Wilsons disease. Indian J Psychiatry 2011; **53 Suppl** 5:S93–S94.
19. Cardinal RN et al. Psychosis and catatonia as a first presentation of antiphospholipid syndrome. Br J Psychiatry 2009; **195**:272.
20. Pustilnik S et al. Catatonia as the presenting symptom in systemic lupus erythematosus. J Psychiatr Pract 2011; **17**:217–221.
21. Sienaert P et al. Adult catatonia: Etiopathogenesis, diagnosis and treatment. Neuropsychiatry (London) 2013; **3**:391–399.
22. Huang TL et al. Lorazepam reduces the serum brain-derived neurotrophic factor level in schizophrenia patients with catatonia. Prog Neuropsychopharmacol Biol Psychiatry 2009; **33**:158–159.
23. Fink M et al. Neuroleptic malignant syndrome is malignant catatonia, warranting treatments efficacious for catatonia. Prog Neuropsychopharmacol Biol Psychiatry 2006; **30**:1182–1183.
24. Rosebush PI et al. Catatonia: re-awakening to a forgotten disorder. Mov Disord 1999; **14**:395–397.
25. Ungvari GS et al. Lorazepam for chronic catatonia: a randomized, double-blind, placebo-controlled cross-over study. Psychopharmacology 1999; **142**:393–398.
26. Dutt A et al. Phenomenology and treatment of catatonia: A descriptive study from north India. Indian J Psychiatry 2011; **53**:36–40.
27. Luchini F et al. Catatonia and neuroleptic malignant syndrome: two disorders on a same spectrum? Four case reports. J Nerv Ment Dis 2013; **201**:36–42.
28. Mishima T et al. [Diazepam-responsive malignant catatonia in a patient with an initial clinical diagnosis of neuroleptic malignant syndrome: a case report]. Brain Nerve 2011; **63**:503–507.
29. Mann SC et al. Catatonia, malignant catatonia, and neuroleptic malignant syndrome. Curr Psychiatry Rev 2013; **9**:111–119.
30. Taylor MA et al. Catatonia in psychiatric classification: a home of its own. Am J Psychiatry 2003; **160**:1233–1241.
31. Bush G et al. Catatonia. II. Treatment with lorazepam and electroconvulsive therapy. Acta Psychiatr Scand 1996; **93**:137–143.
32. Cristancho P et al. Successful use of right unilateral ECT for catatonia: a case series. J ECT 2014; **30**:69–72.
33. Philbin D et al. Catatonic schizophrenia: therapeutic challenges and potentially a new role for electroconvulsive therapy? BMJ Case Rep 2013; 2013.

34. Takebayashi M. [Electroconvulsive therapy in schizophrenia]. Nihon Rinsho 2013; **71**:694–700.

35. Oviedo G et al. Trends in the administration of electroconvulsive therapy for schizophrenia in Colombia. Descriptive study and literature review. Eur Arch Psychiatry Clin Neurosci 2013; **263 Suppl** 1:S98

36. Pompili M et al. Indications for electroconvulsive treatment in schizophrenia: a systematic review. Schizophr Res 2013; **146**:1–9.

37. Ogando Portilla N et al. Electroconvulsive therapy as an effective treatment in neuroleptic malignant syndrome: purposely a case. Eur Psychiatry 2013; **28 Suppl** 1:1.

38. Unal A et al. Effective treatment of catatonia by combination of benzodiazepine and electroconvulsive therapy. J ECT 2013; **29**:206–209.

39. Kaliora SC et al. The practice of electroconvulsive therapy in Greece. J ECT 2013; **29**:219–224.

40. Girardi P et al. Life-saving electroconvulsive therapy in a patient with near-lethal catatonia. Riv Psichiatr 2012; **47**:535–537.

41. Kumar V et al. Electroconvulsive therapy in pregnancy. Indian J Psychiatry 2011; **53 Suppl** 5:S100–S101.

42. Weiss M et al. Treatment of catatonia with electroconvulsive therapy in adolescents. J Child Adolesc Psychopharmacol 2012; **22**:96–100.

43. Bauer J et al. Should the term catatonia be explicitly included in the ICD-10 description of acute transient psychotic disorder F23.0? Nord J Psychiatry 2012; **66**:68–69.

44. Mohammadbeigi H et al. Electroconvulsive therapy in single manic episodes: a case series. Afr J Psychiatry (Johannesbg) 2011; **14**:56–59.

45. Dragasek J. [Utilisation of electroconvulsive therapy in treatment of depression disorders]. Psychiatrie 2011; **15**:1211–9.

46. van Waarde JA et al. Electroconvulsive therapy for catatonia: treatment characteristics and outcomes in 27 patients. J ECT 2010; **26**:248–252.

47. Kellner CH et al. Electroconvulsive therapy for catatonia. Am J Psychiatry 2010; **167**:1127–1128.

48. Van Den EF et al. The use of atypical antipsychotics in the treatment of catatonia. Eur Psychiatry 2005; **20**:422–429.

49. Caroff SN et al. Movement disorders associated with atypical antipsychotic drugs. J Clin Psychiatry 2002; **63 Suppl** 4:12–19.

50. Guzman CS et al. Treatment of periodic catatonia with atypical antipsychotic, olanzapine. Psychiatry Clin Neurosci 2008; **62**:482.

51. Babington PW et al. Treatment of catatonia with olanzapine and amantadine. Psychosomatics 2007; **48**:534–536.

52. Bastiampillai T et al. Catatonia resolution and aripiprazole. Aust N Z J Psychiatry 2008; **42**:907.

53. Strawn JR et al. Successful treatment of catatonia with aripiprazole in an adolescent with psychosis. J Child Adolesc Psychopharmacol 2007; **17**:733–735.

54. Rosebush PI et al. Catatonia and its treatment. Schizophr Bull 2010; **36**:239–242.

55. Voros V et al. [Use of aripiprazole in the treatment of catatonia]. Neuropsychopharmacol Hung 2010; **12**:373–376.

56. Yoshimura B et al. Is quetiapine suitable for treatment of acute schizophrenia with catatonic stupor? A case series of 39 patients. Neuropsychiatr Dis Treat 2013; **9**:1565–1571.

57. Todorova K. Olanzapine in the treatment of catatonic stupor - two case reports and discussion. Eur Neuropsychopharmacol 2012; **22 Suppl** 2:S326.

58. Prakash O et al. Catatonia and mania in patient with AIDS: treatment with lorazepam and risperidone. Gen Hosp Psychiatry 2012; **34**:321–326.

59. Daniels J. Catatonia: clinical aspects and neurobiological correlates. J Neuropsychiatry Clin Neurosci 2009; **21**:371–380.

60. Obregon DF et al. Memantine and catatonia: a case report and literature review. J Psychiatr Pract 2011; **17**:292–299.

61. Hervey WM et al. Treatment of catatonia with amantadine. Clin Neuropharmacol 2012; **35**:86–87.

62. Consoli A et al. Lorazepam, fluoxetine and packing therapy in an adolescent with pervasive developmental disorder and catatonia. J Physiol Paris 2010; **104**:309–314.

63. Lewis AL et al. Malignant catatonia in a patient with bipolar disorder, B12 deficiency, and neuroleptic malignant syndrome: one cause or three? J Psychiatr Pract 2009; **15**:415–422.

64. Padhy SK et al. The catatonia conundrum: controversies and contradictions. Asian J Psychiatr 2014; **7**:6–9.

CHAPTER 2

QT prolongation

Introduction

Many psychotropic drugs are associated with ECG changes and some are causally linked to serious ventricular arrhythmia and sudden cardiac death. Specifically, some antipsychotics block cardiac potassium channels and are linked to prolongation of the cardiac QT interval, a risk factor for the ventricular arrhythmia torsade de pointes, which is often fatal. Case-control studies have suggested that the use of most antipsychotics is associated with an increase in the rate of sudden cardiac death.[1-7] This risk is probably a result of the arrhythmogenic potential of antipsychotics[8,9] although schizophrenia itself may be associated with QT prolongation.[10] Overall risk is probably dose-related and, although the absolute risk is low, it is substantially higher than the, say, risk of fatal agranulocytosis with clozapine.[8]

ECG monitoring of drug-induced changes in mental health settings is complicated by a number of factors. Psychiatrists may have limited expertise in ECG interpretation, for example, and still less expertise in manually measuring QT intervals. Even cardiologists show an interrater reliability in QT measurement of up to 20 msec.[11] Self-reading, computerised ECG devices are available and to some extent compensate for some lack of expertise, but different models use different algorithms and different correction formulae.[12] In addition, ECG machines may not be as readily available in all clinical areas as they are in general medicine. Also, time for ECG determination may not be available in many areas (e.g. out-patients). Lastly, ECG determination may be difficult to perform in acutely disturbed, physically uncooperative patients.

ECG monitoring is essential for all patients prescribed antipsychotics. An estimate of QT_C interval should be made on admission to in-patient units (note that this is recommended in the NICE schizophrenia guideline[13]) and at least yearly thereafter.

QT prolongation

- The cardiac QT interval (usually cited as QTc – QT corrected for heart rate) is a useful, but imprecise indicator of risk of torsade de pointes and of increased cardiac mortality[14]. Different correction factors and methods may give markedly different values.[15]
- The QT interval broadly reflects the duration of cardiac repolarisation. Lengthening of repolarisation duration induces heterogeneity of electrical phasing in different ventricular structures (dispersion), which in turn allows the emergence of early after depolarisations (EADs) which may provoke ventricular extrasystole and torsade de pointes.
- There is some controversy over the exact association between QTc and risk of arrhythmia. Very limited evidence suggests that risk is exponentially related to the extent of prolongation beyond normal limits (440 msec for men; 470 msec for women), although there are well-known exceptions which appear to disprove this theory[16] (some drugs prolong QT without increasing dispersion). Rather stronger evidence links QTc values over 500 msec to a clearly increased risk of arrhythmia.[17]

QT intervals of >650 msec may be more likely than not to induce torsades.[18] Despite some uncertainties, QTc determination remains an important measure in estimating risk of arrhythmia and sudden death.

- QTc measurements and evaluation are complicated by:

  - difficulty in determining the end of the T wave, particularly where U waves are present (this applies both to manual and self-reading ECG machines)
  - normal physiological variation in QTc interval: QT varies with gender, time of day, food intake, alcohol intake, menstrual cycle, ECG lead, etc[15,16]
  - variation in the extent of drug-induced prolongation of QTc because of changes in plasma levels. QTc prolongation is most prominent at peak drug plasma levels and least obvious at trough levels.[15,16]

Other ECG changes

Other reported antipsychotic-induced changes include atrial fibrillation, giant P waves, T-wave changes and heart block.[16]

Quantifying risk

Drugs are categorised in Table 2.23 according to data available on their effects on the cardiac QTc interval (as reported; mostly using Bazett's correction formula). 'No-effect' drugs are those with which QTc prolongation has not been reported either at therapeutic

Table 2.23 Effects of antipsychotics on QTc[15,16,22–45]

No effect	Low effect	Moderate effect	High effect	Unknown effect
Aripiprazole*	Asenapine	Amisulpride[‡]	Any intravenous antipsychotic	Loxapine
Lurasidone	Clozapine	Chlorpromazine	Pimozide	Pipotiazine
	Flupentixol	Haloperidol	Sertindole	Trifluoperazine
	Fluphenazine	Iloperidone	Any drug or combination of drugs used in doses exceeding recommended maximum	Zuclopenthixol
	Perphenazine	Levomepromazine		
	Prochlorperazine	Melperone		
	Olanzapine[†]	Quetiapine		
	Paliperidone	Ziprasidone		
	Risperidone			
	Sulpiride			

*One case of torsades de pointes reported.[46]
[†]Isolated cases of QTc prolongation[26,47] and has effects on cardiac ion channel, I_{Kr},[48] other data suggest no effect on QT_C.[16,24,25,49]
[‡]Torsades de pointes common in overdose.[18]

doses or in overdose. 'Low-effect' drugs are those for which severe QTc prolongation has been reported only following overdose or where only small average increases (<10 msec) have been observed at clinical doses. 'Moderate-effect' drugs are those which have been observed to prolong QTc by >10 msec on average when given at normal clinical doses or where ECG monitoring is officially recommended in some circumstances. 'High-effect' drugs are those for which extensive average QTc prolongation (usually >20 msec at normal clinical doses).

Note that, as outlined above, effect on QTc may not necessarily equate directly to risk of torsade de pointes or sudden death,[19] although this is often assumed. (A good example here is ziprasidone – a drug with a moderate effect on QTc but with no evidence of cardiac toxicity.[20]) Note also that categorisation is inevitably approximate given the problems associated with QTc measurements. Lastly, keep in mind that differences in the effects of different antipsychotics on the QT interval rarely reach statistical significance even in meta-analyses.[21]

Other risk factors

A number of physiological/pathological factors are associated with an increased risk of QT changes and of arrhythmia (Table 2.24) and many non-psychotropic drugs are linked to QT prolongation (Table 2.25). These additional risk factors seem almost always to be present in cases of antipsychotic-induced torsades de pointes.[50]

Table 2.24 Physiological risk factors for QTc prolongation and arrhythmia

Factor	Symptom
Cardiac	Long QT syndrome
	Bradycardia
	Ischaemic heart disease
	Myocarditis
	Myocardial infarction
	Left ventricular hypertrophy
Metabolic	Hypokalaemia
	Hypomagnesaemia
	Hypocalcaemia
Others	Extreme physical exertion
	Stress or shock
	Anorexia nervosa
	Extremes of age – children and elderly may be more susceptible to QT changes
	Female gender

Hypokalaemia-related QTc prolongation is more commonly observed in acute psychotic admissions.[51] Also, be aware that there are number of physical and genetic factors which may not be discovered on routine examination but which probably predispose patients to arrhythmia.[52,53]

Table 2.25 Non-psychotropics associated with QT prolongation

Drug class	Drug
Antibiotics	Erythromycin
	Clarithromycin
	Ampicillin
	Co-trimoxazole
	Pentamidine
	(Some 4 quinolones affect QTc – see manufacturers' literature)
Antimalarials	Chloroquine
	Mefloquine
	Quinine
Antiarrhythmics	Quinidine
	Disopyramide
	Procainamide
	Sotalol
	Amiodarone
	Bretylium
Others	Amantadine
	Cyclosporin
	Diphenhydramine
	Hydroxyzine
	Methadone
	Nicardipine
	Tamoxifen

Beta-2 agonists and sympathomimetics may provoke torsade de pointes in patients with prolonged QTc.

ECG monitoring

Measure QT_C in all patients prescribed antipsychotics:

- on admission
- if previous abnormality or known additional risk factor, at annual physical health check.

Consider measuring QTc within a week of achieving a therapeutic dose of a newly prescribed antipsychotic that is associated with a moderate or high risk of QTc prolongation or of newly prescribed combined antipsychotics. See Table 2.26 for the management of QT prolongation in patients receiving antipsychotic drugs.

Metabolic inhibition

The effect of drugs on the QTc interval is usually plasma level-dependent. Drug interactions are therefore important, especially when metabolic inhibition results in increased plasma levels of the drug affecting QTc. Commonly used metabolic inhibitors include fluvoxamine, fluoxetine, paroxetine and valproate.

CHAPTER 2

Table 2.26 Management of QT prolongation in patients receiving antipsychotic drugs

QTc	Action	Refer to cardiologist
<440 msec (men) or <470 msec (women)	None unless abnormal T-wave morphology	Consider if in doubt
>440 msec (men) or >470 msec (women) but <500 msec	Consider reducing dose or switching to drug of lower effect; repeat ECG	Consider
>500 msec	Repeat ECG. Stop suspected causative drug(s) and switch to drug of lower effect	Immediately
Abnormal T-wave morphology	Review treatment. Consider reducing dose or switching to drug of lower effect	Immediately

Other cardiovascular risk factors

The risk of drug-induced arrhythmia and sudden cardiac death with psychotropics is an important consideration. With respect to cardiovascular disease, note that other risk factors such as smoking, obesity and impaired glucose tolerance, present a much greater risk to patient morbidity and mortality than the uncertain outcome of QT changes. See relevant sections for discussion of these problems.

Summary

- In the absence of conclusive data, assume all antipsychotics are linked to sudden cardiac death.
- Prescribe the lowest dose possible and avoid polypharmacy/metabolic interactions.
- Perform ECG on admission, and, if previous abnormality or additional risk factor, at yearly check-up.
- Consider measuring QTc within a week of achieving a therapeutic dose of a moderate/high risk antipsychotic.

References

1. Reilly JG et al. Thioridazine and sudden unexplained death in psychiatric in-patients. Br J Psychiatry 2002; 180:515–522.
2. Murray-Thomas T et al. Risk of mortality (including sudden cardiac death) and major cardiovascular events in atypical and typical antipsychotic users: a study with the general practice research database. Cardiovasc Psychiatry Neurol 2013; 2013:247486.
3. Ray WA et al. Antipsychotics and the risk of sudden cardiac death. Arch Gen Psychiatry 2001; 58:1161–1167.
4. Hennessy S et al. Cardiac arrest and ventricular arrhythmia in patients taking antipsychotic drugs: cohort study using administrative data. BMJ 2002; 325:1070.
5. Straus SM et al. Antipsychotics and the risk of sudden cardiac death. Arch Intern Med 2004; 164:1293–1297.
6. Liperoti R et al. Conventional and atypical antipsychotics and the risk of hospitalization for ventricular arrhythmias or cardiac arrest. Arch Intern Med 2005; 165:696–701.
7. Ray WA et al. Atypical antipsychotic drugs and the risk of sudden cardiac death. N Engl J Med 2009; 360:225–235.
8. Schneeweiss S et al. Antipsychotic agents and sudden cardiac death--how should we manage the risk? N Engl J Med 2009; 360:294–296.
9. Nakagawa S et al. Antipsychotics and risk of first-time hospitalization for myocardial infarction: a population-based case-control study. J Intern Med 2006; 260:451–458.
10. Fujii K et al. QT is longer in drug-free patients with schizophrenia compared with age-matched healthy subjects. PLoS One 2014; 9:e98555.
11. Goldenberg I et al. QT interval: how to measure it and what is "normal". J Cardiovasc Electrophysiol 2006; 17:333–336.

12. Nielsen J et al. Assessing QT interval prolongation and its associated risks with antipsychotics. CNS Drugs 2011; **25**:473–490.

13. National Institute for Health and Care Excellence. Psychosis and schizophrenia in adults: treatment and management. Clinical Guideline 178, 2014. http://www.nice.org.uk/Guidance/CG178

14. Malik M et al. Evaluation of drug-induced QT interval prolongation: implications for drug approval and labelling. Drug Saf 2001; **24**:323–351.

15. Haddad PM et al. Antipsychotic-related QTc prolongation, torsade de pointes and sudden death. Drugs 2002; **62**:1649–1671.

16. Taylor DM. Antipsychotics and QT prolongation. Acta Psychiatr Scand 2003; **107**:85–95.

17. Botstein P. Is QT interval prolongation harmful? A regulatory perspective. Am J Cardiol 1993; **72**:50B–52B.

18. Joy JP et al. Prediction of torsade de pointes from the QT Interval: analysis of a case series of amisulpride overdoses. Clin Pharmacol Ther 2011; **90**:243–245.

19. Witchel HJ et al. Psychotropic drugs, cardiac arrhythmia, and sudden death. J Clin Psychopharmacol 2003; **23**:58–77.

20. Strom BL et al. Comparative mortality associated with ziprasidone and olanzapine in real-world use among 18,154 patients with schizophrenia: the Ziprasidone Observational Study of Cardiac Outcomes (ZODIAC). Am J Psychiatry 2011; **168**:193–201.

21. Chung AK et al. Effects on prolongation of Bazett's corrected QT interval of seven second-generation antipsychotics in the treatment of schizophrenia: a meta-analysis. J Psychopharmacol 2011; **25**:646–666.

22. Glassman AH et al. Antipsychotic drugs: prolonged QTc interval, torsade de pointes, and sudden death. Am J Psychiatry 2001; **158**:1774–1782.

23. Warner B et al. Investigation of the potential of clozapine to cause torsade de pointes. Adverse Drug React Toxicol Rev 2002; **21**:189–203.

24. Harrigan EP et al. A randomized evaluation of the effects of six antipsychotic agents on QTc, in the absence and presence of metabolic inhibition. J Clin Psychopharmacol 2004; **24**:62–69.

25. Lindborg SR et al. Effects of intramuscular olanzapine vs. haloperidol and placebo on QTc intervals in acutely agitated patients. Psychiatry Res 2003; **119**:113–123.

26. Dineen S et al. QTc prolongation and high-dose olanzapine (Letter). Psychosomatics 2003; **44**:174–175.

27. Gupta S et al. Quetiapine and QTc issues: a case report (Letter). J Clin Psychiatry 2003; **64**:612–613.

28. Su KP et al. A pilot cross-over design study on QTc interval prolongation associated with sulpiride and haloperidol. Schizophr Res 2003; **59**:93–94.

29. Chong SA et al. Prolonged QTc intervals in medicated patients with schizophrenia. Hum Psychopharmacol 2003; **18**:647–649.

30. Stollberger C et al. Antipsychotic drugs and QT prolongation. Int Clin Psychopharmacol 2005; **20**:243–251.

31. Isbister GK et al. Amisulpride deliberate self-poisoning causing severe cardiac toxicity including QT prolongation and torsades de pointes. Med J Aust 2006; **184**:354–356.

32. Ward DI. Two cases of amisulpride overdose: a cause for prolonged QT syndrome. Emerg Med Australas 2005; **17**:274–276.

33. Vieweg WV et al. Torsade de pointes in a patient with complex medical and psychiatric conditions receiving low-dose quetiapine. Acta Psychiatr Scand 2005; **112**:318–322.

34. Huang BH et al. Sulpiride induced torsade de pointes. Int J Cardiol 2007; **118**:e100–e102.

35. Kane JM et al. Long-term efficacy and safety of iloperidone: results from 3 clinical trials for the treatment of schizophrenia. J Clin Psychopharmacol 2008; **28**:S29–S35.

36. Kim MD et al. Blockade of HERG human K+channel and IKr of guinea pig cardiomyocytes by prochlorperazine. Eur J Pharmacol 2006; **544**:82–90.

37. Meltzer H et al. Efficacy and tolerability of oral paliperidone extended-release tablets in the treatment of acute schizophrenia: pooled data from three 6-week placebo-controlled studies. J Clin Psychiatry 2006; **69**:817–829.

38. Chapel S et al. Exposure-response analysis in patients with schizophrenia to assess the effect of asenapine on QTc prolongation. J Clin Pharmacol 2009; **49**:1297–1308.

39. Ozeki Y et al. QTc prolongation and antipsychotic medications in a sample of 1017 patients with schizophrenia. Prog Neuropsychopharmacol Biol Psychiatry 2010; **34**:401–405.

40. Girardin FR et al. Drug-induced long QT in adult psychiatric inpatients: the 5-year cross-sectional ECG Screening Outcome in Psychiatry study. Am J Psychiatry 2013; **170**:1468–1476.

41. Leucht S et al. Comparative efficacy and tolerability of 15 antipsychotic drugs in schizophrenia: a multiple-treatments meta-analysis. Lancet 2013; **382**:951–962.

42. Grande I et al. QTc prolongation: is clozapine safe? Study of 82 cases before and after clozapine treatment. Hum Psychopharmacol 2011.

43. Hong HK et al. Block of hERG K+channel and prolongation of action potential duration by fluphenazine at submicromolar concentration. Eur J Pharmacol 2013; **702**:165–173.

44. Vieweg WV et al. Risperidone, QTc interval prolongation, and torsade de pointes: a systematic review of case reports. Psychopharmacology (Berl) 2013; **228**:515–524.

45. Suzuki Y et al. QT prolongation of the antipsychotic risperidone is predominantly related to its 9-hydroxy metabolite paliperidone. Hum Psychopharmacol 2012; **27**:39–42.

46. Nelson S et al. Torsades de pointes after administration of low-dose aripiprazole. Ann Pharmacother 2013; **47**:e11.

47. Su KP et al. Olanzapine-induced QTc prolongation in a patient with Wolff-Parkinson-White syndrome. Schizophr Res 2004; **66**:191–192.

48. Morissette P et al. Olanzapine prolongs cardiac repolarization by blocking the rapid component of the delayed rectifier potassium current. J Psychopharmacol 2007; **21**:735–741.

49. Bar KJ et al. Influence of olanzapine on QT variability and complexity measures of heart rate in patients with schizophrenia. J Clin Psychopharmacol 2008; **28**:694–698.

50. Hasnain M et al. Quetiapine, QTc interval prolongation, and torsade de pointes: a review of case reports. Ther Adv Psychopharmacol 2014; 4:130–138.

51. Hatta K et al. Prolonged QT interval in acute psychotic patients. Psychiatry Res 2000; 94:279–285.

52. Priori SG et al. Low penetrance in the long-QT syndrome: clinical impact. Circulation 1999; 99:529–533.

53. Frassati D et al. Hidden cardiac lesions and psychotropic drugs as a possible cause of sudden death in psychiatric patients: a report of 14 cases and review of the literature. Can J Psychiatry 2004; 49:100–105.

Further reading

Leonard CE et al. Antipsychotics and the risks of sudden cardiac death and all-cause death: cohort studies in Medicaid and dually-eligible Medicaid-Medicare beneficiaries of five states. J Clin Exp Cardiolog 2013; **Suppl** 10:1–9.

Poluzzi E et al. Antipsychotics and torsadogenic risk: signals emerging from the US FDA Adverse Event Reporting System database. Drug Saf 2013; 36:467–479.

Dyslipidaemia

Morbidity and mortality from cardiovascular disease are higher in people with schizophrenia than in the general population.[1] Dyslipidaemia is an established risk factor for cardiovascular disease along with obesity, hypertension, smoking, diabetes and sedentary lifestyle. The majority of patients with schizophrenia have several of these risk factors and can be considered at 'high risk' of developing cardiovascular disease. Dyslipidaemia is treatable and intervention is known to reduce morbidity and mortality.[2] Aggressive treatment is particularly important in people with diabetes, the prevalence of which is increased two- to three-fold over population norms in people with schizophrenia (see section on 'Diabetes and impaired glucose tolerance' in this chapter).

Effect of antipsychotic drugs on lipids

First-generation antipsychotics

Phenothiazines are known to be associated with increases in triglycerides and low-density lipoprotein (LDL) cholesterol and decreases in high-density lipoprotein (HDL)[3] cholesterol, but the magnitude of these effects is poorly quantified.[4] Haloperidol seems to have minimal effect on lipid profiles.[3]

Second-generation antipsychotics

Although there are relatively more data pertaining to some atypicals, they are derived from a variety of sources and are reported in different ways, making it difficult to compare drugs directly. While cholesterol levels can rise, the most profound effect of these drugs seems to be on triglycerides. Raised triglycerides are in general, associated with obesity and diabetes. From the available data, olanzapine[5] would seem to have the greatest propensity to increase lipids, and quetiapine and risperidone moderate propensity.[6,7] Aripiprazole, lurasidone and ziprasidone have minimal adverse effect on blood lipids[5,8-12] and may even modestly reverse dyslipidaemias associated with previous antipsychotics.[12-14] Iloperidone causes some weight gain but may not adversely affect cholesterol or triglycerides.[15]

Olanzapine has been shown to increase triglyceride levels by 40% over the short (12 weeks) and medium (16 months) term.[16,17] Levels may continue to rise for up to a year.[18] Up to two-thirds of olanzapine-treated patients have raised triglycerides[19] and just under 10% may develop severe hypertriglyceridaemia.[20] While weight gain with olanzapine is generally associated with both increases in cholesterol[17,21] and triglycerides,[20] severe hypertriglyceridaemia can occur independently of weight gain.[20] In one study, patients treated with olanzapine and risperidone gained a similar amount of weight, but in olanzapine patients serum triglyceride levels increased by four times as much (80 mg/dL) as in risperidone patients (20 mg/dL).[20] Quetiapine[22] seems to have more modest effects than olanzapine, although data are conflicting.[23]

A case-control study conducted in the UK found that patients with schizophrenia who were treated with olanzapine were five times more likely to develop hyperlipidaemia than controls and three times more likely to develop hyperlipidaemia than patients receiving typical antipsychotics.[24] Risperidone-treated patients could not be distinguished from controls.

Clozapine

Mean triglyceride levels have been shown to double and cholesterol levels to increase by at least 10% after 5 years' treatment with clozapine.[25] Patients treated with clozapine have triglyceride levels that are almost double those of patients who are treated with FGA drugs.[26,27] Cholesterol levels are also increased.[5]

Particular care should be taken before prescribing clozapine or olanzapine for patients who are obese, diabetic or known to have pre-existing hyperlipidaemia.[28]

Screening

All patients should have their lipids measured at baseline, 3 months after starting treatment with a new antipsychotic, and then annually. Those prescribed clozapine and olanzapine should ideally have their serum lipids measured every 3 months for the first year of treatment, and then annually. Clinically significant changes in cholesterol are unlikely over the short term but triglycerides can increase dramatically.[29] In practice, dyslipidaemia is widespread in patients taking long-term antipsychotics irrespective of drug prescribed or of diagnosis.[30–32] Screening for this potentially serious side-effect of antipsychotics is not yet routine in clinical practice,[33] but is strongly recommended by NICE.[34]

Severe hypertriglyceridemia (fasting level of >5 mmol/L) is a risk factor for pancreatitis. Note that antipsychotic-induced dyslipidaemia can occur independent of weight gain.[35]

Treatment of dyslipidaemia

If moderate to severe hyperlipidaemia develops during antipsychotic treatment, a switch to another antipsychotic less likely to cause this problem should be considered in the first instance. Although not recommended as a strategy in patients with treatment-resistant illness, clozapine-induced hypertriglyceridaemia has been shown to reverse after a switch to risperidone.[36] This may hold true with other switching regimens but data are scarce.[37] Aripiprazole (or ziprasidone outside the UK) seems at present to be the treatment of choice in those with prior antipsychotic-induced dyslipidaemia.[14,38]

Patients with raised cholesterol may benefit from dietary advice, lifestyle changes and/or treatment with statins.[39] Statins seem to be effective in this patient group but interactions are possible.[40] Risk tables and treatment guidelines can be found in the *British National Formulary (BNF)*. Evidence supports the treatment of cholesterol concentrations as low as 4 mmol/L in high-risk patients[41] and this is the highest level recommended by NICE for secondary prevention of cardiovascular events.[42] NICE makes no recommendations on target levels for primary prevention but recent advice promotes the use of statins for anyone with a >10% ten year risk of cardiovascular disease.[42] Coronary heart disease and stroke risk can be reduced by one-third by

Table 2.27 Monitoring lipid concentrations in patients on antipsychotic drugs

Drug	Suggested monitoring
Clozapine Olanzapine	Fasting lipids at baseline then every 3 months for a year, then annually
Other antipsychotics	Fasting lipids at baseline and at 3 months, and then annually

reducing cholesterol to as low as 3.5 mmol/L.[2] When triglycerides alone are raised, diets low in saturated fats, and the taking of fish oil and fibrates are effective treatments[18,43] although there is no proof that mortality is reduced. Such patients should be screened for impaired glucose tolerance and diabetes.

The recommended procedure for monitoring lipid levels in patients on antipsychotics is summarised in Table 2.27.

References

1. Brown S et al. Causes of the excess mortality of schizophrenia. Br J Psychiatry 2000; 177:212–217.
2. Durrington P. Dyslipidaemia. Lancet 2003; 362:717–731.
3. Sasaki J et al. Lipids and apolipoproteins in patients treated with major tranquilizers. Clin Pharmacol Ther 1985; 37:684–687.
4. Henkin Y et al. Secondary dyslipidemia. Inadvertent effects of drugs in clinical practice. JAMA 1992; 267:961–968.
5. Chaggar PS et al. Effect of antipsychotic medications on glucose and lipid levels. J Clin Pharmacol 2011; 51:631–638.
6. Smith RC et al. Effects of olanzapine and risperidone on lipid metabolism in chronic schizophrenic patients with long-term antipsychotic treatment: a randomized five month study. Schizophr Res 2010; 120:204–209.
7. Perez-Iglesias R et al. Glucose and lipid disturbances after 1 year of antipsychotic treatment in a drug-naive population. Schizophr Res 2009; 107:115–121.
8. Olfson M et al. Hyperlipidemia following treatment with antipsychotic medications. Am J Psychiatry 2006; 163:1821–1825.
9. L'Italien GJ et al. Comparison of metabolic syndrome incidence among schizophrenia patients treated with aripiprazole versus olanzapine or placebo. J Clin Psychiatry 2007; 68:1510–1516.
10. Fenton WS et al. Medication-induced weight gain and dyslipidemia in patients with schizophrenia. Am J Psychiatry 2006; 163:1697–1704.
11. Meyer JM et al. Change in metabolic syndrome parameters with antipsychotic treatment in the CATIE Schizophrenia Trial: prospective data from phase 1. Schizophr Res 2008; 101:273–286.
12. Potkin SG et al. Double-blind comparison of the safety and efficacy of lurasidone and ziprasidone in clinically stable outpatients with schizophrenia or schizoaffective disorder. Schizophr Res 2011; 132:101–117.
13. Fleischhacker WW et al. Effects of adjunctive treatment with aripiprazole on body weight and clinical efficacy in schizophrenia patients treated with clozapine: a randomized, double-blind, placebo-controlled trial. Int J Neuropsychopharmacol 2010; 13:1115–1125.
14. Chen Y et al. Comparative effectiveness of switching antipsychotic drug treatment to aripiprazole or ziprasidone for improving metabolic profile and atherogenic dyslipidemia: a 12-month, prospective, open-label study. J Psychopharmacol 2012; 26:1201–1210.
15. Citrome L. Iloperidone: chemistry, pharmacodynamics, pharmacokinetics and metabolism, clinical efficacy, safety and tolerability, regulatory affairs, and an opinion. Expert Opin Drug Metab Toxicol 2010; 6:1551–1564.
16. Sheitman BB et al. Olanzapine-induced elevation of plasma triglyceride levels. Am J Psychiatry 1999; 156:1471–1472.
17. Osser DN et al. Olanzapine increases weight and serum triglyceride levels. J Clin Psychiatry 1999; 60:767–770.
18. Meyer JM. Effects of atypical antipsychotics on weight and serum lipid levels. J Clin Psychiatry 2001; 62 Suppl 27:27–34.
19. Melkersson KI et al. Elevated levels of insulin, leptin, and blood lipids in olanzapine-treated patients with schizophrenia or related psychoses. J Clin Psychiatry 2000; 61:742–749.
20. Meyer JM. Novel antipsychotics and severe hyperlipidemia. J Clin Psychopharmacol 2001; 21:369–374.
21. Kinon BJ et al. Long-term olanzapine treatment: weight change and weight-related health factors in schizophrenia. J Clin Psychiatry 2001; 62:92–100.
22. Atmaca M et al. Serum leptin and triglyceride levels in patients on treatment with atypical antipsychotics. J Clin Psychiatry 2003; 64:598–604.
23. de Leon J et al. A clinical study of the association of antipsychotics with hyperlipidemia. Schizophr Res 2007; 92:95–102.
24. Koro CE et al. An assessment of the independent effects of olanzapine and risperidone exposure on the risk of hyperlipidemia in schizophrenic patients. Arch Gen Psychiatry 2002; 59:1021–1026.
25. Henderson DC et al. Clozapine, diabetes mellitus, weight gain, and lipid abnormalities: A five-year naturalistic study. Am J Psychiatry 2000; 157:975–981.

26. Ghaeli P et al. Serum triglyceride levels in patients treated with clozapine. Am J Health Syst Pharm 1996; 53:2079–2081.

27. Spivak B et al. Diminished suicidal and aggressive behavior, high plasma norepinephrine levels, and serum triglyceride levels in chronic neuroleptic-resistant schizophrenic patients maintained on clozapine. Clin Neuropharmacol 1998; 21:245–250.

28. Baptista T et al. Novel antipsychotics and severe hyperlipidemia: comments on the Meyer paper. J Clin Psychopharmacol 2002; 22:536–537.

29. Meyer JM et al. The effects of antipsychotic therapy on serum lipids: a comprehensive review. Schizophr Res 2004; 70:1–17.

30. Paton C et al. Obesity, dyslipidaemias and smoking in an inpatient population treated with antipsychotic drugs. Acta Psychiatr Scand 2004; 110:299–305.

31. De Hert M et al. The METEOR study of diabetes and other metabolic disorders in patients with schizophrenia treated with antipsychotic drugs. I. Methodology. Int J Methods Psychiatr Res 2010; 19:195–210.

32. Jin H et al. Comparison of longer-term safety and effectiveness of 4 atypical antipsychotics in patients over age 40: a trial using equipoise-stratified randomization. J Clin Psychiatry 2013; 74:10–18.

33. Barnes TR et al. Screening for the metabolic syndrome in community psychiatric patients prescribed antipsychotics: a quality improvement programme. Acta Psychiatr Scand 2008; 118:26–33.

34. National Institute for Health and Care Excellence. Psychosis and schizophrenia in adults: treatment and management. Clinical Guideline 178, 2014. http://www.nice.org.uk/Guidance/CG178

35. Birkenaes AB et al. Dyslipidemia independent of body mass in antipsychotic-treated patients under real-life conditions. J Clin Psychopharmacol 2008; 28:132–137.

36. Ghaeli P et al. Elevated serum triglycerides in clozapine resolve with risperidone. Pharmacotherapy 1995; 15:382–385.

37. Weiden PJ. Switching antipsychotics as a treatment strategy for antipsychotic-induced weight gain and dyslipidemia. J Clin Psychiatry 2007; 68 Suppl 4:34–39.

38. Newcomer JW et al. A multicenter, randomized, double-blind study of the effects of aripiprazole in overweight subjects with schizophrenia or schizoaffective disorder switched from olanzapine. J Clin Psychiatry 2008; 69:1046–1056.

39. Ojala K et al. Statins are effective in treating dyslipidemia among psychiatric patients using second-generation antipsychotic agents. J Psychopharmacol 2008; 22:33–38.

40. Tse L et al. Pharmacological treatment of antipsychotic-induced dyslipidemia and hypertension. Int Clin Psychopharmacol 2014; 29:125–137.

41. Heart Protection Study Collaborative Group. MRC/BHF Heart Protection Study of cholesterol lowering with simvastatin in 20,536 high-risk individuals: a randomised placebo-controlled trial. Lancet 2002; 360:7–22.

42. National Institute for Health and Care Excellence. Lipid modification: cardiovascular risk assessment and the modification of blood lipids for the primary and secondary prevention of cardiovascular disease. Clinical Guideline 181, 2014. http://www.nice.org.uk/Guidance/CG181

43. Caniato RN et al. Effect of omega-3 fatty acids on the lipid profile of patients taking clozapine. Aust N Z J Psychiatry 2006; 40:691–697.

Diabetes and impaired glucose tolerance

Schizophrenia

Schizophrenia is associated with relatively high rates of insulin resistance and diabetes[1,2] – an observation that predates the discovery and widespread use of antipsychotics.[3-5] Lifestyle interventions (lower weight, more activity) are effective in preventing diabetes[6] and should be considered for all people with a diagnosis of schizophrenia.

Antipsychotics

Data relating to diabetes and antipsychotic use are numerous but less than perfect.[7-10] The main problem is that incidence and prevalence studies assume full or uniform screening for diabetes. Neither assumption is likely to be correct.[7] Many studies do not account for other factors affecting risk of diabetes.[10] Small differences between drugs are therefore difficult to substantiate but may in any case be ultimately unimportant: risk is probably increased for all those with schizophrenia receiving any antipsychotic.

The mechanisms involved in the development of antipsychotic-related diabetes are unclear, but may include $5HT_{2A}/5HT_{2C}$ antagonism, increased plasma lipids, weight gain and leptin resistance.[11] Insulin resistance may occur in the absence of weight gain.[12]

First-generation antipsychotics

Phenothiazine derivatives have long been associated with impaired glucose tolerance and diabetes.[13] Diabetes prevalence rates were reported to have substantially increased following the introduction and widespread use of FGA drugs.[14] The prevalence of impaired glucose tolerance seems to be higher with aliphatic phenothiazines than with fluphenazine or haloperidol.[15] Hyperglycaemia has also been reported with other conventional drugs, such as loxapine,[16] and other data confirm an association with haloperidol.[17] Some studies even suggest that FGAs are no different from SGAs in their propensity to cause diabetes,[18,19] whereas others suggest a modest but statistically significant excess incidence of diabetes with SGAs.[20]

Second-generation antipsychotics

Clozapine

Clozapine is strongly linked to hyperglycaemia, impaired glucose tolerance and diabetic ketoacidosis.[21] The risk of diabetes appears to be higher with clozapine than with other SGAs and conventional drugs, especially in younger patients,[22-25] although this is not a consistent finding.[26,27]

As many as one-third of patients might develop diabetes after 5 years of treatment.[28] Many cases of diabetes are noted in the first 6 months of treatment and some occur within 1 month,[29] some only after many years.[27] Death from ketoacidosis has also been reported.[29] Diabetes associated with clozapine is not necessarily linked to obesity or to family history of diabetes,[21,30] although these factors greatly increase the risk of developing diabetes on clozapine.[31]

CHAPTER 2

Clozapine appears to increase plasma levels of insulin in a clozapine level-dependent fashion.[32,33] It has been shown to be more likely than FGAs to increase plasma glucose and insulin following oral glucose challenge.[34] Testing for diabetes is essential given the high prevalence of diabetes in people receiving clozapine.[35]

Olanzapine

As with clozapine, olanzapine has been strongly linked to impaired glucose tolerance, diabetes and diabetic ketoacidosis.[36] Olanzapine and clozapine appear to directly induce insulin resistance.[37,38] Risk of diabetes has also been reported to be higher with olanzapine than with FGA drugs,[39] again with a particular risk in younger patients.[23] The time course of development of diabetes has not been established but impaired glucose tolerance seems to occur even in the absence of obesity and family history of diabetes.[21,30] Olanzapine is probably more diabetogenic than risperidone.[40–44] Olanzapine is also associated with plasma levels of glucose and insulin higher than those seen with FGAs (after oral glucose load).[34,45]

Risperidone

Risperidone has been linked, mainly in case reports, to impaired glucose tolerance,[46] diabetes[47] and ketoacidosis.[48] The number of reports of such adverse effects is substantially smaller than with either clozapine or olanzapine.[49] At least one study has suggested that changes in fasting glucose are significantly less common with risperidone than with olanzapine[40] but other studies have detected no difference.[50]

Risperidone seems no more likely than FGA drugs to be associated with diabetes,[23,39,41] although there may be an increased risk in patients under 40 years of age.[23] Risperidone has, however, been observed adversely to affect fasting glucose and plasma glucose (following glucose challenge) compared with levels seen in healthy volunteers (but not compared with patients taking conventional drugs).[34]

Quetiapine

Like risperidone, quetiapine has been linked to cases of new-onset diabetes and ketoacidosis.[51,52] Again, the number of reports is much lower than with olanzapine or clozapine. Quetiapine appears to be more likely than FGA drugs to be associated with diabetes.[23,53] Two studies showed quetiapine to be equal to olanzapine in incidence of diabetes.[50,54] Risk with quetiapine may be dose-related, with daily doses of 400 mg or more being clearly linked to changes in HbA_{1C}.[55]

Other SGAs

Amisulpride appears not to elevate plasma glucose[56] and seems not to be associated with diabetes.[57] There is one reported case of ketoacidosis occurring in a patient given the closely related sulpiride.[58] Data for aripiprazole[59–62] and ziprasidone[63,64] suggest that neither drug alters glucose homeostasis. Aripiprazole may even reverse diabetes caused by other drugs[65] (although ketoacidosis has been reported with aripiprazole[66–68]). A large

CHAPTER 2

case-control study has confirmed that neither amisulpride nor aripiprazole increase the risk of diabetes.[69] These three drugs (amisulpride, aripiprazole and ziprasidone) are cautiously recommended for those with a history of or predisposition to diabetes mellitus or as an alternative to other antipsychotics known to be diabetogenic. Limited data suggest neither lurasidone[70] nor asenapine[71,72] has any effect on glucose homeostasis.

Predicting antipsychotic-related diabetes

Risk of diabetes is increased to a much greater extent in younger adults than in the elderly[73] (in which antipsychotics may show no increased risk[74]). First-episode patients seem particularly prone to the development of diabetes when given a variety of antipsychotics.[75-77] During treatment, rapid weight gain and a rise in plasma triglycerides seem to predict the development of diabetes.[78]

Monitoring

Diabetes is a growing problem in western society and has a strong association with obesity, (older) age, (lower) educational achievement and certain racial groups.[79,80] Diabetes markedly increases cardiovascular mortality, largely as a consequence of atherosclerosis.[81] Likewise, the use of antipsychotics also increases cardiovascular mortality.[82-84] Intervention to reduce plasma glucose levels and minimise other risk factors (obesity, hypercholesterolaemia) is therefore essential.[85]

There is no clear consensus on diabetes-monitoring practice for those receiving antipsychotics[86] and recommendations in formal guidelines vary considerably.[87] Given the previous known parlous state of testing for diabetes in the UK[7,88,89] and elsewhere[90,91] arguments over precisely which tests are done and when seem to miss the point. There is an overwhelming need to improve monitoring by any means and so any tests for diabetes are supported – urine glucose and random plasma glucose included (Table 2.28).

Ideally, though, all patients should have oral glucose tolerance tests (OGTT) performed as this is the most sensitive method of detection.[92] Fasting plasma glucose (FPG) tests are less sensitive but recommended.[93] Any abnormality in FPG should provoke an OGTT.

Table 2.28 Recommended monitoring for diabetes in patients receiving antipsychotic drugs

Time	Ideally	Minimum
Baseline	OGTT or FPG HbA$_{1C}$ if fasting not possible	Urine glucose RPG
Continuation	All drugs: OGTT or FPG + HbA$_{1C}$ every 12 months For clozapine and olanzapine or if other risk factors present: OGTT or FPG after one month, then every 4–6 months For on-going regular screening, HbA$_{1C}$ is a suitable test. Note that this test is not suitable for detecting short-term change	Urine glucose or RPG every 12 months, with symptom monitoring

FPG, fasting plasma glucose; OGTT, oral glucose tolerance tests; RPG, random plasma glucose.

Table 2.29 Antipsychotics – risk of diabetes and impaired glucose tolerance

Degree of risk	Antipsychotic drug
High risk	Clozapine, olanzapine
Moderate risk	Quetiapine, risperidone, phenothiazines
Low risk	High potency FGAs (e.g. haloperidol)
Minimal risk	Aripiprazole, amisulpride, asenapine, lurasidone, ziprasidone

FGA, first-generation antipsychotic.

Fasting tests are often difficult to obtain in acutely ill, disorganised patients so measurement of random plasma glucose or glycosylated haemoglobin (HbA_{1C}) may also be used (fasting not required). HbA_{1C} is now recognised as a useful tool in detecting and monitoring diabetes.[94] Frequency of monitoring should then be determined by physical factors (e.g. weight gain) and known risk factors (e.g. family history of diabetes, lipid abnormalities, smoking status). The absolute minimum is yearly testing for diabetes for all patients. In addition, all patients should be asked to look out for and report signs and symptoms of diabetes (fatigue, candida infection, thirst, polyuria).

Treatment of antipsychotic-related diabetes

Switching to a drug of low or minimal risk of diabetes is often effective in reversing changes in glucose tolerance. In this respect the most compelling evidence is for switching to aripiprazole[95,96] but also to ziprasidone.[96] Standard anti-diabetic treatments are otherwise recommended. Pioglitazone[97] may have particular benefit but note the hepatotoxic potential of this drug.

The overall risk of impaired glucose tolerance and diabetes for different antipsychotics is summarised in Table 2.29.

References

1. Schimmelbusch WH et al. The positive correlation between insulin resistance and duration of hospitalization in untreated schizophrenia. Br J Psychiatry 1971; **118**:429–436.
2. Waitzkin L. A survey for unknown diabetics in a mental hospital. I. Men under age fifty. Diabetes 1966; **15**:97–104.
3. Kasanin J. The blood sugar curve in mental disease. II. The schizophrenia (dementia praecox) groups. Arch Neurol Psychiatry 1926; **16**:414–419.
4. Braceland FJ et al. Delayed action of insulin in schizophrenia. Am J Psychiatry 1945; **102**:108–110.
5. Kohen D. Diabetes mellitus and schizophrenia: historical perspective. Br J Psychiatry Suppl 2004; **47**:S64–S66.
6. Knowler WC et al. 10-year follow-up of diabetes incidence and weight loss in the Diabetes Prevention Program Outcomes Study. Lancet 2009; **374**:1677–1686.
7. Taylor D et al. Testing for diabetes in hospitalised patients prescribed antipsychotic drugs. Br J Psychiatry 2004; **185**:152–156.
8. Haddad PM. Antipsychotics and diabetes: review of non-prospective data. Br J Psychiatry Suppl 2004; **47**:S80–S86.
9. Bushe C et al. Association between atypical antipsychotic agents and type 2 diabetes: review of prospective clinical data. Br J Psychiatry 2004; **184**:S87–S93.
10. Gianfrancesco F et al. The influence of study design on the results of pharmacoepidemiologic studies of diabetes risk with antipsychotic therapy. Ann Clin Psychiatry 2006; **18**:9–17.
11. Buchholz S et al. Atypical antipsychotic-induced diabetes mellitus: an update on epidemiology and postulated mechanisms. Intern Med J 2008; **38**:602–606.

12. Teff KL et al. Antipsychotic-induced insulin resistance and postprandial hormonal dysregulation independent of weight gain or psychiatric disease. Diabetes 2013; 62:3232–3240.

13. Arneson GA. Phenothiazine derivatives and glucose metabolism. J Neuropsychiatr 1964; 5:181.

14. Lindenmayer JP et al. Hyperglycemia associated with the use of atypical antipsychotics. J Clin Psychiatry 2001; 62 Suppl 23:30–38.

15. Keskiner A et al. Psychotropic drugs, diabetes and chronic mental patients. Psychosomatics 1973; 14:176–181.

16. Tollefson G et al. Nonketotic hyperglycemia associated with loxapine and amoxapine: case report. J Clin Psychiatry 1983; 44:347–348.

17. Lindenmayer JP et al. Changes in glucose and cholesterol levels in patients with schizophrenia treated with typical or atypical antipsychotics. Am J Psychiatry 2003; 160:290–296.

18. Carlson C et al. Diabetes mellitus and antipsychotic treatment in the United Kingdom. Eur Neuropsychopharmacol 2006; 16:366–375.

19. Ostbye T et al. Atypical antipsychotic drugs and diabetes mellitus in a large outpatient population: a retrospective cohort study. Pharmacoepidemiol Drug Saf 2005; 14:407–415.

20. Smith M et al. First- v. second-generation antipsychotics and risk for diabetes in schizophrenia: systematic review and meta-analysis. Br J Psychiatry 2008; 192:406–411.

21. Mir S et al. Atypical antipsychotics and hyperglycaemia. Int Clin Psychopharmacol 2001; 16:63–74.

22. Lund BC et al. Clozapine use in patients with schizophrenia and the risk of diabetes, hyperlipidemia, and hypertension: a claims-based approach. Arch Gen Psychiatry 2001; 58:1172–1176.

23. Sernyak MJ et al. Association of diabetes mellitus with use of atypical neuroleptics in the treatment of schizophrenia. Am J Psychiatry 2002; 159:561–566.

24. Gianfrancesco FD et al. Differential effects of risperidone, olanzapine, clozapine, and conventional antipsychotics on type 2 diabetes: findings from a large health plan database. J Clin Psychiatry 2002; 63:920–930.

25. Guo JJ et al. Risk of diabetes mellitus associated with atypical antipsychotic use among patients with bipolar disorder: A retrospective, population-based, case-control study. J Clin Psychiatry 2006; 67:1055–1061.

26. Wang PS et al. Clozapine use and risk of diabetes mellitus. J Clin Psychopharmacol 2002; 22:236–243.

27. Sumiyoshi T et al. A comparison of incidence of diabetes mellitus between atypical antipsychotic drugs: a survey for clozapine, risperidone, olanzapine, and quetiapine (Letter). J Clin Psychopharmacol 2004; 24:345–348.

28. Henderson DC et al. Clozapine, diabetes mellitus, weight gain, and lipid abnormalities: A five-year naturalistic study. Am J Psychiatry 2000; 157:975–981.

29. Koller E et al. Clozapine-associated diabetes. Am J Med 2001; 111:716–723.

30. Sumiyoshi T et al. The effect of hypertension and obesity on the development of diabetes mellitus in patients treated with atypical antipsychotic drugs (Letter). J Clin Psychopharmacol 2004; 24:452–454.

31. Zhang R et al. The prevalence and clinical-demographic correlates of diabetes mellitus in chronic schizophrenic patients receiving clozapine. Hum Psychopharmacol 2011; 26:392–396.

32. Melkersson KI et al. Different influences of classical antipsychotics and clozapine on glucose-insulin homeostasis in patients with schizophrenia or related psychoses. J Clin Psychiatry 1999; 60:783–791.

33. Melkersson K. Clozapine and olanzapine, but not conventional antipsychotics, increase insulin release in vitro. Eur Neuropsychopharmacol 2004; 14:115–119.

34. Newcomer JW et al. Abnormalities in glucose regulation during antipsychotic treatment of schizophrenia. Arch Gen Psychiatry 2002; 59:337–345.

35. Lamberti JS et al. Diabetes mellitus among outpatients receiving clozapine: prevalence and clinical-demographic correlates. J Clin Psychiatry 2005; 66:900–906.

36. Wirshing DA et al. Novel antipsychotics and new onset diabetes. Biol Psychiatry 1998; 44:778–783.

37. Engl J et al. Olanzapine impairs glycogen synthesis and insulin signaling in L6 skeletal muscle cells. Mol Psychiatry 2005; 10:1089–1096.

38. Vestri HS et al. Atypical antipsychotic drugs directly impair insulin action in adipocytes: effects on glucose transport, lipogenesis, and antilipolysis. Neuropsychopharmacology 2007; 32:765–772.

39. Koro CE et al. Assessment of independent effect of olanzapine and risperidone on risk of diabetes among patients with schizophrenia: population based nested case-control study. BMJ 2002; 325:243.

40. Meyer JM. A retrospective comparison of weight, lipid, and glucose changes between risperidone- and olanzapine-treated inpatients: metabolic outcomes after 1 year. J Clin Psychiatry 2002; 63:425–433.

41. Gianfrancesco F et al. Antipsychotic-induced type 2 diabetes: evidence from a large health plan database. J Clin Psychopharmacol 2003; 23:328–335.

42. Leslie DL et al. Incidence of newly diagnosed diabetes attributable to atypical antipsychotic medications. Am J Psychiatry 2004; 161:1709–1711.

43. Duncan E et al. Relative risk of glucose elevation during antipsychotic exposure in a Veterans Administration population. Int Clin Psychopharmacol 2007; 22:1–11.

44. Meyer JM et al. Change in metabolic syndrome parameters with antipsychotic treatment in the CATIE Schizophrenia Trial: prospective data from phase 1. Schizophr Res 2008; 101:273–286.

45. Ebenbichler CF et al. Olanzapine induces insulin resistance: results from a prospective study. J Clin Psychiatry 2003; 64:1436–1439.

46. Mallya A et al. Resolution of hyperglycemia on risperidone discontinuation: a case report. J Clin Psychiatry 2002; 63:453–454.

47. Wirshing DA et al. Risperidone-associated new-onset diabetes. Biol Psychiatry 2001; 50:148–149.

48. Croarkin PE et al. Diabetic ketoacidosis associated with risperidone treatment? Psychosomatics 2000; 41:369–370.

49. Koller EA et al. Risperidone-associated diabetes mellitus: a pharmacovigilance study. Pharmacotherapy 2003; 23:735–744.

50. Lambert BL et al. Diabetes risk associated with use of olanzapine, quetiapine, and risperidone in veterans health administration patients with schizophrenia. Am J Epidemiol 2006; 164:672–681.

51. Henderson DC. Atypical antipsychotic-induced diabetes mellitus: how strong is the evidence? CNS Drugs 2002; 16:77–89.

52. Koller EA et al. A survey of reports of quetiapine-associated hyperglycemia and diabetes mellitus. J Clin Psychiatry 2004; 65:857–863.

53. Citrome L et al. Relationship between antipsychotic medication treatment and new cases of diabetes among psychiatric inpatients. Psychiatr Serv 2004; 55:1006–1013.

54. Bushe C et al. Comparison of metabolic and prolactin variables from a six-month randomised trial of olanzapine and quetiapine in schizophrenia. J Psychopharmacol 2010; 24:1001–1009.

55. Guo Z et al. A real-world data analysis of dose effect of second-generation antipsychotic therapy on hemoglobin A1C level. Prog Neuropsychopharmacol Biol Psychiatry 2011; 35:1326–1332.

56. Vanelle JM et al. A double-blind randomised comparative trial of amisulpride versus olanzapine for 2 months in the treatment of subjects with schizophrenia and comorbid depression. Eur Psychiatry 2006; 21:523–530.

57. De Hert MA et al. Prevalence of the metabolic syndrome in patients with schizophrenia treated with antipsychotic medication. Schizophr Res 2006; 83:87–93.

58. Toprak O et al. New-onset type II diabetes mellitus, hyperosmolar non-ketotic coma, rhabdomyolysis and acute renal failure in a patient treated with sulpiride. Nephrol Dial Transplant 2005; 20:662–663.

59. Keck PE, Jr. et al. Aripiprazole: a partial dopamine D2 receptor agonist antipsychotic. Expert Opin Investig Drugs 2003; 12:655–662.

60. Pigott TA et al. Aripiprazole for the prevention of relapse in stabilized patients with chronic schizophrenia: a placebo-controlled 26-week study. J Clin Psychiatry 2003; 64:1048–1056.

61. van WR et al. Major changes in glucose metabolism, including new-onset diabetes, within 3 months after initiation of or switch to atypical antipsychotic medication in patients with schizophrenia and schizoaffective disorder. J Clin Psychiatry 2008; 69:472–479.

62. Baker RA et al. Atypical antipsychotic drugs and diabetes mellitus in the US Food and Drug Administration Adverse Event Database: A Systematic Bayesian Signal Detection Analysis. Psychopharmacol Bull 2009; 42:11–31.

63. Simpson GM et al. Randomized, controlled, double-blind multicenter comparison of the efficacy and tolerability of ziprasidone and olanzapine in acutely ill inpatients with schizophrenia or schizoaffective disorder. Am J Psychiatry 2004; 161:1837–1847.

64. Sacher J et al. Effects of olanzapine and ziprasidone on glucose tolerance in healthy volunteers. Neuropsychopharmacology 2008; 33:1633–1641.

65. De Hert M et al. A case series: evaluation of the metabolic safety of aripiprazole. Schizophr Bull 2007; 33:823–830.

66. Church CO et al. Diabetic ketoacidosis associated with aripiprazole. Diabet Med 2005; 22:1440–1443.

67. Reddymasu S et al. Elevated lipase and diabetic ketoacidosis associated with aripiprazole. JOP 2006; 7:303–305.

68. Campanella LM et al. Severe hyperglycemic hyperosmolar nonketotic coma in a nondiabetic patient receiving aripiprazole. Ann Emerg Med 2009; 53:264–266.

69. Kessing LV et al. Treatment with antipsychotics and the risk of diabetes in clinical practice. Br J Psychiatry 2010; 197:266–271.

70. McEvoy JP et al. Effectiveness of lurasidone in patients with schizophrenia or schizoaffective disorder switched from other antipsychotics: a randomized, 6-week, open-label study. J Clin Psychiatry 2013; 74:170–179.

71. McIntyre RS et al. Asenapine for long-term treatment of bipolar disorder: a double-blind 40-week extension study. J Affect Disord 2010; 126:358–365.

72. McIntyre RS et al. Asenapine versus olanzapine in acute mania: a double-blind extension study. Bipolar Disord 2009; 11:815–826.

73. Hammerman A et al. Antipsychotics and diabetes: an age-related association. Ann Pharmacother 2008; 42:1316–1322.

74. Albert SG et al. Atypical antipsychotics and the risk of diabetes in an elderly population in long-term care: a retrospective nursing home chart review study. J Am Med Dir Assoc 2009; 10:115–119.

75. De HM et al. Typical and atypical antipsychotics differentially affect long-term incidence rates of the metabolic syndrome in first-episode patients with schizophrenia: a retrospective chart review. Schizophr Res 2008; 101:295–303.

76. Saddichha S et al. Metabolic syndrome in first episode schizophrenia - a randomized double-blind controlled, short-term prospective study. Schizophr Res 2008; 101:266–272.

77. Saddichha S et al. Diabetes and schizophrenia - effect of disease or drug? Results from a randomized, double-blind, controlled prospective study in first-episode schizophrenia. Acta Psychiatr Scand 2008; 117:342–347.

78. Reaven GM et al. In search of moderators and mediators of hyperglycemia with atypical antipsychotic treatment. J Psychiatr Res 2009; 43:997–1002.

79. Mokdad AH et al. The continuing increase of diabetes in the US. Diabetes Care 2001; 24:412.

80. Mokdad AH et al. Diabetes trends in the US: 1990-1998. Diabetes Care 2000; 23:1278–1283.

81. Beckman JA et al. Diabetes and atherosclerosis: epidemiology, pathophysiology, and management. JAMA 2002; 287:2570–2581.

82. Henderson DC et al. Clozapine, diabetes mellitus, hyperlipidemia, and cardiovascular risks and mortality: results of a 10-year naturalistic study. J Clin Psychiatry 2005; 66:1116–1121.

83. Lamberti JS et al. Prevalence of the metabolic syndrome among patients receiving clozapine. Am J Psychiatry 2006; 163:1273–1276.

84. Goff DC et al. A comparison of ten-year cardiac risk estimates in schizophrenia patients from the CATIE study and matched controls. Schizophr Res 2005; 80:45–53.

85. Haupt DW et al. Hyperglycemia and antipsychotic medications. J Clin Psychiatry 2001; 62 Suppl 27:15–26.

86. Cohn TA et al. Metabolic monitoring for patients treated with antipsychotic medications. Can J Psychiatry 2006; 51:492–501.

87. De HM et al. Guidelines for screening and monitoring of cardiometabolic risk in schizophrenia: systematic evaluation. Br J Psychiatry 2011; 199:99–105.

88. Barnes TR et al. A UK audit of screening for the metabolic side effects of antipsychotics in community patients. Schizophr Bull 2007; **33**:1397–1403.

89. Barnes TR et al. Screening for the metabolic syndrome in community psychiatric patients prescribed antipsychotics: a quality improvement programme. Acta Psychiatr Scand 2008; **118**:26–33.

90. Barnes TR et al. Screening for the metabolic syndrome in community psychiatric patients prescribed antipsychotics: a quality improvement programme. Acta Psychiatr Scand 2008; **118**:26–33.

91. Morrato EH et al. Metabolic screening after the ADA's Consensus Statement on Antipsychotic Drugs and Diabetes. Diabetes Care 2009; **32**:1037–1042.

92. De Hert M et al. Oral glucose tolerance tests in treated patients with schizophrenia. Data to support an adaptation of the proposed guidelines for monitoring of patients on second generation antipsychotics? Eur Psychiatry 2006; **21**:224–226.

93. Marder SR et al. Physical health monitoring of patients with schizophrenia. Am J Psychiatry 2004; **161**:1334–1349.

94. National Institute for Health and Clinical Excellence. Type 2 diabetes - newer agents (a partial update of CG66). Clinical Guideline 87, 2009. http://guidance.nice.org.uk/CG87

95. Stroup TS et al. Effects of switching from olanzapine, quetiapine, and risperidone to aripiprazole on 10-year coronary heart disease risk and metabolic syndrome status: results from a randomized controlled trial. Schizophr Res 2013; **146**:190–195.

96. Chen Y et al. Comparative effectiveness of switching antipsychotic drug treatment to aripiprazole or ziprasidone for improving metabolic profile and atherogenic dyslipidemia: a 12-month, prospective, open-label study. J Psychopharmacol 2012; **26**:1201–1210.

97. Smith RC et al. Effects of pioglitazone on metabolic abnormalities, psychopathology, and cognitive function in schizophrenic patients treated with antipsychotic medication: a randomized double-blind study. Schizophr Res 2013; **143**:18–24.

Hypertension

There are two ways in which antipsychotic drugs may be associated with the development or worsening of hypertension.

- **Slow steady rise in blood pressure over time.** This may be linked to weight gain. Being overweight increases the risk of developing hypertension. The magnitude of the effect has been modelled using the Framingham data; for every 30 people who gain 4 kg, one will develop hypertension over the next 10 years.[1] Note that this is a very modest weight gain, the majority of patients treated with some antipsychotics gain more than this, increasing further the risk of developing hypertension.
- **Unpredictable rapid sharp increase in blood pressure on starting a new drug or increasing the dose.** Increases in blood pressure occur shortly after starting, ranging from within hours of the first dose to a month. The information below relates to the pharmacological mechanism behind this and the antipsychotic drugs that are most implicated.

Postural hypotension is commonly associated with antipsychotic drugs that are antagonists at postsynaptic α_1-adrenergic receptors. Examples include clozapine, chlorpromazine, quetiapine and risperidone. Some antipsychotics are also antagonists at pre-synaptic α_2-adrenergic receptors; this can lead to increased release of norepinephrine, increased vagal activity and vasoconstriction. As all antipsychotics that are antagonists at α_2-receptors are also antagonists at α_1-receptors, the end result for any given patient can be difficult to predict, but for a very small number the result can be hypertension. Some antipsychotics are more commonly implicated than others, but individual patient factors are undoubtedly also important.

Receptor binding studies have demonstrated that clozapine, olanzapine and risperidone have the highest affinity for α_2-adrenergic receptors[2] so it might be predicted that these drugs would be most likely to cause hypertension. Most case reports implicate clozapine[3–9] with some clearly describing normal blood pressure before clozapine was introduced, a sharp rise during treatment and return to normal when clozapine was discontinued. Blood pressure has also been reported to rise again on re-challenge and increased plasma catecholamines have been noted in some cases. Case reports also implicate aripiprazole,[10–13] sulpiride,[14] risperidone,[8] quetiapine[8] and ziprasidone.[15]

Data available through the Medical and Healthcare Products Regulatory Agency (MHRA) yellow card system indicate that clozapine is the antipsychotic drug most associated with hypertension. There are a very small number of reports with aripiprazole, olanzapine, quetiapine and risperidone.[16] The timing of the onset of hypertension in these reports with respect to antipsychotic initiation is unknown, and likely to be variable.

In long-term treatment, hypertension is seen in around 30–40% of patients regardless of antipsychotic prescribed.[17] A recent cross-sectional study found an increased risk of hypertension only for perphenazine,[18] a finding not readily explained by its pharmacology.

No antipsychotic is contraindicated in essential hypertension but extreme care is needed when clozapine is prescribed. Concomitant treatment with SSRIs may increase risk of hypertension, possibly via inhibition of the metabolism of the antipsychotic.[8] It is also (theoretically) possible that α_2 antagonism may be at least partially responsible for clozapine-induced tachycardia and nausea.[19]

Treatment of antipsychotic-associated hypertension should follow standard protocols. There is specific evidence for the efficacy of valsartan and telmisartan in antipsychotic-related hypertension.[20]

References

1. Fontaine KR et al. Estimating the consequences of anti-psychotic induced weight gain on health and mortality rate. Psychiatry Res 2001; **101**:277–288.

2. Abi-Dargham A et al. Mechanisms of action of second generation antipsychotic drugs in schizophrenia: insights from brain imaging studies. Eur Psychiatry 2005; **20**:15–27.

3. Gupta S et al. Paradoxical hypertension associated with clozapine. Am J Psychiatry 1994; **151**:148.

4. Krentz AJ et al. Drug Points: Pseudophaeochromocytoma syndrome associated with clozapine. BMJ 2001; **322**:1213.

5. George TP et al. Hypertension after initiation of clozapine. Am J Psychiatry 1996; **153**:1368–1369.

6. Prasad SE et al. Pseudophaeochromocytoma associated with clozapine treatment. Ir J Psychol Med 2003; **20**:132–134.

7. Shiwach RS. Treatment of clozapine induced hypertension and possible mechanisms. Clin Neuropharmacol 1998; **21**:139–140.

8. Coulter D. Atypical antipsychotics may cause hypertension. Prescriber Update 2003; **24**:4.

9. Li JK et al. Clozapine: a mimicry of phaeochromocytoma. Aust N Z J Psychiatry 1997; **31**:889–891.

10. Borras L et al. Hypertension and aripiprazole. Am J Psychiatry 2005; **162**:2392.

11. Hsiao YL et al. Aripiprazole augmentation induced hypertension in major depressive disorder: a case report. Prog Neuropsychopharmacol Biol Psychiatry 2011; **35**:305–306.

12. Pitchot W et al. Aripiprazole, hypertension, and confusion. J Neuropsychiatry Clin Neurosci 2010; **22**:123.

13. Yasui-Furukori N et al. Worsened hypertension control induced by aripiprazole. Neuropsychiatr Dis Treat 2013; **9**:505–507.

14. Mayer RD et al. Acute hypertensive episode induced by sulpiride - a case report. Hum Psychopharmacol 1989; **4**:149–150.

15. Villanueva N et al. Probable association between ziprasidone and worsening hypertension. Pharmacotherapy 2006; **26**:1352–1357.

16. Medicines and Healthcare Products Regulatory Agency. Drug Analysis Prints (DAPs). http://www.mhra.gov.uk/, 2014.

17. Kelly AC et al. A naturalistic comparison of the long-term metabolic adverse effects of clozapine versus other antipsychotics for patients with psychotic illnesses. J Clin Psychopharmacol 2014; **34**:441–445.

18. Boden R et al. A comparison of cardiovascular risk factors for ten antipsychotic drugs in clinical practice. Neuropsychiatr Dis Treat 2013; **9**:371–377.

19. Pandharipande P et al. Alpha-2 agonists: can they modify the outcomes in the Postanesthesia Care Unit? Curr Drug Targets 2005; **6**:749–754.

20. Tse L et al. Pharmacological treatment of antipsychotic-induced dyslipidemia and hypertension. Int Clin Psychopharmacol 2014; **29**:125–137.

Hyponatraemia

Hyponatraemia can occur in the context of the following.

- **Water intoxication** where water consumption exceeds the maximal renal clearance capacity. Serum and urine osmolality are low. Cross-sectional studies of chronically ill, hospitalised, psychiatric patients have found the prevalence of water intoxication to be approximately 5%.[1,2] A longitudinal study found that 10% of severely ill patients with a diagnosis of schizophrenia had episodic hyponatraemia secondary to fluid overload.[3] The primary aetiology is poorly understood. It has been postulated that it may be driven, at least in part, by an extreme compensatory response to the anticholinergic side-effects of antipsychotic drugs.[4]

- Drug-induced **syndrome of inappropriate antidiuretic hormone (SIADH)** where the kidney retains an excessive quantity of solute-free water. Serum osmolality is low and urine osmolality relatively high. The prevalence of SIADH has been estimated to be as high as 11% in acutely ill psychiatric patients.[5] Risk factors for antidepressant-induced SIADH (increasing age, female gender, medical co-morbidity and polypharmacy) seem to be less relevant in the population of patients treated with antipsychotic drugs.[6] SIADH usually develops in the first few weeks of treatment with the offending drug. Case reports and case series implicate phenothiazines, haloperidol, pimozide, risperidone, quetiapine, olanzapine, aripiprazole and clozapine.[6-9] A systematic review[10] and a case-control study[11] each suggested a clear increase in risk of hyponatraemia with antipsychotics. Another review[12] confirmed that drug-induced hyponatraemia is associated with concentrated urine and suggested that an antipsychotic was five times more likely than water intoxication to be the cause of hyponatraemia. Overall prevalence of antipsychotic-induced hyponatraemia has been estimated at 0.004%[13] and 26.1%[14] of patients. It is assumed the true figure is somewhere between these two extremes. Desmopressin use (for clozapine-induced enuresis) can also result in hyponatraemia.[15]

- Severe **hyperlipidaemia** and/or **hyperglycaemia** lead to secondary increases in plasma volume and 'pseudohyponatraemia'.[4] Both are more common in people treated with antipsychotic drugs than in the general population and should be excluded as causes.

Mild to moderate hyponatraemia presents as confusion, nausea, headache and lethargy. As the plasma sodium falls, these symptoms become increasingly severe and seizures and coma can develop.

Monitoring of plasma sodium is deisrable for all those receiving antipsychotics. Signs of confusion or lethargy should provoke thorough diagnostic analysis, including plasma sodium determination and urine osmolality.

Standard treatments for antipsychotic-induced hyponatraemia are summarised in Table 2.30. Recently introduced drugs such as tolvaptan,[23] a so-called vaptan (non-peptide arginine-vasopression antagonist – also known as aquaretics because they induce a highly hypotonic diuresis[24]), show promise in the treatment of hyponatraemia of varying aetiology, including that caused by drug-related SIADH.

Table 2.30 Treatment of antipsychotic-induced hyponatraemia

Cause of hyponatraemia	Antipsychotic drugs implicated	Treatment[4,5]
Water intoxication (serum and urine osmolality low)	Only very speculative evidence to support drugs as a cause Core part of illness in a minority of patients (e.g. psychotic polydipsia)	▪ **Fluid restriction** with careful monitoring of serum sodium, particularly diurnal variation (Na drops as the day progresses). Refer to specialist medical care if Na < 125 mmol/L. Note that the use of IV saline to correct hyponatraemia has been reported to precipitate rhabdomyolysis[16] ▪ Consider treatment with **clozapine**: shown to increase plasma osmolality into the normal range and increase urine osmolality (not usually reaching the normal range).[17] These effects are consistent with reduced fluid intake. This effect is not clearly related to improvements in mental state[18] ▪ There are both[6] positive and negative reports for olanzapine[19] and risperidone[20] and one positive case report for quetiapine.[21] Compared with clozapine, the evidence base is weak ▪ There is no evidence that either reducing or increasing the dose of an antipsychotic results in improvements in serum sodium in water-intoxicated patients[22] ▪ **Demeclocycline should not be used** (exerts its effect by interfering with ADH and increasing water excretion, already at capacity in these patients)
SIADH (serum osmolality low; urine osmolality relatively high)	All antipsychotic drugs	▪ If mild, **fluid restriction** with careful monitoring of serum sodium. Refer to specialist medical care if Na < 125 mmol/L ▪ **Switching to a different antipsychotic drug**. There are insufficient data available to guide choice. Be aware that cross-sensitivity may occur (the individual may be predisposed and the choice of drug relatively less important) ▪ Consider **demeclocycline** (see formal prescribing instruction for details) ▪ Lithium may be effective[6] but is a potentially toxic drug. Remember that hyponatraemia predisposes to lithium toxicity

ADH, antidiuretic hormone; IV, intravenous; SIADH, syndrome of inappropriate antidiuretic hormone.

CHAPTER 2

References

1. de Leon J et al. Polydipsia and water intoxication in psychiatric patients: a review of the epidemiological literature. Biol Psychiatry 1994; 35:408–419.
2. Patel JK. Polydipsia, hyponatremia, and water intoxication among psychiatric patients. Hosp Community Psychiatry 1994; 45:1073–1074.
3. de Leon J. Polydipsia--a study in a long-term psychiatric unit. Eur Arch Psychiatry Clin Neurosci 2003; 253:37–39.
4. Siegel AJ et al. Primary and drug-induced disorders of water homeostasis in psychiatric patients: principles of diagnosis and management. Harv Rev Psychiatry 1998; 6:190–200.
5. Siegler EL et al. Risk factors for the development of hyponatremia in psychiatric inpatients. Arch Intern Med 1995; 155:953–957.
6. Madhusoodanan S et al. Hyponatraemia associated with psychotropic medications. A review of the literature and spontaneous reports. Adverse Drug React Toxicol Rev 2002; 21:17–29.
7. Bachu K et al. Aripiprazole-induced syndrome of inappropriate antidiuretic hormone secretion (SIADH). Am J Ther 2006; 13:370–372.
8. Dudeja SJ et al. Olanzapine induced hyponatraemia. Ulster Med J 2010; 79:104–105.
9. Yam FK et al. Syndrome of inappropriate antidiuretic hormone associated with aripiprazole. Am J Health Syst Pharm 2013; 70:2110–2114.
10. Meulendijks D et al. Antipsychotic-induced hyponatraemia: a systematic review of the published evidence. Drug Saf 2010; 33:101–114.
11. Mannesse CK et al. Hyponatraemia as an adverse drug reaction of antipsychotic drugs: a case-control study in VigiBase. Drug Saf 2010; 33:569–578.
12. Atsariyasing W et al. A systematic review of the ability of urine concentration to distinguish antipsychotic- from psychosis-induced hyponatremia. Psychiatry Res 2014; 217:129–133.
13. Letmaier M et al. Hyponatraemia during psychopharmacological treatment: results of a drug surveillance programme. Int J Neuropsychopharmacol 2012; 15:739–748.
14. Serrano A et al. Safety of long-term clozapine administration. Frequency of cardiomyopathy and hyponatraemia: two cross-sectional, naturalistic studies. Aust N Z J Psychiatry 2014; 48:183–192.
15. Sarma S et al. Severe hyponatraemia associated with desmopressin nasal spray to treat clozapine-induced nocturnal enuresis. Aust N Z J Psychiatry 2005; 39:949.
16. Zaidi AN. Rhabdomyolysis after correction of hyponatremia in psychogenic polydipsia possibly complicated by ziprasidone. Ann Pharmacother 2005; 39:1726–1731.
17. Canuso CM et al. Clozapine restores water balance in schizophrenic patients with polydipsia-hyponatremia syndrome. J Neuropsychiatry Clin Neurosci 1999; 11:86–90.
18. Spears NM et al. Clozapine treatment in polydipsia and intermittent hyponatremia. J Clin Psychiatry 1996; 57:123–128.
19. Littrell KH et al. Effects of olanzapine on polydipsia and intermittent hyponatremia. J Clin Psychiatry 1997; 58:549.
20. Kawai N et al. Risperidone failed to improve polydipsia-hyponatremia of the schizophrenic patients. Psychiatry Clin Neurosci 2002; 56:107–110.
21. Montgomery JH et al. Adjunctive quetiapine treatment of the polydipsia, intermittent hyponatremia, and psychosis syndrome: a case report. J Clin Psychiatry 2003; 64:339–341.
22. Canuso CM et al. Does minimizing neuroleptic dosage influence hyponatremia? Psychiatry Res 1996; 63:227–229.
23. Josiassen RC et al. Tolvaptan: a new tool for the effective treatment of hyponatremia in psychotic disorders. Expert Opin Pharmacother 2010; 11:637–648.
24. Decaux G et al. Non-peptide arginine-vasopressin antagonists: the vaptans. Lancet 2008; 371:1624–1632.

Hyperprolactinaemia

Dopamine inhibits prolactin release and so dopamine antagonists can be expected to increase prolactin plasma levels. All antipsychotics cause measurable changes in prolactin but some do not increase prolactin above the normal range at standard doses. These drugs are asenapine, clozapine, olanzapine, quetiapine, lurasidone, aripiprazole and ziprasidone.[1-6] Even with these drugs (particularly olanzapine and ziprasidone), raised prolactin and prolactin-related symptoms are occasionally reported.[7-10] Aripiprazole usually decreases plasma prolactin.[11] With all drugs, the degree of prolactin elevation is probably dose-related,[12] and for most the threshold activity (D_2 occupancy) for increased prolactin is very close to that of therapeutic efficacy.[13]

Hyperprolactinaemia is often superficially asymptomatic (that is, the patient does not spontaneously report problems) and there is some evidence that hyperprolactinaemia does not affect subjective quality of life.[14] Nonetheless, persistent elevation of plasma prolactin is associated with a number of adverse consequences. These include sexual dysfunction[15-18] (but note that other pharmacological activities also give rise to sexual dysfunction), reductions in bone mineral density,[19-22] menstrual disturbances,[2,23] breast growth and galactorrhoea,[23] suppression of the hypothalamic-pituitary-gonadal axis[24] and a possible increase in the risk of breast cancer.[2,25-27]

Monitoring

All patients should have a prolactin level measured before starting any antipsychotic known to be associated with raised prolactin. This gives a baseline measure against which any change can be gauged. At 3 months, all patients should be asked about prolactin-related symptoms (sexual dysfunction, amenorrhoea, etc.). If hyperprolactinaemia is suspected, another prolactin level should be obtained. Where prolactin is high and the patient is symptomatic, switching to an antipsychotic that is less likely to raise prolactin (see Box 2.1) should be considered. Where prolactin is high but the patient is not symptomatic, the clinical implications of the test results should be discussed with the patient and a joint decision taken on whether to continue current treatment with annual monitoring or switch to another antipsychotic.

Prolactin-elevating drugs (amisulpride, sulpiride, risperidone, paliperidone, FGAs) should, if possible, be avoided in the following patient groups:

- patients under 25 years of age (i.e. before peak bone mass)
- patients with osteoporosis
- patients with a history of hormone-dependent breast cancer.

> **Box 2.1** Established antipsychotics not usually associated with hyperprolactinaemia
>
> - Aripiprazole
> - Asenapine
> - Clozapine
> - Lurasidone
> - Olanzapine
> - Quetiapine
> - Ziprasidone

Long-term use of prolactin-elevating drugs should probably be avoided in young women, given the possible increased risk of breast cancer and the known risk of decreased bone mineral density.

Prolactin concentration interpretation[28]

- Take blood sample at least 1 hour after waking or eating.
- Minimise stress during venepuncture (stress elevates plasma prolactin).
- Treatment of hyperprolactinaemia depends more on symptoms and long-term risk than on measured plasma level.

Normal	Women	0–25 ng/mL	~0–530 mIU/L
	Men	0–20 ng/mL	~0–424 mIU/L

- Need systematic assessment of prolactin-related side-effects and discussion of clinical consequences of prolonged raised prolactin if prolactin concentration **25–118 ng/mL (530–2500 mIU/L)**
- Need referral for tests to rule out prolactinoma if prolactin concentration **>118 ng/mL (>2500 mIU/L)**

Symptoms (reduced libido, infertility) are usually seen with prolactin levels are above 31–50 ng/mL (~660–1060 mIU/L). When levels exceed 100 ng/mL (~2120 mIU/L) there is usually galactorrhoea and amenorrhoea.[29]

Treatment

For most patients with symptomatic hyperprolactinaemia, a switch to a non prolactin-elevating drug (see Box 2.1) is the first choice.[2,18,30,31] (Limited data[32–34] suggest asenapine and lurasidone have minimal effects on prolactin.) An alternative is to add aripiprazole to existing treatment[35–39] – hyperprolactinaemia and related symptoms are reported to improve fairly promptly following the addition of aripiprazole. The effect of co-administered aripiprazole on prolactin is dose-dependent: 3 mg/day is effective but 6 mg/day more so. Higher doses appear unnecessary.[40] When switching, symptoms tend to resolve slowly and symptom severity does not always reflect prolactin changes.[30] Genetic differences may play a part.[41] Where aripiprazole augmentation has been successful, consideration should be given to slowly reducing the dose of the antipsychotic responsible for raising prolactin, with the aim of maintaining the patient on aripiprazole as the sole antipsychotic. Only if this strategy fails should long-term combined antipsychotics be considered.

For patients who need to remain on a prolactin-elevating antipsychotic and who cannot tolerate aripiprazole, dopamine agonists may be effective.[3,42,43] Amantadine, carbergoline and bromocriptine have all been used, but each has the potential to worsen psychosis (although this has not been reported in trials). A herbal remedy – Peony Glycyrrhiza Decoction – has also been shown to be effective.[44]

References

1. David SR et al. The effects of olanzapine, risperidone, and haloperidol on plasma prolactin levels in patients with schizophrenia. Clin Ther 2000; 22:1085–1096.
2. Haddad PM et al. Antipsychotic-induced hyperprolactinaemia: mechanisms, clinical features and management. Drugs 2004; 64:2291–2314.
3. Hamner MB et al. Hyperprolactinaemia in antipsychotic-treated patients: guidelines for avoidance and management. CNS Drugs 1998; 10:209–222.
4. Bushe C et al. Comparison of metabolic and prolactin variables from a six-month randomised trial of olanzapine and quetiapine in schizophrenia. J Psychopharmacol 2010; 24:1001–1009.
5. Byerly MJ et al. Effects of aripiprazole on prolactin levels in subjects with schizophrenia during cross-titration with risperidone or olanzapine: Analysis of a randomized, open-label study. Schizophr Res 2009; 107:218–222.
6. Leucht S et al. Comparative efficacy and tolerability of 15 antipsychotic drugs in schizophrenia: a multiple-treatments meta-analysis. Lancet 2013; 382:951–962.
7. Melkersson K. Differences in prolactin elevation and related symptoms of atypical antipsychotics in schizophrenic patients. J Clin Psychiatry 2005; 66:761–767.
8. Kopecek M et al. Ziprasidone-induced galactorrhea: a case report. Neuro Endocrinol Lett 2005; 26:69–70.
9. Buhagiar K et al. Quetiapine-Induced Hyperprolactinemic Galactorrhea in an Adolescent Male. German J Psychiatry 2006; 9:118–120.
10. Johnsen E et al. Antipsychotic-induced hyperprolactinemia: a cross-sectional survey. J Clin Psychopharmacol 2008; 28:686–690.
11. Suzuki Y et al. Differences in plasma prolactin levels in patients with schizophrenia treated on monotherapy with five second-generation antipsychotics. Schizophr Res 2013; 145:116–119.
12. Staller J. The effect of long-term antipsychotic treatment on prolactin. J Child Adolesc Psychopharmacol 2006; 16:317–326.
13. Tsuboi T et al. Hyperprolactinemia and estimated dopamine D2 receptor occupancy in patients with schizophrenia: analysis of the CATIE data. Prog Neuropsychopharmacol Biol Psychiatry 2013; 45:178–182.
14. Kaneda Y. The impact of prolactin elevation with antipsychotic medications on subjective quality of life in patients with schizophrenia. Clin Neuropharmacol 2003; 26:182–184.
15. Bobes J et al. Frequency of sexual dysfunction and other reproductive side-effects in patients with schizophrenia treated with risperidone, olanzapine, quetiapine, or haloperidol: the results of the EIRE study. J Sex Marital Ther 2003; 29:125–147.
16. Smith S. Effects of antipsychotics on sexual and endocrine function in women: implications for clinical practice. J Clin Psychopharmacol 2003; 23:S27–S32.
17. Spollen JJ, III et al. Prolactin levels and erectile function in patients treated with risperidone. J Clin Psychopharmacol 2004; 24:161–166.
18. Knegtering R et al. A randomized open-label study of the impact of quetiapine versus risperidone on sexual functioning. J Clin Psychopharmacol 2004; 24:56–61.
19. Becker D et al. Risperidone, but not olanzapine, decreases bone mineral density in female premenopausal schizophrenia patients. J Clin Psychiatry 2003; 64:761–766.
20. Meaney AM et al. Reduced bone mineral density in patients with schizophrenia receiving prolactin raising anti-psychotic medication. J Psychopharmacol 2003; 17:455–458.
21. Meaney AM et al. Effects of long-term prolactin-raising antipsychotic medication on bone mineral density in patients with schizophrenia. Br J Psychiatry 2004; 184:503–508.
22. Kishimoto T et al. Antipsychotic-induced hyperprolactinemia inhibits the hypothalamo-pituitary-gonadal axis and reduces bone mineral density in male patients with schizophrenia. J Clin Psychiatry 2008; 69:385–391.
23. Wieck A et al. Antipsychotic-induced hyperprolactinaemia in women: pathophysiology, severity and consequences. Selective literature review. Br J Psychiatry 2003; 182:199–204.
24. Smith S et al. The effects of antipsychotic-induced hyperprolactinaemia on the hypothalamic-pituitary-gonadal axis. J Clin Psychopharmacol 2002; 22:109–114.
25. Halbreich U et al. Are chronic psychiatric patients at increased risk for developing breast cancer? Am J Psychiatry 1996; 153:559–560.
26. Wang PS et al. Dopamine antagonists and the development of breast cancer. Arch Gen Psychiatry 2002; 59:1147–1154.
27. Harvey PW et al. Adverse effects of prolactin in rodents and humans: breast and prostate cancer. J Psychopharmacol 2008; 22:20–27.
28. Walters J et al. Clinical questions and uncertainty--prolactin measurement in patients with schizophrenia and bipolar disorder. J Psychopharmacol 2008; 22:82–89.
29. Serri O et al. Diagnosis and management of hyperprolactinemia. CMAJ 2003; 169:575–581.
30. Duncan D et al. Treatment of psychotropic-induced hyperprolactinaemia. Psychiatr Bull 1995; 19:755–757.
31. Anghelescu I et al. Successful switch to aripiprazole after induction of hyperprolactinemia by ziprasidone: a case report. J Clin Psychiatry 2004; 65:1286–1287.
32. McIntyre RS et al. Asenapine in the treatment of acute mania in bipolar I disorder: a randomized, double-blind, placebo-controlled trial. J Affect Disord 2010; 122:27–38.
33. Stahl SM et al. Effectiveness of lurasidone for patients with schizophrenia following 6 weeks of acute treatment with lurasidone, olanzapine, or placebo: a 6-month, open-label, extension study. J Clin Psychiatry 2013; 74:507–515.
34. McEvoy JP et al. Effectiveness of lurasidone in patients with schizophrenia or schizoaffective disorder switched from other antipsychotics: a randomized, 6-week, open-label study. J Clin Psychiatry 2013; 74:170–179.

CHAPTER 2

35. Shim JC et al. Adjunctive treatment with a dopamine partial agonist, aripiprazole, for antipsychotic-induced hyperprolactinemia: a placebo-controlled trial. Am J Psychiatry 2007; **164**:1404–1410.

36. Lorenz RA et al. Resolution of haloperidol-induced hyperprolactinemia with aripiprazole. J Clin Psychopharmacol 2007; **27**:524–525.

37. Lu ML et al. Time course of the changes in antipsychotic-induced hyperprolactinemia following the switch to aripiprazole. Prog Neuropsychopharmacol Biol Psychiatry 2008; **32**:1978–1981.

38. Mir A et al. Change in sexual dysfunction with aripiprazole: a switching or add-on study. J Psychopharmacol 2008; **22**:244–253.

39. van KM et al. Preliminary report: a naturalistic study of the effect of aripiprazole addition on risperidone-related hyperprolactinemia in patients treated with risperidone long-acting injection. J Clin Psychopharmacol 2011; **31**:126–128.

40. Yasui-Furukori N et al. Dose-dependent effects of adjunctive treatment with aripiprazole on hyperprolactinemia induced by risperidone in female patients with schizophrenia. J Clin Psychopharmacol 2010; **30**:596–599.

41. Young RM et al. Prolactin levels in antipsychotic treatment of patients with schizophrenia carrying the DRD2*A1 allele. Br J Psychiatry 2004; **185**:147–151.

42. Duncan D et al. Treatment of psychotropic-induced hyperprolactinaemia. Psychiatr Bull 1995; **19**:755–757.

43. Cavallaro R et al. Cabergoline treatment of risperidone-induced hyperprolactinemia: a pilot study. J Clin Psychiatry 2004; **65**:187–190.

44. Yuan HN et al. A randomized, crossover comparison of herbal medicine and bromocriptine against risperidone-induced hyperprolactinemia in patients with schizophrenia. J Clin Psychopharmacol 2008; **28**:264–370.

Sexual dysfunction

Primary sexual disorders are common, although reliable normative data are lacking.[1] Physical illness, psychiatric illness, substance misuse and prescribed drug treatment can all cause sexual dysfunction.[2] It has been estimated that 50–60% of people with schizophrenia have problems with sexual dysfunction compared with 30% of the general population,[3] but note that in both groups reported prevalence rates vary depending on the method of data collection (low numbers with spontaneous reports, increasing with confidential questionnaires and further still with direct questioning[2]). In one study of patients with psychosis, 37% spontaneously reported sexual problems but 46% were found to be experiencing difficulties when directly questioned.[4]

Baseline sexual functioning should be determined if possible (questionnaires may be useful) because sexual function can affect quality of life[5] and compliance with medication (sexual dysfunction is one of the major causes of treatment dropout).[6] Complaints of sexual dysfunction may also indicate progression or inadequate treatment of underlying medical or psychiatric conditions.[7,8] Sexual problems may also be caused by drug treatment where intervention may greatly improve quality of life.[9]

There are four phases of the human sexual response, as detailed in Table 2.31.[2,10,11]

Effects of psychosis

Sexual dysfunction is already known to be a problem in first-episode schizophrenia[12] and up to 82% of men and 96% of women with established illness report problems, with associated reductions in quality of life.[5] Men[13] complain of reduced desire, inability to achieve an erection and premature ejaculation, whereas women complain more generally about reduced enjoyment.[13,14] Women with psychosis are known to have reduced fertility.[15] People with psychosis are less able to develop good psychosexual relationships and,

Table 2.31 The human sexual response

Desire	■ Related to testosterone levels in men
	■ Possibly increased by dopamine and decreased by prolactin
	■ Psychosocial context and conditioning significantly affect desire
Arousal	■ Influenced by testosterone in men and oestrogen in women
	■ Other potential mechanisms include: central dopamine stimulation, modulation of the cholinergic/adrenergic balance, peripheral α_1 agonism and nitric oxide pathways
	■ Physical pathology such as hypertension or diabetes can have a significant effect
Orgasm	■ May be related to oxytocin
	■ Inhibition of orgasm may be caused by an increase in serotonin activity and raised prolactin, as well as α_1 blockade
Resolution	■ Occurs passively after orgasm

Note: Many other hormones and neurotransmitters may interact in a complex way at each phase.

for some, treatment with an antipsychotic can improve sexual functioning.[16] Assessment of sexual functioning can clearly be difficult in someone who is psychotic. The Arizona Sexual Experience Scale (ASEX) may be useful in this respect.[17]

Effects of antipsychotic drugs

Sexual dysfunction has been reported as a side-effect of all antipsychotics, and up to 45% of people taking older or conventional antipsychotics experience sexual dysfunction.[18] Individual susceptibility varies and all effects are reversible. Note though that physical illness and drugs other than antipsychotics can cause sexual dysfunction and many studies do not control for either, making the prevalence of sexual dysfunction with different antipsychotics difficult to compare.[19]

Antipsychotics decrease dopaminergic transmission, which in itself can decrease libido but may also increase prolactin levels via negative feedback. It has been estimated that prolactin elevation explains 40% of the sexual dysfunction that is associated with antipsychotic medication.[3] Hyperprolactinaemia can also cause amenorrhoea in women, and breast enlargement and galactorrhoea in both men and women.[20] Although it has been suggested that the overall propensity of an antipsychotic to cause sexual dysfunction is related to propensity to raise prolactin, i.e. risperidone > haloperidol > olanzapine > quetiapine > aripiprazole,[7,19,21] it should be noted that in the CUtLASS-1 study, FGAs (primarily sulpiride, but also other FGAs known to be associated with prolactin elevation) did not fare any worse than SGAs (70% of patients in this arm were prescribed an antipsychotic not associated with prolactin elevation) with respect to worsening sexual dysfunction. In fact, sexual functioning improved in both arms over the one year duration of the study.[16] Aripiprazole is relatively free of sexual side-effects when used as monotherapy[22] and possibly also in combination with another antipsychotic.[23,24]

Anticholinergic effects can cause disorders of arousal[25] and drugs that block peripheral α_1-receptors cause particular problems with erection and ejaculation in men.[9] Drugs that are antagonists at both peripheral α_1-receptors and cholinergic receptors can cause priapism.[26] Antipsychotic-induced sedation and weight gain may reduce sexual desire.[26] These principles can be used to predict the sexual side-effects of different antipsychotic drugs (Table 2.32).

Treatment

Before attempting to treat sexual dysfunction, a thorough assessment is essential to determine the most likely cause. Assuming that physical pathology (diabetes, hypertension, cardiovascular disease, etc.) has been excluded, the following principles apply.

Spontaneous remission may occasionally occur.[26] The most obvious first step is to decrease the dose or discontinue the offending drug where appropriate. The next step is to switch to a different drug that is less likely to cause the specific sexual problem experienced (see Table 2.32). Another option is to add 5–10 mg aripiprazole – this can normalise prolactin and improve sexual function.[27-29] If this fails or is not practicable, 'antidote' drugs can be tried: for example, cyproheptadine (a $5HT_2$ antagonist at doses of 4–16 mg/day) has been used to treat SSRI-induced sexual dysfunction but sedation is a common side-effect. Amantadine, bupropion, buspirone, bethanechol and

Table 2.32 Sexual adverse effects of antipsychotics

Drug	Type of problem
Phenothiazines (e.g. chlorpromazine)	■ Hyperprolactinaemia and anticholinergic effects. Reports of delayed orgasm at lower doses followed by normal orgasm but without ejaculation at higher doses[14] ■ Most problems occur with thioridazine (which can also reduce testosterone levels)[30] ■ Priapism has been reported with thioridazine, risperidone and chlorpromazine (probably due to α_1 blockade)[31–33]
Thioxanthenes (e.g. flupentixol)	■ Arousal problems and anorgasmia[34]
Haloperidol	■ Similar problems to the phenothiazines[35] but anticholinergic effects reduced[31] ■ Prevalence of sexual dysfunction reported to be up to 70%[36]
Olanzapine	■ Possibly less sexual dysfunction due to relative lack of prolactin-related effects[35] ■ Priapism reported rarely[37,38] ■ Prevalence of sexual dysfunction reported to be >50%[36]
Risperidone	■ Potent elevator of serum prolactin ■ Less anticholinergic ■ Specific peripheral α_1-adrenergic blockade leads to a moderately high reported incidence of ejaculatory problems such as retrograde ejaculation[39,40] ■ Priapism reported rarely[26] ■ Prevalence of sexual dysfunction reported to be 60–70%[36]
Sulpiride/amisulpride	■ Potent elevators of serum prolactin[18] but note that sulpiride (as the main FGA prescribed in the study) was not associated with greater sexual dysfunction than SGAs (with variable ability to raise prolactin) in the CUtLASS-1 study.[16]
Quetiapine	■ No effect on serum prolactin[41] ■ Possibly associated with low risk of sexual dysfunction,[42–45] but studies are conflicting[46,47]
Clozapine	■ Significant α_1-adrenergic blockade and anticholinergic effects.[48] No effect on prolactin[49] ■ Probably fewer problems than with typical antipsychotics[50]
Aripiprazole	■ No effect on prolactin or α_1-receptors. No reported adverse effects on sexual function. Improves sexual function in those switched from other antipsychotics[22,24,51] Case reports of aripiprazole-induced hypersexuality have been published[52]

FGA, first-generation antipsychotic; SGA, second-generation antipsychotic.

yohimbine have all been used with varying degrees of success but have a number of unwanted side-effects and interactions with other drugs (Table 2.33). Given that hyperprolactinaemia may contribute to sexual dysfunction, selegiline (enhances dopamine activity) has been tested in an RCT. This was negative.[53] Testosterone patches have been shown to increase libido in women, although note though that breast cancer risk may be significantly increased.[54,55] The evidence base supporting the use of 'antidotes' is poor.[26]

CHAPTER 2

Table 2.33 Remedial treatments for psychotropic-induced sexual dysfunction

Drug	Pharmacology	Potential treatment for	Side-effects
Alprostadil[1,11]	Prostaglandin	Erectile dysfunction	Pain, fibrosis, hypotension, priapism
Amantadine[1,56]	Dopamine agonist	Prolactin-induced reduction in desire and arousal (dopamine increases libido and facilitates ejaculation)	Return of psychotic symptoms, GI effects, nervousness, insomnia, rash
Bethanechol[57]	Cholinergic or cholinergic potentiation of adrenergic neurotransmission	Anticholinergic induced arousal problems and anorgasmia (from TCAs, antipsychotics, etc)	Nausea and vomiting, colic, bradycardia, blurred vision, sweating
Bromocriptine[9]	Dopamine agonist	Prolactin-induced reduction in desire and arousal	Return of psychotic symptoms, GI effects
Bupropion[58]	Noradrenaline and dopamine reuptake inhibitor	SSRI-induced sexual dysfunction (evidence poor)	Concentration problems, reduced sleep, tremor
Buspirone[59]	$5HT_{1a}$ partial agonist	SSRI-induced sexual dysfunction, particularly decreased libido and anorgasmia	Nausea, dizziness, headache
Cyproheptadine[1,59,60]	$5HT_2$ antagonist	Sexual dysfunction caused by increased serotonin transmission (e.g. SSRIs), particularly anorgasmia	Sedation and fatigue. Reversal of the therapeutic effect of antidepressants
Sildenafil[11,61–64]	Phosphodiesterase inhibitor	Erectile dysfunction of any aetiology Anorgasmia in women. Effective when prolactin raised	Mild headaches, dizziness, nasal congestion
Yohimbine[1,11,65–67]	Central and peripheral α_2 adrenoceptor antagonist	SSRI-induced sexual dysfunction, particularly erectile dysfunction, decreased libido and anorgasmia (evidence poor)	Anxiety, nausea, fine tremor, increased blood pressure, sweating, fatigue

Note: The use of the drugs listed above should ideally be under the care or supervision of a specialist in sexual dysfunction.
GI, gastrointestinal; SSRI, selective serotonin reuptake inhibitor; TCA, tricyclic antidepressant.

Drugs such as sildenafil (Viagra) or alprostadil (Caverject) are effective only in the treatment of erectile dysfunction. Psychological approaches used by sexual dysfunction clinics may be difficult for clients with mental health problems to engage in.[9]

References

1. Baldwin DS et al. Effects of antidepressant drugs on sexual function. Int J Psychiatry Clin Pract 1997; 1:47–58.
2. Pollack MH et al. Genitourinary and sexual adverse effects of psychotropic medication. Int J Psychiatry Med 1992; 22:305–327.
3. Nunes LV et al. Strategies for the treatment of antipsychotic-induced sexual dysfunction and/or hyperprolactinemia among patients of the schizophrenia spectrum: a review. J Sex Marital Ther 2012; 38:281–301.

4. Montejo AL et al. Frequency of sexual dysfunction in patients with a psychotic disorder receiving antipsychotics. J Sex Med 2010; 7:3404–3413.

5. Olfson M et al. Male sexual dysfunction and quality of life in schizophrenia. J Clin Psychiatry 2005; 66:331–338.

6. Montejo AL et al. Incidence of sexual dysfunction associated with antidepressant agents: a prospective multicenter study of 1022 outpatients. Spanish Working Group for the Study of Psychotropic-Related Sexual Dysfunction. J Clin Psychiatry 2001; 62 Suppl 3:10–21.

7. Baggaley M. Sexual dysfunction in schizophrenia: focus on recent evidence. Hum Psychopharmacol 2008; 23:201–209.

8. Ucok A et al. Sexual dysfunction in patients with schizophrenia on antipsychotic medication. Eur Psychiatry 2007; 22:328–333.

9. Segraves RT. Effects of psychotropic drugs on human erection and ejaculation. Arch Gen Psychiatry 1989; 46:275–284.

10. Stahl SM. The psychopharmacology of sex, Part 1: Neurotransmitters and the 3 phases of the human sexual response. J Clin Psychiatry 2001; 62:80–81.

11. Garcia-Reboll L et al. Drugs for the treatment of impotence. Drugs Aging 1997; 11:140–151.

12. Bitter I et al. Antipsychotic treatment and sexual functioning in first-time neuroleptic-treated schizophrenic patients. Int Clin Psychopharmacol 2005; 20:19–21.

13. Macdonald S et al. Nithsdale Schizophrenia Surveys 24: sexual dysfunction. Case-control study. Br J Psychiatry 2003; 182:50–56.

14. Smith S. Effects of antipsychotics on sexual and endocrine function in women: implications for clinical practice. J Clin Psychopharmacol 2003; 23:S27–S32.

15. Howard LM et al. The general fertility rate in women with psychotic disorders. Am J Psychiatry 2002; 159:991–997.

16. Peluso MJ et al. Non-neurological and metabolic side effects in the Cost Utility of the Latest Antipsychotics in Schizophrenia Randomised Controlled Trial (CUtLASS-1). Schizophr Res 2013; 144:80–86.

17. Byerly MJ et al. An empirical evaluation of the Arizona sexual experience scale and a simple one-item screening test for assessing antipsychotic-related sexual dysfunction in outpatients with schizophrenia and schizoaffective disorder. Schizophr Res 2006; 81:311–316.

18. Smith SM et al. Sexual dysfunction in patients taking conventional antipsychotic medication. Br J Psychiatry 2002; 181:49–55.

19. Serretti A et al. A meta-analysis of sexual dysfunction in psychiatric patients taking antipsychotics. Int Clin Psychopharmacol 2011; 26:130–140.

20. Anon. Adverse effects of the atypical antipsychotics. Collaborative Working Group on Clinical Trial Evaluations. J Clin Psychiatry 1998; 59 Suppl 12:17–22.

21. Knegtering H et al. Are sexual side effects of prolactin-raising antipsychotics reducible to serum prolactin? Psychoneuroendocrinology 2008; 33:711–717.

22. Hanssens L et al. The effect of antipsychotic medication on sexual function and serum prolactin levels in community-treated schizophrenic patients: results from the Schizophrenia Trial of Aripiprazole (STAR) study (NCT00237913). BMC Psych 2008; 8:95.

23. Mir A et al. Change in sexual dysfunction with aripiprazole: a switching or add-on study. J Psychopharmacol 2008; 22:244–253.

24. Byerly MJ et al. Effects of aripiprazole on prolactin levels in subjects with schizophrenia during cross-titration with risperidone or olanzapine: Analysis of a randomized, open-label study. Schizophr Res 2009; 107:218–222.

25. Aldridge SA. Drug-induced sexual dysfunction. Clin Pharm 1982; 1:141–147.

26. Baldwin D et al. Sexual side-effects of antidepressant and antipsychotic drugs. Adv Psychiatr Treat 2003; 9:202–210.

27. Shim JC et al. Adjunctive treatment with a dopamine partial agonist, aripiprazole, for antipsychotic-induced hyperprolactinemia: a placebo-controlled trial. Am J Psychiatry 2007; 164:1404–1410.

28. Yasui-Furukori N et al. Dose-dependent effects of adjunctive treatment with aripiprazole on hyperprolactinemia induced by risperidone in female patients with schizophrenia. J Clin Psychopharmacol 2010; 30:596–599.

29. Trives MZ et al. Effect of the addition of aripiprazole on hyperprolactinemia associated with risperidone long-acting injection. J Clin Psychopharmacol 2013; 33:538–541.

30. Kotin J et al. Thioridazine and sexual dysfunction. Am J Psychiatry 1976; 133:82–85.

31. Mitchell JE et al. Antipsychotic drug therapy and sexual dysfunction in men. Am J Psychiatry 1982; 139:633–637.

32. Loh C et al. Risperidone-induced retrograde ejaculation: case report and review of the literature. Int Clin Psychopharmacol 2004; 19:111–112.

33. Thompson JW, Jr. et al. Psychotropic medication and priapism: a comprehensive review. J Clin Psychiatry 1990; 51:430–433.

34. Aizenberg D et al. Sexual dysfunction in male schizophrenic patients. J Clin Psychiatry 1995; 56:137–141.

35. Crawford AM et al. The acute and long-term effect of olanzapine compared with placebo and haloperidol on serum prolactin concentrations. Schizophr Res 1997; 26:41–54.

36. Serretti A et al. Sexual side effects of pharmacological treatment of psychiatric diseases. Clin Pharmacol Ther 2011; 89:142–147.

37. Dossenbach M et al. Effects of atypical and typical antipsychotic treatments on sexual function in patients with schizophrenia: 12-month results from the Intercontinental Schizophrenia Outpatient Health Outcomes (IC-SOHO) study. Eur Psychiatry 2006; 21:251–258.

38. Aurobindo Pharma - Milpharm Ltd. Summary of Product Characteristics. Olanzapine 10 mg tablets. 2013. http://www.medicines.org.uk/emc/medicine/27661/SPC/Olanzapine++10+mg+tablets/

39. Tran PV et al. Double-blind comparison of olanzapine versus risperidone in the treatment of schizophrenia and other psychotic disorders. J Clin Psychopharmacol 1997; 17:407–418.

40. Raja M. Risperidone-induced absence of ejaculation. Int Clin Psychopharmacol 1999; 14:317–319.

41. Peuskens J et al. A comparison of quetiapine and chlorpromazine in the treatment of schizophrenia. Acta Psychiatr Scand 1997; 96:265–273.

42. Bobes J et al. Frequency of sexual dysfunction and other reproductive side-effects in patients with schizophrenia treated with risperidone, olanzapine, quetiapine, or haloperidol: the results of the EIRE study. J Sex Marital Ther 2003; 29:125–147.

43. Byerly MJ et al. An open-label trial of quetiapine for antipsychotic-induced sexual dysfunction. J Sex Marital Ther 2004; 30:325–332.

44. Knegtering R et al. A randomized open-label study of the impact of quetiapine versus risperidone on sexual functioning. J Clin Psychopharmacol 2004; 24:56–61.

CHAPTER 2

45. Montejo Gonzalez AL et al. A 6-month prospective observational study on the effects of quetiapine on sexual functioning. J Clin Psychopharmacol 2005; 25:533–538.

46. Atmaca M et al. A new atypical antipsychotic: quetiapine-induced sexual dysfunctions. Int J Impot Res 2005; 17:201–203.

47. Kelly DL et al. A randomized double-blind 12-week study of quetiapine, risperidone or fluphenazine on sexual functioning in people with schizophrenia. Psychoneuroendocrinology 2006; 31:340–346.

48. Coward DM. General pharmacology of clozapine. Br J Psychiatry 1992; 160:5–11.

49. Meltzer HY et al. Effect of clozapine on human serum prolactin levels. Am J Psychiatry 1979; 136:1550–1555.

50. Aizenberg D et al. Comparison of sexual dysfunction in male schizophrenic patients maintained on treatment with classical antipsychotics versus clozapine. J Clin Psychiatry 2001; 62:541–544.

51. Rykmans V et al. A comparision of switching strategies from risperidone to aripiprazole in patients with schizophrenia with insufficient efficacy/tolerability on risperidone (cn138-169). Eur Psychiatry 2008; 23:S111.

52. Chen CY et al. Improvement of serum prolactin and sexual function after switching to aripiprazole from risperidone in schizophrenia: a case series. Psychiatry Clin Neurosci 2011; 65:95–97.

53. Kodesh A et al. Selegiline in the treatment of sexual dysfunction in schizophrenic patients maintained on neuroleptics: a pilot study. Clin Neuropharmacol 2003; 26:193–195.

54. Davis SR et al. Testosterone for low libido in postmenopausal women not taking estrogen. N Engl J Med 2008; 359:2005–2017.

55. Schover LR. Androgen therapy for loss of desire in women: is the benefit worth the breast cancer risk? Fertil Steril 2008; 90:129–140.

56. Valevski A et al. Effect of amantadine on sexual dysfunction in neuroleptic-treated male schizophrenic patients. Clin Neuropharmacol 1998; 21:355–357.

57. Gross MD. Reversal by bethanechol of sexual dysfunction caused by anticholinergic antidepressants. Am J Psychiatry 1982; 139:1193–1194.

58. Masand PS et al. Sustained-release bupropion for selective serotonin reuptake inhibitor-induced sexual dysfunction: a randomized, double-blind, placebo-controlled, parallel-group study. Am J Psychiatry 2001; 158:805–807.

59. Rothschild AJ. Sexual side effects of antidepressants. J Clin Psychiatry 2000; 61 Suppl 11:28–36.

60. Lauerma H. Successful treatment of citalopram-induced anorgasmia by cyproheptadine. Acta Psychiatr Scand 1996; 93:69–70.

61. Nurnberg HG et al. Sildenafil for women patients with antidepressant-induced sexual dysfunction. Psychiatr Serv 1999; 50:1076–1078.

62. Salerian AJ et al. Sildenafil for psychotropic-induced sexual dysfunction in 31 women and 61 men. J Sex Marital Ther 2000; 26:133–140.

63. Nurnberg HG et al. Treatment of antidepressant-associated sexual dysfunction with sildenafil: a randomized controlled trial. JAMA 2003; 289:56–64.

64. Gopalakrishnan R et al. Sildenafil in the treatment of antipsychotic-induced erectile dysfunction: a randomized, double-blind, placebo-controlled, flexible-dose, two-way crossover trial. Am J Psychiatry 2006; 163:494–499.

65. Jacobsen FM. Fluoxetine-induced sexual dysfunction and an open trial of yohimbine. J Clin Psychiatry 1992; 53:119–122.

66. Michelson D et al. Mirtazapine, yohimbine or olanzapine augmentation therapy for serotonin reuptake-associated female sexual dysfunction: a randomized, placebo controlled trial. J Psychiatr Res 2002; 36:147–152.

67. Woodrum ST et al. Management of SSRI-induced sexual dysfunction. Ann Pharmacother 1998; 32:1209–1215.

Pneumonia

A Dutch database study published in 2008[1] found that current use of antipsychotics was associated with a 60% increased risk of pneumonia in an elderly population. Risk was highest in the first week of treatment and an increased risk was seen with SGAs but not FGAs. Another study[2] found a higher rate of chest infection in people taking SGAs. Three further studies found a dose-related increased risk of pneumonia in older people taking both FGAs and SGAs.[3-5] The risk was again noted to be highest in the first week(s) of treatment. More recently, a study of patients with bipolar affective disorder found that clozapine, olanzapine and haloperidol were linked to increased rates of pneumonia while lithium was protective.[6] Another recent study suggests amisulpride is not linked to pneumonia.[7] Schizophrenia itself seems to afford a higher risk of complications (e.g. admission to intensive care) in people diagnosed with pneumonia.[8]

The mechanism by which antipsychotics increase the risk of pneumonia is not known. Possibilities include sedation (risk seems to be highest with drugs that show greatest H_1 antagonism[3,7]); dystonia or dyskinesia; dry mouth causing poor bolus transport and so increasing the risk of aspiration; general poor physical health;[7] or perhaps some ill-defined effect on immune response.[1,3] With clozapine, pneumonia may also be secondary to constipation.[9]

An increased risk of pneumonia should be assumed for all patients (regardless of age) taking any antipsychotic for any period. All patients should be very carefully monitored for signs of chest infection and effective treatment started promptly. Early referral to general medical services should be considered where there is any doubt about the severity or type of chest infection.

Summary

- Assume the use of all antipsychotics increase the risk of pneumonia.
- Monitor all patients for signs of chest infection and treat promptly.

References

1. Knol W et al. Antipsychotic drug use and risk of pneumonia in elderly people. J Am Geriatr Soc 2008; 56:661–666.
2. Star K et al. Pneumonia following antipsychotic prescriptions in electronic health records: a patient safety concern? Br J Gen Pract 2010; 60:e385–e394.
3. Trifiro G et al. Association of community-acquired pneumonia with antipsychotic drug use in elderly patients: a nested case-control study. Ann Intern Med 2010; 152:418–440.
4. Pratt N et al. Risk of hospitalization for hip fracture and pneumonia associated with antipsychotic prescribing in the elderly: a self-controlled case-series analysis in an Australian health care claims database. Drug Saf 2011; 34:567–575.
5. Aparasu RR et al. Risk of pneumonia in elderly nursing home residents using typical versus atypical antipsychotics. Ann Pharmacother 2013; 47:464–474.
6. Yang SY et al. Antipsychotic drugs, mood stabilizers, and risk of pneumonia in bipolar disorder: a nationwide case-control study. J Clin Psychiatry 2013; 74:e79–e86.
7. Kuo CJ et al. Second-generation antipsychotic medications and risk of pneumonia in schizophrenia. Schizophr Bull 2013; 39:648–657.
8. Chen YH et al. Poor clinical outcomes among pneumonia patients with schizophrenia. Schizophr Bull 2011; 37:1088–1094.
9. Galappathie N et al. Clozapine-associated pneumonia and respiratory arrest secondary to severe constipation. Med Sci Law 2014; 54:105–109.

Switching antipsychotics

General recommendations for switching antipsychotics because of poor tolerability are shown in Table 2.34.

Table 2.34 General recommendations for switching antipsychotic drugs

Adverse effect	Suggested drugs	Alternatives
Acute EPS[1-6]	Aripiprazole Olanzapine Quetiapine	Clozapine Lurasidone Ziprasidone
Dyslipidaemia[7-12]	Amisulpride Aripiprazole[42] Lurasidone Ziprasidone	Asenapine
Impaired glucose tolerance[11,13-16]	Amisulpride Aripiprazole[42] Lurasidone Ziprasidone	Risperidone Haloperidol
Hyperprolactinaemia[11,17-22]	Aripiprazole* Lurasidone Quetiapine	Clozapine Olanzapine Ziprasidone
Postural hypotension[11]	Amisulpride Aripiprazole Lurasidone	Haloperidol Sulpiride Trifluoperazine
QT prolongation[22-27]	Aripiprazole Lurasidone Paliperidone (with ECG monitoring)	Low dose monotherapy of any drug not formally contra-indicated in QT prolongation (with ECG monitoring)
Sedation[22]	Amisulpride Aripiprazole Risperidone Sulpiride	Haloperidol Trifuoperazine Ziprasidone
Sexual dysfuction[28-34]	Aripiprazole Quetiapine	Clozapine Lurasidone
Tardive dyskinesia[35-38]	Clozapine	Aripiprazole Olanzapine Quetiapine
Weight gain[12,39-45]	Amisulpride Aripiprazole[42] Haloperidol Lurasidone Ziprasidone	Asenapine Trifluoperazine

*There is evidence that both switching to and co-prescription of aripiprazole are effective in reducing weight, prolactin and dyslipidaemia and in reversing impaired glucose tolerance.[46-48]
ECG, electrocardiogram; EPS, extrapyramidal side-effects.

References

1. Stanniland C et al. Tolerability of atypical antipsychotics. Drug Saf 2000; **22**:195–214.
2. Tarsy D et al. Effects of newer antipsychotics on extrapyramidal function. CNS Drugs 2002; **16**:23–45.
3. Caroff SN et al. Movement disorders associated with atypical antipsychotic drugs. J Clin Psychiatry 2002; 63 Suppl 4:12–19.
4. Lemmens P et al. A combined analysis of double-blind studies with risperidone vs. placebo and other antipsychotic agents: factors associated with extrapyramidal symptoms. Acta Psychiatr Scand 1999; **99**:160–170.
5. Taylor DM. Aripiprazole: a review of its pharmacology and clinical use. Int J Clin Pract 2003; **57**:49–54.
6. Meltzer HY et al. Lurasidone in the treatment of schizophrenia: a randomized, double-blind, placebo- and olanzapine-controlled study. Am J Psychiatry 2011; **168**:957–967.
7. Rettenbacher MA et al. Early changes of plasma lipids during treatment with atypical antipsychotics. Int Clin Psychopharmacol 2006; **21**:369–372.
8. Ball MP et al. Clozapine-induced hyperlipidemia resolved after switch to aripiprazole therapy. Ann Pharmacother 2005; **39**:1570–1572.
9. Chrzanowski WK et al. Effectiveness of long-term aripiprazole therapy in patients with acutely relapsing or chronic, stable schizophrenia: a 52-week, open-label comparison with olanzapine. Psychopharmacology 2006; **189**:259–266.
10. De Hert M et al. A case series: evaluation of the metabolic safety of aripiprazole. Schizophr Bull 2007; **33**:823–830.
11. Citrome L et al. Long-term safety and tolerability of lurasidone in schizophrenia: a 12-month, double-blind, active-controlled study. Int Clin Psychopharmacol 2012; **27**:165–176.
12. Kemp DE et al. Weight change and metabolic effects of asenapine in patients with schizophrenia and bipolar disorder. J Clin Psychiatry 2014; **75**:238–245.
13. Haddad PM. Antipsychotics and diabetes: review of non-prospective data. Br J Psychiatry Suppl 2004; **47**:S80–S86.
14. Berry S et al. Improvement of insulin indices after switch from olanzapine to risperidone. Eur Neuropsychopharmacol 2002; **12**:316.
15. Gianfrancesco FD et al. Differential effects of risperidone, olanzapine, clozapine, and conventional antipsychotics on type 2 diabetes: findings from a large health plan database. J Clin Psychiatry 2002; **63**:920–930.
16. Mir S et al. Atypical antipsychotics and hyperglycaemia. Int Clin Psychopharmacol 2001; **16**:63–74.
17. Turrone P et al. Elevation of prolactin levels by atypical antipsychotics. Am J Psychiatry 2002; **159**:133–135.
18. David SR et al. The effects of olanzapine, risperidone, and haloperidol on plasma prolactin levels in patients with schizophrenia. Clin Ther 2000; **22**:1085–1096.
19. Hamner MB et al. Hyperprolactinaemia in antipsychotic-treated patients: guidelines for avoidance and management. CNS Drugs 1998; **10**:209–222.
20. Trives MZ et al. Effect of the addition of aripiprazole on hyperprolactinemia associated with risperidone long-acting injection. J Clin Psychopharmacol 2013; **33**:538–541.
21. Suzuki Y et al. Differences in plasma prolactin levels in patients with schizophrenia treated on monotherapy with five second-generation antipsychotics. Schizophr Res 2013; **145**:116–119.
22. Leucht S et al. Comparative efficacy and tolerability of 15 antipsychotic drugs in schizophrenia: a multiple-treatments meta-analysis. Lancet 2013; **382**:951–962.
23. Glassman AH et al. Antipsychotic drugs: prolonged QTc interval, torsade de pointes, and sudden death. Am J Psychiatry 2001; **158**:1774–1782.
24. Taylor D. Antipsychotics and QT prolongation. Acta Psychiatr Scand 2003; **107**:85–95.
25. Titier K et al. Atypical antipsychotics: from potassium channels to torsade de pointes and sudden death. Drug Saf 2005; **28**:35–51.
26. Ray WA et al. Atypical antipsychotic drugs and the risk of sudden cardiac death. N Engl J Med 2009; **360**:225–235.
27. Loebel A et al. Efficacy and safety of lurasidone 80 mg/day and 160 mg/day in the treatment of schizophrenia: a randomized, double-blind, placebo- and active-controlled trial. Schizophr Res 2013; **145**:101–109.
28. Byerly MJ et al. An open-label trial of quetiapine for antipsychotic-induced sexual dysfunction. J Sex Marital Ther 2004; **30**:325–332.
29. Byerly MJ et al. Sexual dysfunction associated with second-generation antipsychotics in outpatients with schizophrenia or schizoaffective disorder: an empirical evaluation of olanzapine, risperidone, and quetiapine. Schizophr Res 2006; **86**:244–250.
30. Montejo Gonzalez AL et al. A 6-month prospective observational study on the effects of quetiapine on sexual functioning. J Clin Psychopharmacol 2005; **25**:533–538.
31. Dossenbach M et al. Effects of atypical and typical antipsychotic treatments on sexual function in patients with schizophrenia: 12-month results from the Intercontinental Schizophrenia Outpatient Health Outcomes (IC-SOHO) study. Eur Psychiatry 2006; **21**:251–258.
32. Kerwin R et al. A multicentre, randomized, naturalistic, open-label study between aripiprazole and standard of care in the management of community-treated schizophrenic patients Schizophrenia Trial of Aripiprazole: (STAR) study. Eur Psychiatry 2007; **22**:433–443.
33. Hanssens L et al. The effect of antipsychotic medication on sexual function and serum prolactin levels in community-treated schizophrenic patients: results from the Schizophrenia Trial of Aripiprazole (STAR) study (NCT00237913). BMC Psych 2008; **8**:95.
34. Loebel A et al. Effectiveness of lurasidone vs. quetiapine XR for relapse prevention in schizophrenia: a 12-month, double-blind, noninferiority study. Schizophr Res 2013; **147**:95–102.
35. Lieberman J et al. Clozapine pharmacology and tardive dyskinesia. Psychopharmacology 1989; 99 Suppl 1:S54–S59.
36. O'Brien J et al. Marked improvement in tardive dyskinesia following treatment with olanzapine in an elderly subject. Br J Psychiatry 1998; **172**:186.
37. Sacchetti E et al. Quetiapine, clozapine, and olanzapine in the treatment of tardive dyskinesia induced by first-generation antipsychotics: a 124-week case report. Int Clin Psychopharmacol 2003; **18**:357–359.

CHAPTER 2

38. Witschy JK et al. Improvement in tardive dyskinesia with aripiprazole use. Can J Psychiatry 2005; **50**:188.

39. Taylor DM et al. Atypical antipsychotics and weight gain - a systematic review. Acta Psychiatr Scand 2000; **101**:416–432.

40. Allison D et al. Antipsychotic-induced weight gain: A comprehensive research synthesis. Am J Psychiatry 1999; **156**:1686–1696.

41. Brecher M et al. The long term effect of quetiapine (SeroquelTM) monotherapy on weight in patients with schizophrenia. Int J Psychiatry Clin Pract 2000; **4**:287–291.

42. Casey DE et al. Switching patients to aripiprazole from other antipsychotic agents: a multicenter randomized study. Psychopharmacology 2003; **166**:391–399.

43. Newcomer JW et al. A multicenter, randomized, double-blind study of the effects of aripiprazole in overweight subjects with schizophrenia or schizoaffective disorder switched from olanzapine. J Clin Psychiatry 2008; **69**:1046–1056.

44. McEvoy JP et al. Effectiveness of lurasidone in patients with schizophrenia or schizoaffective disorder switched from other antipsychotics: a randomized, 6-week, open-label study. J Clin Psychiatry 2013; **74**:170–179.

45. McEvoy JP et al. Effectiveness of paliperidone palmitate vs haloperidol decanoate for maintenance treatment of schizophrenia: a randomized clinical trial. JAMA 2014; **311**:1978–1987.

46. Shim JC et al. Adjunctive treatment with a dopamine partial agonist, aripiprazole, for antipsychotic-induced hyperprolactinemia: a placebo-controlled trial. Am J Psychiatry 2007; **164**:1404–1410.

47. Fleischhacker WW et al. Weight change on aripiprazole-clozapine combination in schizophrenic patients with weight gain and suboptimal response on clozapine: 16-week double-blind study. Eur Psychiatry 2008; **23 Suppl** 2:S114–S115.

48. Henderson DC et al. Aripiprazole added to overweight and obese olanzapine-treated schizophrenia patients. J Clin Psychopharmacol 2009; **29**:165–169.

REFRACTORY SCHIZOPHRENIA AND CLOZAPINE

Clozapine – dosing regimen

Many of the adverse effects of clozapine are dose-dependent and associated with speed of titration. Adverse effects also tend to be more common and severe at the beginning of therapy. Standard maintenance doses may even prove fatal in clozapine-naïve subjects.[1] To minimise these problems, it is important to start treatment at a low dose and to increase dosage slowly.

Clozapine should normally be started at a dose of 12.5 mg once a day, at night. Blood pressure should be monitored hourly for 6 hours because of the hypotensive effect of clozapine. This monitoring is not usually necessary if the first dose is given at night. On day 2, the dose can be increased to 12.5 mg twice daily. If the patient is tolerating clozapine, the dose can be increased by 25–50 mg a day, until a dose of 300 mg a day is reached. This can usually be achieved in 2–3 weeks. Further dosage increases should be

Table 2.35 Suggested starting regime for clozapine (in-patients)

Day	Morning dose (mg)	Evening dose (mg)
1	–	12.5
2	12.5	12.5
3	25	25
4	25	25
5	25	50
6	25	50
7	50	50
8	50	75
9	75	75
10	75	100
11	100	100
12	100	125
13	125	125*
14	125	150
15	150	150
18	150	200†
21	200	200
28	200	250‡

*Target dose for female non smokers (250 mg/day)
†Target dose for male non smokers (350 mg/day)
‡Target dose for female smokers (450 mg/day)

made slowly in increments of 50–100 mg each week. A plasma level of 350 µg/L should be aimed for to ensure an adequate trial, but response may occur at lower plasma level. The **average** (there is substantial variation) dose at which this plasma level is reached varies according to gender and smoking status. The range is approximately 250 mg/day (female non-smoker) to 550 mg/day (male smoker).[2] The total clozapine dose should be divided (usually twice daily) and, if sedation is a problem, the larger portion of the dose can be given at night.

Table 2.34 shows a suggested starting regime for clozapine. This is a cautious regimen – more rapid increases have been used. Slower titration may be necessary where sedation or other dose-related side-effects are severe, in the elderly, the very young, those who are physically compromised or those who have poorly tolerated other antipsychotics. If the patient is not tolerating a particular dose, decrease to one that was previously tolerated. If the adverse effect resolves, increase the dose again but at a slower rate.

If for any reason a patient misses fewer than 2 days' clozapine, restart at the dose prescribed before the event. Do not administer extra tablets to catch up. If more than 2 days are missed, restart and increase slowly (but at a faster rate than in drug-naïve patients). See section on 'Restarting clozapine after a break in treatment' in this chapter.

References

1. Stanworth D et al. Clozapine - a dangerous drug in a clozapine-naive subject. Forensic Sci Int 2011; **214**:e23–e25.
2. Rostami-Hodjegan A et al. Influence of dose, cigarette smoking, age, sex, and metabolic activity on plasma clozapine concentrations: a predictive model and nomograms to aid clozapine dose adjustment and to assess compliance in individual patients. J Clin Psychopharmacol 2004; **24**:70–78.

Optimising clozapine treatment

Using clozapine alone

Target dose – note that dose is best adjusted according to patient tolerability and plasma level.

- Average dose in UK is around 450 mg/day.[1]
- Response usually seen in the range 150–900 mg/day.[2]
- Lower doses required in the elderly, females and non-smokers, and in those prescribed certain enzyme inhibitors[3,4] (see Table 2.35).

Plasma levels

- Most studies indicate that threshold for response is in the range 350–420 µg/L.[5,6] Threshold may be as high as 500 µg/L[7] (see Chapter 1).
- In male smokers who cannot achieve therapeutic plasma levels, metabolic inhibitors (fluvoxamine or cimetidine for example[8,9]) can be co-prescribed but extreme caution is required.
- Importance of norclozapine levels not established but clozapine/norclozapine ratio may aid assessment of recent compliance.

Clozapine augmentation

Clozapine 'augmentation' has become common practice because inadequate response to clozapine alone is a frequent clinical event. The evidence base supporting augmentation strategies is growing but remains insufficient to allow the development of any algorithm or schedule of treatment options. In practice, the result of clozapine augmentation is often disappointing and substantial changes in symptom severity are rarely observed. This clinical impression is supported by the equivocal results of many studies, which suggests a small effect size at best. Meta-analyses of antipsychotic augmentation suggest no effect,[10] a small effect in long-term studies[11] or, in the largest meta-analysis, a very small effect overall.[12] An update on this last study[13] confirmed this small effect size. Recent investigations into dopaminergic activity in refractory schizophrenia suggest there is no overproduction of dopamine.[14,15] Dopamine antagonists are thus unlikely to be effective.

It is recommended that all augmentation attempts are carefully monitored and, if no clear benefit is forthcoming, abandoned after 3–6 months. The addition of another drug to clozapine treatment must be expected to worsen overall adverse effect burden and so continued ineffective treatment is not appropriate. In some cases, the addition of an augmenting agent may reduce the severity of some adverse effects (e.g. weight gain, dyslipidaemia) or allow a reduction in clozapine dose. The addition of aripiprazole to clozapine may be particularly effective in reversing metabolic effects.[16,17]

Table 2.36 shows suggested treatment options (in alphabetical order) where 3–6 months of optimised clozapine alone has provided unsatisfactory benefit.

Table 2.36 Suggested options for augmenting clozapine

Option	Comment
Add amisulpride[18–23] (400–800 mg/day)	▪ Some evidence and experience suggests amisulpride augmentation may be worthwhile. One small RCT. May allow clozapine dose reduction.[24] Large study – AMICUS – in progress
Add aripiprazole[16,25–27] (15–30 mg/day)	▪ Very limited evidence of therapeutic benefit. Improves metabolic parameters
Add haloperidol[27–29] (2–3 mg/day)	▪ Modest evidence of benefit
Add lamotrigine[30–32] (25–300 mg/day)	▪ May be useful in partial or non-responders. May reduce alcohol consumption.[33] Several equivocal reports[34–36] but meta-analysis suggests moderate effect size[37]
Add omega-3 triglycerides[38,39] (2–3 g EPA daily)	▪ Modest, and somewhat contested, evidence to support efficacy in non- or partial responders to antipsychotics, including clozapine
Add risperidone[40,41] (2–6 mg/day)	▪ Supported by an RCT but there are also two negative RCTs each with minuscule response rates[42,43] Small number of reports of increases in clozapine plasma levels. Long-term injection also an option[44]
Add sulpiride[45] (400 mg/day)	▪ May be useful in partial or non-responders. Supported by a single randomised trial in English and three in Chinese.[46] Overall effect modest
Add topiramate[47–51] (50–300 mg/day)	▪ Two positive RCTs, two negative. Can worsen psychosis in some.[31,52] Causes weight loss but impairs cognitive function (especially at doses >200 mg/day). Not recommended
Add ziprasidone[53–56] (80–160 mg/day)	▪ Supported by two RCTs.[56,57] Associated with QTc prolongation. Rarely used

Notes:
- Always consider the use of mood stabilisers and/or antidepressants especially where mood disturbance is thought to contribute to symptoms.[58–60]
- Other options include adding **pimozide**, **olanzapine** or **sertindole**. None is recommended: pimozide and sertindole have important cardiac toxicity and the addition of olanzapine is poorly supported[61] and likely to exacerbate metabolic adverse effects. Several studies of pimozide[62,63] and sertindole[64] have shown no effect. One small RCT supports the use of **Ginkgo biloba**,[65] another supports the use of **memantine.**[66]

References

1. Taylor D et al. A prescription survey of the use of atypical antipsychotics for hospital patients in the UK. Int J Psychiatry Clin Pract 2000; 4:41–46.
2. Murphy B et al. Maintenance doses for clozapine. Psychiatr Bull 1998; 22:12–14.
3. Taylor D. Pharmacokinetic interactions involving clozapine. Br J Psychiatry 1997; 171:109–112.
4. Lane HY et al. Effects of gender and age on plasma levels of clozapine and its metabolites: analyzed by critical statistics. J Clin Psychiatry 1999; 60:36–40.
5. Taylor D et al. The use of clozapine plasma levels in optimising therapy. Psychiatr Bull 1995; 19:753–755.
6. Spina E et al. Relationship between plasma concentrations of clozapine and norclozapine and therapeutic response in patients with schizophrenia resistant to conventional neuroleptics. Psychopharmacology 2000; 148:83–89.
7. Perry PJ. Therapeutic drug monitoring of antipsychotics. Psychopharmacol Bull 2001; 35:19–29.
8. Papetti F et al. [Clozapine-resistant schizophrenia related to an increased metabolism and benefit of fluvoxamine: four case reports]. Encephale 2007; 33:811–818.

9. Watras M et al. A therapeutic interaction between cimetidine and clozapine: case study and review of the literature. Ther Adv Psychopharmacol 2013; 3:294–297.

10. Barbui C et al. Does the addition of a second antipsychotic drug improve clozapine treatment? Schizophr Bull 2009; 35:458–468.

11. Paton C et al. Augmentation with a second antipsychotic in patients with schizophrenia who partially respond to clozapine: a meta-analysis. J Clin Psychopharmacol 2007; 27:198–204.

12. Taylor DM et al. Augmentation of clozapine with a second antipsychotic - a meta-analysis of randomized, placebo-controlled studies. Acta Psychiatr Scand 2009; 119:419–425.

13. Taylor D et al. Augmentation of clozapine with a second antipsychotic. A meta analysis. Acta Psychiatr Scand 2012; 125:15–24.

14. Demjaha A et al. Dopamine synthesis capacity in patients with treatment-resistant schizophrenia. Am J Psychiatry 2012; 169:1203–1210.

15. Demjaha A et al. Antipsychotic treatment resistance in schizophrenia associated with elevated glutamate levels but normal dopamine function. Biol Psychiatry 2014; 75:e11–e13.

16. Fleischhacker WW et al. Effects of adjunctive treatment with aripiprazole on body weight and clinical efficacy in schizophrenia patients treated with clozapine: a randomized, double-blind, placebo-controlled trial. Int J Neuropsychopharmacol 2010; 13:1115–1125.

17. Correll CU et al. Selective effects of individual antipsychotic cotreatments on cardiometabolic and hormonal risk status: results from a systematic review and meta-analysis. Schizophr Bull 2013; 39 (Suppl 1):S29–S30.

18. Matthiasson P et al. Relationship between dopamine D2 receptor occupancy and clinical response in amisulpride augmentation of clozapine non-response. J Psychopharmacol 2001; 15:S41.

19. Munro J et al. Amisulpride augmentation of clozapine: an open non-randomized study in patients with schizophrenia partially responsive to clozapine. Acta Psychiatr Scand 2004; 110:292–298.

20. Zink M et al. Combination of clozapine and amisulpride in treatment-resistant schizophrenia--case reports and review of the literature. Pharmacopsychiatry 2004; 37:26–31.

21. Ziegenbein M et al. Augmentation of clozapine with amisulpride in patients with treatment-resistant schizophrenia. An open clinical study. German J Psychiatry 2006; 9:17–21.

22. Kampf P et al. Augmentation of clozapine with amisulpride: a promising therapeutic approach to refractory schizophrenic symptoms. Pharmacopsychiatry 2005; 38:39–40.

23. Assion HJ et al. Amisulpride augmentation in patients with schizophrenia partially responsive or unresponsive to clozapine. A randomized, double-blind, placebo-controlled trial. Pharmacopsychiatry 2008; 41:24–28.

24. Croissant B et al. Reduction of side effects by combining clozapine with amisulpride: case report and short review of clozapine-induced hypersalivation-a case report. Pharmacopsychiatry 2005; 38:38–39.

25. Chang JS et al. Aripiprazole augmentation in clozapine-treated patients with refractory schizophrenia: an 8-week, randomized, double-blind, placebo-controlled trial. J Clin Psychiatry 2008; 69:720–731.

26. Muscatello MR et al. Effect of aripiprazole augmentation of clozapine in schizophrenia: a double-blind, placebo-controlled study. Schizophr Res 2011; 127:93–99.

27. Cipriani A et al. Aripiprazole versus haloperidol in combination with clozapine for treatment-resistant schizophrenia: a 12-month, randomized, naturalistic trial. J Clin Psychopharmacol 2013; 33:533–537.

28. Rajarethinam R et al. Augmentation of clozapine partial responders with conventional antipsychotics. Schizophr Res 2003; 60:97–98.

29. Barbui C et al. Aripiprazole versus haloperidol in combination with clozapine for treatment-resistant schizophrenia in routine clinical care: a randomized, controlled trial. J Clin Psychopharmacol 2011; 31:266–273.

30. Dursun SM et al. Clozapine plus lamotrigine in treatment-resistant schizophrenia. Arch Gen Psychiatry 1999; 56:950.

31. Dursun SM et al. Augmenting antipsychotic treatment with lamotrigine or topiramate in patients with treatment-resistant schizophrenia: a naturalistic case-series outcome study. J Psychopharmacol 2001; 15:297–301.

32. Tiihonen J et al. Lamotrigine in treatment-resistant schizophrenia: a randomized placebo-controlled crossover trial. Biol Psychiatry 2003; 54:1241–1248.

33. Kalyoncu A et al. Use of lamotrigine to augment clozapine in patients with resistant schizophrenia and comorbid alcohol dependence: a potent anti-craving effect? J Psychopharmacol 2005; 19:301–305.

34. Goff DC et al. Lamotrigine as add-on therapy in schizophrenia: results of 2 placebo-controlled trials. J Clin Psychopharmacol 2007; 27:582–589.

35. Heck AH et al. Addition of lamotrigine to clozapine in inpatients with chronic psychosis. J Clin Psychiatry 2005; 66:1333.

36. Vayisoglu S et al. Lamotrigine augmentation in patients with schizophrenia who show partial response to clozapine treatment. Schizophr Res 2013; 143:207–214.

37. Tiihonen J et al. The efficacy of lamotrigine in clozapine-resistant schizophrenia: a systematic review and meta-analysis. Schizophr Res 2009; 109:10–14.

38. Peet M et al. Double-blind placebo controlled trial of N-3 polyunsaturated fatty acids as an adjunct to neuroleptics. Schizophr Res 1998; 29:160–161.

39. Puri BK et al. Sustained remission of positive and negative symptoms of schizophrenia following treatment with eicosapentaenoic acid. Arch Gen Psychiatry 1998; 55:188–189.

40. Josiassen RC et al. Clozapine augmented with risperidone in the treatment of schizophrenia: a randomized, double-blind, placebo-controlled trial. Am J Psychiatry 2005; 162:130–136.

41. Raskin S et al. Clozapine and risperidone: combination/augmentation treatment of refractory schizophrenia: a preliminary observation. Acta Psychiatr Scand 2000; 101:334–336.

42. Anil Yagcioglu AE et al. A double-blind controlled study of adjunctive treatment with risperidone in schizophrenic patients partially responsive to clozapine: efficacy and safety. J Clin Psychiatry 2005; 66:63–72.

CHAPTER 2

43. Honer WG et al. Clozapine alone versus clozapine and risperidone with refractory schizophrenia. N Engl J Med 2006; **354**:472–482.
44. Se HK et al. The combined use of risperidone long-acting injection and clozapine in patients with schizophrenia non-adherent to clozapine: a case series. J Psychopharmacol 2010; **24**:981–986.
45. Shiloh R et al. Sulpiride augmentation in people with schizophrenia partially responsive to clozapine. A double-blind, placebo-controlled study. Br J Psychiatry 1997; **171**:569–573.
46. Wang J et al. Sulpiride augmentation for schizophrenia. Schizophr Bull 2010; **36**:229–230.
47. Tiihonen J et al. Topiramate add-on in treatment-resistant schizophrenia: a randomized, double-blind, placebo-controlled, crossover trial. J Clin Psychiatry 2005; **66**:1012–1015.
48. Afshar H et al. Topiramate add-on treatment in schizophrenia: a randomised, double-blind, placebo-controlled clinical trial. J Psychopharmacol 2009; **23**:157–162.
49. Muscatello MR et al. Topiramate augmentation of clozapine in schizophrenia: a double-blind, placebo-controlled study. J Psychopharmacol 2011; **25**:667–674.
50. Hahn MK et al. Topiramate augmentation in clozapine-treated patients with schizophrenia: clinical and metabolic effects. J Clin Psychopharmacol 2010; **30**:706–710.
51. Behdani F et al. Effect of topiramate augmentation in chronic schizophrenia: a placebo-controlled trial. Arch Iran Med 2011; **14**:270–275.
52. Millson RC et al. Topiramate for refractory schizophrenia. Am J Psychiatry 2002; **159**:675.
53. Zink M et al. Combination of ziprasidone and clozapine in treatment-resistant schizophrenia. Hum Psychopharmacol 2004; **19**:271–273.
54. Ziegenbein M et al. Clozapine and ziprasidone: a useful combination in patients with treatment-resistant schizophrenia. J Neuropsychiatry Clin Neurosci 2006; **18**:246–247.
55. Ziegenbein M et al. Combination of clozapine and ziprasidone in treatment-resistant schizophrenia: an open clinical study. Clin Neuropharmacol 2005; **28**:220–224.
56. Zink M et al. Efficacy and tolerability of ziprasidone versus risperidone as augmentation in patients partially responsive to clozapine: a randomised controlled clinical trial. J Psychopharmacol 2009; **23**:305–314.
57. Muscatello MR et al. Augmentation of clozapine with ziprasidone in refractory schizophrenia: a double-blind, placebo-controlled study. J Clin Psychopharmacol 2014; **34**:129–133.
58. Citrome L. Schizophrenia and valproate. Psychopharmacol Bull 2003; **37 Suppl** 2:74–88.
59. Tranulis C et al. Somatic augmentation strategies in clozapine resistance--what facts? Clin Neuropharmacol 2006; **29**:34–44.
60. Suzuki T et al. Augmentation of atypical antipsychotics with valproic acid. An open-label study for most difficult patients with schizophrenia. Hum Psychopharmacol 2009; **24**:628–638.
61. Gupta S et al. Olanzapine augmentation of clozapine. Ann Clin Psychiatry 1998; **10**:113–115.
62. Friedman JI et al. Pimozide augmentation of clozapine inpatients with schizophrenia and schizoaffective disorder unresponsive to clozapine monotherapy. Neuropsychopharmacology 2011; **36**:1289–1295.
63. Gunduz-Bruce H et al. Efficacy of pimozide augmentation for clozapine partial responders with schizophrenia. Schizophr Res 2013; **143**:344–347.
64. Nielsen J et al. Augmenting clozapine with sertindole: a double-blind, randomized, placebo-controlled study. J Clin Psychopharmacol 2012; **32**:173–178.
65. Doruk A et al. A placebo-controlled study of extract of ginkgo biloba added to clozapine in patients with treatment-resistant schizophrenia. Int Clin Psychopharmacol 2008; **23**:223–227.
66. de Lucena D et al. Improvement of negative and positive symptoms in treatment-refractory schizophrenia: a double-blind, randomized, placebo-controlled trial with memantine as add-on therapy to clozapine. J Clin Psychiatry 2009; **70**:1416–1423.

Further reading

Nielsen J et al. Optimizing clozapine treatment. Acta Psychiatr Scand 2011; **123**:411–422.
Porcelli S et al. Clozapine resistance: augmentation strategies. Eur Neuropsychopharmacol 2012; **22**:165–182.
Remington G et al. Augmenting strategies in clozapine-resistant schizophrenia. CNS Drugs 2006;**20**:171.
Sommer IE et al. Pharmacological augmentation strategies for schizophrenia patients with insufficient response to clozapine: a quantitative literature review. Schizophr Bull 2011; **38**:1003–1111.

Alternatives to clozapine

Clozapine is the treatment of choice in refractory schizophrenia. Where treatment resistence is established, clozapine treatment should not normally be delayed or withheld. The practice of using successive antipsychotics (or the latest) instead of clozapine is widespread but not supported by any cogent research. Where clozapine cannot be used (because of toxicity or patient refusal) other drugs or drug combinations may be tried (Table 2.37) but outcome is usually disappointing. Available data do not allow the drawing of any distinction between treatment regimens, but it seems wise to use single drugs before trying multiple drug regimens. In practice, olanzapine is most often used, usually in above licensed doses. If this fails, then the addition of a second antipsychotic (amisulpride, for example) is a reasonable next step. Amongst unconventional agents, minocycline and ondansetron have the advantage of low toxcity and very good tolerability. Depot medication is an option where adherence is in doubt. Many of the treatments listed below are somewhat experimental and some of the compounds difficult to obtain (e.g. glycine, D-serine, sarcosine, etc). Before using any of the regimens outlined, readers should consult the primary literature cited. Particular care should be taken to inform patients where prescribing is off-label and to ensure they understand the potential side-effects of more experimental treatments.

Table 2.37 Alternatives to clozapine. Treatments are listed in alphabetical order: no preference is implied by position in table

Treatment	Comments
Allopurinol 300–600 mg/day **(+antipsychotic)**[1–4]	Increases adenosinergic transmission which may reduce effects of dopamine. Three positive RCTs[1,2,4]
Amisulpride[5] (up to 1200 mg/day)	Single, small open study. Not usually a treatment option in practice
Aripiprazole[6,7] (15–30 mg/day)	Single randomized controlled study indicating moderate effect in patients resistant to risperidone or olanzapine (+others). Higher doses (60 mg/day) have been used[8]
Bexarotene 75 mg/day[9] **(+antipsychotic)**	Retinoid receptor agonist. One RCT (n = 90) in non-refractory but suboptimally treated patients suggest worthwhile effect on positive symptoms.
CBT[10]	Non-drug therapies should always be considered
Celexcoxib + risperidone[11] (400 mg + 6 mg/day)	COX-2 inhibitors modulate immune response and may prevent glutamate-related cell death. One RCT showed useful activity in all main symptom domains. Associated with increased caardiovascular mortality
Donepezil 5–10 mg/day **(+antipsychotic)**[12–14]	Three RCTs, one negative,[13] two positive,[12,14] suggesting a small effect on cognitive and negative symptoms
D-Alanine 100 mg/kg/day **(+antipsychotic)**[15]	Glycine (NMDA) agonist. One positive RCT

Continued

Table 2.37 (Continued)

Treatment	Comments
D-Serine 30 mg/kg/day (+olanzapine)[16]	Glycine (NMDA) agonist. One positive RCT
D-serine up to 3 g as monotherapy[17]	Improved negative symptoms in one RCT, but inferior to high dose olanzapine for treatment of positive symptoms
ECT[18-21]	Open studies suggest moderate effect. Often reserved for last-line treatment in practice but can be successful in the short[22] and long[23] term
Famotidine 100 mg bd + antipsychotic[24]	H₂ antagonist. One short (4 week) RCT suggested some benefit in overall PANSS and CGI scores
Ginkgo biloba **(+antipsychotic)**[25,26]	Possibly effective in combination with haloperidol. Unlikely to give rise to additional adverse effects but clinical experience limited
Memantine 20 mg/day (+antipsychotic)[27-29]	Memantine is an NMDA antagonist. Two RCTs. The larger of the two (n = 138) was negative. In the smaller (n = 21), memantine improved positive and negative symptoms when added to clozapine. In another study in non-refractory schizophrenia, memantine improved negative symptoms when added to risperidone
Mianserin + FGA 30 mg/day[30]	5HT₂ antagonist. One, small positive RCT
Minocycline 200 mg/day (+antipsychotic)[31,32]	May be anti-inflammatory and neuroprotective. One open study (n = 22) and one RCT (n = 54) suggest good effect on negative and cognitive symptoms. Also two cases of augmentation of clozapine.[33] RCT evidence of neuroprotective effect in early psychosis[34]
Mirtazapine 30 mg/day (+antipsychotic)[35-37]	5HT₂ antagonist. Two RCTs, one negative,[36] one positive.[35] Effect seems to be mainly on positive symptoms
N-acetylcysteine 2 g/day (+antipsychotic)[38]	One RCT suggests small benefits in negative symptoms and rates of akathisia. Case study of successful use of 600 mg a day[39]
Olanzapine[40-45] 5–25 mg/day	Supported by some well conducted trials but clinical experience disappointing. Some patients show moderate response
Olanzapine[46-52] 30–60 mg/day	Contradictory findings in the literature but possibly effective. High dose olanzapine is not atypical[53] and can be poorly tolerated[54] with gross metabolic changes[52]
Olanzapine + amisulpride[55] (up to 800 mg/day)	Small open study suggests benefit
Olanzapine + aripiprazole[56]	Single case report suggests benefit. Probably reduces metabolic toxicity
Olanzapine + glycine[57] (0.8 g/kg/day)	Small, double-blind crossover trial suggests clinically relevant improvement in negative symptoms
Olanzapine + lamotrigine[58,59] (up to 400 mg/day)	Reports contradictory and rather unconvincing. Reasonable theoretical basis for adding lamotrigine which is usually well tolerated
Olanzapine + risperidone[60] (various doses)	Small study suggests some patients may benefit from combined therapy after sequential failure of each drug alone
Olanzapine + sulpiride[61] (600 mg/day)	Some evidence that this combination improves mood symptoms

Table 2.37 (*Continued*)

Treatment	Comments
Omega-3-triglycerides[62,63]	Suggested efficacy but data very limited
Ondansetron 8 mg/day (**+antipsychotic**)[64,65]	Two RCTs. Both show improvements in negative and cognitive symptoms
Propentofylline + risperidone[66] (900 mg + 6 mg/day)	One RCT suggests some activity against postive symptoms
Quetiapine[67–70]	Very limited evidence and clinical experience not encouraging. High doses (>1200 mg/day) have been used but are no more effective[71]
Quetiapine + amisulpride[72]	Single naturalistic observation of 19 patients suggested useful benefit. Doses averaged 700 mg quetiapine and 950 mg amisulpride
Quetiapine + haloperidol[73]	Two case reports
Riluzole 100 mg/day + **risperidone** up to 6 mg/day[74]	Glutamate modulating agent. One RCT demonstrated improvement in negative symptoms
Risperidone[75–77] 4–8 mg/day	Doubtful efficacy in true treatment-refractory schziophrenia but some supporting evidence. May also be tried in combination with glycine[57] or lamotrigine[58] or indeed with other atypicals[78]
Risperidone 50/100 mg 2/52[79]	One RCT showing good response for both doses in refractory schizophrenia. Plasma levels for 100 mg dose similar to 6–8 mg/day oral risperidone
Ritanserin + risperidone (12 mg + 6 mg/day)[80]	$5HT_{2A/2C}$ antagonist. One RCT suggests small effect on negative symptoms
Sarcosine (2 g/day)[81,82] (**+antipsychotic**)	Enhances glycine action. Supported by two RCTs
Sertindole[83] (12–24 mg/day)	One large RCT (conducted in 1996–8 but published in 2011) suggested good effect and equivalence to risperidone. Around half of subjects responded. Another RCT[84] showed no effect at all when added to clozapine. Little experience in practice
Topiramate (300 mg/day) (**+antipsychotic**)[85]	Small effect shown in single RCT. Induces weight loss. Cognitive adverse effects likely
Transcranial magnetic stimulation[86,87]	Probably not effective
Valproate[88]	Doubtful effect but may be useful where there is a clear affective component
Ziprasidone 80–160 mg/day[89–91]	Two good RCTs. One[91] suggests superior efficacy to chlorpromazine in refractory schziophrenia, the other[89] suggests equivalence to clozapine in subjects with treatment intolerance/resistance. Disappointing results in practice, however. Supratherapeutic doses offer no advantage[92]

CBT, cognitive behavioural therapy; CGI, clinical global impression; COX, cyclo-oxgenase; ECT, electroconvulsive therapy; FGA, first-generation antipsychotic; NMDA, N-methyl-D-aspartate; PANSS, positive and negative syndrome scale; RCT, randomised controlled trial.

CHAPTER 2

References

1. Akhondzadeh S et al. Beneficial antipsychotic effects of allopurinol as add-on therapy for schizophrenia: a double blind, randomized and placebo controlled trial. Prog Neuropsychopharmacol Biol Psychiatry 2005; 29:253–259.
2. Brunstein MG et al. A clinical trial of adjuvant allopurinol therapy for moderately refractory schizophrenia. J Clin Psychiatry 2005; 66:213–219.
3. Buie LW et al. Allopurinol as adjuvant therapy in poorly responsive or treatment refractory schizophrenia. Ann Pharmacother 2006; 40:2200–2204.
4. Dickerson FB et al. A double-blind trial of adjunctive allopurinol for schizophrenia. Schizophr Res 2009; 109:66–69.
5. Kontaxakis VP et al. Switching to amisulpride monotherapy for treatment-resistant schizophrenia. Eur Psychiatry 2006; 21:214–217.
6. Kane JM et al. Aripiprazole for treatment-resistant schizophrenia: results of a multicenter, randomized, double-blind, comparison study versus perphenazine. J Clin Psychiatry 2007; 68:213–223.
7. Hsu WY et al. Aripiprazole in treatment-refractory schizophrenia. J Psychiatr Pract 2009; 15:221–226.
8. Crossman AM et al. Tolerability of high-dose aripiprazole in treatment-refractory schizophrenic patients. J Clin Psychiatry 2006; 67:1158–1159.
9. Lerner V et al. The retinoid X receptor agonist bexarotene relieves positive symptoms of schizophrenia: a 6-week, randomized, double-blind, placebo-controlled multicenter trial. J Clin Psychiatry 2013; 74:1224–1232.
10. Valmaggia LR et al. Cognitive-behavioural therapy for refractory psychotic symptoms of schizophrenia resistant to atypical antipsychotic medication. Randomised controlled trial. Br J Psychiatry 2005; 186:324–330.
11. Akhondzadeh S et al. Celecoxib as adjunctive therapy in schizophrenia: a double-blind, randomized and placebo-controlled trial. Schizophr Res 2007; 90:179–185.
12. Lee BJ et al. A 12-week, double-blind, placebo-controlled trial of donepezil as an adjunct to haloperidol for treating cognitive impairments in patients with chronic schizophrenia. J Psychopharmacol 2007; 21:421–427.
13. Keefe RSE et al. Efficacy and safety of donepezil in patients with schizophrenia or schizoaffective disorder: significant placebo/practice effects in a 12-week, randomized, double-blind, placebo-controlled trial. Neuropsychopharmacology 2007; 33:1217–1228.
14. Akhondzadeh S et al. A 12-week, double-blind, placebo-controlled trial of donepezil adjunctive treatment to risperidone in chronic and stable schizophrenia. Prog Neuropsychopharmacol Biol Psychiatry 2008; 32:1810–1815.
15. Tsai GE et al. D-alanine added to antipsychotics for the treatment of schizophrenia. Biol Psychiatry 2006; 59:230–234.
16. Heresco-Levy U et al. D-serine efficacy as add-on pharmacotherapy to risperidone and olanzapine for treatment-refractory schizophrenia. Biol Psychiatry 2005; 57:577–585.
17. Ermilov M et al. A pilot double-blind comparison of d-serine and high-dose olanzapine in treatment-resistant patients with schizophrenia. Schizophr Res 2013; 150:604–605.
18. Chanpattana W et al. Combined ECT and neuroleptic therapy in treatment-refractory schizophrenia: prediction of outcome. Psychiatry Res 2001; 105:107–115.
19. Tang WK et al. Efficacy of electroconvulsive therapy in treatment-resistant schizophrenia: a prospective open trial. Prog Neuropsychopharmacol Biol Psychiatry 2003; 27:373–379.
20. Chanpattana W et al. Acute and maintenance ECT with flupenthixol in refractory schizophrenia: sustained improvements in psychopathology, quality of life, and social outcomes. Schizophr Res 2003; 63:189–193.
21. Chanpattana W et al. ECT for treatment-resistant schizophrenia: a response from the far East to the UK. NICE report. J ECT 2006; 22:4–12.
22. Chanpattana W et al. Electroconvulsive therapy in treatment-resistant schizophrenia: prediction of response and the nature of symptomatic improvement. J ECT 2010; 26:289–298.
23. Ravanic DB et al. Long-term efficacy of electroconvulsive therapy combined with different antipsychotic drugs in previously resistant schizophrenia. Psychiatr Danub 2009; 21:179–186.
24. Meskanen K et al. A randomized clinical trial of histamine 2 receptor antagonism in treatment-resistant schizophrenia. J Clin Psychopharmacol 2013; 33:472–478.
25. Zhou D et al. The effects of classic antipsychotic haloperidol plus the extract of ginkgo biloba on superoxide dismutase in patients with chronic refractory schizophrenia. Chin Med J 1999; 112:1093–1096.
26. Zhang XY et al. A double-blind, placebo-controlled trial of extract of Ginkgo biloba added to haloperidol in treatment-resistant patients with schizophrenia. J Clin Psychiatry 2001; 62:878–883.
27. Lieberman JA et al. A randomized, placebo-controlled study of memantine as adjunctive treatment in patients with schizophrenia. Neuropsychopharmacology 2009; 34:1322–1329.
28. de Lucena D et al. Improvement of negative and positive symptoms in treatment-refractory schizophrenia: a double-blind, randomized, placebo-controlled trial with memantine as add-on therapy to clozapine. J Clin Psychiatry 2009; 70:1416–1423.
29. Rezaei F et al. Memantine add-on to risperidone for treatment of negative symptoms in patients with stable schizophrenia: randomized, double-blind, placebo-controlled study. J Clin Psychopharmacol 2013; 33:336–342.
30. Shiloh R et al. Mianserin or placebo as adjuncts to typical antipsychotics in resistant schizophrenia. Int Clin Psychopharmacol 2002; 17:59–64.
31. Levkovitz Y et al. A double-blind, randomized study of minocycline for the treatment of negative and cognitive symptoms in early-phase schizophrenia. J Clin Psychiatry 2010; 71:138–149.
32. Miyaoka T et al. Minocycline as adjunctive therapy for schizophrenia: an open-label study. Clin Neuropharmacol 2008; 31:287–292.

33. Kelly DL et al. Adjunct minocycline to clozapine treated patients with persistent schizophrenia symptoms. Schizophr Res 2011; **133**:257–258.

34. Chaudhry IB et al. Minocycline benefits negative symptoms in early schizophrenia: a randomised double-blind placebo-controlled clinical trial in patients on standard treatment. J Psychopharmacol 2012; **26**:1185–1193.

35. Joffe G et al. Add-on mirtazapine enhances antipsychotic effect of first generation antipsychotics in schizophrenia: A double-blind, randomized, placebo-controlled trial. Schizophr Res 2009; **108**:245–251.

36. Berk M et al. Mirtazapine add-on therapy in the treatment of schizophrenia with atypical antipsychotics: a double-blind, randomised, placebo-controlled clinical trial. Hum Psychopharmacol 2009; **24**:233–238.

37. Delle CR et al. Add-on mirtazapine enhances effects on cognition in schizophrenic patients under stabilized treatment with clozapine. Exp Clin Psychopharmacol 2007; **15**:563–568.

38. Berk M et al. N-acetyl cysteine as a glutathione precursor for schizophrenia--a double-blind, randomized, placebo-controlled trial. Biol Psychiatry 2008; **64**:361–368.

39. Bulut M et al. Beneficial effects of N-acetylcysteine in treatment resistant schizophrenia. World J Biol Psychiatry 2009; **10**:626–628.

40. Breier A et al. Comparative efficacy of olanzapine and haloperidol for patients with treatment-resistant schizophrenia. Biol Psychiatry 1999; **45**:403–411.

41. Conley RR et al. Olanzapine compared with chlorpromazine in treatment-resistant schizophrenia. Am J Psychiatry 1998; **155**:914–920.

42. Sanders RD et al. An open trial of olanzapine in patients with treatment-refractory psychoses. J Clin Psychopharmacol 1999; **19**:62–66.

43. Taylor D et al. Olanzapine in practice: a prospective naturalistic study. Psychiatr Bull 1999; **23**:178–180.

44. Bitter I et al. Olanzapine versus clozapine in treatment-resistant or treatment-intolerant schizophrenia. Prog Neuropsychopharmacol Biol Psychiatry 2004; **28**:173–180.

45. Tollefson GD et al. Double-blind comparison of olanzapine versus clozapine in schizophrenic patients clinically eligible for treatment with clozapine. Biol Psychiatry 2001; **49**:52–63.

46. Sheitman BB et al. High-dose olanzapine for treatment-refractory schizophrenia. Am J Psychiatry 1997; **154**:1626.

47. Fanous A et al. Schizophrenia and schizoaffective disorder treated with high doses of olanzapine. J Clin Psychopharmacol 1999; **19**:275–276.

48. Dursun SM et al. Olanzapine for patients with treatment-resistant schizophrenia: a naturalistic case-series outcome study. Can J Psychiatry 1999; **44**:701–704.

49. Conley RR et al. The efficacy of high-dose olanzapine versus clozapine in treatment-resistant schizophrenia: a double-blind crossover study. J Clin Psychopharmacol 2003; **23**:668–671.

50. Kumra S et al. Clozapine and "high-dose" olanzapine in refractory early-onset schizophrenia: a 12-week randomized and double-blind comparison. Biol Psychiatry 2008; **63**:524–529.

51. Kumra S et al. Clozapine versus "high-dose" olanzapine in refractory early-onset schizophrenia: an open-label extension study. J Child Adolesc Psychopharmacol 2008; **18**:307–316.

52. Meltzer HY et al. A randomized, double-blind comparison of clozapine and high-dose olanzapine in treatment-resistant patients with schizophrenia. J Clin Psychiatry 2008; **69**:274–285.

53. Bronson BD et al. Adverse effects of high-dose olanzapine in treatment-refractory schizophrenia. J Clin Psychopharmacol 2000; **20**:382–384.

54. Kelly DL et al. Adverse effects and laboratory parameters of high-dose olanzapine vs. clozapine in treatment-resistant schizophrenia. Ann Clin Psychiatry 2003; **15**:181–186.

55. Zink M et al. Combination of amisulpride and olanzapine in treatment-resistant schizophrenic psychoses. Eur Psychiatry 2004; **19**:56–58.

56. Duggal HS. Aripirazole-olanzapine combination for treatment of schizophrenia. Can J Psychiatry 2004; **49**:151.

57. Heresco-Levy U et al. High-dose glycine added to olanzapine and risperidone for the treatment of schizophrenia. Biol Psychiatry 2004; **55**:165–171.

58. Kremer I et al. Placebo-controlled trial of lamotrigine added to conventional and atypical antipsychotics in schizophrenia. Biol Psychiatry 2004; **56**:441–446.

59. Dursun SM et al. Augmenting antipsychotic treatment with lamotrigine or topiramate in patients with treatment-resistant schizophrenia: a naturalistic case-series outcome study. J Psychopharmacol 2001; **15**:297–301.

60. Suzuki T et al. Effectiveness of antipsychotic polypharmacy for patients with treatment refractory schizophrenia: an open-label trial of olanzapine plus risperidone for those who failed to respond to a sequential treatment with olanzapine, quetiapine and risperidone. Hum Psychopharmacol 2008; **23**:455–463.

61. Kotler M et al. Sulpiride augmentation of olanzapine in the management of treatment-resistant chronic schizophrenia: evidence for improvement of mood symptomatology. Int Clin Psychopharmacol 2004; **19**:23–26.

62. Mellor JE et al. Omega-3 fatty acid supplementation in schizophrenic patients. Hum Psychopharmacol 1996; **11**:39–46.

63. Puri BK et al. Sustained remission of positive and negative symptoms of schizophrenia following treatment with eicosapentaenoic acid. Arch Gen Psychiatry 1998; **55**:188–189.

64. Zhang ZJ et al. Beneficial effects of ondansetron as an adjunct to haloperidol for chronic, treatment-resistant schizophrenia: a double-blind, randomized, placebo-controlled study. Schizophr Res 2006; **88**:102–110.

65. Akhondzadeh S et al. Added ondansetron for stable schizophrenia: A double blind, placebo controlled trial. Schizophr Res 2009; **107**:206–212.

66. Salimi S et al. A placebo controlled study of the propentofylline added to risperidone in chronic schizophrenia. Prog Neuropsychopharmacol Biol Psychiatry 2008; **32**:726–732.

67. Reznik I et al. Long-term efficacy and safety of quetiapine in treatment-refractory schizophrenia: A case report. Int J Psychiatry Clin Pract 2000; 4:77–80.

68. De Nayer A et al. Efficacy and tolerability of quetiapine in patients with schizophrenia switched from other antipsychotics. Int J Psychiatry Clin Pract 2003; 7:59–66.

69. Larmo I et al. Efficacy and tolerability of quetiapine in patients with schizophrenia who switched from haloperidol, olanzapine or risperidone. Hum Psychopharmacol 2005; 20:573–581.

70. Boggs DL et al. Quetiapine at high doses for the treatment of refractory schizophrenia. Schizophr Res 2008; 101:347–348.

71. Lindenmayer JP et al. A randomized, double-blind, parallel-group, fixed-dose, clinical trial of quetiapine at 600 versus 1200 mg/d for patients with treatment-resistant schizophrenia or schizoaffective disorder. J Clin Psychopharmacol 2011; 31:160–168.

72. Quintero J et al. The effectiveness of the combination therapy of amisulpride and quetiapine for managing treatment-resistant schizophrenia: a naturalistic study. J Clin Psychopharmacol 2011; 31:240–242.

73. Aziz MA et al. Remission of positive and negative symptoms in refractory schizophrenia with a combination of haloperidol and quetiapine: Two case studies. J Psychiatr Pract 2006; 12:332–336.

74. Farokhnia M et al. A double-blind, placebo controlled, randomized trial of riluzole as an adjunct to risperidone for treatment of negative symptoms in patients with chronic schizophrenia. Psychopharmacology (Berl) 2014; 231:533–542.

75. Breier AF et al. Clozapine and risperidone in chronic schizophrenia: effects on symptoms, parkinsonian side effects, and neuroendocrine response. Am J Psychiatry 1999; 156:294–298.

76. Bondolfi G et al. Risperidone versus clozapine in treatment-resistant chronic schizophrenia: a randomized double-blind study. The Risperidone Study Group. Am J Psychiatry 1998; 155:499–504.

77. Conley RR et al. Risperidone, quetiapine, and fluphenazine in the treatment of patients with therapy-refractory schizophrenia. Clin Neuropharmacol 2005; 28:163–168.

78. Lerner V et al. Combination of "atypical" antipsychotic medication in the management of treatment-resistant schizophrenia and schizoaffective disorder. Prog Neuropsychopharmacol Biol Psychiatry 2004; 28:89–98.

79. Meltzer HY et al. A six month randomized controlled trial of long acting injectable risperidone 50 and 100 mg in treatment resistant schizophrenia. Schizophr Res 2014; 154:14–22.

80. Akhondzadeh S et al. Effect of ritanserin, a 5HT2A/2C antagonist, on negative symptoms of schizophrenia: a double-blind randomized placebo-controlled study. Prog Neuropsychopharmacol Biol Psychiatry 2008; 32:1879–1883.

81. Lane HY et al. Sarcosine or D-serine add-on treatment for acute exacerbation of schizophrenia: a randomized, double-blind, placebo-controlled study. Arch Gen Psychiatry 2005; 62:1196–1204.

82. Tsai G et al. Glycine transporter I inhibitor, N-methylglycine (sarcosine), added to antipsychotics for the treatment of schizophrenia. Biol Psychiatry 2004; 55:452–456.

83. Kane JM et al. A double-blind, randomized study comparing the efficacy and safety of sertindole and risperidone in patients with treatment-resistant schizophrenia. J Clin Psychiatry 2011; 72:194–204.

84. Nielsen J et al. Augmenting clozapine with sertindole: a double-blind, randomized, placebo-controlled study. J Clin Psychopharmacol 2012; 32:173–178.

85. Tiihonen J et al. Topiramate add-on in treatment-resistant schizophrenia: a randomized, double-blind, placebo-controlled, crossover trial. J Clin Psychiatry 2005; 66:1012–1015.

86. Franck N et al. Left temporoparietal transcranial magnetic stimulation in treatment-resistant schizophrenia with verbal hallucinations. Psychiatry Res 2003; 120:107–109.

87. Fitzgerald PB et al. A double-blind sham-controlled trial of repetitive transcranial magnetic stimulation in the treatment of refractory auditory hallucinations. J Clin Psychopharmacol 2005; 25:358–362.

88. Basan A et al. Valproate as an adjunct to antipsychotics for schizophrenia: a systematic review of randomized trials. Schizophr Res 2004; 70:33–37.

89. Sacchetti E et al. Ziprasidone vs clozapine in schizophrenia patients refractory to multiple antipsychotic treatments: the MOZART study. Schizophr Res 2009; 110:80–89.

90. Loebel AD et al. Ziprasidone in treatment-resistant schizophrenia: a 52-week, open-label continuation study. J Clin Psychiatry 2007; 68:1333–1338.

91. Kane JM et al. Efficacy and tolerability of ziprasidone in patients with treatment-resistant schizophrenia. Int Clin Psychopharmacol 2006; 21:21–28.

92. Goff DC et al. High-dose oral ziprasidone versus conventional dosing in schizophrenia patients with residual symptoms: the ZEBRAS study. J Clin Psychopharmacol 2013; 33:485–490.

Re-starting clozapine after a break in treatment

Re-titration of clozapine is somewhat constrained by the manufacturer's recommendation that re-titration should be the same as initial titration if more than 48 hours' clozapine is missed. This recommendation does not seem to be based on any research but it certainly recognises the dangers of giving clozapine to those not tolerant to its effects. However, there is evidence that faster titrations are safe in both those naïve to clozapine and those re-starting it.[93] Table 2.38 gives some broad recommendations on re-starting clozapine after gaps of various lengths. The advice takes into account the need to regain antipsychotic activity with clozapine while ensuring safety during titration. The key feature is that of flexibility: the dose given to the patient depends upon their ability to tolerate prior doses.

Table 2.38 Re-starting clozapine

Time since last clozapine dose	Action to re-start
Up to 48 hours	**Restart at previous dose** – no re-titration required
48–72 hours	**Begin rapid re-titration as soon as possible** Restart with half of the previously prescribed total daily dose on day one (in divided doses 12 hours apart). Then give 75% of previous daily dose on day two and, if tolerated, the whole of the previous daily dose in the normal dosing schedule on day three
72 hours – one week	**Begin re-titration with 12.5 mg or 25 mg clozapine** Increase according to patient tolerability over at least 3 days
More than one week	**Re-titrate as if new patient** Aim to reach previously prescribed dose within 3–4 weeks

Reference

1. Ifteni P et al. Effectiveness and safety of rapid clozapine titration in schizophrenia. Acta Psychiatr Scand 2014;130:25–29.

Initiation of clozapine for community-based patients

Contraindications to community initiation

- History of seizures, significant cardiac disease, unstable diabetes, paralytic ileus, blood dyscrasia, neuroleptic malignant syndrome or other disorder that increases the risk of serious side-effects (initiation with close monitoring in hospital may still be possible).
- Unreliable or chaotic life-style that may affect adherence to the medication or the monitoring regimen.
- Significant abuse of alcohol or other drugs likely to increase the risk of side-effects (e.g. cocaine).

Suitability for community initiation

All the answers should be yes.

- Is the patient likely to be adherent with oral medication and to monitoring requirements?
- Has the patient understood the need for regular physical monitoring and blood tests?
- Has the patient understood the possible side-effects and what to do about them (particularly the rare but serious ones)?
- Is the patient readily contactable (e.g. in the event of a result that needs follow-up)?
- Is it possible for the patient to be seen every day during the early titration phase?
- Is the patient able to collect medication every week or can medication be delivered to their home?
- Is the patient likely to be able to seek help out-of-hours if they experience potentially serious side-effects (eg: indicators of myocarditis or infection such as fever, malaise, chest pain)?

Initial work-up

To screen for risk factors and provide a baseline, carry out:

- physical examination, FBC (see below), LFTs, U&E, lipids, glucose/HbA1c. Consider troponin, CRP, beta-naturietic peptide, ESR (as baseline for further tests)
- ECG – particularly to screen for evidence of past myocardial infarction or ventricular abnormality
- echocardiogram if clinically indicated.

Mandatory blood monitoring and registration

- Register with the relevant monitoring service.
- Perform baseline blood tests (WCC and differential count) before starting clozapine.
- Further blood testing continues weekly for the first 18 weeks and then every 2 weeks for the remainder of the year. After that, the blood monitoring is usually done monthly.
- Inform the patient's GP.

Dosing

Starting clozapine in the community requires a slow and flexible titration schedule. Prior antipsychotics should be slowly discontinued during the titration phase (depots can usually be stopped at the start of titration). Clozapine can cause marked postural hypotension. The initial monitoring is partly aimed at detecting and managing this.

There are two basic methods for starting clozapine in the community. One is to give the first dose in the morning in clinic and then monitor the patient for at least three hours. If the dose is well tolerated, the patient is then allowed home with a dose to take before going to bed. This dosing schedule is described in Table 2.39. This is a very cautious schedule: most patients will tolerate faster titration. The second method involves giving the patient the first dose to take immediately before bed, so avoiding the need for close physical monitoring immediately after administration. Subsequent doses and monitoring is as for the first method. All initiations should take place early in the week (e.g. on a Monday) so that adequate staffing and monitoring are assured.

Adverse effects

Sedation, hypersalivation and hypotension are common at the start of treatment. These effects can usually be managed (see section on 'Common adverse effects' in this chapter) but require particular attention in community titration.

The formal carer (usually the Community Psychiatric Nurse) should inform the prescriber if:

- **temperature rises above 38 °C** (this is very common and is not a good reason, on its own, for stopping clozapine)
- **pulse is >100 bpm** (also common and not, on its own a reason for stopping, but may sometimes be linked to myocarditis)
- **postural drop of >30 mmHg**
- **patient is clearly over-sedated**
- **any other adverse effect is intolerable.**

A doctor should see the patient at least once a week for the first month to assess mental and physical state. Recommended additional monitoring is summarised in Table 2.40.

Consider monitoring plasma troponin, beta-natriuretic peptide and C-reactive protein weekly in the first 6 weeks of treatment, particularly where there is any suspicion of myocarditis (see section on 'Myocarditis' in this chapter).

Switching from other antipsychotics

- The switching regime will be largely dependent on the patient's mental state.
- Consider potential additive side-effects of antipsychotics (e.g. hypotension, sedation, effect on QTc interval).
- Consider drug interactions (e.g. some SSRIs may increase clozapine levels).
- All depots, sertindole, pimozide and ziprasidone should be stopped before clozapine is started.

Table 2.39 Suggested titration regime for initiation of clozapine in the community. Note that much faster titrations can be undertaken in many patients where tolerability allows

Day	Day of the week	Morning dose (mg)	Evening dose (mg)	Monitoring	Percentage dose of previous antipsychotic
1	Monday	6.25	6.25	A	100*
2	Tuesday	6.25	6.25	A	
3	Wednesday	6.25	6.25	A	
4	Thursday	6.25	12.5	A, B, FBC	
5	Friday	12.5	12.5	A Check results from day 4. Remind patient of out-of-hours arrangements for week-end	
6	Saturday	12.5	12.5	No routine monitoring unless clinically indicated	
7	Sunday	12.5	12.5	No routine monitoring unless clinically indicated	
8	Monday	12.5	25	A	75*
9	Tuesday	12.5	25	A	
10	Wednesday	25	25	A	
11	Thursday	25	37.5	A, B, FBC	
12	Friday	25	37.5	A Check results from day 1. Remind patient of out-of-hours arrangements for week-end	
13	Saturday	25	37.5	No routine monitoring unless clinically indicated	
14	Sunday	25	37.5	No routine monitoring unless clinically indicated	
15	Monday	37.5	37.5	A	50*
16	Tuesday	37.5	37.5	Not seen unless problems	
17	Wednesday	37.5	50	A	
18	Thursday	37.5	50	Not seen unless problems	
19	Friday	50	50	A, B, FBC	
20	Saturday	50	50	No routine monitoring unless clinically indicated	
21	Sunday	50	50	No routine monitoring unless clinically indicated	
22	Monday	50	75	A	25*

Table 2.39 *Continued*

Day	Day of the week	Morning dose (mg)	Evening dose (mg)	Monitoring	Percentage dose of previous antipsychotic
23	Tuesday	50	75	Not seen unless problems	
24	Wednesday	75	75	A	
25	Thursday	75	75	Not seen unless problems	
26	Friday	75	100	A, B, FBC	
27	Saturday	75	100	No routine monitoring unless clinically indicated	
28	Sunday	75	100	No routine monitoring unless clinically indicated	

Futher increments should be 25–50 mg/day (generally 25 mg/day) until target dose is reached (use plasma levels). Beware sudden increase in plasma levels due to saturation of first pass metabolism (watch for increase in sedation/ other side-effects).

A, pulse, postural blood pressure, temperature, enquire about side-effects.
B, mental state, weight, review and actively manage side-effects (e.g. behavioural advice, slow clozapine titration or reduce dose of other antipsychotic, start adjunctive treatments – see sections on clozapine adverse effects in this chapter). Consider troponin, C-reactive protein, beta-naturietic peptide.
*May need to be adjusted depending on side-effects and mental state.
FBC, full blood count.

Table 2.40 Recommended additional monitoring

Baseline	1 month	3 months	4-6 months	12 months
Weight/BMI/waist	Weight/BMI/waist	Weight/BMI/waist	Weight/BMI/waist	Weight/BMI/waist
Plasma glucose and lipids	Plasma glucose and lipids		Plasma glucose and lipids	Plasma glucose and lipids
LFTs			LFTs	

BMI, body mass index; LFTs, liver function tests.

- Other antipsychotics and clozapine may be cross-tapered with varying degrees of caution. ECG monitoring is prudent when clozapine is co-prescribed with other drugs known to affect QT interval.

Serious cardiac adverse effects

Patients should be closely observed for signs or symptoms of myocarditis, particularly during the first 2 months, and advised to inform staff if they experience these, and to seek out-of-hours review if necessary. These include persistent tachycardia (although commonly benign), palpitations, shortness of breath, fever, arrhythmia, symptoms mimicking myocardial infarction, chest pain and other unexplained symptoms of heart failure. (See section on 'Serious haematological and cardiovascular adverse effects' in this chapter.)

Further reading

Beck K et al. The practical management of refractory schizophrenia - the Maudsley Treatment Review and Assessment Team service approach. Acta Psychiatr Scand 2014; 130:427–438.

Lovett L. Initiation of clozapine treatment at home. Prog Neurol Psychiatry 2004; 8:19–21.

O'Brien A. Starting clozapine in the community: a UK perspective. CNS Drugs 2004;18:845–52.

CLOZAPINE – ADVERSE EFFECTS

Common adverse effects

Clozapine has a wide range of adverse effects many of which are serious or potentially life-threatening. Table 2.41 describes some more common adverse effects; Table 2.42 deals with rare and serious events.

Table 2.41 Common adverse effects of clozapine

Adverse effect	Time course	Action
Sedation	First few months May persist, but usually wears off to some extent	Give smaller dose in the morning Reduce dose if possible
Hypersalivation	First few months May persist, but sometimes wears off Often very troublesome at night	Give hyoscine 300 µg (Kwells) sucked and swallowed up to three times a day. Many other options (see section on 'Hypersalivation' in this chapter). Note: anticholinergics worsen constipation and cognition
Constipation	First 4 months are the highest risk[1] Usually persists	Advise patients of the risks before starting, screen regularly, ensure adequate fibre, fluid and exercise. Bulk forming laxatives are usually first line, but have a low threshold for adding osmotic and/or stimulant laxatives early. Stop other medicines that may be contributing and reduce clozapine dose if possible. Effective treatment or prevention of constipation is essential as death may result[1–5]
Hypotension	First 4 weeks	Advise patient to take time when standing up. Reduce dose or slow down rate of increase. If severe, consider moclobemide and Bovril,[6] or fludrocortisone. Over longer term, weight gain may lead to hypertension
Hypertension	First 4 weeks, sometimes longer	Monitor closely and increase dose as slowly as is necessary. Hypotensive therapy (e.g. atenolol 25 mg/day) is sometimes necessary[7]
Tachycardia	First 4 weeks, but sometimes persists	Very common in early stages of treatment but usually benign. Tachycardia, if persistent at rest and associated with fever, hypotension or chest pain, may indicate myocarditis[8,9] (see section on 'Serious adverse effects of clozapine' in this chapter). Referral to a cardiologist is advised. Clozapine should be stopped if tachycardia occurs in the context of chest pain or heart failure. Benign sinus tachycardia can be treated with bisoprolol or atenolol.[10] Ivabradine may be used if hypotension or contraindications limit the use of beta-blockers.[11] Note that prolonged tachycardia can itself precipitate cardiomyopathy[12]
Weight gain	Usually during the first year of treatment	Dietary counselling is essential. Advice may be more effective if given before weight gain occurs. Weight gain is common and often profound (>10 lb). Many treatments available (see section on 'Weight gain' in this chapter)

Continued

Table 2.41 (Continued)

Adverse effect	Time course	Action
Fever	First 3 weeks	Clozapine induces inflammatory response (increased CRP and interleukin-6).[13,14] Give paracetamol but check FBC for neutropenia. Reduce rate of dose titration.[15] This fever is not usually related to blood dyscrasias[16,17] but beware myocarditis and NMS (see section on 'Serious adverse effects of clozapine' in this chapter)
Seizures	May occur at any time[18]	Related to dose, plasma level and rapid dose escalation.[19] Consider prophylactic, lamotrigine, gabapentin or valproate* if on high dose (≥500 mg/day) or with high plasma level (≥500 μg/L). Note that some suggest risk of seizures below 1300 μg/L (about 1 in 20 people) is not enough to support primary prophylaxis.[20] After a seizure: withhold clozapine for one day; restart at half previous dose; give anticonvulsant.†EEG abnormalities are common in those on clozapine[21]
Nausea	First 6 weeks	May give anti-emetic. Avoid prochlorperazine and metoclopramide if previous EPS. Avoid domperidone if underlying cardiac risk or QTc prolongation. Ondansetron is a good choice
Nocturnal enuresis	May occur at any time	Try reducing the dose or manipulating dose schedule to avoid periods of deep sedation. Avoid fluids before bedtime. May resolve spontaneously,[22] but may persist for months or years.[23] May affect one in five people on clozapine.[24] In severe cases, desmopressin nasal spray (10–20 μg nocte) is usually effective[25] but is not without risk: hyponatraemia may result.[26] Anticholinergic agents may be effective[27] but support for this approach is weak and constipation and sedation may worsen
Neutropenia/agranulocytosis	First 18 weeks (but may occur at any time)	Stop clozapine; admit to hospital if agranulocytosis confirmed
Gastro-oesophageal reflux disease (GORD)[28]	Any time	Proton pump inhibitors often prescribed. Reasons for GORD association unclear – clozapine is an H_2 antagonist[29]

*Usual dose is 1000–2000 mg/day. Plasma levels may be useful as a rough guide to dosing – aim for 50–100 mg/L. Use of modified-release preparation (Epilim Chrono) may aid compliance: can be given once-daily and may be better tolerated.
†Use valproate if schizoaffective; lamotrigine if poor response to clozapine or continued negative symptoms; topiramate if weight loss required (but beware cognitive adverse effects); gabapentin if other anticonvulsants are poorly tolerated.[19]
CRP, C-reactive protein; EEG, electroencephalogram; EPS, extrapyramidal side-effects; FBC, full blood count; NMS, neuroleptic malignant syndrome.

References

1. Palmer SE et al. Life-threatening clozapine-induced gastrointestinal hypomotility: an analysis of 102 cases. J Clin Psychiatry 2008; **69**:759–768.
2. Townsend G et al. Case report: rapidly fatal bowel ischaemia on clozapine treatment. BMC Psych 2006; **6**:43.
3. Rege S et al. Life-threatening constipation associated with clozapine. Australas Psychiatry 2008; **16**:216–219.
4. Leung JS et al. Rapidly fatal clozapine-induced intestinal obstruction without prior warning signs. Aust N Z J Psychiatry 2008; **42**:1073–1074.
5. Flanagan RJ et al. Gastrointestinal hypomotility: an under-recognised life-threatening adverse effect of clozapine. Forensic Sci Int 2011; **206**:e31–e36.
6. Taylor D et al. Clozapine-induced hypotension treated with moclobemide and Bovril. Br J Psychiatry 1995; **167**:409–410.
7. Henderson DC et al. Clozapine and hypertension: a chart review of 82 patients. J Clin Psychiatry 2004; **65**:686–689.
8. Committee on Safety of Medicines. Clozapine and cardiac safety: updated advice for prescribers. Curr Probl Pharmacovigil 2002; **28**:8.
9. Hagg S et al. Myocarditis related to clozapine treatment. J Clin Psychopharmacol 2001; **21**:382–388.
10. Stryjer R et al. Beta-adrenergic antagonists for the treatment of clozapine-induced sinus tachycardia: a retrospective study. Clin Neuropharmacol 2009; **32**:290–292.
11. Lally J et al. Ivabradine, a novel treatment for clozapine-induced sinus tachycardia: a case series. Ther Adv Psychopharmacol 2014; **4**:117–122.
12. Shinbane JS et al. Tachycardia-Induced Cardiomyopathy: A Review of Animal Models and Clinical Studies. J Am Coll Cardiol 1997; **29**:709–715.
13. Kohen I et al. Increases in C-reactive protein may predict recurrence of clozapine-induced fever. Ann Pharmacother 2009; **43**:143–146.
14. Kluge M et al. Effects of clozapine and olanzapine on cytokine systems are closely linked to weight gain and drug-induced fever. Psychoneuroendocrinology 2009; **34**:118–128.
15. Chung J.P.U. et al. The incidence and characteristics of clozapine- induced fever in a local psychiatric unit in Hong Kong. Can J Psychiatry 2008; **53**:857–862.
16. Tham JC et al. Clozapine-induced fevers and 1-year clozapine discontinuation rate. J Clin Psychiatry 2002; **63**:880–884.
17. Tremeau F et al. Spiking fevers with clozapine treatment. Clin Neuropharmacol 1997; **20**:168–170.
18. Pacia SV et al. Clozapine-related seizures: experience with 5,629 patients. Neurology 1994; **44**:2247–2249.
19. Varma S et al. Clozapine-related EEG changes and seizures: dose and plasma-level relationships. Ther Adv Psychopharmacol 2011; **1**:47–66.
20. Caetano D. Use of anticonvulsants as prophylaxis for seizures in patients on clozapine. Australas Psychiatry 2014; **22**:78–83.
21. Centorrino F et al. EEG abnormalities during treatment with typical and atypical antipsychotics. Am J Psychiatry 2002; **159**:109–115.
22. Warner JP et al. Clozapine and urinary incontinence. Int Clin Psychopharmacol 1994; **9**:207–209.
23. Jeong SH et al. A 2-year prospective follow-up study of lower urinary tract symptoms in patients treated with clozapine. J Clin Psychopharmacol 2008; **28**:618–624.
24. Harrison-Woolrych M et al. Nocturnal enuresis in patients taking clozapine, risperidone, olanzapine and quetiapine: comparative cohort study. Br J Psychiatry 2011; **199**:140–144.
25. Steingard S. Use of desmopressin to treat clozapine-induced nocturnal enuresis. J Clin Psychiatry 1994; **55**:315–316.
26. Sarma S et al. Severe hyponatraemia associated with desmopressin nasal spray to treat clozapine-induced nocturnal enuresis. Aust N Z J Psychiatry 2005; **39**:949.
27. Praharaj SK et al. Amitriptyline for clozapine-induced nocturnal enuresis and sialorrhoea. Br J Clin Pharmacol 2007; **63**:128–129.
28. Taylor D et al. Use of antacid medication in patients receiving clozapine: a comparison with other second-generation antipsychotics. J Clin Psychopharmacol 2010; **30**:460–461.
29. Humbert-Claude M et al. Involvement of histamine receptors in the atypical antipsychotic profile of clozapine: a reassessment in vitro and in vivo. Psychopharmacology (Berl) 2011; **220**:225–241.

Further reading

Iqbal MM et al. Clozapine: a clinical review of adverse effects and management. Ann Clin Psychiatry 2003; **15**: 33–48.
Lieberman JA. Maximizing clozapine therapy: managing side-effects. J Clin Psychiatry 1998; **59** (Suppl. 3): 38–43.

Clozapine: uncommon or unusual adverse effects

Pharmacoepidemiological monitoring of clozapine is more extensive than with any other drug used in psychiatry. Awareness of adverse effects related to clozapine treatment is therefore enhanced. Table 2.42 gives brief details of unusual or uncommon adverse effects of clozapine reported since its relaunch in 1990.

Table 2.42 Uncommon or unusual adverse effects of clozapine

Adverse effect	Comment
Agranulocytosis/ neutropenia (delayed)[1–3]	Occasional reports of apparent clozapine-related blood dyscrasia even after 1 year of treatment. It is possible that clozapine is not the causative agent in some cases[4,5]
Colitis[6–8]	A few reports in the literature, but clear causative link to clozapine not determined. Any severe or chronic diarrhoea should prompt specialist referral as there is a substantial risk of death. Anticholinergic use probably increases risk of colitis and necrosis[9]
Delirium[10,11]	Reported to be fairly common, but rarely seen in practice if dose is titrated slowly and plasma level determinations are used
Eosinophilia[12,13]	Reasonably common but significance unclear. Some suggestion that eosinophilia predicts neutropenia but this is disputed. May be associated with colitis and related symptoms.[14] Occasional reports linking eosinophilia with myocarditis[15]
Heat stroke[16]	Occasional case reported. May be mistaken for neuroleptic malignant syndrome
Hepatic failure/enzyme abnormalities[17–20]	Benign changes in liver function tests are common (up to 50% of patients) but worth monitoring because of the very small risk of fulminant hepatic failure.[21] Rash may be associated with clozapine-related hepatitis[22]
Interstitial nephritis[23,24]	A handful of reports implicating clozapine. May occur after only a few doses
Ocular pigmentation[25]	Single case report
Pancreatitis[26,27]	Rare reports of asymptomatic and symptomatic pancreatitis sometimes associated with eosinophilia. Some authors recommend monitoring serum amylase in all patients treated with clozapine. No cases of successful re-challenge after pancreatitis[28]
Parotid gland swelling[29]	A few case reports. Unclear mechanism, possibly immunological. May be recurrent. Treatment of hypersalivation with terazosin in combination with benzatropine may be helpful
Pericardial effusion[30,31]	Several reports in the literature. Symptoms include fatigue, dyspnoea and tachycardia. Use echocardiogram to confirm/rule out effusion
Pneumonia[32,33]	Very rarely results from saliva aspiration. Pneumonia is a common cause of death in people on clozapine.[33] Infections in general may be more common in those on clozapine[34] and use of antibiotics is also increased.[35] Note that respiratory infections may give rise to elevated clozapine levels.[36,37] (Possibly an artefact: smoking usually ceases during an infection)
Reflux oesophagitis[38]	Those treated with clozapine are more than three times as likely to be treated with antacids than those on other antipsychotics. Reasons unclear
Stuttering[39,40]	Case reports. May be a result of extrapyramidal side-effects or epileptiform activity. Check plasma levels, consider dose reduction and/or anticonvulsant drug
Thrombocytopenia[41]	Few data but apparently fairly common. Probably transient and clinically unimportant
Vasculitis[42]	One report in the literature in which patient developed confluent erythematous rash on lower limbs

References

1. Thompson A et al. Late onset neutropenia with clozapine. Can J Psychiatry 2004; 49:647–648.
2. Bhanji NH et al. Late-onset agranulocytosis in a patient with schizophrenia after 17 months of clozapine treatment. J Clin Psychopharmacol 2003; 23:522–523.
3. Sedky K et al. Clozapine-induced agranulocytosis after 11 years of treatment (Letter). Am J Psychiatry 2005; 162:814.
4. Panesar N et al. Late onset neutropenia with clozapine. Aust N Z J Psychiatry 2011; 45:684.
5. Tourian L et al. Late-onset agranulocytosis in a patient treated with clozapine and lamotrigine. J Clin Psychopharmacol 2011; 31:665–667.
6. Hawe R et al. Response to clozapine-induced microscopic colitis: a case report and review of the literature. J Clin Psychopharmacol 2008; 28:454–455.
7. Shah V et al. Clozapine-induced ischaemic colitis. BMJ Case Rep 2013; 2013.
8. Linsley KR et al. Clozapine-associated colitis: case report and review of the literature. J Clin Psychopharmacol 2012; 32:564–566.
9. Peyriere H et al. Antipsychotics-induced ischaemic colitis and gastrointestinal necrosis: a review of the French pharmacovigilance database. Pharmacoepidemiol Drug Saf 2009; 18:948–955.
10. Centorrino F et al. Delirium during clozapine treatment: incidence and associated risk factors. Pharmacopsychiatry 2003; 36:156–160.
11. Shankar BR. Clozapine-induced delirium. J Neuropsychiatry Clin Neurosci 2008; 20:239–240.
12. Hummer M et al. Does eosinophilia predict clozapine induced neutropenia? Psychopharmacology 1996; 124:201–204.
13. Ames D et al. Predictive value of eosinophilia for neutropenia during clozapine treatment. J Clin Psychiatry 1996; 57:579–581.
14. Karmacharya R et al. Clozapine-induced eosinophilic colitis (Letter). Am J Psychiatry 2005; 162:1386–1387.
15. Chatterton R. Eosinophilia after commencement of clozapine treatment. Aust N Z J Psychiatry 1997; 31:874–876.
16. Kerwin RW et al. Heat stroke in schizophrenia during clozapine treatment: rapid recognition and management. J Psychopharmacol 2004; 18:121–123.
17. Erdogan A et al. Management of marked liver enzyme increase during clozapine treatment: a case report and review of the literature. Int J Psychiatry Med 2004; 34:83–89.
18. Macfarlane B et al. Fatal acute fulminant liver failure due to clozapine: a case report and review of clozapine-induced hepatotoxicity. Gastroenterology 1997; 112:1707–1709.
19. Chang A et al. Clozapine-induced fatal fulminant hepatic failure: a case report. Can J Gastroenterol 2009; 23:376–378.
20. Chaplin AC et al. Re: Recent case report of clozapine-induced acute hepatic failure. Can J Gastroenterol 2010; 24:739–740.
21. Tucker P. Liver toxicity with clozapine. Aust N Z J Psychiatry 2013; 47:975–976.
22. Fong SY et al. Clozapine-induced toxic hepatitis with skin rash. J Psychopharmacol 2005; 19:107.
23. Hunter R et al. Clozapine-induced interstitial nephritis - a rare but important complication: a case report. J Med Case Reports 2009; 3:8574.
24. Elias TJ et al. Clozapine-induced acute interstitial nephritis. Lancet 1999; 354:1180–1181.
25. Borovik AM et al. Ocular pigmentation associated with clozapine. Med J Aust 2009; 190:210–211.
26. Bergemann N et al. Asymptomatic pancreatitis associated with clozapine. Pharmacopsychiatry 1999; 32:78–80.
27. Raja M et al. A case of clozapine-associated pancreatitis. Open Neuropsychopharmacol J 2011; 4:5–7.
28. Huang YJ et al. Recurrent pancreatitis without eosinophilia on clozapine rechallenge. Prog Neuropsychopharmacol Biol Psychiatry 2009; 33:1561–1562.
29. Immadisetty V et al. A successful treatment strategy for clozapine-induced parotid swelling: a clinical case and systematic review. Ther Adv Psychopharmacol 2012; 2:235–239.
30. Raju P et al. Pericardial effusion in patients with schizophrenia: are they on clozapine? Emerg Med J 2008; 25:383–384.
31. Dauner DG et al. Clozapine-induced pericardial effusion. J Clin Psychopharmacol 2008; 28:455–456.
32. Hinkes R et al. Aspiration pneumonia possibly secondary to clozapine-induced sialorrhea. J Clin Psychopharmacol 1996; 16:462–463.
33. Taylor DM et al. Reasons for discontinuing clozapine: matched, case-control comparison with risperidone long-acting injection. Br J Psychiatry 2009; 194:165–167.
34. Landry P et al. Increased use of antibiotics in clozapine-treated patients. Int Clin Psychopharmacol 2003; 18:297–298.
35. Nielsen J et al. Increased use of antibiotics in patients treated with clozapine. Eur Neuropsychopharmacol 2009; 19:483–486.
36. Raaska K et al. Bacterial pneumonia can increase serum concentration of clozapine. Eur J Clin Pharmacol 2002; 58:321–322.
37. de Leon J et al. Serious respiratory infections can increase clozapine levels and contribute to side effects: a case report. Prog Neuropsychopharmacol Biol Psychiatry 2003; 27:1059–1063.
38. Taylor D et al. Use of antacid medication in patients receiving clozapine: a comparison with other second-generation antipsychotics. J Clin Psychopharmacol 2010; 30:460–461.
39. Kumar T et al. Dose dependent stuttering with clozapine: a case report. Asian J Psychiatr 2013; 6:178–179.
40. Grover S et al. Clozapine-induced stuttering: a case report and analysis of similar case reports in the literature. Gen Hosp Psychiatry 2012; 34:703.
41. Jagadheesan K et al. Clozapine-induced thrombocytopenia: a pilot study. Hong Kong J Psychiatry 2003; 13:12–15.
42. Penaskovic KM et al. Clozapine-induced allergic vasculitis (Letter). Am J Psychiatry 2005; 162:1543–1542.

Clozapine: serious haematological and cardiovascular adverse effects

Agranulocytosis, thromboembolism, cardiomyopathy and myocarditis

Clozapine is a somewhat toxic drug, but it may reduce overall mortality in schizophrenia, largely because of a reduction in the rate of suicide.[1,2] Clozapine can cause serious, life-threatening adverse effects, of which **agranulocytosis** is the best known. In the UK, the risk of death from agranulocytosis is probably less than 1 in 10,000 patients exposed (Novartis report 4 deaths from 47,000 exposed).[3] Risk is well managed by the approved clozapine-monitoring systems.

Thromboembolism

A possible association between clozapine and **thromboembolism** has been suggested.[4] Initially, Walker et al.[1] uncovered a risk of fatal pulmonary embolism of 1 in 4500 – about 20 times the risk in the population as a whole. Following a case report of non-fatal pulmonary embolism possibly related to clozapine,[5] data from the Swedish authorities were published.[6] Twelve cases of venous thromboembolism were described, of which five were fatal. The risk of thromboembolism was estimated to be 1 in 2000 to 1 in 6000 patients treated. Thromboembolism may be related to clozapine's observed effects on antiphospholipid antibodies[7] and platelet aggregation.[8] It seems most likely to occur in the first 3 months of treatment but can occur at any time. Other antipsychotics are also strongly linked to thromboembolism[9–15] although clozapine appears to have the most reports.[16]

With all drugs, the causes of thromboembolism are probably multifactorial.[10] Encouraging exercise and ensuring good hydration are essential precautionary measures.[17]

Myocarditis and cardiomyopathy

It has also been suggested that clozapine is associated with **myocarditis** and **cardiomyopathy**. Australian data initially identified 23 cases (15 myocarditis, eight cardiomyopathy), of which six were fatal.[18] Risk of death from either cause was estimated from these data to be 1 in 1300. Similar findings were reported in New Zealand.[19] Myocarditis seems to occur within 6–8 weeks of starting clozapine (median 3 weeks[20]); cardiomyopathy may occur later in treatment (median 9 months[20]) but both may occur at any time. It is notable that other data sources give rather different risk estimates: in Canada the risk of fatal myocarditis was estimated to be 1 in 12,500; in the USA, 1 in 67,000.[21] Conversely, another Australian study identified nine cases of possible (non-fatal) myocarditis in 94 patients treated.[22] A later Australian study estimated the risk of myocarditis to be around 1% of those treated (in whom 1 in 10 died).[23]

Despite this uncertainty over incidence, patients should be closely monitored for signs of myocarditis especially in the first few months of treatment.[24] Symptoms include hypotension, tachycardia, fever, flu-like symptoms, fatigue, dyspnoea (with increased respiratory rate) and chest pain.[25] Signs include ECG changes (ST depression), enlarged heart on radiography/echo and eosinophilia. Many of these symptoms occur in patients on clozapine not developing myocarditis[26] and conversely, their absence does not rule out myocarditis.[27] Nonetheless, signs of heart failure should provoke immediate cessation of clozapine. Re-challenge has been successfully completed[22] (the use of beta-blockers and angiotensin-converting enzyme [ACE] inhibitors may help[28,29]) but recurrence is possible.[30–32] Use of echocardiography, CRP and troponin are essential in cases of re-challenge.[33–35]

Autopsy findings suggest that fatal myocarditis can occur in the absence of clear cardiac symptoms, although tachycardia and fever are usually present.[36] A group from Melbourne, Australia has put forward a monitoring programme which is said to detect 100% of symptomatic cases of myocarditis[37] using measurement of troponin I or T- and C-reactive protein (Table 2.43).

Factors that may increase the risk of developing myocarditis include rapid dose increases, concurrent use of sodium valproate, and older age (31% increased risk for each additional decade).[38] Other psychotropics, including lithium, risperidone, haloperidol, chlorpromazine and fluphenazine have also been associated with myocarditis.[39] It is probably preferable to avoid concomitant use of other medicines that may contribute to the risk, but this may be practically difficult. Any pre-existing cardiac disorder, previous cardiac event or family history of cardiac disease should provoke extra caution.

Cardiomyopathy should be suspected in any patient showing signs of heart failure, which should provoke immediate cessation of clozapine and referral. Presentation of cardiomyopathy varies somewhat[40,41] so any reported symptoms of palpitations, chest pain, syncope, sweating, decreased exercise capacity or breathing difficulties should be closely investigated.

Note also that, despite an overall reduction in mortality, younger patients may have an increased risk of sudden death,[42] perhaps because of clozapine-induced ECG changes.[43]

Table 2.43 Suggested monitoring for myocarditis[36,37,46]

Time/condition	Signs/symptoms to monitor
Baseline	Pulse, blood pressure, temperature, respiratory rate Full blood count (FBC) C-reactive protein (CRP) Troponin Echocardiography (if available)
Daily, if possible	Pulse, blood pressure, temperature, respiratory rate Ask about: chest pain, fever, cough, shortness of breath, exercise capacity
On days 7, 14, 21, and 28	CRP Troponin FBC ECG if possible
If CRP > 100 mg/L or troponin > twice upper limit of normal	Stop clozapine; repeat echo
If fever + tachycardia + raised CRP or troponin (but not as above)	Daily CRP and troponin measures

ECG, electrocardiogram.

CHAPTER 2

The overall picture remains very unclear but caution is required. There may, of course, be similar problems with other antipsychotics.[44,39,45]

Summary

- Overall mortality may be lower for those on clozapine than in schizophrenia as a whole.
- Risk of fatal agranulocytosis is less than 1 in 10 000 patients treated in the UK.
- Risk of fatal pulmonary embolism is estimated to be around 1 in 4500 patients treated.
- Risk of fatal myocarditis or cardiomyopathy may be as high as 1 in 1000 patients.
- Careful monitoring is essential during clozapine treatment, particularly during the first 3 months (see Table 2.39).

References

1. Walker AM et al. Mortality in current and former users of clozapine. Epidemiology 1997; 8:671–677.
2. Munro J et al. Active monitoring of 12760 clozapine recipients in the UK and Ireland. Br J Psychiatry 1999; 175:576–580.
3. Thuillier S. Clozapine and agranulocytosis. 2006. Personal Communication
4. Paciullo CA. Evaluating the association between clozapine and venous thromboembolism. Am J Health Syst Pharm 2008; 65:1825–1829.
5. Lacika S et al. Pulmonary embolus possibly associated with clozapine treatment (Letter). Can J Psychiatry 1999; 44:396–397.
6. Hagg S et al. Association of venous thromboembolism and clozapine. Lancet 2000; 355:1155–1156.
7. Davis S et al. Antiphospholipid antibodies associated with clozapine treatment. Am J Hematol 1994; 46:166–167.
8. Axelsson S et al. In vitro effects of antipsychotics on human platelet adhesion and aggregation and plasma coagulation. Clin Exp Pharmacol Physiol 2007; 34:775–780.
9. Liperoti R et al. Venous thromboembolism among elderly patients treated with atypical and conventional antipsychotic agents. Arch Intern Med 2005; 165:2677–2682.
10. Lacut K. Association between antipsychotic drugs, antidepressant drugs, and venous thromboembolism. Clin Adv Hematol Oncol 2008; 6:887–890.
11. Borras L et al. Pulmonary thromboembolism associated with olanzapine and risperidone. J Emerg Med 2008; 35:159–161.
12. Maly R et al. Four cases of venous thromboembolism associated with olanzapine. Psychiatry Clin Neurosci 2009; 63:116–118.
13. Hagg S et al. Associations between venous thromboembolism and antipsychotics. A study of the WHO database of adverse drug reactions. Drug Saf 2008; 31:685–694.
14. Lacut K et al. Association between antipsychotic drugs, antidepressant drugs and venous thromboembolism: results from the EDITH case-control study. Fundam Clin Pharmacol 2007; 21:643–650.
15. Zink M et al. A case of pulmonary thromboembolism and rhabdomyolysis during therapy with mirtazapine and risperidone. J Clin Psychiatry 2006; 67:835.
16. Allenet B et al. Antipsychotic drugs and risk of pulmonary embolism. Pharmacoepidemiol Drug Saf 2012; 21:42–48.
17. Maly R et al. Assessment of risk of venous thromboembolism and its possible prevention in psychiatric patients. Psychiatry Clin Neurosci 2008; 62:3–8.
18. Killian JG et al. Myocarditis and cardiomyopathy associated with clozapine. Lancet 1999; 354:1841–1845.
19. Hill GR et al. Clozapine and myocarditis: a case series from the New Zealand Intensive Medicines Monitoring Programme. N Z Med J 2008; 121:68–75.
20. La Grenade L et al. Myocarditis and cardiomyopathy associated with clozapine use in the United States (Letter). N Engl J Med 2001; 345:224–225.
21. Warner B et al. Clozapine and sudden death. Lancet 2000; 355:842.
22. Reinders J et al. Clozapine-related myocarditis and cardiomyopathy in an Australian metropolitan psychiatric service. Aust N Z J Psychiatry 2004; 38:915–922.
23. Haas SJ et al. Clozapine-associated myocarditis: a review of 116 cases of suspected myocarditis associated with the use of clozapine in Australia during 1993-2003. Drug Saf 2007; 30:47–57.
24. Marder SR et al. Physical health monitoring of patients with schizophrenia. Am J Psychiatry 2004; 161:1334–1349.
25. Annamraju S et al. Early recognition of clozapine-induced myocarditis. J Clin Psychopharmacol 2007; 27:479–483.
26. Wehmeier PM et al. Chart review for potential features of myocarditis, pericarditis, and cardiomyopathy in children and adolescents treated with clozapine. J Child Adolesc Psychopharmacol 2004; 14:267–271.
27. McNeil JJ et al. Clozapine-induced myocarditis: characterisation using case-control design. Eur Heart J 2013; 34 (Suppl 1):688–.
28. Rostagno C et al. Beta-blocker and angiotensin-converting enzyme inhibitor may limit certain cardiac adverse effects of clozapine. Gen Hosp Psychiatry 2008; 30:280–283.

29. Floreani J et al. Successful re-challenge with clozapine following development of clozapine-induced cardiomyopathy. Aust N Z J Psychiatry 2008; **42**:747–748.

30. Roh S et al. Cardiomyopathy associated with clozapine. Exp Clin Psychopharmacol 2006; **14**:94–98.

31. Masopust J et al. Repeated occurrence of clozapine-induced myocarditis in a patient with schizoaffective disorder and comorbid Parkinson's disease. Neuro Endocrinol Lett 2009; **30**:19–21.

32. Ronaldson KJ et al. Observations from 8 cases of clozapine rechallenge after development of myocarditis. J Clin Psychiatry 2012; **73**:252–254.

33. Hassan I et al. Monitoring in clozapine rechallenge after myocarditis. Australas Psychiatry 2011; **19**:370–371.

34. Bray A et al. Successful clozapine rechallenge after acute myocarditis. Aust N Z J Psychiatry 2011; **45**:90.

35. Rosenfeld AJ et al. Successful clozapine retrial after suspected myocarditis. Am J Psychiatry 2010; **167**:350–351.

36. Ronaldson KJ et al. Clinical course and analysis of ten fatal cases of clozapine-induced myocarditis and comparison with 66 surviving cases. Schizophr Res 2011; **128**:161–165.

37. Ronaldson KJ et al. A new monitoring protocol for clozapine-induced myocarditis based on an analysis of 75 cases and 94 controls. Aust N Z J Psychiatry 2011; **45**:458–465.

38. Ronaldson KJ et al. Rapid clozapine dose titration and concomitant sodium valproate increase the risk of myocarditis with clozapine: a case-control study. Schizophr Res 2012; **141**:173–178.

39. Coulter DM et al. Antipsychotic drugs and heart muscle disorder in international pharmacovigilance: data mining study. BMJ 2001; **322**:1207–1209.

40. Pastor CA et al. Masked clozapine-induced cardiomyopathy. J Am Board Fam Med 2008; **21**:70–74.

41. Sagar R et al. Clozapine-induced cardiomyopathy presenting as panic attacks. J Psychiatr Pract 2008; **14**:182–185.

42. Modai I et al. Sudden death in patients receiving clozapine treatment: a preliminary investigation. J Clin Psychopharmacol 2000; **20**:325–327.

43. Kang UG et al. Electrocardiographic abnormalities in patients treated with clozapine. J Clin Psychiatry 2000; **61**:441–446.

44. Thomassen R et al. Antipsychotic drugs and venous thromboembolism (Letter). Lancet 2000; **356**:252.

45. Hagg S et al. Antipsychotic-induced venous thromboembolism: a review of the evidence. CNS Drugs 2002; **16**:765–776.

46. Ronaldson KJ et al. Diagnostic characteristics of clozapine-induced myocarditis identified by an analysis of 38 cases and 47 controls. J Clin Psychiatry 2010; **71**:976–981.

Further reading

Caforio AL et al. Current state of knowledge on aetiology, diagnosis, management, and therapy of myocarditis: a position statement of the European Society of Cardiology Working Group on Myocardial and Pericardial Diseases. Eur Heart J 2013; **34**:2636–2648d.

Razminia M et al. Clozapine induced myopericarditis: early recognition improves clinical outcome. Am J Ther 2006;**13**:274–6.

Wehmeier PM et al. Myocarditis, pericarditis and cardiomyopathy in patients treated with clozapine. J Clin Pharm Ther 2005;**30**:91–6.

Clozapine-induced hypersalivation

Clozapine is well known to be causally associated with apparent hypersalivation (drooling, particularly at night). This seems to be chiefly problematic in the early stages of treatment and is probably dose-related. Clinical observation suggests that hypersalivation reduces in severity over time (usually several months) but may persist. Clozapine-induced hypersalivation is socially embarrassing and potentially life-threatening,[1] so treatment is a matter of some urgency.

The pharmacological basis of clozapine-related hypersalivation remains unclear.[2] Suggested mechanisms include muscarinic M_4 agonism, α_2-adrenergic antagonism and inhibition of the swallowing reflex.[3,4] The last of these is supported by trials which suggest that saliva production is not increased in clozapine-treated patients,[5,6] although at least one study has observed marked increases in salivary flow in the first 3 weeks of treatment.[7]

Whatever the mechanism, drugs which reduce saliva production are likely to diminish the severity of this adverse effect. Non-drug treatments may be used if appropriate – these include chewing gum, elevating pillows and placing a towel on the pillow to prevent soaking of clothes.[2] Table 2.44 describes drug treatments so far examined.

Table 2.44 Clozapine-related hypersalivation

Treatment	Comments
Amisulpride 100–400 mg/day[8,9]	Supported by a positive RCT compared with placebo, one other in which it was compared with moclobemide and numerous case studies.[10–13] May allow dose reduction of clozapine
Amitriptyline 25–100 mg/day[14,15]	Limited literature support. Adverse effects may be troublesome. Worsens constipation
Atropine eye drops (1%) given sublingually[16,17] or as solution (1 mg/10 mL) used as a mouthwash	Limited literature support. Rarely used
Benzhexol (trihexyphenidyl) 5–15 mg/day[18]	Small, open study suggests useful activity. Used in some centres but may impair cognitive function. Lower doses (2 mg) may be effective[19]
Benztropine 2 mg/day **+ terazosin** 2 mg/day[20]	Combination shown to be better than either drug alone. Terazosin is an α_1-antagonist so may cause hypotension
Botulinum toxin[21–23] (Botox) Bilateral parotid gland injections (150 IU into each gland)	Effective in treating sialorrhoea associated with neurological disorders. Five cases of successful treatment of clozapine-related hypersalivation in the literature
Bupropion 100–150 mg/day[24]	Single case report. May lower seizure threshold
Clonidine 0.1–0.2 mg patch weekly or 0.1 mg orally at night[25,26]	α_2-partial agonist. Limited literature support. May exacerbate psychosis, depression and cause hypotension

Table 2.44 (*Continued*)

Treatment	Comments
Glycopyrrolate 0.5–4 mg twice daily[27–29]	One RCT showed glycopyrrolate to be more effective than biperiden without worsening cognitive function
Guanfacine 1 mg daily[30]	α_2-agonist. Single case report. May cause hypotension
Hyoscine 0.3 mg tablet sucked or chewed up to 3 times daily or 1.5 mg/72 hour patch[31,32]	Peripheral and central anticholinergic. Very widely used but no published data available on oral treatment. May cause cognitive impairment, drowsiness and worsens constipation.
Ipratropium Nasal spray (0.03% or 0.06%) – given sublingually[33,34] up to 2 sprays three times a day of the 0.06% or intranasally[30] 1 spray into each nostril daily of the 0.03%	Limited literature support. The only placebo-controlled RCT conducted was negative[35]
Lofexidine 0.2 mg twice daily[36]	α_2-agonist. Very few data. May exacerbate psychosis, depression and cause hypotension
Moclobemide 150–300 mg/day[37]	Effective in 9 out of 14 patients treated in one open study. Appears to be as effective as amisupride (see above)
Oxybutynin 5 mg up to twice daily[38]	Single case report
Pirenzepine 50–150 mg/day[39–41]	Selective M_1, M_4 antagonist. Extensive clinical experience suggests efficacy in some but one RCT suggested no effect. Still widely used. Does not have a UK licence for any indication. May cause constipation
Propantheline 7.5 mg at night[42]	Peripheral anticholinergic. No central effects. Two Chinese RCTs (one positive). May worsen constipation
Quetiapine[43]	May reduce hypersalivation by allowing lower doses of clozapine to be used
Sulpiride 150–300 mg/day[44,45]	Supported by one, small positive RCT and a Cochrane Review of clozapine augmentation with sulpiride (at higher sulpiride doses). May allow dose reduction of clozapine

RCT, randomised controlled trial.

References

1. Hinkes R et al. Aspiration pneumonia possibly secondary to clozapine-induced sialorrhea. J Clin Psychopharmacol 1996; **16**:462–463.
2. Praharaj SK et al. Clozapine-induced sialorrhea: pathophysiology and management strategies. Psychopharmacology 2006; **185**:265–273.
3. Davydov L et al. Clozapine-induced hypersalivation. Ann Pharmacother 2000; **34**:662–665.
4. Rogers DP et al. Therapeutic options in the treatment of clozapine-induced sialorrhea. Pharmacotherapy 2000; **20**:1092–1095.
5. Rabinowitz T et al. The effect of clozapine on saliva flow rate: a pilot study. Biol Psychiatry 1996; **40**:1132–1134.
6. Ben Aryeh H et al. Salivary flow-rate and composition in schizophrenic patients on clozapine: subjective reports and laboratory data. Biol Psychiatry 1996; **39**:946–949.
7. Praharaj SK et al. Salivary flow rate in patients with schizophrenia on clozapine. Clin Neuropharmacol 2010; **33**:176–178.
8. Kreinin A et al. Amisulpride treatment of clozapine-induced hypersalivation in schizophrenia patients: a randomized, double-blind, placebo-controlled cross-over study. Int Clin Psychopharmacol 2006; **21**:99–103.
9. Kreinin A et al. Amisulpride versus moclobemide in treatment of clozapine-induced hypersalivation. World J Biol Psychiatry 2010; **12**:620–626.
10. Praharaj SK et al. Amisulpride treatment for clozapine-induced sialorrhea. J Clin Psychopharmacol 2009; **29**:189–190.
11. Aggarwal A et al. Amisulpride for clozapine induced sialorrhea. Psychopharmacol Bull 2009; **42**:69–71.

12. Croissant B et al. Reduction of side effects by combining clozapine with amisulpride: case report and short review of clozapine-induced hypersalivation-a case report. Pharmacopsychiatry 2005; **38**:38–39.
13. Praharaj SK et al. Amisulpride improved debilitating clozapine-induced sialorrhea. Am J Ther 2011; **18**:e84–e85.
14. Copp P et al. Amitriptyline in clozapine-induced sialorrhoea. Br J Psychiatry 1991; **159**:166.
15. Praharaj SK et al. Amitriptyline for clozapine-induced nocturnal enuresis and sialorrhoea. Br J Clin Pharmacol 2007; **63**:128–129.
16. Antonello C et al. Clozapine and sialorrhea: a new intervention for this bothersome and potentially dangerous side effect. J Psychiatry Neurosci 1999; **24**:250.
17. Mustafa FA et al. Sublingual atropine for the treatment of severe and hyoscine-resistant clozapine-induced sialorrhea. Afr J Psychiatry (Johannesbg) 2013; **16**:242.
18. Spivak B et al. Trihexyphenidyl treatment of clozapine-induced hypersalivation. Int Clin Psychopharmacol 1997; **12**:213–215.
19. Praharaj SK et al. Complete resolution of clozapine-induced sialorrhea with low dose trihexyphenidyl. Psychopharmacol Bull 2010; **43**:73–75.
20. Reinstein M et al. Comparative efficacy and tolerability of benzatropine and terazosin in the treatment of hypersalivation secondary to clozapine. Clin Drug Invest 1999; **17**:97–102.
21. Kahl KG et al. Botulinum toxin as an effective treatment of clozapine-induced hypersalivation. Psychopharmacology 2004; **173**:229–230.
22. Steinlechner S et al. Botulinum toxin B as an effective and safe treatment for neuroleptic-induced sialorrhea. Psychopharmacology (Berl) 2010; **207**:593–597.
23. Kahl KG et al. [Pharmacological strategies for clozapine-induced hypersalivation: treatment with botulinum toxin B in one patient and review of the literature]. Nervenarzt 2005; **76**:205–208.
24. Stern RG et al. Clozapine-induced sialorrhea alleviated by bupropion--a case report. Prog Neuropsychopharmacol Biol Psychiatry 2009; **33**:1578–1580.
25. Grabowski J. Clonidine treatment of clozapine-induced hypersalivation. J Clin Psychopharmacol 1992; **12**:69–70.
26. Praharaj SK et al. Is clonidine useful for treatment of clozapine-induced sialorrhea? J Psychopharmacol 2005; **19**:426–428.
27. Duggal HS. Glycopyrrolate for clozapine-induced sialorrhea. Prog Neuropsychopharmacol Biol Psychiatry 2007; **31**:1546–1547.
28. Robb AS et al. Glycopyrrolate for treatment of clozapine-induced sialorrhea in three adolescents. J Child Adolesc Psychopharmacol 2008; **18**:99–107.
29. Liang CS et al. Comparison of the efficacy and impact on cognition of glycopyrrolate and biperiden for clozapine-induced sialorrhea in schizophrenic patients: a randomized, double-blind, crossover study. Schizophr Res 2010; **119**:138–144.
30. Webber MA et al. Guanfacine treatment of clozapine-induced sialorrhea. J Clin Psychopharmacol 2004; **24**:675–676.
31. McKane JP et al. Hyoscine patches in clozapine-induced hypersalivation. Psychiatr Bull 2001; **25**:277.
32. Gaftanyuk O et al. Scolpolamine patch for clozapine-induced sialorrhea. Psychiatr Serv 2004; **55**:318.
33. Calderon J et al. Potential use of ipatropium bromide for the treatment of clozapine-induced hypersalivation: a preliminary report. Int Clin Psychopharmacol 2000; **15**:49–52.
34. Freudenreich O et al. Clozapine-induced sialorrhea treated with sublingual ipratropium spray: a case series. J Clin Psychopharmacol 2004; **24**:98–100.
35. Sockalingam S et al. Treatment of clozapine-induced hypersalivation with ipratropium bromide: a randomized, double-blind, placebo-controlled crossover study. J Clin Psychiatry 2009; **70**:1114–1119.
36. Corrigan FM et al. Clozapine-induced hypersalivation and the alpha 2 adrenoceptor. Br J Psychiatry 1995; **167**:412.
37. Kreinin A et al. Moclobemide treatment of clozapine-induced hypersalivation: pilot open study. Clin Neuropharmacol 2009; **32**:151–153.
38. Leung JG et al. Immediate-release oxybutynin for the treatment of clozapine-induced sialorrhea. Ann Pharmacother 2011; **45**:e45.
39. Fritze J et al. Pirenzepine for clozapine-induced hypersalivation. Lancet 1995; **346**:1034.
40. Bai YM et al. Therapeutic effect of pirenzepine for clozapine-induced hypersalivation: a randomized, double-blind, placebo-controlled, crossover study. J Clin Psychopharmacol 2001; **21**:608–611.
41. Schneider B et al. Reduction of clozapine-induced hypersalivation by pirenzepine is safe. Pharmacopsychiatry 2004; **37**:43–45.
42. Syed Sheriff RJ et al. Pharmacological interventions for clozapine-induced hypersalivation. Schizophr Bull 2008; **34**:611–612.
43. Reinstein MJ et al. Use of quetiapine to manage patients who experienced adverse effects with clozapine. Clin Drug Invest 2003; **23**:63–67.
44. Kreinin A et al. Sulpiride addition for the treatment of clozapine-induced hypersalivation: preliminary study. Isr J Psychiatry Relat Sci 2005; **42**:61–63.
45. Wang J et al. Sulpiride augmentation for schizophrenia. Cochrane Database Syst Rev 2010; CD008125.

Further reading

Bird AM et al. Current treatment strategies for clozapine-induced sialorrhea. Ann Pharmacother 2011; **45**:667–675.

Clozapine-induced gastrointestinal hypomotility (CIGH)

Constipation is a common adverse effect of clozapine treatment with a prevalence of up to 60%.[1] The mechanism of action is not completely understood but is thought to be a combination of the drug's anticholinergic[2,3] and antihistaminergic properties[4] which are further complicated by antagonism at 5-HT$_3$ receptors.[2,3,5] In addition, clozapine-induced sedation can result in a sedentary lifestyle,[4] which is itself a risk factor for constipation. Essentially clozapine causes constipation by slowing transit time through the gut.

Clozapine-induced constipation is much more common than blood dyscrasias, and mortality rates are also higher;[4] when constipation is severe, the fatality rate (calculated from severe cases reported in the literature) is around 20–30%.[4,6,7] Enhanced monitoring for CIGH is urgently needed to reduce constipation-related fatalities.

A gastrointestinal history and abdominal examination is recommended prior to starting treatment and if the patient is constipated, clozapine should not be initiated until this has resolved.[7] CIGH is most severe during the first 4 months of treatment[7] and so weekly assessments are recommended during this time frame.[8] Adopting the Rome III criteria[9] at routine FBCs might be a successful strategy to combat preventable deaths due to CIGH.

Opinions differ on the relationship between clozapine dose and constipation, and clozapine plasma level and constipation,[7,10,11] however, the deaths that have occurred as a result of CIGH were in people taking higher daily doses (mean 535 mg/day)[7].

The risk factors for developing clozapine-induced constipation are summarised in Box 2.2.

Prevention and simple management of CIGH

A slower clozapine titration may reduce the risk of developing constipation with dose increments not exceeding 25 mg/day or 100 mg/week.[1] Increasing dietary fibre intake to at least 20–25 g per day can increase stool weight and decrease gut transit time.[14,15]

Box 2.2 Risk factors for developing clozapine-induced constipation[7,8,12–14]

- Increasing age
- Female sex
- Anticholinergic medication
- Hypersalivation
- Higher clozapine dose/plasma level
- Hypercalcaemia
- Gastrointestinal disease
- Obesity
- Diaphoresis
- Low fibre diet
- Poor bowel habit
- Dehydration
- Diabetes
- Hypothyroidism
- Parkinson's disease
- Multiple sclerosis

If fibre intake is increased it is important that adequate fluid intake (1.5–2 L/day) is also maintained to avoid intestinal obstruction.[7,14,16] Daily food and fluid charts would be ideal to monitor fibre and fluid intake especially during the titration phase of clozapine. Regular exercise (150 minutes/week)[17] in addition to a high fibre diet and increased fluid intake also assist in the prevention of CIGH.[18,19]

Weekly stool charts,[14,20] should be used for all patients starting clozapine. If there is a change from usual baseline bowel habit or fewer than three bowel movements (BM) per week[9] an abdominal examination is indicated.[7] Where this excludes intestinal obstruction, both a stimulant and stool-softening laxative should be started (for example senna and docusate[7,21]). Bulk forming laxatives are not effective in slow-transit constipation[2,22] and therefore should be avoided. There is some evidence that lactulose and polyethylene glycol (for example Movicol) are effective[2,23] and could be considered as second line options or alternatives to the stimulant and softener combination. Choice of laxative should also be guided by the patients' previous response to certain agents in association with the required speed of action.[24] It would not be appropriate for example to start lactulose treatment (takes up to 72 hours of regular use to work[25]) for someone in need of urgent treatment.

Management of suspected acute CIGH

Signs and symptoms that warrant immediate medical attention are abdominal pain, distension, vomiting, overflow diarrhoea, absent bowel sounds, acute abdomen, feculent vomitus and symptoms of sepsis,[7] [1,6,26–33] There have been case reports of fatalities occurring only hours after first symptoms present,[34] which emphasises the urgency for prompt assessment and management. There should therefore be a low threshold for referral to a gastroenterologist when conservative management fails or constipation is severe and acute.[7,35]

Physicians may not be familiar with clozapine-induced constipation and may welcome information on the associated morbidity and mortality; a copy of this section of the guidelines may facilitate timely treatment. The following may be helpful to communicate to staff in emergency departments.

1. Stop clozapine,[7] and all other anti-muscarinic medicines.
2. Assess for bowel obstruction.
3. If obstruction is not present, consider use of an enema or digital disimpaction.[7]
   In some cases, the off-label use of neostigmine or physostigmine has been employed to accelerate gastrointestinal transit time and has shown good results for acute colonic pseudo-obstruction.[7,36,37]
4. If obstruction is present, consider urgent surgical referral.

Clozapine re-challenge following severe constipation

Some patients have been successfully re-challenged following severe cases of CIGH, however, this does not come without risk. Prophylactic measures should therefore be considered for those with a history of CIGH or who are deemed high risk of developing CIGH. Where conventional laxatives have not been tried in regular and adequate doses, this should be done. However, when this approach has previously failed, a number of more experimental options are available. Prescribers must familiarise themselves with the literature (at the very least by reading the SPC) before using any of these treatments.

The prostaglandin E1 analogue **lubiprostone** is licensed in the UK for the treatment of chronic idiopathic constipation and associated symptoms in adults, when response to diet and other non-pharmacological measures (e.g. educational measures, physical activity) are inappropriate.[38] The recommended dose for the licensed indication is 24 µg twice daily for a maximum of 2 weeks duration.[38] Lubiprostone has been reported to be effective in obviating the need for other laxatives in a clozapine re-challenge following a severe case of CIGH,[39] and is used in some centres for this indication.[39]

Orlistat, a drug used to aid weight loss, is also known to have a laxative effect particularly when a high-fat diet is consumed. It has been successfully used for three patients with severe constipation associated with opioid use (hypomotility-induced constipation).[40] A small, randomised placebo controlled study of orlistat for clozapine-induced constipation found a statistically significant favourable difference at study endpoint (week 16) for the prevalence of constipation, diarrhoea, and normal stools for orlistat compared with placebo;[41] note that 47 of the 54 participants required conventional laxatives. Note also that orlistat is known to reduce the absorption of some drugs from the GI tract. It is therefore important to monitor plasma clozapine levels if starting treatment with orlistat.

Bethanechol, a cholinergic agonist, has been described as being effective in reducing the amount of laxatives and enemas required to maintain regular bowel movements for a patient diagnosed with CIGH.[42] Bethanechol in this scenario was used at a dose of 10 mg three times daily. Bethanechol should only ever be initiated after other options have failed and in consultation with a gastroenterologist.[42]

References

1. Hayes G et al. Clozapine-induced constipation. Am J Psychiatry 1995; **152**:298.
2. Hibbard KR et al. Fatalities associated with clozapine-related constipation and bowel obstruction: a literature review and two case reports. Psychosomatics 2009; **50**:416–419.
3. Rege S et al. Life-threatening constipation associated with clozapine. Australas Psychiatry 2008; **16**:216–219.
4. De Hert M et al. Second-generation antipsychotics and constipation: a review of the literature. Eur Psychiatry 2011; **26**:34–44.
5. Meltzer HY et al. Effects of antipsychotic drugs on serotonin receptors. Pharmacol Rev 1991; **43**:587–604.
6. Cohen D et al. Beyond white blood cell monitoring: screening in the initial phase of clozapine therapy. J Clin Psychiatry 2012; **73**:1307–1312.
7. Palmer SE et al. Life-threatening clozapine-induced gastrointestinal hypomotility: an analysis of 102 cases. J Clin Psychiatry 2008; **69**:759–768.
8. Nielsen J et al. Termination of clozapine treatment due to medical reasons: when is it warranted and how can it be avoided? J Clin Psychiatry 2013; **74**:603–613; quiz 613.
9. Rome Foundation. Rome III Disorders and Criteria. http://www.theromefoundation.org/criteria/, 2006.
10. Chengappa KN et al. Anticholinergic differences among patients receiving standard clinical doses of olanzapine or clozapine. J Clin Psychopharmacol 2000; **20**:311–316.
11. Vella-Brincat J et al. Clozapine-induced gastrointestinal hypomotility. Australas Psychiatry 2011; **19**:450–451.
12. Nielsen J et al. Risk factors for ileus in patients with schizophrenia. Schizophr Bull 2012; **38**:592–598.
13. Longmore M et al. Oxford Handbook of Clinical Medicine Oxford, UK: OUP Oxford, 2010.
14. ZTAS. Zaponex Fact Sheet - Constipation. https://www.ztas.com/Manuals/ZFS_Constipation2.pdf, 2013.
15. Muller-Lissner SA. Effect of wheat bran on weight of stool and gastrointestinal transit time: a meta analysis. Br Med J (Clin Res Ed) 1988; **296**:615–617.
16. National Prescribing Centre. The management of constipation. MedRec Bulletin 2011; **21**:1–8.
17. NHS Choices. Physical activity guidelines for adults. http://www.nhs.uk/Livewell/fitness/Pages/physical-activity-guidelines-for-adults.aspx, 2013.
18. Fitzsimons J et al. A review of clozapine safety. Expert Opin Drug Saf 2005; **4**:731–744.
19. Young CR et al. Management of the adverse effects of clozapine. Schizophr Bull 1998; **24**:381–390.
20. Lewis SJ et al. Stool form scale as a useful guide to intestinal transit time. Scand J Gastroenterol 1997; **32**:920–924.

21. Swegle JM et al. Management of common opioid-induced adverse effects. Am Fam Physician 2006; 74:1347–1354.
22. Voderholzer WA et al. Clinical response to dietary fiber treatment of chronic constipation. Am J Gastroenterol 1997; 92:95–98.
23. Brandt LJ et al. Systematic review on the management of chronic constipation in North America. Am J Gastroenterol 2005; 100 Suppl 1:S5–s21.
24. Bleakley S et al. Clozapine Handbook. Warwickshire, UK: Lloyd-Reinhold Communications LLP, 2013.
25. Intrapharm Laboratories Limited. Summary of Product Characteristics. Lactulose 10 g / 15 ml oral solution sachets. https://www.medicines.org.uk/, 2013.
26. Leong QM et al. Necrotising colitis related to clozapine? A rare but life threatening side effect. World J Emerg Surg 2007; 2:21.
27. Shammi CM et al. Clozapine-induced necrotizing colitis. J Clin Psychopharmacol 1997; 17:230–232.
28. Rondla S et al. A case of clozapine-induced paralytic ileus. Emerg Med J 2007; 24:e12.
29. Levin TT et al. Death from clozapine-induced constipation: case report and literature review. Psychosomatics 2002; 43:71–73.
30. Townsend G et al. Case report: rapidly fatal bowel ischaemia on clozapine treatment. BMC Psychiatry 2006; 6:43.
31. Karmacharya R et al. Clozapine-induced eosinophilic colitis. Am J Psychiatry 2005; 162:1386–1387.
32. Erickson B et al. Clozapine-associated postoperative ileus: case report and review of the literature. Arch Gen Psychiatry 1995; 52:508–509.
33. Schwartz BJ et al. A case report of clozapine-induced gastric outlet obstruction. Am J Psychiatry 1993; 150:1563.
34. Drew L et al. Clozapine and constipation: a serious issue. Aust N Z J Psychiatry 1997; 31:149.
35. Ikai S et al. Reintroduction of clozapine after perforation of the large intestine--a case report and review of the literature. Ann Pharmacother 2013; 47:e31.
36. Loftus CG et al. Assessment of predictors of response to neostigmine for acute colonic pseudo-obstruction. Am J Gastroenterol 2002; 97:3118–3122.
37. Saunders MD et al. Systematic review: acute colonic pseudo-obstruction. Aliment Pharmacol Ther 2005; 22:917–925.
38. Sucampo Pharma Europe Ltd. AMITIZA 24 microgram soft capsules. https://www.medicines.org.uk/, 2013.
39. Meyer,JM et al. Lubiprostone for treatment-resistant constipation associated with clozapine use. Acta Psychiatr Scand 2014; 130:71–72.
40. Guarino AH. Treatment of intractable constipation with orlistat: a report of three cases. Pain Med 2005; 6:327–328.
41. Chukhin E et al. In a randomized placebo-controlled add-on study orlistat significantly reduced clozapine-induced constipation. Int Clin Psychopharmacol 2013; 28:67–70.
42. Poetter CE et al. Treatment of clozapine-induced constipation with bethanechol. J Clin Psychopharmacol 2013; 33:713–714.

CHAPTER 2

Clozapine, neutropenia and lithium

Risk of clozapine-induced neutropenia

Around 2.7% of patients treated with clozapine develop neutropenia. Of these, half do so within the first 18 weeks of treatment and three-quarters by the end of the first year.[1] Risk factors[1] include being Afro-Caribbean (77% increase in risk) and young (17% decrease in risk per decade increase in age), and having a low baseline white cell count (WCC) (31% increase in risk for each 1×10^9/L drop). Risk is not dose-related. Approximately 0.8% will develop agranulocytosis. The mechanism of clozapine-induced neutropenia/ agranulocytosis is unclear and it is possible that immune-mediated and direct cytotoxic effects may both be important. The mechanism may differ between individuals and also between mild and severe forms of marrow suppression.[2] One-third of patients who stop clozapine because they have developed neutropenia or agranulocytosis will develop a blood dyscrasia on re-challenge. In almost all cases, the second reaction will occur more rapidly, be more severe and last longer than the first.[3]

Benign ethnic neutropenia (BEN)

After being released from the bone marrow, neutrophils can either circulate freely in the bloodstream or be deposited next to vessel walls (margination).[4] All of these neutrophils are available to fight infection. The proportion of marginated neutrophils is greater in people of Afro-Caribbean or African origin than in Caucasians, leading to lower apparent white cell counts (WCC) in the former. This is benign ethnic neutropenia. Many countries allow registration of BEN status with the clozapine supplier whereby different (lower) limits are set for neutrophil counts in these patients.

Many patients develop neutropenia on clozapine but not all are clozapine-related or even pathological. Benign ethnic neutropenia very probably accounts for a proportion of observed or apparent clozapine-associated neutropenias (hence higher rates among Afro-Caribbeans). Distinguishing between true clozapine toxicity and neutropenia unrelated to clozapine is not possible with certainty but some factors are important. True clozapine-induced neutropenia generally occurs early in treatment. White cell counts are normal to begin with but then fall precipitously (over 1–2 weeks or less) and recover slowly once clozapine is withdrawn. In benign ethnic neutropenia, WCCs are generally low and may frequently fall below the lower limit of normal. This pattern may be observed before, during and after the use of clozapine. Of course, true clozapine-induced neutropenia can occur in the context of benign ethnic neutropenia. Partly because of this, **any iatrogenic manipulation of WCCs in benign ethnic neutropenia carries significant risk.**

Effect of lithium on the WCC

Lithium increases the neutrophil count and total WCC both acutely[5] and chronically.[6,7] The magnitude of this effect is poorly quantified, but a mean neutrophil count of 11.9×10^9/L has been reported in lithium-treated patients[5] and a mean rise in neutrophil count of 2×10^9/L was seen in clozapine-treated patients after the addition of lithium.[8] This effect does not seem to be clearly dose-related[5,6] although a minimum lithium serum level of 0.4mmol/L may be required.[9] The mechanism is not completely understood: both stimulation of granulocyte-macrophage colony-stimulating factor (GM-CSF)[10] and demargination[8] have been suggested. Lithium has been successfully used to raise the WCC during cancer chemotherapy.[11–13] White cells are fully formed and function normally – there is no 'left shift'.

Case reports

Lithium has been used to increase the WCC in patients who have developed neutropenia whilst taking clozapine, allowing clozapine treatment to continue. Several case reports in adults[9,14–18] and in children[19,20] have been published. Almost all patients had serum lithium levels of >0.6mmol/L. Lithium has also been reported to speed the recovery of the WCC when prescribed after the development of clozapine-induced agranulocytosis.[9] In a case series (n = 25) of patients who had stopped clozapine because of a blood dyscrasia and were re-challenged in the presence of lithium, only one developed a subsequent dyscrasia; a far lower proportion than would be expected[21] (see above).

Other potential benefits of lithium–clozapine combinations

Combinations of clozapine and lithium may improve symptoms in schizoaffective patients[8] and refractory bipolar illness.[22,23] There are no data pertaining to schizophrenia.

Agranulocytosis

At least 0.8% of clozapine-treated patients develop agranulocytosis, which is potentially fatal. Over 80% of cases develop within the first 18 weeks of treatment.[1] Risk factors include increasing age and Asian race.[1] Some patients may be genetically predisposed.[24] Although the timescale and individual risk factors for the development of agranulocytosis are different from those associated with neutropenia, it is impossible to be certain in any given patient that neutropenia is not a precursor to agranulocytosis. Lithium does not seem to protect against true clozapine-induced agranulocytosis: one case of fatal agranulocytosis has occurred with this combination[25] and a second case of agranulocytosis has been reported where the bone marrow was resistant to treatment with granulocyte-colony stimulating factor (G-CSF).[26] Note also that up to 20% of patients who receive clozapine–lithium combinations develop neurological symptoms typical of lithium toxicity despite lithium levels being maintained well within the therapeutic range.[8,27]

Management options

The use of iatrogenic agents to elevate WCC in patients with clear prior clozapine-induced neutropenia is not recommended. Lithium or other medicines should only be used to elevate WCC where it is strongly felt that prior neutropenic episodes were unrelated to clozapine. **Patients who have had a previous clear *clozapine-induced* agranulocytosis should not be re-challenged with clozapine.**

The patient's individual clinical circumstances should be considered. In particular, patients in whom the first dyscrasia:

- was inconsistent with previous WCCs (i.e. not part of a pattern of repeated low WCCs)
- occurred within the first 18 weeks of treatment
- was severe (neutrophils $< 0.5 \times 10^9$/L), and
- was prolonged

should be considered to be very high risk if re-challenged with clozapine. Generally re-exposure to clozapine should not be attempted.

Management of patients with either of the following conditions:

- low initial WCC ($<4 \times 10^9$/L) or neutrophils ($<2.5 \times 10^9$/L), or
- leucopenia (WCC $< 3 \times 10^9$/L) or neutropenia (neutrophils $< 1.5 \times 10^9$/L) thought to be linked to benign ethnic neutropenia. Such patients may be of African or Middle Eastern

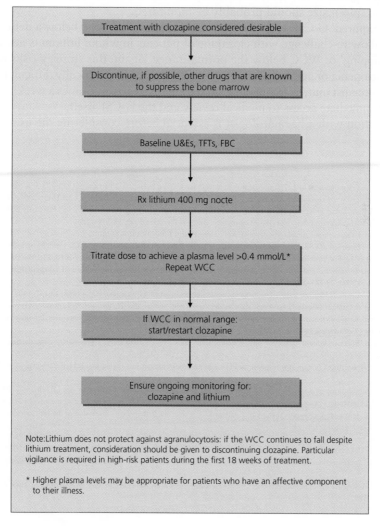

Note:Lithium does not protect against agranulocytosis: if the WCC continues to fall despite lithium treatment, consideration should be given to discontinuing clozapine. Particular vigilance is required in high-risk patients during the first 18 weeks of treatment.

* Higher plasma levels may be appropriate for patients who have an affective component to their illness.

Figure 2.6 The use of lithium with clozapine.

descent, have no history of susceptibility to infection and have morphologically normal white blood cells.

should be treated as outlined in Figure 2.6.

Granulocyte-colony stimulating factor

The use of granulocyte-colony stimulating factor (G-CSF) to facilitate uninterrupted clozapine therapy in patients with previous neutropenia is a strategy that is attracting increasing interest, but is somewhat controversial. There are both successful[28-30] and unsuccessful[30,31] case reports of patients receiving regular long-term G-CSF to enable clozapine therapy. As well as the commonly reported side-effects of bone pain[32] and neutrophil dysplasia,[33] the administration of G-CSF in the face of a low or declining neutrophil count may mask an impending neutropenia or agranulocytosis, leading to severe consequences. The long term safety of G-CSF has not been determined – bone density and spleen size should probably be monitored.

'When required' G-CSF, to be administered if neutrophils drop below a defined threshold, may allow re-challenge with clozapine of patients in whom lithium is insufficient to prevent 'dipping' of WCC below the normal range. Again, this strategy risks masking a severe neutropenia or agranulocytosis. It is also likely to be practically difficult to manage outside a specialist unit, as frequent blood testing (twice to three times a week) is required, as well as immediate access to medical review and the G-CSF itself.

Consultation with a haematologist is essential before considering the use of G-CSF.

References

1. Munro J et al. Active monitoring of 12760 clozapine recipients in the UK and Ireland. Br J Psychiatry 1999; **175**:576–580.
2. Whiskey E et al. Restarting clozapine after neutropenia: evaluating the possibilities and practicalities. CNS Drugs 2007; **21**:25–35.
3. Dunk LR et al. Rechallenge with clozapine following leucopenia or neutropenia during previous therapy. Br J Psychiatry 2006; **188**:255–263.
4. Abramson N et al. Leukocytosis: basics of clinical assessment. Am Fam Physician 2000; **62**:2053–2060.
5. Lapierre G et al. Lithium carbonate and leukocytosis. Am J Hosp Pharm 1980; **37**:1525–1528.
6. Carmen J et al. The effects of lithium therapy on leukocytes: a 1-year follow-up study. J Natl Med Assoc 1993; **85**:301–303.
7. Palominao A et al. Leukocytosis after lithium and clozapine combination therapy. Ann Clin Psychiatry 2010; **22**:205–206.
8. Small JG et al. Tolerability and efficacy of clozapine combined with lithium in schizophrenia and schizoaffective disorder. J Clin Psychopharmacol 2003; **23**:223–228.
9. Blier P et al. Lithium and clozapine-induced neutropenia/agranulocytosis. Int Clin Psychopharmacol 1998; **13**:137–140.
10. Ozdemir MA et al. Lithium-induced hematologic changes in patients with bipolar affective disorder. Biol Psychiatry 1994; **35**:210–213.
11. Johnke RM et al. Accelerated marrow recovery following total-body irradiation after treatment with vincristine, lithium or combined vincristine-lithium. Int J Cell Cloning 1991; **9**:78–88.
12. Greco FA et al. Effect of lithium carbonate on the neutropenia caused by chemotherapy: a preliminary clinical trial. Oncology 1977; **34**:153–155.
13. Ridgway D et al. Enhanced lymphocyte response to PHA among leukopenia patients taking oral lithium carbonate. Cancer Invest 1986; **4**:513–517.
14. Adityanjee A. Modification of clozapine-induced leukopenia and neutropenia with lithium carbonate. Am J Psychiatry 1995; **152**:648–649.
15. Silverstone PH. Prevention of clozapine-induced neutropenia by pretreatment with lithium. J Clin Psychopharmacol 1998; **18**:86–88.
16. Boshes RA et al. Initiation of clozapine therapy in a patient with preexisting leukopenia: a discussion of the rationale of current treatment options. Ann Clin Psychiatry 2001; **13**:233–237.
17. Papetti F et al. Treatment of clozapine-induced granulocytopenia with lithium (two observations). Encephale 2004; **30**:578–582.
18. Kutscher EC et al. Clozapine-induced leukopenia successfully treated with lithium. Am J Health Syst Pharm 2007; **64**:2027–2031.
19. Sporn A et al. Clozapine-induced neutropenia in children: management with lithium carbonate. J Child Adolesc Psychopharmacol 2003; **13**:401–404.
20. Mattai A et al. Adjunctive use of lithium carbonate for the management of neutropenia in clozapine-treated children. Hum Psychopharmacol 2009; **24**:584–589.

21. Kanaan RA et al. Lithium and clozapine rechallenge: a restrospective case analysis. J Clin Psychiatry 2006; **67**:756–760.

22. Suppes T et al. Clozapine treatment of nonpsychotic rapid cycling bipolar disorder: a report of three cases. Biol Psychiatry 1994; **36**:338–340.

23. Puri BK et al. Low-dose maintenance clozapine treatment in the prophylaxis of bipolar affective disorder. Br J Clin Pract 1995; **49**:333–334.

24. Dettling M et al. Further evidence of human leukocyte antigen-encoded susceptibility to clozapine-induced agranulocytosis independent of ancestry. Pharmacogenetics 2001; **11**:135–141.

25. Gerson SL et al. Polypharmacy in fatal clozapine-asscoaited agranulocytosis. Lancet 1991; **338**:262–263.

26. Valevski A et al. Clozapine-lithium combined treatment and agranulocytosis. Int Clin Psychopharmacol 1993; **8**:63–65.

27. Blake LM et al. Reversible neurologic symptoms with clozapine and lithium. J Clin Psychopharmacol 1992; **12**:297–299.

28. Spencer BW et al. Granulocyte colony stimulating factor (G-CSF) can allow treatment with clozapine in a patient with severe benign ethnic neutropaenia (BEN): a case report. J Psychopharmacol 2012; **26**:1280–1282.

29. Hagg S et al. Long-term combination treatment with clozapine and filgrastim in patients with clozapine-induced agranulocytosis. Int Clin Psychopharmacol 2003; **18**:173–174.

30. Joffe G et al. Add-on filgrastim during clozapine rechallenge in patients with a history of clozapine-related granulocytopenia/agranulocytosis. Am J Psychiatry 2009; **166**:236.

31. Mathewson KA et al. Clozapine and granulocyte colony-stimulating factor: potential for long-term combination treatment for clozapine-induced neutropenia. J Clin Psychopharmacol 2007; **27**:714–715.

32. Puhalla S et al. Hematopoietic growth factors: personalization of risks and benefits. Mol Oncol 2012; **6**:237–241.

33. Bain BJ et al. Neutrophil dysplasia induced by granulocyte colony-stimulating factor. Am J Hematol 2010; **85**:354.

Further reading

Paton C et al. Managing clozapine-induced neutropenia with lithium. Psychiatr Bull 2005;**29**:186–8.

Clozapine and chemotherapy

The use of clozapine with agents that cause neutropenia is formally contraindicated. Most chemotherapy treatments cause significant bone marrow suppression. When the white blood cell count drops below $3.0 \times 10^9/L$ clozapine is usually discontinued; this is an important safety precaution outlined in the formal licence/labelling. In many regimens it can be predicted that chemotherapy will reduce the white blood cell count below this level, irrespective of the use of clozapine.

If possible clozapine should be discontinued before chemotherapy. However, this will place most patients at high risk of relapse or deterioration which may affect their capacity to consent to chemotherapy. This poses a therapeutic dilemma in patients prescribed clozapine and requiring chemotherapy. Many patients, perhaps even a majority, continue clozapine during chemotherapy.

There are a number of case reports supporting the continued use of clozapine during chemotherapy.[1–13] Before initiating chemotherapy in a patient who takes clozapine, it is essential to put in place a treatment plan that is agreed with all relevant staff involved in the patient's care, and of course, the patient themself; this will include the oncologist/physician, psychiatrist, pharmacist and the clozapine monitoring service. Plans should be made in advance for the action that should be taken when the white blood count drops below the normally accepted minimum. This plan should cover the frequency of haematological monitoring, increased vigilance regarding the clinical consequences of neutropenia/agranulocytosis, if and when clozapine should be stopped, and the place of 'antidote' medication such as lithium and G-CSF.

In the UK, the clozapine monitoring service will normally ask for the psychiatrist to sign an 'unlicensed use' form and will request additional blood monitoring. Complications appear to be rare, but there is one case report of neutropenia persisting for 6 months after doxorubicin, radiotherapy and clozapine.[7] G-CSF has been used to treat agranulocytosis associated with chemotherapy and clozapine in combination.[8] Risks of life-threatening blood dyscrasia are probably lowest in those who have received clozapine for longer than a year in whom clozapine-induced neutropenia would be highly unusual.

Summary

- If possible clozapine should be discontinued before starting chemotherapy. For most patients withdrawal is not possible.
- The risk of relapse or deterioration must be considered before discontinuing clozapine.
- If the patient's mental state deteriorates they may retract their consent for chemotherapy.
- When clozapine is continued during chemotherapy a collaborative approach between the oncologist, psychiatrist, pharmacy, patient and clozapine monitoring service is strongly recommended.

References

1. Wesson ML et al. Continuing clozapine despite neutropenia. Br J Psychiatry 1996; **168**:217–220.
2. Bareggi C et al. Clozapine and full-dose concomitant chemoradiation therapy in a schizophrenic patient with nasopharyngeal cancer. Tumori 2002; **88**:59–60.
3. Avnon M et al. Clozapine, cancer, and schizophrenia. Am J Psychiatry 1993; **150**:1562–1563.

4. Hundertmark J et al. Reintroduction of clozapine after diagnosis of lymphoma. Br J Psychiatry 2001; **178**:576.

5. McKenna RC et al. Clozapine and chemotherapy. Hosp Community Psychiatry 1994; **45**:831.

6. Haut FA. Clozapine and chemotherapy. J Drug Dev Clin Pract 1995; **7**:237–239.

7. Rosenstock J. Clozapine therapy during cancer treatment. Am J Psychiatry 2004; **161**:175.

8. Lee SY et al. Combined antitumor chemotherapy in a refractory schizophrenic receiving clozapine (Korean). J Korean Neuropsychiatr Assoc 2000; **39**:234–239.

9. Rosenberg I et al. Restarting clozapine treatment during ablation chemotherapy and stem cell transplant for Hodgkin's lymphoma. Am J Psychiatry 2007; **164**:1438–1439.

10. Goulet K et al. Case report: clozapine given in the context of chemotherapy for lung cancer. Psychooncology 2008; **17**:512–516.

11. Frieri T et al. Maintaining clozapine treatment during chemotherapy for non-Hodgkin's lymphoma. Prog Neuropsychopharmacol Biol Psychiatry 2008; **32**:1611–1612.

12. Sankaranarayanan A et al. Clozapine, cancer chemotherapy and neutropenia - dilemmas in management. Psychiatr Danub 2013; **25**:419–422.

13. De Berardis D et al. Safety and efficacy of combined clozapine-azathioprine treatment in a case of resistant schizophrenia associated with Behcet's disease: a 2-year follow-up. Gen Hosp Psychiatry 2013; **35**:213–11.

CHAPTER 2

Bipolar affective disorder

Lithium

Mechanism of action

Lithium is an element that the body handles in a similar way to sodium. The ubiquitous nature of sodium in the human body, its involvement in a wide range of biological processes, and the potential for lithium to alter these processes, has made it extremely difficult to ascertain the key mechanism(s) of action of lithium in regulating mood. For example, there is some evidence that people with bipolar illness have higher intracellular concentrations of sodium and calcium than controls, and that lithium can reduce these. Reduced activity of sodium-dependent intracellular second messenger systems has been demonstrated, as have modulation of dopamine and serotonin neurotransmitter pathways, reduced activity of protein kinase C and reduced turnover of arachidonic acid. Lithium may also have neuroprotective effects, possibly mediated through its effects on N-methyl-D-aspartate (NMDA) pathways. For a review see Marmol (2008).[1] It is notable that, with the exception of a database study linking lithium use with a reduced risk of developing dementia,[2] literature pertaining to the possible neuroprotective effect of lithium reports largely on either *in vitro* or animal studies. The clinical literature is rather more dominated by reports of neurotoxicity.[3]

Indications

Lithium is effective in the treatment of *moderate to severe mania* with a number needed to treat (NNT) of 6.[4] Its use for this indication is limited by the fact that it usually takes at least a week to achieve a response[5] and that the co-administration of antipsychotics may increase the risk of neurological side-effects. It can also be difficult to achieve therapeutic plasma levels rapidly and monitoring can be problematic if the patient is uncooperative.

The Maudsley Prescribing Guidelines in Psychiatry, Twelfth Edition. David Taylor, Carol Paton and Shitij Kapur.
© 2015 David Taylor, Carol Paton and Shitij Kapur. Published 2015 by John Wiley & Sons, Ltd.

The main indication for lithium is in the *prophylaxis of bipolar affective disorder* where it reduces both the number and the severity of relapses.[6] Lithium is more effective at preventing manic than depressive relapse;[7] the NNT to prevent relapse into mania or depression has been calculated to be 10 and 14 respectively.[7] Lithium also offers some protection against antidepressant-induced hypomania. It is generally clinically appropriate to initiate prophylactic treatment: (1) after a single manic episode that was associated with significant risk and adverse consequences; (2) in the case of bipolar I illness, two or more acute episodes; or (3) in the case of bipolar II illness, significant functional impairment, frequent episodes or significant risk of suicide.[8] NICE supports the use of lithium as a first-line mood stabiliser; lithium alone is probably more effective than valproate alone,[9] with the combination being better still.[10] The earlier in the course of the illness that lithium treatment is started, the better the response is likely to be.[11]

Lithium *augmentation of an antidepressant* in patients with unipolar depression is recommended by NICE as a next-step treatment in patients who have not responded to standard antidepressant drugs.[12] A recent meta-analysis found lithium to be three times as effective as placebo for this indication with a NNT of 5,[13] although the response rate in STAR-D was more modest (see section on 'Refractory depression' in Chapter 4).

The effectiveness of lithium in treating mood disorders does not go unchallenged. For a review, see Moncrieff.[14]

Lithium is also used to treat aggressive[15] and self-mutilating behaviour, to both prevent and treat steroid-induced psychosis,[16] and to raise the white blood cell count in patients receiving clozapine.

Lithium and suicide

It is estimated that 15% of people with bipolar affective disorder take their own life.[17] A meta-analysis of clinical trials concluded that lithium reduced by 80% the risk of both attempted and completed suicide in patients with bipolar illness,[18,19] and two large database studies have shown that lithium-treated patients were less likely to complete suicide than patients treated with divalproex[20] or with other mood stabilising drugs (valproate, gabapentin, carbamazepine).[21]

In patients with unipolar depression, lithium also seems to protect against suicide; the effect size being slightly smaller than that seen in bipolar illness.[19,22] The mechanism of this protective effect is unknown.

Plasma levels

A recent systematic review of the relationship between plasma levels and response in patients with bipolar illness concluded that the minimum effective plasma level for prophylaxis is 0.4 mmol/L, with the optimal range being 0.6–0.75 mmol/L. Levels above 0.75 mmol/L offer additional protection only against manic symptoms.[8,23] Changes in plasma levels seem to worsen the risk of relapse.[24] The optimal plasma level range in patients who have unipolar depression is less clear.[13]

Children and adolescents may require higher plasma levels than adults to ensure that an adequate concentration of lithium is present in the central nervous system (CNS).[25]

Lithium is rapidly absorbed from the gastrointestinal tract but has a long distribution phase. Blood samples for plasma lithium level estimations should be taken 10–14 hours (ideally 12) post dose in patients who are prescribed a single daily dose of a prolonged-release preparation at bedtime.[26]

Formulations

There is no clinically significant difference in the pharmacokinetics of the two most widely prescribed brands of lithium in the UK: Priadel and Camcolit. Other preparations should not be assumed to be bioequivalent and should be prescribed by brand.

- Lithium carbonate 400 mg tablets each contain 10.8 mmol/lithium.
- Lithium citrate liquid is available in two strengths and should be administered twice daily:
  - 5.4 mmol/5mLs is equivalent to 200 mg lithium carbonate
  - 10.8 mmol/5mLs is equivalent to 400 mg lithium carbonate.

Lack of clarity over which liquid preparation is intended when prescribing can lead to the patient receiving a sub-therapeutic or toxic dose.

Adverse effects

Most side-effects are dose- (and therefore plasma level) related. These include mild gastro-intestinal upset, fine tremor, polyuria and polydipsia. Polyuria may occur more frequently with twice-daily dosing.[27] Propranolol can be useful in lithium-induced tremor. Some skin conditions such as psoriasis and acne can be aggravated by lithium therapy. Lithium can also cause a metallic taste in the mouth, ankle oedema and weight gain.

Lithium can cause a reduction in urinary concentrating capacity – nephrogenic diabetes insipidus – hence the occurrence of thirst and polyuria. This effect is usually reversible in the short to medium term but may be irreversible after long-term treatment (>15 years).[26,27] Lithium treatment can also lead to a reduction in the glomerular filtration rate (GFR);[28] the magnitude of the risk is uncertain.[29,30] One large cross-sectional study found that one-third of young people prescribed lithium had an e-GFR of <60 mLs/minute (chronic kidney disease stage 3).[28] A very small number of patients may develop interstitial nephritis. Lithium levels of >0.8 mmol/L are associated with a higher risk of renal toxicity.[23]

In the longer term, lithium increases the risk of hypothyroidism;[31] in middle-aged women, the risk may be up to 20%.[32] A case has been made for testing thyroid autoantibodies in this group before starting lithium (to better estimate risk) and for measuring thyroid function tests (TFTs) more frequently in the first year of treatment.[33] Hypothyroidism is easily treated with thyroxine. TFTs usually return to normal when lithium is discontinued. Lithium also increases the risk of hyperparathyroidism, and some recommend that calcium levels should be monitored in patients on long-term treatment.[33] Clinical consequences of chronically increased serum calcium include renal stones, osteoporosis, dyspepsia, hypertension and renal impairment.[33]

For a review of the toxicity profile of lithium, see McKnight et al.[34]

Lithium toxicity

Toxic effects reliably occur at levels >1.5 mmol/L and usually consist of gastro-intestinal effects (increasing anorexia, nausea and diarrhoea) and CNS effects (muscle weakness, drowsiness, ataxia, course tremor and muscle twitching). Above 2 mmol/L, increased disorientation and seizures usually occur, which can progress to coma, and ultimately death. In the presence of more severe symptoms, osmotic or forced alkaline diuresis should be used (note NEVER thiazide or loop diuretics). Above 3 mmol/L peritoneal or haemodialysis is often used. These plasma levels are only a guide and individuals vary in their susceptibility to symptoms of toxicity.

Most *risk factors for toxicity* involve changes in sodium levels or the way the body handles sodium. For example low salt diets, dehydration, drug interactions (see Table 3.1) and some uncommon physical illnesses such as Addison's disease.

Information relating to the symptoms of toxicity and the common risk factors should always be given to patients when treatment with lithium is initiated.[35] This information should be repeated at appropriate intervals to make sure that it is clearly understood.

Pre-treatment tests

Before prescribing lithium, renal, thyroid and cardiac function should be checked. As a minimum, e-GRF[36] and TFTs should be checked. An electrocardiogram (ECG) is also recommended in patients who have risk factors for, or existing, cardiovascular disease. A baseline measure of weight is also desirable.

Lithium is a human teratogen. Women of child-bearing age should be advised to use a reliable form of contraception. See section on 'Pregnancy' in Chapter 7.

Table 3.1 Lithium: prescribing and monitoring

Indications	Mania, hypomania, prophylaxis of bipolar affective disorder and recurrent depression. Reduces aggression and suicidality
Pre-lithium work up	e-GRF and TFTs. ECG recommended in patients who have risk factors for, or existing cardiovascular disease. Baseline measure of weight desirable
Prescribing	Start at 400 mg at night (200 mg in the elderly). Plasma level after 7 days, then 7 days after every dose change until the desired level is reached (0.4 mmol/L may be effective in unipolar depression, 0.6–1.0 mmol/L in bipolar illness, slightly higher levels in difficult to treat mania). Blood should be taken 12 hours after the last dose. Take care when prescribing liquid preparations to clearly specify the strength required
Monitoring	Plasma lithium every 6 months (more frequent monitoring is necessary in those prescribed interacting drugs, the elderly and those with established renal impairment or other relevant physical illness). e-GFR and TFTs every 6 months. Weight (or BMI) should also be monitored
Stopping	Reduce slowly over at least 1 month. Avoid incremental reductions in plasma levels of >0.2 mmol/L

BMI, body mass index; ECG, electrocardiogram; e-GFR, estimated glomerular filtration rate; TFT, thyroid function test.

On-treatment monitoring[8]

NICE recommend that plasma lithium, e-GFR and TFTs should be checked every 6 months. More frequent tests may be required in those who are prescribed interacting drugs, elderly or have established chronic kidney disease (CKD). A patient safety alert related to the importance of biochemical monitoring in patients prescribed lithium has been issued by the National Patient Safety Agency.[37] Weight (or BMI) should also be monitored. Lithium monitoring in clinical practice in the UK is known to be suboptimal,[38] although there has been a modest improvement over time.[39] The use of automated reminder systems has been shown to improve monitoring rates.[40]

Discontinuation

Intermittent treatment with lithium may worsen the natural course of bipolar illness. A much greater than expected incidence of manic relapse is seen in the first few months after discontinuing lithium,[41] even in patients who have been symptom free for as long as 5 years.[42] This has led to recommendations that lithium treatment should not be started unless there is a clear intention to continue it for at least 3 years.[43] This advice has obvious implications for initiating lithium treatment against a patient's will (or in a patient known to be non-compliant with medication) during a period of acute illness.

The risk of relapse is reduced by decreasing the dose gradually over a period of at least a month,[44] and avoiding decremental serum level reductions of >0.2 mmol/L.[23] The course of illness may, however, still be adversely affected: a recent naturalistic study found that, in patients who had been in remission for at least 2 years and had discontinued lithium very slowly, the recurrence rate was at least three times greater than in patients who continued lithium; significant survival differences persisted for many years. Patients maintained on high lithium levels prior to discontinuation were particularly prone to relapse.[45]

One large US study based on prescription records found that half of those prescribed lithium took almost all of their prescribed doses, a quarter took between 50 and 80%, and the remaining quarter took less than 50%. In addition one-third of patients took lithium for less than 6 months in total.[46] A large audit found that one in ten patients prescribed long-term lithium treatment had a plasma level below the therapeutic range.[47] It is clear that sub-optimal adherence limits the effectiveness of lithium in clinical practice. One database study suggested the extent to which lithium was taken was directly related to the risk of suicide (more prescriptions = lower suicide rate).[48]

Less convincing data support the emergence of depressive symptoms in patients with bipolar illness after lithium discontinuation.[41] There are few data relating to patients with unipolar depression.

Interactions with other drugs[49,50]

Because of lithium's relatively narrow therapeutic index, pharmacokinetic interactions with other drugs can precipitate lithium toxicity. Most clinically significant interactions are with drugs that alter renal sodium handling; see Table 3.2.

Table 3.2 Lithium: clinically relevant drug interactions

Drug group	Magnitude of effect	Timescale of effect	Additional information
ACE inhibitors	Unpredictable Up to four-fold increases in [Li]	Develops over several weeks	Seven-fold increased risk of hospitalisation for lithium toxicity in the elderly **Angiotensin II receptor antagonists** may be associated with similar risk
Thiazide diuretics	Unpredictable Up to four-fold increases in [Li]	Usually apparent in first 10 days	Loop diuretics are safer Any effect will be apparent in the first month
NSAIDs	Unpredictable From 10% to > four-fold increases in [Li]	Variable; few days to several months	NSAIDs are widely used on a prn basis Can be bought without a prescription

ACE, angiotensin converting enzyme; [Li], lithium; NSAIDs, non-steroidal anti-inflammatory drugs.

Angiotensin converting enzyme inhibitors

Angiotensin converting enzyme (ACE) inhibitors can (1) reduce thirst which can lead to mild dehydration, and (2) increase renal sodium loss leading to increased sodium re-absorption by the kidney, resulting in an increase in lithium plasma levels. The magnitude of this effect is variable; from no increase to a four-fold increase. The full effect can take several weeks to develop. The risk seems to be increased in patients with heart failure, dehydration and renal impairment (presumably because of changes in fluid balance/handling). In the elderly, ACE inhibitors increase seven-fold the risk of hospitalisation due to lithium toxicity. ACE inhibitors can also precipitate renal failure so, if co-prescribed with lithium, more frequent monitoring of e-GFR and plasma lithium is required.

The following drugs are ACE inhibitors: captopril, cilazapril enalapril, fosinopril, imidapril, lisinopril, moexipril, perindopril, quinapril, ramipril and trandolapril.

Care is also required with **angiotensin II receptor antagonists;** candesartan, eprosartan, irbesartan, losartan, olmesartan, telmisartan and valsartan.

Diuretics

Diuretics can reduce the renal clearance of lithium, the magnitude of this effect being greater with thiazide than loop diuretics. Lithium levels usually rise within 10 days of a *thiazide diuretic* being prescribed; the magnitude of the rise is unpredictable and can vary from an increase of 25% to 400%.

The following drugs are thiazide (or related) diuretics: bendroflumethiazide, chlortalidone, cyclopenthiazide, indapamide, metolazone and xipamide.

Although there are case reports of lithium toxicity induced by *loop diuretics*, many patients receive this combination of drugs without apparent problems. The risk of an interaction seems to be greatest in the first month after the loop diuretic has been prescribed and extra lithium plasma level monitoring during this time is recommended if these drugs are co-prescribed. Loop diuretics can increase sodium loss and subsequent re-absorption by the kidney. Patients taking loop diuretics may also have been advised to restrict their salt intake; this may contribute to the risk of lithium toxicity in these individuals.

The following drugs are loop diuretics: bumetanide, furosemide and torasemide.

Non-steroidal anti-inflammatory drugs

Non-steroidal anti-inflammatory drugs (NSAIDs) inhibit the synthesis of renal prosta-glandins, thereby reducing renal blood flow and possibly increasing renal re-absorption of sodium and therefore lithium. The magnitude of the rise is unpredictable for any given patient; case reports vary from increases of around 10% to over 400%. The onset of effect also seems to be variable; from a few days to several months. Risk appears to be increased in those patients who have impaired renal function, renal artery stenosis or heart failure and who are dehydrated or on a low salt diet. There are a growing number of case reports of an interaction between lithium and cyclo-oxygenase (COX)-2 inhibitors.

NSAIDs (or COX-2 inhibitors) can be combined with lithium, but (1) they should be prescribed regularly NOT prn, and (2) more frequent plasma lithium monitoring is essential.

Some NSAIDs can be purchased without a prescription, so it is particularly important that patients are aware of the potential for interaction.

The following drugs are NSAIDs or COX-2 inhibitors: aceclofenac, acemetacin, celecoxib, dexibuprofen, dexketoprofen, diclofenac, diflunisal, etodolac, etoricoxib, fenbufen, fenoprofen, flurbiprofen, ibuprofen, indometacin, ketoprofen, lumiracoxib, mefenamic acid, meloxicam, nabumetone, naproxen, piroxicam, sulindac, tenoxicam and tiaprofenic acid.

Carbamazepine

There are rare reports of neurotoxicity when carbamazepine is combined with lithium. Most are old and in the context of treatment involving high plasma lithium levels. It is of note though that carbamazepine can cause hyponatraemia, which may in turn lead to lithium retention and toxicity. Similarly, rare reports of CNS toxicity implicate **selective serotonin reuptake inhibitors** (SSRIs), another group of drugs that can cause hyponatraemia.

References

1. Marmol F. Lithium: Bipolar disorder and neurodegenerative diseases Possible cellular mechanisms of the therapeutic effects of lithium. Prog Neuropsychopharmacol Biol Psychiatry 2008; **32**:1761–1771.

2. Kessing LV et al. Does lithium protect against dementia? Bipolar Disord 2010; **12**:87–94.

3. Fountoulakis KN et al. A systematic review of existing data on long-term lithium therapy: neuroprotective or neurotoxic? Int J Neuropsychopharmacol 2008; **11**:269–287.

4. Storosum JG et al. Magnitude of effect of lithium in short-term efficacy studies of moderate to severe manic episode. Bipolar Disord 2007; **9**:793–798.

5. Ferrier IN et al. Lithium therapy. Adv Psychiatr Treat 1995; **1**:102–110.

6. Tondo L et al. Long-term clinical effectiveness of lithium maintenance treatment in types I and II bipolar disorders. Br J Psychiatry Suppl 2001; **41**:s184–s190.

7. Geddes JR et al. Long-term lithium therapy for bipolar disorder: systematic review and meta-analysis of randomized controlled trials. Am J Psychiatry 2004; **161**:217–222.

8. National Institute for Health and Care Excellence. Bipolar disorder: the assessment and management of bipolar disorder in adults, children and young people in primary and secondary care. Draft for consultation, April 2014. http://www.nice.org.uk/

9. Kessing LV et al. Valproate v. lithium in the treatment of bipolar disorder in clinical practice: observational nationwide register-based cohort study. Br J Psychiatry 2011; **199**:57–63.

CHAPTER 3

10. Geddes JR et al. Lithium plus valproate combination therapy versus monotherapy for relapse prevention in bipolar I disorder (BALANCE): a randomised open-label trial. Lancet 2010; 375:385–395.

11. Kessing LV et al. Starting lithium prophylaxis early v. late in bipolar disorder. Br J Psychiatry 2014; 205:214–220.

12. National Institute for Health and Clinical Excellence. Depression in adults: The treatment and management of depression in adults. Clinical Guideline 90, 2009. http://www.nice.org.uk/Guidance/cg90

13. Crossley NA et al. Acceleration and augmentation of antidepressants with lithium for depressive disorders: two meta-analyses of randomized, placebo-controlled trials. J Clin Psychiatry 2007; 68:935–940.

14. Moncrieff J. Lithium: evidence reconsidered. Br J Psychiatry 1997; 171:113–119.

15. Tyrer SP. Lithium and treatment of aggressive behaviour. Eur Neuropsychopharmacol 1994; 4:234–236.

16. Falk WE et al. Lithium prophylaxis of corticotropin-induced psychosis. JAMA 1979; 241:1011–1012.

17. Harris EC et al. Excess mortality of mental disorder. Br J Psychiatry 1998; 173:11–53.

18. Baldessarini RJ et al. Decreased risk of suicides and attempts during long-term lithium treatment: a meta-analytic review. Bipolar Disord 2006; 8:625–639.

19. Cipriani A et al. Lithium in the prevention of suicide in mood disorders: updated systematic review and meta-analysis. BMJ 2013; 346:f3646.

20. Goodwin FK et al. Suicide risk in bipolar disorder during treatment with lithium and divalproex. JAMA 2003; 290:1467–1473.

21. Collins JC et al. Divalproex, lithium and suicide among Medicaid patients with bipolar disorder. J Affect Disord 2008; 107:23–28.

22. Guzzetta F et al. Lithium treatment reduces suicide risk in recurrent major depressive disorder. J Clin Psychiatry 2007; 68:380–383.

23. Severus WE et al. What is the optimal serum lithium level in the long-term treatment of bipolar disorder–a review? Bipolar Disord 2008; 10:231–237.

24. Perlis RH et al. Effect of abrupt change from standard to low serum levels of lithium: a reanalysis of double-blind lithium maintenance data. Am J Psychiatry 2002; 159:1155–1159.

25. Moore CM et al. Brain-to-serum lithium ratio and age: an in vivo magnetic resonance spectroscopy study. Am J Psychiatry 2002; 159:1240–1242.

26. Anon. Using lithium safely. Drug Ther Bull 1999; 37:22–24.

27. Bowen RC et al. Less frequent lithium administration and lower urine volume. Am J Psychiatry 1991; 148:189–192.

28. Bassilios N et al. Monitoring of glomerular filtration rate in lithium-treated outpatients–an ambulatory laboratory database surveillance. Nephrol Dial Transplant 2008; 23:562–565.

29. Paul R et al. Meta-analysis of the effects of lithium usage on serum creatinine levels. J Psychopharmacol 2010; 24:1425–1431.

30. Kripalani M et al. Lithium and chronic kidney disease. BMJ 2009; 339:b2452.

31. Frye MA et al. Depressive relapse during lithium treatment associated with increased serum thyroid-stimulating hormone: results from two placebo-controlled bipolar I maintenance studies. Acta Psychiatr Scand 2009; 120:10–13.

32. Johnston AM et al. Lithium-associated clinical hypothyroidism. Prevalence and risk factors. Br J Psychiatry 1999; 175:336–339.

33. Livingstone C et al. Lithium: a review of its metabolic adverse effects. J Psychopharmacol 2006; 20:347–355.

34. McKnight RF et al. Lithium toxicity profile: a systematic review and meta-analysis. Lancet 2012; 379:721–728.

35. Gerrett D et al. Prescribing and monitoring lithium therapy: summary of a safety report from the National Patient Safety Agency. BMJ 2010; 341:c6258.

36. Morriss R et al. Lithium and eGFR: a new routinely available tool for the prevention of chronic kidney disease. Br J Psychiatry 2008; 193:93–95.

37. National Patient Safety Agency. Safer lithium therapy. NPSA/2009/PSA005. 2009. http://www.nrls.npsa.nhs.uk/

38. Collins N et al. Standards of lithium monitoring in mental health trusts in the UK. BMC Psych 2010; 10:80.

39. Paton C et al. Monitoring lithium therapy: the impact of a quality improvement programme in the UK. Bipolar Disord 2013; 15:865–875.

40. Kirkham E et al. Impact of active monitoring on lithium management in Norfolk. Ther Adv Psychopharmacol 2013; 3:260–265.

41. Cavanagh J et al. Relapse into mania or depression following lithium discontinuation: a 7-year follow-up. Acta Psychiatr Scand 2004; 109:91–95.

42. Yazici O et al. Controlled lithium discontinuation in bipolar patients with good response to long-term lithium prophylaxis. J Affect Disord 2004; 80:269–271.

43. Goodwin GM. Recurrence of mania after lithium withdrawal. Implications for the use of lithium in the treatment of bipolar affective disorder. Br J Psychiatry 1994; 164:149–152.

44. Baldessarini RJ et al. Effects of the rate of discontinuing lithium maintenance treatment in bipolar disorders. J Clin Psychiatry 1996; 57:441–448.

45. Biel MG et al. Continuation versus discontinuation of lithium in recurrent bipolar illness: a naturalistic study. Bipolar Disord 2007; 9:435–442.

46. Sajatovic M et al. Treatment adherence with lithium and anticonvulsant medications among patients with bipolar disorder. Psychiatr Serv 2007; 58:855–863.

47. Paton C et al. Lithium in bipolar and other affective disorders: prescribing practice in the UK. J Psychopharmacol 2010; 24:1739–1746.

48. Kessing LV et al. Suicide risk in patients treated with lithium. Arch Gen Psychiatry 2005; 62:860–866.

49. Stockley's Drug Interactions. London: Pharamceutical Press; 2014. https://www.medicinescomplete.com/

50. Juurlink DN et al. Drug-induced lithium toxicity in the elderly: a population-based study. J Am Geriatr Soc 2004; 52:794–798.

Valproate

Mechanism of action[1]

Valproate is a simple branched-chain fatty acid. Its mechanism of action is complex and not fully understood. Valproate inhibits the catabolism of gamma-aminobutyric acid (GABA), reduces the turnover of arachidonic acid, activates the extracellular signal-regulated kinase (ERK) pathway thus altering synaptic plasticity, interferes with intra-cellular signaling, promotes brain-derived neurotrophic factor (BDNF) expression and reduces levels of protein kinase C. Recent research has focused on the ability of valproate to alter the expression of multiple genes that are involved in transcription regulation, cytoskeletal modifications and ion homeostasis. Other mechanisms that have been proposed include depletion of inositol, and indirect effects on non-GABA pathways through inhibition of voltage-gated sodium channels.

There is a growing literature relating to the potential use of valproate as an adjunctive treatment in several types of cancer; the relevant mechanism of action being inhibition of histone deacetylase.[2–4]

Formulations

Valproate is available in the UK in three forms: sodium valproate and valproic acid (licensed for the treatment of epilepsy), and semi-sodium valproate, licensed for the treatment of acute mania. Both semi-sodium and sodium valproate are metabolised to valproic acid, which is responsible for the pharmacological activity of all three preparations.[5] Clinical studies of the treatment of affective disorders variably use sodium valproate, semi-sodium valproate, 'valproate' or valproic acid. The great majority have used semi-sodium valproate (divalproex in the US).

In the US, valproic acid is widely used in the treatment of bipolar illness,[6] and in the UK sodium valproate is widely used. It is important to remember that doses of sodium valproate and semi-sodium valproate are not equivalent; a slightly higher (approximately 10%) dose is required if sodium valproate is used to allow for the extra sodium content.

It is unclear if there is any difference in efficacy between valproic acid, valproate semi-sodium and sodium valproate. One large US quasi-experimental study found that inpatients who initially received the semi-sodium preparation had a hospital stay that was a third longer than patients who initially received valproic acid.[7] Note that sodium valproate controlled release (Epilim Chrono) can be administered as a once-daily dose whereas other sodium and semi-sodium valproate preparations require at least twice-daily administration.

Indications

Randomised controlled trials (RCTs) have shown valproate to be effective in the treatment of **mania**,[8,9] with a response rate of 50% and a NNT of 2–4,[10] although large negative studies do exist.[11] One RCT found lithium to be more effective overall than valproate[9] but a large (n = 300) randomized open trial of 12 weeks duration found lithium and valproate to be equally effective in the treatment of acute mania.[12] Valproate may be effective in patients who have failed to respond to lithium; in a small placebo controlled RCT (n = 36) in patients who had failed to respond to or could not tolerate lithium, the median decrease in Young Mania Rating Scale scores was 54% in the valproate group and 5% in the placebo group.[13] It may be less effective than olanzapine, both as monotherapy[14] as an adjunctive treatment to lithium[12] in acute mania. A network meta-analysis reported that valproate was less effective but better tolerated than lithium.[15]

A meta-analysis of four small RCTs concluded that valproate is effective in **bipolar depression** with a small to medium effect size,[16] although further data are required.[10]

Although open label studies suggest that valproate is effective in the **prophylaxis** of bipolar affective disorder,[17] RCT data are limited.[18,19] Bowden et al.[20] found no difference between lithium, valproate and placebo in the primary outcome measure, time to any mood episode, although valproate was superior to lithium and placebo on some secondary outcome measures. This study can be criticised for including patients who were 'not ill enough' and for not lasting 'long enough' (1 year). In another RCT,[18] which lasted for 47 weeks, there was no difference in relapse rates between valproate and olanzapine. The study had no placebo arm and the attrition rate was high, so is difficult to interpret. A post-hoc analysis of data from this study found that patients with rapid cycling illness had a better very early response to valproate than to olanzapine but that this advantage was not maintained.[19] Outcomes with respect to manic symptoms for those who did not have a rapid cycling illness were better at 1 year with olanzapine than valproate. In a further 20 month RCT of lithium versus valproate in patients with rapid cycling illness, both the relapse and attrition rate were high, and no difference in efficacy between valproate and lithium was apparent.[21] More recently, the BALANCE study found lithium to be numerically superior to valproate, and the combination of lithium and valproate statistically superior to valproate alone.[22] Aripiprazole in combination with valproate is superior to valproate alone.[23]

NICE recommends valproate as a first-line option for the treatment of acute episodes of mania, in combination with an antidepressant for the treatment of acute episodes of depression, and for prophylaxis,[24] but importantly NOT in women of child-bearing potential.[24,25] Cochrane conclude that the evidence supporting the use of valproate as prophylaxis is limited,[26] yet use for this indication has substantially increased in recent years.[27]

Valproate is sometimes used to treat aggressive behaviours of variable aetiology.[28] One small RCT (n = 16) failed to detect any advantage for risperidone augmented with valproate over risperidone alone in reducing hostility in patients with schizophrenia.[29] A mirror-image study found that, in patients with schizophrenia or bipolar disorder in a secure setting, valproate decreased agitation.[30]

There is a small positive placebo controlled RCT of valproate in generalised anxiety disorder.[31]

Plasma levels

The pharmacokinetics of valproate are complex, following a three-compartmental model and showing protein-binding saturation. Plasma level monitoring is supposedly of more limited use than with lithium or carbamazepine.[32] There may be a linear association between valproate serum levels and response in acute mania, with serum levels <55 mg/L being no more effective than placebo and levels >94 mg/L being associated with the most robust response,[33] although these data are weak.[32] Note that this is the top of the reference range (for epilepsy) that is quoted on laboratory forms. Optimal serum levels during the maintenance phase are unknown, but are likely to be at least 50 mg/L.[34] Achieving therapeutic plasma levels rapidly using a loading dose regimen is generally well tolerated. Plasma levels can also be used to detect non-compliance or toxicity.

Adverse effects

Valproate can cause both gastric irritation and hyperammonaemia,[35] both of which can lead to nausea. Lethargy and confusion can occasionally occur with starting doses above 750 mg/day. Weight gain can be significant,[36] particularly when valproate is used in combination with clozapine. Valproate causes dose related tremor in up to one-quarter of patients.[37] In the majority of these patients it is intention/postural tremor that is problematic, but a very small proportion develop parkinsonism associated with cognitive decline; these symptoms are reversible when valproate is discontinued.[38]

Hair loss with curly regrowth and peripheral oedema can occur, as can thrombocytopenia, leucopenia, red cell hypoplasia and pancreatitis.[39] Valproate can cause hyperandrogenism in women[40] and has been linked with the development of polycystic ovaries; the evidence supporting this association is conflicting. Valproate is a major human teratogen (see section on 'Pregnancy' in Chapter 7). Valproate may very rarely cause fulminant hepatic failure. Young children receiving multiple anticonvulsants are most at risk. Any patient with raised liver function tests (LFTs) (common in early treatment[41]) should be evaluated clinically and other markers of hepatic function, such as albumin and clotting time, should be checked.

Many side-effects of valproate are dose-related (peak plasma-level related) and increase in frequency and severity when the plasma level is >100 mg/L. The once daily chrono form of sodium valproate does not produce as high peak plasma levels as the conventional formulation, and so may be better tolerated.

Valproate and other anticonvulsant drugs have been associated with an increased risk of suicidal behaviour,[42] but this finding is not consistent across studies.[43] Patients with depression[44] or who take another anticonvulsant drug that increases the risk of developing depression may be a sub-group at greater risk.[45]

Note that valproate is eliminated mainly through the kidneys, partly in the form of ketone bodies, and may give a false positive urine test for ketones.

Pre-treatment tests

Baseline full blood count (FBC), LFTs, and weight or BMI, are recommended by NICE.

On-treatment monitoring

NICE recommend that a FBC and LFTs should be repeated after 6 months, and that BMI should be monitored. Valproate summary of product characteristics (SPCs) recommend more frequent LFTs during the first 6 months, with albumin and clotting measured if enzyme levels are abnormal.

Discontinuation

It is unknown if abrupt discontinuation of valproate worsens the natural course of bipolar illness in the same way that discontinuation of lithium does. One small naturalistic retrospective study suggests that it might.[46] Until further data are available, if valproate is to be discontinued, it should be done slowly over at least a month.

Use in women of child-bearing age

Valproate is an established human teratogen. NICE recommend that alternative anti-convulsants are preferred in women with epilepsy[47] and that valproate should not be used to treat bipolar illness in women of child-bearing age.[24]

The SPCs for sodium valproate and semi-sodium valproate[48,49] state that:

- these drugs should not be initiated in women of child-bearing potential without specialist advice (from a neurologist or psychiatrist)
- women who are trying to conceive and require valproate, should be prescribed prophylactic folate.

Women who have mania are likely to be sexually disinhibited. The risk of unplanned pregnancy is likely to be above population norms (where 50% of pregnancies are unplanned). If valproate cannot be avoided, adequate contraception should be ensured and prophylactic folate prescribed.

The teratogenic potential of valproate is not widely appreciated and many women of child-bearing age are not advised of the need for contraception or prophylactic folate.[50,51] Valproate may also cause impaired cognitive function in children exposed to valproate *in utero*.[52] See section on 'Pregnancy' in Chapter 7.

Interactions with other drugs

Valproate is highly protein bound and can be displaced by other protein-bound drugs, such as aspirin, leading to toxicity. Aspirin also inhibits the metabolism of valproate; a dose of at least 300 mg aspirin is required.[53] Other, less strongly protein-bound drugs, such as warfarin, can be displaced by valproate, leading to higher free levels and toxicity.

Valproate is hepatically metabolised; drugs that inhibit CYP enzymes can increase valproate levels (e.g. erythromycin, fluoxetine and cimetidine). Valproate can increase the plasma levels of some drugs, possibly by inhibition/competitive inhibition of their metabolism. Examples include tricyclic antidepressants (TCAs) (particularly clomipramine[54]), lamotrigine,[55] quetiapine,[56] warfarin[57] and phenobarbital. Valproate may also significantly lower plasma olanzapine concentrations; the mechanism is unknown.[58]

Pharmacodynamic interactions also occur. The anticonvulsant effect of valproate is antagonised by drugs that lower the seizure threshold (e.g. antipsychotics). Weight gain can be exacerbated by other drugs such as clozapine and olanzapine.

The prescribing and monitoring of valproate are summarised in Table 3.3.

Table 3.3 Valproate: prescribing and monitoring

Indications	Mania, hypomania, bipolar depression and prophylaxis of bipolar affective disorder May reduce aggression in a range of psychiatric disorders (data weak) Note that sodium valproate is licensed only for epilepsy and semi-sodium valproate only for acute mania
Pre-valproate work up	FBC and LFTs. Baseline measure of weight desirable
Prescribing	Titrate dose upwards against response and side-effects. Loading doses can be used and are generally well tolerated Note that controlled release sodium valproate (Epilim Chrono) can be given once daily. All other formulations must be administered at least twice daily Plasma levels can be used to ensure adequate dosing and treatment compliance. Blood should be taken immediately before the next dose
Monitoring	FBC and LFTs if clinically indicated Weight (or BMI)
Stopping	Reduce slowly over at least 1 month

BMI, body mass index; FBC, full blood count; LFT, liver function test.

References

1. Rosenberg G. The mechanisms of action of valproate in neuropsychiatric disorders: can we see the forest for the trees? Cell Mol Life Sci 2007; **64**:2090–2103.
2. Kuendgen A et al. Valproic acid for the treatment of myeloid malignancies. Cancer 2007; **110**:943–954.
3. Atmaca A et al. Valproic acid (VPA) in patients with refractory advanced cancer: a dose escalating phase I clinical trial. Br J Cancer 2007; **97**:177–182.
4. Hallas J et al. Cancer risk in long-term users of valproate: a population-based case-control study. Cancer Epidemiol Biomarkers Prev 2009; **18**:1714–1719.
5. Fisher C et al. Sodium valproate or valproate semisodium: is there a difference in the treatment of bipolar disorder? Psychiatr Bull 2003; **27**:446–448.
6. Iqbal SU et al. Divalproex sodium vs. valproic acid: drug utilization patterns, persistence rates and predictors of hospitalization among VA patients diagnosed with bipolar disorder. J Clin Pharm Ther 2007; **32**:625–632.
7. Wassef AA et al. Lower effectiveness of divalproex versus valproic acid in a prospective, quasi-experimental clinical trial involving 9,260 psychiatric admissions. Am J Psychiatry 2005; **162**:330–339.
8. Bowden CL et al. Efficacy of divalproex vs lithium and placebo in the treatment of mania. The Depakote Mania Study Group. JAMA 1994; **271**:918–924.
9. Freeman TW et al. A double-blind comparison of valproate and lithium in the treatment of acute mania. Am J Psychiatry 1992; **149**:108–111.
10. Nasrallah HA et al. Carbamazepine and valproate for the treatment of bipolar disorder: a review of the literature. J Affect Disord 2006; **95**:69–78.
11. Hirschfeld RM et al. A randomized, placebo-controlled, multicenter study of divalproex sodium extended-release in the acute treatment of mania. J Clin Psychiatry 2010; **71**:426–432.
12. Bowden C et al. A 12-week, open, randomized trial comparing sodium valproate to lithium in patients with bipolar I disorder suffering from a manic episode. Int Clin Psychopharmacol 2008; **23**:254–262.
13. Pope HG, Jr. et al. Valproate in the treatment of acute mania. A placebo-controlled study. Arch Gen Psychiatry 1991; **48**:62–68.
14. Novick D et al. Translation of randomised controlled trial findings into clinical practice: comparison of olanzapine and valproate in the EMBLEM study. Pharmacopsychiatry 2009; **42**:145–152.
15. Cipriani A et al. Comparative efficacy and acceptability of antimanic drugs in acute mania: a multiple-treatments meta-analysis. Lancet 2011; **378**:1306–1315.
16. Smith LA et al. Valproate for the treatment of acute bipolar depression: systematic review and meta-analysis. J Affect Disord 2010; **122**:1–9.
17. Calabrese JR et al. Spectrum of efficacy of valproate in 55 patients with rapid-cycling bipolar disorder. Am J Psychiatry 1990; **147**:431–434.
18. Tohen M et al. Olanzapine versus divalproex sodium for the treatment of acute mania and maintenance of remission: a 47-week study. Am J Psychiatry 2003; **160**:1263–1271.
19. Suppes T et al. Rapid versus non-rapid cycling as a predictor of response to olanzapine and divalproex sodium for bipolar mania and maintenance of remission: post hoc analyses of 47-week data. J Affect Disord 2005; **89**:69–77.
20. Bowden CL et al. A randomized, placebo-controlled 12-month trial of divalproex and lithium in treatment of outpatients with bipolar I disorder. Divalproex Maintenance Study Group. Arch Gen Psychiatry 2000; **57**:481–489.

21. Calabrese JR et al. A 20-month, double-blind, maintenance trial of lithium versus divalproex in rapid-cycling bipolar disorder. Am J Psychiatry 2005; **162**:2152–2161.

22. Geddes JR et al. Lithium plus valproate combination therapy versus monotherapy for relapse prevention in bipolar I disorder (BALANCE): a randomised open-label trial. Lancet 2010; **375**:385–395.

23. Marcus R et al. Efficacy of aripiprazole adjunctive to lithium or valproate in the long-term treatment of patients with bipolar I disorder with an inadequate response to lithium or valproate monotherapy: a multicenter, double-blind, randomized study. Bipolar Disord 2011; **13**: 133–144.

24. National Institute for Health and Care Excellence. Bipolar disorder: the assessment and management of bipolar disorder in adults, children and young people in primary and secondary care. Draft for consultation, April 2014. http://www.nice.org.uk/

25. National Institute for Health and Care Excellence. Antenatal and postnatal mental health (update): full version. Clinical management and service 5 guidance. Draft for consultation. 2014. http://www.nice.org.uk/

26. Cipriani A et al. Valproic acid, valproate and divalproex in the maintenance treatment of bipolar disorder. Cochrane Database Syst Rev 2013; **10**: CD003196.

27. Hayes J et al. Prescribing trends in bipolar disorder: cohort study in the United Kingdom THIN primary care database 1995–2009. PLoS One 2011; **6**:e28725.

28. Lindenmayer JP et al. Use of sodium valproate in violent and aggressive behaviors: a critical review. J Clin Psychiatry 2000; **61**:123–128.

29. Citrome L et al. Risperidone alone versus risperidone plus valproate in the treatment of patients with schizophrenia and hostility. Int Clin Psychopharmacol 2007; **22**:356–362.

30. Gobbi G et al. Efficacy of topiramate, valproate, and their combination on aggression/agitation behavior in patients with psychosis. J Clin Psychopharmacol 2006; **26**:467–473.

31. Aliyev NA et al. Valproate (depakine-chrono) in the acute treatment of outpatients with generalized anxiety disorder without psychiatric comorbidity: randomized, double-blind placebo-controlled study. Eur Psychiatry 2008; **23**:109–114.

32. Haymond J et al. Does valproic acid warrant therapeutic drug monitoring in bipolar affective disorder? Ther Drug Monit 2010; **32**:19–29.

33. Allen MH et al. Linear relationship of valproate serum concentration to response and optimal serum levels for acute mania. Am J Psychiatry 2006; **163**:272–275.

34. Taylor D et al. Doses of carbamazepine and valproate in bipolar affective disorder. Psychiatr Bull 1997; **21**:221–223.

35. Segura-Bruna N et al. Valproate-induced hyperammonemic encephalopathy. Acta Neurol Scand 2006; **114**:1–7.

36. El-Khatib F et al. Valproate, weight gain and carbohydrate craving: a gender study. Seizure 2007; **16**:226–232.

37. Zadikoff C et al. Movement disorders in patients taking anticonvulsants. J Neurol Neurosurg Psychiatry 2007; **78**:147–151.

38. Ristic AJ et al. The frequency of reversible parkinsonism and cognitive decline associated with valproate treatment: a study of 364 patients with different types of epilepsy. Epilepsia 2006; **47**:2183–2185.

39. Gerstner T et al. Valproic acid-induced pancreatitis: 16 new cases and a review of the literature. J Gastroenterol 2007; **42**:39–48.

40. Joffe H et al. Valproate is associated with new-onset oligoamenorrhea with hyperandrogenism in women with bipolar disorder. Biol Psychiatry 2006; **59**:1078–1086.

41. Bjornsson E. Hepatotoxicity associated with antiepileptic drugs. Acta Neurol Scand 2008; **118**:281–290.

42. Patorno E et al. Anticonvulsant medications and the risk of suicide, attempted suicide, or violent death. JAMA 2010; **303**:1401–1409.

43. Gibbons RD et al. Relationship between antiepileptic drugs and suicide attempts in patients with bipolar disorder. Arch Gen Psychiatry 2009; **66**:1354–1360.

44. Arana A et al. Suicide-related events in patients treated with antiepileptic drugs. N Engl J Med 2010; **363**:542–551.

45. Andersohn F et al. Use of antiepileptic drugs in epilepsy and the risk of self-harm or suicidal behavior. Neurology 2010; **75**:335–340.

46. Franks MA et al. Bouncing back: is the bipolar rebound phenomenon peculiar to lithium? A retrospective naturalistic study. J Psychopharmacol 2008; **22**:452–456.

47. National Institute for Health and Clinical Excellence. The epilepsies: the diagnosis and management of the epilepsies in adults and children in primary and secondary care. Clinical Guideline 137, 2012. http://guidance.nice.org.uk/CG137

48. Sanofi. Summary of Product Characteristics. Epilim Chrono 500 mg. 2013. http://www.medicines.org.uk/

49. Sanofi. Summary of Product Characteristics. Depakote 250 mg Tablets. 2013. http://www.medicines.org.uk/

50. James L et al. Informing patients of the teratogenic potential of mood stabilising drugs; a case notes review of the practice of psychiatrists. J Psychopharmacol 2007; **21**:815–819.

51. James L et al. Mood stabilizers and teratogenicity – prescribing practice and awareness amongst practising psychiatrists. J Ment Health 2009; **18**:137–143.

52. Meador KJ et al. Cognitive function at 3 years of age after fetal exposure to antiepileptic drugs. N Engl J Med 2009; **360**:1597–1605.

53. Sandson NB et al. An interaction between aspirin and valproate: the relevance of plasma protein displacement drug-drug interactions. Am J Psychiatry 2006; **163**:1891–1896.

54. Fehr C et al. Increase in serum clomipramine concentrations caused by valproate. J Clin Psychopharmacol 2000; **20**:493–494.

55. Morris RG et al. Clinical study of lamotrigine and valproic acid in patients with epilepsy: using a drug interaction to advantage? Ther Drug Monit 2000; **22**:656–660.

56. Aichhorn W et al. Influence of age, gender, body weight and valproate comedication on quetiapine plasma concentrations. Int Clin Psychopharmacol 2006; **21**:81–85.

57. Gunes A et al. Inhibitory effect of valproic acid on cytochrome P450 2C9 activity in epilepsy patients. Basic Clin Pharmacol Toxicol 2007; **100**:383–386.

58. Bergemann N et al. Valproate lowers plasma concentration of olanzapine. J Clin Psychopharmacol 2006; **26**:432–434.

Carbamazepine

Mechanism of action[1]

Carbamazepine blocks voltage-dependent sodium channels thus inhibiting repetitive neuronal firing. It reduces glutamate release and decreases the turnover of dopamine and nor-adrenaline. Carbamazepine has a similar molecular structure to TCAs.

As well as blocking voltage-dependent sodium channels, oxcarbazepine also increases potassium conductance and modulates high-voltage activated calcium channels.

Formulations

Carbamazepine is available as a liquid, chewable, immediate-release and controlled-release tablets. Conventional formulations generally have to be administered two- to three-times daily. The controlled release preparation can be given once or twice daily, and the reduced fluctuation in serum levels usually leads to improved tolerability. This preparation has a lower bioavailability and an increase in dose of 10–15% may be required.

Indications

Carbamazepine is primarily used as an anticonvulsant in the treatment of grand mal and focal seizures. It is also used in the treatment of trigeminal neuralgia and, in the UK, is licensed for the treatment of bipolar illness in patients who do not respond to lithium.

With respect to the treatment of *mania*, two placebo-controlled randomised studies have found the extended-release formulation of carbamazepine to be effective; in both studies, the response rate in the carbamazepine arm was twice that in the placebo arm.[2,3] Carbamazepine was not particularly well tolerated; the incidence of dizziness, somnolence and nausea was high. Another study found carbamazepine alone to be as effective as carbamazepine plus olanzapine.[4] NICE does not recommend carbamazepine as a first-line treatment for mania.[5]

Open studies suggest that carbamazepine monotherapy has some efficacy in *bipolar depression*;[6] note that the evidence base supporting other strategies is stronger (see section on 'Bipolar depression' in this chapter). Carbamazepine may also be useful in *unipolar depression* either alone[7] or as an augmentation strategy.[8]

Carbamazepine is generally considered to be less effective than lithium in the *prophylaxis* of bipolar illness;[9] several published studies report a low response rate and high drop-out rate. A meta-analysis (n = 464) failed to find a significant difference in efficacy between lithium and carbamazepine, but those who received carbamazepine were more likely to drop out of treatment because of side-effects.[10] Lithium is considered to be superior to carbamazepine in reducing suicidal behaviour,[11] although data are not consistent.[12] NICE considers carbamazepine to be a third-line prophylactic agent.[5] Three small studies suggest the related oxcarbazepine may have some prophylactic efficacy when used in combination with other mood stabilising drugs.[13–15]

There are data supporting the use of carbamazepine in the management of alcohol withdrawal symptoms,[16] although the high doses required initially are often poorly tolerated. Cochrane does not consider the evidence strong enough to support the use of carbamazepine for this indication.[17] Carbamazepine has also been used to manage aggressive behaviour in patients with schizophrenia;[18] the quality of data is weak and the mode of action unknown. There are a number of case reports and open case series that report on the use of carbamazepine in various psychiatric illnesses such as panic disorder, borderline personality disorder and episodic dyscontrol syndrome.

Plasma levels

When carbamazepine is used as an anticonvulsant, the therapeutic range is generally considered to be 4–12 mg/L, although the supporting evidence is not strong. In patients with affective illness, a dose of at least 600 mg/day and a plasma level of at least 7 mg/L may be required,[19] although this is not a consistent finding.[4,7,20] Levels above 12 mg/L are associated with a higher side-effect burden.

Carbamazepine serum levels vary markedly within a dosage interval. It is therefore important to sample at a point in time where levels are likely to be reproducible for any given individual. The most appropriate way of monitoring is to take a trough level before the first dose of the day.

Carbamazepine is a hepatic enzyme inducer that induces its own metabolism as well as that of other drugs. An initial plasma half-life of around 30 hours is reduced to around 12 hours on chronic dosing. For this reason, plasma levels should be checked 2–4 weeks after an increase in dose to ensure that the desired level is still being obtained.

Most published clinical trials that demonstrate the efficacy of carbamazepine as a mood stabiliser use doses that are significantly higher (800–1200 mg/day) than those commonly prescribed in UK clinical practice.[21]

Adverse effects[1]

The main side-effects associated with carbamazepine therapy are dizziness, diplopia, drowsiness, ataxia, nausea and headaches. They can sometimes be avoided by starting with a low dose and increasing slowly. Avoiding high peak blood levels by splitting the dose throughout the day, or using a controlled release formulation, may also help. Dry mouth, oedema and hyponatraemia are also common. Sexual dysfunction can occur, probably mediated through reduced testosterone levels.[22] Around 3% of patients treated with carbamazepine develop a generalised erythematous rash. Serious exfoliative dermatological reactions can rarely occur; vulnerability is genetically determined,[23] and genetic testing of people of Han Chinese or Thai origin is recommended before carbamazepine is prescribed. Carbamazepine is a known human teratogen (see section on 'Pregnancy' in Chapter 7).

Carbamazepine commonly causes a chronic low white blood cell (WBC) count. One patient in 20,000 develops agranulocytosis and/or aplastic anaemia.[24] Raised alkaline phosphatase (ALP) and gamma-glutamyl transferase (GGT) are common (a GGT of 2–3 times normal is rarely a cause for concern[25]). A delayed multi-organ hypersensitivity reaction rarely occurs, mainly manifesting itself as various skin reactions, a low WBC count, and abnormal LFTs. Fatalities have been reported.[25,26] There is no clear timescale for these events.

Some anticonvulsant drugs have been associated with an increased risk of suicidal behaviour. Carbamazepine has not been implicated, either in general,[27,28] or more specifically, in those with bipolar illness.[29]

Pre-treatment tests

Baseline U&Es, FBC and LFTs are recommended by NICE. A baseline measure of weight is also desirable.

On-treatment monitoring

NICE recommend that U&Es, FBC and LFTs should be repeated after 6 months, and that weight (or BMI) should also be monitored.

Discontinuation

It is not known if abrupt discontinuation of carbamazepine worsens the natural course of bipolar illness in the same way that abrupt cessation of lithium does. In one small case series (n = 6), one patient developed depression within 1 month of discontinuation,[30] while in another small case series (n = 4), three patients had a recurrence of their mood disorder within 3 months.[31] Until further data are available, if carbamazepine is to be discontinued, it should be done slowly (over at least a month).

Use in women of child-bearing age

Carbamazepine is an established human teratogen (see section on 'Pregnancy' in Chapter 7).

Women who have mania are likely to be sexually disinhibited. The risk of unplanned pregnancy is likely to be above population norms (where 50% of pregnancies are unplanned). If carbamazepine cannot be avoided, adequate contraception should be ensured (note the interaction between carbamazepine and oral contraceptives outlined below) and prophylactic folate prescribed.

Interactions with other drugs[32-35]

Carbamazepine is a potent inducer of hepatic cytochrome enzymes and is metabolised by CYP3A4. Plasma levels of most **antidepressants**, most **antipsychotics, benzodiazepines**, some **cholinesterase inhibitors, methadone, thyroxine, theophylline, oestrogens** and other steroids may be reduced by carbamazepine, resulting in treatment failure. Patients requiring contraception should either receive a preparation containing not less than 50 μg oestrogen or use a non-hormonal method. Drugs that inhibit CYP3A4 will increase carbamazepine plasma levels and may precipitate toxicity. Examples include cimetidine, diltiazem, verapamil, erythromycin and some selective serotonin reuptake inhibitors (SSRIs).

Pharmacodynamic interactions also occur. The anticonvulsant activity of carbamazepine is reduced by drugs that lower the seizure threshold (e.g. antipsychotics and

CHAPTER 3

Table 3.4 Carbamazepine: prescribing and monitoring

Indications	Mania (not first line), bipolar depression (evidence weak), unipolar depression (evidence weak), and prophylaxis of bipolar disorder (third line after antipsychotics and valproate). Alcohol withdrawal (may be poorly tolerated) Carbamazepine is licensed for the treatment of bipolar illness in patients who do not respond to lithium
Pre-carbamazepine work up	U&Es, FBC and LFTs. Baseline measure of weight desirable
Prescribing	Titrate dose upwards against response and side effects; start with 100–200 mg bd and aim for 400 mg bd (some patients will require higher doses) Note that the modified release formulation (Tegretol Retard) can be given once to twice daily, is associated with less severe fluctuations in serum levels, and is generally better tolerated Plasma levels can be used to assure adequate dosing and treatment compliance. Blood should be taken immediately before the next dose. Carbamazepine induces its own metabolism; serum levels (if used) should be re-checked a month after an increase in dose
Monitoring	U&Es, FBC and LFTs if clinically indicated Weight (or BMI)
Stopping	Reduce slowly over at least 1 month

bd, *bis in die* (twice a day); BMI, body mass index; FBC, full blood count; LFT, liver function test; U&E, urea and electrolytes.

antidepressants), the potential for carbamazepine to cause neutropenia may be increased by other drugs that have the potential to depress the bone marrow (e.g. clozapine), and the risk of hyponatraemia may be increased by other drugs that have the potential to deplete sodium (e.g. diuretics). Neurotoxicity has been reported when carbamazepine is used in combination with lithium. This is rare.

As carbamazepine is structurally similar to TCAs, in theory it should not be given within 14 days of discontinuing a monoamine oxidase inhibitor (MAOI).

The prescribing and monitoring of carbamazepine is summarised in Table 3.4.

References

1. Novartis Pharmaceuticals UK Ltd. Summary of Product Characteristics. Tegretol Prolonged Release 200 mg and 400 mg Tablets (formerly Tegretol retard). 2014. http://www.medicines.org.uk/
2. Weisler RH et al. A multicenter, randomized, double-blind, placebo-controlled trial of extended-release carbamazepine capsules as monotherapy for bipolar disorder patients with manic or mixed episodes. J Clin Psychiatry 2004; 65:478–484.
3. Weisler RH et al. Extended-release carbamazepine capsules as monotherapy for acute mania in bipolar disorder: a multicenter, randomized, double-blind, placebo-controlled trial. J Clin Psychiatry 2005; 66:323–330.
4. Tohen M et al. Olanzapine plus carbamazepine v. carbamazepine alone in treating manic episodes. Br J Psychiatry 2008; 192:135–143.
5. National Institute for Health and Care Excellence. Bipolar disorder: the assessment and management of bipolar disorder in adults, children and young people in primary and secondary care. Draft for consultation, April 2014. https://www.nice.org.uk/
6. Dilsaver SC et al. Treatment of bipolar depression with carbamazepine: results of an open study. Biol Psychiatry 1996; 40:935–937.
7. Zhang ZJ et al. The effectiveness of carbamazepine in unipolar depression: a double-blind, randomized, placebo-controlled study. J Affect Disord 2008; 109:91–97.
8. Kramlinger KG et al. The addition of lithium to carbamazepine. Antidepressant efficacy in treatment-resistant depression. Arch Gen Psychiatry 1989; 46:794–800.
9. Nasrallah HA et al. Carbamazepine and valproate for the treatment of bipolar disorder: a review of the literature. J Affect Disord 2006; 95:69–78.

10. Ceron-Litvoc D et al. Comparison of carbamazepine and lithium in treatment of bipolar disorder: a systematic review of randomized controlled trials. Hum Psychopharmacol 2009; **24**:19–28.

11. Kleindienst N et al. Differential efficacy of lithium and carbamazepine in the prophylaxis of bipolar disorder: results of the MAP study. Neuropsychobiology 2000; **42 Suppl 1**:2–10.

12. Yerevanian BI et al. Bipolar pharmacotherapy and suicidal behavior. Part I: Lithium, divalproex and carbamazepine. J Affect Disord 2007; **103**:5–11.

13. Vieta E et al. A double-blind, randomized, placebo-controlled prophylaxis trial of oxcarbazepine as adjunctive treatment to lithium in the long-term treatment of bipolar I and II disorder. Int J Neuropsychopharmacol 2008; **11**:445–452.

14. Conway CR et al. An open-label trial of adjunctive oxcarbazepine for bipolar disorder. J Clin Psychopharmacol 2006; **26**:95–97.

15. Juruena MF et al. Bipolar I and II disorder residual symptoms: oxcarbazepine and carbamazepine as add-on treatment to lithium in a double-blind, randomized trial. Prog Neuropsychopharmacol Biol Psychiatry 2009; **33**:94–99.

16. Malcolm R et al. The effects of carbamazepine and lorazepam on single versus multiple previous alcohol withdrawals in an outpatient randomized trial. J Gen Intern Med 2002; **17**:349–355.

17. Minozzi S et al. Anticonvulsants for alcohol withdrawal. Cochrane Database Syst Rev 2010;CD005064.

18. Brieden T et al. Psychopharmacological treatment of aggression in schizophrenic patients. Pharmacopsychiatry 2002; **35**:83–89.

19. Taylor D et al. Doses of carbamazepine and valproate in bipolar affective disorder. Psychiatr Bull 1997; **21**:221–223.

20. Simhandl C et al. The comparative efficacy of carbamazepine low and high serum level and lithium carbonate in the prophylaxis of affective disorders. J Affect Disord 1993; **28**:221–231.

21. Taylor DM et al. Prescribing and monitoring of carbamazepine and valproate – a case note review. Psychiatr Bull 2000; **24**:174–177.

22. Lossius MI et al. Reversible effects of antiepileptic drugs on reproductive endocrine function in men and women with epilepsy–a prospective randomized double-blind withdrawal study. Epilepsia 2007; **48**:1875–1882.

23. Hung SI et al. Genetic susceptibility to carbamazepine-induced cutaneous adverse drug reactions. Pharmacogenet Genomics 2006; **16**:297–306.

24. Kaufman DW et al. Drugs in the aetiology of agranulocytosis and aplastic anaemia. Eur J Haematol Suppl 1996; **60**:23–30.

25. Bjornsson E. Hepatotoxicity associated with antiepileptic drugs. Acta Neurol Scand 2008; **118**:281–290.

26. Ganeva M et al. Carbamazepine-induced drug reaction with eosinophilia and systemic symptoms (DRESS) syndrome: report of four cases and brief review. Int J Dermatol 2008; **47**:853–860.

27. Patorno E et al. Anticonvulsant medications and the risk of suicide, attempted suicide, or violent death. JAMA 2010; **303**:1401–1409.

28. Andersohn F et al. Use of antiepileptic drugs in epilepsy and the risk of self-harm or suicidal behavior. Neurology 2010; **75**:335–340.

29. Gibbons RD et al. Relationship between antiepileptic drugs and suicide attempts in patients with bipolar disorder. Arch Gen Psychiatry 2009; **66**:1354–1360.

30. Macritchie KA et al. Does 'rebound mania' occur after stopping carbamazepine? A pilot study. J Psychopharmacol 2000; **14**:266–268.

31. Franks MA et al. Bouncing back: is the bipolar rebound phenomenon peculiar to lithium? A retrospective naturalistic study. J Psychopharmacol 2008; **22**:452–456.

32. Spina E et al. Clinical significance of pharmacokinetic interactions between antiepileptic and psychotropic drugs. Epilepsia 2002; **43 Suppl 2**: 37–44.

33. Patsalos PN et al. The importance of drug interactions in epilepsy therapy. Epilepsia 2002; **43**:365–385.

34. Crawford P. Interactions between antiepileptic drugs and hormonal contraception. CNS Drugs 2002; **16**:263–272.

35. Citrome L et al. Pharmacokinetics of aripiprazole and concomitant carbamazepine. J Clin Psychopharmacol 2007; **27**:279–283.

CHAPTER 3

Antipsychotics in bipolar disorder

It is unhelpful to think of antipsychotic drugs as having only 'antipsychotic' actions. Individual antipsychotics variously possess sedative, anxiolytic, antimanic, mood-stabilising and antidepressant properties. Some antipsychotics (quetiapine and olanzapine) show all of these activities.

First-generation antipsychotics (FGAs) have long been used in mania and several studies support their use in a variety of hypomanic and manic presentations.[1–3] Their effectiveness seems to be enhanced by the addition of a mood stabiliser.[4,5] In the longer-term treatment of bipolar affective disorder, FGAs are widely used (presumably as prophylaxis)[6] but robust supporting data are absent.[7] The observation that typical antipsychotics are associated with both depression and tardive dyskinesia in bipolar patients militates against their long-term use.[7–9] Certainly the use of second-generation antipsychotics (SGAs) seems less likely to cause depression than treatment with halo-peridol.[10] The use of FGA depots is common in practice but poorly supported and seems to be associated with a high risk of depression.[11]

Among newer antipsychotics, olanzapine, risperidone, quetiapine, aripiprazole and asenapine have been most robustly evaluated and are licensed in many countries for the treatment of mania. Olanzapine is more effective than placebo in mania,[12,13] and at least as effective as valproate semi-sodium[14,15] and lithium.[16,17] As with FGAs, olanzapine may be most effective when used in combination with a mood-stabiliser[18,19] (although in one study, olanzapine + carbamazepine was no better than carbamazepine alone[20]). Data suggest olanzapine may offer benefits in longer-term treatment;[21,22] it may be more effective than lithium,[23] and it is formally licensed as prophylaxis.

Data relating to quetiapine[24–26] suggest robust efficacy in all aspects of bipolar affective disorder including prevention of bipolar depression.[27] Aripiprazole is effective in mania both alone[28–30] and as an add-on agent,[31] and in long-term prophylaxis.[32,33] Clozapine seems to be effective in refractory bipolar conditions, including refractory mania.[34–37] Risperidone has shown efficacy in mania,[38] particularly in combination with a mood-stabiliser.[2,39] Risperidone long acting injection is also effective[40] (note though that the pharmacokinetics of this formulation generally render it an unsuitable choice for the acute treatment of mania). There are few data for amisulpride[41] rather more for ziprasidone[42] and effectively none for lurasidone (notwithstanding its effect as an acute treatment for bipolar depression[43,44]) or iloperidone.

Asenapine is given by the sublingual route and is effective in mania.[45,46] Efficacy seems to be maintained in the longer term.[47] Asenapine is less sedative than olanzapine with a similar (low) propensity for akathisia and other movement disorders[46,47] and is less likely than olanzapine to cause weight gain and metabolic disturbance.[48]

Overall, antipsychotics (particularly haloperidol, olanzapine and risperidone) may be more effective than traditional mood stabilisers in the treatment of mania,[49] and quetiapine is similarly effective but better tolerated than aripiprazole or lithium.[49]

References

1. Prien RF et al. Comparison of lithium carbonate and chlorpromazine in the treatment of mania. Report of the Veterans Administration and National Institute of Mental Health Collaborative Study Group. Arch Gen Psychiatry 1972; 26:146–153.
2. Sachs GS et al. Combination of a mood stabilizer with risperidone or haloperidol for treatment of acute mania: a double-blind, placebo-controlled comparison of efficacy and safety. Am J Psychiatry 2002; 159:1146–1154.

3. McElroy SL et al. A randomized comparison of divalproex oral loading versus haloperidol in the initial treatment of acute psychotic mania. J Clin Psychiatry 1996; 57:142–146.

4. Chou JC et al. Acute mania: haloperidol dose and augmentation with lithium or lorazepam. J Clin Psychopharmacol 1999; 19:500–505.

5. Small JG et al. A placebo-controlled study of lithium combined with neuroleptics in chronic schizophrenic patients. Am J Psychiatry 1975; 132:1315–1317.

6. Soares JC et al. Adjunctive antipsychotic use in bipolar patients: an open 6-month prospective study following an acute episode. J Affect Disord 1999; 56:1–8.

7. Keck PE, Jr. et al. Anticonvulsants and antipsychotics in the treatment of bipolar disorder. J Clin Psychiatry 1998; 59 Suppl 6:74–81.

8. Tohen M et al. Antipsychotic agents and bipolar disorder. J Clin Psychiatry 1998; 59 Suppl 1:38–48.

9. Zarate CA, Jr. et al. Double-blind comparison of the continued use of antipsychotic treatment versus its discontinuation in remitted manic patients. Am J Psychiatry 2004; 161:169–171.

10. Goikolea JM et al. Lower rate of depressive switch following antimanic treatment with second-generation antipsychotics versus haloperidol. J Affect Disord 2013; 144:191–198.

11. Gigante AD et al. Long-acting injectable antipsychotics for the maintenance treatment of bipolar disorder. CNS Drugs 2012; 26:403–420.

12. Tohen M et al. Olanzapine versus placebo in the treatment of acute mania. Olanzapine HGEH Study Group. Am J Psychiatry 1999; 156:702–709.

13. Tohen M et al. Efficacy of olanzapine in acute bipolar mania: a double-blind, placebo-controlled study. The Olanzipine HGGW Study Group. Arch Gen Psychiatry 2000; 57:841–849.

14. Tohen M et al. Olanzapine versus divalproex in the treatment of acute mania. Am J Psychiatry 2002; 159:1011–1017.

15. Tohen M et al. Olanzapine versus divalproex versus placebo in the treatment of mild to moderate mania: a randomized, 12-week, double-blind study. J Clin Psychiatry 2008; 69:1776–1789.

16. Berk M et al. Olanzapine compared to lithium in mania: a double-blind randomized controlled trial. Int Clin Psychopharmacol 1999; 14:339–343.

17. Niufan G et al. Olanzapine versus lithium in the acute treatment of bipolar mania: a double-blind, randomized, controlled trial. J Affect Disord 2008; 105:101–108.

18. Tohen M et al. Efficacy of olanzapine in combination with valproate or lithium in the treatment of mania in patients partially nonresponsive to valproate or lithium monotherapy. Arch Gen Psychiatry 2002; 59:62–69.

19. Tohen M et al. Relapse prevention in bipolar I disorder: 18-month comparison of olanzapine plus mood stabiliser v. mood stabiliser alone. Br J Psychiatry 2004; 184:337–345.

20. Tohen M et al. Olanzapine plus carbamazepine v. carbamazepine alone in treating manic episodes. Br J Psychiatry 2008; 192:135–143.

21. Sanger TM et al. Long-term olanzapine therapy in the treatment of bipolar I disorder: an open-label continuation phase study. J Clin Psychiatry 2001; 62:273–281.

22. Vieta E et al. Olanzapine as long-term adjunctive therapy in treatment-resistant bipolar disorder. J Clin Psychopharmacol 2001; 21:469–473.

23. Tohen M et al. Olanzapine versus lithium in the maintenance treatment of bipolar disorder: a 12-month, randomized, double-blind, controlled clinical trial. Am J Psychiatry 2005; 162:1281–1290.

24. Ghaemi SN et al. The use of quetiapine for treatment-resistant bipolar disorder: a case series. Ann Clin Psychiatry 1999; 11:137–140.

25. Sachs G et al. Quetiapine with lithium or divalproex for the treatment of bipolar mania: a randomized, double-blind, placebo-controlled study. Bipolar Disord 2004; 6:213–223.

26. Altamura AC et al. Efficacy and tolerability of quetiapine in the treatment of bipolar disorder: preliminary evidence from a 12-month open label study. J Affect Disord 2003; 76:267–271.

27. Young AH et al. A randomised, placebo-controlled 52-week trial of continued quetiapine treatment in recently depressed patients with bipolar I and bipolar II disorder. World J Biol Psychiatry 2014; 15:96–112.

28. Sachs G et al. Aripiprazole in the treatment of acute manic or mixed episodes in patients with bipolar I disorder: a 3-week placebo-controlled study. J Psychopharmacol 2006; 20:536–546.

29. Keck PE et al. Aripiprazole monotherapy in the treatment of acute bipolar I mania: a randomized, double-blind, placebo- and lithium-controlled study. J Affect Disord 2009; 112:36–49.

30. Young AH et al. Aripiprazole monotherapy in acute mania: 12-week randomised placebo- and haloperidol-controlled study. The British Journal of Psychiatry 2009; 194:40–48.

31. Vieta E et al. Efficacy of adjunctive aripiprazole to either valproate or lithium in bipolar mania patients partially nonresponsive to valproate/lithium monotherapy: a placebo-controlled study. Am J Psychiatry 2008; 165:1316–1325.

32. Keck PE, Jr. et al. Aripiprazole monotherapy for maintenance therapy in bipolar I disorder: a 100-week, double-blind study versus placebo. J Clin Psychiatry 2007; 68:1480–1491.

33. Vieta E et al. Assessment of safety, tolerability and effectiveness of adjunctive aripiprazole to lithium/valproate in bipolar mania: a 46-week, open-label extension following a 6-week double-blind study. Curr Med Res Opin 2010; 26:1485–1496.

34. Calabrese JR et al. Clozapine for treatment-refractory mania. Am J Psychiatry 1996; 153:759–764.

35. Green AI et al. Clozapine in the treatment of refractory psychotic mania. Am J Psychiatry 2000; 157:982–986.

36. Kimmel SE et al. Clozapine in treatment-refractory mood disorders. J Clin Psychiatry 1994; 55 Suppl B:91–93.

37. Chang JS et al. The effects of long-term clozapine add-on therapy on the rehospitalization rate and the mood polarity patterns in bipolar disorders. J Clin Psychiatry 2006; 67:461–467.

38. Segal J et al. Risperidone compared with both lithium and haloperidol in mania: a double-blind randomized controlled trial. Clin Neuropharmacol 1998; 21:176–180.

39. Vieta E et al. Risperidone in the treatment of mania: efficacy and safety results from a large, multicentre, open study in Spain. J Affect Disord 2002; 72:15–19.

40. Quiroz JA et al. Risperidone long-acting injectable monotherapy in the maintenance treatment of bipolar I disorder. Biol Psychiatry 2010; 68:156–162.

41. Vieta E et al. An open-label study of amisulpride in the treatment of mania. J Clin Psychiatry 2005; 66:575–578.

42. Vieta E et al. Ziprasidone in the treatment of acute mania: a 12-week, placebo-controlled, haloperidol-referenced study. J Psychopharmacol 2010; 24:547–558.

43. Loebel A et al. Lurasidone monotherapy in the treatment of bipolar I depression: a randomized, double-blind, placebo-controlled study. Am J Psychiatry 2014; 171:160–168.

44. Loebel A et al. Lurasidone as adjunctive therapy with lithium or valproate for the treatment of bipolar I depression: a randomized, double-blind, placebo-controlled study. Am J Psychiatry 2014; 171:169–177.

45. McIntyre RS et al. Asenapine in the treatment of acute mania in bipolar I disorder: a randomized, double-blind, placebo-controlled trial. J Affect Disord 2010; 122:27–38.

46. McIntyre RS et al. Asenapine versus olanzapine in acute mania: a double-blind extension study. Bipolar Disord 2009; 11:815–826.

47. McIntyre RS et al. Asenapine for long-term treatment of bipolar disorder: a double-blind 40-week extension study. J Affect Disord 2010; 126:358–365.

48. Kemp DE et al. Weight change and metabolic effects of asenapine in patients with schizophrenia and bipolar disorder. J Clin Psychiatry 2014; 75:238–245.

49. Cipriani A et al. Comparative efficacy and acceptability of antimanic drugs in acute mania: a multiple-treatments meta-analysis. Lancet 2011; 378:1306–1315.

CHAPTER 3

Treatment of acute mania or hypomania

Drug treatment is the mainstay of therapy for mania and hypomania. Both antipsychotics and so-called mood stabilisers are effective. Sedative and anxiolytic drugs (e.g. benzodiazepines) may add to the effects of these drugs. Drug choice is made difficult by the dearth of direct comparisons and so no drug can be recommended over another on efficacy grounds. However, a multiple treatments meta-analysis[1] (which allows indirect comparison)

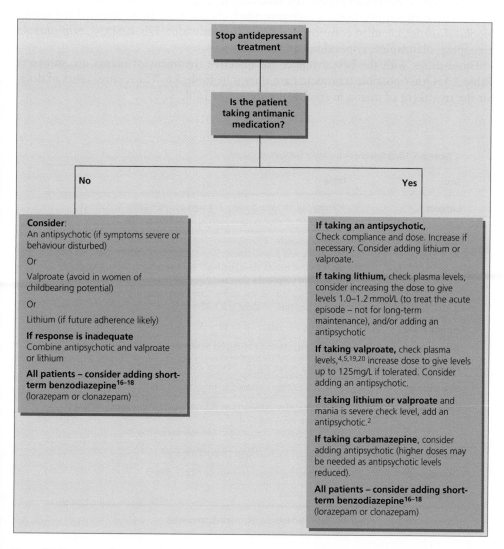

Figure 3.1 Treatment of acute mania or hypomania.[2–15] Note that lithium may be relatively less effective in mixed states[21] or substance misuse.[22]

suggested that olanzapine, risperidone haloperidol and quetiapine had the best combination of efficacy and acceptability. The added benefit of antipsychotic–mood stabiliser combinations (compared with mood-stabiliser alone) is established for those relapsing while on mood stabilisers, but unclear for those presenting on no treatment.[2–6]

Figure 3.1 outlines a treatment strategy for mania and hypomania. These recommendations are based on UK NICE guidelines,[3] the British Association of Psychopharmacology guidelines,[4] American Psychiatric Association guidelines[5] and individual references cited. Where an antipsychotic is recommended, choose from those licensed for mania/bipolar disorder, i.e. most conventional drugs (see individual labels/SPCs), aripiprazole, asenapine, olanzapine, risperidone and quetiapine.

Those drugs with the best evidence for effective treatment of mania are shown in Table 3.5. Other possible treatments are shown in Table 3.6. The relative costs of drugs for the treatment of mania in the UK are shown in Table 3.7.

Table 3.5 Drug treatment of mania: suggested doses

Drug	Dose
Lithium	400 mg/day, increasing every 3–4 days according to plasma levels. At least one study has used 800 mg as a starting dose[23]
Valproate	As **semi-sodium**: 250 mg three-times daily increasing according to tolerability and plasma levels. Slow release semi-sodium valproate may also be effective (at 15–30 mg/kg)[24] but there is one failed study[25] As **sodium valproate** slow release – 500 mg/day increasing as above Higher, so-called loading doses, have been used, both oral[26–28] and intravenous.[29,30] Dose is 20–30 mg/kg/day
Aripiprazole	15 mg/day increasing up to 30 mg/day as required[31,32]
Asenapine	5 mg bd increasing to 10 mg bd as required
Olanzapine	10 mg/day increasing to 15 mg or 20 mg as required
Risperidone	2 mg or 3 mg/day increased to 6 mg/day as required
Quetiapine	**IR** – 100 mg/day increasing to 800 mg as required. Higher starting doses have been used[33] **ER** – 300 mg/day increasing to 600 mg/day on day 2
Haloperidol	5–10 mg/day increasing to 15 mg if required
Lorazepam[17,18]	Up to 4 mg/day (some centres use higher doses)
Clonazepam[16,18]	Up to 8 mg/day

bd, bis in die (twice a day); ER, extended release; IR, immediate release.

Table 3.6 Other possible drug treatments for mania (listed in alphabetical order)

Treatment	Comments
Allopurinol[34] (600 mg/day)	Clear therapeutic effect when added to lithium in one RCT (n = 120), but no effect in a smaller recent study[35]
Clozapine[36,37]	Established treatment option for refractory mania/bipolar disorder
Gabapentin[38–40] (up to 2.4 g/day)	Probably only effective by virtue of an anxiolytic effect. Rarely used. Possibly useful as prophylaxis[41]
Lamotrigine[42,43] (up to 200 mg/day)	Possibly effective but better evidence for bipolar depression
Levetiracetam[44,45] (up to 4000 mg/day)	Possibly effective but controlled studies required
Memantine[46] (10–30 mg/day)	Small open study
Oxcarbazepine[47–53] (around 300–3000 mg/day)	Probably effective acutely and as prophylaxis although one controlled study conducted (in youths) was negative[54]
Phenytoin[55] (300–400 mg/day)	Rarely used. Limited data. Complex kinetics with narrow therapeutic range
Ritanserin[56] (10 mg/day)	Supported by a single RCT. Well tolerated. May protect against EPS
Tamoxifen[57–59] (10–140 mg/day)	Possibly effective. Three small RCTs. Dose–response relationship unclear, but 80 mg/day clearly effective when added to lithium
Topiramate[60–63] (up to 300 mg/day)	Possibly effective. Causes weight loss but poorly tolerated
Tryptophan depletion[64]	Supported by a small RCT
Ziprasidone[65–67]	Supported by three RCTs

Consult specialist and primary literature before using any treatment listed.
EPS, extrapyramidal side-effects; RCT, randomised controlled trial.

Table 3.7 Drugs for acute mania: relative costs

Drug	Cost	Comments
Lithium (Priadel) 800 mg/day	£+	Add cost of plasma level monitoring
Carbamazepine (Tegretol Retard) 800 mg/day	£++	Self-induction complicates acute treatment; reduces plasma levels of other drugs
Sodium valproate (Epilim Chrono) 1500 mg/day	£++	Not licensed for mania, but may be given once daily
Valproate semi-sodium (Depakote) 1500 mg/day	£++	Licensed for mania, but given two or three times daily
Aripiprazole (Abilify) 15 mg/day	£+++	Non-sedative, but effective. Patent near expiration in most countries
Haloperidol (generic) 10 mg/day	£+	Most widely used typical antipsychotic in mania
Asenapine (Sycrest) 20 mg/day	£+++	Sublingual only. Licensed for mania only
Olanzapine (generic) 15 mg/day	£+	Velotabs or equivalent may be more expensive
Quetiapine (generic - IR) 600 mg/day	£+	ER preparation branded in some countries
Risperidone (generic) 4 mg/day	£+	Non-sedative but effective

ER, extended release; IR, immediate release.

References

1. Cipriani A et al. Comparative efficacy and acceptability of antimanic drugs in acute mania: a multiple-treatments meta-analysis. Lancet 2011; 378:1306–1315.
2. Smith LA et al. Acute bipolar mania: a systematic review and meta-analysis of co-therapy vs. monotherapy. Acta Psychiatr Scand 2007; 115:12–20.
3. National Institute for Health and Care Excellence. Bipolar disorder: the assessment and management of bipolar disorder in adults, children and young people in primary and secondary care. Draft for consultation, April 2014. https://www.nice.org.uk/
4. Goodwin GM. Evidence-based guidelines for treating bipolar disorder: revised second edition–recommendations from the British Association for Psychopharmacology. J Psychopharmacol 2009; 23:346–388.
5. American Psychiatric Association. Guideline Watch: Practice guideline for the treatment of patients with bipolar disorder, 2nd edn. Washington DC: American Psychiatric Association; 2005. DOI: 10.1176/appi.books.9780890423363.148430.
6. Sachs GS. Decision tree for the treatment of bipolar disorder. J Clin Psychiatry 2003; 64 Suppl 8:35–40.
7. Tohen M et al. A 12-week, double-blind comparison of olanzapine vs haloperidol in the treatment of acute mania. Arch Gen Psychiatry 2003; 60:1218–1226.
8. Baldessarini RJ et al. Olanzapine versus placebo in acute mania treatment responses in subgroups. J Clin Psychopharmacol 2003; 23:370–376.
9. Sachs G et al. Quetiapine with lithium or divalproex for the treatment of bipolar mania: a randomized, double-blind, placebo-controlled study. Bipolar Disord 2004; 6:213–223.
10. Yatham LN et al. Quetiapine versus placebo in combination with lithium or divalproex for the treatment of bipolar mania. J Clin Psychopharmacol 2004; 24:599–606.
11. Yatham LN et al. Risperidone plus lithium versus risperidone plus valproate in acute and continuation treatment of mania. Int Clin Psychopharmacol 2004; 19:103–109.
12. Bowden CL et al. Risperidone in combination with mood stabilizers: a 10-week continuation phase study in bipolar I disorder. J Clin Psychiatry 2004; 65:707–714.
13. Hirschfeld RM et al. Rapid antimanic effect of risperidone monotherapy: a 3-week multicenter, double-blind, placebo-controlled trial. Am J Psychiatry 2004; 161:1057–1065.
14. Bowden CL et al. A randomized, double-blind, placebo-controlled efficacy and safety study of quetiapine or lithium as monotherapy for mania in bipolar disorder. J Clin Psychiatry 2005; 66:111–121.
15. Khanna S et al. Risperidone in the treatment of acute mania: double-blind, placebo-controlled study. Br J Psychiatry 2005; 187:229–234.
16. Sachs GS et al. Adjunctive clonazepam for maintenance treatment of bipolar affective disorder. J Clin Psychopharmacol 1990; 10:42–47.
17. Modell JG et al. Inpatient clinical trial of lorazepam for the management of manic agitation. J Clin Psychopharmacol 1985; 5:109–113.
18. Curtin F et al. Clonazepam and lorazepam in acute mania: a Bayesian meta-analysis. J Affect Disord 2004; 78:201–208.
19. Taylor D et al. Doses of carbamazepine and valproate in bipolar affective disorder. Psychiatr Bull 1997; 21:221–223.
20. Allen MH et al. Linear relationship of valproate serum concentration to response and optimal serum levels for acute mania. Am J Psychiatry 2006; 163:272–275.
21. Swann AC et al. Lithium treatment of mania: clinical characteristics, specificity of symptom change, and outcome. Psychiatry Res 1986; 18:127–141.
22. Goldberg JF et al. A history of substance abuse complicates remission from acute mania in bipolar disorder. J Clin Psychiatry 1999; 60:733–740.
23. Bowden CL et al. Efficacy of valproate versus lithium in mania or mixed mania: a randomized, open 12-week trial. Int Clin Psychopharmacol 2010; 25:60–67.
24. McElroy SL et al. Randomized, double-blind, placebo-controlled study of divalproex extended release loading monotherapy in ambulatory bipolar spectrum disorder patients with moderate-to-severe hypomania or mild mania. J Clin Psychiatry 2010; 71:557–565.
25. Hirschfeld RM et al. A randomized, placebo-controlled, multicenter study of divalproex sodium extended-release in the acute treatment of mania. J Clin Psychiatry 2010; 71:426–432.
26. McElroy SL et al. A randomized comparison of divalproex oral loading versus haloperidol in the initial treatment of acute psychotic mania. J Clin Psychiatry 1996; 57:142–146.
27. Hirschfeld RM et al. Safety and tolerability of oral loading divalproex sodium in acutely manic bipolar patients. J Clin Psychiatry 1999; 60:815–818.
28. Hirschfeld RM et al. The safety and early efficacy of oral-loaded divalproex versus standard-titration divalproex, lithium, olanzapine, and placebo in the treatment of acute mania associated with bipolar disorder. J Clin Psychiatry 2003; 64:841–846.
29. Jagadheesan K et al. Acute antimanic efficacy and safety of intravenous valproate loading therapy: an open-label study. Neuropsychobiology 2003; 47:90–93.
30. Sekhar S et al. Efficacy of sodium valproate and haloperidol in the management of acute mania: a randomized open-label comparative study. J Clin Pharmacol 2010; 50:688–692.
31. Young AH et al. Aripiprazole monotherapy in acute mania: 12-week randomised placebo- and haloperidol-controlled study. Br J Psychiatry 2009; 194:40–48.
32. Keck PE et al. Aripiprazole monotherapy in the treatment of acute bipolar I mania: a randomized, double-blind, placebo- and lithium-controlled study. J Affect Disord 2009; 112:36–49.
33. Pajonk FG et al. Rapid dose titration of quetiapine for the treatment of acute schizophrenia and acute mania: a case series. J Psychopharmacol 2006; 20:119–124.

34. Machado-Vieira R et al. A double-blind, randomized, placebo-controlled 4-week study on the efficacy and safety of the purinergic agents allopurinol and dipyridamole adjunctive to lithium in acute bipolar mania. J Clin Psychiatry 2008; 69:1237–1245.

35. Fan A et al. Allopurinol augmentation in the outpatient treatment of bipolar mania: a pilot study. Bipolar Disord 2012; 14:206–210.

36. Mahmood T et al. Clozapine in the management of bipolar and schizoaffective manic episodes resistant to standard treatment. Aust N Z J Psychiatry 1997; 31:424–426.

37. Green AI et al. Clozapine in the treatment of refractory psychotic mania. Am J Psychiatry 2000; 157:982–986.

38. Macdonald KJ et al. Newer antiepileptic drugs in bipolar disorder: rationale for use and role in therapy. CNS Drugs 2002; 16:549–562.

39. Cabras PL et al. Clinical experience with gabapentin in patients with bipolar or schizoaffective disorder: results of an open-label study. J Clin Psychiatry 1999; 60:245–248.

40. Pande AC et al. Gabapentin in bipolar disorder: a placebo-controlled trial of adjunctive therapy. Gabapentin Bipolar Disorder Study Group. Bipolar Disord 2000; 2 (3 Pt 2):249–255.

41. Vieta E et al. A double-blind, randomized, placebo-controlled, prophylaxis study of adjunctive gabapentin for bipolar disorder. J Clin Psychiatry 2006; 67:473–477.

42. Calabrese JR et al. Spectrum of activity of lamotrigine in treatment-refractory bipolar disorder. Am J Psychiatry 1999; 156:1019–1023.

43. Bowden CL et al. A placebo-controlled 18-month trial of lamotrigine and lithium maintenance treatment in recently manic or hypomanic patients with bipolar I disorder. Arch Gen Psychiatry 2003; 60:392–400.

44. Grunze H et al. Levetiracetam in the treatment of acute mania: an open add-on study with an on-off-on design. J Clin Psychiatry 2003; 64:781–784.

45. Goldberg JF et al. Levetiracetam for acute mania (Letter). Am J Psychiatry 2002; 159:148.

46. Koukopoulos A et al. Antimanic and mood-stabilizing effect of memantine as an augmenting agent in treatment-resistant bipolar disorder. Bipolar Disord 2010; 12:348–349.

47. Benedetti A et al. Oxcarbazepine as add-on treatment in patients with bipolar manic, mixed or depressive episode. J Affect Disord 2004; 79:273–277.

48. Lande RG. Oxcarbazepine: Efficacy, safety, and tolerability in the treatment of mania. Int J Psychiatry Clin Pract 2004; 8:37–40.

49. Ghaemi SN et al. Oxcarbazepine treatment of bipolar disorder. J Clin Psychiatry 2003; 64:943–945.

50. Pratoomsri W et al. Oxcarbazepine in the treatment of bipolar disorder: a review. Can J Psychiatry 2006; 51:540–545.

51. Juruena MF et al. Bipolar I and II disorder residual symptoms: oxcarbazepine and carbamazepine as add-on treatment to lithium in a double-blind, randomized trial. Prog Neuropsychopharmacol Biol Psychiatry 2009; 33:94–99.

52. Suppes T et al. Comparison of two anticonvulsants in a randomized, single-blind treatment of hypomanic symptoms in patients with bipolar disorder. Aust N Z J Psychiatry 2007; 41:397–402.

53. Vieta E et al. A double-blind, randomized, placebo-controlled prophylaxis trial of oxcarbazepine as adjunctive treatment to lithium in the long-term treatment of bipolar I and II disorder. Int J Neuropsychopharmacol 2008; 11:445–452.

54. Wagner KD et al. A double-blind, randomized, placebo-controlled trial of oxcarbazepine in the treatment of bipolar disorder in children and adolescents. Am J Psychiatry 2006; 163:1179–1186.

55. Mishory A et al. Phenytoin as an antimanic anticonvulsant: a controlled study. Am J Psychiatry 2000; 157:463–465.

56. Akhondzadeh S et al. Ritanserin as an adjunct to lithium and haloperidol for the treatment of medication-naive patients with acute mania: a double blind and placebo controlled trial. BMC Psych 2003; 3:7.

57. Zarate CA, Jr. et al. Efficacy of a protein kinase C inhibitor (tamoxifen) in the treatment of acute mania: a pilot study. Bipolar Disord 2007; 9:561–570.

58. Yildiz A et al. Protein kinase C inhibition in the treatment of mania: a double-blind, placebo-controlled trial of tamoxifen. Arch Gen Psychiatry 2008; 65:255–263.

59. Amrollahi Z et al. Double-blind, randomized, placebo-controlled 6-week study on the efficacy and safety of the tamoxifen adjunctive to lithium in acute bipolar mania. J Affect Disord 2011; 129:327–331.

60. Grunze HC et al. Antimanic efficacy of topiramate in 11 patients in an open trial with an on-off-on design. J Clin Psychiatry 2001; 62:464–468.

61. Yatham LN et al. Third generation anticonvulsants in bipolar disorder: a review of efficacy and summary of clinical recommendations. J Clin Psychiatry 2002; 63:275–283.

62. Vieta E et al. 1-year follow-up of patients treated with risperidone and topiramate for a manic episode. J Clin Psychiatry 2003; 64:834–839.

63. Vieta E et al. Use of topiramate in treatment-resistant bipolar spectrum disorders. J Clin Psychopharmacol 2002; 22:431–435.

64. Applebaum J et al. Rapid tryptophan depletion as a treatment for acute mania: a double-blind, pilot-controlled study. Bipolar Disord 2007; 9:884–887.

65. Keck PE, Jr. et al. Ziprasidone in the treatment of acute bipolar mania: a three-week, placebo-controlled, double-blind, randomized trial. Am J Psychiatry 2003; 160:741–748.

66. Potkin SG et al. Ziprasidone in acute bipolar mania: a 21-day randomized, double-blind, placebo-controlled replication trial. J Clin Psychopharmacol 2005; 25:301–310.

67. Vieta E et al. Ziprasidone in the treatment of acute mania: a 12-week, placebo-controlled, haloperidol-referenced study. J Psychopharmacol 2010; 24:547–558.

CHAPTER 3

Bipolar depression

Bipolar depression is a common and debilitating disorder which differs from unipolar disorder in severity, time course, recurrence and response to drug treatment. Episodes of bipolar depression are, compared with unipolar depression, more rapid in onset, more frequent, more severe, shorter and more likely to involve delusions and reverse neurovegetative symptoms such as hyperphagia and hypersomnia.[1-3] Around 15% of people with bipolar affective disorder commit suicide,[4] a statistic which aptly reflects the severity and frequency of depressive episodes. Bipolar depression affords greater socio-economic burden than either mania and unipolar depression[5] and represents the majority of symptomatic illness in bipolar affective disorder in respect to time.[6,7]

The drug treatment of bipolar depression is somewhat controversial for two reasons. First, until recently there were few well-conducted, randomised, controlled trials specifically in bipolar depression and second, the condition entails consideration of lifelong outcome rather than simply discrete episode response.[8] We have some knowledge of the therapeutic effects of drugs in bipolar depressive episodes but more limited awareness of the therapeutic or deleterious effects of drugs in the longer term. In the UK, NICE recommends the initial use of fluoxetine combined with olanzapine or quetiapine on its own (assuming an antipsychotic is not already prescribed).[9] Lamotrigine is considered to be second-line treatment (although we consider the evidence for lamotrigine rather weak). Tables 3.8, 3.9 and 3.10 give some broad guidance on treatment options in bipolar depression.

Table 3.8 Established treatments for bipolar depression (listed in alphabetical order)

Drug/regime	Comments
Lamotrigine[1,10,11–16]	Lamotrigine appears to be effective both as a treatment for bipolar depression and as prophylaxis against further episodes. It does not induce switching or rapid cycling. It is as effective as citalopram and causes less weight gain than lithium. Overall, the effect of lamotrigine is modest, with numerous failed trials.[17,18] It may be useful as an adjunct to lithium[19] or as an alternative to it in pregnancy[20]
	Treatment is somewhat complicated by the small risk of rash, which is associated with speed of dose titration. The necessity for titration may limit clinical utility
	A further complication is the question of dose: 50 mg/day has efficacy, but 200 mg/day is probably better. In the USA doses of up to 1200 mg/day have been used (mean around 250 mg/day)
Lithium and antidepressant[21–28]	Antidepressants are still widely used in bipolar depression, particularly for breakthrough episodes occurring in those on mood stabilisers. They have been assumed to be effective, although there is a risk of cycle acceleration and/or switching. Studies suggest mood stabilisers alone are just as effective as mood stabilisers/antidepressant combination.[29,30] Tricyclic antidepressants and MAOIs are usually avoided. SSRIs are generally recommended if an antidepressant is to be prescribed. Venlafaxine and bupropion (amfebutamone) have also been used. Venlafaxine may be more likely to induce a switch to mania.[31,32] There is controversial evidence that antidepressants are effective only when lithium plasma levels are below 0.8 mmol/L
	Continuing antidepressant treatment after resolution of symptoms may protect against depressive relapse,[33,34] although only in the absence of a mood stabiliser.[35] At the time of writing, there is no consensus on whether or not to continue antidepressants long term[36]
Lithium[1,10,37–39]	Lithium is probably effective in treating bipolar depression but supporting data are methodologically questionable.[40] There is some evidence that lithium prevents depressive relapse but its effects on manic relapse are considered more robust. Fairly strong support for lithium in reducing suicidality in bipolar affectivedisorder[41,42]
Lurasidone	Two RCTs show good effect for lurasidone either alone[43] or as an adjunct to mood stabilisers.[44] Not licensed for bipolar depression in the UK at the time of writing.
Olanzapine +/– fluoxetine[10,40,45–48]	This combination (Symbyax®) is more effective than both placebo and olanzapine alone in treating bipolar depression. The dose is 6 mg and 25 mg or 12 mg and 50 mg/day (so presumably 5/20 mg and 10/40 mg are effective). May be more effective than lamotrigine. Reasonable evidence of prophylactic effect. Recommended as first-line treatment by NICE[9]
	Olanzapine alone is effective when compared with placebo,[49] but the combination with fluoxetine is more effective. (This is possibly the strongest evidence for a beneficial effect for an antidepressant in bipolar depression.)
Quetiapine[50–54]	Five large RCTs have demonstrated clear efficacy for doses of 300 mg and 600 mg daily (as monotherapy) in bipolar I and bipolar II depression. May be superior to both lithium and paroxetine
	Quetiapine also prevents relapse into depression and mania[55,56] and so one of the treatments of choice in bipolar depression.[57] It appears not to be associated with switching to mania
Valproate[1,10,57–61]	Limited evidence of efficacy as monotherapy but recommended in some guidelines. Several very small RCTs but many negative. Probably protects against depressive relapse but database is small

MAOI, monoamine oxidase inhibitor; RCT, randomised controlled trial; SSRI. Selective serotonin reuptake inhibitor.

Table 3.9 Alternative drug treatments for bipolar depression

Drug/regime	Comments
Antidepressants[62–70]	'Unopposed' antidepressants (i.e. without mood-stabiliser protection) are generally avoided in bipolar depression because of the risk of switching. There is also evidence that they are relatively less effective (perhaps not effective at all) in bipolar depression than in unipolar depression. Nonetheless short-term use of fluoxetine, venlafaxine and moclobemide seems reasonably effective and safe even as monotherapy. Overall, however, unopposed antidepressant treatment should be avoided, especially in bipolar I disorder[36]
Carbamazepine[1,10,71]	Occasionally recommended but database is poor and effect modest. May have useful activity when added to other mood-stabilisers
Pramipexole[72,73]	Pramipexole is a dopamine agonist which is widely used in Parkinson's disease. Two small placebo-controlled trials suggest useful efficacy in bipolar depression. Effective dose averages around 1.7 mg/day. Both studies used pramipexole as an adjunct to existing mood-stabiliser treatment. Neither study detected an increased risk of switching to mania/hypomania (a theoretical consideration) but data are insufficient to exclude this possibility. Probably best reserved for specialist centres

Refer to primary literature before using.

Table 3.10 Other possible treatments for bipolar depression

Drug/regime	Comments
Aripiprazole[74–77]	Limited support from open studies as add-on treatment. RCT negative. Possibly not effective
Gabapentin[1,78,79]	Open studies suggest modest effect when added to mood-stabilisers or antipsychotics. Doses average around 1750 mg/day. Anxiolytic effect may account for apparent effect in bipolar depression
Inositol[80]	Small, randomised, pilot study suggests that 12 g/day inositol is effective in bipolar depression
Ketamine[81–83]	A single IV dose of 0.5 mg/kg is effective in refractory bipolar depression. Very high response rate. Dissociative symptoms common but brief. Risk of ulcerative cystitis if repeatedly used
Mifepristone[84,85]	Some evidence of mood-elevating properties in bipolar depression. May also improve cognitive function. Dose is 600 mg/day
Modafinil[86,87]	One positive RCT as adjunct to mood-stabiliser. Dose is 100–200 mg/day. Positive RCT with amodafinil 150 mg/day
Omega-3 fatty acids[88,89]	One positive RCT (1 g/2 g a day) and one negative (6 g a day)
Riluzole[90,91]	Riluzole shares some pharmacological characteristics with lamotrigine. Database is limited to a single case report supporting use in bipolar depression
Thyroxine[92]	Limited evidence of efficacy as augmentation. Doses average around 300 µg/day. One failed RCT[93]
Zonisamide[94–97]	Supported by several open-label studies. Dose is 100–300 mg a day

Seek specialist advice before using.
IV, intravenous; RCT, randomised controlled trial.

Meta-analysis in bipolar depression

Meta-analytic studies in bipolar depression are constrained by the variety of methods used to assess efficacy. This means that many scientifically robust studies cannot be included in some meta-analyses because their parameters (outcomes, duration, etc.) do not match, and so cannot be compared with other studies. Early lithium studies are an important example – their short duration and cross-over design precludes their inclusion in meta-analysis. A meta-analysis of five trials (906 participants) revealed that antidepressants were no better than placebo in respect to response or remission, although results approached statistical significance.[76] Another analysis of trials not involving antidepressants[98] (7,307 participants) found a statistical advantage over placebo for olanzapine + fluoxetine, valproate, quetiapine, lurasidone, olanzapine, aripiprazole and carbamazepine (in order of effect size, highest first).

The largest analysis is a multiple treatments meta-analysis of 29 studies including 8,331 subjects.[99] Overall olanzapine + fluoxetine, lurasidone, olanzapine, valproate, SSRIs and quetiapine were ranked highest in terms of effect size and response with olanzapine + fluoxetine ranked first for both.

Summary of drug choice

The combination of olanzapine + fluoxetine is probably the most effective treatment available for bipolar depression (other SSRIs may be effective but should be avoided unless clear individual benefit is obvious[36]). Other first-line choices are quetiapine, olanzapine, lurasidone and valproate. These drugs differ substantially in adverse effect profile, tolerability and cost, each of which needs to be considered when prescribing for an individual. Lithium and lamotrigine are also effective but supporting evidence is relatively weak (although clinical experience is, in contrast, vast). Aripiprazole, risperidone, ziprasidone, tricyclics and MAOIs are probably not effective and should not be used.[99]

References

1. Malhi GS et al. Bipolar depression: management options. CNS Drugs 2003; **17**:9–25.
2. Perlis RH et al. Clinical features of bipolar depression versus major depressive disorder in large multicenter trials. Am J Psychiatry 2006; **163**:225–231.
3. Mitchell PB et al. Comparison of depressive episodes in bipolar disorder and in major depressive disorder within bipolar disorder pedigrees. Br J Psychiatry 2011; **199**:303–309.
4. Haddad P et al. Pharmacological management of bipolar depression. Acta Psychiatr Scand 2002; **105**:401–403.
5. Hirschfeld RM. Bipolar depression: the real challenge. Eur Neuropsychopharmacol 2004; **14 Suppl 2**:S83–S88.
6. Judd LL et al. The long-term natural history of the weekly symptomatic status of bipolar I disorder. Arch Gen Psychiatry 2002; **59**:530–537.
7. Judd LL et al. A prospective investigation of the natural history of the long-term weekly symptomatic status of bipolar II disorder. Arch Gen Psychiatry 2003; **60**:261–269.
8. Baldassano CF et al. Rethinking the treatment paradigm for bipolar depression: the importance of long-term management. CNS Spectr 2004; **9**:11–18.
9. National Institute for Health and Care Excellence. Bipolar disorder: the assessment and management of bipolar disorder in adults, children and young people in primary and secondary care. Clinical Guideline 185, 2014. https://www.nice.org.uk/
10. Yatham LN et al. Bipolar depression: criteria for treatment selection, definition of refractoriness, and treatment options. Bipolar Disord 2003; **5**:85–97.
11. Calabrese JR et al. A double-blind placebo-controlled study of lamotrigine monotherapy in outpatients with bipolar I depression. Lamictal 602 Study Group. J Clin Psychiatry 1999; **60**:79–88.

CHAPTER 3

12. Bowden CL et al. Lamotrigine in the treatment of bipolar depression. Eur Neuropsychopharmacol 1999; **9 Suppl 4**:S113–S117.

13. Marangell LB et al. Lamotrigine treatment of bipolar disorder: data from the first 500 patients in STEP-BD. Bipolar Disord 2004; **6**:139–143.

14. Schaffer A et al. Randomized, double-blind pilot trial comparing lamotrigine versus citalopram for the treatment of bipolar depression. J Affect Disord 2006; **96**:95–99.

15. Bowden CL et al. Impact of lamotrigine and lithium on weight in obese and nonobese patients with bipolar I disorder. Am J Psychiatry 2006; **163**:1199–1201.

16. Suppes T et al. A single blind comparison of lithium and lamotrigine for the treatment of bipolar II depression. J Affect Disord 2008; **111**:334–343.

17. Geddes JR et al. Lamotrigine for treatment of bipolar depression: independent meta-analysis and meta-regression of individual patient data from five randomised trials. Br J Psychiatry 2009; **194**:4–9.

18. Calabrese JR et al. Lamotrigine in the acute treatment of bipolar depression: results of five double-blind, placebo-controlled clinical trials. Bipolar Disord 2008; **10**:323–333.

19. van der Loos ML et al. Efficacy and safety of lamotrigine as add-on treatment to lithium in bipolar depression: a multicenter, double-blind, placebo-controlled trial. J Clin Psychiatry 2009; **70**:223–231.

20. Newport DJ et al. Lamotrigine in bipolar disorder: efficacy during pregnancy. Bipolar Disord 2008; **10**:432–436.

21. Montgomery SA et al. Pharmacotherapy of depression and mixed states in bipolar disorder. J Affect Disord 2000; **59 Suppl 1**:S39–S56.

22. Calabrese JR et al. International Consensus Group on Bipolar I Depression Treatment Guidelines. J Clin Psychiatry 2004; **65**:571–579.

23. Nemeroff CB et al. Double-blind, placebo-controlled comparison of imipramine and paroxetine in the treatment of bipolar depression. Am J Psychiatry 2001; **158**:906–912.

24. Vieta E et al. A randomized trial comparing paroxetine and venlafaxine in the treatment of bipolar depressed patients taking mood stabilizers. J Clin Psychiatry 2002; **63**:508–512.

25. Young LT et al. Double-blind comparison of addition of a second mood stabilizer versus an antidepressant to an initial mood stabilizer for treatment of patients with bipolar depression. Am J Psychiatry 2000; **157**:124–126.

26. Fawcett JA. Lithium combinations in acute and maintenance treatment of unipolar and bipolar depression. J Clin Psychiatry 2003; **64 Suppl 5**: 32–37.

27. Altshuler L et al. The impact of antidepressant discontinuation versus antidepressant continuation on 1-year risk for relapse of bipolar depression: a retrospective chart review. J Clin Psychiatry 2001; **62**:612–616.

28. Erfurth A et al. Bupropion as add-on strategy in difficult-to-treat bipolar depressive patients. Neuropsychobiology 2002; **45 Suppl 1**:33–36.

29. Sachs GS et al. Effectiveness of adjunctive antidepressant treatment for bipolar depression. N Engl J Med 2007; **356**:1711–1722.

30. Goldberg JF et al. Adjunctive antidepressant use and symptomatic recovery among bipolar depressed patients with concomitant manic symptoms: findings from the STEP-BD. Am J Psychiatry 2007; **164**:1348–1355.

31. Post RM et al. Mood switch in bipolar depression: comparison of adjunctive venlafaxine, bupropion and sertraline. Br J Psychiatry 2006; **189**:124–131.

32. Leverich GS et al. Risk of switch in mood polarity to hypomania or mania in patients with bipolar depression during acute and continuation trials of venlafaxine, sertraline, and bupropion as adjuncts to mood stabilizers. Am J Psychiatry 2006; **163**:232–239.

33. Salvi V et al. The use of antidepressants in bipolar disorder. J Clin Psychiatry 2008; **69**:1307–1318.

34. Altshuler LL et al. Impact of antidepressant continuation after acute positive or partial treatment response for bipolar depression: a blinded, randomized study. J Clin Psychiatry 2009; **70**:450–457.

35. Ghaemi SN et al. Long-term antidepressant treatment in bipolar disorder: meta-analyses of benefits and risks. Acta Psychiatr Scand 2008; **118**:347–356.

36. Pacchiarotti I et al. The International Society for Bipolar Disorders (ISBD) task force report on antidepressant use in bipolar disorders. Am J Psychiatry 2013; **170**:1249–1262.

37. Geddes JR et al. Long-term lithium therapy for bipolar disorder: systematic review and meta-analysis of randomized controlled trials. Am J Psychiatry 2004; **161**:217–222.

38. Calabrese JR et al. A placebo-controlled 18-month trial of lamotrigine and lithium maintenance treatment in recently depressed patients with bipolar I disorder. J Clin Psychiatry 2003; **64**:1013–1024.

39. Prien RF et al. Lithium carbonate and imipramine in prevention of affective episodes. A comparison in recurrent affective illness. Arch Gen Psychiatry 1973; **29**:420–425.

40. Grunze H et al. The World Federation of Societies of Biological Psychiatry (WFSBP) Guidelines for the Biological Treatment of Bipolar Disorders: Update 2010 on the treatment of acute bipolar depression. World J Biol Psychiatry 2010; **11**:81–109.

41. Goodwin FK et al. Suicide risk in bipolar disorder during treatment with lithium and divalproex. JAMA 2003; **290**:1467–1473.

42. Kessing LV et al. Suicide risk in patients treated with lithium. Arch Gen Psychiatry 2005; **62**:860–866.

43. Loebel A et al. Lurasidone monotherapy in the treatment of bipolar I depression: a randomized, double-blind, placebo-controlled study. Am J Psychiatry 2014; **171**:160–168.

44. Loebel A et al. Lurasidone as adjunctive therapy with lithium or valproate for the treatment of bipolar I depression: a randomized, double-blind, placebo-controlled study. Am J Psychiatry 2014; **171**:169–177.

45. Tohen M et al. Efficacy of olanzapine and olanzapine-fluoxetine combination in the treatment of bipolar I depression. Arch Gen Psychiatry 2003; **60**:1079–1088.

46. Brown EB et al. A 7-week, randomized, double-blind trial of olanzapine/fluoxetine combination versus lamotrigine in the treatment of bipolar I depression. J Clin Psychiatry 2006; **67**:1025–1033.

47. Corya SA et al. A 24-week open-label extension study of olanzapine-fluoxetine combination and olanzapine monotherapy in the treatment of bipolar depression. J Clin Psychiatry 2006; **67**:798–806.

48. Dube S et al. Onset of antidepressant effect of olanzapine and olanzapine/fluoxetine combination in bipolar depression. Bipolar Disord 2007; **9**:618–627.

49. Tohen M et al. Randomised, double-blind, placebo-controlled study of olanzapine in patients with bipolar I depression. BrJPsychiatry 2012; **201**:376–382.

50. Calabrese JR et al. A randomized, double-blind, placebo-controlled trial of quetiapine in the treatment of bipolar I or II depression. Am J Psychiatry 2005; **162**:1351–1360.

51. Thase ME et al. Efficacy of quetiapine monotherapy in bipolar I and II depression: a double-blind, placebo-controlled study (the BOLDER II study). J Clin Psychopharmacol 2006; **26**:600–609.

52. Suppes T et al. Effectiveness of the extended release formulation of quetiapine as monotherapy for the treatment of acute bipolar depression. J Affect Disord 2010; **121**:106–115.

53. Young AH et al. A double-blind, placebo-controlled study of quetiapine and lithium monotherapy in adults in the acute phase of bipolar depression (EMBOLDEN I). J Clin Psychiatry 2010; **71**:150–162.

54. McElroy SL et al. A double-blind, placebo-controlled study of quetiapine and paroxetine as monotherapy in adults with bipolar depression (EMBOLDEN II). J Clin Psychiatry 2010; **71**:163–174.

55. Vieta E et al. Efficacy and safety of quetiapine in combination with lithium or divalproex for maintenance of patients with bipolar I disorder (international trial 126). J Affect Disord 2008; **109**:251–263.

56. Suppes T et al. Maintenance treatment for patients with bipolar I disorder: results from a north american study of quetiapine in combination with lithium or divalproex (trial 127). Am J Psychiatry 2009; **166**:476–488.

57. Goodwin GM. Evidence-based guidelines for treating bipolar disorder: revised second edition–recommendations from the British Association for Psychopharmacology. J Psychopharmacol 2009; **23**:346–388.

58. Davis LL et al. Divalproex in the treatment of bipolar depression: a placebo-controlled study. J Affect Disord 2005; **85**:259–266.

59. Ghaemi SN et al. Divalproex in the treatment of acute bipolar depression: a preliminary double-blind, randomized, placebo-controlled pilot study. J Clin Psychiatry 2007; **68**:1840–1844.

60. Smith LA et al. Valproate for the treatment of acute bipolar depression: systematic review and meta-analysis. J Affect Disord 2010; **122**:1–9.

61. Muzina DJ et al. Acute efficacy of divalproex sodium versus placebo in mood stabilizer-naive bipolar I or II depression: a double-blind, randomized, placebo-controlled trial. J Clin Psychiatry 2011; **72**:813–819.

62. Amsterdam JD et al. Short-term fluoxetine monotherapy for bipolar type II or bipolar NOS major depression – low manic switch rate. Bipolar Disord 2004; **6**:75–81.

63. Amsterdam JD et al. Efficacy and safety of fluoxetine in treating bipolar II major depressive episode. J Clin Psychopharmacol 1998; **18**:435–440.

64. Amsterdam J. Efficacy and safety of venlafaxine in the treatment of bipolar II major depressive episode. J Clin Psychopharmacol 1998; **18**:414–417.

65. Amsterda, JD et al. Venlafaxine monotherapy in women with bipolar II and unipolar major depression. J Affect Disord 2000; **59**:225–229.

66. Silverstone T. Moclobemide vs. imipramine in bipolar depression: a multicentre double-blind clinical trial. Acta Psychiatr Scand 2001; **104**:104–109.

67. Ghaemi SN et al. Antidepressant treatment in bipolar versus unipolar depression. Am J Psychiatry 2004; **161**:163–165.

68. Post RM et al. A re-evaluation of the role of antidepressants in the treatment of bipolar depression: data from the Stanley Foundation Bipolar Network. Bipolar Disord 2003; **5**:396–406.

69. Amsterdam JD et al. Comparison of fluoxetine, olanzapine, and combined fluoxetine plus olanzapine initial therapy of bipolar type I and type II major depression–lack of manic induction. J Affect Disord 2005; **87**:121–130.

70. Amsterdam JD et al. Fluoxetine monotherapy of bipolar type II and bipolar NOS major depression: a double-blind, placebo-substitution, continuation study. Int Clin Psychopharmacol 2005; **20**:257–264.

71. Dilsaver SC et al. Treatment of bipolar depression with carbamazepine: results of an open study. Biol Psychiatry 1996; **40**:935–937.

72. Goldberg JF et al. Preliminary randomized, double-blind, placebo-controlled trial of pramipexole added to mood stabilizers for treatment-resistant bipolar depression. Am J Psychiatry 2004; **161**:564–566.

73. Zarate CA, Jr. et al. Pramipexole for bipolar II depression: a placebo-controlled proof of concept study. Biol Psychiatry 2004; **56**:54–60.

74. Ketter TA et al. Adjunctive aripiprazole in treatment-resistant bipolar depression. Ann Clin Psychiatry 2006; **18**:169–172.

75. Mazza M et al. Beneficial acute antidepressant effects of aripiprazole as an adjunctive treatment or monotherapy in bipolar patients unresponsive to mood stabilizers: results from a 16-week open-label trial. Expert Opin Pharmacother 2008; **9**:3145–3149.

76. Sidor MM et al. Antidepressants for the acute treatment of bipolar depression: a systematic review and meta-analysis. J Clin Psychiatry 2011; **72**:156–167.

77. Cruz N et al. Efficacy of modern antipsychotics in placebo-controlled trials in bipolar depression: a meta-analysis. Int J Neuropsychopharmacol 2010; **13**:5–14 .

78. Wang PW et al. Gabapentin augmentation therapy in bipolar depression. Bipolar Disord 2002; **4**:296–301.

79. Ashton H et al. GABA-ergic drugs: exit stage left, enter stage right. J Psychopharmacol 2003; **17**:174–178.

80. Chengappa KN et al. Inositol as an add-on treatment for bipolar depression. Bipolar Disord 2000; **2**:47–55.

81. Diazgranados N et al. A randomized add-on trial of an N-methyl-D-aspartate antagonist in treatment-resistant bipolar depression. Arch Gen Psychiatry 2010; **67**:793–802.

CHAPTER 3

82. Shahani R et al. Ketamine-associated ulcerative cystitis: a new clinical entity. Urology 2007; **69**:810–812.

83. Zarate CA, Jr. et al. Replication of ketamine's antidepressant efficacy in bipolar depression: a randomized controlled add-on trial. Biol Psychiatry 2012; **71**:939–946.

84. Young AH et al. Improvements in neurocognitive function and mood following adjunctive treatment with mifepristone (RU-486) in bipolar disorder. Neuropsychopharmacology 2004; **29**:1538–1545.

85. Watson S et al. A randomized trial to examine the effect of mifepristone on neuropsychological performance and mood in patients with bipolar depression. Biol Psychiatry 2012; **72**:943–949.

86. Frye MA et al. A placebo-controlled evaluation of adjunctive modafinil in the treatment of bipolar depression. Am J Psychiatry 2007; **164**:1242–1249.

87. Calabrese JR et al. Adjunctive armodafinil for major depressive episodes associated with bipolar I disorder: a randomized, multicenter, double-blind, placebo-controlled, proof-of-concept study. J Clin Psychiatry 2010; **71**:1363–1370.

88. Frangou S et al. Efficacy of ethyl-eicosapentaenoic acid in bipolar depression: randomised double-blind placebo-controlled study. Br J Psychiatry 2006; **188**:46–50.

89. Keck PE, Jr. et al. Double-blind, randomized, placebo-controlled trials of ethyl-eicosapentanoate in the treatment of bipolar depression and rapid cycling bipolar disorder. Biol Psychiatry 2006; **60**:1020–1022.

90. Singh J et al. Case report: Successful riluzole augmentation therapy in treatment-resistant bipolar depression following the development of rash with lamotrigine. Psychopharmacology (Berl) 2004; **173**:227–228.

91. Brennan BP et al. Rapid enhancement of glutamatergic neurotransmission in bipolar depression following treatment with riluzole. Neuropsychopharmacology 2010; 35:834–846.

92. Bauer M. Thyroid hormone augmentation with levothyroxine in bipolar depression. Bipolar Disord 2002; **4 Suppl 1**:109–110.

93. Stamm TJ et al. Supraphysiologic doses of levothyroxine as adjunctive therapy in bipolar depression: a randomized, double-blind, placebo-controlled study. J Clin Psychiatry 2014; **75**:162–168.

94. Ghaemi SN et al. An open prospective study of zonisamide in acute bipolar depression. J Clin Psychopharmacol 2006; **26**:385–388.

95. Anand A et al. A preliminary open-label study of zonisamide treatment for bipolar depression in 10 patients. J Clin Psychiatry 2005; **66**:195–198.

96. Wilson MS et al. Zonisamide for bipolar depression. Expert Opin Pharmacother 2007; **8**:111–113.

97. McElroy SL et al. Open-label adjunctive zonisamide in the treatment of bipolar disorders: a prospective trial. J Clin Psychiatry 2005; **66**:617–624.

98. Selle V et al. Treatments for acute bipolar depression: meta-analyses of placebo-controlled, monotherapy trials of anticonvulsants, lithium and antipsychotics. Pharmacopsychiatry 2014; **47**:43–52.

99. Taylor DM et al. Comparative efficacy and acceptability of drug treatments for bipolar depression: a multiple-treatments meta-analysis. *Acta Psychiatr Scand* 2014:in press.

CHAPTER 3

Rapid-cycling bipolar affective disorder

Rapid cycling is usually defined as bipolar affective disorder in which four or more episodes of (hypo) mania or depression occur in a 12-month period. It is generally held to be less responsive to drug treatment than non-rapid-cycling bipolar illness[1,2] and entails considerable depressive morbidity and suicide risk.[3] Table 3.11 outlines a treatment strategy for rapid cycling based on rather limited data and very few direct comparisons of drugs.[4,5] This strategy is broadly in line with the findings of a recent systematic review.[5] NICE conclude that there is no evidence to support rapid-cycling illness being managed any differently from that with a more conventional course.[6] Lithium, alone or in combination with valproate, would therefore be first-line treatment. An alternative would be to add an antipsychotic with proven activity in bipolar affective disorder and/or rapid cycling (see below).

In practice, response to treatment is sometimes idiosyncratic: individuals may show significant response only to one or two drugs. Spontaneous or treatment-related remissions occur in around one-third of rapid-cyclers[7] and rapid cycling may come and go in most patients.[8] Non-drug methods may also be considered.[9,10]

Table 3.11 Recommended treatment strategy for rapid-cycling bipolar affective disorder

Step	Suggested treatment
Step 1	**Withdraw antidepressants** in all patients[11–15] (some controversial evidence supports continuation of SSRIs[16,17])
Step 2	**Evaluate possible precipitants** (e.g. alcohol, thyroid dysfunction, external stressors) [2]
Step 3	**Optimise mood stabiliser treatment**[18–21] (using plasma levels), and **Consider combining mood-stabilisers**, e.g. lithium + valproate; lithium + lamotrigine
Step 4	**Consider other (usually adjunct) treatment options** (alphabetical order; preferred treatment options in bold) **Aripiprazole**[23,24] (15–30 mg/day) Clozapine[25] (usual doses) Lamotrigine[26–28] (up to 225 mg/day) Levetiracetam[29] (up to 2000 mg/day) Nimodipine[30,31] (180 mg/day) **Olanzapine**[18] (usual doses) **Quetiapine**[32–35] (300–600 mg/day) Risperidone[36–38] (up to 6 mg/day) Thyroxine[39,40] (150–400 µg/day) Topiramate[41] (up to 300 mg/day)

Choice of drug is determined by patient factors – few comparative efficacy data to guide choice at the time of writing. **Quetiapine** probably has best supporting data[32–34] and may be considered treatment of choice. **Olanzapine** is probably second choice.[5] Conversely, supporting data for levetiracetam, nimodipine, thyroxine and topiramate are rather limited.

References

1. Calabrese JR et al. Current research on rapid cycling bipolar disorder and its treatment. J Affect Disord 2001; **67**:241–255.
2. Kupka RW et al. Rapid and non-rapid cycling bipolar disorder: a meta-analysis of clinical studies. J Clin Psychiatry 2003; **64**:1483–1494.
3. Coryell W et al. The long-term course of rapid-cycling bipolar disorder. Arch Gen Psychiatry 2003; **60**:914–920.
4. Tondo L et al. Rapid-cycling bipolar disorder: effects of long-term treatments. Acta Psychiatr Scand 2003; **108**:4–14 .
5. Fountoulakis KN et al. A systematic review of the evidence on the treatment of rapid cycling bipolar disorder. Bipolar Disord 2013; **15**:115–137.
6. National Institute for Health and Care Excellence. Bipolar disorder: the assessment and management of bipolar disorder in adults, children and young people in primary and secondary care. Clinical Guidance 185, 2014. https://www.nice.org.uk/
7. Koukopoulos A et al. Duration and stability of the rapid-cycling course: a long-term personal follow-up of 109 patients. J Affect Disord 2003; **73**:75–85.
8. Carvalho AF et al. Rapid cycling in bipolar disorder: a systematic review. J Clin Psychiatry 2014; **75**:e578–586.
9. Dell'osso B et al. Augmentative transcranial magnetic stimulation (TMS) combined with brain navigation in drug-resistant rapid cycling bipolar depression: a case report of acute and maintenance efficacy. World J Biol Psychiatry 2009; **10**:673–676.
10. Marangell LB et al. A 1-year pilot study of vagus nerve stimulation in treatment-resistant rapid-cycling bipolar disorder. J Clin Psychiatry 2008; **69**:183–189.
11. Wehr TA et al. Can antidepressants cause mania and worsen the course of affective illness? Am J Psychiatry 1987; **144**:1403–1411.
12. Altshuler LL et al. Antidepressant-induced mania and cycle acceleration: a controversy revisited. Am J Psychiatry 1995; **152**:1130–1138.
13. Association AP. Practice guideline for the treatment of patients with bipolar disorder. Am J Psychiatry 2002; **159 Suppl 4**:1–50.
14. Ghaemi SN et al. Antidepressant discontinuation in bipolar depression: a Systematic Treatment Enhancement Program for Bipolar Disorder (STEP-BD) randomized clinical trial of long-term effectiveness and safety. J Clin Psychiatry 2010; **71**:372–380.
15. Ghaemi SN. Treatment of rapid-cycling bipolar disorder: are antidepressants mood destabilizers? Am J Psychiatry 2008; **165**:300–302.
16. Amsterdam JD et al. Efficacy and mood conversion rate during long-term fluoxetine v. lithium monotherapy in rapid- and non-rapid-cycling bipolar II disorder. Br J Psychiatry 2013; **202**:301–306.
17. Amsterdam JD et al. Effectiveness and mood conversion rate of short-term fluoxetine monotherapy in patients with rapid cycling bipolar II depression versus patients with nonrapid cycling bipolar II depression. J Clin Psychopharmacol 2013; **33**:420–424.
18. Sanger TM et al. Olanzapine in the acute treatment of bipolar I disorder with a history of rapid cycling. J Affect Disord 2003; **73**:155–161.
19. Kemp DE et al. A 6-month, double-blind, maintenance trial of lithium monotherapy versus the combination of lithium and divalproex for rapid-cycling bipolar disorder and Co-occurring substance abuse or dependence. J Clin Psychiatry 2009; **70**:113–121.
20. da Rocha FF et al. Addition of lamotrigine to valproic acid: a successful outcome in a case of rapid-cycling bipolar affective disorder. Prog Neuropsychopharmacol Biol Psychiatry 2007; **31**:1548–1549.
21. Woo YS et al. Lamotrigine added to valproate successfully treated a case of ultra-rapid cycling bipolar disorder. Psychiatry Clin Neurosci 2007; **61**:130–131.
22. Calabrese JR et al. A 20-month, double-blind, maintenance trial of lithium versus divalproex in rapid-cycling bipolar disorder. Am J Psychiatry 2005; **162**:2152–2161.
23. Suppes T et al. Efficacy and safety of aripiprazole in subpopulations with acute manic or mixed episodes of bipolar I disorder. J Affect Disord 2008; **107**:145–154.
24. Muzina DJ et al. Aripiprazole monotherapy in patients with rapid-cycling bipolar I disorder: an analysis from a long-term, double-blind, placebo-controlled study. Int J Clin Pract 2008; **62**:679–687.
25. Calabrese JR et al. Clozapine prophylaxis in rapid cycling bipolar disorder. J Clin Psychopharmacol 1991; **11**:396–397.
26. Fatemi SH et al. Lamotrigine in rapid-cycling bipolar disorder. J Clin Psychiatry 1997; **58**:522–527.
27. Calabrese JR et al. A double-blind, placebo-controlled, prophylaxis study of lamotrigine in rapid-cycling bipolar disorder. Lamictal 614 Study Group. J Clin Psychiatry 2000; **61**:841–850.
28. Wang Z et al. Lamotrigine adjunctive therapy to lithium and divalproex in depressed patients with rapid cycling bipolar disorder and a recent substance use disorder: a 12-week, double-blind, placebo-controlled pilot study. Psychopharmacol Bull 2010; **43**:5–21.
29. Braunig P et al. Levetiracetam in the treatment of rapid cycling bipolar disorder. J Psychopharmacol 2003; **17**:239–241.
30. Goodnick PJ. Nimodipine treatment of rapid cycling bipolar disorder. J Clin Psychiatry 1995; **56**:330.
31. Pazzaglia PJ et al. Preliminary controlled trial of nimodipine in ultra-rapid cycling affective dysregulation. Psychiatry Res 1993; **49**:257–272.
32. Goldberg JF et al. Effectiveness of quetiapine in rapid cycling bipolar disorder: a preliminary study. J Affect Disord 2008; **105**:305–310.
33. Vieta E et al. Quetiapine monotherapy in the treatment of patients with bipolar I or II depression and a rapid-cycling disease course: a randomized, double-blind, placebo-controlled study. Bipolar Disord 2007; **9**:413–425.
34. Langosch JM et al. Efficacy of quetiapine monotherapy in rapid-cycling bipolar disorder in comparison with sodium valproate. J Clin Psychopharmacol 2008; **28**:555–560.
35. Vieta E et al. Quetiapine in the treatment of rapid cycling bipolar disorder. Bipolar Disord 2002; **4**:335–340.
36. Jacobsen FM. Risperidone in the treatment of affective illness and obsessive-compulsive disorder. J Clin Psychiatry 1995; **56**:423–429.
37. Bobo WV et al. A randomized open comparison of long-acting injectable risperidone and treatment as usual for prevention of relapse, rehospitalization, and urgent care referral in community-treated patients with rapid cycling bipolar disorder. Clin Neuropharmacol 2011; **34**:224–233.
38. Vieta E et al. Treatment of refractory rapid cycling bipolar disorder with risperidone. J Clin Psychopharmacol 1998; **18**:172–174.
39. Weeston TF et al. High-dose T4 for rapid-cycling bipolar disorder. J Am Acad Child Adolesc Psychiatry 1996; **35**:131–132 .
40. Extein IL. High doses of levothyroxine for refractory rapid cycling. Am J Psychiatry 2000; **157**:1704–1705.
41. Chen CK et al. Combination treatment of clozapine and topiramate in resistant rapid-cycling bipolar disorder. Clin Neuropharmacol 2005; **28**:136–138.

Prophylaxis in bipolar affective disorder

The median duration of mood episodes in people with bipolar affective disorder has been reported to be 13 weeks, with a quarter of patients remaining unwell at 1 year.[1] Most people with bipolar affective disorder spend much more time depressed than manic,[2] and bipolar depression can be very difficult to treat. The suicide rate in bipolar illness is increased 25-fold over population norms and the vast majority of suicides occur during episodes of depression.[3] Mixed states are also common and present an increased risk of suicide.[4]

Note that residual symptoms after an acute episode are a strong predictor of recurrence.[1,5] Most evidence supports the efficacy of lithium[6-10] in preventing episodes of mania and depression. Carbamazepine is somewhat less effective[10,11] and the long-term efficacy of valproate is uncertain,[8,9,12-14] although it too may protect against relapse both into depression and mania.[10,15] Lithium has the advantage of a proven anti-suicidal effect[16-18] but perhaps, relative to other mood stabilisers, the disadvantage of a worsened outcome following abrupt discontinuation.[19-22]

The BALANCE study found that valproate as monotherapy was relatively less effective than lithium or the combination of lithium and valproate,[13] casting doubt on its use as a first-line single treatment. Also, a large observational study has shown that lithium is much more effective than valproate in preventing relapse to any condition and in preventing rehospitalisation.[23] Given this and the fact that valproate is not licensed for prophylaxis, it should now be considered a second-line treatment.

Conventional antipsychotics have traditionally been used and are perceived to be effective although the objective evidence base is, again, weak.[24,25] FGA depots protect against mania but may worsen depression.[26] Evidence supports the efficacy of some SGAs, particularly olanzapine,[9,27] quetiapine,[28] aripiprazole[29] and risperidone.[30] Olanzapine, quetiapine and aripiprazole are licensed for prophylaxis and appear to protect against both mania and depression. Whether SGAs are more effective than FGAs, or are truly associated with a reduced overall side-effect burden, remains untested.

NICE recommendations[27]

- When planning long-term pharmacological interventions to prevent relapse, take into account drugs that have been effective during episodes of mania or bipolar depression. Discuss with the person whether they prefer to continue this treatment or switch to lithium, and explain that lithium is the most effective long-term treatment for bipolar affective disorder.
- Offer lithium as a first-line, long-term pharmacological treatment for bipolar affective disorder and: if lithium is insufficiently effective, consider adding valproate; if lithium is poorly tolerated, consider valproate or olanzapine instead, or if it has been effective during an episode of mania or bipolar depression, quetiapine.
- Do not offer valproate to women of child-bearing age.
- Discuss with the person the possible benefits and risks of each drug for them.
- The secondary care team should maintain responsibility for monitoring the efficacy and tolerability of antipsychotic medication until the person's condition has stabilised.
- Before stopping medication, discuss with the person how to recognise early signs of relapse and what to do if symptoms recur.

- If stopping medication, do so gradually and monitor for signs of relapse.
- Continue monitoring symptoms, mood and mental state for 2 years after stopping medication. This may be undertaken in primary care.

A significant proportion of patients with bipolar illness fail to be treated adequately with a single mood-stabiliser,[13] so combinations of mood-stabilisers[31,32] or a mood-stabiliser and an antipsychotic[32,33] are commonly used.[34] Also, there is evidence that where combination treatments are effective in mania or depression, then continuation with the same combination provides optimal prophylaxis.[28,33] The use of polypharmacy needs to be balanced against the likely increased side-effect burden. Combinations of olanzapine, risperidone, quetiapine or haloperidol with lithium or valproate are recommend by NICE.[27] Alternative antipsychotics are also options in combinations with lithium or valproate, particularly if these have been found to be effective during the treatment of an acute episode of mania or depression[28,35] Carbamazepine is considered to be third line. Lamotrigine may be useful in bipolar II disorder[27] but seems only to prevent recurrence of depression.[36] Extrapolation of currently available data suggests that lithium plus a SGA is probably the polypharmacy regimen of choice.

A meta-analysis of long-term antidepressant treatment found that the number needed to treat (NNT) to prevent a new episode of depression was larger than the number needed to harm (NNH) related to precipitating a new episode of mania.[37] The STEP-BD study found no significant benefit for continuing (compared with discontinuing) an antidepressant and worse outcomes in those with rapid-cycling illness.[38] There is thus essentially no support for long-term use of antidepressants in bipolar illness, although they continue to be widely used.

Substance misuse increases the risk of switching into mania.[39]

Summary: prophylaxis in bipolar affective disorder

First line: lithium
Second line: valproate (NOT in women of child-bearing age), olanzapine, or quetiapine
Third line: alternative antipsychotic that has been effective during an acute episode, carbamazepine, lamotrigine

- Always maintain successful acute treatment regimens (e.g. mood stabiliser + antipsychotic) prophylaxis.
- Avoid long-term antidepressants.

References

1. Solomon DA et al. Longitudinal course of bipolar I disorder: duration of mood episodes. Arch Gen Psychiatry 2010; 67:339–347.
2. Judd LL et al. A prospective investigation of the natural history of the long-term weekly symptomatic status of bipolar II disorder. Arch Gen Psychiatry 2003; 60:261–269.
3. Rihmer Z. Suicide and Bipolar Disorder. In: Zarate C, Jr., Manji HK, eds. Bipolar Depression: Molecular Neurobiology, Clinical Diagnosis and Pharmacotherapy (Milestones in Drug Therapy). Switzerland: Birkhäuser Basel; 2009. pp. 47–58.
4. Houston JP et al. Reduced suicidal ideation in bipolar I disorder mixed-episode patients in a placebo-controlled trial of olanzapine combined with lithium or divalproex. J Clin Psychiatry 2006; 67:1246–1252.
5. Perlis RH et al. Predictors of recurrence in bipolar disorder: primary outcomes from the Systematic Treatment Enhancement Program for Bipolar Disorder (STEP-BD). Am J Psychiatry 2006; 163:217–224.
6. Young AH et al. Lithium in mood disorders: increasing evidence base, declining use? Br J Psychiatry 2007; 191:474–476.

7. Biel MG et al. Continuation versus discontinuation of lithium in recurrent bipolar illness: a naturalistic study. Bipolar Disord 2007; **9**: 435–442.

8. Bowden CL et al. A randomized, placebo-controlled 12-month trial of divalproex and lithium in treatment of outpatients with bipolar I disorder. Divalproex Maintenance Study Group. Arch Gen Psychiatry 2000; **57**:481–489.

9. Tohen M et al. Olanzapine versus divalproex sodium for the treatment of acute mania and maintenance of remission: a 47-week study. Am J Psychiatry 2003; **160**:1263–1271.

10. Goodwin G. Evidence-based guidelines for treating bipolar disorder: revised second edition–recommendations from the British Association for Psychopharmacology. J Psychopharmacol 2009; **23**:346–388.

11. Hartong EG et al. Prophylactic efficacy of lithium versus carbamazepine in treatment-naive bipolar patients. J Clin Psychiatry 2003; **64**:144–151.

12. Cipriani A et al. Valproic acid, valproate and divalproex in the maintenance treatment of bipolar disorder. Cochrane Database Syst Rev 2013; **10**: CD003196.

13. Geddes JR et al. Lithium plus valproate combination therapy versus monotherapy for relapse prevention in bipolar I disorder (BALANCE): a randomised open-label trial. Lancet 2010; **375**:385–395.

14. Kemp DE et al. A 6-month, double-blind, maintenance trial of lithium monotherapy versus the combination of lithium and divalproex for rapid-cycling bipolar disorder and Co-occurring substance abuse or dependence. J Clin Psychiatry 2009; **70**:113–121.

15. Smith LA et al. Effectiveness of mood stabilizers and antipsychotics in the maintenance phase of bipolar disorder: a systematic review of randomized controlled trials. Bipolar Disord 2007; **9**:394–412.

16. Cipriani A et al. Lithium in the prevention of suicidal behavior and all-cause mortality in patients with mood disorders: a systematic review of randomized trials. Am J Psychiatry 2005; **162**:1805–1819.

17. Kessing LV et al. Suicide risk in patients treated with lithium. Arch Gen Psychiatry 2005; **62**:860–866.

18. Young AH et al. Lithium in maintenance therapy for bipolar disorder. J Psychopharmacol 2006; **20**:17–22.

19. Mander AJ et al. Rapid recurrence of mania following abrupt discontinuation of lithium. Lancet 1988; **2**:15–17.

20. Faedda GL et al. Outcome after rapid vs gradual discontinuation of lithium treatment in bipolar disorders. Arch Gen Psychiatry 1993; **50**:448–455.

21. Macritchie KA et al. Does 'rebound mania' occur after stopping carbamazepine? A pilot study. J Psychopharmacol 2000; **14**:266–268.

22. Franks MA et al. Bouncing back: is the bipolar rebound phenomenon peculiar to lithium? A retrospective naturalistic study. J Psychopharmacol 2008; **22**:452–456.

23. Kessing LV et al. Valproate v. lithium in the treatment of bipolar disorder in clinical practice: observational nationwide register-based cohort study. Br J Psychiatry 2011; **199**:57–63.

24. Gao K et al. Typical and atypical antipsychotics in bipolar depression. J Clin Psychiatry 2005; **66**:1376–1385.

25. Hellewell JS. A review of the evidence for the use of antipsychotics in the maintenance treatment of bipolar disorders. J Psychopharmacol 2006; **20**:39–45.

26. Gigante AD et al. Long-acting injectable antipsychotics for the maintenance treatment of bipolar disorder. CNS Drugs 2012; **26**:403–420.

27. National Institute for Health and Care Excellence. Bipolar disorder: the assessment and management of bipolar disorder in adults, children and young people in primary and secondary care. Draft for consultation, April 2014. https://www.nice.org.uk/

28. Vieta E et al. Efficacy and safety of quetiapine in combination with lithium or divalproex for maintenance of patients with bipolar I disorder (international trial 126). J Affect Disord 2008; **109**:251–263.

29. McIntyre RS. Aripiprazole for the maintenance treatment of bipolar I disorder: A review. Clin Ther 2010; **32 Suppl 1**:S32–S38.

30. Ghaemi SN et al. Long-term risperidone treatment in bipolar disorder: 6-month follow up. Int Clin Psychopharmacol 1997; **12**:333–338.

31. Freeman MP et al. Mood stabilizer combinations: a review of safety and efficacy. Am J Psychiatry 1998; **155**:12–21.

32. Muzina DJ et al. Maintenance therapies in bipolar disorder: focus on randomized controlled trials. Aust N Z J Psychiatry 2005; **39**:652–661.

33. Tohen M et al. Relapse prevention in bipolar I disorder: 18-month comparison of olanzapine plus mood stabiliser v. mood stabiliser alone. Br J Psychiatry 2004; **184**:337–345.

34. Paton C et al. Lithium in bipolar and other affective disorders: prescribing practice in the UK. J Psychopharmacol 2010; **24**:1739–1746.

35. Marcus R et al. Efficacy of aripiprazole adjunctive to lithium or valproate in the long-term treatment of patients with bipolar I disorder with an inadequate response to lithium or valproate monotherapy: a multicenter, double-blind, randomized study. Bipolar Disord 2011; **13**:133–144.

36. Bowden CL et al. A placebo-controlled 18-month trial of lamotrigine and lithium maintenance treatment in recently manic or hypomanic patients with bipolar I disorder. Arch Gen Psychiatry 2003; **60**:392–400.

37. Ghaemi SN et al. Long-term antidepressant treatment in bipolar disorder: meta-analyses of benefits and risks. Acta Psychiatr Scand 2008; **118**:347–356.

38. Ghaemi SN et al. Antidepressant discontinuation in bipolar depression: a Systematic Treatment Enhancement Program for Bipolar Disorder (STEP-BD) randomized clinical trial of long-term effectiveness and safety. J Clin Psychiatry 2010; **71**:372–380.

39. Ostacher MJ et al. Impact of substance use disorders on recovery from episodes of depression in bipolar disorder patients: prospective data from the Systematic Treatment Enhancement Program for Bipolar Disorder (STEP-BD). Am J Psychiatry 2010; **167**:289–297.

CHAPTER 3

Physical monitoring for people with bipolar affective disorder

Table 3.12 Physical monitoring for people with bipolar affective disorder*

Test or measurement	Monitoring for all patients		Additional monitoring for specific drugs				
	Initial health check	Annual check up	Antipsychotics	Lithium	Valproate	Carbamazepine
Thyroid function	Yes	Yes		At start and every 6 months; more often if evidence of deterioration		
Liver function	Yes	Yes			At start and periodically during treatment if clinically indicated	At start and periodically during treatment if clinically indicated
Renal function (e-GFR)	Yes	Yes		At start and every 6 months; more often if there is evidence of deterioration of the patient starts taking interacting drugs		
Urea and electrolytes	Yes	Yes		At start and then every 6 months (include serum calcium)		Every 6 months. More often if clinically indicated
Full blood count	Yes	Yes		Only if clinically indicated		At start and at 6 months
Blood (plasma) glucose	Yes	Yes, as part of a routine physical health check	At start and then every 4–6 months (and at 1 month if taking olanzapine); more often if evidence of elevated levels		At start and 6 months	At start and 6 months
Lipid profile	Yes	Yes, as part of a routine physical health check	At start and at 3 months; more often initially if evidence of elevated levels			

Blood pressure	Yes	Yes, as part of a routine physical health check	During dosage titration if antipsychotic prescribed is associated with postural hypotension	
Prolactin	Children and adolescents only	At start and if symptoms of raised prolactin develop	Raised prolactin unlikely with quetiapine or aripiprazole. Very occasionally seen with olanzapine and asenapine. Very common with risperidone and FGAs	
ECG	If indicated by history or clinical picture	At start if there are risk factors for, or existing, cardiovascular disease (or haloperidol is prescribed). If relevant abnormalities are detected, as a minimum recheck after each dose increase	At start if risk factors for or existing cardiovascular disease. If relevant abnormalities are detected, as a minimum recheck after each dose increase	At start if risk factors for or existing cardiovascular disease. If relevant abnormalities are detected, as a minimum recheck after each dose increase
Weight (and height in adolescents onlyn)	Yes, as part of a routine physical health check	At start then frequently for first 3 months then three monthly for first year. Thereafter, at least annually	At start, and when needed if the patient gains weight rapidly	At start and when needed if the patient gains weight rapidly
Plasma levels of drug		At least 3–4 days after initiation and 3–4 days after every dose change until levels stable, then **every 3 months** in the first year, then every 6 months for most patients (see NICE[1])	Titrate by effect and tolerability. Do not routinely measure unless there is evidence of lack of effectiveness, poor adherence or toxicity	Two weeks after initiation and two weeks after dose change. Thereafter, do not routinely measure unless there is evidence of lack of effectiveness, poor adherence or toxicity

For patients on **lamotrigine**, do an annual health check, but no special monitoring tests are needed

*Based on NICE Guidelines[1] and NPSA advice.[2]

ECG, electrocardiogram; eGFR, estimated glomerular filtration rate; FGA, first-generation antipsychotics.

References

1. National Institute for Health and Care Excellence. Bipolar disorder: the assessment and management of bipolar disorder in adults, children and young people in primary and secondary care. Clinical Guideline 185, 2014. https://www.nice.org.uk/

2. National Patient Safety Agency. Safer lithium therapy. NPSA/2009/PSA005, 2009. http://www.nrls.npsa.nhs.uk/

Chapter 4

Depression and anxiety

Introduction

Depression is, of course, widely recognised as a major public health problem around the world. The mainstay of treatment is the prescription of antidepressants although, of late, psychological treatments have found a place as an alternative to antidepressants in milder forms of depression.[1] Other methods of treating depression (vagal nerve stimulation [VNS],[2] transcranial magnetic stimulation [TMS],[3] etc.) have also emerged but remain somewhat experimental and are not widely available. The basic principles of prescribing are described below along with a summary of National Institute of Health and Care Excellence (NICE) guidance.

Basic principles of prescribing in depression

- Discuss with the patient choice of drug and utility/availability of other, non-pharmacological treatments.
- Discuss with the patient likely outcomes, such as gradual relief from depressive symptoms over several weeks.
- Prescribe a dose of antidepressant (after titration, if necessary) that is likely to be effective.
- For a single episode, continue treatment for at least 6–9 months after resolution of symptoms (multiple episodes may require longer).
- Withdraw antidepressants gradually; always inform patients of the risk and nature of discontinuation symptoms.

The Maudsley Prescribing Guidelines in Psychiatry, Twelfth Edition. David Taylor, Carol Paton and Shitij Kapur.
© 2015 David Taylor, Carol Paton and Shitij Kapur. Published 2015 by John Wiley & Sons, Ltd.

Official guidance on the treatment of depression

NICE guidelines:[1] a summary

- Antidepressants are not recommended as a first-line treatment in recent-onset, mild depression – active monitoring, individual guided self-help, cognitive behavioural therapy (CBT) or exercise are preferred.
- Antidepressants are recommended for the treatment of moderate to severe depression and for dysthymia.
- When an antidepressant is prescribed, a generic selective serotonin reuptake inhibitor (SSRI) is recommended.
- All patients should be informed about the withdrawal (discontinuation) effects of antidepressants.
- For treatment-resistant depression, recommended strategies include augmentation with lithium or an antipsychotic or the addition of a second antidepressant (see section on 'Refractory depression' in this chapter).
- Patients with two prior episodes and functional impairment should be treated for at least 2 years.
- The use of electroconvulsive therapy (ECT) is supported in severe and treatment-resistant depression.

This chapter concentrates on the use of antidepressants and offers advice on drug choice, dosing, switching strategies and sequencing of treatments. The near exclusion of other treatment modalities does not imply any lack of confidence in their efficacy but simply reflects the need (in a prescribing guideline) to concentrate on medicines-related subjects.

References

1. National Institute for Health and Clinical Excellence. Depression: the treatment and management of depression in adults (update). Clinical Guideline 90, 2009. http://www.nice.org.uk/
2. George MS et al. Vagus nerve stimulation for the treatment of depression and other neuropsychiatric disorders. Expert Rev Neurother 2007; 7:63–74.
3. Loo CK et al. A review of the efficacy of transcranial magnetic stimulation (TMS) treatment for depression, and current and future strategies to optimize efficacy. J Affect Disord 2005; 88:255–267.

Antidepressants: general overview

Effectiveness

The *severity* of depression at which antidepressants show consistent benefits over placebo is poorly defined. Although it is generally accepted that the more severe the symptoms, the greater the benefit from antidepressant treatment[1-3], there is some evidence to support the view that response may be independent of symptom severity.[4] Antidepressants are normally recommended as first-line treatment in patients whose depression is of at least moderate severity. Of this patient group, approximately 20% will recover with no treatment at all, 30% will respond to placebo and 50% will respond to antidepressant drug treatment.[5] This gives a number needed to treat (NNT) of 3 for antidepressant over true no-treatment control and an NNT of 5 for antidepressant over placebo. Note though that response in clinical trials is generally defined as a 50% reduction in depression rating scale scores, a somewhat arbitrary dichotomy, and that change measured using continuous scales tends to show a relatively small mean difference between active treatment and placebo (which itself is an effective treatment for depression). Drug–placebo differences have diminished over time largely because of methodological changes.[6]

In patients with sub-syndromal depression, it is difficult to separate the response rate to antidepressants from that to placebo; antidepressant treatment is not indicated unless the patient has a history of severe depression (where less severe symptoms may indicate the onset of another episode), or if symptoms persist. Patients with dysthymia (symptom *duration* of at least 2 years) benefit from antidepressant treatment; the minimum duration of symptoms associated with benefit is unknown. In other patients, the side-effects associated with antidepressant treatment may outweigh any small benefit seen.

Onset of action

It is widely held that antidepressants do not exert their effects for 2–4 weeks. This is a myth. All antidepressants show a pattern of response where the rate of improvement is highest during weeks 1–2 and lowest during weeks 4–6. Statistical separation from placebo is seen at 2–4 weeks in single trials (hence the idea of a lag effect) but after only 1–2 weeks in (statistically more powerful) meta-analyses[7,8]. Thus, where large numbers of patients are treated and detailed rating scales are used, an antidepressant effect is statistically evident at 1 week. In clinical practice using simple observations, an antidepressant effect in an individual is usually seen by 2 weeks.[9] It follows that in individuals where *no* antidepressant effect is evident after 3–4 weeks' treatment, a change in dose or drug may be indicated. It is important, however, to be clear about what constitutes 'no effect'. Different patterns of response have been identified[10] and, in some, response is slow to emerge. However, in those ultimately responsive to treatment, all will have begun to show at least minor improvement at 3 weeks. Thus, those showing no discernible improvement at this time will very probably never respond to the prescribed drug at that dose. In contrast, those showing small improvements at 3 weeks (that is, improvement not meeting criteria for 'response') may well go on to respond fully.[11]

CHAPTER 4

Choice of antidepressant and relative side-effects

Selective serotonin reuptake inhibitors (SSRIs) (Table 4.1) are well tolerated compared with the older tricyclic antidepressants (TCAs) (Table 4.2) and monoamine oxidase inhibitors (MAOIs) (Table 4.3), and are generally recommended as *first-line* pharmacological treatment for depression.[1] There is a suggestion from a network meta-analysis[12] that some antidepressants may be more effective overall than others but this has not been consistently demonstrated in head to head studies, and should therefore be treated with caution. Side-effect profiles of antidepressants do differ. For example, paroxetine has been associated with more weight gain and a higher incidence of sexual dysfunction, and sertraline with a higher incidence of diarrhoea than other SSRIs.[13] Dual reuptake inhibitors such as venlafaxine and duloxetine tend to be tolerated less well than SSRIs but better than TCAs (Table 4.4). With all drugs there is marked interindividual variation in tolerability which is not easily predicted by knowledge of a drug's likely adverse effects. A flexible approach is usually required to find the right drug for a particular patient.

As well as *headache* and *GI symptoms*, **SSRIs** as a class are associated with a range of other side-effects including *sexual dysfunction* (see section on 'Antidepressants and sexual dysfunction' in this chapter), *hyponatraemia* (see section on 'Antidepressant-induced hyponatraemia' in this chapter) and *GI bleeds* (see section on 'SSRIs and bleeding' in this chapter). **TCAs** have a number of *adverse cardiovascular effects* (hypotension, tachycardia and QTc prolongation), and are particularly *toxic in overdose*[14] (see section on 'Overdose' in Chapter 8). The now rarely used **MAOIs** have the potential to interact with tyramine-containing foods to cause *hypertensive crisis*. All antidepressant drugs can cause *discontinuation symptoms* with short half-life drugs being most problematic in this respect (see section on 'Antidepressant discontinuation symptoms' in this chapter).

Drug interactions

Some SSRIs are potent *inhibitors* of individual or multiple *hepatic cytochrome P450 (CYP)* pathways and the magnitude of these effects is dose related. A number of clinically significant drug interactions can therefore be predicted. For example, fluvoxamine is a potent inhibitor of CYP1A2 which can result in increased theophylline serum levels, fluoxetine is a potent inhibitor of CYP2D6 which can result in increased seizure risk with clozapine, and paroxetine is a potent inhibitor of CYP2D6 which can result in treatment failure with tamoxifen (a pro-drug) leading to increased mortality.[15]

Antidepressants can also cause pharmacodynamic interactions. For example, the cardiotoxicity of TCAs may be exacerbated by drugs such as diuretics that can cause electrolyte disturbances. A summary of clinically relevant drug interactions with antidepressants can be found in Table 4.16.

Potential **pharmacokinetic** and **pharmacodynamic** interactions between antidepressants have to be considered when **switching** from one antidepressant to another (see section on 'Swapping and stopping' in this chapter).

Table 4.1 Antidepressant drugs: SSRIs*

SSRI	Licensed indication	Licensed doses (elderly doses not included)	Main adverse effects	Major interactions	Approx. half-life (h)	Cost
Citalopram	Depression – treatment of the initial phase and as maintenance therapy against potential relapse or recurrence Panic disorder ± agoraphobia	20–40 mg/day Use lowest dose – evidence for higher doses poor 10 mg for 1 week, increasing up to 40 mg/day	Nausea, vomiting, dyspepsia, abdominal pain, diarrhoea, rash, sweating, agitation, anxiety, headache, insomnia, tremor, sexual dysfunction (male and female), hyponatraemia, cutaneous bleeding disorders Discontinuation symptoms may occur	Not a potent inhibitor of most cytochrome enzymes Avoid – MAOIs Avoid – St John's wort Caution with alcohol (although no interaction seen) NSAIDs/tryptophan/warfarin	~33 Has weak active metabolites	Tabs – low Drops – moderate
Escitalopram	Depression Panic disorder ± agoraphobia Social anxiety Generalised anxiety disorder OCD	10–20 mg/day 5 mg/day for 1 week, increasing up to 20 mg/day 10–20 mg/day 10–20 mg/day 10–20 mg/day	As for citalopram	As for citalopram	~30 Has weak active metabolites	High
Fluoxetine	Depression OCD Bulimia nervosa All indications higher doses possible – see SPC	20–60 mg/day 8–18 years:10–20 mg/day 20–60 mg/day (long-term efficacy >24 months has not been demonstrated in OCD) 60 mg/day (long-term efficacy >3 months has not been demonstrated in OCD) (up to 80 mg/day)	As for citalopram but insomnia and agitation possibly more common Rash may occur more frequently May alter insulin requirements	Inhibits CYP2D6, CYP3A4. Increases plasma levels of some antipsychotics/some benzos/ carbamazepine/ ciclosporin/ phenytoin/tricyclics MAOIs – never Avoid – selegiline/St John's wort Caution – alcohol (although no interaction seen)/NSAIDs/ tryptophan/warfarin	4–6 days 4–16 days active metabolite (norfluoxetine)	Low

Continued

CHAPTER 4

Table 4.1 (Continued)

SSRI	Licensed indication	Licensed doses (elderly doses not included)	Main adverse effects	Major interactions	Approx. half-life (h)	Cost
Fluvoxamine	Depression	100–300 mg/day bd if >150 mg	As for citalopram but nausea more common	Inhibits CYP1A2/2C9/3A4 Increases plasma levels of some benzos/ carbamazepine/ ciclosporin/ methadone/olanzapine/ clozapine/ phenytoin/ propranolol/ theophylline/some tricyclics/ warfarin	17–22	Moderate
	OCD	100–300 mg/day (start at 50 mg/day) bd if >150 mg		MAOIs – never Caution – alcohol/lithium/ NSAIDs/St John's wort/ tryptophan/warfarin		
		8–18 years:100–200 mg/day (given bd if >150 mg)				
Paroxetine	Depression	20–50 mg/day Use lowest dose – evidence for higher doses poor	As for citalopram but antimuscarinic effects and sedation more common	Potent inhibitor of CYP2D6 Increases plasma level of some antipsychotics/ tricyclics	~24 (non-linear kinetics)	Low
	OCD	20–60 mg/day	EPS rare but more common than with other SSRIs	MAOIs – never		
	Panic disorder ± agoraphobia	10–60 mg/day	Discontinuation symptoms common – withdraw slowly	Avoid – St John's wort		
	Social phobia/social anxiety disorders	20–50 mg/day		Caution – alcohol/lithium/ NSAIDs/ tryptophan/warfarin		
	PTSD	20–50 mg/day				
	Generalised anxiety disorder	20–50 mg/day				

Drug	Indication	Dose	Side-effects / Interactions	Half-life (h)	Inhibitory potential
Sertraline	Depression ± anxiety and prevention of relapse or recurrence of depression ± anxiety	50–200 mg/day Use 50–100 mg – evidence for higher doses poor	As for citalopram	Inhibits CYP2D6 (more likely to occur at doses ≥100 mg/day). Increases plasma levels of some antipsychotics/ tricyclics	~26 Has a weak active metabolite	Low
	Panic disorder ± agoraphobia	25–200 mg/day		Avoid – St John's wort		
	Social anxiety disorder	25–200 mg/day		Caution – alcohol (although no interaction seen)/lithium/ NSAIDs/ tryptophan/warfarin		
	OCD (under specialist supervision in children)	50–200 mg/day (adults) 6–12 years: 25–50 mg/day				
	PTSD	13–17 years: 50–200 mg/day; may be increased in steps of 50 mg at intervals of 1 week 25–200 mg/day				
Vortioxetine	Major depressive episodes in adults	Starting dose is 10 mg/day. Dose may be adjusted in the range 5–20 mg/day	Nausea, decreased appetite, abnormal dreams, dizziness, pruritus, diarrhoea	Metabolised by CYP2D6	~66	High
				No effect on enzyme activity. No active metabolites		
				Avoid MAOIs, caution with selegiline, tramadol, triptans		
				When used with CYP2D6 inhibitors, reduce dose		
				Increase dose if used with CYP2D6 inducers		
				No observed interaction with alcohol		

*For full details refer to the manufacturer's information.
bd, twice a day; EPS, extrapyramidal side-effects; MAOI, monoamine oxidase inhibitor; NSAID, non-steroidal anti-inflammatory drug; OCD, obsessive compulsive disorder; PTSD, post-traumatic stress disorder; SPC, summary of product characteristics; SSRI, selective serotonin reuptake inhibitor.

Table 4.2 Antidepressant drugs: tricyclics*

Tricyclic	Licensed indication	Licensed doses (elderly doses not included)	Main adverse effects	Major interactions	Approx. half-life(h)	Cost
Amitriptyline	Depression	50–200 mg/day	Sedation, often with hangover; postural hypotension; tachycardia/arrhythmia; dry mouth, blurred vision, constipation, urinary retention	SSRIs (except escitalopram/ citalopram), phenothiazines, Alcohol Antimuscarinics Antipsychotics MAOIs Antiarrhythmics	9–25	Low
	Nocturnal enuresis in children	7–10 yr: 10–20 mg 11–16 yr: 25–50 mg at night for maximum of 3 months. The dose should be given 30 minutes before bedtime	As doses used for nocturnal enuresis are lower, side-effects are less frequent; sedation and anticholinergic side-effects are most common		18–96 active metabolite (nortriptyline)	Liquid available
Clomipramine	Depression	30–250 mg/day	As for amitriptyline	As for amitriptyline	12–36	Low
	Phobic and obsessional states	100–150 mg/day			36 active metabolite (desmethyl-clomipramine)	
	Adjunctive treatment of cataplexy associated with narcolepsy	10–75 mg/day				
Dosulepin (dothiepin)	Depression	75–225 mg/day	As for amitriptyline	As for amitriptyline	14–45 22–60 active metabolite (desmethyldosulepin)	Low
Doxepin	Depression	30–300 mg/day (up to 100 mg as a single dose)	As for amitriptyline	As for amitriptyline	8–24 33–80 active metabolite (desmethyldoxepin)	Low

Drug	Indication	Dose	Side effects	Cautions	Half-life (hours)	Toxicity in overdose	Notes
Imipramine	Depression Nocturnal enuresis in children	50–200 mg/day (up to 100 mg as a single dose; up to 300 mg in hospital patients) 6–7 yr (20–25 kg): 25 mg 8–11 yr (25–35 kg): 25–50 mg >11 yr (>35 kg): 50–75 mg at night for maximum of 3 months. The dose should be given 30 minutes before bedtime	As for amitriptyline but less sedative	As for amitriptyline	~19 12–36 active metabolite(desipramine)	Low	
Lofepramine	Depression	140–210 mg/day	As for amitriptyline but less sedative/ anticholinergic/ cardiotoxic Constipation common	As for amitriptyline	1.5–6 ? 12–24 active metabolite (desipramine)	Low	Liquid available
Nortriptyline	Depression Nocturnal enuresis in children	Adults: 75–150 mg/day Adolescents: 30–50 mg/day in divided doses 6–7 yr (20–25 kg): 10 mg 8–11 yr (25–35 kg): 10–20 mg >11 yr (>35 kg): 25–35 mg at night for max. 3 months. The dose should be given 30 minutes before bedtime	As for amitriptyline but less sedative/anticholinergic/ hypotensive Constipation may be problematic	As for amitriptyline	15–39	Low	
Trimipramine	Depression	50–300 mg/day	As for amitriptyline but more sedative	As for amitriptyline Safer with MAOIs than other tricyclics	7–23 ~23	Low	

*For full details refer to the manufacturer's information.
MAOI, monoamine oxidase inhibitor; SSRI, selective serotonin reuptake inhibitor.

Table 4.3 Antidepressant drugs: monoamine oxidase inhibitors*

MAOI	Licensed indication	Licensed doses (elderly doses not included)	Main adverse effects	Major interactions	Approx. half-life (h)	Cost
Isocarboxazid	Depression	30 mg/day in single or divided doses (increased after 4 weeks if necessary to max. 60 mg/day for 4–6 weeks) then reduce to usual maintenance dose 10–20 mg/day (but up to 40 mg/day may be required)	Postural hypotension, dizziness, drowsiness, insomnia, headaches, oedema, anticholinergic adverse effects, nervousness, paraesthesia, weight gain, hepatotoxicity, leucopenia, hypertensive crisis	Tyramine in food, sympathomimetics, alcohol, opioids, antidepressants, levadopa, 5HT$_1$ agonists (buspirone)	36 (reduces MAO function for up to 2 weeks)	Low
Phenelzine	Depression. Usually used in patients with 'atypical' or 'non-endogenous' depression	15 mg tds – qid (hospital patients: max. 30 mg tds) Consider reducing to lowest possible maintenance dose	As for isocarboxazid but more postural hypotension, less hepatotoxicity	As for isocarboxazid. Probably safest of MAOIs and the one that should be used if combinations are considered	~1 (reduces MAO function for up to 2 weeks)	Low
Tranylcypromine	Depression. Used especially where phobic symptoms are present and where other antidepressants have failed	10 mg bd. Doses >30 mg/day under close supervision only Usual maintenance: 10 mg/day Last dose no later than 3 pm	As for isocarboxazid but insomnia, nervousness, hypertensive crisis more common than with other MAOIs; hepatotoxicity less common than phenelzine. Mild dependence as amfetamine-like structure	As for isocarboxazid but interactions more severe. Never use in combination therapy with other antidepressants	2.5 (reduces MAO function for up to 2 weeks)	Low

Moclobemide (reversible inhibitor of *MAO-A)	Major depression	150–600 mg/day (given bd after food)	Sleep disturbances, nausea, agitation, confusion	Tyramine interactions rare and mild but possible if high doses (>600 mg/day) used or if large quantities of tyramine ingested: CNS excitation/depression with dextromethorphan/pethidine	2–4	Low
	Social phobia	300–600 mg/day (given bd after food)				
				Avoid: clomipramine/levodopa/ selegiline/sympathomimetics/ SSRIs		
				Caution with fentanyl/morphine/ tricyclics		
				Cimetidine – use half-dose of moclobemide		

*For full details refer to the manufacturer's information and BNF.

bd, twice a day; CNS, central nervous system; MAOI, monoamine oxidase inhibitor; qid, four times a day; SSRI, selective serotonin reuptake inhibitor; tds, three times a day.

Table 4.4 Antidepressant drugs: others*

Antidepressant	Licensed indication	Licensed doses (elderly doses not included)	Main adverse effects	Major interactions	Approx. half-life (h)	Cost
Agomelatine	Major depression	25–50 mg/day at bedtime	Nausea, dizziness, headache, insomnia, somnolence, migraine, changes in LFTs especially AST and ALT LFTs should be done at initiation, 3, 6, 12 and 24 weeks and when clinically indicated. Discontinue drug if AST and ALT exceeds 3× the normal range	Metabolised by CYP1A2 (90%) and CYP2C19/9 (10%) Fluvoxamine and ciprofloxacin contraindicated Caution with oestrogens, propranolol and any drugs acting on either enzyme Caution – alcohol	1–2	High
Duloxetine	Depression (and other non-psychiatric indications) Generalised anxiety disorder	60–120 mg/day. Limited data to support advantage of doses above 60 mg/day 60–120 mg/day	Nausea, insomnia, headache, dizziness, dry mouth, somnolence, constipation, anorexia. Very small increases in heart rate and blood pressure, including hypertensive crisis	Metabolised by CYP1A2 and CYP2D6. Inhibitor of CYP2D6 Caution with drugs acting on either enzyme MAOIs – avoid Caution – alcohol (although no interaction seen)	12 (metabolites inactive)	High
Mianserin	Depression, particularly where sedation required	30–90 mg daily	Sedation, rash; rarely: blood dyscrasia, jaundice, arthralgia. No anticholinergic effects. Sexual dysfunction uncommon. Low cardiotoxicity	Other sedatives, alcohol MAOIs – avoid Effect on hepatic enzymes unclear, so caution is required	10–20 2-desmethyl-mianserin is major metabolite (?activity)	Moderate
Mirtazapine	Major depression	15–45 mg/day	Increased appetite, weight gain, drowsiness, oedema, dizziness, headache, blood dyscrasia. Nausea/sexual dysfunction relatively uncommon	Minimal effect on CYP2D6/1A2/3A Caution – alcohol/sedatives	20–40 25 active metabolite (demethyl-mirtazapine)	Tabs – low Soltab – moderate

Drug	Indication	Dose	Side effects	Interactions/Metabolism	Half-life (h)	Toxicity in overdose
Reboxetine	Depression – acute and maintenance	8–12 mg/day (given bd)	Insomnia, sweating, dizziness, dry mouth, constipation, nausea, tachycardia, urinary hesitancy, headache. Erectile dysfunction may occur rarely	Metabolised by CYP3A4 – avoid drugs inhibiting this enzyme (e.g. erythromycin ketoconazole). Minimal effect on CYP2D6/3A4 MAOIs – avoid No interaction with alcohol	13	Moderate
Trazodone	Depression ± anxiety Anxiety	150–300 mg/day (up to 600 mg/day in hospitalised patients). Twice daily dosing above 300 mg/day 75–300 mg/day	Sedation, dizziness, headache, nausea, vomiting, tremor, postural hypotension, tachycardia, priapism. Not anticholinergic, less cardiotoxic than tricyclics	Caution – sedatives/alcohol/ other antidepressants/digoxin/ phenytoin MAOIs – avoid	5–13 (biphasic) 4–9 active metabolite (mCPP)	Tabs – low Liquid – high
Venlafaxine	Depression ± anxiety and prevention of relapse or recurrence of depression (tablets, ER preps) Social anxiety (prolonged release caps and ER) Generalised anxiety disorder (prolonged release caps and ER prep only) Panic disorder (ER prep only)	75–375 mg/day (bd) with food 75–375 mg ER/day (od) with food 75–225 mg PR/ER/day 75–225 mg PR/ER/day 75–225 mg ER/day	Nausea, insomnia, dry mouth, somnolence, dizziness, sweating, nervousness, headache, sexual dysfunction, constipation. Elevation of blood pressure at higher doses. Avoid if at risk of arrhythmia. Discontinuation symptoms common – withdraw slowly	Metabolised by CYP2D6/3A4– caution with drugs known to inhibit both isozymes Minimal inhibitory effects on CYP2D6 No effects on CYP1A2/2C9/3A4 MAOIs – avoid Caution – alcohol (although no interaction seen)/ cimetidine/ clozapine/warfarin	5 11 active metabolite (O-desmethyl-venlafaxine)	Low

*For full details refer to the manufacturer's information.

ALT, alanine aminotransferase; AST, aspartate aminotransferase; bd, twice a day; ER, extended release; LFT, liver function test; MAOI, monoamine oxidase inhibitor; od, once a day; PR, prolonged release capsules.

Suicidality

Antidepressant treatment has been associated with an increased risk of suicidal thoughts and acts, particularly in adolescents and young adults,[16,17] leading to the recommendation that patients should be warned of this potential adverse effect during the early weeks of treatment and know how to seek help if required. All antidepressants have been implicated,[18] including those that are marketed for an indication other than depression (e.g. atomoxetine). It should be noted that:

- although the relative risk may be elevated above placebo rates in some patient groups, the absolute risk remains very small
- the most effective way to prevent suicidal thoughts and acts is to treat depression[19–21]
- antidepressant drugs are the most effective treatment currently available.[5,22]

For the most part, suicidality is greatly reduced by the use of antidepressants.[23–25] Note, however, that those who experience treatment-emergent or worsening suicidal ideation with one antidepressant may be more likely to have a similar experience with subsequent treatments.[26]

Toxicity in overdose varies both between and within groups of antidepressants.[27] See section on 'Psychotropics in overdose' in Chapter 8.

Duration of treatment

Antidepressants relieve the symptoms of depression but do not treat the underlying cause. They should therefore be taken **for 6–9 months after recovery from a single episode** (to cover the assumed duration of most single untreated episodes). In those patients who have had multiple episodes, there is evidence of benefit from maintenance treatment for at least 2 years; no upper duration of treatment has been identified (see section on 'Antidepressant prophylaxis' in this chapter). There are few data on which to base recommendations about the duration of treatment of augmentation regimens.

Next step treatments

Approximately a third of patients do not respond to the first antidepressant that is prescribed. Options in this group include dose escalation, switching to a different drug and a number of augmentation strategies. The lessons from STAR*D (Sequenced Treatment Alternatives to Relieve Depression) are that a small proportion of non-responders will respond with each treatment change, but that **effect sizes are modest** and there is no clear difference in effectiveness between strategies. See section on 'Treatment of refractory depression' in this chapter.

Use of antidepressants in anxiety spectrum disorders

Antidepressants are first-line treatments in a number of anxiety spectrum disorders. See section on 'Anxiety spectrum disorders' in this chapter.

References

1. National Institute for Health and Clinical Excellence. Depression in adults: the treatment and management of depression in adults. Clinical Guideline 90, 2009. http://www.nice.org.uk/Guidance/cg90

2. Kirsch I et al. Initial severity and antidepressant benefits: a meta-analysis of data submitted to the Food and Drug Administration. PLoS Med 2008; 5:e45.

3. Fournier JC et al. Antidepressant drug effects and depression severity: a patient-level meta-analysis. JAMA 2010; 303:47–53.

4. Gibbons RD et al. Benefits from antidepressants: synthesis of 6-week patient-level outcomes from double-blind placebo-controlled randomized trials of fluoxetine and venlafaxine. Arch Gen Psychiatry 2012; 69:572–579.

5. Anderson IM et al. Evidence-based guidelines for treating depressive disorders with antidepressants: a revision of the 2000 British Association for Psychopharmacology guidelines. J Psychopharmacol 2008; 22:343–396.

6. Khan A et al. Why has the antidepressant-placebo difference in antidepressant clinical trials diminished over the past three decades? CNS Neurosci Ther 2010; 16:217–226.

7. Taylor MJ et al. Early onset of selective serotonin reuptake inhibitor antidepressant action: systematic review and meta-analysis. Arch Gen Psychiatry 2006; 63:1217–1223.

8. Papakostas GI et al. A meta-analysis of early sustained response rates between antidepressants and placebo for the treatment of major depressive disorder. J Clin Psychopharmacol 2006; 26:56–60.

9. Szegedi A et al. Early improvement in the first 2 weeks as a predictor of treatment outcome in patients with major depressive disorder: a meta-analysis including 6562 patients. J Clin Psychiatry 2009; 70:344–353.

10. Uher R et al. Early and delayed onset of response to antidepressants in individual trajectories of change during treatment of major depression: a secondary analysis of data from the Genome-Based Therapeutic Drugs for Depression (GENDEP) study. J Clin Psychiatry 2011; 72: 1478–1484.

11. Posternak MA et al. Response rates to fluoxetine in subjects who initially show no improvement. J Clin Psychiatry 2011; 72:949–954.

12. Cipriani A et al. Comparative efficacy and acceptability of 12 new-generation antidepressants: a multiple-treatments meta-analysis. Lancet 2009; 373:746–758.

13. Gartlehner G et al. Comparative benefits and harms of second-generation antidepressants: background paper for the American College of Physicians. Ann Intern Med 2008; 149:734–750.

14. Flanagan RJ. Fatal toxicity of drugs used in psychiatry. Hum Psychopharmacol 2008; 23 Suppl 1:43–51.

15. Kelly CM et al. Selective serotonin reuptake inhibitors and breast cancer mortality in women receiving tamoxifen: a population based cohort study. BMJ 2010; 340:c693.

16. Stone M et al. Risk of suicidality in clinical trials of antidepressants in adults: analysis of proprietary data submitted to US Food and Drug Administration. BMJ 2009; 339:b2880.

17. Carpenter DJ et al. Meta-analysis of efficacy and treatment-emergent suicidality in adults by psychiatric indication and age subgroup following initiation of paroxetine therapy: a complete set of randomized placebo-controlled trials. J Clin Psychiatry 2011; 72:1503–1514.

18. Schneeweiss S et al. Variation in the risk of suicide attempts and completed suicides by antidepressant agent in adults: a propensity score-adjusted analysis of 9 years' data. Arch Gen Psychiatry 2010; 67:497–506.

19. Isacsson G et al. The increased use of antidepressants has contributed to the worldwide reduction in suicide rates. Br J Psychiatry 2010; 196:429–433.

20. Gibbons RD et al. Suicidal thoughts and behavior with antidepressant treatment: reanalysis of the randomized placebo-controlled studies of fluoxetine and venlafaxine. Arch Gen Psychiatry 2012; 69:580–587.

21. Lu CY et al. Changes in antidepressant use by young people and suicidal behavior after FDA warnings and media coverage: quasi-experimental study. BMJ 2014; 348:g3596.

22. Isacsson G et al. Antidepressant medication prevents suicide in depression. Acta Psychiatr Scand 2010; 122:454–460.

23. Simon GE et al. Suicide risk during antidepressant treatment. Am J Psychiatry 2006; 163:41–47.

24. Mulder RT et al. Antidepressant treatment is associated with a reduction in suicidal ideation and suicide attempts. Acta Psychiatr Scand 2008; 118:116–122.

25. Tondo L et al. Suicidal status during antidepressant treatment in 789 Sardinian patients with major affective disorder. Acta Psychiatr Scand 2008; 118:106–115.

26. Perlis RH et al. Do suicidal thoughts or behaviors recur during a second antidepressant treatment trial? J Clin Psychiatry 2012; 73:1439–1442.

27. Hawton K et al. Toxicity of antidepressants: rates of suicide relative to prescribing and non-fatal overdose. Br J Psychiatry 2010; 196:354–358.

CHAPTER 4

St John's wort

St John's wort (SJW) is the popular name for the plant *Hypericum perforatum*. It contains a combination of at least 10 different components, including hypericins, flavonoids and xanthons.[1] Preparations of SJW are often unstandardised and this has complicated the interpretation of clinical trials.

The active ingredient(s) and mechanism(s) of action of SJW are unclear. Constituents of SJW may inhibit MAO,[2] inhibit the reuptake of noradrenaline and serotonin,[3] upregulate serotonin receptors[3] and decrease serotonin receptor expression.[4]

Some preparations of SJW have been granted a traditional herbal registration certificate; note that this is based on traditional use rather than proven efficacy and tolerability. SJW is licensed in Germany for the treatment of depression.

Evidence for SJW in the treatment of depression

A number of trials have examined the efficacy of SJW in the treatment of depression. They have been extensively reviewed[1,5,6] and most authors conclude that SJW is likely to be effective in the treatment of dysthymia[7] and mild to moderate depression,[4,5,8] e.g. Cochrane concludes that SJW is more effective than placebo in the treatment of mild to moderate depression, and is as effective as, and better tolerated than, standard antidepressants.[6] Studies in German-speaking countries showed more favourable results than studies elsewhere. Efficacy in severe depression remains uncertain.[6] A reanalysis of data from a large negative randomised controlled trial (RCT) of SJW found that subjects who guessed that they had been randomised to active treatment fared better than those who guessed that they had received placebo: patient guess regarding receiving active treatment was associated with improvement while actual treatment allocation was not.[9]

It should be noted that:

- the active component of SJW for treating depression has not yet been determined. Trials used different preparations of SJW which were standardised according to their total content of hypericins. However, evidence suggests that hypericins alone do not treat depression[10]
- published studies are generally acute treatment studies. There are fewer data to support the effectiveness of SJW in the medium term[11] or for prophylaxis.[8]

On balance, SJW should not be prescribed: we lack understanding of what the active ingredient is or what constitutes a therapeutic dose. Most preparations of SJW are unlicensed.

Adverse effects

St John's wort appears to be well tolerated.[12] Pooled data from 35 RCTS show that drop-out rates and adverse effects were less than with older antidepressants, slightly less than SSRIs and similar to placebo.[13] The most common, if infrequent, side-effects are dry mouth, nausea, constipation, fatigue, dizziness, headache and restlessness.[14–17]

In addition, SJW contains a red pigment that can cause photosensitivity reactions.[18] It has been suggested that hypericin may be phototoxic to the retina, and contribute to the early development of macular degeneration.[19] SJW may also share the propensity of SSRIs to increase the risk of bleeding; a case report describes prolonged epistaxis after nasal insertion of SJW.[20] In common with other antidepressant drugs, SJW has been known to precipitate hypomania in people with bipolar affective disorder.[21]

Drug interactions

St John's wort is a potent inducer of intestinal and hepatic CYP3A4, CYP2C9, CYP2C19, CYP2E1 and intestinal p-glycoprotein.[22–24] Hyperforin is responsible for this effect.[25] The hyperforin content of SJW preparations varies 50-fold, which will result in a different propensity for drug interactions between brands. Preparations with <1 mg/dose hyperforin do not induce CYP enzymes.[22] CYP3A4 activity is induced over 1–2 weeks and returns to normal approximately 7 days after SJW is discontinued.[26]

Studies have shown that SJW significantly reduces plasma concentrations of digoxin and indinavir[27,28] (a drug used in the treatment of HIV). According to case reports, SJW has lowered the plasma concentrations of clozapine,[29] theophylline, ciclosporin, warfarin, gliclazide, atorvastatin and the combined oral contraceptive pill and has led to treatment failure.[23,24,30,31] There is a theoretical risk that SJW may interact with some anticonvulsant drugs[32]. It has also been reported that SJW can increase the effects of clopidogrel (a pro-drug).[33] Serotonin syndrome has been reported when SJW was taken together with sertraline, paroxetine, nefazodone and the triptans[32,34] (a group of serotonin agonists used to treat migraine). SJW should not be taken with any drugs that have a predominantly serotonergic action.

Key points that patients should know

- Evidence suggests that SJW may be effective in the treatment of mild to moderate depression, but we do not know enough about how much should be taken or what the side-effects are. There is less evidence of benefit in severe depression.
- SJW is not a licensed medicine.
- SJW can interact with other medicines, resulting in serious side-effects. Some important drugs may be metabolised more rapidly and therefore become ineffective with serious consequences (e.g. increased viral load in HIV, failure of oral contraceptives leading to unwanted pregnancy, reduced anticoagulant effect with warfarin leading to thrombosis).
- The symptoms of depression can sometimes be caused by other physical or mental illness. It is important that these possible causes are investigated.
- It is always best to consult the doctor if any herbal or natural remedy is being taken or the patient is thinking of taking one.

Many people regard herbal remedies as 'natural' and therefore harmless.[35] Many are not aware of the potential of such remedies for causing side-effects or interacting with other drugs. A large study from Germany (n = 588), where SJW is a licensed

CHAPTER 4

antidepressant, found that for every prescription written for SJW, one person purchased SJW without seeking the advice of a doctor.[36] Many of these people had severe or persistent depression but few told their doctor that they took SJW. A small US study (n = 22) found that people tend to take SJW because it is easy to obtain alternative medicines and also because they perceive herbal medicines as being purer and safer than prescription medicines. Few would discuss this medication with their conventional healthcare provider.[17] Clinicians need to be proactive in asking patients if they use such treatments and try to dispel the myth that natural is the same as safe.

References

1. Linde K et al. St John's Wort for depression: meta-analysis of randomised controlled trials. Br J Psychiatry 2005; **186**:99–107.
2. Cott JM. In vitro receptor binding and enzyme inhibition by Hypericum perforatum extract. Pharmacopsychiatry 1997; **30 Suppl** 2:108–112.
3. Muller WE et al. Effects of *Hypericum* extract (LI 160) in biochemical models of antidepressant activity. Pharmacopsychiatry 1997; **30 Suppl** 2:102–107.
4. Kasper S et al. Superior efficacy of St John's wort extract WS 5570 compared to placebo in patients with major depression: a randomized, double-blind, placebo-controlled, multi-center trial [ISRCTN77277298]. BMC Med 2006; **4**:14.
5. National Institute for Health and Clinical Excellence. Depression: the treatment and management of depression in adults (update). Clinical Guideline 90, 2009. http://www.nice.org.uk/
6. Linde K et al. St John's Wort for major depression. Cochrane Database Syst Rev 2008; 4:CD000448.
7. Randlov C et al. The efficacy of St. John's Wort in patients with minor depressive symptoms or dysthymia – a double-blind placebo-controlled study. Phytomedicine 2006; **13**:215–221.
8. Kasper S et al. Continuation and long-term maintenance treatment with Hypericum extract WS 5570 after recovery from an acute episode of moderate depression – a double-blind, randomized, placebo controlled long-term trial. Eur Neuropsychopharmacol 2008; **18**:803–813.
9. Chen JA et al. Association between patient beliefs regarding assigned treatment and clinical response: reanalysis of data from the Hypericum Depression Trial Study Group. J Clin Psychiatry 2011; **72**:1669–1676.
10. Teufel-Mayer R et al. Effects of long-term administration of *Hypericum* extracts on the affinity and density of the central serotonergic 5-HT1 A and 5-HT2 A receptors. Pharmacopsychiatry 1997; **30 Suppl** 2:113–116.
11. Anghelescu IG et al. Comparison of Hypericum extract WS 5570 and paroxetine in ongoing treatment after recovery from an episode of moderate to severe depression: results from a randomized multicenter study. Pharmacopsychiatry 2006; **39**:213–219.
12. Kasper S et al. Better tolerability of St. John's wort extract WS 5570 compared to treatment with SSRIs: a reanalysis of data from controlled clinical trials in acute major depression. Int Clin Psychopharmacol 2010; **25**:204–213.
13. Knuppel L et al. Adverse effects of St. John's Wort: a systematic review. J Clin Psychiatry 2004; **65**:1470–1479.
14. Volz HP. Controlled clinical trials of *Hypericum* extracts in depressed patients – an overview. Pharmacopsychiatry 1997; **30 Suppl** 2:72–76.
15. Gaster B et al. St John's Wort for depression: a systematic review. Arch Intern Med 2000; **160**:152–156.
16. Woelk H. Comparison of St John's Wort and imipramine for treating depression: randomised controlled trial. BMJ 2000; **321**:536–539.
17. Wagner PJ et al. Taking the edge off: why patients choose St. John's Wort. J Fam Pract 1999; **48**:615–619.
18. Bove GM. Acute neuropathy after exposure to sun in a patient treated with St John's Wort. Lancet 1998; **352**:1121–1122.
19. Wielgus AR et al. Phototoxicity in human retinal pigment epithelial cells promoted by hypericin, a component of St. John's wort. Photochem Photobiol 2007; **83**:706–713.
20. Crampsey DP et al. Nasal insertion of St John's wort: an unusual cause of epistaxis. J Laryngol Otol 2007; **121**:279–280.
21. Nierenberg AA et al. Mania associated with St. John's wort. Biol Psychiatry 1999; **46**:1707–1708.
22. Rahimi R et al. An update on the ability of St. John's wort to affect the metabolism of other drugs. Expert Opin Drug Metab Toxicol 2012; **8**:691–708.
23. Xu H et al. Effects of St John's wort and CYP2C9 genotype on the pharmacokinetics and pharmacodynamics of gliclazide. Br J Pharmacol 2008; **153**:1579–1586.
24. Russo E et al. Hypericum perforatum: pharmacokinetic, mechanism of action, tolerability, and clinical drug-drug interactions. Phytother Res 2014; **28**:643–655.
25. Madabushi R et al. Hyperforin in St. John's wort drug interactions. Eur J Clin Pharmacol 2006; **62**:225–233.
26. Imai H et al. The recovery time-course of CYP3A after induction by St John's wort administration. Br J Clin Pharmacol 2008; **65**:701–707.
27. Johne A et al. Pharmacokinetic interaction of digoxin with an herbal extract from St John's Wort (*Hypericum perforatum*). Clin Pharmacol Ther 1999; **66**:338–345.
28. Piscitelli SC et al. Indinavir concentrations and St John's Wort. Lancet 2000; **355**:547–548.
29. Van Strater AC et al. Interaction of St John's wort (Hypericum perforatum) with clozapine. Int Clin Psychopharmacol 2012; **27**:121–124.
30. Ernst E. Second thoughts about safety of St John's Wort. Lancet 1999; **354**:2014–2016.

31. Andren L et al. Interaction between a commercially available St. John's wort product (Movina) and atorvastatin in patients with hypercholesterolemia. Eur J Clin Pharmacol 2007; **63**:913–916.

32. Anon. Reminder: St John's Wort (*Hypericum perforatum*) interactions. Curr Probl Pharmacovigilance 2000; **26**:6–7.

33. Lau WC et al. The effect of St. John's wort on the pharmacodynamic response of clopidogrel in hyporesponsive volunteers and patients: increased platelet inhibition by enhancement of CYP 3A4 metabolic activity. J Cardiovasc Pharmacol 2011; **57**:86–93.

34. Lantz MS et al. St. John's wort and antidepressant drug interactions in the elderly. J Geriatr Psychiatry Neurol 1999; **12**:7–10.

35. Barnes J et al. Different standards for reporting ADRs to herbal remedies and conventional OTC medicines: face-to-face interviews with 515 users of herbal remedies. Br J Clin Pharmacol 1998; **45**:496–500.

36. Linden M et al. Self medication with St. John's wort in depressive disorders: an observational study in community pharmacies. J Affect Disord 2008; **107**:205–210.

Recognised minimum effective doses of antidepressants

The recommended minimum effective doses of antidepressants are summarised in Table 4.5.

Table 4.5 The recommended minimum effective doses of antidepressants

Antidepressant	Dose
Tricyclics	Unclear; at least 75–100 mg/day,[1] possibly 125 mg/day[2]
Lofepramine	140 mg/day[3]
SSRIs	
Citalopram	20 mg/day[4]
Escitalopram	10 mg/day[5]
Fluoxetine	20 mg/day[6]
Fluvoxamine	50 mg/day[7]
Paroxetine	20 mg/day[8]
Sertraline	50 mg/day[9]
Others	
Agomelatine	25 mg/day[10]
Duloxetine	60 mg/day[11,12]
Mirtazapine	30 mg/day[13]
Moclobemide	300 mg/day[14]
Reboxetine	8 mg/day[15]
Trazodone	150 mg/day[16]
Venlafaxine	75 mg/day[17]
Vortioxetine	10 mg/day[18,19]

References

1. Furukawa TA et al. Meta-analysis of effects and side effects of low dosage tricyclic antidepressants in depression: systematic review. BMJ 2002; **325**:991.
2. Donoghue J et al. Suboptimal use of antidepressants in the treatment of depression. CNS Drugs 2000; **13**:365–368.
3. Lancaster SG et al. Lofepramine. A review of its pharmacodynamic and pharmacokinetic properties, and therapeutic efficacy in depressive illness. Drugs 1989; **37**:123–140.
4. Montgomery SA et al. The optimal dosing regimen for citalopram – a meta-analysis of nine placebo-controlled studies. Int Clin Psychopharmacol 1994; **9 Suppl** 1:35–40.
5. Burke WJ et al. Fixed-dose trial of the single isomer SSRI escitalopram in depressed outpatients. J Clin Psychiatry 2002; **63**:331–336.
6. Altamura AC et al. The evidence for 20mg a day of fluoxetine as the optimal dose in the treatment of depression. Br J Psychiatry 1988; **3 Suppl**: 109–112.
7. Walczak DD et al. The oral dose-effect relationship for fluvoxamine: a fixed-dose comparison against placebo in depressed outpatients. Ann Clin Psychiatry 1996; **8**:139–151.
8. Dunner DL et al. Optimal dose regimen for paroxetine. J Clin Psychiatry 1992; **53 Suppl**:21–26.

9. Moon CAL et al. A double-blind comparison of sertraline and clomipramine in the treatment of major depressive disorder and associative anxiety in general practice. J Psychopharmacol 1994; **8**:171–176.

10. Loo H et al. Determination of the dose of agomelatine, a melatoninergic agonist and selective 5-HT(2C) antagonist, in the treatment of major depressive disorder: a placebo-controlled dose range study. Int Clin Psychopharmacol 2002; **17**:239–247.

11. Goldstein DJ et al. Duloxetine in the treatment of depression: a double-blind placebo-controlled comparison with paroxetine. J Clin Psychopharmacol 2004; **24**:389–399.

12. Detke MJ et al. Duloxetine, 60 mg once daily, for major depressive disorder: a randomized double-blind placebo-controlled trial. J Clin Psychiatry 2002; **63**:308–315.

13. van Moffaert M et al. Mirtazapine is more effective than trazodone: a double-blind controlled study in hospitalized patients with major depression. Int Clin Psychopharmacol 1995; **10**:3–9.

14. Priest RG et al. Moclobemide in the treatment of depression. Rev Contemp Pharmacother 1994; **5**:35–43.

15. Schatzberg AF. Clinical efficacy of reboxetine in major depression. J Clin Psychiatry 2000; **61 Suppl** 10:31–38.

16. Brogden RN et al. Trazodone: a review of its pharmacological properties and therapeutic use in depression and anxiety. Drugs 1981; **21**:401–429.

17. Feighner JP et al. Efficacy of once-daily venlafaxine extended release (XR) for symptoms of anxiety in depressed outpatients. J Affect Disord 1998; **47**:55–62.

18. Mahableshwarkar AR et al. A randomized, double-blind, fixed-dose study comparing the efficacy and tolerability of vortioxetine 2.5 and 10 mg in acute treatment of adults with generalized anxiety disorder. Hum Psychopharmacol 2014; **29**:64–72.

19. Takeda Pharmaceuticals America Inc. Highlights of Prescribing Information. Brintellix (vortioxetine) tablets. http://www.us.brintellix.com/

Drug treatment of depression

The drug treatment of depression is summarised in Figure 4.1.

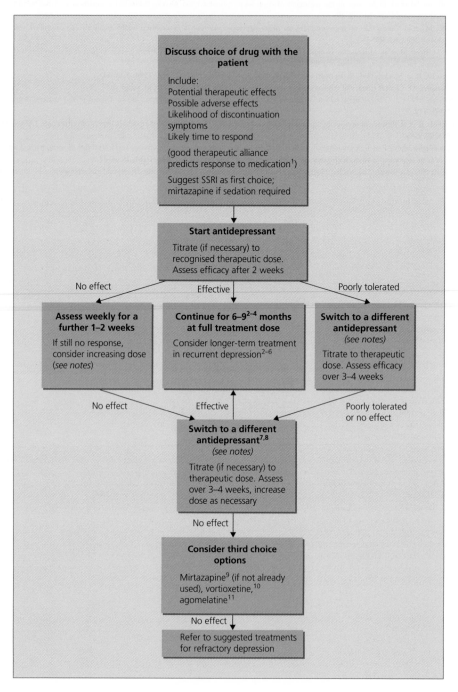

Figure 4.1 Drug treatment of depression. SSRI, selective serotonin reuptake inhibitor.

Notes to Figure 4.1

- Tools such as the Montgomery–Asberg Depression Rating Scale (MADRS)[12] and the Hamilton Depression Rating Scale (HAM-D)[13] are used in trials to assess drug effect. The HAM-D is now somewhat anachronistic and few clinicians are familiar with the MADRS (although it is probably the best scale to measure severity and change). The PHQ-9[14] is simple to use and is recommended for assessing symptom change in depression (although it better measures frequency rather than severity of symptoms).
- Switching between drug classes in cases of poor tolerability is not clearly supported by published studies but has a strong theoretical basis. Having said that, in practice, many patients who cannot tolerate one SSRI will readily tolerate another
- In cases of non-response, there is some evidence that switching within a drug class is effective,[8,15–18] but switching between classes is, in practice, the most common option and is supported by some analyses.[19] NICE and the American Psychological Association (APA) recommend both options.[2,9]
- There is minimal evidence to support increasing the dose of most SSRIs in depression.[20] Slightly better evidence suggests that increasing the dose of venlafaxine, escitalopram and tricyclics may be helpful.[3]
- Switch treatments early (e.g. after a week or two) if adverse effects intolerable or if no improvement *at all* is seen by 3–4 weeks. Opinions on when to switch vary somewhat but it is clear that antidepressants have a fairly prompt onset of action[21–23] and that non-response at 2–6 weeks is a good predictor of overall non-response.[24–26] The absence of any improvement at all at 3–4 weeks should normally provoke a change in treatment (British Association for Psychopharmacology [BAP] guidelines suggest 4 weeks[3]). If there is some improvement at this time, continue and assess for a further 2–3 weeks (see section on 'Antidepressants: general overview' in this chapter).

References

1. Leuchter AF et al. Role of pill-taking, expectation and therapeutic alliance in the placebo response in clinical trials for major depression. Br J Psychiatry 2014; 205:443–449.
2. American Psychiatric Association. *Practice Guideline for the Treatment of Patients with Major Depressive Disorder*, 3rd edn. Washington, DC: American Psychiatric Association.doi: 10.1176/appi.books.9780890423387.654001, 2010
3. Anderson IM et al. Evidence-based guidelines for treating depressive disorders with antidepressants: a revision of the 2000 British Association for Psychopharmacology guidelines. J Psychopharmacol 2008; 22:343–396.
4. Crismon ML et al. The Texas Medication Algorithm Project: report of the Texas Consensus Conference Panel on Medication Treatment of Major Depressive Disorder. J Clin Psychiatry 1999; 60:142–156.
5. Kocsis JH et al. Maintenance therapy for chronic depression. A controlled clinical trial of desipramine. Arch Gen Psychiatry 1996; 53:769–774.
6. Dekker J et al. The use of antidepressants after recovery from depression. Eur J Psychiatry 2000; 14:207–212.
7. Nelson JC. Treatment of antidepressant nonresponders: augmentation or switch? J Clin Psychiatry 1998; 59 Suppl 15:35–41.
8. Joffe RT. Substitution therapy in patients with major depression. CNS Drugs 1999; 11:175–180.
9. National Institute for Health and Clinical Excellence. Depression in adults: the treatment and management of depression in adults. Clinical Guideline 90, 2009. http://www.nice.org.uk/Guidance/cg90
10. Montgomery SA et al. A randomised, double-blind study in adults with major depressive disorder with an inadequate response to a single course of selective serotonin reuptake inhibitor or serotonin-noradrenaline reuptake inhibitor treatment switched to vortioxetine or agomelatine. Hum Psychopharmacol 2014; 29:470–482.
11. Sparshatt A et al. A naturalistic evaluation and audit database of agomelatine: clinical outcome at 12 weeks. Acta Psychiatr Scand 2013; 128:203–211.
12. Montgomery SA et al. A new depression scale designed to be sensitive to change. Br J Psychiatry 1979; 134:382–389.
13. Hamilton M. Development of a rating scale for primary depressive illness. Br J Soc Clin Psychol 1967; 6:278–296.
14. Kroenke K et al. The PHQ-9: validity of a brief depression severity measure. J Gen Intern Med 2001; 16:606–613.
15. Thase ME et al. Citalopram treatment of fluoxetine nonresponders. J Clin Psychiatry 2001; 62:683–687.
16. Rush AJ et al. Bupropion-SR, sertraline, or venlafaxine-XR after failure of SSRIs for depression. N Engl J Med 2006; 354:1231–1242.
17. Ruhe HG et al. Switching antidepressants after a first selective serotonin reuptake inhibitor in major depressive disorder: a systematic review. J Clin Psychiatry 2006; 67:1836–1855.
18. Brent D et al. Switching to another SSRI or to venlafaxine with or without cognitive behavioral therapy for adolescents with SSRI-resistant depression: the TORDIA Randomized Controlled Trial. JAMA 2008; 299:901–913.
19. Papakostas GI et al. Treatment of SSRI-resistant depression: a meta-analysis comparing within- versus across-class switches. Biol Psychiatry 2008; 63:699–704.
20. Adli M et al. Is dose escalation of antidepressants a rational strategy after a medium-dose treatment has failed? A systematic review. Eur Arch Psychiatry Clin Neurosci 2005; 255:387–400.
21. Papakostas GI et al. A meta-analysis of early sustained response rates between antidepressants and placebo for the treatment of major depressive disorder. J Clin Psychopharmacol 2006; 26:56–60.

22. Taylor MJ et al. Early onset of selective serotonin reuptake inhibitor antidepressant action: systematic review and meta-analysis. Arch Gen Psychiatry 2006; **63**:1217–1223.

23. Posternak MA et al. Is there a delay in the antidepressant effect? A meta-analysis. J Clin Psychiatry 2005; **66**:148–158.

24. Szegedi A et al. Early improvement in the first 2 weeks as a predictor of treatment outcome in patients with major depressive disorder: a meta-analysis including 6562 patients. J Clin Psychiatry 2009; **70**:344–353.

25. Baldwin DS et al. How long should a trial of escitalopram treatment be in patients with major depressive disorder, generalised anxiety disorder or social anxiety disorder? An exploration of the randomised controlled trial database. Hum Psychopharmacol 2009; **24**:269–275.

26. Nierenberg AA et al. Early nonresponse to fluoxetine as a predictor of poor 8-week outcome. Am J Psychiatry 1995; **152**:1500–1503.

Further reading

Barbui C et al. Amitriptyline v. the rest: still the leading antidepressant after 40 years of randomised controlled trials. Br J Psychiatry 2001;**178**:129–144.

Preskorn SH. The use of biomarkers in psychiatric research: how serotonin transporter occupancy explains the dose-response curves of SSRIs. J Psychiatr Pract 2012; **18**:38–45.

Rubinow DR. Treatment strategies after SSRI failure – good news and bad news. N Engl J Med 2006;**354**:1305–1307.

Smith D et al. Efficacy and tolerability of venlafaxine compared with selective serotonin reuptake inhibitors and other antidepressants: a meta-analysis. Br J Psychiatry 2002;**180**:396–404.

CHAPTER 4

Treatment of refractory depression

Refractory depression is difficult to treat successfully and outcomes are poor,[1-3] especially if evidence-based protocols are not followed.[4] Refractory depression is not a uniform entity but a complex spectrum of severity which can be graded[5] and in which outcome is closely linked to grading.[6] A significant minority of apparently resistant unipolar depression may in fact be bipolar-type depression[7,8] which is often unresponsive to antidepressants[9,10] (see section on 'Bipolar depression' in Chapter 3).

Treatment of refractory depression is to some extent informed by results of the STAR*D programme (Sequenced Treatment Alternatives to Relieve Depression). This was a pragmatic effectiveness study which used remission of symptoms as its main outcome. At stage 1,[11] 2786 subjects received citalopram (mean dose 41.8 mg/day) for 14 weeks; remission was seen in 28% (response [50% reduction in symptoms score] 47%). Subjects who failed to remit were entered into the continued study of sequential treatments.[12-16] Remission rates are given in Figure 4.2. Very few statistically significant

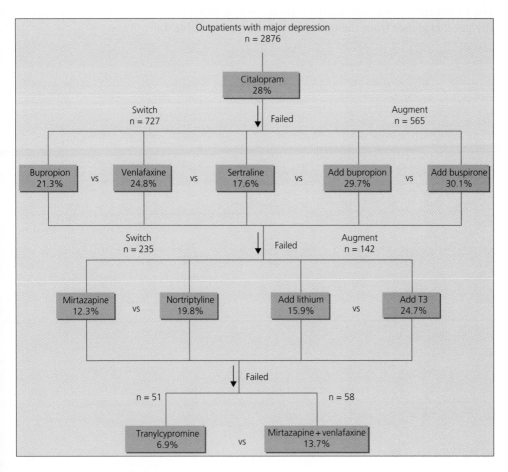

Figure 4.2 Remission rates in STAR*D.

differences were noted from this point on. At stage 3,[15] T_3 was found to be significantly better tolerated than lithium. At stage 4,[16] tranylcypromine was less effective and less well tolerated than the mirtazapine/venlafaxine combination. Overall, remission rates, as can be seen, were worryingly low for individual treatments, although it should be noted that the trial consisted of subjects with long histories of recurrent depression, and the majority ultimately responded.

STAR*D demonstrated that the treatment of refractory depression requires a flexible approach and that response to a particular treatment option is not readily predicted by pharmacology or previous treatments. The programme established bupropion and buspirone augmentation as worthwhile options and resurrected from some obscurity the use of T_3 augmentation and of nortriptyline. It also, to some extent, confirmed the safety and (to a lesser extent) efficacy of the combination of mirtazapine and venlafaxine.

Treatment of refractory depression: first choice

The treatments commonly used in the treatment of refractory depression, with generally good evidence from the literature, are shown in Table 4.6.

Table 4.6 First choice: commonly used treatments generally well supported by published literature (no preference implied by order)

Treatment	Advantages	Disadvantages	Refs
Add **lithium**. Aim for plasma level of 0.4–0.8 mmol/L initially, increasing to up to 1.0 mmol/L if sub-optimal response	■ Well established ■ Well supported in the literature ■ Recommended by NICE[17]	■ Sometimes poorly tolerated at higher plasma levels ■ Potentially toxic (NICE recommends ECG) ■ Usually needs specialist referral ■ Plasma level monitoring is essential (and TFTs; eGFR) ■ May not be effective in patients refractory to multiple treatments	15,18–21
Electroconvulsive therapy	■ Well established ■ Effective ■ Well supported in the literature	■ Poor reputation in public domain ■ Necessitates general anaesthetic ■ Needs specialist referral ■ Usually reserved for last-line treatment or if rapid response needed ■ Best used with other treatments to prevent relapse	22–24
Add **tri-iodothyronine** (20–50 µg/day) Higher doses have been safely used	■ Usually well tolerated ■ Good literature support (including STAR*D)	■ TFT monitoring required ■ Usually needs specialist referral ■ Some negative studies ■ No advantage over antidepressant alone in non-refractory illness[25]	15,26–30
*Combine **olanzapine** and **fluoxetine** (12.5 mg + 50 mg daily)	■ Well researched ■ Usually well tolerated ■ Olanzapine + TCA may also be effective	■ Risk of weight gain ■ Limited clinical experience in UK ■ Most data relate to bipolar depression	31–35
*Add **quetiapine** (150 mg or 300 mg a day) to SSRI/SNRI	■ Good evidence base ■ Usually well tolerated ■ Plausible explanation for antidepressant effect ■ Possibly more effective than lithium	■ Dry mouth, sedation, constipation can be problematic ■ Weight gain risk in the longer term	36–41
Add **risperidone** (0.5–3 mg/day) to antidepressant	■ Small evidence base ■ Usually well tolerated	■ Hypotension ■ Hyperprolactinaemia	42–47
Add **aripiprazole** (2–20 mg/day) to antidepressant	■ Good evidence base ■ Usually well tolerated and safe ■ Low doses (2–10 mg/day) may be effective	■ Akathisia and restlessness common at standard doses (≥10 mg/day)	48–55
SSRI + bupropion up to 400 mg/day	■ Supported by STAR*D ■ Well tolerated	■ Not licensed for depression in the UK	13,56–60
SSRI or venlafaxine + mianserin (30 mg/day) or **mirtazapine** (30–45 mg/day)	■ Recommended by NICE ■ Usually well tolerated ■ Excellent literature support ■ Widely used	■ Theoretical risk of serotonin syndrome (inform patient) ■ Risk of blood dyscrasia with mianserin ■ Weight gain with mirtazapine	16,61–63

Always consider non-drug approaches (e.g. cognitive behavioural therapy).

*Strategies recommended by NICE for the treatment of bipolar depression (see section on 'Bipolar depression' in Chapter 3).

ECG, electrocardiogram; eGFR, estimated glomerular filtration rate; NICE, National Institute for Health and Care Excellence; SNRI, selective noradrenaline reuptake inhibitor; SSRI, selective serotonin reuptake inhibitor; STAR*D, Sequenced Treatment Alternatives to Relieve Depression; TCA, tricyclic antidepressant; TFT, thyroid function test.

References

1. Dunner DL et al. Prospective, long-term, multicenter study of the naturalistic outcomes of patients with treatment-resistant depression. J Clin Psychiatry 2006; 67:688–695.

2. Wooderson SC et al. Prospective evaluation of specialist inpatient treatment for refractory affective disorders. J Affect Disord 2011; 131:92–103.

3. Fekadu A et al. What happens to patients with treatment-resistant depression? A systematic review of medium to long term outcome studies. J Affect Disord 2009; 116:4–11.

4. Trivedi MH et al. Clinical results for patients with major depressive disorder in the Texas Medication Algorithm Project. Arch Gen Psychiatry 2004; 61:669–680.

5. Fekadu A et al. A multidimensional tool to quantify treatment resistance in depression: the Maudsley staging method. J Clin Psychiatry 2009; 70:177–184.

6. Fekadu A et al. The Maudsley Staging Method for treatment-resistant depression: prediction of longer-term outcome and persistence of symptoms. J Clin Psychiatry 2009; 70:952–957.

7. Angst J et al. Toward a re-definition of subthreshold bipolarity: epidemiology and proposed criteria for bipolar-II, minor bipolar disorders and hypomania. J Affect Disord 2003; 73:133–146.

8. Smith DJ et al. Unrecognised bipolar disorder in primary care patients with depression. Br J Psychiatry 2011; 199:49–56.

9. Sidor MM et al. Antidepressants for the acute treatment of bipolar depression: a systematic review and meta-analysis. J Clin Psychiatry 2011; 72:156–167.

10. Taylor DM et al. Comparative efficacy and acceptability of drug treatments for bipolar depression: a multiple-treatments meta-analysis. Acta Psychiatr Scand 2014; 130:452–469.

11. Trivedi MH et al. Evaluation of outcomes with citalopram for depression using measurement-based care in STAR*D: implications for clinical practice. Am J Psychiatry 2006; 163:28–40.

12. Rush AJ et al. Bupropion-SR, sertraline, or venlafaxine-XR after failure of SSRIs for depression. N Engl J Med 2006; 354:1231–1242.

13. Trivedi MH et al. Medication augmentation after the failure of SSRIs for depression. N Engl J Med 2006; 354:1243–1252.

14. Fava M et al. A comparison of mirtazapine and nortriptyline following two consecutive failed medication treatments for depressed outpatients: a STAR*D report. Am J Psychiatry 2006; 163:1161–1172.

15. Nierenberg AA et al. A comparison of lithium and T(3) augmentation following two failed medication treatments for depression: a STAR*D report. Am J Psychiatry 2006; 163:1519–1530.

16. McGrath PJ et al. Tranylcypromine versus venlafaxine plus mirtazapine following three failed antidepressant medication trials for depression: a STAR*D report. Am J Psychiatry 2006; 163:1531–1541.

17. National Institute for Health and Clinical Excellence. Depression: the treatment and management of depression in adults (update). Clinical Guideline 90, 2009. http://www.nice.org.uk/

18. Fava M et al. Lithium and tricyclic augmentation of fluoxetine treatment for resistant major depression: a double-blind, controlled study. Am J Psychiatry 1994; 151:1372–1374.

19. Bauer M et al. Lithium augmentation in treatment-resistant depression: meta-analysis of placebo-controlled studies. J Clin Psychopharmacol 1999; 19:427–434.

20. Crossley NA et al. Acceleration and augmentation of antidepressants with lithium for depressive disorders: two meta-analyses of randomized, placebo-controlled trials. J Clin Psychiatry 2007; 68:935–940.

21. Nierenberg AA et al. Lithium augmentation of nortriptyline for subjects resistant to multiple antidepressants. J Clin Psychopharmacol 2003; 23:92–95.

22. Folkerts HW et al. Electroconvulsive therapy vs. paroxetine in treatment-resistant depression – a randomized study. Acta Psychiatr Scand 1997; 96:334–342.

23. Gonzalez-Pinto A et al. Efficacy and safety of venlafaxine-ECT combination in treatment-resistant depression. J Neuropsychiatry Clin Neurosci 2002; 14:206–209.

24. Eranti S et al. A randomized, controlled trial with 6-month follow-up of repetitive transcranial magnetic stimulation and electroconvulsive therapy for severe depression. Am J Psychiatry 2007; 164:73–81.

25. Garlow SJ et al. The combination of triiodothyronine (T3) and sertraline is not superior to sertraline monotherapy in the treatment of major depressive disorder. J Psychiatr Res 2012; 46:1406–1413.

26. Joffe RT et al. A comparison of triiodothyronine and thyroxine in the potentiation of tricyclic antidepressants. Psychiatry Res 1990; 32:241–251.

27. Anderson IM. Drug treatment of depression: reflections on the evidence. Adv Psychiatr Treat 2003; 9:11–20.

28. Iosifescu DV et al. An open study of triiodothyronine augmentation of selective serotonin reuptake inhibitors in treatment-resistant major depressive disorder. J Clin Psychiatry 2005; 66:1038–1042.

29. Abraham G et al. T3 augmentation of SSRI resistant depression. J Affect Disord 2006; 91:211–215.

30. Kelly TF et al. Long term augmentation with T3 in refractory major depression. J Affect Disord 2009; 115:230–233.

31. Shelton RC et al. Olanzapine/fluoxetine combination for treatment-resistant depression: a controlled study of SSRI and nortriptyline resistance. J Clin Psychiatry 2005; 66:1289–1297.

32. Corya SA et al. A randomized, double-blind comparison of olanzapine/fluoxetine combination, olanzapine, fluoxetine, and venlafaxine in treatment-resistant depression. Depress Anxiety 2006; 23:364–372.

33. Takahashi H et al. Augmentation with olanzapine in TCA-refractory depression with melancholic features: a consecutive case series. Hum Psychopharmacol 2008; 23:217–220.

34. Thase ME et al. A randomized, double-blind comparison of olanzapine/fluoxetine combination, olanzapine, and fluoxetine in treatment-resistant major depressive disorder. J Clin Psychiatry 2007; 68:224–236.

35. Trivedi MH et al. An integrated analysis of olanzapine/fluoxetine combination in clinical trials of treatment-resistant depression. J Clin Psychiatry 2009; 70:387–396.

36. Jensen NH et al. N-desalkylquetiapine, a potent norepinephrine reuptake inhibitor and partial 5-HT1A agonist, as a putative mediator of quetiapine's antidepressant activity. Neuropsychopharmacology 2008; 33:2303–2312.

37. El-Khalili N et al. Extended-release quetiapine fumarate (quetiapine XR) as adjunctive therapy in major depressive disorder (MDD) in patients with an inadequate response to ongoing antidepressant treatment: a multicentre, randomized, double-blind, placebo-controlled study. Int J Neuropsychopharmacol 2010; 13:917–932.

38. Bauer M et al. Extended-release quetiapine as adjunct to an antidepressant in patients with major depressive disorder: results of a randomized, placebo-controlled, double-blind study. J Clin Psychiatry 2009; 70:540–549.

39. Bauer M et al. A pooled analysis of two randomised, placebo-controlled studies of extended release quetiapine fumarate adjunctive to antidepressant therapy in patients with major depressive disorder. J Affect Disord 2010; 127:19–30.

40. Montgomery S et al. P01-75 – Quetiapine XR or lithium combination with antidepressants in treatment resistant depression. Eur Psychiatry 2010; 25:296–296.

41. Doree JP et al. Quetiapine augmentation of treatment-resistant depression: a comparison with lithium. Curr Med Res Opin 2007; 23:333–341.

42. Yoshimura R et al. Addition of risperidone to sertraline improves sertraline-resistant refractory depression without influencing plasma concentrations of sertraline and desmethylsertraline. Hum Psychopharmacol 2008; 23:707–713.

43. Mahmoud RA et al. Risperidone for treatment-refractory major depressive disorder: a randomized trial. Ann Intern Med 2007; 147:593–602.

44. Ostroff RB et al. Risperidone augmentation of selective serotonin reuptake inhibitors in major depression. J Clin Psychiatry 1999; 60:256–259.

45. Rapaport MH et al. Effects of risperidone augmentation in patients with treatment-resistant depression: results of open-label treatment followed by double-blind continuation. Neuropsychopharmacology 2006; 31:2505–2513.

46. Stoll AL et al. Tranylcypromine plus risperidone for treatment-refractory major depression. J Clin Psychopharmacol 2000; 20:495–496.

47. Keitner GI et al. A randomized, placebo-controlled trial of risperidone augmentation for patients with difficult-to-treat unipolar, non-psychotic major depression. J Psychiatr Res 2009; 43:205–214.

48. Marcus RN et al. The efficacy and safety of aripiprazole as adjunctive therapy in major depressive disorder: a second multicenter, randomized, double-blind, placebo-controlled study. J Clin Psychopharmacol 2008; 28:156–165.

49. Hellerstein DJ et al. Aripiprazole as an adjunctive treatment for refractory unipolar depression. Prog Neuropsychopharmacol Biol Psychiatry 2008; 32:744–750.

50. Simon JS et al. Aripiprazole augmentation of antidepressants for the treatment of partially responding and nonresponding patients with major depressive disorder. J Clin Psychiatry 2005; 66:1216–1220.

51. Papakostas GI et al. Aripiprazole augmentation of selective serotonin reuptake inhibitors for treatment-resistant major depressive disorder. J Clin Psychiatry 2005; 66:1326–1330.

52. Berman RM et al. Aripiprazole augmentation in major depressive disorder: a double-blind, placebo-controlled study in patients with inadequate response to antidepressants. CNS Spectr 2009; 14:197–206.

53. Fava M et al. A double-blind, placebo-controlled study of aripiprazole adjunctive to antidepressant therapy among depressed outpatients with inadequate response to prior antidepressant therapy (ADAPT-A Study). Psychother Psychosom 2012; 81:87–97.

54. Jon DI et al. Augmentation of aripiprazole for depressed patients with an inadequate response to antidepressant treatment: a 6-week prospective, open-label, multicenter study. Clin Neuropharmacol 2013; 36:157–161.

55. Yoshimura R et al. Comparison of the efficacy between paroxetine and sertraline augmented with aripiprazole in patients with refractory major depressive disorder. Prog Neuropsychopharmacol Biol Psychiatry 2012; 39:355–357.

56. Zisook S et al. Use of bupropion in combination with serotonin reuptake inhibitors. Biol Psychiatry 2006; 59:203–210.

57. Fatemi SH et al. Venlafaxine and bupropion combination therapy in a case of treatment-resistant depression. Ann Pharmacother 1999; 33:701–703.

58. Pierre JM et al. Bupropion-tranylcypromine combination for treatment-refractory depression. J Clin Psychiatry 2000; 61:450–451.

59. Lam RW et al. Citalopram and bupropion-SR: combining versus switching in patients with treatment-resistant depression. J Clin Psychiatry 2004; 65:337–340.

60. Papakostas GI et al. The combination of duloxetine and bupropion for treatment-resistant major depressive disorder. Depress Anxiety 2006; 23:178–181.

61. Carpenter LL et al. A double-blind, placebo-controlled study of antidepressant augmentation with mirtazapine. Biol Psychiatry 2002; 51:183–188.

62. Carpenter LL et al. Mirtazapine augmentation in the treatment of refractory depression. J Clin Psychiatry 1999; 60:45–49.

63. Ferreri M et al. Benefits from mianserin augmentation of fluoxetine in patients with major depression non-responders to fluoxetine alone. Acta Psychiatr Scand 2001; 103:66–72.

Treatment of refractory depression: second choice

Treatments that may be used in the treatment of refractory depression, although less commonly and with less support from published evaluations, are shown in Table 4.7.

Table 4.7 Second choice: less commonly used, variably supported by published evaluations (no preference implied by order)

Treatment	Advantages	Disadvantages	Refs
Add **ketamine** (0.5 mg/kg IV over 40 minutes)	▪ Very rapid response (within hours) ▪ Very high remission rate ▪ Some evidence of maintained response if repeated doses given ▪ Usually well tolerated at this sub-anaesthetic dose	▪ Needs to be administered in hospital ▪ Cognitive effects (confusion, dissociation, etc.) do occasionally occur ▪ Associated with transient increased in BP, tachycardia and arrhythmias. Pre-treatment ECG required[1] ▪ Repeated infusions necessary to maintain effect (beware bladder problems) ▪ Not widely available	2–6
*Add **lamotrigine** (200 mg and 400 mg a day have been used)	▪ Reasonably well researched ▪ Quite widely used	▪ Slow titration ▪ Risk of rash ▪ Appropriate dosing unclear. High doses often needed ▪ Two failed RCTs	7–11
SSRI + buspirone up to 60 mg/day	▪ Supported by STAR*D	▪ Higher doses required poorly tolerated (dizziness common) ▪ Not widely used	12,13
Venlafaxine (>200 mg/day)	▪ Usually well tolerated ▪ Can be initiated in primary care ▪ Recommended by NICE[14] ▪ Supported by STAR-D	▪ Limited support in literature ▪ Nausea and vomiting more common ▪ Discontinuation reactions common ▪ Can increase BP: monitoring essential	15–18

*Recommended by NICE for the treatment of bipolar depression (see section on 'Bipolar depression' in Chapter 3).
BP, blood pressure; ECG, electrocardiogram; NICE, National Institute for Health and Care Excellence; STAR*D, Sequenced Treatment Alternatives to Relieve Depression.

References

1. aan het Rot M et al. Safety and efficacy of repeated-dose intravenous ketamine for treatment-resistant depression. Biol Psychiatry 2010; 67:139–145.
2. Ibrahim L et al. Course of improvement in depressive symptoms to a single intravenous infusion of ketamine vs add-on riluzole: results from a 4-week, double-blind, placebo-controlled study. Neuropsychopharmacology 2012; 37:1526–1533.
3. Murrough JW et al. Rapid and longer-term antidepressant effects of repeated ketamine infusions in treatment-resistant major depression. Biol Psychiatry 2013; 74:250–256.
4. Murrough JW et al. Antidepressant efficacy of ketamine in treatment-resistant major depression: a two-site randomized controlled trial. Am J Psychiatry 2013; 170:1134–1142.
5. Segmiller F et al. Repeated S-ketamine infusions in therapy resistant depression: a case series. J Clin Pharmacol 2013; 53:996–998.
6. Diamond PR et al. Ketamine infusions for treatment resistant depression: a series of 28 patients treated weekly or twice weekly in an ECT clinic. J Psychopharmacol 2014; 28:536–544.
7. Normann C et al. Lamotrigine as adjunct to paroxetine in acute depression: a placebo-controlled, double-blind study. J Clin Psychiatry 2002; 63:337–344.
8. Barbosa L et al. A double-blind, randomized, placebo-controlled trial of augmentation with lamotrigine or placebo in patients concomitantly treated with fluoxetine for resistant major depressive episodes. J Clin Psychiatry 2003; 64:403–407.
9. Santos MA et al. Efficacy and safety of antidepressant augmentation with lamotrigine in patients with treatment-resistant depression: a randomized, placebo-controlled, double-blind study. Prim Care Companion J Clin Psychiatry 2008; 10:187–190.
10. Barbee JG et al. Lamotrigine as an augmentation agent in treatment-resistant depression. J Clin Psychiatry 2002; 63:737–741.
11. Barbee JG et al. A double-blind placebo-controlled trial of lamotrigine as an antidepressant augmentation agent in treatment-refractory unipolar depression. J Clin Psychiatry 2011; 72:1405–1412.
12. Trivedi MH et al. Medication augmentation after the failure of SSRIs for depression. N Engl J Med 2006; 354:1243–1252.
13. Appelberg BG et al. Patients with severe depression may benefit from buspirone augmentation of selective serotonin reuptake inhibitors: results from a placebo-controlled, randomized, double-blind, placebo wash-in study. J Clin Psychiatry 2001; 62:448–452.
14. National Institute for Health and Clinical Excellence. Depression: the treatment and management of depression in adults (update). Clinical Guideline 90, 2009. http://www.nice.org.uk/
15. Poirier MF et al. Venlafaxine and paroxetine in treatment-resistant depression. Double-blind, randomised comparison. Br J Psychiatry 1999; 175:12–16.
16. Nierenberg AA et al. Venlafaxine for treatment-resistant unipolar depression. J Clin Psychopharmacol 1994; 14:419–423.
17. Smith D et al. Efficacy and tolerability of venlafaxine compared with selective serotonin reuptake inhibitors and other antidepressants: a meta-analysis. Br J Psychiatry 2002; 180:396–404.
18. Rush AJ et al. Bupropion-SR, sertraline, or venlafaxine-XR after failure of SSRIs for depression. N Engl J Med 2006; 354:1231–1242.

Treatment of refractory depression: other reported treatments

Other pharmacological treatments have been reported in the literature, but the evidence is sparse (Table 4.8). Prescribers *must* familiarise themselves with the primary literature before using these strategies.

Table 4.8 Other reported treatments (no preference implied by order)

Treatment	Comments	Refs
Add amantadine (up to 300 mg/day)	Limited data	1
Add carbergoline 2 mg/day	Very limited data	2
Add D-cycloserine (1000 mg/day)	One small RCT showing useful effect	3
Add mecamylamine (up to 10 mg/day)	One pilot study of 21 patients	4,5
Add pindolol (5 mg tds or 7.5 mg once daily)	Well tolerated, can be initiated in primary care, reasonably well researched, but data mainly relate to acceleration of response. Refractory data contradictory	6–10
Add tianeptine (25–50 mg/day)	Tiny database. Tianeptine not available in many countries	11,12
Add tryptophan 2–3 g tds	Long history of successful use	13–16
Add zinc (25 mg Zn+/day)	One RCT (n = 60) showed good results in refractory illness	17
Add ziprasidone up to 160 mg/day	Poorly supported. Probably has no antidepressant effects	18–20
Combine MAOI and TCA, e.g. trimipramine and phenelzine	Formerly widely used, but great care needed	21–23
Dexamethasone 3–4 mg/day	Use for 4 days only. Limited data	24,25
Hyoscine (scopolomine 4 µg/kg IV)	Growing evidence base of prompt and sizeable effect	26
Ketoconazole 400–800 mg/day	Rarely used. Risk of hepatotoxicity	27
Modafinil 100–400 mg/day	Data mainly relate to non-refractory illness. Usually added to antidepressant treatment. May worsen anxiety (see section on stimulants in depression this chapter)	28–31
Nemifitide (40–240 mg/day SC)	One pilot study in 25 patients	32
Nortriptyline ± lithium	Re-emergent treatment option	33–36
Oestrogens (various regimens)	Limited data	37

Table 4.8 (*Continued*)

Treatment	Comments	Refs
Omega-3-triglycerides EPA 1–2 g/day	Usually added to antidepressant treatment	38,39
Pramipexole 0.125–5 mg/day	One good RCT showing clear effect	40,41
Riluzole 100–200 mg/day	Very limited data. Costly	42
S-adenosyl-L-methionine 400 mg/day IM; 1600 mg/day oral	Limited data in refractory depression	43,44
SSRI + TCA	Formerly widely used	45
Stimulants: amfetamine; methylphenidate	Varied outcomes	See section on 'Psychostimulants in depression' in this chapter
TCA – high dose	Formerly widely used. Cardiac monitoring essential	46
Testosterone gel	Effective in those with low testosterone levels	47
Venlafaxine – very high dose (up to 600 mg/day)	Cardiac monitoring essential	48
Venlafaxine + IV clomipramine	Cardiac monitoring essential	49

Note: Other non-drug treatments are available. Discussion of these is beyond the scope of this book.
EPA, eicosapentanoic acid; IM, intramuscular; IV, intravenous; MAOI, monoamine oxidase inhibitor; RCT, randomised controlled trial; SC, sub-cutaneous; SSRI, selective serotonin reuptake inhibitor; TCA, tricyclic antidepressant; tds, three times a day.

References

1. Stryjer R et al. Amantadine as augmentation therapy in the management of treatment-resistant depression. Int Clin Psychopharmacol 2003; **18**:93–96.
2. Takahashi H et al. Addition of a dopamine agonist, cabergoline, to a serotonin-noradrenalin reuptake inhibitor, milnacipran as a therapeutic option in the treatment of refractory depression: two case reports. Clin Neuropharmacol 2003; **26**:230–232.
3. Heresco-Levy U et al. A randomized add-on trial of high-dose D-cycloserine for treatment-resistant depression. Int J Neuropsychopharmacol 2013; **16**:501–506.
4. George TP et al. Nicotinic antagonist augmentation of selective serotonin reuptake inhibitor-refractory major depressive disorder: a preliminary study. J Clin Psychopharmacol 2008; **28**:340–344.
5. Bacher I et al. Mecamylamine – a nicotinic acetylcholine receptor antagonist with potential for the treatment of neuropsychiatric disorders. Expert Opin Pharmacother 2009; **10**:2709–2721.
6. McAskill R et al. Pindolol augmentation of antidepressant therapy. Br J Psychiatry 1998; **173**:203–208.
7. Rasanen P et al. Mitchell B. Balter Award – 1998. Pindolol and major affective disorders: a three-year follow-up study of 30,485 patients. J Clin Psychopharmacol 1999; **19**:297–302.
8. Perry EB et al. Pindolol augmentation in depressed patients resistant to selective serotonin reuptake inhibitors: a double-blind, randomized, controlled trial. J Clin Psychiatry 2004; **65**:238–243.
9. Sokolski KN et al. Once-daily high-dose pindolol for SSRI-refractory depression. Psychiatry Res 2004; **125**:81–86.
10. Whale R et al. Pindolol augmentation of serotonin reuptake inhibitors for the treatment of depressive disorder: a systematic review. J Psychopharmacol 2010; **24**:513–520.
11. Tobe EH et al. Possible usefulness of tianeptine in treatment-resistant depression. Int J Psychiatry Clin Pract 2013; **17**:313–316.
12. Woo YS et al. Tianeptine combination for partial or non-response to selective serotonin re-uptake inhibitor monotherapy. Psychiatry Clin Neurosci 2013; **67**:219–227.

CHAPTER 4

13. Angst J et al. The treatment of depression with L-5-hydroxytryptophan versus imipramine. Results of two open and one double-blind study. Arch Psychiatr Nervenkr 1977; **224**:175–186.
14. Alino JJ et al. 5-Hydroxytryptophan (5-HTP) and a MAOI (nialamide) in the treatment of depressions. A double-blind controlled study. Int Pharmacopsychiatry 1976; **11**:8–15.
15. Hale AS et al. Clomipramine, tryptophan and lithium in combination for resistant endogenous depression: seven case studies. Br J Psychiatry 1987; **151**:213–217.
16. Young SN. Use of tryptophan in combination with other antidepressant treatments: a review. J Psychiatry Neurosci 1991; **16**:241–246.
17. Siwek M et al. Zinc supplementation augments efficacy of imipramine in treatment resistant patients: a double blind, placebo-controlled study. J Affect Disord 2009; **118**:187–195.
18. Papakostas GI et al. Ziprasidone augmentation of selective serotonin reuptake inhibitors (SSRIs) for SSRI-resistant major depressive disorder. J Clin Psychiatry 2004; **65**:217–221.
19. Dunner DL et al. Efficacy and tolerability of adjunctive ziprasidone in treatment-resistant depression: a randomized, open-label, pilot study. J Clin Psychiatry 2007; **68**:1071–1077.
20. Papakostas GI et al. A 12-week, randomized, double-blind, placebo-controlled, sequential parallel comparison trial of ziprasidone as monotherapy for major depressive disorder. J Clin Psychiatry 2012; **73**:1541–1547.
21. White K et al. The combined use of MAOIs and tricyclics. J Clin Psychiatry 1984; **45**:67–69.
22. Kennedy N et al. Treatment and response in refractory depression: results from a specialist affective disorders service. J Affect Disord 2004; **81**:49–53.
23. Connolly KR et al. If at first you don't succeed: a review of the evidence for antidepressant augmentation, combination and switching strategies. Drugs 2011; **71**:43–64.
24. Dinan TG et al. Dexamethasone augmentation in treatment-resistant depression. Acta Psychiatr Scand 1997; **95**:58–61.
25. Bodani M et al. The use of dexamethasone in elderly patients with antidepressant-resistant depressive illness. J Psychopharmacol 1999; **13**:196–197.
26. Drevets WC et al. Antidepressant effects of the muscarinic cholinergic receptor antagonist scopolamine: a review. Biol Psychiatry 2013; **73**:1156–1163.
27. Wolkowitz OM et al. Antiglucocorticoid treatment of depression: double-blind ketoconazole. Biol Psychiatry 1999; **45**:1070–1074.
28. DeBattista C et al. A prospective trial of modafinil as an adjunctive treatment of major depression. J Clin Psychopharmacol 2004; **24**:87–90.
29. Ninan PT et al. Adjunctive modafinil at initiation of treatment with a selective serotonin reuptake inhibitor enhances the degree and onset of therapeutic effects in patients with major depressive disorder and fatigue. J Clin Psychiatry 2004; **65**:414–420.
30. Menza MA et al. Modafinil augmentation of antidepressant treatment in depression. J Clin Psychiatry 2000; **61**:378–381.
31. Taneja I et al. A randomized, double-blind, crossover trial of modafinil on mood. J Clin Psychopharmacol 2007; **27**:76–78.
32. Feighner JP et al. Clinical effect of nemifitide, a novel pentapeptide antidepressant, in the treatment of severely depressed refractory patients. Int Clin Psychopharmacol 2008; **23**:29–35.
33. Nierenberg AA et al. Nortriptyline for treatment-resistant depression. J Clin Psychiatry 2003; **64**:35–39.
34. Nierenberg AA et al. Lithium augmentation of nortriptyline for subjects resistant to multiple antidepressants. J Clin Psychopharmacol 2003; **23**:92–95.
35. Fava M et al. A comparison of mirtazapine and nortriptyline following two consecutive failed medication treatments for depressed outpatients: a STAR*D report. Am J Psychiatry 2006; **163**:1161–1172.
36. Shelton RC et al. Olanzapine/fluoxetine combination for treatment-resistant depression: a controlled study of SSRI and nortriptyline resistance. J Clin Psychiatry 2005; **66**:1289–1297.
37. Stahl SM. Basic psychopharmacology of antidepressants, part 2: Oestrogen as an adjunct to antidepressant treatment. J Clin Psychiatry 1998; **59** Suppl 4:15–24.
38. Nemets B et al. Addition of omega-3 fatty acid to maintenance medication treatment for recurrent unipolar depressive disorder. Am J Psychiatry 2002; **159**:477–479.
39. Appleton KM et al. Updated systematic review and meta-analysis of the effects of n-3 long-chain polyunsaturated fatty acids on depressed mood. Am J Clin Nutr 2010; **91**:757–770.
40. Whiskey E et al. Pramipexole in unipolar and bipolar depression. Psychiatr Bull 2004; **28**:438–440.
41. Cusin C et al. A randomized, double-blind, placebo-controlled trial of pramipexole augmentation in treatment-resistant major depressive disorder. J Clin Psychiatry 2013; **74**:e636–641.
42. Zarate CA Jr et al. An open-label trial of riluzole in patients with treatment-resistant major depression. Am J Psychiatry 2004; **161**:171–174.
43. Pancheri P et al. A double-blind, randomized parallel-group, efficacy and safety study of intramuscular S-adenosyl-L-methionine 1,4-butanedisulphonate (SAMe) versus imipramine in patients with major depressive disorder. Int J Neuropsychopharmacol 2002; **5**:287–294.
44. Alpert JE et al. S-adenosyl-L-methionine (SAMe) as an adjunct for resistant major depressive disorder: an open trial following partial or nonresponse to selective serotonin reuptake inhibitors or venlafaxine. J Clin Psychopharmacol 2004; **24**:661–664.
45. Taylor D. Selective serotonin reuptake inhibitors and tricyclic antidepressants in combination – interactions and therapeutic uses. Br J Psychiatry 1995; **167**:575–580.
46. Malhi GS et al. Management of resistant depression. Int J Psychiatry Clin Pract 1997; **1**:269–276.
47. Pope HG Jr et al. Testosterone gel supplementation for men with refractory depression: a randomized, placebo-controlled trial. Am J Psychiatry 2003; **160**:105–111.
48. Harrison CL et al. Tolerability of high-dose venlafaxine in depressed patients. J Psychopharmacol 2004; **18**:200–204.
49. Fountoulakis KN et al. Combined oral venlafaxine and intravenous clomipramine-A: successful temporary response in a patient with extremely refractory depression. Can J Psychiatry 2004; **49**:73–74.

Treatment of refractory depression: sequence of treatments – summary

Figure 4.3 outlines the sequence of treatment options for refractory depression.

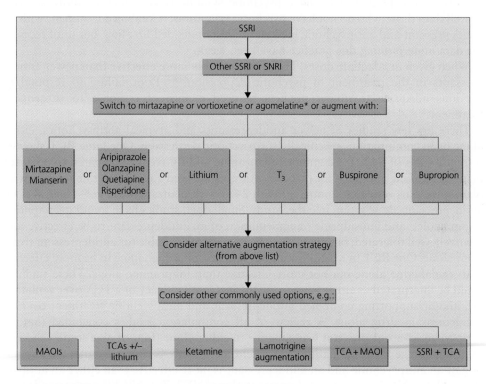

Figure 4.3 Treatment sequence options for refractory depression.
*Some may consider the closely supervised use of older antidepressants – TCAs (e.g. amitriptyline or nortriptyline) or MAOIs (e.g. phenelzine) at this point. MAOI, monoamine oxidase inhibitor; SNRI, selective noradrenaline reuptake inhibitor; SSRI, selective serotonin reuptake inhibitor; TCA, tricyclic antidepressant.

CHAPTER 4

Psychotic depression

Although psychotic symptoms can occur across the whole spectrum of depression severity,[1] those patients who have psychotic symptoms are generally more severely unwell than those who do not have psychotic symptoms.[2] Combined treatment with an antidepressant and antipsychotic is often the recommended first line[3] but until recently the data underpinning this practice have been weak.[4,5]

When given in adequate doses, TCAs are probably more effective than newer antidepressants in the treatment of psychotic depression.[4,6,7] Prior failure to respond to previous adequate treatment predicts reduced chance of response to subsequent treatment.[8]

There are few studies of newer antidepressants and atypical antipsychotics, either alone or in combination, specifically for psychotic depression. One large RCT showed response rates of 64% for combined olanzapine and fluoxetine compared to 35% for olanzapine alone and 28% for placebo.[9] Another showed a remission rate of 42% with olanzapine plus sertraline compared with 24% with olanzapine alone.[10] There was no antidepressant-alone group in either study. Small open studies have found quetiapine,[11] aripiprazole[12] and amisulpride[13] augmentation of an antidepressant to be effective and relatively well tolerated, but again there were no data available for antidepressant treatment alone. One RCT (n = 122)[7] found venlafaxine plus quetiapine to be more effective than venlafaxine alone but not more effective than imipramine alone. These findings could be interpreted as either supporting the increased efficacy of a TCA over venlafaxine, and/or supporting combined antidepressant and antipsychotic treatment over an antidepressant drug alone. A review of all combination studies concluded that an antipsychotic+antidepressant was superior to either alone (four of nine studies showed some advantage for combination[14]). A recent meta-analysis concluded that a combination of an antipsychotic and an antidepressant is more effective than either an antipsychotic alone (NNT 5) or an antidepressant alone (NNT 7).[15] NICE[16] recommends that consideration should be given to augmenting an antidepressant with an antipsychotic in the treatment of an acute episode of psychotic depression. Cochrane is in agreement but with reservations.[17] Note that these data relate to acute treatment.

Virtually nothing is known of the optimum duration of treatment with a combination of an antidepressant and antipsychotic. NICE recommends augmentation of an antidepressant with an antipsychotic in non-psychotic depression that does not respond adequately to an antidepressant alone and states that if one agent is to be stopped during the maintenance phase, it should usually be the augmenting agent. It would seem reasonable to use the same approach in psychotic depression.

In clinical practice, at least until recent years, only a small proportion of patients with psychotic depression received an antipsychotic drug,[18] perhaps reflecting clinicians' uncertainty regarding the risk–benefit ratio of this treatment strategy and the lack of consensus across published guidelines.[19] Under-diagnosis (and hence inadequacy of treatment) of psychotic symptoms in depression is also a significant problem.[20] Nonetheless, some antipsychotic drugs such as quetiapine and olanzapine have useful antidepressant effects (as well as being antipsychotic) and so there is an empirical basis (in addition to the trial outcomes above) for their use as additive agents to antidepressant treatment.

Long-term outcome is generally poorer for psychotic than non-psychotic depression.[21,22] Patients with psychotic depression may also have a poorer response to combined pharmacological and psychological treatment than those with non-psychotic depression.[23]

Psychotic depression is one of the indications for ECT. Not only is ECT effective, it may also be more protective against relapse in psychotic depression than in non-psychotic depression.[24] One small RCT demonstrated superiority of maintenance ECT plus nortriptyline over nortriptyline alone at 2 years.[25]

Novel approaches being developed include those based on antiglucocorticoid strategies, since hypothalamic-pituitary-adrenal (HPA) axis hyperactivity is more common in psychotic depression; one small open study found rapid effects of the glucocorticoid receptor antagonist mifepristone,[26] although these findings have been criticised.[27] Response may be related to mifepristone plasma levels (>1800 ng/mL).[28] There is an anecdotal report of the successful use of methylphenidate in a patient who did not respond to robust doses of an antidepressant and antipsychotic combined.[29] Minocycline has also shown good effect in an open study.[30]

There is no specific indication for other therapies or augmentation strategies in psychotic depression over and above that for resistant depression or psychosis described elsewhere.

Summary

- TCAs are probably the drugs of first choice in psychotic depression.
- SSRIs/SNRIs are a second-line alternative when TCAs are poorly tolerated.
- Augmentation of an antidepressant with olanzapine or quetiapine is recommended.
- The optimum dose and duration of antipsychotic augmentation are unknown. If one treatment is to be stopped during the maintenance phase, this should usually be the antipsychotic.
- ECT should always be considered where a rapid response is required or where other treatments have failed.

References

1. Forty L et al. Is depression severity the sole cause of psychotic symptoms during an episode of unipolar major depression? A study both between and within subjects. J Affect Disord 2009; **114**:103–109.

2. Gaudiano BA et al. Depressive symptom profiles and severity patterns in outpatients with psychotic vs nonpsychotic major depression. Compr Psychiatry 2008; **49**:421–429.

3. Anderson IM et al. Evidence-based guidelines for treating depressive disorders with antidepressants: a revision of the 2000 British Association for Psychopharmacology guidelines. J Psychopharmacol 2008; **22**:343–396.

4. Wijkstra W et al. Pharmacological treatment for unipolar psychotic depression: systematic review and meta-analysis. Br J Psychiatry 2006; **188**:410–415.

5. Mulsant BH et al. A double-blind randomized comparison of nortriptyline plus perphenazine versus nortriptyline plus placebo in the treatment of psychotic depression in late life. J Clin Psychiatry 2001; **62**:597–604.

6. Birkenhager TK et al. Efficacy of imipramine in psychotic versus nonpsychotic depression. J Clin Psychopharmacol 2008; **28**:166–170.

7. Wijkstra J et al. Treatment of unipolar psychotic depression: a randomized, double-blind study comparing imipramine, venlafaxine, and venlafaxine plus quetiapine. Acta Psychiatr Scand 2010; **121**:190–200.

8. Blumberger DM et al. Impact of prior pharmacotherapy on remission of psychotic depression in a randomized controlled trial. J Psychiatr Res 2011; **45**:896–901.

9. Rothschild AJ et al. A double-blind, randomized study of olanzapine and olanzapine/fluoxetine combination for major depression with psychotic features. J Clin Psychopharmacol 2004; **24**:365–373.

CHAPTER 4

10. Meyers BS et al. A double-blind randomized controlled trial of olanzapine plus sertraline vs olanzapine plus placebo for psychotic depression: the study of pharmacotherapy of psychotic depression (STOP-PD). Arch Gen Psychiatry 2009; 66:838–847.

11. Konstantinidis A et al. Quetiapine in combination with citalopram in patients with unipolar psychotic depression. Prog Neuropsychopharmacol Biol Psychiatry 2007; 31:242–247.

12. Matthews JD et al. An open study of aripiprazole and escitalopram for psychotic major depressive disorder. J Clin Psychopharmacol 2009; 29:73–76.

13. Politis AM et al. Combination therapy with amisulpride and antidepressants: clinical observations in case series of elderly patients with psychotic depression. Prog Neuropsychopharmacol Biol Psychiatry 2008; 32:1227–1230.

14. Rothschild AJ. Challenges in the treatment of major depressive disorder with psychotic features. Schizophr Bull 2013; 39:787–796.

15. Farahani A et al. Are antipsychotics or antidepressants needed for psychotic depression? A systematic review and meta-analysis of trials comparing antidepressant or antipsychotic monotherapy with combination treatment. J Clin Psychiatry 2012; 73:486–496.

16. National Institute for Health and Care Excellence. Depression in adults: the treatment and management of depression in adults. Clinical Guideline 90, 2009. http://www.nice.org.uk/Guidance/cg90

17. Wijkstra J et al. Pharmacological treatment for psychotic depression. Cochrane Database Syst Rev 2013; 11:CD004044.

18. Andreescu C et al. Persisting low use of antipsychotics in the treatment of major depressive disorder with psychotic features. J Clin Psychiatry 2007; 68:194–200.

19. Leadholm AK et al. The treatment of psychotic depression: is there consensus among guidelines and psychiatrists? J Affect Disord 2013; 145:214–220.

20. Rothschild AJ et al. Missed diagnosis of psychotic depression at 4 academic medical centers. J Clin Psychiatry 2008; 69:1293–1296.

21. Flint AJ et al. Two-year outcome of psychotic depression in late life. Am J Psychiatry 1998; 155:178–183.

22. Maj M et al. Phenomenology and prognostic significance of delusions in major depressive disorder: a 10-year prospective follow-up study. J Clin Psychiatry 2007; 68:1411–1417.

23. Gaudiano BA et al. Differential response to combined treatment in patients with psychotic versus nonpsychotic major depression. J Nerv Ment Dis 2005; 193:625–628.

24. Birkenhager TK et al. One-year outcome of psychotic depression after successful electroconvulsive therapy. J ECT 2005; 21:221–226.

25. Navarro V et al. Continuation/maintenance treatment with nortriptyline versus combined nortriptyline and ECT in late-life psychotic depression: a two-year randomized study. Am J Geriatr Psychiatry 2008; 16:498–505.

26. Belanoff JK et al. An open label trial of C-1073 (mifepristone) for psychotic major depression. Biol Psychiatry 2002; 52:386–392.

27. Rubin RT. Dr. Rubin replies (letter). Am J Psychiatry 2004; 161:1722.

28. Blasey CM et al. A multisite trial of mifepristone for the treatment of psychotic depression: a site-by-treatment interaction. Contemp Clin Trials 2009; 30:284–288.

29. Huang CC et al. Adjunctive use of methylphenidate in the treatment of psychotic unipolar depression. Clin Neuropharmacol 2008; 31:245–247.

30. Miyaoka T et al. Minocycline as adjunctive therapy for patients with unipolar psychotic depression: an open-label study. Prog Neuropsychopharmacol Biol Psychiatry 2012; 37:222–226.

Electroconvulsive therapy and psychotropic drugs

Psychotropics are often continued during ECT and some agents (particularly antide-pressants[1,2]) enhance its efficacy.

Table 4.9 summarises the effect of various psychotropics on seizure duration during ECT. Note that there are few well-controlled studies in this area and so recommendations should be viewed with this in mind. Note also that choice of anaesthetic agent profoundly affects seizure duration,[3–8] post-ictal confusion and ECT efficacy.[9] Besides concurrent medication, there are many factors that influence seizure threshold and duration.[10]

Table 4.9 Effect of psychotropic drugs on seizure duration in ECT

Drug	Effect on ECT seizure duration	Comments[11–15]
Benzodiazepines	Reduced	All may raise seizure threshold and so should be avoided where possible. Many are long-acting and may need to be discontinued some days before ECT. Benzodiazepines may also complicate anaesthesia and may reduce efficacy of ECT
		If sedation is required, consider hydroxyzine. If benzodiazepine use is very long term and essential, continue and use higher stimulus
SSRIs[2,16–19]	Minimal effect; small increase possible	Generally considered safe to use during ECT. Beware complex pharmacokinetic interactions with anaesthetic agents
Venlafaxine[20]	Minimal effect at standard doses	Limited data suggest no effect on seizure duration but possibility of increased risk of asystole with doses above 300 mg/day. Clearly epileptogenic in higher doses. ECG advised
Mirtazapine[2,21]	Minimal effect – small increase	Apparently safe in ECT and, like other antidepressants, may enhance ECT efficacy. May reduce post-ECT nausea and headache
Duloxetine[22,23]	Not known	One case report suggests duloxetine does not complicate ECT. Another links its use to ventricular tachycardia
TCAs[2,17]	Possibly increased	Few data relevant to ECT but many TCAs lower seizure threshold. TCAs are associated with arrhythmia following ECT and should be avoided in elderly patients and those with cardiac disease. In others, it is preferable to continue TCA treatment during ECT. Close monitoring is essential. Beware hypotension and risk of prolonged seizures
MAOIs[24]	Minimal effect	Data relating to ECT very limited but long history of ECT use during MAOI therapy. MAOIs probably do not affect seizure duration but interactions with sympathomimetics occasionally used in anaesthesia are possible and may lead to hypertensive crisis. MAOIs may be continued during ECT but the anaesthetist must be informed. Beware hypotension
Lithium[25–27]	Possibly increased	Conflicting data on lithium and ECT. The combination may be more likely to lead to delirium and confusion, and some authorities suggest discontinuing lithium 48 hours before ECT. In the UK, ECT is often used during lithium therapy but starting with a low stimulus and with very close monitoring. The combination is generally well tolerated
		Note that lithium potentiates the effects of non-depolarising neuromuscular blockers such as suxamethonium

Continued

CHAPTER 4

Table 4.9 (Continued)

Drug	Effect on ECT seizure duration	Comments[11-15]
Antipsychotics[28-32]	Variable – increased with phenothiazines and clozapine Others – no obvious effect reported	Few published data but widely used. Phenothiazines and clozapine are perhaps most likely to prolong seizures, and some suggest withdrawal before ECT. However, safe concurrent use has been reported (particularly with clozapine,[33,34] which is now usually continued). ECT and antipsychotics appear generally to be a safe combination. Few data on aripiprazole, quetiapine and ziprasidone, but they too appear to be safe. One case series[35] suggests antipsychotics increase post-ictal cognitive dysfunction
Anticonvulsants[36-39]	Reduced	If used as a mood stabiliser, continue but be prepared to use higher energy stimulus (not always required). If used for epilepsy, their effect is to normalise seizure threshold. Interactions are possible. Valproate may prolong the effect of thiopental; carbamazepine may inhibit neuromuscular blockade. Lamotrigine is reported to cause no problems
Barbiturates	Reduced	All barbiturates reduce seizure duration in ECT but are widely used as sedative anaesthetic agents Thiopental and methohexital may be associated with cardiac arrhythmia

ECG, electrocardiogram; ECT, electroconvulsive therapy; MAOI, monoamine oxidase inhibitor; SSRI, selective serotonin reuptake inhibitor; TCA, tricyclic antidepressant.

For drugs known to lower seizure threshold, treatment is best begun with a low-energy stimulus (50 mC). Staff should be alerted to the possibility of prolonged seizures and intravenous (IV) diazepam should be available. With drugs known to elevate seizure threshold, higher stimuli may, of course, be required. Methods are available to lower seizure threshold or prolong seizures,[40] but discussion of these is beyond the scope of this book.

Electroconvulsive therapy frequently causes confusion and disorientation; more rarely, it causes delirium. Close observation is essential. Very limited data support the use of thiamine (200 mg daily) in reducing post-ECT confusion.[41] Nortriptyline seems to enhance ECT efficacy and reduce cognitive adverse effects.[1] Donepezil has been shown to improve recovery time post ECT (and appears to be safe).[42] Ibuprofen may be used to prevent headache,[43] and intranasal sumatriptan[44] can be used to treat it.

References

1. Sackeim HA et al. Effect of concomitant pharmacotherapy on electroconvulsive therapy outcomes: short-term efficacy and adverse effects. Arch Gen Psychiatry 2009; 66:729–737.
2. Baghai TC et al. The influence of concomitant antidepressant medication on safety, tolerability and clinical effectiveness of electroconvulsive therapy. World J Biol Psychiatry 2006; 7:82–90.
3. Avramov MN et al. The comparative effects of methohexital, propofol, and etomidate for electroconvulsive therapy. Anesth Analg 1995; 81:596–602.
4. Stadtland C et al. A switch from propofol to etomidate during an ECT course increases EEG and motor seizure duration. J ECT 2002; 18:22–25.
5. Gazdag G et al. Etomidate versus propofol for electroconvulsive therapy in patients with schizophrenia. J ECT 2004; 20:225–229.
6. Conca A et al. Etomidate vs. thiopentone in electroconvulsive therapy. An interdisciplinary challenge for anesthesiology and psychiatry. Pharmacopsychiatry 2003; 36:94–97.
7. Rasmussen KG et al. Seizure length with sevoflurane and thiopental for induction of general anesthesia in electroconvulsive therapy: a randomized double-blind trial. J ECT 2006; 22:240–242.

8. Bundy BD et al. Influence of anesthetic drugs and concurrent psychiatric medication on seizure adequacy during electroconvulsive therapy. J Clin Psychiatry 2010; **71**:775–777.

9. Eser D et al. The influence of anaesthetic medication on safety, tolerability and clinical effectiveness of electroconvulsive therapy. World J Biol Psychiatry 2010; **11**:447–456.

10. van Waarde JA et al. Clinical predictors of seizure threshold in electroconvulsive therapy: a prospective study. Eur Arch Psychiatry Clin Neurosci 2013; **263**:167–175.

11. Royal College of Psychiatrists. *The ECT Handbook – Council Report 176*, 3rd edn. London: RCPsych Publications, 2013.

12. Kellner CH et al. ECT–drug interactions: a review. Psychopharmacol Bull 1991; **27**:595–609.

13. Creelman W et al. Electroconvulsive Therapy. In: Ciraulo DA, Shader RI, Greenblatt DJ et al., eds. *Drug Interactions in Psychiatry*, 3rd edn. Philadelphia: Lippincott Williams and Wilkins; 2005, 337–389.

14. Naguib M et al. Interactions between psychotropics, anaesthetics and electroconvulsive therapy: implications for drug choice and patient management. CNS Drugs 2002; **16**:229–247.

15. Maidment I. The interaction between psychiatric medicines and ECT. Hosp Pharm 1997; **4**:102–105.

16. Masdrakis VG et al. The safety of the electroconvulsive therapy-escitalopram combination. J ECT 2008; **24**:289–291.

17. Dursun SM et al. Effects of antidepressant treatments on first-ECT seizure duration in depression. Prog Neuropsychopharmacol Biol Psychiatry 2001; **25**:437–443.

18. Jarvis MR et al. Novel antidepressants and maintenance electroconvulsive therapy: a review. Ann Clin Psychiatry 1992; **4**:275–284.

19. Papakostas YG et al. Administration of citalopram before ECT: seizure duration and hormone responses. J ECT 2000; **16**:356–360.

20. Gonzalez-Pinto A et al. Efficacy and safety of venlafaxine-ECT combination in treatment-resistant depression. J Neuropsychiatry Clin Neurosci 2002; **14**:206–209.

21. Li TC et al. Mirtazapine relieves post-electroconvulsive therapy headaches and nausea: a case series and review of the literature. J ECT 2011; **27**:165–167.

22. Hanretta AT et al. Combined use of ECT with duloxetine and olanzapine: a case report. J ECT 2006; **22**:139–141.

23. Heinz B et al. Postictal ventricular tachycardia after electroconvulsive therapy treatment associated with a lithium-duloxetine combination. J ECT 2013; **29**:e33–35.

24. Dolenc TJ et al. Electroconvulsive therapy in patients taking monoamine oxidase inhibitors. J ECT 2004; **20**:258–261.

25. Jha AK et al. Negative interaction between lithium and electroconvulsive therapy – a case-control study. Br J Psychiatry 1996; **168**:241–243.

26. Rucker J et al. A case of prolonged seizure after ECT in a patient treated with clomipramine, lithium, L-tryptophan, quetiapine, and thyroxine for major depression. J ECT 2008; **24**:272–274.

27. Dolenc TJ et al. The safety of electroconvulsive therapy and lithium in combination: a case series and review of the literature. J ECT 2005; **21**:165–170.

28. Havaki-Kontaxaki BJ et al. Concurrent administration of clozapine and electroconvulsive therapy in clozapine-resistant schizophrenia. Clin Neuropharmacol 2006; **29**:52–56.

29. Nothdurfter C et al. The influence of concomitant neuroleptic medication on safety, tolerability and clinical effectiveness of electroconvulsive therapy. World J Biol Psychiatry 2006; **7**:162–170.

30. Gazdag G et al. The impact of neuroleptic medication on seizure threshold and duration in electroconvulsive therapy. Ideggyogy Sz 2004; **57**:385–390.

31. Masdrakis VG et al. The safety of the electroconvulsive therapy-aripiprazole combination: four case reports. J ECT 2008; **24**:236–238.

32. Oulis P et al. Corrected QT interval changes during electroconvulsive therapy-antidepressants-atypical antipsychotics coadministration: safety issues. J ECT 2011; **27**:e4–e6.

33. Biedermann F et al. Combined clozapine and electroconvulsive therapy in clozapine-resistant schizophrenia: clinical and cognitive outcomes. J ECT 2011; **27**:e61–62.

34. Flamarique I et al. Electroconvulsive therapy and clozapine in adolescents with schizophrenia spectrum disorders: is it a safe and effective combination? J Clin Psychopharmacol 2012; **32**:756–766.

35. van Waarde JA et al. Patient, treatment, and anatomical predictors of outcome in electroconvulsive therapy: a prospective study. J ECT 2013; **29**:113–121.

36. Penland HR et al. Combined use of lamotrigine and electroconvulsive therapy in bipolar depression: a case series. J ECT 2006; **22**:142–147.

37. Zarate CA Jr et al. Combined valproate or carbamazepine and electroconvulsive therapy. Ann Clin Psychiatry 1997; **9**:19–25.

38. Sienaert P et al. Concurrent use of lamotrigine and electroconvulsive therapy. J ECT 2011; **27**:148–152.

39. Jahangard L et al. Comparing efficacy of ECT with and without concurrent sodium valproate therapy in manic patients. J ECT 2012; **28**:118–123.

40. Datto C et al. Augmentation of seizure induction in electroconvulsive therapy: a clinical reappraisal. J ECT 2002; **18**:118–125.

41. Linton CR et al. Using thiamine to reduce post-ECT confusion. Int J Geriatr Psychiatry 2002; **17**:189–192.

42. Prakash J et al. Therapeutic and prophylactic utility of the memory-enhancing drug donepezil hydrochloride on cognition of patients undergoing electroconvulsive therapy: a randomized controlled trial. J ECT 2006; **22**:163–168.

43. Leung M et al. Pretreatment with ibuprofen to prevent electroconvulsive therapy-induced headache. J Clin Psychiatry 2003; **64**:551–553.

44. Markowitz JS et al. Intranasal sumatriptan in post-ECT headache: results of an open-label trial. J ECT 2001; **17**:280–283.

Psychostimulants in depression

Psychostimulants reduce fatigue, promote wakefulness and are mood elevating (as distinct from antidepressant). Amfetamines have been used as treatments for depression since the 1930s[1] and more recently, modafinil has been evaluated as an adjunct to standard antidepressants.[2] Amfetamines are now rarely used in depression because of their propensity for the development of tolerance and dependence. Prolonged use of high doses is associated with paranoid psychosis.[3] Methylphenidate is now more widely used but may have similar shortcomings. Modafinil seems not to induce tolerance, dependence or psychosis but lacks the euphoric effects of amfetamines. Armodafinil, the longer acting isomer of modafinil, is available in some countries.

Psychostimulants differ importantly from standard antidepressants in that their effects are usually seen within a few hours. Amfetamines and methylphenidate may thus be useful where a prompt effect is required and where dependence would not be problematic (e.g. in depression associated with terminal illness) although ketamine might also be considered. Their use might also be justified in severe, prolonged depression unresponsive to standard treatments (e.g. in those considered for psychosurgery). Modafinil might justifiably be used as an adjunct to antidepressants in a wider range of patients and as a specific treatment for hypersomnia and fatigue.[4]

Table 4.10 outlines support (or the absence of it) for the use of psychostimulants in various clinical situations. Generally speaking, data relating to stimulants in depression are poor and inconclusive.[5,6] Careful consideration should be given to any use of any psychostimulant in depression since their short- and long-term safety have not been clearly established. Inclusion of individual drugs in Table 4.10 should not in itself be considered a recommendation for their use.

Table 4.10 Psychostimulants in depression

Clinical use	Regimens evaluated	Comments	Recommendations
Monotherapy in uncomplicated depression	Modafinil 100–200 mg/day[7,8]	Case reports only – efficacy unproven	Standard antidepressants preferred. Avoid psychostimulants as monotherapy in uncomplicated depression
	Methylphenidate 20–40 mg/day[9,10]	Minimal efficacy	
	Dexamfetamine 20 mg/day[9]	Minimal efficacy	
Adjunctive therapy to accelerate or improve response	SSRI + methylphenidate 10–20 mg/day[11,12]	No clear effect on time to response	Psychostimulants in general not recommended, but modafinil may be useful
	SSRI + modafinil 400 mg/day[13]	Improved response over SSRI alone	
	Tricyclic + methylphenidate 5–15 mg/day[14]	Single open-label trial suggests faster response	
Adjunctive treatment of depression with fatigue and hypersomnia	SSRI + modafinil 200 mg/day[15,16]	Beneficial effect only on hypersomnia. Modafinil may induce suicidal ideation	Possible effect on fatigue, but weak evidence base. An option where fatigue is prominent and otherwise unresponsive
	SSRI + methylphenidate 10–40 mg/day[17]	Clear effect on fatigue in hospice patients	
Adjunctive therapy in refractory depression	SSRI + modafinil 100–400 mg/day[18–23]	Effect mainly on fatigue and daytime sleepiness	Data limited. Modafinil may be useful for fatigue
	MAOI + dexamfetamine 7.5–40 mg/day[24]	Support from single case series	Stimulants an option in refractory illness but other options better supported
	Methylphenidate or dexamfetamine +/– antidepressant[25]	Large case series (n = 50) suggests benefit in the majority	
	Lisdexamfetamine + escitalopram 20–50 mg/day[26]	RCT shows significant effect on depression	
	Lisdexamfetamine + antidepressant 20–30 mg/day[27]	RCT shows significant benefit on executive functioning and depression	
Adjunctive treatment in bipolar depression	Mood stabiliser and/or antidepressants + modafinil 100–200 mg/day[28]	Significantly superior to placebo. No evidence of switching to mania	Possible treatment option where other standard treatments fail
	Mood stabiliser + armodafinil 150 mg/day[29]	Superior to placebo on some measures	
	Mood stabiliser + methylphenidate 10–40 mg/day[30]	Mixed results, mainly positive	
Monotherapy or add-on treatment in late-stage terminal cancer	Methylphenidate 5–30 mg/day[31–35]	Case series and open prospective studies	Useful treatment options in those expected to live only for a few weeks. Best reserved for hospices and other specialist units
	Dexamfetamine 2.5–20 mg/day[36,37]	Beneficial effects seen on mood, fatigue and pain	
	Methylphenidate 20 mg/day + mirtazapine 30 mg/day[38]	RCT shows benefit for combination from third day of treatment	

Continued

Table 4.10 (Continued)

Clinical use	Regimens evaluated	Comments	Recommendations
Monotherapy for depression in the very old	Methylphenidate 1.25–20 mg/day[39,40]	Use supported by two placebo-controlled studies. Rapid effect observed on mood and activity	Recommended only where patients fail to tolerate standard antidepressants or where contraindications apply
Monotherapy in post-stroke depression	Methylphenidate 5–40 mg/day[41–44]	Variable support but including two placebo-controlled trials.[41,44] Effect on mood evident after a few days	Standard antidepressants preferred. Further investigation required; stimulants may improve cognition and motor function
	Modafinil 100 mg/day[45]	Single case report	
Monotherapy in depression secondary to medical illness	Methylphenidate 5–20 mg/day[46]	Limited data	Psychostimulants now not appropriate therapy. Standard antidepressant preferred
	Dexamfetamine 2.5–30 mg/day[47,48]		
Monotherapy in depression and fatigue associated with HIV	Dexamfetamine 2.5–40 mg/day[49,50]	Supported by one good, controlled study[50]	Possible treatment option where fatigue is not responsive to standard antidepressants
		Beneficial effect on mood and fatigue	

HIV, human immunodeficiency virus; MAOI, monoamine oxidase inhibitor; RCT, randomised controlled trial; SSRI, selective serotonin reuptake inhibitor.

References

1. Satel SL et al. Stimulants in the treatment of depression: a critical overview. J Clin Psychiatry 1989; 50:241–249.
2. Menza MA et al. Modafinil augmentation of antidepressant treatment in depression. J Clin Psychiatry 2000; 61:378–381.
3. Warneke L. Psychostimulants in psychiatry. Can J Psychiatry 1990; 35:3–10.
4. Goss AJ et al. Modafinil augmentation therapy in unipolar and bipolar depression: a systematic review and meta-analysis of randomized controlled trials. J Clin Psychiatry 2013; 74:1101–1107.
5. Candy M et al. Psychostimulants for depression. Cochrane Database Syst Rev 2008: 2:CD006722.
6. Hardy SE. Methylphenidate for the treatment of depressive symptoms, including fatigue and apathy, in medically ill older adults and terminally ill adults. Am J Geriatr Pharmacother 2009; 7:34–59.
7. Lundt L. Modafinil treatment in patients with seasonal affective disorder/winter depression: an open-label pilot study. J Affect Disord 2004; 81:173–178.
8. Kaufman KR et al. Modafinil monotherapy in depression. Eur Psychiatry 2002; 17:167–169.
9. Little KY. d-Amphetamine versus methylphenidate effects in depressed inpatients. J Clin Psychiatry 1993; 54:349–355.
10. Robin AA et al. A controlled trial of methylphenidate (ritalin) in the treatment of depressive states. J Neurol Neurosurg Psychiatry 1958; 21:55–57.
11. Lavretsky H et al. Combined treatment with methylphenidate and citalopram for accelerated response in the elderly: an open trial. J Clin Psychiatry 2003; 64:1410–1414.
12. Postolache TT et al. Early augmentation of sertraline with methylphenidate. J Clin Psychiatry 1999; 60:123–124.
13. Abolfazli R et al. Double-blind randomized parallel-group clinical trial of efficacy of the combination fluoxetine plus modafinil versus fluoxetine plus placebo in the treatment of major depression. Depress Anxiety 2011; 28:297–302.
14. Gwirtsman HE et al. The antidepressant response to tricyclics in major depressives is accelerated with adjunctive use of methylphenidate. Psychopharmacol Bull 1994; 30:157–164.
15. Dunlop BW et al. Coadministration of modafinil and a selective serotonin reuptake inhibitor from the initiation of treatment of major depressive disorder with fatigue and sleepiness: a double-blind, placebo-controlled study. J Clin Psychopharmacol 2007; 27:614–619.

16. Fava M et al. Modafinil augmentation of selective serotonin reuptake inhibitor therapy in MDD partial responders with persistent fatigue and sleepiness. Ann Clin Psychiatry 2007; **19**:153–159.

17. Kerr CW et al. Effects of methylphenidate on fatigue and depression: a randomized, double-blind, placebo-controlled trial. J Pain Symptom Manage 2012; **43**:68–77.

18. DeBattista C et al. Adjunct modafinil for the short-term treatment of fatigue and sleepiness in patients with major depressive disorder: a preliminary double-blind, placebo-controlled study. J Clin Psychiatry 2003; **64**:1057–1064.

19. Fava M et al. A multicenter, placebo-controlled study of modafinil augmentation in partial responders to selective serotonin reuptake inhibitors with persistent fatigue and sleepiness. J Clin Psychiatry 2005; **66**:85–93.

20. Rasmussen NA et al. Modafinil augmentation in depressed patients with partial response to antidepressants: a pilot study on self-reported symptoms covered by the major depression inventory (MDI) and the symptom checklist (SCL-92). Nordic J Psychiatry 2005; **59**:173–178.

21. DeBattista C et al. A prospective trial of modafinil as an adjunctive treatment of major depression. J Clin Psychopharmacol 2004; **24**:87–90.

22. Markovitz PJ et al. An open-label trial of modafinil augmentation in patients with partial response to antidepressant therapy. J Clin Psychopharmacol 2003; **23**:207–209.

23. Ravindran AV et al. Osmotic-release oral system methylphenidate augmentation of antidepressant monotherapy in major depressive disorder: results of a double-blind, randomized, placebo-controlled trial. J Clin Psychiatry 2008; **69**:87–94.

24. Fawcett J et al. CNS stimulant potentiation of monoamine oxidase inhibitors in treatment refractory depression. J Clin Psychopharmacol 1991; **11**:127–132.

25. Parker G et al. Do the old psychostimulant drugs have a role in managing treatment-resistant depression? Acta Psychiatr Scand 2010; **121**:308–314.

26. Trivedi MH et al. A randomized controlled trial of the efficacy and safety of lisdexamfetamine dimesylate as augmentation therapy in adults with residual symptoms of major depressive disorder after treatment with escitalopram. J Clin Psychiatry 2013; **74**:802–809.

27. Madhoo M et al. Lisdexamfetamine dimesylate augmentation in adults with persistent executive dysfunction after partial or full remission of major depressive disorder. Neuropsychopharmacology 2014; **39**:1388–1398.

28. Frye MA et al. A placebo-controlled evaluation of adjunctive modafinil in the treatment of bipolar depression. Am J Psychiatry 2007; **164**:1242–1249.

29. Calabrese JR et al. Adjunctive armodafinil for major depressive episodes associated with bipolar I disorder: a randomized, multicenter, double-blind, placebo-controlled, proof-of-concept study. J Clin Psychiatry 2010; **71**:1363–1370.

30. Dell'Osso B et al. Assessing the roles of stimulants/stimulant-like drugs and dopamine-agonists in the treatment of bipolar depression. Curr Psychiatr Rep 2013; **15**:378.

31. Fernandez F et al. Methylphenidate for depressive disorders in cancer patients. Psychosomatics 1987; **28**:455–461.

32. Macleod AD. Methylphenidate in terminal depression. J Pain Symptom Manage 1998; **16**:193–198.

33. Homsi J et al. Methylphenidate for depression in hospice practice. Am J Hosp Palliat Care 2000; **17**:393–398.

34. Sarhill N et al. Methylphenidate for fatigue in advanced cancer: a prospective open-label pilot study. Am J Hosp Palliat Care 2001; **18**:187–192.

35. Homsi J et al. A phase II study of methylphenidate for depression in advanced cancer. Am J Hosp Palliat Care 2001; **18**:403–407.

36. Burns MM et al. Dextroamphetamine treatment for depression in terminally ill patients. Psychosomatics 1994; **35**:80–83.

37. Olin J et al. Psychostimulants for depression in hospitalized cancer patients. Psychosomatics 1996; **37**:57–62.

38. Ng CG et al. Rapid response to methylphenidate as an add-on therapy to mirtazapine in the treatment of major depressive disorder in terminally ill cancer patients: a four-week, randomized, double-blinded, placebo-controlled study. Eur Neuropsychopharmacol 2014; **24**:491–498.

39. Kaplitz SE. Withdrawn, apathetic geriatric patients responsive to methylphenidate. J Am Geriatr Soc 1975; **23**:271–276.

40. Wallace AE et al. Double-blind, placebo-controlled trial of methylphenidate in older, depressed, medically ill patients. Am J Psychiatry 1995; **152**:929–931.

41. Grade C et al. Methylphenidate in early poststroke recovery: a double-blind, placebo-controlled study. Arch Phys Med Rehabil 1998; **79**:1047–1050.

42. Lazarus LW et al. Efficacy and side effects of methylphenidate for poststroke depression. J Clin Psychiatry 1992; **53**:447–449.

43. Lingam VR et al. Methylphenidate in treating poststroke depression. J Clin Psychiatry 1988; **49**:151–153.

44. Delbari A et al. Effect of methylphenidate and/or levodopa combined with physiotherapy on mood and cognition after stroke: a randomized, double-blind, placebo-controlled trial. Eur Neurol 2011; **66**:7–13.

45. Sugden SG et al. Modafinil monotherapy in poststroke depression. Psychosomatics 2004; **45**:80–81.

46. Rosenberg PB et al. Methylphenidate in depressed medically ill patients. J Clin Psychiatry 1991; **52**:263–267.

47. Woods SW et al. Psychostimulant treatment of depressive disorders secondary to medical illness. J Clin Psychiatry 1986; **47**:12–15.

48. Kaufmann MW et al. The use of d-amphetamine in medically ill depressed patients. J Clin Psychiatry 1982; **43**:463–464.

49. Wagner GJ et al. Dexamphetamine as a treatment for depression and low energy in AIDS patients: a pilot study. J Psychosom Res 1997; **42**:407–411.

50. Wagner GJ et al. Effects of dextroamphetamine on depression and fatigue in men with HIV: a double-blind, placebo-controlled trial. J Clin Psychiatry 2000; **61**:436–440.

CHAPTER 4

Post-stroke depression

Depression itself is a well-established risk factor for stroke.[1-3] In addition, depression is seen in at least 30–40% of survivors of stroke[4,5] and post-stroke depression is known to slow functional rehabilitation.[6] Antidepressants may reduce depressive symptoms and thereby facilitate faster rehabilitation.[7] They may also improve global cognitive functioning[8] and enhance motor recovery.[9] Despite these benefits, most post-stroke depression goes untreated.[10]

Prophylaxis

The high incidence of depression after stroke makes prophylaxis worthy of considera-tion. Pooled data suggest a robust prophylactic effect for antidepressants.[11] Nortriptyline, fluoxetine, escitalopram, duloxetine and sertraline appear to prevent post-stroke depression.[12-16] Mirtazapine may both protect against depressive episodes and treat them.[17] Note, though, that a large cohort study that examined adverse outcomes in elderly patients treated with antidepressants reported that mirtazapine (and venlafax-ine) may be associated with an increased risk of a new stroke compared with SSRIs or TCAs.[18] Mianserin seems ineffective in the treatment of post-stroke depression.[19] Amitriptyline is effective in treating central post-stroke pain.[20]

Treatment

Treatment is complicated by medical co-morbidity and by the potential for interaction with other co-prescribed drugs (especially warfarin – see below). Contraindication to antidepressant treatment is more likely with tricyclics than with SSRIs.[21] Fluoxetine,[9,22,23] citalopram[8,24] and nortriptyline[25,26] are probably the most studied[27] and seem to be effective and safe.[28] SSRIs and nortriptyline are widely recommended for post-stroke depression. Reboxetine (which does not affect platelet activity) may also be effective and well tolerated[29] although its effects overall are doubtful.[30]

Despite fears, SSRIs seem not to increase risk of stroke[31] (post-stroke), although some doubt remains.[32,33] (Stroke can be embolic or haemorrhagic – SSRIs may protect against the former and provoke the latter[34,35] – see section on 'SSRIs and bleeding' in this chap-ter). Antidepressants are clearly effective in post-stroke depression[28,36] and treatment should not usually be withheld (although Cochrane is rather lukewarm about the benefits of antidepressants[37]).

Post-stroke depression – recommended drugs

- SSRIs*
- Nortriptyline

*Caution is clearly required if the index stroke was known to be haemorrhagic because SSRIs increase the risk of *de novo* haemorrhagic stroke (absolute risk is low) when combined with warfarin or other antiplatelet drugs.[38] If the patient is also tak-ing warfarin, suggest citalopram or escitalopram (probably lowest interaction potential[39]). Where SSRIs are given in any anticoagulated or aspirin-treated patient, consideration should be given to the prescription of a proton pump inhibitor for gastric protection.

References

1. Pan A et al. Depression and risk of stroke morbidity and mortality: a meta-analysis and systematic review. JAMA 2011; **306**:1241–1249.
2. Pequignot R et al. Depressive symptoms, antidepressants and disability and future coronary heart disease and stroke events in older adults: the Three City Study. Eur J Epidemiol 2013; **28**:249–256.
3. Li CT et al. Major depressive disorder and stroke risks: a 9-year follow-up population-based, matched cohort study. PLoS One 2012; **7**:e46818.
4. Gainotti G et al. Relation between depression after stroke, antidepressant therapy, and functional recovery. J Neurol Neurosurg Psychiatry 2001; **71**:258–261.
5. Hayee MA et al. Depression after stroke-analysis of 297 stroke patients. Bangladesh Med Res Counc Bull 2001; **27**:96–102.
6. Paolucci S et al. Post-stroke depression, antidepressant treatment and rehabilitation results. A case-control study. Cerebrovasc Dis 2001; **12**:264–271.
7. Gainotti G et al. Determinants and consequences of post-stroke depression. Curr Opin Neurol 2002; **15**:85–89.
8. Jorge RE et al. Escitalopram and enhancement of cognitive recovery following stroke. Arch Gen Psychiatry 2010; **67**:187–196.
9. Chollet F et al. Fluoxetine for motor recovery after acute ischaemic stroke (FLAME): a randomised placebo-controlled trial. Lancet Neurol 2011; **10**:123–130.
10. El Husseini N et al. Depression and antidepressant use after stroke and transient ischemic attack. Stroke 2012; **43**:1609–1616.
11. Chen Y et al. Antidepressant prophylaxis for poststroke depression: a meta-analysis. Int Clin Psychopharmacol 2007; **22**:159–166.
12. Narushima K et al. Preventing poststroke depression: a 12-week double-blind randomized treatment trial and 21-month follow-up. J Nerv Ment Dis 2002; **190**:296–303.
13. Rasmussen A et al. A double-blind, placebo-controlled study of sertraline in the prevention of depression in stroke patients. Psychosomatics 2003; **44**:216–221.
14. Robinson RG et al. Escitalopram and problem-solving therapy for prevention of poststroke depression: a randomized controlled trial. JAMA 2008; **299**:2391–2400.
15. Almeida OP et al. Preventing depression after stroke: results from a randomized placebo-controlled trial. J Clin Psychiatry 2006; **67**:1104–1109.
16. Zhang LS et al. Prophylactic effects of duloxetine on post-stroke depression symptoms: an open single-blind trial. Eur Neurol 2013; **69**:336–343.
17. Niedermaier N et al. Prevention and treatment of poststroke depression with mirtazapine in patients with acute stroke. J Clin Psychiatry 2004; **65**:1619–1623.
18. Coupland C et al. Antidepressant use and risk of adverse outcomes in older people: population based cohort study. BMJ 2011; **343**:d4551.
19. Palomaki H et al. Prevention of poststroke depression: 1 year randomised placebo controlled double blind trial of mianserin with 6 month follow up after therapy. J Neurol Neurosurg Psychiatry 1999; **66**:490–494.
20. Lampl C et al. Amitriptyline in the prophylaxis of central poststroke pain. Preliminary results of 39 patients in a placebo-controlled, long-term study. Stroke 2002; **33**:3030–3032.
21. Cole MG et al. Feasibility and effectiveness of treatments for post-stroke depression in elderly inpatients: systematic review. J Geriatr Psychiatry Neurol 2001; **14**:37–41.
22. Wiart L et al. Fluoxetine in early poststroke depression: a double-blind placebo-controlled study. Stroke 2000; **31**:1829–1832.
23. Choi-Kwon S et al. Fluoxetine improves the quality of life in patients with poststroke emotional disturbances. Cerebrovasc Dis 2008; **26**:266–271.
24. Andersen G et al. Effective treatment of poststroke depression with the selective serotonin reuptake inhibitor citalopram. Stroke 1994; **25**:1099–1104.
25. Robinson RG et al. Nortriptyline versus fluoxetine in the treatment of depression and in short-term recovery after stroke: a placebo-controlled, double-blind study. Am J Psychiatry 2000; **157**:351–359.
26. Zhang W et al. Nortriptyline protects mitochondria and reduces cerebral ischemia/hypoxia injury. Stroke 2008; **39**:455–462.
27. Starkstein SE et al. Antidepressant therapy in post-stroke depression. Expert Opin Pharmacother 2008; **9**:1291–1298.
28. Mead GE et al. Selective serotonin reuptake inhibitors for stroke recovery. JAMA 2013; **310**:1066–1067.
29. Rampello L et al. An evaluation of efficacy and safety of reboxetine in elderly patients affected by 'retarded' post-stroke depression. A random, placebo-controlled study. Arch Gerontol Geriatr 2005; **40**:275–285.
30. Eyding D et al. Reboxetine for acute treatment of major depression: systematic review and meta-analysis of published and unpublished placebo and selective serotonin reuptake inhibitor controlled trials. BMJ 2010; **341**:c4737.
31. Douglas I et al. The use of antidepressants and the risk of haemorrhagic stroke: a nested case control study. Br J Clin Pharmacol 2011; **71**:116–120.
32. Ramasubbu R. SSRI treatment-associated stroke: causality assessment in two cases. Ann Pharmacother 2004; **38**:1197–1201.
33. Hackam DG et al. Selective serotonin reuptake inhibitors and brain hemorrhage: a meta-analysis. Neurology 2012; **79**:1862–1865.

CHAPTER 4

34. Trifiro G et al. Risk of ischemic stroke associated with antidepressant drug use in elderly persons. J Clin Psychopharmacol 2010; 30:252–258.

35. Wu CS et al. Association of cerebrovascular events with antidepressant use: a case-crossover study. Am J Psychiatry 2011; **168**:511–521.

36. Chen Y et al. Treatment effects of antidepressants in patients with post-stroke depression: a meta-analysis. Ann Pharmacother 2006; 40:2115–2122.

37. Hackett ML et al. Interventions for treating depression after stroke. Cochrane Database Syst Rev 2008: 4:CD003437.

38. Quinn GR et al. Effect of selective serotonin reuptake inhibitors on bleeding risk in patients with atrial fibrillation taking warfarin. Am J Cardiol 2014; **114**:583–586.

39. Sayal KS et al. Psychotropic interactions with warfarin. Acta Psychiatr Scand 2000; **102**:250–255.

Further reading

Robinson RG et al. Poststroke depression: a review. Can J Psychiatry 2010; 55:341–349.

Treatment of depression in the elderly

The prevalence of most physical illnesses increases with age. Many physical problems such as cardiovascular disease, chronic pain, diabetes and Parkinson's disease are associated with a high risk of depressive illness.[1,2] The morbidity and mortality associated with depression are increased in the elderly[3] as they are more likely to be physically frail and therefore vulnerable to serious consequences from self-neglect (e.g. life-threatening dehydration or hypothermia) and immobility (e.g. venous stasis). Almost 20% of completed suicides occur in the elderly.[4] Mortality is reduced by effective treatment of depression.

In common with placebo-controlled studies in younger adults, at least some adequately powered studies in elderly patients have failed to find 'active' antidepressants to be more effective than placebo,[5–8] although it is commonly perceived that the elderly may take longer to respond to antidepressants than younger adults.[9] Even in the elderly, it may still be possible to identify non-responders as early as 4 weeks into treatment.[10] Two studies have found that in elderly people who had recovered from an episode of depression and had received antidepressants for 2 years, 60% relapsed within 2 years if antidepressant treatment was withdrawn.[11,12] This finding held true for first-episode patients. Lower doses of antidepressants may be effective as prophylaxis. Dothiepin (dosulepin) 75 mg/day has been shown to be effective in this regard.[13] Note that NICE recommends that dosulepin should not be used as it is particularly cardiotoxic in overdose.[14] There is no evidence to suggest that the response to antidepressants is reduced in the physically ill,[15] although outcome in the elderly in general is often suboptimal.[16,17]

There is no ideal antidepressant in the elderly. All are associated with problems (Table 4.11). SSRIs are generally better tolerated than TCAs;[18] they do, however, increase the risk of gastrointestinal (GI) bleeds, particularly in the very elderly and those with established risk factors such as a history of bleeds or treatment with a non-steroidal anti-inflammatory drug (NSAID), steroid or warfarin. The risk of other types of bleed such as haemorrhagic stroke may also be increased[19] (see section on 'SSRIs and bleeding' in this chapter). The elderly are also particularly prone to develop hyponatraemia[20] with SSRIs (see section on 'Antidepressant-induced hyponatraemia' in this chapter), as well as postural hypotension and falls (the clinical consequences of which may be increased by SSRI-induced osteopenia[21]). Agomelatine is effective in older patients, is well tolerated and has not been linked to hyponatraemia.[22,23] Its use is limited by the need for frequent blood sampling to check liver function tests (LFTs). Vortioxetine and duloxetine have also been shown to be effective and reasonably well tolerated in the elderly[24] but caveats related to SSRIs, above, are relevant here. A general practice database study found that, compared with SSRIs, 'other antidepressants' (venlafaxine, mirtazapine, etc.) were associated with a greater risk of a number of potentially serious side-effects in the elderly (stroke/transient ischaemic attack (TIA), fracture, seizures, attempted suicide/self-harm) as well as increased all-cause mortality;[20] the study was observational and so could not separate the effect of antidepressants from any increased risk inherent in the group of patients treated with these antidepressants. Polyunsaturated fatty acids (fish oils) are probably not effective.[25]

Ultimately, choice is determined by the individual clinical circumstances of each patient, particularly physical co-morbidity and concomitant medication (both prescribed and 'over the counter') (see section on 'Drug interactions with antidepressants' in this chapter).

CHAPTER 4

Table 4.11 Antidepressants and the elderly

	Anticholinergic side-effects (urinary retention, dry mouth, blurred vision, constipation)	Postural hypotension	Sedation	Weight gain	Safety in overdose	Other side-effects	Drug interactions
Older tricyclics[26]	Variable: moderate with nortriptyline, imipramine and dosulepin (dothiepin) Marked with others	All can cause postural hypotension Dosage titration is required	Variable: from minimal with imipramine to profound with trimipramine	All tricyclics can cause weight gain	Dothiepin and amitriptyline are the most toxic (seizures and cardiac arrhythmia)	Seizures, anticholinergic-induced cognitive impairment Increased risk of bleeds with serotonergic drugs	Mainly pharmacodynamic: increased sedation with benzodiazepines, increased hypotension with diuretics, increased constipation with other anticholinergic drugs, etc.
Lofepramine	Moderate, although constipation/sweating can be severe	Can be a problem but generally better tolerated than the older tricyclics	Minimal	Few data, but lack of spontaneous reports may indicate less potential than the older tricyclics	Relatively safe	Raised LFTs	
SSRIs[26,27]	Dry mouth can be a problem with paroxetine	Much less of a problem, but an increased risk of falls is documented with SSRIs	Can be a problem with paroxetine and fluvoxamine Unlikely with the other SSRIs	Paroxetine and possibly citalopram may cause weight gain Others are weight neutral	Safe with the possible exception of citalopram; one minor metabolite can cause QTc prolongation. Significance unknown	GI effects and headaches, hyponatraemia, increased risk of bleeds in the elderly, orofacial dyskinesia with paroxetine	Fluvoxamine, fluoxetine and paroxetine are potent inhibitors of several hepatic cytochrome enzymes (see section on 'Drug interactions with antidepressants' in this chapter). Sertraline is safer and citalopram, escitalopram and vortioxetine are safest

Others[28,29]	Minimal with mirtazapine and venlafaxine*	Venlafaxine can cause hypotension at lower doses, but it can increase BP at higher doses, as can duloxetine	Mirtazapine, mianserin and trazodone are sedative	Greatest problem is with mirtazapine, although the elderly are not particularly prone to weight gain	Venlafaxine is more toxic in overdose than SSRIs, but safer than TCAs	Insomnia and hypokalaemia with reboxetine	Duloxetine inhibits CYP2D6
	Can be rarely a problem with reboxetine*		Venlafaxine, duloxetine – neutral effects		Others are relatively safe	Nausea with venlafaxine and duloxetine	Moclobemide and venlafaxine inhibit CYP450 enzymes. Check for potential interactions
	Duloxetine* – few effects	Dizziness common with agomelatine	Agomelatine aids sleep	Low incidence with agomelatine		Weight loss and nausea with duloxetine	Reboxetine is safe
	Very low incidence with agomelatine					Possibly hepatotoxicity with agomelatine. Monitor LFTs	Agomelatine should be avoided in patients who take potent CYP1A2 inhibitors

*Noradrenergic drugs may produce 'anticholinergic' effects via noradrenaline reuptake inhibition.
BP, blood pressure; GI, gastrointestinal; LFT, liver function test; SSRI, selective serotonin reuptake inhibitor; TCA, tricyclic antidepressant.

References

1. Katona C et al. Impact of screening old people with physical illness for depression? Lancet 2000; **356**:91–92.
2. Lyketsos CG. Depression and diabetes: more on what the relationship might be. Am J Psychiatry 2010; **167**:496–497.
3. Gallo JJ et al. Long term effect of depression care management on mortality in older adults: follow-up of cluster randomized clinical trial in primary care. BMJ 2013; **346**:f2570.
4. Cattell H et al. One hundred cases of suicide in elderly people. Br J Psychiatry 1995; **166**:451–457.
5. Schatzberg A et al. A double-blind, placebo-controlled study of venlafaxine and fluoxetine in geriatric outpatients with major depression. Am J Geriatr Psychiatry 2006; **14**:361–370.
6. Wilson K et al. Antidepressant versus placebo for depressed elderly. Cochrane Database Syst Rev 2001; **2**:CD000561.
7. O'Connor CM et al. Safety and efficacy of sertraline for depression in patients with heart failure: results of the SADHART-CHF (Sertraline Against Depression and Heart Disease in Chronic Heart Failure) trial. J Am Coll Cardiol 2010; **56**:692–699.
8. Seitz DP et al. Citalopram versus other antidepressants for late-life depression: a systematic review and meta-analysis. Int J Geriatr Psychiatry 2010; **25**:1296–1305.
9. Paykel ES et al. Residual symptoms after partial remission: an important outcome in depression. Psychol Med 1995; **25**:1171–1180.
10. Mulsant BH et al. What is the optimal duration of a short-term antidepressant trial when treating geriatric depression? J Clin Psychopharmacol 2006; **26**:113–120.
11. Flint AJ et al. Recurrence of first-episode geriatric depression after discontinuation of maintenance antidepressants. Am J Psychiatry 1999; **156**:943–945.
12. Reynolds CF III et al. Maintenance treatment of major depression in old age. N Engl J Med 2006; **354**:1130–1138.
13. Old Age Depression Interest Group. How long should the elderly take antidepressants? A double-blind placebo-controlled study of continuation/prophylaxis therapy with dothiepin. Br J Psychiatry 1993; **162**:175–182.
14. National Institute for Health and Care Excellence. Depression in adults: the treatment and management of depression in adults. Clinical Guideline 90, 2009. http://www.nice.org.uk/Guidance/cg90
15. Evans M et al. Placebo-controlled treatment trial of depression in elderly physically ill patients. Int J Geriatr Psychiatry 1997; **12**:817–824.
16. Calati R et al. Antidepressants in elderly: metaregression of double-blind, randomized clinical trials. J Affect Disord 2013; **147**:1–8.
17. Tedeschini E et al. Efficacy of antidepressants for late-life depression: a meta-analysis and meta-regression of placebo-controlled randomized trials. J Clin Psychiatry 2011; **72**:1660–1668.
18. Mottram P et al. Antidepressants for depressed elderly. Cochrane Database Syst Rev 2006; **1**:CD003491.
19. Smoller JW et al. Antidepressant use and risk of incident cardiovascular morbidity and mortality among postmenopausal women in the Women's Health Initiative study. Arch Intern Med 2009; **169**:2128–2139.
20. Coupland C et al. Antidepressant use and risk of adverse outcomes in older people: population based cohort study. BMJ 2011; **343**:d4551.
21. Williams LJ et al. Selective serotonin reuptake inhibitor use and bone mineral density in women with a history of depression. Int Clin Psychopharmacol 2008; **23**:84–87.
22. Heun R et al. The efficacy of agomelatine in elderly patients with recurrent Major Depressive Disorder: a placebo-controlled study. J Clin Psychiatry 2013; **74**:587–594.
23. Laux G. The antidepressant efficacy of agomelatine in daily practice: results of the non-interventional study VIVALDI. Eur Psychiatry 2011; **26 Suppl 1**:647.
24. Katona C et al. A randomized, double-blind, placebo-controlled, duloxetine-referenced, fixed-dose study comparing the efficacy and safety of Lu AA21004 in elderly patients with major depressive disorder. Int Clin Psychopharmacol 2012; **27**:215–223.
25. Sinn N et al. Effects of n-3 fatty acids, EPA v. DHA, on depressive symptoms, quality of life, memory and executive function in older adults with mild cognitive impairment: a 6-month randomised controlled trial. Br J Nutr 2012; **107**:1682–1693.
26. Draper B et al. Tolerability of selective serotonin reuptake inhibitors: issues relevant to the elderly. Drugs Aging 2008; **25**:501–519.
27. Bose A et al. Escitalopram in the acute treatment of depressed patients aged 60 years or older. Am J Geriatr Psychiatry 2008; **16**:14–20.
28. Raskin J et al. Safety and tolerability of duloxetine at 60 mg once daily in elderly patients with major depressive disorder. J Clin Psychopharmacol 2008; **28**:32–38.
29. Johnson EM et al. Cardiovascular changes associated with venlafaxine in the treatment of late-life depression. Am J Geriatr Psychiatry 2006; **14**:796–802.

Further reading

National Institute for Health and Clinical Excellence. Depression with a chronic physical health problem. Clinical Guideline 91, 2009. http://www.nice.org.uk/CG91

Pinquart M et al. Treatments for later-life depressive conditions: a meta-analytic comparison of pharmacotherapy and psychotherapy. Am J Psychiatry 2006; **163**:1493–1501.

Van der Wurff FB et al. Electroconvulsive therapy for the depressed elderly. Cochrane Database Syst Rev 2003; **2**:CD003593.

Antidepressant discontinuation symptoms

What are discontinuation symptoms?

The term 'discontinuation symptoms' is used to describe symptoms experienced on stopping prescribed drugs that are not drugs of dependence. There is an important semantic difference between 'discontinuation' and 'withdrawal' symptoms – the latter implies addiction; the former does not. While this distinction is important for precise medical terminology, it may be irrelevant to patient experience. Discontinuation symptoms may occur after stopping many drugs, including antidepressants, and can sometimes be explained in the context of 'receptor rebound'[1,2] – e.g. an antidepressant with potent anticholinergic side-effects may be associated with diarrhoea on discontinuation.

Discontinuation symptoms may be entirely new or similar to some of the original symptoms of the illness, and so cannot be attributed to other causes. They can be broadly divided into six categories; affective (e.g. irritability); gastrointestinal (e.g. nausea); neuromotor (e.g. ataxia); vasomotor (e.g. diaphoresis); neurosensory (e.g. paraesthesia); and other neurological (e.g. increased dreaming).[2] Rarely, mania may occur.[4] Discontinuation symptoms are experienced by at least a third of patients[5-8] and are seen to some extent with all antidepressants,[9] with the possible exceptions of agomelatine[10] and vortioxetine.[11]

The onset of symptoms is usually within 5 days of stopping treatment (depending on the half-life of the antidepressant) or occasionally during taper or after missed doses[12,13] (short half-life drugs only). Symptoms can vary in form and intensity and occur in any combination. They are usually mild and self-limiting, but can occasionally be severe and prolonged. The perception of symptom severity is probably made worse by the absence of forewarnings. Some symptoms are more likely with individual drugs (Table 4.12). Symptoms can be quantified using the Discontinuation–Emergent Signs and Symptoms (DESS) scale.[6]

Agomelatine seems to be associated with a very low, if any, risk of discontinuation symptoms.[10] Mirtazapine withdrawal seems to be characterised by anxiety, insomnia and nausea.[15-17] Bupropion withdrawal syndrome is similar to that seen with SSRIs. Limited data suggest vortioxetine has a low potential for withdrawal symtpoms[11] and its Summary of Product Characteristics (SPC) suggests abrupt withdrawal is possible.[18]

Clinical relevance[19]

The symptoms of a discontinuation reaction may be mistaken for a relapse of illness or the emergence of a new physical illness,[20] leading to unnecessary investigations or reintroduction of the antidepressant. Symptoms may be severe enough to interfere with daily functioning and those who have experienced discontinuation symptoms may reason (perhaps appropriately) that antidepressants are 'addictive' and not wish to accept treatment. There is also evidence of emergent suicidal thoughts on discontinuation with paroxetine.[8]

CHAPTER 4

Table 4.12 Antidepressant discontinuation symptoms

Symptoms	MAOIs	TCAs	SSRIs and related
	Common	**Common**	**Common**
	Agitation, irritability, ataxia, movement disorders, insomnia, somnolence, vivid dreams, cognitive impairment, slowed speech, pressured speech	Flu-like symptoms (chills, myalgia, excessive sweating, headache, nausea), insomnia, excessive dreaming	Flu-like symptoms, 'shock-like' sensations, dizziness exacerbated by movement, insomnia, excessive (vivid) dreaming, irritability, crying spells
	Occasionally	**Occasionally**	**Occasionally**
	Hallucinations, paranoid delusions	Movement disorders, mania, cardiac arrhythmia	Movement disorders, problems with concentration and memory
Drugs most commonly associated with discontinuation symptoms	All	Amitriptyline Imipramine	Paroxetine Venlafaxine
	Tranylcypromine is partly metabolised to amfetamine and is therefore associated with a true 'withdrawal syndrome'. Delirium is common[14]		

Who is most at risk?[19,20]

Although anyone can experience discontinuation symptoms, the risk is increased in those prescribed short half-life drugs[6,12,21–24] (e.g. paroxetine, venlafaxine), particularly if they do not take them regularly. Two-thirds of patients prescribed antidepressants skip a few doses from time to time,[25] and many patients stop their antidepressant abruptly.[5] The risk is also increased in those who have been taking antidepressants for 8 weeks or longer,[26] those who have developed anxiety symptoms at the start of antidepressant therapy (particularly with SSRIs), those receiving other centrally acting medication (e.g. antihypertensives, antihistamines, antipsychotics), children and adolescents, and those who have experienced discontinuation symptoms before.

Antidepressant discontinuation symptoms are common in neonates born to women taking antidepressants (see section on 'Pregnancy' in Chapter 7).

How to avoid discontinuation symptoms[19–21]

Generally, antidepressant therapy should be discontinued over at least a 4-week period (this is not required with fluoxetine).[12] The shorter the half-life of the drug, the more important that this rule is followed. The end of the taper may need to be slower, as symptoms may not appear until the reduction in the total daily dosage of the antidepressant is (proportionately) substantial. Patients receiving MAOIs may need to be tapered over a longer period. Tranylcypromine may be particularly difficult to stop.[14] At-risk patients (see above) may need a slower taper. Agomelatine and vortioxetine can probably be stopped abruptly.

Many people suffer symptoms despite slow withdrawal and even if they have received adequate education regarding discontinuation symptoms.[8,23] For these patients, the option of abrupt withdrawal should be discussed. Some may prefer to face a week or two of intense symptoms rather than months of less severe discontinuation effects.

How to treat discontinuation symptoms[19,20]

There are few systematic studies in this area. Treatment is pragmatic. If symptoms are mild, reassure the patient that these symptoms are common after discontinuing an antidepressant and will pass in a few days. If symptoms are severe, reintroduce the original antidepressant (or another with a longer half-life from the same class) and taper gradually while monitoring for symptoms.

Some evidence supports the use of anticholinergic agents in tricyclic withdrawal[27] and fluoxetine for symptoms associated with stopping clomipramine[28] or venlafaxine[29] – fluoxetine, having a longer plasma half-life, seems to be associated with a lower incidence of discontinuation symptoms than other similar drugs.[30]

Key points that patients should know

- Antidepressants are not addictive (a survey of 1946 people across the UK conducted in 1997 found that 74% thought that antidepressants were addictive[3]). Note, however, that the semantic and categorical distinctions between addiction and the withdrawal symptoms seen with antidepressants may be unimportant to patients.
- Patients should be informed that they may experience discontinuation symptoms (and the most likely symptoms associated with the drug that they are taking) when they stop their antidepressant.
- Short half-life antidepressants should not generally be stopped abruptly, although some patients may prefer to risk a short period of intense symptoms rather than a prolonged period of milder symptoms.
- Discontinuation symptoms can occur after missed doses if the antidepressant prescribed has a short half-life. A very few patients experience pre-dose discontinuation symptoms which provoke the taking of the antidepressant at an earlier time each day.

References

1. Blier P et al. Physiologic mechanisms underlying the antidepressant discontinuation syndrome. J Clin Psychiatry 2006; **67 Suppl 4**:8–13.
2. Delgado PL. Monoamine depletion studies: implications for antidepressant discontinuation syndrome. J Clin Psychiatry 2006; **67 Suppl 4**: 22–26.
3. Paykel ES et al. Changes in public attitudes to depression during the Defeat Depression Campaign. Br J Psychiatry 1998; **173**:519–522.
4. Narayan V et al. Antidepressant discontinuation manic states: a critical review of the literature and suggested diagnostic criteria. J Psychopharmacol 2011; **25**:306–313.
5. van Geffen, EC et al. Discontinuation symptoms in users of selective serotonin reuptake inhibitors in clinical practice: tapering versus abrupt discontinuation. Eur J Clin Pharmacol 2005; **61**:303–307.
6. Fava M. Prospective studies of adverse events related to antidepressant discontinuation. J Clin Psychiatry 2006; **67 Suppl 4**:14–21.

CHAPTER 4

7. Perahia DG et al. Symptoms following abrupt discontinuation of duloxetine treatment in patients with major depressive disorder. J Affect Disord 2005; **89**:207–212.

8. Tint A et al. The effect of rate of antidepressant tapering on the incidence of discontinuation symptoms: a randomised study. J Psychopharmacol 2008; **22**:330–332.

9. Taylor D et al. Antidepressant withdrawal symptoms – telephone calls to a national medication helpline. J Affect Disord 2006; **95**:129–133.

10. Goodwin GM et al. Agomelatine prevents relapse in patients with major depressive disorder without evidence of a discontinuation syndrome: a 24-week randomized, double-blind, placebo-controlled trial. J Clin Psychiatry 2009; **70**:1128–1137.

11. Jain R et al. A randomized, double-blind, placebo-controlled 6-wk trial of the efficacy and tolerability of 5 mg vortioxetine in adults with major depressive disorder. Int J Neuropsychopharmacol 2013; **16**:313–321.

12. Rosenbaum JF et al. Selective serotonin reuptake inhibitor discontinuation syndrome: a randomized clinical trial. Biol Psychiatry 1998; **44**:77–87.

13. Michelson D et al. Interruption of selective serotonin reuptake inhibitor treatment. Double-blind, placebo-controlled trial. Br J Psychiatry 2000; **176**:363–368.

14. Gahr M et al. Withdrawal and discontinuation phenomena associated with tranylcypromine: a systematic review. Pharmacopsychiatry 2013; **46**:123–129.

15. Berigan TR. Mirtazapine-associated withdrawal symptoms: a case report. Prim Care Companion J Clin Psychiatry 2001; **3**:143.

16. Benazzi F. Mirtazapine withdrawal symptoms. Can J Psychiatry 1998; **43**:525.

17. Berigan TR et al. Bupropion-associated withdrawal symptoms: a case report. Prim Care Companion J Clin Psychiatry 1999; **1**:50–51.

18. Takeda Pharmaceuticals America Inc. Highlights of Prescribing Information. Brintellix (vortioxetine) tablets. http://www.us.brintellix.com/

19. Lejoyeux M et al. Antidepressant withdrawal syndrome: recognition, prevention and management. CNS Drugs 1996; **5**:278–292.

20. Haddad PM. Antidepressant discontinuation syndromes. Drug Saf 2001; **24**:183–197.

21. Sir A et al. Randomized trial of sertraline versus venlafaxine XR in major depression: efficacy and discontinuation symptoms. J Clin Psychiatry 2005; **66**:1312–1320.

22. Baldwin DS et al. A double-blind, randomized, parallel-group, flexible-dose study to evaluate the tolerability, efficacy and effects of treatment discontinuation with escitalopram and paroxetine in patients with major depressive disorder. Int Clin Psychopharmacol 2006; **21**:159–169.

23. Fava GA et al. Effects of gradual discontinuation of selective serotonin reuptake inhibitors in panic disorder with agoraphobia. Int J Neuropsychopharmacol 2007; **10**:835–838.

24. Montgomery SA et al. Discontinuation symptoms and taper/poststudy-emergent adverse events with desvenlafaxine treatment for major depressive disorder. Int Clin Psychopharmacol 2009; **24**:296–305.

25. Meijer WE et al. Spontaneous lapses in dosing during chronic treatment with selective serotonin reuptake inhibitors. Br J Psychiatry 2001; **179**:519–522.

26. Kramer JC et al. Withdrawal symptoms following discontinuation of imipramine therapy. Am J Psychiatry 1961; **118**:549–550.

27. Dilsaver, SC et al. Antidepressant withdrawal symptoms treated with anticholinergic agents. Am J Psychiatry 1983; **140**:249–251

28. Benazzi F. Fluoxetine for clomipramine withdrawal symptoms. Am J Psychiatry 1999; **156**:661–662.

29. Giakas WJ et al. Intractable withdrawal from venlafaxine treated with fluoxetine. Psychiatr Ann 1997; **27**:85–93.

30. Coupland NJ et al. Serotonin reuptake inhibitor withdrawal. J Clin Psychopharmacol 1996; **16**:356–362.

Further reading

Blier P et al. Physiologic mechanisms underlying the antidepressant discontinuation syndrome. J Clin Psychiatry 2006; **67** Suppl 4:8–13.

Haddad PM et al. Recognising and managing antidepressant discontinuation symptoms. Adv Psychiatr Treat 2007; **13**:447–457.

Schatzberg AF et al. Antidepressant discontinuation syndrome: consensus panel recommendations for clinical management and additional research. J Clin Psychiatry 2006; **67** Suppl 4:27–30.

Shelton RC. The nature of the discontinuation syndrome associated with antidepressant drugs. J Clin Psychiatry 2006; **67** Suppl 4:3–7.

CHAPTER 4

Antidepressant prophylaxis

First episode

A single episode of depression should be treated for at least 6–9 months after full remission.[1] If antidepressant therapy is stopped immediately on recovery, 50% of patients experience a return of their depressive symptoms within 3–6 months.[1,2] Even non-continuous use of antidepressants during the first 6 months of treatment predicts higher rates of relapse.[3]

Recurrent depression

Of those patients who have one episode of major depression, 50–85% will go on to have a second episode, and 80–90% of those who have a second episode will have a third.[4] Many factors are known to increase the risk of recurrence, including a family history of depression, recurrent dysthymia, concurrent non-affective psychiatric illness, female gender, long episode duration, degree of treatment resistance,[5] chronic medical illness and social factors (e.g. lack of confiding relationships and psychosocial stressors). Some prescription drugs may precipitate depression.[5,6]

Figure 4.4 outlines the risk of recurrence for multiple-episode patients: those recruited to the study had already experienced at least three episodes of depression, with 3 years or less between episodes.[7,8] People with depression are at increased risk of cardiovascular disease.[9] Suicide mortality is significantly increased over population norms.

A meta-analysis of antidepressant continuation studies[10] concluded that continuing treatment with antidepressants reduces the odds of depressive relapse by around two-thirds, which is approximately equal to halving the absolute risk. A later meta-analysis of 54 studies produced almost exactly the same results: odds of relapse were reduced by 65%.[11] The risk of relapse is greatest in the first few months after discontinuation; this holds true irrespective of the duration of prior treatment.[12] Benefits persist at 36 months and beyond and seem to be similar across heterogeneous patient groups (first episode, multiple episode and chronic), although none of the studies included first-episode

CHAPTER 4

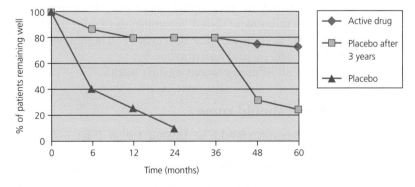

Figure 4.4 The risk of recurrence of depression in multi-episode patients. Patients had experienced at least three episodes of depression with 3 years or less between episodes.

patients only. Specific studies in first-episode patients are required to confirm that treatment beyond 6–9 months confers additional benefit in this patient group. Most data are for adults.

An RCT of maintenance treatment in elderly patients, many of whom were first episode, found continuation treatment with antidepressants beneficial over 2 years with a similar effect size to that seen in adults.[13] One small RCT (n = 22) demonstrated benefit from prophylactic antidepressants in adolescents.[14]

Many patients who might benefit from maintenance treatment with antidepressants do not receive them.[15] Assuring optimal management of long-term depression vastly reduces mortality associated with the condition.[16]

Potential disadvantages of long-term antidepressants include an increased risk of GI and cerebral haemorrhage (see section on 'SSRIs and bleeding' in this chapter) and an additional risk of interaction with co-prescribed drugs likely to increase risk of bleeding or hyponatraemia.

NICE recommends that:[17]

- patients who have had two or more episodes of depression in the recent past, and who have experienced significant functional impairment during these episodes, should be advised to continue antidepressants for at least 2 years
- patients on maintenance treatment should be re-evaluated, taking into account age, co-morbid conditions and other risk factors in the decision to continue maintenance treatment beyond 2 years.

Dose for prophylaxis

Adults should receive the same dose as used for acute treatment.[1] There is some evidence to support the use of lower doses in elderly patients: dosulepin 75 mg/day offers effective prophylaxis[18] but is now rarely used. There is no evidence to support the use of lower than standard doses of SSRIs.[19]

Relapse rates after ECT are similar to those after stopping antidepressants.[20] Antidepressant prophylaxis will be required, ideally with a different drug from the one that failed to get the patient well in the first instance, although good data in this area are lacking.

Lithium also has some efficacy in the prophylaxis of unipolar depression; efficacy relative to antidepressants is unknown.[21] NICE recommends that lithium should not be used as the sole prophylactic drug in unipolar depression.[17] There is some support for the use of a combination of lithium and nortriptyline.[22]

Maintenance treatment with lithium protects against suicide.[1]

Key points that patients should know

- A single episode of depression should be treated for at least 6–9 months after remission.
- The risk of recurrence of depressive illness is high and increases with each episode.
- Those who have had multiple episodes may require treatment for many years.
- The chances of staying well are greatly increased by taking antidepressants.

- Antidepressants are:
  - effective
  - not addictive
  - not known to lose their efficacy over time
  - not known to cause new long-term side-effects.

- Medication needs to be continued at the treatment dose. If side-effects are intolerable, it may be possible to find a more suitable alternative.

- If patients decide to stop their medication, this must not be done abruptly, as this may lead to unpleasant discontinuation effects (see section on 'Antidepressant discontinuation symptoms' in this chapter) and confers a higher risk of relapse.[23] The medication needs to be reduced slowly under the supervision of a doctor.

References

1. Anderson IM et al. Evidence-based guidelines for treating depressive disorders with antidepressants: a revision of the 2000 British Association for Psychopharmacology guidelines. J Psychopharmacol 2008; **22**:343–396.
2. Reimherr FW et al. Optimal length of continuation therapy in depression: a prospective assessment during long-term fluoxetine treatment. Am J Psychiatry 1998; **155**:1247–1253.
3. Kim KH et al. The effects of continuous antidepressant treatment during the first 6 months on relapse or recurrence of depression. J Affect Disord 2011; **132**:121–129.
4. Forshall S et al. Maintenance pharmacotherapy of unipolar depression. Psychiatr Bull 1999; **23**:370–373.
5. National Institute for Health and Clinical Excellence. Depression in adults with a chronic physical health problem: treatment and management. Clinical Guideline 91, 2009. http://www.nice.org.uk/CG91
6. Patten SB et al. Drug-induced depression. Psychother Psychosom 1997; **66**:63–73.
7. Frank E et al. Three-year outcomes for maintenance therapies in recurrent depression. Arch Gen Psychiatry 1990; **47**:1093–1099.
8. Kupfer DJ et al. Five-year outcome for maintenance therapies in recurrent depression. Arch Gen Psychiatry 1992; **49**:769–773.
9. Taylor D. Antidepressant drugs and cardiovascular pathology: a clinical overview of effectiveness and safety. Acta Psychiatr Scand 2008; **118**:434–442.
10. Geddes JR et al. Relapse prevention with antidepressant drug treatment in depressive disorders: a systematic review. Lancet 2003; **361**:653–661.
11. Glue P et al. Meta-analysis of relapse prevention antidepressant trials in depressive disorders. Aust NZ J Psychiatry 2010; **44**:697–705.
12. Keller MB et al. The Prevention of Recurrent Episodes of Depression with Venlafaxine for Two Years (PREVENT) Study: outcomes from the 2-year and combined maintenance phases. J Clin Psychiatry 2007; **68**:1246–1256.
13. Reynolds CF III et al. Maintenance treatment of major depression in old age. N Engl J Med 2006; **354**:1130–1138.
14. Cheung A et al. Maintenance study for adolescent depression. J Child Adolesc Psychopharmacol 2008; **18**:389–394.
15. Holma IA et al. Maintenance pharmacotherapy for recurrent major depressive disorder: 5-year follow-up study. Br J Psychiatry 2008; **193**:163–164.
16. Gallo JJ et al. Long term effect of depression care management on mortality in older adults: follow-up of cluster randomized clinical trial in primary care. BMJ 2013; **346**:f2570.
17. National Institute for Health and Clinical Excellence. Depression: the treatment and management of depression in adults (update). Clinical Guideline 90, 2009. http://www.nice.org.uk/
18. Old Age Depression Interest Group. How long should the elderly take antidepressants? A double-blind placebo-controlled study of continuation/prophylaxis therapy with dothiepin. Br J Psychiatry 1993; **162**:175–182.
19. Franchini L et al. Dose-response efficacy of paroxetine in preventing depressive recurrences: a randomized, double-blind study. J Clin Psychiatry 1998; **59**:229–232.
20. Nobler MS et al. Refractory depression and electroconvulsive therapy. In: Nolen WA, Zohar J, Roose SP, eds. Refractory Depression: Current Strategies and Future Directions. Chichester: John Wiley & Sons Ltd; 1994, p.69–81.
21. Cipriani A et al. Lithium versus antidepressants in the long-term treatment of unipolar affective disorder. Cochrane Database Syst Rev 2006; **4**:CD003492.
22. Sackeim HA et al. Continuation pharmacotherapy in the prevention of relapse following electroconvulsive therapy: a randomized controlled trial. JAMA 2001; **285**:1299–1307.
23. Baldessarini RJ et al. Illness risk following rapid versus gradual discontinuation of antidepressants. Am J Psychiatry 2010; **167**:934–941.

Antidepressants: alternative routes of administration

In rare cases, patients may be unable or unwilling to take antidepressants orally, and alternative treatments including psychological interventions and ECT are either impractical or contraindicated.

One such scenario is depression in the medically ill,[1] particularly in those who have undergone surgical resection procedures affecting the GI tract. Where the intra-gastric (IG) route is used, antidepressants can usually be crushed and administered. If an intra-jejunal (IJ) tube is used then more care is required because of changes in pharmacokinetics; there are few data on the exact site of absorption for the majority of antidepressants. In clinical practice it is often assumed (perhaps wrongly) that administration via the IJ route is likely to result in the same absorption characteristics as via the oral or IG route.

Very few non-oral formulations are available as commercial products. Most formulations do not have UK licences and may be very difficult to obtain, being available only through pharmaceutical importers or from Specials manufacturers. In addition, the use of these preparations beyond their licence or in the absence of a licence usually means that accountability for adverse effects lies with the prescriber. As a consequence, non-oral administration of antidepressants should be undertaken only when absolutely necessary. Table 4.13 shows possible alternative formulations and routes of administration.

Alternative antidepressant delivery methods

Sublingual

There are a small number of case reports supporting the effectiveness of **fluoxetine** liquid used sublingually in depressed, medically compromised patients.[2] In these reports doses of up to 60 mg a day produced plasma fluoxetine and norfluoxetine levels towards the lower end of the proposed therapeutic range.[2] There are no published data supporting the use of other (low-volume) liquid antidepressant formulations sublingually. If other antidepressants were to be used then it would be advisable to carry out plasma level monitoring of the antidepressant to assess the extent of sublingual absorption.

Intravenous and intramuscular injections

Intravenous **citalopram** followed by maintenance oral citalopram is a clinically useful treatment strategy for severely depressed, hospitalised patients.[3] The IV preparation appears to be well tolerated with the most common adverse events being nausea, headache, tremor and somnolence, similar to oral administration.[4,5] A case report of a 65-year-old man describes acute hyperkinetic delirium associated with IV citalopram.[6] Intravenous **escitalopram** also exists although studies reported to date are pharmacokinetic studies.[7] Note that oral citalopram is associated with a higher risk of QTc prolongation than other SSRIs; if used IV in a medically compromised patient, electrocardiogram (ECG) monitoring is recommended.

Table 4.13 Alternative formulations and routes of administration of antidepressants

Drug name and route	Dosing information	Manufacturer	Notes
Sublingual fluoxetine	Doses up to 60 mg a day	Use liquid fluoxetine preparation	Plasma levels may be slightly lower compared with oral dosing
Intravenous amitriptyline	25–100 mg given in 250 mL NaCl 0.9% by slow infusion over 120 minutes	Contact local importer	Adverse effects tend to be dose-related and are largely similar to the oral formulation. At higher doses drowsiness and dizziness occur.
	The intramuscular preparation has been used intravenously by dissolving in 5% glucose and given by slow infusion.	Elavil® Zeneca	Bradycardia may occur with doses around 100 mg. ECG monitoring recommended
Intravenous clomipramine	25 mg/2 mL injection. Starting dose is 25 mg diluted in 500 mL NaCL 0.9% by slow infusion over 90 minutes. Increased to 250–300 mg in increments of 25 mg/day over 10–14 days[43,44]	Novartis Defiante	The most common reported side-effects are similar to the oral formulation, which included nausea, sweating, restlessness, flushing, drowsiness, fatigue, abdominal distress and nervousness. ECG monitoring recommended
Intravenous citalopram	40 mg/mL injection. Doses from 20 to 40 mg in 250 mL NaCL 0.9% or glucose 5%. Doses up to 80 mg have been used for OCD. Rate of infusion is 20 mg per hour	Lundbeck	The most commonly reported side-effects are nausea, headache, tremor and somnolence similar to adverse effects of the oral preparation. A case of acute hyperkinetic delirium has also been reported. ECG monitoring recommended
Intravenous escitalopram	10 mg slow infusion over 60 minutes	Lundbeck	Studies to date have only looked at pharmacokinetic profile. ECG monitoring recommended
Intravenous mirtazapine	6 mg/2 mL infusion solution. 15 mg/5 mL infusion solution. Dose 15 mg in glucose 5% over 60 minutes	Contact local importer	The most common reported side-effects are nausea, sedation and dizziness similar to side-effects of the oral preparation
Intramuscular amitriptyline	Amitriptyline 10 mg/mL. Elavil®	Zeneca	IM preparations are very rarely used because of the requirement of a high volume. Many preparations have been discontinued
Amitriptyline gel	50 mmol/L or 100 mmol/L gel 5% amitriptyline 5% lidocaine gel	Prepared by manufacturing pharmacies	No data on plasma amitriptyline levels. This preparation has been used for pain relief rather than antidepressant activity
Nortriptyline patches	25–75 mg per 24 hour patch	Clinical trial use only	This preparation has been used for smoking cessation rather than antidepressant activity
Imipramine or doxepin nanoemulsion	Unknown. Antidepressant concentration 3% (w/w)	Clinical trial use only	Formulated for potential analgesic therapy rather than antidepressant activity

CHAPTER 4

Continued

Table 14.13 (*Continued*)

Drug name and route	Dosing information	Manufacturer	Notes
Transdermal selegiline	6 mg/24 hours, 9 mg/24 hours, 12 mg/24 hours. Starting dose is 6 mg/24 hours. Titration to higher doses in 3 mg/24 hours increments at ≥2-week intervals, up to a maximum dose of 12 mg/24 hours[35]	Bristol Myers Squibb	The 6 mg/24 hour dose does not require a tyramine-restricted diet. At higher doses, although no hypertensive crisis reactions have been reported, the manufacturer recommends avoiding high tyramine content food substances. Application site reactions and insomnia are the most common reported side-effects
Rectal amitriptyline	Doses up to 50 mg bd	Suppositories have been manufactured by pharmacies	Very little information on rectal administration. Largely in the form of case reports
Rectal clomipramine	No detailed information available		
Rectal imipramine	No detailed information available		
Rectal doxepin	No detailed information available	Capsules have been used rectally	
Rectal trazodone	No detailed information available	Suppositories have been manufactured by pharmacies	Trazodone in the rectal formulation has been used for post-operative or cancer pain control rather than antidepressant activity

bd, twice a day; ECG, electrocardiogram; IM, intramuscular; OCD, obsessive compulsive disorder.

Mirtazapine is also available as an intravenous preparation. It has been administered by slow infusion at a dose of 15 mg a day for 14 days in two studies and was well tolerated in depressed patients.[8,9] There are reports of IV mirtazapine 6–30 mg/day being used to treat hyperemesis gravidarum.[10,11]

Amitriptyline is available as both an IV and IM injection (IM injection has been given IV) and both routes have been used in the treatment of post-operative pain and depression.[12] The concentration of the IM preparation (10 mg/mL) necessitates a high-volume injection to achieve antidepressant doses; this clearly discourages its use intramuscularly.[13] **Clomipramine** is the most widely studied IV antidepressant. Pulse loading doses of intravenous clomipramine have been shown to produce a larger, more rapid decrease in obsessive compulsive disorder symptoms compared with oral doses.[14,15] The potential for serious cardiac side-effects when using any tricyclic antidepressant intravenously necessitates monitoring of pulse, blood pressure and ECG.

The primary rationale for IV administration of antidepressants is the more rapid onset of antidepressant action. However, most trials have generally not supported this assumption.[16] Intravenous formulations also avoid the first-pass effect, leading to higher drug plasma levels[14,17] and perhaps greater response.[17,18] However, negative reports also exist.[3,18,19] The placebo effect associated with IV administration is known to be large.[20]

Note that calculating the correct parenteral dose of antidepressants is difficult given the variable first-pass effect to which oral drugs are usually subjected. Parenteral doses can be expected to be much lower than oral doses and give the same effect.

Extensive studies of IV **ketamine**, a glutamate N-methyl-D-aspartate (NMDA) receptor antagonist, have demonstrated rapid, albeit short-lived antidepressant effects; however, more information is required on safety, dosing and duration of response before implementation into clinical practice.[21] Intravenous **scopolamine (hyoscine)** as an antidepressant has also been investigated and has produced rapid antidepressant effects within 72 hours in both unipolar and bipolar depression.[22-24] Again, further investigation is needed before use in clinical practice.

Transdermal

Amitriptyline usually in the form of a gel preparation is used in pain clinics as an adjuvant in the treatment of a variety of chronic pain conditions.[25,26] It is usually prepared as a 50 mmol/L or 100 mmol/L gel with or without lidocaine and although it has proven analgesic activity, there are no published data on the plasma levels attained via this route. **Nortriptyline** hydrochloride has been formulated as a transdermal patch for the use in smoking cessation.[27] Nanoemulsion formulations of **imipramine** and of **doxepin** have also been formulated for transdermal delivery for use as an analgesic.[28] At the time of writing, there are no published studies on nortriptyline patches or imipramine or doxepin nanoemulsions in depression.

Oral selegiline at doses greater than 20 mg/day may be an effective antidepressant, but enzyme selectivity is lost at these doses, necessitating a tyramine-restricted diet.[29,30] **Selegiline** can be administered transdermally; it is efficacious and tolerable and delivers 25–30% of the selegiline content over 24 hours and steady-state plasma concentrations are achieved within 5 days of daily dosing.[31] This route bypasses first-pass metabolism, thereby providing a higher, more sustained plasma concentration of selegiline while being relatively sparing of the gastrointestinal MAO-A system;[32,33] there seems to be no need for tyramine restriction when the lower dose patch (6 mg/24 hour) is used and there have been no reports of hypertensive reactions even with the higher dose patch. However, because safety experience with the higher selegiline transdermal system (STS) doses (9 mg/24 hour and 12 mg/24 hour) is more limited, it is recommended that patients using these patches should avoid very high tyramine content food substances.[34] Age and gender do not affect the pharmacokinetics of the STS.[35,36] When administered transdermally, application site reactions and insomnia are the two most commonly reported adverse effects; both are dose related, usually mild or moderate in intensity and do not lead to dropout from treatment.[34,35,37,38] There appear to be no clinically significant effects of the STS on sexual function or weight gain.[35,38] Advantages of the STS include once-daily dosing, visual indicator of adherence and its potential in dysphagic patients.[36]

Rectal

The rectal mucosa lacks the extensive villi and microvilli of other parts of the gastrointestinal tract, limiting its surface area. Therefore rectal agents need to be in a formulation that maximises the extent of contact the active ingredient will have with the

CHAPTER 4

mucosa. There are no readily available antidepressant suppositories, but extemporaneous preparation is possible. For example, **amitriptyline** (in cocoa butter) suppositories have been manufactured by a hospital pharmacy and administered in a dose of 50 mg twice daily with some subjective success.[39,40] **Doxepin** capsules have been administered via the rectal route directly in the treatment of cancer-related pain (without a special formulation) and produced plasma concentrations within the supposed therapeutic range.[41] Similarly, it has been reported that extemporaneously manufactured **imipramine** and **clomipramine** suppositories produced plasma levels comparable with the oral route of administration.[42] **Trazodone** has also been successfully administered in a suppository formulation post-operatively for a patient who was stable on the oral formulation prior to surgery.[40,41]

References

1. Cipriani A et al. Metareview on short-term effectiveness and safety of antidepressants for depression: an evidence-based approach to inform clinical practice. Can J Psychiatry 2007; 52:553–562.
2. Pakyurek M et al. Sublingually administered fluoxetine for major depression in medically compromised patients. Am J Psychiatry 1999; 156:1833–1834.
3. Baumann P et al. A double-blind double-dummy study of citalopram comparing infusion versus oral administration. J Affect Disord 1998; 49:203–210.
4. Guelfi JD et al. Efficacy of intravenous citalopram compared with oral citalopram for severe depression. Safety and efficacy data from a double-blind, double-dummy trial. J Affect Disord 2000; 58:201–209.
5. Kasper S et al. Intravenous antidepressant treatment: focus on citalopram. Eur Arch Psychiatry Clin Neurosci 2002; 252:105–109.
6. Delic M et al. Delirium during i. v. citalopram treatment: a case report. Pharmacopsychiatry 2013; 46:37–38.
7. Sogaard B et al. The pharmacokinetics of escitalopram after oral and intravenous administration of single and multiple doses to healthy subjects. J Clin Pharmacol 2005; 45:1400–1406.
8. Konstantinidis A et al. Intravenous mirtazapine in the treatment of depressed inpatients. Eur Neuropsychopharmacol 2002; 12:57–60.
9. Muhlbacher M et al. Intravenous mirtazapine is safe and effective in the treatment of depressed inpatients. Neuropsychobiology 2006; 53:83–87.
10. Guclu S et al. Mirtazapine use in resistant hyperemesis gravidarum: report of three cases and review of the literature. Arch Gynecol Obstet 2005; 272:298–300.
11. Schwarzer V et al. Treatment resistant hyperemesis gravidarum in a patient with type 1 diabetes mellitus: neonatal withdrawal symptoms after successful antiemetic therapy with mirtazapine. Arch Gynecol Obstet 2008; 277:67–69.
12. Collins JJ et al. Intravenous amitriptyline in pediatrics. J Pain Symptom Manage 1995; 10:471–475.
13. Elavil. http://www.rxlist.com
14. Deisenhammer EA et al. Intravenous versus oral administration of amitriptyline in patients with major depression. J Clin Psychopharmacol 2000; 20:417–422.
15. Koran LM et al. Pulse loading versus gradual dosing of intravenous clomipramine in obsessive-compulsive disorder. Eur Neuropsychopharmacol 1998; 8:121–126.
16. Moukaddam NJ et al. Intravenous antidepressants: a review. Depress Anxiety 2004; 19:1–9.
17. Koran LM et al. Rapid benefit of intravenous pulse loading of clomipramine in obsessive-compulsive disorder. Am J Psychiatry 1997; 154:396–401.
18. Svestka J et al. [Citalopram (Seropram) in tablet and infusion forms in the treatment of major depression]. Cesk Psychiatr 1993; 89:331–339.
19. Pollock BG et al. Acute antidepressant effect following pulse loading with intravenous and oral clomipramine. Arch Gen Psychiatry 1989; 46:29–35.
20. Sallee FR et al. Pulse intravenous clomipramine for depressed adolescents: double-blind, controlled trial. Am J Psychiatry 1997; 154:668–673.
21. Murrough JW et al. Antidepressant efficacy of ketamine in treatment-resistant major depression: a two-site randomized controlled trial. Am J Psychiatry 2013; 170:1134–1142.
22. Jaffe RJ et al. Scopolamine as an antidepressant: a systematic review. Clin Neuropharmacol 2013; 36:24–26.
23. Furey ML et al. Pulsed intravenous administration of scopolamine produces rapid antidepressant effects and modest side effects. J Clin Psychiatry 2013; 74:850–851.
24. Drevets WC et al. Replication of scopolamine's antidepressant efficacy in major depressive disorder: a randomized, placebo-controlled clinical trial. Biol Psychiatry 2010; 67:432–438.
25. Gerner P et al. Topical amitriptyline in healthy volunteers. Reg Anesth Pain Med 2003; 28:289–293.

26. Ho KY et al. Topical amitriptyline versus lidocaine in the treatment of neuropathic pain. Clin J Pain 2008; **24**:51–55.

27. Melero A et al. Nortriptyline for smoking cessation: release and human skin diffusion from patches. Int J Pharmacol 2009; **378**:101–107.

28. Sandig AG et al. Transdermal delivery of imipramine and doxepin from newly oil-in-water nanoemulsions for an analgesic and anti-allodynic activity: development, characterization and in vivo evaluation. Colloids Surf B Biointerfaces 2013; **103**:558–565.

29. Sunderland T et al. High-dose selegiline in treatment-resistant older depressive patients. Arch Gen Psychiatry 1994; **51**:607–615.

30. Mann JJ et al. A controlled study of the antidepressant efficacy and side effects of (-)-deprenyl. A selective monoamine oxidase inhibitor. Arch Gen Psychiatry 1989; **46**:45–50.

31. Mylan Specialty LP. Highlights of Prescribing Information: EMSAM®(Selegiline Transdermal System) Continous Delivery for Once-Daily Application. http://www.emsam.com/

32. Wecker L et al. Transdermal selegiline: targeted effects on monoamine oxidases in the brain. Biol Psychiatry 2003; **54**:1099–1104.

33. Azzaro AJ et al. Pharmacokinetics and absolute bioavailability of selegiline following treatment of healthy subjects with the selegiline transdermal system (6 mg/24 h): a comparison with oral selegiline capsules. J Clin Pharmacol 2007; **47**:1256–1267.

34. Amsterdam JD et al. Selegiline transdermal system in the prevention of relapse of major depressive disorder: a 52-week, double-blind, placebo-substitution, parallel-group clinical trial. J Clin Psychopharmacol 2006; **26**:579–586.

35. Nandagopal JJ et al. Selegiline transdermal system: a novel treatment option for major depressive disorder. Expert Opin Pharmacother 2009; **10**:1665–1673.

36. VanDenBerg CM. The transdermal delivery system of monoamine oxidase inhibitors. J Clin Psychiatry 2012; **73** Suppl 1:25–30.

37. Robinson DS et al. The selegiline transdermal system in major depressive disorder: a systematic review of safety and tolerability. J Affect Disord 2008; **105**:15–23.

38. Citrome L et al. Placing transdermal selegiline for major depressive disorder into clinical context: number needed to treat, number needed to harm, and likelihood to be helped or harmed. J Affect Disord 2013; **151**:409–417.

39. Adams S. Amitriptyline suppositories. N Engl J Med 1982; **306**:996.

40. Mirassou MM. Rectal antidepressant medication in the treatment of depression. J Clin Psychiatry 1998; **59**:29.

41. Storey P et al. Rectal doxepin and carbamazepine therapy in patients with cancer. N Engl J Med 1992; **327**:1318–1319.

42. Chaumeil JC et al. Formulation of suppositories containing imipramine and clomipramine chlorhydrates. Drug Dev Ind Pharm 1988; **15-17**:2225–2239.

43. Lopes R et al. The utility of intravenous clomipramine in a case of Cotard's syndrome. Rev Bras Psiquiatr 2013; **35**:212–213.

44. Fallon BA et al. Intravenous clomipramine for obsessive-compulsive disorder refractory to oral clomipramine: a placebo-controlled study. Arch Gen Psychiatry 1998; **55**:918–924.

CHAPTER 4

Antidepressants: swapping and stopping

General guidelines

- All antidepressants have the potential to cause withdrawal phenomena.[1] When taken continuously *for 6 weeks or longer*, antidepressants should not be stopped abruptly unless a serious adverse event has occurred (e.g. cardiac arrhythmia with a tricyclic). (See section on 'Antidepressant discontinuation symptoms' in this chapter.)
- Although abrupt cessation is generally not recommended, slow tapering may not reduce the incidence or severity of discontinuation reactions.[2] Some patients may therefore prefer abrupt cessation and a shorter discontinuation syndrome.
- When changing from one antidepressant to another, abrupt withdrawal should usually be avoided. Cross-tapering is preferred, in which the dose of the ineffective or poorly tolerated drug is slowly reduced while the new drug is slowly introduced. See Table 4.14 for an example.
- The speed of cross-tapering is best judged by monitoring patient tolerability. Few studies have been done, so caution is required.
- Note that the co-administration of some antidepressants, even when cross-tapering, is absolutely contraindicated. In other cases, theoretical risks or lack of experience preclude recommending cross-tapering.
- In some cases cross-tapering may not be considered necessary. An example is when switching from one SSRI to another: their effects are so similar that administration of the second drug is likely to ameliorate withdrawal effects of the first. In fact, the use of fluoxetine has been advocated as an abrupt switch treatment for SSRI discontinuation symptoms.[3] Abrupt cessation may also be acceptable when switching to a drug with a similar, but not identical, mode of action.[4] Thus, in some cases, abruptly stopping one antidepressant and starting another antidepressant at the usual dose may not only be well tolerated, but may also reduce the risk of discontinuation symptoms.
- Potential dangers of simultaneously administering two antidepressants include pharmacodynamic interactions (serotonin syndrome,[5–8] hypotension, drowsiness) and pharmacokinetic interactions (e.g. elevation of tricyclic plasma levels by some SSRIs). See Figure 4.5.
- The advice given in Table 4.15 should be treated with caution and patients should be very carefully monitored when switching.

Table 4.14 Changing from citalopram to mirtazapine

Example		Week 1	Week 2	Week 3	Week 4
Withdrawing citalopram	40 mg od	20 mg od	10 mg od	5 mg od	Nil
Introducing mirtazapine	Nil	15 mg od	30 mg od	30 mg od	45 mg od (if required)

od, once a day.

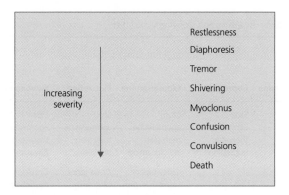

Figure 4.5 Serotonin syndrome: symptoms.[5,6]

- Agomelatine can be started immediately while tapering the dosage of a SSRI/SNRI. Early discontinuation symptoms that arise upon cessation of SSRI/SNRI can alter the patient's perception of the clinical benefit of the new antidepressant. Agomelatine should also be stopped completely before beginning another antidepressant. It does not seem to be associated with a discontinuation syndrome.[10] Given agomelatine's mode of action (melatonin agonism; $5HT_{2c}$ antagonism), it is not expected to mitigate discontinuation reactions of other antidepressants. Agomelatine can be co-administrated with other antidepressants (except co-administration with fluvoxamine which is contraindicated)
- Similarly, little information is available for switching to or from vortioxetine. See following table for suggestions on switching.

CHAPTER 4

Table 4.15 Antidepressants: swapping and stopping*

From	To Agomelatine	Bupropion	Clomipramine	Fluoxetine	Fluvoxamine	MAOIs Phenelzine Tranylcypromine Selegiline
Agomelatine[†]		Stop agomelatine then start bupropion	Stop agomelatine then start clomipramine	Stop agomelatine then start fluoxetine	Stop agomelatine then start fluvoxamine	Stop agomelatine then start MAOIs
Bupropion[‡]	Cross-taper cautiously		Cross-taper cautiously with low dose clomipramine	Cross-taper cautiously	Cross-taper cautiously	Taper and stop then wait for 2 weeks then start MAOIs
Clomipramine	Cross-taper cautiously	Cross-taper cautiously		Taper and stop then start fluoxetine at 10 mg/day	Taper and stop then start low dose fluvoxamine	Taper and stop then wait for 3 weeks then start MAOIs
Fluoxetine[§]	Cross-taper cautiously	Cross-taper cautiously	Taper and stop fluoxetine. Wait 2 weeks. Start low dose clomipramine		Taper and stop. Wait 2 weeks then start low dose fluvoxamine	Taper and stop then wait for 5–6 weeks then start MAOIs
Fluvoxamine[¶]	Taper and stop then wait for 1 week	Cross-taper cautiously	Taper and stop then start low dose clomipramine	Taper and stop then start fluoxetine at 10 mg/day		Taper and stop then wait for 1 week then start MAOIs
MAOIs Phenelzine Tranylcypromine Selegiline	Cross-taper cautiously	Taper and stop then wait for 2 weeks	Taper and stop then wait for 3 weeks	Taper and stop then wait for 2 weeks	Taper and stop then wait for 2 weeks	Taper and stop then wait for 2 weeks
Moclobemide	Cross-taper cautiously	Taper and stop then wait 24 hours	Taper and stop then wait 24 hours	Taper and stop then wait 24 hours	Taper and stop then wait 24 hours	Taper and stop, wait 24 hours then start MAOIs
Mirtazapine	Cross-taper cautiously	Cross-taper cautiously	Cross-taper cautiously	Cross-taper cautiously	Cross-taper cautiously	Taper and stop then wait for 2 weeks then start MAOIs
Reboxetine**	Cross-taper cautiously	Cross-taper cautiously	Cross-taper cautiously	Cross-taper cautiously	Cross-taper cautiously	Taper and stop then wait for 1 week then start MAOIs
Trazodone	Cross-taper cautiously	Cross-taper cautiously	Cross-taper cautiously with low dose clomipramine	Cross-taper cautiously	Cross-taper cautiously	Taper and stop then wait for 1 week

Table 4.15 (*Continued*)

Moclobemide	Mirtazapine	Reboxetine	Trazodone	Other SSRIs,†† vortioxetine	SNRIs Duloxetine Venlafaxine Desvenlafaxine	TCAs (except clomipramine)
Stop agomelatine then start moclobemide	Stop agomelatine then start mirtazapine	Stop agomelatine then start reboxetine	Stop agomelatine then start trazodone	Stop agomelatine then start SSRI	Stop agomelatine then start SNRI	Stop agomelatine then start TCA
Taper and stop then start moclobemide	Cross-taper cautiously	Cross-taper cautiously	Cross-taper cautiously	Cross-taper cautiously	Cross-taper cautiously	Cross-taper cautiously with low dose TCA
Taper and stop then wait for 1 week then start moclobemide	Cross-taper cautiously	Cross-taper cautiously	Cross-taper cautiously starting with low dose trazodone	Taper and stop then start low dose.	Taper and stop. Start low dose SNRI	Cross-taper cautiously
Taper and stop then wait for 5–6 weeks then start moclobemide	Cross-taper cautiously	Cross-taper cautiously	Cross-taper cautiously starting with low dose trazodone	Taper and stop fluoxetine. Wait 4–7 days then start low dose	Taper and stop. Start low dose SNRI¶¶	Taper and stop fluoxetine. Wait 4–7 days then start low dose
Taper and stop then wait for 1 week then start moclobemide	Cross-taper cautiously. Start mirtazapine at 15 mg	Cross-taper cautiously	Cross-taper cautiously starting with low dose trazodone	Taper and stop then start low dose SSRI	Taper and stop then start low dose SNRI¶¶	Cross-taper cautiously with low dose TCA
Taper and stop then wait for 2 weeks then start moclobemide	Taper and stop then wait for 2 weeks	Taper and stop then wait for 2 weeks	Taper and stop then wait for 2 weeks	Taper and stop then wait for 2 weeks	Taper and stop then wait for 2 weeks	Taper and stop then wait for 2 weeks†††
	Taper and stop then wait 24 hours	Taper and stop then wait 24 hours	Taper and stop then wait 24 hours	Taper and stop then wait 24 hours	Taper and stop then wait 24 hours	Taper and stop then wait 24 hours
Taper and stop then wait for 1 week then start moclobemide		Cross-taper cautiously	Cross-taper cautiously	Cross-taper cautiously	Cross-taper cautiously	Cross-taper cautiously
Taper and stop then wait for 1 week then start moclobemide	Cross-taper cautiously		Cross-taper cautiously	Cross-taper cautiously	Cross-taper cautiously	Cross-taper cautiously
Taper and stop then wait for 1 week then start moclobemide	Cross-taper cautiously	Cross-taper cautiously		Cross-taper cautiously	Cross-taper cautiously	Cross-taper cautiously with low dose TCA

CHAPTER 4

Continued

Table 4.15 (Continued)

From	To Agomelatine	Bupropion	Clomipramine	Fluoxetine	Fluvoxamine	MAOIs Phenelzine Tranylcypromine Selegiline
Other SSRIs,[†] vortioxetine[‡‡,‡‡‡]	Cross-taper cautiously	Cross-taper cautiously starting with low dose bupropion	Taper and stop then start low dose clomipramine	Taper and stop then start fluoxetine at 10 mg/day	Taper and stop then start low dose fluvoxamine	Taper and stop then wait for 1 week[§§]
SNRI Duloxetine[¶¶] Venlafaxine Desvenlafaxine	Cross-taper cautiously	Cross-taper cautiously starting with low dose bupropion	Taper and stop then start low dose clomipramine	Taper and stop then start fluoxetine at 10 mg/day	Taper and stop then start low dose fluvoxamine	Taper and stop then wait for 1 week
Tricyclics	Cross-taper cautiously	Halve dose and add bupropion and then slow withdrawal	Cross-taper cautiously	Halve dose and add fluoxetine and then slow withdrawal	Cross-taper cautiously	Taper and stop then wait for 2 weeks***
Stopping[†††]	Can be stopped abruptly	Reduce over 4 weeks	Reduce over 4 weeks	At 20 mg/day just stop. At higher doses reduce over 2 weeks	Reduce over 4 weeks	Reduce over 4 weeks or longer if necessary

Notes

*Advice given in this table is partly derived from manufacturers' information and available published data and partly theoretical. There are several factors that affect individual drug handling and caution is required in every instance.

[†]Agomelatine has no effect on monoamine uptake and no affinity for α, β adrenergic, histaminergic, cholinergic, dopaminergic and benzodiazepine receptors. The potential for interactions between agomelatine and other antidepressants is low (except contraindication with concomitant use of fluvoxamine) and it is not expected to mitigate discontinuation reactions of other antidepressants.

[§]Beware: interactions with fluoxetine may still occur for 5 weeks after stopping fluoxetine because of its long half-life.

[¶]Fluvoxamine is a potent inhibitor of CYP1A2, and to a lesser extent of CYP2C and CYP3A4, and has a high potential for interactions hence extra caution is required

**Switching to reboxetine as antidepressant monotherapy is no longer recommended.

[††]Citalopram, escitalopram, paroxetine and sertraline.

[‡‡]Limited experience with vortioxetine and extra precaution required. Particular care when switching to or from bupropion and other 2D6 inhibitors such as fluoxetine and paroxetine.[11]

[§§]Wait 3 weeks in the case of vortioxetine.[12]

[¶¶]Abrupt switch from SSRIs and venlafaxine to duloxetine is possible starting at 60 mg/day.[4]

***Wait 3 weeks in the case of imipramine.

[†††]See general guidance at the beginning of this section.

[‡‡‡]Reduce over 1 week to 10 mg/day, then stop.

MAOI, monoamine oxidase inhibitor; SNRI, selective noradrenaline reuptake inhibitor; SSRI, selective serotonin reuptake inhibitor; TCA, tricyclic antidepressant.

Table 4.15 *(Continued)*

Moclobemide	Mirtazapine	Reboxetine	Trazodone	Other SSRIs,[††] vortioxetine	SNRIs Duloxetine Venlafaxine Desvenlafaxine	TCAs (except clomipramine)
Taper and stop then wait for 1 week then start moclobemide	Cross-taper cautiously	Cross-taper cautiously	Cross-taper cautiously starting with low dose trazodone	Cross-taper cautiously starting with low dose	Cross-taper cautiously with low dose SNRI[¶¶]	Cross-taper cautiously with low dose TCA
Taper and stop then wait for 1 week then start moclobemide	Cross-taper cautiously	Cross-taper cautiously	Cross-taper cautiously	Cross-taper cautiously starting with low dose	Cross-taper cautiously with low dose SNRI[¶¶]	Cross-taper cautiously with low dose TCA
Taper and stop then wait for 1 week then start moclobemide	Cross-taper cautiously	Cross-taper cautiously	Halve dose and add trazodone and then slow withdrawal	Halve dose and add SSRI then slow withdrawal	Cross-taper cautiously starting with low dose SNRI	Cross-taper cautiously
Reduce over 4 weeks	Reduce over 4 weeks	Reduce over 4 weeks	Reduce over 4 weeks	Reduce over 4 weeks or longer if necessary[‡‡‡]	Reduce over 4 weeks or longer if necessary	Reduce over 4 weeks

CHAPTER 4

References

1. Taylor D et al. Antidepressant withdrawal symptoms – telephone calls to a national medication helpline. J Affect Disord 2006; **95**:129–133.
2. Tint A et al. The effect of rate of antidepressant tapering on the incidence of discontinuation symptoms: a randomised study. J Psychopharmacol 2008; **22**:330–332.
3. Benazzi F. Fluoxetine for the treatment of SSRI discontinuation syndrome. Int J Neuropsychopharmacol 2008; **11**:725–726.
4. Perahia DG et al. Switching to duloxetine from selective serotonin reuptake inhibitor antidepressants: a multicenter trial comparing 2 switching techniques. J Clin Psychiatry 2008; **69**:95–105.
5. Sternbach H. The serotonin syndrome. Am J Psychiatry 1991; **148**:705–713.
6. Mir S et al. Serotonin syndrome. Psychiatr Bull 1999; **23**:742–747.
7. Pan JJ et al. Serotonin syndrome induced by low-dose venlafaxine. Ann Pharmacother 2003; **37**:209–211.
8. Houlihan DJ. Serotonin syndrome resulting from coadministration of tramadol, venlafaxine, and mirtazapine. Ann Pharmacother 2004; **38**:411–413.
9. Dolder CR et al. Agomelatine treatment of major depressive disorder. Ann Pharmacother 2008; **42**:1822–1831.
10. Goodwin GM et al. Agomelatine prevents relapse in patients with major depressive disorder without evidence of a discontinuation syndrome: a 24-week randomized, double-blind, placebo-controlled trial. J Clin Psychiatry 2009; **70**:1128–1137.
11. Chen G et al. Pharmacokinetic drug interactions involving vortioxetine (Lu AA21004), a multimodal antidepressant. Clin Drug Invest 2013; **33**:727–736.
12. Citrome L. Vortioxetine for major depressive disorder: a systematic review of the efficacy and safety profile for this newly approved antidepressant – what is the number needed to treat, number needed to harm and likelihood to be helped or harmed? Int J Clin Pract 2014; **68**:60–82.

Drug interactions with antidepressants

Drugs can interact with each other in two different ways.

- **Pharmacokinetic interactions** where one drug interferes with the absorption, distribution, metabolism or elimination of another drug. This may result in a subtherapeutic effect or toxicity. The largest group of pharmacokinetic interactions involves drugs that inhibit or induce hepatic CYP450 enzymes (see Table 4.16 and Table 7.35). Other enzyme systems include FMO[1] and UGT.[2] While both of these latter enzyme systems are involved in the metabolism of psychotropic drugs, the potential for drugs to inhibit or induce these enzyme systems has been poorly studied.

  The clinical consequences of pharmacokinetic interactions in an individual patient can be difficult to predict. Some are highly clinically significant; for example when paroxetine is taken with tamoxifen, up to one extra woman in 20 will die within 5 years of stopping tamoxifen.[3] The following factors affect outcome of interactions: the degree of enzyme inhibition or induction, the pharmacokinetic properties of the affected drug and other co-administered drugs, the relationship between plasma level and pharmacodynamic effect for the affected drug, and patient-specific factors such as variability in the role of primary and secondary metabolic pathways and the presence of co-morbid physical illness.[4]

- **Pharmacodynamic interactions** where the effects of one drug are altered by another drug via physiological mechanisms such as direct competition at receptor sites (e.g. dopamine agonists with dopamine blockers negate any therapeutic effect), augmentation of the same neurotransmitter pathway (e.g. fluoxetine with tramadol or a triptan can lead to serotonin syndrome) or an effect on the physiological functioning of an organ/organ system in different ways (e.g. SSRIs impair clotting and NSAIDs irritate the gastric mucosa; when these drugs are used together, the risk of GI bleeds is increased). Most of these interactions can be easily predicted by a sound knowledge of pharmacology. An up-to-date list of important interactions can be found at the back of the BNF.

Pharmacodynamic interactions

Tricyclic antidepressants:[5,6]

- are H_1 blockers (sedative). This effect can be exacerbated by other sedative drugs or alcohol. Beware respiratory depression
- are anticholinergic (dry mouth, blurred vision, constipation). This effect can be exacerbated by other anticholinergic drugs such as antihistamines or antipsychotics. Beware cognitive impairment and GI obstruction
- are adrenergic α_1 blockers (postural hypotension). This effect can be exacerbated by other drugs that block α_1-receptors and by antihypertensive drugs in general. Beware falls. Adrenaline in combination with α_1-blockers can lead to hypertension
- are arrhythmogenic. Caution is required with other drugs that can alter cardiac conduction directly (e.g. antiarrhythmics or phenothiazines) or indirectly through a potential to cause electrolyte disturbance (e.g. diuretics)

CHAPTER 4

Table 4.16 Pharmacokinetic interactions of antidepressants with cytochromes[3,7,20]

p4501A2	p4502C	p4502D6	p4503A
Genetic polymorphism Ultra-rapid metabolisers occur	5–10% of Caucasians poor metabolisers	3–5% of Caucasians poor metabolisers	60% p450 content
Induced by:	*Induced by:*	*Induced by:*	*Induced by:*
cigarette smoke	phenytoin	carbamazepine	carbamazepine
charcoal cooking	rifampicin	phenytoin	phenytoin
carbamazepine			prednisolone
omeprazole			rifampicin
phenobarbitone			
phenytoin			
Inhibited by:	*Inhibited by:*	*Inhibited by:*	*Inhibited by:*
cimetidine	cimetidine	chlorpromazine	erythromycin
ciprofloxacin	fluoxetine	duloxetine	grapefruit juice
erythromycin	fluvoxamine	fluoxetine	norfluoxetine
fluvoxamine	sertraline	fluphenazine	fluoxetine
paroxetine		haloperidol	fluvoxamine
		paroxetine	ketoconazole
		sertraline	paroxetine
		tricyclics	sertraline
			tricyclics
Metabolises:	*Metabolises:*	*Metabolises:*	*Metabolises:*
agomelatine	agomelatine	clozapine	atorvastatin
benzodiazepines	diazepam	codeine	calcium blockers
caffeine	omeprazole	donepezil	carbamazepine
clozapine	phenytoin	haloperidol	cimetidine
haloperidol	tolbutamide	phenothiazines	clozapine
mirtazapine	tricyclics	risperidone	codeine
olanzapine	warfarin	TCA secondary amines	donepezil
theophylline		tramadol	erythromycin
tricyclics		trazodone	galantamine
warfarin		venlafaxine	methadone
		vortioxetine	mirtazapine

Table 4.16 (*Continued*)

p4501A2	p4502C	p4502D6	p4503A
		tamoxifen	risperidone
			simvastatin
			steroids
			terfenadine
			tricyclics
			valproate
			venlafaxine
			vortioxetine
			Z-hypnotics

- lower the seizure threshold. Caution is required with other proconvulsive drugs (e.g. antipsychotics) and particularly if the patient is being treated for epilepsy (higher doses of anticonvulsants may be required)
- may be serotonergic (e.g. amitriptyline, clomipramine). There is the potential for these drugs to interact with other serotonergic drugs (e.g. tramadol, SSRIs, selegiline, triptans) to cause serotonin syndrome.

SSRIs/SNRIs:[7,8–12]

- increase serotonergic neurotransmission. The main concern when co-prescribed with other serotonergic drugs is serotonin syndrome
- inhibit platelet aggregation and increase the risk of bleeding, particularly of the upper GI tract. This effect is exacerbated by aspirin and NSAIDs (see section on 'SSRIs and bleeding' in this chapter)
- may be more likely than other antidepressants to cause hyponatraemia (see section on 'Antidepressant-induced hyponatraemia' in this chapter). This may exacerbate electrolyte disturbances caused by other drugs such as diuretics
- may cause osteopenia. This adds to the negative effects prolactin elevating drugs have on bone mineral density and increases the risks of clinical harm should the patient have a fall.

MAOIs:[13,14]

- prevent the destruction of monoamine neurotransmitters. Sympathomimetic and dopaminergic drugs can lead to monoamine overload and hypertensive crisis. Pethidine and fermented foods can have the same effect
- can interact with serotonergic drugs to cause serotonin syndrome.

Avoid/minimise problems by:

- where antidepressant polypharmacy is used, select drugs that are safer to use together and monitor carefully for side-effects when the second antidepressant is initiated (see section on 'Treatment of refractory depression' in this chapter)

CHAPTER 4

- avoiding the co-prescription of other drugs with a similar pharmacology but not marketed as antidepressants (e.g. atomoxetine, bupropion)
- knowing your pharmacology (most interactions can be easily predicted).

References

1. Cashman JR. Human flavin-containing monooxygenase: substrate specificity and role in drug metabolism. Curr Drug Metab 2000; 1:181–191.
2. Anderson GD. A mechanistic approach to antiepileptic drug interactions. Ann Pharmacother 1998; 32:554–563.
3. Kelly CM et al. Selective serotonin reuptake inhibitors and breast cancer mortality in women receiving tamoxifen: a population based cohort study. BMJ 2010; 340:c693.
4. Devane CL. Antidepressant-drug interactions are potentially but rarely clinically significant. Neuropsychopharmacology 2006; 31: 1594–1604.
5. Watsky EJ et al. Psychotropic drug interactions. Hosp Community Psychiatry 1991; 42:247–256.
6. Joint Formulary Committee. BNF 67 March-September 2014 (online). London: Pharmaceutical Press; 2014. http://www.medicinescomplete.com/mc/bnf/current/
7. Mitchell PB. Drug interactions of clinical significance with selective serotonin reuptake inhibitors. Drug Saf 1997; 17:390–406.
8. Edwards JG et al. Systematic review and guide to selection of selective serotonin reuptake inhibitors. Drugs 1999; 57:507–533.
9. Loke YK et al. Meta-analysis: gastrointestinal bleeding due to interaction between selective serotonin uptake inhibitors and non-steroidal anti-inflammatory drugs. Aliment Pharmacol Ther 2008; 27:31–40.
10. Williams LJ et al. Selective serotonin reuptake inhibitor use and bone mineral density in women with a history of depression. Int Clin Psychopharmacol 2008; 23:84–87.
11. Spina E et al. Clinically relevant pharmacokinetic drug interactions with second-generation antidepressants: an update. Clin Ther 2008; 30:1206–1227.
12. Montastruc F et al. The importance of drug-drug interactions as a cause of adverse drug reactions: a pharmacovigilance study of serotonin-ergic reuptake inhibitors in France. Eur J Clin Pharmacol 2012; 68:767–775.
13. Livingston MG et al. Monoamine oxidase inhibitors. An update on drug interactions. Drug Saf 1996; 14:219–227.
14. Wimbiscus M et al. MAO inhibitors: risks, benefits, and lore. Cleve Clin J Med 2010; 77:859–882.
15. Lin JH et al. Inhibition and induction of cytochrome P450 and the clinical implications. Clin Pharmacokinet 1998; 35:361–390.
16. Richelson E. Pharmacokinetic interactions of antidepressants. J Clin Psychiatry 1998; 59 Suppl 10:22–26.
17. Greenblatt DJ et al. Drug interactions with newer antidepressants: role of human cytochromes P450. J Clin Psychiatry 1998; 59 Suppl 15:19–27.
18. Taylor D. Pharmacokinetic interactions involving clozapine. Br J Psychiatry 1997; 171:109–112.
19. Dolder CR et al. Agomelatine treatment of major depressive disorder. Ann Pharmacother 2008; 42:1822–1831.
20. Chen G et al. Pharmacokinetic drug interactions involving vortioxetine (Lu AA21004), a multimodal antidepressant. Clin Drug Invest 2013; 33:727–736.

Cardiac effects of antidepressants

Selective serotonin reuptake inhibitors are generally recommended in cardiac disease but beware antiplatelet activity and cytochrome-medicated interactions with co-administered cardiac drugs. Mirtazapine is a suitable alternative.[28] SSRIs may protect against myocardial infarction,[53,54] and untreated depression worsens prognosis in cardiovascular disease.[55] Post myocardial infarction (MI), SSRIs and mirtazapine have either a neutral or beneficial effect on mortality.[56] Treatment of depression with SSRIs should not therefore be withheld post MI. Protective effects of treatment of depression post MI appear to relate to antidepressant administration possibly because of an anti-coagulant effect or because of indirect reduction in arrhythmia frequency.[41,57] CBT may be ineffective in this respect.[58] Note that the antiplatelet effect of SSRIs may have adverse consequences too: upper GI bleeding is more common in those taking SSRIs.[59] See Table 4.17 for an overview.

Table 4.17 Summary of cardiac effects of antidepressants

Drug	Heart rate	Blood pressure	QTc	Arrhythmia	Conduction disturbance	Licensed restrictions post MI	Comments
Agomelatine[1,2]	No changes reported	No changes reported	Single case of QTc prolongation	No arrhythmia reported	Unclear	See SPC	Limited data – not recommended
Bupropion*[3-6]	Slight increase	Slight increases in blood pressure but can sometimes be significant. Rarely postural hypotension	QTc shortening, but prolongation has been reported in cases of overdose	No effect. Rare reports in overdose	None	Well tolerated for smoking cessation in post-MI patients	Be aware of interaction potential. Monitor blood pressure
Citalopram[7-11] (assume same for escitalopram)	Small decrease in heart rate	Slight drop in systolic blood pressure	Dose-related increase in QTc	Torsades de pointes reported, mainly in overdose	None	Caution but some evidence of safety in cardiovascular disease	Minor metabolite which may ↑ QTc interval. No clear evidence of increased risk of arrhythmia at any licensed dose
Duloxetine[12-17]	Slight increase	Important effect (see SPC). Caution in hypertension	Isolated reports of QTc prolongation	Isolated reports of toxicity	Isolated reports of toxicity	Caution in patients with recent MI	Limited clinical experience – not recommended
Fluoxetine[18-21]	Small decrease in mean heart rate	Minimal effect on blood pressure	No effect on QTc interval	None	None	Caution. Clinical experience is limited	Evidence of safety post MI
Fluvoxamine[22,23]	Minimal effect on heart rate	Small drop in systolic blood pressure	No significant effect on QTc	None	None	Caution	Limited changes in ECG have been observed
Lofepramine[24,25]	Modest increase in heart rate	Less decrease in postural blood pressure compared with other TCAs	Can possibly prolong QTc interval at higher doses	May occur at higher doses, but rare	Unclear	CI in patients with recent MI	Less cardiotoxic than other TCAs. Reasons unclear
MAOIs[24,26]	Decrease in heart rate	Postural hypotension Risk of hypertensive crisis	Unclear but may shorten QTc interval	May cause arrhythmia and decrease LVF	No clear effect on cardiac conduction	Use with caution in patients with cardiovascular disease	Not recommended in cardiovascular disease
Mirtazapine[27,28]	Minimal change in heart rate	Minimal effect on blood pressure	No effect on QTc	None	None	Caution in patients with recent MI	Evidence of safety post MI. Good alternative to SSRIs

Drug	Effect on heart rate	Effect on blood pressure	Effect on QTc/ECG	Arrhythmia	Cardiac conduction	Contraindications/cautions	Notes
Moclobemide[29–31]	Marginal decrease in heart rate	Minimal effect on blood pressure. Isolated cases of hypertensive episodes	No effect on QTc interval in normal doses. Prolongation in overdose	None	None	None	Possibly arrhythmogenic in overdose
Paroxetine[32,33]	Small decrease in mean heart rate	Minimal effect on blood pressure	No effect on QTc interval	None	None	General caution in cardiac patients	Probably safe post MI
Reboxetine[34–36]	Significant increase in heart rate	Marginal increase in both systolic and diastolic blood pressure. Postural decrease at higher doses	No effect on QTc	Rhythm abnormalities may occur	Atrial and ventricular ectopic beats, especially in the elderly	Caution in patient with cardiac disease	Probably best avoided in coronary disease
Sertraline[37–41]	Minimal effect on heart rate	Minimal effect on blood pressure	No effect on QTc interval	None	None	None – drug of choice	Safe post MI and in heart failure
Trazodone[24,42,43]	Decrease in heart rate more common, although increase can also occur	Can cause significant postural hypotension	Can prolong QTc interval	Several case reports of prolonged QT and arrhythmia	Unclear	Care in patients with severe cardiac disease	May be arrhythmogenic in patients with pre-existing cardiac disease
Tricyclics[24,44–46]	Increase in heart rate	Postural hypotension	Prolongation of QTc interval and QRS interval	Ventricular arrhythmia common in overdose. Torsades de pointes reported	Slows cardiac conduction – blocks cardiac Na/K channels	CI in patients with recent MI	TCAs affect cardiac contractility. Some TCAs linked to ischaemic heart disease and sudden cardiac death. Avoid in coronary artery disease
Venlafaxine[15,47–50] (assume same for desvenlafaxine)	Marginally increased	Some increase in postural blood pressure. At higher doses increase in blood pressure	Possible prolongation in overdose, but very rare	Rare reports of cardiac arrhythmia in overdose	Rare reports of conduction abnormalities	Has not been evaluated in post-MI patients. Avoid	Evidence for arrhythmogenic potential is slim, but avoid in coronary disease
Vortioxetine[51,52]	No effect, but data limited	No effect, but data limited	No effect, but data limited	No effect, but data limited	No effect, but data limited	No specific contraindication	Trial data suggest no effect on QTc or on coagulation parameters

CI, contraindicated; ECG, electrocardiogram; LVF, left ventricular fraction; MAOI, monoamine oxidase inhibitor; MI, myocardial infarction; SPC, summary of product characteristics; SSRI, selective serotonin reuptake inhibitor; TCA, tricyclic antidepressant.

References

1. Dolder CR et al. Agomelatine treatment of major depressive disorder. Ann Pharmacother 2008; **42**:1822–1831.
2. Kozian R et al. [QTc prolongation during treatment with agomelatine]. Psychiatr Prax 2010; **37**:405–407.
3. Roose SP et al. Pharmacologic treatment of depression in patients with heart disease. Psychosom Med 2005; **67** Suppl 1:S54–S57.
4. Dwoskin LP et al. Review of the pharmacology and clinical profile of bupropion, an antidepressant and tobacco use cessation agent. CNS Drug Rev 2006; **12**:178–207.
5. Castro VM et al. QT interval and antidepressant use: a cross sectional study of electronic health records. BMJ 2013; **346**:f288.
6. Eisenberg MJ et al. Bupropion for smoking cessation in patients hospitalized with acute myocardial infarction: a randomized, placebo-controlled trial. J Am Coll Cardiol 2013; **61**:524–532.
7. Rasmussen SL et al. Cardiac safety of citalopram: prospective trials and retrospective analyses. J Clin Psychopharmacol 1999; **19**:407–415.
8. Catalano G et al. QTc interval prolongation associated with citalopram overdose: a case report and literature review. Clin Neuropharmacol 2001; **24**:158–162.
9. Lesperance F et al. Effects of citalopram and interpersonal psychotherapy on depression in patients with coronary artery disease: the Canadian Cardiac Randomized Evaluation of Antidepressant and Psychotherapy Efficacy (CREATE) trial. JAMA 2007; **297**:367–379.
10. Astrom-Lilja C et al. Drug-induced torsades de pointes: a review of the Swedish pharmacovigilance database. Pharmacoepidemiol Drug Saf 2008; **17**:587–592.
11. Zivin K et al. Evaluation of the FDA warning against prescribing citalopram at doses exceeding 40 mg. Am J Psychiatry 2013; **170**: 642–650.
12. Sharma A et al. Pharmacokinetics and safety of duloxetine, a dual-serotonin and norepinephrine reuptake inhibitor. J Clin Pharmacol 2000; **40**:161–167.
13. Schatzberg,AF. Efficacy and tolerability of duloxetine, a novel dual reuptake inhibitor, in the treatment of major depressive disorder. J Clin Psychiatry 2003; **64** Suppl 13:30–37.
14. Detke MJ et al. Duloxetine, 60 mg once daily, for major depressive disorder: a randomized double-blind placebo-controlled trial. J Clin Psychiatry 2002; **63**:308–315.
15. Colucci VJ et al. Heart failure worsening and exacerbation after venlafaxine and duloxetine therapy. Ann Pharmacother 2008; **42**:882–887.
16. Stuhec M. Duloxetine-induced life-threatening long QT syndrome. Wien Klin Wochenschr 2013; **125**:165–166.
17. Orozco BS et al. Duloxetine: an uncommon cause of fatal ventricular arrhythmia. Clin Toxicol 2014; **51**:672–672.
18. Fisch C. Effect of fluoxetine on the electrocardiogram. J Clin Psychiatry 1985; **46**:42–44.
19. Ellison JM et al. Fluoxetine-induced bradycardia and syncope in two patients. J Clin Psychiatry 1990; **51**:385–386.
20. Roose SP et al. Cardiovascular effects of fluoxetine in depressed patients with heart disease. Am J Psychiatry 1998; **155**:660–665.
21. Strik JJ et al. Efficacy and safety of fluoxetine in the treatment of patients with major depression after first myocardial infarction: findings from a double-blind, placebo-controlled trial. Psychosom Med 2000; **62**:783–789.
22. Strik JJ et al. Cardiac side-effects of two selective serotonin reuptake inhibitors in middle-aged and elderly depressed patients. Int Clin Psychopharmacol 1998; **13**:263–267.
23. Stirnimann G et al. Brugada syndrome ECG provoked by the selective serotonin reuptake inhibitor fluvoxamine. Europace 2010; **12**:282–283.
24. Warrington SJ et al. The cardiovascular effects of antidepressants. Psychol Med Monogr Suppl 1989; **16**:i–40.
25. Stern H et al. Cardiovascular effects of single doses of the antidepressants amitriptyline and lofepramine in healthy subjects. Pharmacopsychiatry 1985; **18**:272–277.
26. Waring WS et al. Acute myocarditis after massive phenelzine overdose. Eur J Clin Pharmacol 2007; **63**:1007–1009.
27. Montgomery SA. Safety of mirtazapine: a review. Int Clin Psychopharmacol 1995; **10** Suppl 4:37–45.
28. Honig A et al. Treatment of post-myocardial infarction depressive disorder: a randomized, placebo-controlled trial with mirtazapine. Psychosom Med 2007; **69**:606–613.
29. Moll E et al. Safety and efficacy during long-term treatment with moclobemide. Clin Neuropharmacol 1994; **17** Suppl 1:S74–S87.
30. Hilton S et al. Moclobemide safety: monitoring a newly developed product in the 1990s. J Clin Psychopharmacol 1995; **15**:76S–83S.
31. Downes MA et al. QTc abnormalities in deliberate self-poisoning with moclobemide. Intern Med J 2005; **35**:388–391.
32. Kuhs H et al. Cardiovascular effects of paroxetine. Psychopharmacology (Berl) 1990; **102**:379–382.
33. Roose SP et al. Comparison of paroxetine and nortriptyline in depressed patients with ischemic heart disease. JAMA 1998; **279**:287–291.
34. Mucci M. Reboxetine: a review of antidepressant tolerability. J Psychopharmacol 1997; **11**:S33–S37.
35. Holm KJ et al. Reboxetine: a review of its use in depression. CNS Drugs 1999; **12**:65–83.
36. Fleishaker JC et al. Lack of effect of reboxetine on cardiac repolarization. Clin Pharmacol Ther 2001; **70**:261–269.
37. Shapiro PA. An open-label preliminary trial of sertraline for treatment of major depression after acute myocardial infarction (the SADHAT Trial).Sertraline Anti-Depressant Heart Attack Trial. Am Heart J 1999; **137**:1100–1106.
38. Glassman AH et al. Sertraline treatment of major depression in patients with acute MI or unstable angina. JAMA 2002; **288**:701–709.
39. Winkler D et al. Trazodone-induced cardiac arrhythmias: a report of two cases. Hum Psychopharmacol 2006; **21**:61–62.
40. Jiang W et al. Safety and efficacy of sertraline for depression in patients with CHF (SADHART-CHF): a randomized, double-blind, placebo-controlled trial of sertraline for major depression with congestive heart failure. Am Heart J 2008; **156**:437–444.
41. Leftheriotis D et al. The role of the selective serotonin re-uptake inhibitor sertraline in nondepressive patients with chronic ischemic heart failure: a preliminary study. Pacing Clin Electrophysiol 2010; **33**:1217–1223.

42. Service JA et al. QT prolongation and delayed atrioventricular conduction caused by acute ingestion of trazodone. Clin Toxicol (Phila) 2008; 46:71–73.

43. Dattilo PB et al. Prolonged QT associated with an overdose of trazodone. J Clin Psychiatry 2007; 68:1309–1310.

44. Hippisley-Cox J et al. Antidepressants as risk factor for ischaemic heart disease: case-control study in primary care. BMJ 2001; 323:666–669.

45. Whyte IM et al. Relative toxicity of venlafaxine and selective serotonin reuptake inhibitors in overdose compared to tricyclic antidepressants. QJM 2003; 96:369–374.

46. van Noord C et al. Psychotropic drugs associated with corrected QT interval prolongation. J Clin Psychopharmacol 2009; 29:9–15.

47. Khawaja IS et al. Cardiovascular effects of selective serotonin reuptake inhibitors and other novel antidepressants. Heart Dis 2003; 5:153–160.

48. Pfizer Limited. Summary of Product Characteristics. Efexor XL 75 mg hard prolonged release capsules. https://www.medicines.org.uk/

49. Letsas K et al. QT interval prolongation associated with venlafaxine administration. Int J Cardiol 2006; 109:116–117.

50. Taylor D et al. Volte-face on venlafaxine – reasons and reflections. J Psychopharmacol 2006; 20:597–601.

51. Citrome L. Vortioxetine for major depressive disorder: a systematic review of the efficacy and safety profile for this newly approved antidepressant – what is the number needed to treat, number needed to harm and likelihood to be helped or harmed? Int J Clin Pract 2014; 68:60–82.

52. Takeda Pharmaceuticals America Inc. Highlights of Prescribing Information. Brintellix (vortioxetine) tablets. http://www.us.brintellix.com/

53. Sauer WH et al. Selective serotonin reuptake inhibitors and myocardial infarction. Circulation 2001; 104:1894–1898.

54. Sauer WH et al. Effect of antidepressants and their relative affinity for the serotonin transporter on the risk of myocardial infarction. Circulation 2003; 108:32–36.

55. Davies SJ et al. Treatment of anxiety and depressive disorders in patients with cardiovascular disease. BMJ 2004; 328:939–943.

56. Taylor D et al. Pharmacological interventions for people with depression and chronic physical health problems: systematic review and meta-analyses of safety and efficacy. Br J Psychiatry 2011; 198:179–188.

57. Chen S et al. Serotonin and catecholaminergic polymorphic ventricular tachycardia: a possible therapeutic role for SSRIs? Cardiovasc J Afr 2010; 21:225–228.

58. Berkman LF et al. Effects of treating depression and low perceived social support on clinical events after myocardial infarction: the Enhancing Recovery in Coronary Heart Disease Patients (ENRICHD) Randomized Trial. JAMA 2003; 289:3106–3116.

59. Dalton SO et al. Use of selective serotonin reuptake inhibitors and risk of upper gastrointestinal tract bleeding: a population-based cohort study. Arch Intern Med 2003; 163:59–64.

Further reading

Tousoulis D et al. Role of depression in heart failure – choosing the right antidepressive treatment. Int J Cardiol 2010; 140:12–18.

CHAPTER 4

Antidepressant-induced arrhythmia

Depression confers an increased of risk of cardiovascular disease[1] and sudden cardiac death,[2] perhaps because of platelet activation,[3] decreased heart rate variability,[4] reduced physical activity,[5] an association with an increased risk of diabetes and/or other factors.

Tricyclic antidepressants have established arrhythmogenic activity which arises as a result of potent blockade of cardiac sodium channels and variable activity at potassium channels.[6] ECG changes produced include PR, QRS and QT prolongation and the Brugada syndrome.[7] Nortriptyline has been associated in one study with an increased risk of cardiac arrest[8] although a large cohort study did not confirm this finding.[9] In patients taking tricyclics, ECG monitoring is a more meaningful and useful measure of toxicity than plasma level monitoring. **Lofepramine,** for reasons unknown, seems to lack the arrhythmogenicity of other TCAs, despite its major metabolite, desipramine, being a potent potassium channel blocker.[10]

There is limited evidence that **venlafaxine** is a sodium channel antagonist[11] and a weak antagonist at hERG potassium channels. Arrhythmia is a rare occurrence even after massive overdose[12–15] and ECG changes no more common than with SSRIs.[16] No ECG changes are seen in therapeutic dosing[17] and sudden cardiac death is no more common than with fluoxetine or citalopram.[9,18] **Moclobemide,**[19] **citalopram,**[20,21] **escitalopram,**[22] **bupropion** (amfebutamone),[23] **trazodone**[24,25] and **sertraline,**[26] amongst others,[1] have been reported to prolong the QTc interval in overdose but the clinical consequences of this are uncertain. QT changes are not usually seen at normal clinical doses.[27,28] An association between SSRIs and QT changes in normal dosing can be shown[29] but this seems largely to be driven by the effects of citalopram and escitalopram[30]. The effect is dose related[30] but modest.[29] Neither a large database study[9] nor a large cohort study[31] found any association between citalopram treatment and arrhythmia or cardiac mortality in routine clinical practice; in fact, higher doses of citalopram (>40 mg) were associated with fewer adverse outcomes than lower doses.[31] Vortioxetine seems to have no effect on QT;[32,33] similarly, agomelatine has no effect, even at supratherapeutic doses.[34]

There is clear evidence for the safety of sertraline[35] and mirtazapine[36] (and to a lesser extent, citalopram,[36] fluoxetine[37] and bupropion[38]) in subjects at risk of arrhythmia due to recent myocardial infarction. Another study supports the safety of citalopram in patients with coronary artery disease[39] (although citalopram is linked to a risk of torsades de pointes[40]).

Relative cardiotoxicity of antidepressants is difficult to establish with any precision. Yellow Card (ADROIT) data suggest that all marketed antidepressants are associated with arrhythmia (ranging from clinically insignificant to life threatening) and sudden cardiac death. For a substantial proportion of drugs, these figures are more likely to reflect coincidence rather than causation. The Fatal Toxicity Index (FTI) may provide some means for comparison. This is a measure of the number of overdose deaths per million (FP10) prescriptions issued. FTI figures suggest high toxicity for tricyclic drugs (especially dosulepin but not lofepramine), medium toxicity for venlafaxine and moclobemide, and low toxicity for SSRIs, mirtazapine and reboxetine.[41–45] However,

FTI does not necessarily reflect only cardiotoxicity (antidepressants variously cause serotonin syndrome, seizures and coma) and is, in any case, open to other influences. This is best evidenced in the change in FTI over time. A good example here is nortriptyline, the FTI of which has been estimated at 0.6[16] and 39.2[12] and several values in between.[41,42,44] This change probably reflects changes in the type of patient prescribed nortriptyline. There is good evidence that venlafaxine is relatively more often prescribed to patients with more severe depression and who are relatively more likely to attempt suicide.[46–48] This is likely to inflate venlafaxine's FTI and erroneously suggest greater inherent toxicity. On the other hand, drugs with consistently low FTIs can probably be assumed to have very low risk of arrhythmias.

Citalopram and escitalopram have very low overdose toxicity despite QT prolongation occurring in about one-third of reported overdoses.[49] Standard doses of citalopram may be linked to an increased risk of cardiac arrest[8] but other data suggest no increased risk of arrhythmia or death with standard and higher licensed doses of citalopram and escitalopram.[31] Citalopram and escitalopram are probably the most cardiotoxic of the SSRIs but their toxicity is modest at worst, insignificant at best.

Summary

- Tricyclics (but not lofepramine) have an established link to ion channel blockade and cardiac arrhythmia.
- Non-tricyclics generally have a very low risk of inducing arrhythmia.
- Sertraline is recommended post MI, but other SSRIs and mirtazapine are also likely to be safe.
- Bupropion, citalopram, escitalopram, moclobemide, lofepramine and venlafaxine should be used with caution or avoided in those at risk of serious arrhythmia (those with heart failure, left ventricular hypertrophy, previous arrhythmia or MI). An ECG should be performed at baseline and 1 week after every increase in dose if any of these drugs are used in at-risk patients.
- TCAs (with the exception of lofepramine) are best avoided completely in patients at risk of serious arrhythmia. If use of a TCA cannot be avoided, an ECG should be performed at baseline, 1 week after each increase in dose and periodically throughout treatment. Frequency will be determined by the stability of the cardiac disorder and the TCA (and dose) being used; advice from cardiology should be sought.
- The arrhythmogenic potential of TCAs and other antidepressants is dose-related. Consideration should be given to ECG monitoring of all patients prescribed doses towards the top of the licensed range and those who are prescribed other drugs that through pharmacokinetic (e.g. fluoxetine) or pharmacodynamic (e.g. diuretics) mechanisms may add to the risk posed by the TCA.

References

1. Taylor D. Antidepressant drugs and cardiovascular pathology: a clinical overview of effectiveness and safety. Acta Psychiatr Scand 2008; 118:434–442.
2. Whang W et al. Depression and risk of sudden cardiac death and coronary heart disease in women: results from the Nurses' Health Study. J Am Coll Cardiol 2009; 53:950–958.

CHAPTER 4

3. Ziegelstein RC et al. Platelet function in patients with major depression. Intern Med J 2009; **39**:38–43.

4. Glassman AH et al. Heart rate variability in acute coronary syndrome patients with major depression: influence of sertraline and mood improvement. Arch Gen Psychiatry 2007; **64**:1025–1031.

5. Whooley MA et al. Depressive symptoms, health behaviors, and risk of cardiovascular events in patients with coronary heart disease. JAMA 2008; **300**:2379–2388.

6. Thanacoody HK et al. Tricyclic antidepressant poisoning : cardiovascular toxicity. Toxicol Rev 2005; **24**:205–214.

7. Sicouri S et al. Sudden cardiac death secondary to antidepressant and antipsychotic drugs. Expert Opin Drug Saf 2008; **7**:181–194.

8. Weeke P et al. Antidepressant use and risk of out-of-hospital cardiac arrest: a nationwide case-time-control study. Clin Pharmacol Ther 2012; **92**:72–79.

9. Leonard CE et al. Antidepressants and the risk of sudden cardiac death and ventricular arrhythmia. Pharmacoepidemiol Drug Saf 2011; **20**:903–913.

10. Hong HK et al. Block of the human ether-a-go-go-related gene (hERG) K+ channel by the antidepressant desipramine. Biochem Biophys Res Commun 2010; **394**:536–541.

11. Khalifa M et al. Mechanism of sodium channel block by venlafaxine in guinea pig ventricular myocytes. J Pharmacol Exp Ther 1999; **291**:280–284.

12. Colbridge MG et al. Venlafaxine in overdose – experience of the National Poisons Information Service (London centre). J Toxicol Clin Toxicol 1999; **37**:383.

13. Blythe D et al. Cardiovascular and neurological toxicity of venlafaxine. Hum Exp Toxicol 1999; **18**:309–313.

14. Combes A et al. Conduction disturbances associated with venlafaxine. Ann Intern Med 2001; **134**:166–167.

15. Isbister GK. Electrocardiogram changes and arrhythmias in venlafaxine overdose. Br J Clin Pharmacol 2009; **67**:572–576.

16. Whyte IM et al. Relative toxicity of venlafaxine and selective serotonin reuptake inhibitors in overdose compared to tricyclic antidepressants. QJM 2003; **96**:369–374.

17. Feighner JP. Cardiovascular safety in depressed patients: focus on venlafaxine. J Clin Psychiatry 1995; **56**:574–579.

18. Martinez C et al. Use of venlafaxine compared with other antidepressants and the risk of sudden cardiac death or near death: a nested case-control study. BMJ 2010; **340**:c249.

19. Downes MA et al. QTc abnormalities in deliberate self-poisoning with moclobemide. Intern Med J 2005; **35**:388–391.

20. Kelly CA et al. Comparative toxicity of citalopram and the newer antidepressants after overdose. J Toxicol Clin Toxicol 2004; **42**:67–71.

21. Grundemar L et al. Symptoms and signs of severe citalopram overdose. Lancet 1997; **349**:1602.

22. Mohammed R et al. Prolonged QTc interval due to escitalopram overdose. J Miss State Med Assoc 2010; **51**:350–353.

23. Isbister GK et al. Bupropion overdose: QTc prolongation and its clinical significance. Ann Pharmacother 2003; **37**:999–1002.

24. Service JA et al. QT prolongation and delayed atrioventricular conduction caused by acute ingestion of trazodone. Clin Toxicol (Phila) 2008; **46**:71–73.

25. Dattilo PB et al. Prolonged QT associated with an overdose of trazodone. J Clin Psychiatry 2007; **68**:1309–1310.

26. de Boer RA et al. QT interval prolongation after sertraline overdose: a case report. BMC Emerg Med 2005; **5**:5.

27. van Noord C et al. Psychotropic drugs associated with corrected QT interval prolongation. J Clin Psychopharmacol 2009; **29**:9–15.

28. van Haelst IM et al. QT interval prolongation in users of selective serotonin reuptake inhibitors in an elderly surgical population: a cross-sectional study. J Clin Psychiatry 2014; **75**:15–21.

29. Beach SR et al. Meta-analysis of selective serotonin reuptake inhibitor-associated QTc prolongation. J Clin Psychiatry 2014; **75**:e441–449.

30. Castro VM et al. QT interval and antidepressant use: a cross sectional study of electronic health records. BMJ 2013; **346**:f288.

31. Zivin K et al. Evaluation of the FDA warning against prescribing citalopram at doses exceeding 40 mg. Am J Psychiatry 2013; **170**:642–650.

32. Dubovsky SL. Pharmacokinetic evaluation of vortioxetine for the treatment of major depressive disorder. Expert Opin Drug Metab Toxicol 2014; **10**:759–766.

33. Alam MY et al. Safety, tolerability, and efficacy of vortioxetine (Lu AA21004) in major depressive disorder: results of an open-label, flexible-dose, 52-week extension study. Int Clin Psychopharmacol 2014; **29**:36–44.

34. Donazzolo Y et al. Evaluation of the effects of therapeutic and supra-therapeutic doses of agomelatine on the QT/QTc interval – A phase I, randomised, double-blind, placebo-controlled and positive-controlled, cross-over thorough QT/QTc study conducted in healthy volunteers. J Cardiovasc Pharmacol 2014; **64**:440–451.

35. Glassman AH et al. Sertraline treatment of major depression in patients with acute MI or unstable angina. JAMA 2002; **288**:701–709.

36. van Melle JP et al. Effects of antidepressant treatment following myocardial infarction. Br J Psychiatry 2007; **190**:460–466.

37. Strik JJ et al. Efficacy and safety of fluoxetine in the treatment of patients with major depression after first myocardial infarction: findings from a double-blind, placebo-controlled trial. Psychosom Med 2000; **62**:783–789.

38. Rigotti NA et al. Bupropion for smokers hospitalized with acute cardiovascular disease. Am J Med 2006; **119**:1080–1087.

39. Lesperance F et al. Effects of citalopram and interpersonal psychotherapy on depression in patients with coronary artery disease: the Canadian Cardiac Randomized Evaluation of Antidepressant and Psychotherapy Efficacy (CREATE) trial. JAMA 2007; **297**:367–379.

40. Astrom-Lilja C et al. Drug-induced torsades de pointes: a review of the Swedish pharmacovigilance database. Pharmacoepidemiol Drug Saf 2008; **17**:587–592.

41. Crome P. The toxicity of drugs used for suicide. Acta Psychiatr Scand Suppl 1993; **371**:33–37.

42. Cheeta S et al. Antidepressant-related deaths and antidepressant prescriptions in England and Wales, 1998-2000. Br J Psychiatry 2004; **184**:41–47.

43. Buckley NA et al. Fatal toxicity of serotoninergic and other antidepressant drugs: analysis of United Kingdom mortality data. BMJ 2002; **325**:1332–1333.

44. Buckley NA et al. Greater toxicity in overdose of dothiepin than of other tricyclic antidepressants. Lancet 1994; **343**:159–162.

45. Morgan O et al. Fatal toxicity of antidepressants in England and Wales, 1993-2002. Health Stat Q **2004**:18–24.

46. Egberts ACG et al. Channeling of three newly introduced antidepressants to patients not responding satisfactorily to previous treatment. J Clin Psychopharmacol 1997; **17**:149–155.

47. Mines D et al. Prevalence of risk factors for suicide in patients prescribed venlafaxine, fluoxetine, and citalopram. Pharmacoepidemiol Drug Saf 2005; **14**:367–372.

48. Chan AN et al. A comparison of venlafaxine and SSRIs in deliberate self-poisoning. J Med Toxicol 2010; **6**:116–121.

49. Hasnain M et al. Escitalopram and QTc prolongation. J Psychiatry Neurosci 2013; **38**:E11.

Antidepressant-induced hyponatraemia

Most antidepressants have been associated with hyponatraemia; the onset is usually within 30 days (median 11 days) of starting treatment[1-3] and is probably not dose-related.[1,4] The most likely mechanism of this adverse effect is the syndrome of inappropriate secretion of antidiuretic hormone (SIADH). Hyponatraemia is a potentially serious adverse effect of antidepressants that demands careful monitoring,[5] particularly in those patients at greatest risk (see 'Monitoring' below).

Antidepressants

No antidepressant has been shown *not* to be associated with hyponatraemia and most have a reported association.[6] It has been suggested that serotonergic drugs are relatively more likely to cause hyponatraemia,[7,8] although this is disputed.[9] The most recent analyses suggest SSRIs are more likely to cause hyponatraemia than TCAs or mirtazapine,[10] and that older women who are co-prescribed other medication known to reduce plasma sodium are at greatest risk.[11] Only one (agomelatine) of the more recently introduced serotonergic drugs appears to be free of this effect – cases of hyponatraemia have been described with mirtazapine[12-14] (although the reported incidence is very low[11]), escitalopram[15,16] and duloxetine.[4] Vortioxetine has also been linked to hyponatraemia,[17] as has desvenlafaxine[18]. Noradrenergic antidepressants are also clearly linked to hyponatraemia[19-25] (albeit at a lower frequency). There are notably few reports for MAOIs[26,27] and none for agomelatine. CYP2D6 poor metabolisers may be at increased risk[28] of antidepressant-induced hyponatraemia although evidence is somewhat inconsistent.[29]

Monitoring[1,11,30-34]

All patients taking antidepressants should be observed for signs of hyponatraemia (dizziness, nausea, lethargy, confusion, cramps, seizures). Serum sodium should be determined (at baseline and 2 and 4 weeks, and then 3-monthly[35]) for those at high risk of drug-induced hyponatraemia. High-risk factors are as follows:

- extreme old age (>80 years)
- female gender
- history of hyponatraemia/low baseline Na concentration
- co-therapy with other drugs known to be associated with hyponatraemia (e.g. diuretics, NSAIDs, carbamazepine, cancer chemotherapy, calcium antagonists, angiotensin converting enzyme [ACE] inhibitors)
- reduced renal function (glomerular filtration rate [GFR] <50 mL/minute)
- medical co-morbidity (e.g. hypothyroidism, diabetes, chronic obstructive pulmonary disease [COPD], hypertension, head injury, congestive cardiac failure [CCF], cerebrovascular accident [CVA], various cancers).

Note that hyponatraemia is common in elderly patients so monitoring is essential.[11,36,37]

Treatment[37]

It may be possible to manage mild hyponatraemia with fluid restriction.[31] Some suggest increasing sodium intake,[4] although this is likely to be impractical. If symptoms persist, the antidepressant should be discontinued.

- The normal range for serum sodium is 136–145 mmol/L.
- If serum sodium is >125 mmol/L, monitor sodium daily until normal. Symptoms include headache, nausea, vomiting, muscle cramps, restlessness, lethargy, confusion and disorientation. Consider withdrawing the offending antidepressant.
- If serum sodium is <125 mmol/L, refer to specialist medical care. There is an increased risk of life-threatening symptoms such as seizures, coma and respiratory arrest. The antidepressant should be discontinuted immediately. (Note risk of discontinuation symptoms which may complicate the clinical picture.) Note also that rapid correction of hyponatraemia may be harmful.[14]

Restarting treatment

- For those who develop hyponatraemia with an SSRI, there are many case reports of recurrent hyponatraemia on rechallenge with the same or a different SSRI, and relatively fewer reports of recurrence occurring with an antidepressant from another class.[11,12] There are also case reports of successful rechallenge.[1]
- Consider withdrawing other drugs associated with hyponatraemia (risk increases exponentially when antidepressants are combined with diruetics, etc.[3]).
- Prescribe a drug from a different class. Consider noradrenergic drugs such as nortriptyline and lofepramine, mirtazapine or an MAOI such as moclobemide. Agomelatine is also an option. Begin with a low dose, increasing slowly, and monitor closely. If hyponatraemia recurs and continued antidepressant use is essential, consider water restriction and/or careful use of demeclocycline (see BNF).
- Consider ECT.

Other prescribed drugs

Carbamazepine has a well-known association with SIADH. Note also that antipsychotic use has been linked to hyponatraemia[38–40] (see section on 'Antipsychotics and hyponatraemia' in Chapter 2). Other commonly prescribed drugs such as thiazide diuretics, NSAIDs, tramadol, omeprazole and trimethoprim can also cause hyponatraemia.[2,32]

References

1. Egger C et al. A review on hyponatremia associated with SSRIs, reboxetine and venlafaxine. Int J Psychiatry Clin Pract 2006; 10:17–26.
2. Liamis G et al. A review of drug-induced hyponatremia. Am J Kidney Dis 2008; 52:144–153.
3. Letmaier M et al. Hyponatraemia during psychopharmacological treatment: results of a drug surveillance programme. Int J Neuropsychopharmacol 2012; 15:739–748.
4. Kruger S et al. Duloxetine and hyponatremia: a report of 5 cases. J Clin Psychopharmacol 2007; 27:101–104.
5. Mohan S et al. Prevalence of hyponatremia and association with mortality: results from NHANES. Am J Med 2013; 126:1127–1137.
6. Thomas A et al. Hyponatraemia and the syndrome of inappropriate antidiuretic hormone secretion associated with drug therapy in psychiatric patients. CNS Drugs 1995; 5:357–369.

CHAPTER 4

7. Movig KL et al. Serotonergic antidepressants associated with an increased risk for hyponatraemia in the elderly. Eur J Clin Pharmacol 2002; 58:143–148.

8. Movig KL et al. Association between antidepressant drug use and hyponatraemia: a case-control study. Br J Clin Pharmacol 2002; 53:363–369.

9. Kirby D et al. Hyponatraemia and selective serotonin re-uptake inhibitors in elderly patients. Int J Geriatr Psychiatry 2001; 16:484–493.

10. De Picker L et al. Antidepressants and the risk of hyponatremia: a class-by-class review of literature. Psychosomatics 2014; April 21 (epub ahead of print).

11. Dirks AC et al. Recurrent hyponatremia after substitution of citalopram with duloxetine. J Clin Psychopharmacol 2007; 27:313.

12. Bavbek N et al. Recurrent hyponatremia associated with citalopram and mirtazapine. Am J Kidney Dis 2006; 48:e61–e62.

13. Ladino M et al. Mirtazapine-induced hyponatremia in an elderly hospice patient. J Palliat Med 2006; 9:258–260.

14. Cheah CY et al. Mirtazapine associated with profound hyponatremia: two case reports. Am J Geriatr Pharmacother 2008; 6:91–95.

15. Grover S et al. Escitalopram-associated hyponatremia. Psychiatry Clin Neurosci 2007; 61:132–133.

16. Covyeou JA et al. Hyponatremia associated with escitalopram. N Engl J Med 2007; 356:94–95.

17. Takeda Pharmaceuticals America Inc. Highlights of Prescribing Information. Brintellix (vortioxetine) tablets. http://www.us.brintellix.com/

18. Lee G et al. Syndrome of inappropriate secretion of antidiuretic hormone due to desvenlafaxine. Gen Hosp Psychiatry 2013; 35:574.e571–573.

19. O'Sullivan D et al. Hyponatraemia and lofepramine. Br J Psychiatry 1987; 150:720–721.

20. Wylie KR et al. Lofepramine-induced hyponatraemia. Br J Psychiatry 1989; 154:419–420.

21. Ranieri P et al. Reboxetine and hyponatremia. N Engl J Med 2000; 342:215–216.

22. Miller MG. Tricyclics as a possible cause of hyponatremia in psychiatric patients. Am J Psychiatry 1989; 146:807.

23. Colgate R. Hyponatraemia and inappropriate secretion of antidiuretic hormone associated with the use of imipramine. Br J Psychiatry 1993; 163:819–822.

24. Koelkebeck K et al. A case of non-SIADH-induced hyponatremia in depression after treatment with reboxetine. World J Biol Psychiatry 2009; 10:609–611.

25. Kate N et al. Bupropion-induced hyponatremia. Gen Hosp Psychiatry 2013; 35:681.

26. Mercier S et al. Severe hyponatremia induced by moclobemide (in French). Therapie 1997; 52:82–83.

27. Peterson JC et al. Inappropriate antidiuretic hormone secondary to a monamine oxidase inhibitor. JAMA 1978; 239:1422–1423.

28. Kwadijk-de GS et al. Variation in the CYP2D6 gene is associated with a lower serum sodium concentration in patients on antidepressants. Br J Clin Pharmacol 2009; 68:221–225.

29. Stedman CA et al. Cytochrome P450 2D6 genotype does not predict SSRI (fluoxetine or paroxetine) induced hyponatraemia. Hum Psychopharmacol 2002; 17:187–190.

30. Jacob S et al. Hyponatremia associated with selective serotonin-reuptake inhibitors in older adults. Ann Pharmacother 2006; 40:1618–1622.

31. Roxanas M et al. Venlafaxine hyponatraemia: incidence, mechanism and management. Aust NZ J Psychiatry 2007; 41:411–418.

32. Reddy P et al. Diagnosis and management of hyponatraemia in hospitalised patients. Int J Clin Pract 2009; 63:1494–1508.

33. Siegler EL et al. Risk factors for the development of hyponatremia in psychiatric inpatients. Arch Intern Med 1995; 155:953–957.

34. Mannesse CK et al. Characteristics, prevalence, risk factors, and underlying mechanism of hyponatremia in elderly patients treated with antidepressants: a cross-sectional study. Maturitas 2013; 76:357–363.

35. Arinzon ZH et al. Delayed recurrent SIADH associated with SSRIs. Ann Pharmacother 2002; 36:1175–1177.

36. Fabian TJ et al. Paroxetine-induced hyponatremia in the elderly due to the syndrome of inappropriate secretion of antidiuretic hormone (SIADH). J Geriatr Psychiatry Neurol 2003; 16:160–164.

37. Sharma H et al. Antidepressant-induced hyponatraemia in the aged. Avoidance and management strategies. Drugs Aging 1996; 8:430–435.

38. Ohsawa H et al. An epidemiological study on hyponatremia in psychiatric patients in mental hospitals in Nara Prefecture. Jpn J Psychiatry Neurol 1992; 46:883–889.

39. Leadbetter RA et al. Differential effects of neuroleptic and clozapine on polydipsia and intermittent hyponatremia. J Clin Psychiatry 1994; 55 Suppl B:110–113.

40. Collins A et al. SIADH induced by two atypical antipsychotics. Int J Geriatr Psychiatry 2000; 15:282–283.

Further reading

Spasovski G et al. Clinical practice guideline on diagnosis and treatment of hyponatraemia. Eur J Endocrinol 2014; 170:G1–47.

Antidepressants and hyperprolactinaemia

Prolactin release is controlled by endogenous dopamine but is also indirectly modulated by serotonin via stimulation of $5HT_{1c}$ and $5HT_2$ receptors.[1,2] Long-standing increased plasma prolactin (with or without symptoms) is very occasionally seen with antidepressant use.[3] Where antidepressant-induced hyperprolactinaemia does occur, rises in prolactin are usually small and short-lived[4] and so symptoms are very rare. There is no association between SSRI use and breast cancer.[5] Routine monitoring of prolactin is not recommended but where symptoms suggest the possibility of hyperprolactinaemia then measurement of plasma prolactin is essential. Where symptomatic hyperprolactinaemia is confirmed, a switch to mirtazapine is recommended (see Table 4.18 below), although there is also evidence that switching to an alternative SSRI can resolve symptoms.[6,7]

Some details of associations between antidepressants and increased prolactin are given in Table 4.18.

Table 4.18 Reported associations between antidepressants and increased prolactin

Drug/group	Prospective studies	Case reports/series
Agomelatine	No mention of prolactin changes in clinical trials[8] Melatonin itself may inhibit prolactin production[9]	None
Bupropion (amfebutamone)	Single doses of up to 100 mg seem not to affect prolactin[10]	None
MAOIs	Small mean changes observed with phenelzine[11] and tranylcypromine[12]	None
Mirtazapine	Strong evidence that mirtazapine has *no* effect on prolactin[13–15]	None
Reboxetine	Small, transient elevation of prolactin observed after reboxetine administration[16]	None
SNRIs	Clear association observed between venlafaxine and prolactin elevation[17]	Galactorrhoea reported with venlafaxine[18,19] and duloxetine[20,21]
SSRIs	Prospective studies generally show no change in prolactin.[22–24] Some evidence from prescription event monitoring that SSRIs are associated with higher risk of non-puerperal lactation.[25] In a French study, 1.6% of adverse event reports for SSRIs were of hyperprolactinaemia[3]	Galactorrhoea reported with fluoxetine[6,26] and paroxetine[27] Euprolactinaemic galactorrhoea reported with escitalopram[28] Hyperprolactinaemia reported with sertraline[7]
Tricyclics	Small mean changes seen in some studies[11,29,30] but no changes in others[11,31]	Symptomatic hyperprolactinaemia reported with imipramine,[28] dosulepin[32] and clomipramine[33,34]
Vortioxetine	No mention of prolactin changes in clinical trials[35,36]	None, although clinical experience is limited

MAOI, monoamine oxidase inhibitor; SNRI, selective noradrenaline reuptake inhibitor; SSRI, selective serotonin reuptake inhibitor.

CHAPTER 4

References

1. Emiliano AB et al. From galactorrhea to osteopenia: rethinking serotonin-prolactin interactions. Neuropsychopharmacology 2004; **29**:833–846.
2. Rittenhouse PA et al. Neurons in the hypothalamic paraventricular nucleus mediate the serotonergic stimulation of prolactin secretion via 5-HT1c/2 receptors. Endocrinology 1993; **133**:661–667.
3. Trenque T et al. Serotonin reuptake inhibitors and hyperprolactinaemia: a case/non-case study in the French pharmacovigilance database. Drug Saf 2011; **34**:1161–1166.
4. Voicu V et al. Drug-induced hypo- and hyperprolactinemia: mechanisms, clinical and therapeutic consequences. Expert Opin Drug Metab Toxicol 2013; **9**:955–968.
5. Ashbury JE et al. Selective serotonin reuptake inhibitor (SSRI) antidepressants, prolactin and breast cancer. Front Oncol 2012; **2**:177.
6. Mondal S et al. A new logical insight and putative mechanism behind fluoxetine-induced amenorrhea, hyperprolactinemia and galactorrhea in a case series. Therapeut Adv Psychopharmacol 2013; **3**:322–334.
7. Strzelecki D et al. Hyperprolactinemia and bleeding following use of sertraline but not use of citalopram and paroxetine: a case report. Arch Psychiatry Psychother 2012; **1**:45–48.
8. Taylor D et al. Antidepressant efficacy of agomelatine: meta-analysis of published and unpublished studies. BMJ 2014; **348**:g1888.
9. Chu YS et al. Stimulatory and entraining effect of melatonin on tuberoinfundibular dopaminergic neuron activity and inhibition on prolactin secretion. J Pineal Res 2000; **28**:219–226.
10. Whiteman PD et al. Bupropion fails to affect plasma prolactin and growth hormone in normal subjects. Br J Clin Pharmacol 1982; **13**:745.
11. Meltzer HY et al. Effect of antidepressants on neuroendocrine axis in humans. Adv Biochem Psychopharmacol 1982; **32**:303–316.
12. Price LH et al. Effects of tranylcypromine treatment on neuroendocrine, behavioral, and autonomic responses to tryptophan in depressed patients. Life Sci 1985; **37**:809–818.
13. Laakmann G et al. Effects of mirtazapine on growth hormone, prolactin, and cortisol secretion in healthy male subjects. Psychoneuroendocrinology 1999; **24**:769–784.
14. Laakmann G et al. Mirtazapine: an inhibitor of cortisol secretion that does not influence growth hormone and prolactin secretion. J Clin Psychopharmacol 2000; **20**:101–103.
15. Schule C et al. The influence of mirtazapine on anterior pituitary hormone secretion in healthy male subjects. Psychopharmacology (Berl) 2002; **163**:95–101.
16. Schule C et al. Reboxetine acutely stimulates cortisol, ACTH, growth hormone and prolactin secretion in healthy male subjects. Psychoneuroendocrinology 2004; **29**:185–200.
17. Daffner-Bugia C et al. The neuroendocrine effects of venlafaxine in healthy subjects. Hum Psychopharmacol 1996; **11**:1–9.
18. Sternbach H. Venlafaxine-induced galactorrhea. J Clin Psychopharmacol 2003; **23**:109–110.
19. Demir EY et al. Hyperprolactinemia connected with venlafaxine: a case report. Anatol J Psychiatry 2014; **15**:S10–S14.
20. Ashton AK et al. Hyperprolactinemia and galactorrhea induced by serotonin and norepinephrine reuptake inhibiting antidepressants. Am J Psychiatry 2007; **164**:1121–1122.
21. Korkmaz S et al. Galactorrhea during duloxetine treatment: a case report. Turk J Psychiatry 2011; **22**:200–201.
22. Sagud M et al. Effects of sertraline treatment on plasma cortisol, prolactin and thyroid hormones in female depressed patients. Neuropsychobiology 2002; **45**:139–143.
23. Schlosser R et al. Effects of subchronic paroxetine administration on night-time endocrinological profiles in healthy male volunteers. Psychoneuroendocrinology 2000; **25**:377–388.
24. Nadeem HS et al. Comparison of the effects of citalopram and escitalopram on 5-Ht-mediated neuroendocrine responses. Neuropsychopharmacology 2004; **29**:1699–1703.
25. Egberts AC et al. Non-puerperal lactation associated with antidepressant drug use. Br J Clin Pharmacol 1997; **44**:277–281.
26. Peterson MC. Reversible galactorrhea and prolactin elevation related to fluoxetine use. Mayo Clin Proc 2001; **76**:215–216.
27. Morrison J et al. Galactorrhea induced by paroxetine. Can J Psychiatry 2001; **46**:88–89.
28. Mahasuar R et al. Euprolactinemic galactorrhea associated with use of imipramine and escitalopram in a postmenopausal woman. Gen Hosp Psychiatry 2010; **32**:341–343.
29. Fava GA et al. Prolactin, cortisol, and antidepressant treatment. Am J Psychiatry 1988; **145**:358–360.
30. Orlander H et al. Imipramine induced elevation of prolactin levels in patients with HIV/AIDS improved their immune status. West Indian Med J 2009; **58**:207–213.
31. Meltzer HY et al. Lack of effect of tricyclic antidepressants on serum prolactin levels. Psychopharmacology (Berl) 1977; **51**:185–187.
32. Gadd EM et al. Antidepressants and galactorrhoea. Int Clin Psychopharmacol 1987; **2**:361–363.
33. Anand VS. Clomipramine-induced galactorrhoea and amenorrhoea. Br J Psychiatry 1985; **147**:87–88.
34. Fowlie S et al. Hyperprolactinaemia and nonpuerperal lactation associated with clomipramine. Scott Med J 1987; **32**:52.
35. Mahableshwarkar AR et al. A randomized, double-blind, fixed-dose study comparing the efficacy and tolerability of vortioxetine 2.5 and 10 mg in acute treatment of adults with generalized anxiety disorder. Hum Psychopharmacol 2014; **29**:64–72.
36. Baldwin DS et al. Vortioxetine (Lu AA21004) in the long-term open-label treatment of major depressive disorder. Curr Med Res Opin 2012; **28**:1717–1724.

Further reading

Coker F et al. Antidepressant-induced hyperprolactinaemia: incidence, mechanisms and management. CNS Drugs 2010; **24**:563–574.

CHAPTER 4

Antidepressants and diabetes mellitus

There is an established link between diabetes and depression.[1] Prevalence rates of co-morbid depressive symptoms in diabetic patients have been reported to range from 9% to 60% depending on the screening method used. A diagnosis of diabetes is linked to an increased likelihood of antidepressant prescription.[2,3] Having diabetes doubles the odds of co-morbid depression.[4] Patients with depression and diabetes have a high number of cardiovascular risk factors and increased mortality.[5,6] The presence of depression has a negative impact on metabolic control and likewise poor metabolic control may worsen depression.[7]

Considering all of this, the treatment of co-morbid depression in patients with diabetes is of vital importance and drug choice should take into account likely effects on metabolic control (see Table 4.19). Cochrane[8] suggests that antidepressants are effective and moderately improve glycaemic control. Be aware, however, that the prescribing of antidepressants may be associated with reduced adherence to antidiabetic medication.[9]

Table 4.19 Effect of antidepressants on glucose homeostasis and weight

Antidepressant class	Effect on glucose homeostasis and weight
SSRIs[10–23]	▪ Studies indicate that SSRIs have a favourable effect on diabetic parameters in patients with type II diabetes. Insulin requirements may be decreased ▪ Fluoxetine has been associated with improvement in HbA_{1c} levels, reduced insulin requirements, weight loss and enhanced insulin sensitivity. Its effect on insulin sensitivity is independent of is effect on weight loss. Sertraline may also reduce HbA_{1c} ▪ Escitalopram also seems to improve glycaemic control ▪ Some evidence that long-term SSRIs may increase the risk of diabetes to a modest extent but also evidence of no effect
TCAs[16,18,24–26]	▪ TCAs are associated with increased appetite, weight gain and hyperglycaemia ▪ Nortriptyline improved depression but worsened glycaemic control in diabetic patients in one study. Overall improvement in depression had a beneficial effect on HbA_{1c}. Clomipramine reported to precipitate diabetes ▪ Long-term use of TCAs seems to increase risk of diabetes
MAOIs[27,28]	▪ Irreversible MAOIs have a tendency to cause extreme hypoglycaemic episodes and weight gain ▪ No known effects with moclobemide
SNRIs[25,29,30]	▪ SNRIs do not appear to disrupt glycaemic control and have minimal impact on weight ▪ Studies of duloxetine in the treatment of diabetic neuropathy show that it has little influence on glycaemic control. No data in depression and diabetes ▪ Limited data on venlafaxine
Mirtazapine, reboxetine and trazodone[2,31]	▪ Mirtazapine is associated with weight gain but little is known about its effect in diabetes ▪ Mirtazapine does not appear to impair glucose tolerance in non-diabetic depressed patients ▪ No data with trazodone and reboxetine
Agomelatine[32]	▪ One small, open study suggests agomelatine is effective without changing glycaemic parameters

MAOI, monoamine oxidase inhibitor; SNRI, selective noradrenaline reuptake inhibitor; SSRI, selective serotonin reuptake inhibitor; TCA, tricyclic antidepressant.

CHAPTER 4

Recommendation: all patients with a diagnosis of depression should be screened for diabetes. In those who are diabetic:

- use SSRIs first line; most data support fluoxetine
- SNRIs are also likely to be safe but there are fewer supporting data
- avoid TCAs and MAOIs if possible due to their effects on weight and glucose homeostasis
- monitor blood glucose and HbA_{1c} carefully when antidepressant treatment is initiated, when the dose is changed and after discontinuation.

References

1. Katon WJ. The comorbidity of diabetes mellitus and depression. Am J Med 2008; **121 Suppl** 2:S8–15.
2. Musselman DL et al. Relationship of depression to diabetes types 1 and 2: epidemiology, biology, and treatment. Biol Psychiatry 2003; 54:317–329.
3. Knol MJ et al. Antidepressant use before and after initiation of diabetes mellitus treatment. Diabetologia 2009; 52:425–432.
4. Anderson RJ et al. The prevalence of comorbid depression in adults with diabetes: a meta-analysis. Diabetes Care 2001; 24:1069–1078.
5. Katon WJ et al. Cardiac risk factors in patients with diabetes mellitus and major depression. J Gen Intern Med 2004; 19:1192–1199.
6. Katon WJ et al. The association of comorbid depression with mortality in patients with type 2 diabetes. Diabetes Care 2005; **28:** 2668–2672.
7. Lustman PJ et al. Depression in diabetic patients: the relationship between mood and glycemic control. J Diabetes Complications 2005; 19:113–122.
8. Baumeister H et al. Psychological and pharmacological interventions for depression in patients with diabetes mellitus and depression. Cochrane Database Syst Rev 2012; 12:CD008381.
9. Caughey GE et al. Does antidepressant medication use affect persistence with diabetes medicines? Pharmacoepidemiol Drug Saf 2013; 22:615–622.
10. Maheux P et al. Fluoxetine improves insulin sensitivity in obese patients with non-insulin-dependent diabetes mellitus independently of weight loss. Int J Obes Relat Metab Disord 1997; 21:97–102.
11. Gulseren L et al. Comparison of fluoxetine and paroxetine in type II diabetes mellitus patients. Arch Med Res 2005; 36:159–165.
12. Lustman PJ et al. Sertraline for prevention of depression recurrence in diabetes mellitus: a randomized, double-blind, placebo-controlled trial. Arch Gen Psychiatry 2006; 63:521–529.
13. Gray DS et al. A randomized double-blind clinical trial of fluoxetine in obese diabetics. Int J Obes Relat Metab Disord 1992; 16 Suppl 4:S67–S72.
14. Knol MJ et al. Influence of antidepressants on glycaemic control in patients with diabetes mellitus. Pharmacoepidemiol Drug Saf 2008; 17:577–586.
15. Briscoe VJ et al. Effects of a selective serotonin reuptake inhibitor, fluoxetine, on counterregulatory responses to hypoglycemia in healthy individuals. Diabetes 2008; 57:2453–2460.
16. Andersohn F et al. Long-term use of antidepressants for depressive disorders and the risk of diabetes mellitus. Am J Psychiatry 2009; 166:591–598.
17. Derijks HJ et al. Influence of antidepressant use on glycemic control in patients with diabetes mellitus: an open-label comparative study. J Clin Psychopharmacol 2009; 29:405–408.
18. Kivimaki M et al. Antidepressant medication use, weight gain, and risk of type 2 diabetes: a population-based study. Diabetes Care 2010; 33:2611–2616.
19. Rubin RR et al. Antidepressant medicine use and risk of developing diabetes during the diabetes prevention program and diabetes prevention program outcomes study. Diabetes Care 2010; 33:2549–2551.
20. Echeverry D et al. Effect of pharmacological treatment of depression on A1C and quality of life in low-income Hispanics and African Americans with diabetes: a randomized, double-blind, placebo-controlled trial. Diabetes Care 2009; 32:2156–2160.
21. Gehlawat P et al. Diabetes with comorbid depression: role of SSRI in better glycemic control. Asian J Psychiatr 2013; 6:364–368.
22. Dhavale HS et al. Depression and diabetes: impact of antidepressant medications on glycaemic control. J Assoc Physicians India 2013; 61:896–899.
23. Mojtabai R. Antidepressant use and glycemic control. Psychopharmacology (Berl) 2013; 227:467–477.
24. Lustman PJ et al. Effects of nortriptyline on depression and glycemic control in diabetes: results of a double-blind, placebo-controlled trial. Psychosom Med 1997; 59:241–250.
25. McIntyre RS et al. The effect of antidepressants on glucose homeostasis and insulin sensitivity: synthesis and mechanisms. Expert Opin drug Saf 2006; 5:157–168.
26. Mumoli N et al. Clomipramine-induced diabetes. Ann Intern Med 2008; 149:595–596.

27. Goodnick PJ. Use of antidepressants in treatment of comorbid diabetes mellitus and depression as well as in diabetic neuropathy. Ann Clin Psychiatry 2001; **13**:31–41.

28. McIntyre RS et al. Mood and psychotic disorders and type 2 diabetes: a metabolic triad. Can J Diabetes 2005; **29**:122–132.

29. Raskin J et al. Duloxetine versus routine care in the long-term management of diabetic peripheral neuropathic pain. J Palliat Med 2006; **9**:29–40.

30. Crucitti A et al. Duloxetine treatment and glycemic controls in patients with diagnoses other than diabetic peripheral neuropathic pain: a meta-analysis. Curr Med Res Opin 2010; **26**:2579–2588.

31. Himmerich H et al. Changes in weight and glucose tolerance during treatment with mirtazapine. Diabetes Care 2006; **29**:170.

32. Karaiskos D et al. Agomelatine and sertraline for the treatment of depression in type 2 diabetes mellitus. Int J Clin Pract 2013; **67**:257–260.

Antidepressants and sexual dysfunction

Primary sexual disorders are common, although reliable normative data are lacking.[1] Reported prevalence rates vary depending on the method of data collection (low numbers with spontaneous reports, increasing with confidential questionnaires and further still with direct questioning).[1,2] Physical illness, psychiatric illness, substance misuse and prescribed drug treatment can all cause sexual dysfunction.[1,2] People with depression are more likely to be obese,[3] have diabetes,[4] and have cardiovascular disease than the general population, making them more likely to suffer sexual dysfunction.

Baseline sexual functioning should be determined, if possible (questionnaires may be useful), because sexual function affects quality of life and compliance (sexual dysfunction is one of the major causes of treatment dropout[5]). Complaints of sexual dysfunction may also indicate progression or inadequate treatment of underlying medical or psychiatric conditions. It may also be the result of drug treatment and intervention may greatly improve quality of life.[6]

Effects of depression

Both depression and the drugs used to treat it can cause disorders of desire, arousal and orgasm. The precise nature of the sexual dysfunction may indicate whether depression or treatment is the more likely cause. For example, 40–50% of people with depression report diminished libido and problems regarding sexual arousal in the month before diagnosis, but only 15–20% experience orgasm problems before taking an antidepressant.[7] In general, the prevalence and severity of sexual dysfunction increase with the severity of depression.[8] In some patients reporting sexual dysfunction before diagnosis, sexual functioning improves on treatment with antidepressants.[9] A post hoc analysis of data from the STAR*D study revealed that sexual dysfunction was problematic in 21% of patients whose depression remitted with citalopram treatment compared with 61% of those whose depression did not remit.[10] In any cohort of people with depression there will be some who do not have sexual dysfunction, and some who develop sexual dysfunction on antidepressants. Amongst those presenting with sexual dysfunction, some will see an improvement, some no change and some a worsening when taking on antidepressant.[11]

Effects of antidepressant drugs

Antidepressants can cause sedation, hormonal changes, disturbance of cholinergic/adrenergic balance, peripheral α-adrenergic antagonism, inhibition of nitric oxide and increased serotonin neurotransmission, all of which can result in sexual dysfunction.[12] Sexual dysfunction has been reported as a side-effect of all antidepressants, although rates vary (see Table 4.20). The impact of antidepressants on sexual function is likely to be dose dependent. Individual susceptibility also varies and may be at least partially genetically determined.[13,14] All effects are reversible.

Not all of the sexual side-effects of antidepressants are undesirable:[1] serotonergic antidepressants including clomipramine are effective in the treatment of premature ejaculation[15] and may also be beneficial in paraphilias.

Table 4.20 Sexual adverse effects of antidepressant drugs

Drug	Approximate prevalence	Type of problem
Tricyclics[16–19]	30%	Decreased libido, erectile dysfunction, delayed orgasm, impaired ejaculation. Prevalence of delayed orgasm with clomipramine may be at least double that with other TCAs. Painful ejaculation reported rarely
Trazodone[5,20–22]	Unknown	Impaired ejaculation and both increases and decreases in libido reported. Used in some cases to promote erection. Priapism occurs in approximately 0.01%
MAOIs[5,23]	40%	Similar to TCAs, although prevalence may be higher.[1] Moclobemide much less likely to cause problems than older MAOIs (4% versus 40%)
SSRIs[5,24–27]	60–70%	Affect all phases of the sexual response; decreased libido and delayed orgasm most commonly reported.[28] Paroxetine is associated with more erectile dysfunction and decreased vaginal lubrication than the other SSRIs. Difficult to determine relative prevalence but there is evidence that ejaculatory delay is worse with paroxetine than citalopram[29]
		Penile and vaginal anaesthesia has been reported rarely with fluoxetine and other SSRIs.[30] Painful ejaculation reported rarely,[31] as is priapism[32]
Venlafaxine[5]	70%	Decreased libido and delayed orgasm common. Erectile dysfunction less common. Rare reports of painfal ejaculation[31] and priapism[32]
Mirtazapine[5,25,33]	25%	Decreased libido and delayed orgasm possible. Erectile dysfunction and absence of orgasm less common
Reboxetine[34]	5–10%	Various abnormalities of orgasmic function
Duloxetine[35]	46%	Any sexual dysfunction with a score ≥5 on the ASEX scale, with a statistical significance seen for the specific item 'ease of orgasm' in male patients
Agomelatine[36,37]	<20%	No clear effect on orgasm, erection or libido. Sexual dysfunction incidence similar to placebo. Note that the antidepressant efficacy of agomelatine has been questioned[38] but is now not in doubt

MAOI, monoamine oxidase inhibitor; SSRI, selective serotonin reuptake inhibitor; TCA, tricyclic antidepressant.

Sexual side-effects can be minimised by careful selection of the antidepressant drug – see Table 4.20.

Treatment

A thorough assessment is essential to exclude physical causes such as diabetes and cardiovascular disease, and psychological and relationship difficulties. Spontaneous remission occurs in approximately 10% of cases and partial remission in a further 11%.[5] If this does not happen, the dose may be reduced or the antidepressant discontinued where appropriate.

Drug 'holidays' or delayed dosing may be used,[39] as may dose reduction. This approach is problematic as the patient may relapse or experience antidepressant discontinuation symptoms. More logical is a switch to a different drug that is less likely to cause the specific sexual problem experienced (see Table 4.20). Note that agomelatine[40,41] and amfebutamone (bupropion – not licensed for depression in UK)[42,43] have probably the lowest risk of sexual dysfunction. Bupropion is widely used in the USA as a first-line antidepressant with minimal risk of sexual side-effects, and as an adjunct (antidote) in patients with SSRI-induced sexual dysfunction.[44] Preliminary data support the reduction of sexual side-effects in patients treated with duloxetine or SSRIs when mirtazapine is added.[45,46] Trazodone may have similar effects.[47] Selegiline transdermal patches (licensed for the treatment of depression in the USA) seem to be associated with a low risk of sexual side-effects.[48]

Adjunctive or 'antidote' drugs may also be used (see section on 'Antipsychotics and sexual dysfunction' in Chapter 2 for further information).

Sildenafil is more effective than placebo at improving erectile function in men,[49] and in improving sexual function in women taking SSRIs.[50] Small RCTs support the modest efficacy of maca root[51] and saffron.[52,53]

A Cochrane review of the 'strategies for managing sexual dysfunction induced by antidepressant medication' found that the addition of sildenafil or tadalafil may improve sexual function in men and bupropion may be useful in women.[54]

References

1. Baldwin DS et al. Effects of antidepressant drugs on sexual function. Int J Psychiatry Clin Pract 1997; 1:47–58.
2. Pollack MH et al. Genitourinary and sexual adverse effects of psychotropic medication. Int J Psychiatry Med 1992; 22:305–327.
3. Luppino FS et al. Overweight, obesity, and depression: a systematic review and meta-analysis of longitudinal studies. Arch Gen Psychiatry 2010; 67:220–229.
4. Kivimaki M et al. Antidepressant medication use, weight gain, and risk of type 2 diabetes: a population-based study. Diabetes Care 2010; 33:2611–2616.
5. Montejo AL et al. Incidence of sexual dysfunction associated with antidepressant agents: a prospective multicenter study of 1022 outpatients. Spanish Working Group for the Study of Psychotropic-Related Sexual Dysfunction. J Clin Psychiatry 2001; 62 Suppl 3:10–21.
6. Segraves RT. Effects of psychotropic drugs on human erection and ejaculation. Arch Gen Psychiatry 1989; 46:275–284.
7. Kennedy SH et al. Sexual dysfunction before antidepressant therapy in major depression. J Affect Disord 1999; 56:201–208.
8. Cheng JY et al. Depressive symptomatology and male sexual functions in late life. J Affect Disord 2007; 104:225–229.
9. Saiz-Ruiz J et al. Assessment of sexual functioning in depressed patients treated with mirtazapine: a naturalistic 6-month study. Hum Psychopharmacol 2005; 20:435–440.
10. Ishak WW et al. Sexual satisfaction and quality of life in major depressive disorder before and after treatment with citalopram in the STAR*D study. J Clin Psychiatry 2013; 74:256–261.
11. Werneke U et al. Antidepressants and sexual dysfunction. Acta Psychiatr Scand 2006; 114:384–397.
12. Clayton AH. Recognition and assessment of sexual dysfunction associated with depression. J Clin Psychiatry 2001; 62 Suppl 3:5–9.
13. Bishop JR et al. Serotonin 2A -1438 G/A and G-protein Beta3 subunit C825T polymorphisms in patients with depression and SSRI-associated sexual side-effects. Neuropsychopharmacology 2006; 31:2281–2288.
14. Bishop JR et al. The association of serotonin transporter genotypes and selective serotonin reuptake inhibitor (SSRI)-associated sexual side effects: possible relationship to oral contraceptives. Hum Psychopharmacol 2009; 24:207–215.
15. Waldinger MD. Premature ejaculation: definition and drug treatment. Drugs 2007; 67:547–568.
16. Harrison WM et al. Effects of antidepressant medication on sexual function: a controlled study. J Clin Psychopharmacol 1986; 6:144–149.
17. Beaumont G. Sexual side-effects of clomipramine (Anafranil). J Int Med Res 1977; 5:37–44.
18. Rickels K et al. Nefazodone: aspects of efficacy. J Clin Psychiatry 1995; 56 Suppl 6:43–46.
19. Sovner R. Anorgasmia associated with imipramine but not desipramine: case report. J Clin Psychiatry 1983; 44:345–346.
20. Gartrell N. Increased libido in women receiving trazodone. Am J Psychiatry 1986; 143:781–782.
21. Sullivan G. Increased libido in three men treated with trazodone. J Clin Psychiatry 1988; 49:202–203.
22. Thompson JW Jr. et al. Psychotropic medication and priapism: a comprehensive review. J Clin Psychiatry 1990; 51:430–433.
23. Lesko LM et al. Three cases of female anorgasmia associated with MAOIs. Am J Psychiatry 1982; 139:1353–1354.
24. Herman JB et al. Fluoxetine-induced sexual dysfunction. J Clin Psychiatry 1990; 51:25–27.
25. Gelenberg AJ et al. Mirtazapine substitution in SSRI-induced sexual dysfunction. J Clin Psychiatry 2000; 61:356–360.
26. Jacobsen FM. Fluoxetine-induced sexual dysfunction and an open trial of yohimbine. J Clin Psychiatry 1992; 53:119–122.

CHAPTER 4

27. Lauerma H. Successful treatment of citalopram-induced anorgasmia by cyproheptadine. Acta Psychiatr Scand 1996; **93**:69–70.

28. Demyttenaere K et al. Review: Bupropion and SSRI-induced side effects. J Psychopharmacol 2008; **22**:792–804.

29. Waldinger MD et al. SSRIs and ejaculation: a double-blind, randomized, fixed-dose study with paroxetine and citalopram. J Clin Psychopharmacol 2001; **21**:556–560.

30. Praharaj SK. Serotonin reuptake inhibitor induced sensory disturbances. Br J Clin Pharmacol 2004; **58**:673–674.

31. Ilie CP et al. Painful ejaculation. BJU Int 2007; **99**:1335–1339.

32. Tran QT et al. Priapism, ecstasy, and marijuana: is there a connection? Adv Urol 2008; **1**. DOI:10.1155/2008/193694

33. Lee KU et al. Antidepressant-induced sexual dysfunction among newer antidepressants in a naturalistic setting. Psychiatry Invest 2010; **7**:55–59.

34. Haberfellner EM. Sexual dysfunction caused by reboxetine. Pharmacopsychiatry 2002; **35**:77–78.

35. Delgado PL et al. Sexual functioning assessed in 4 double-blind placebo- and paroxetine-controlled trials of duloxetine for major depressive disorder. J Clin Psychiatry 2005; **66**:686–692.

36. Kennedy SH et al. A double-blind comparison of sexual functioning, antidepressant efficacy, and tolerability between agomelatine and venlafaxine XR. J Clin Psychopharmacol 2008; **28**:329–333.

37. Montejo A et al. The effects of agomelatine on sexual function in depressed patients and healthy volunteers. Hum Psychopharmacol 2011; **26**:537–542.

38. Koesters M et al. Agomelatine efficacy and acceptability revisited: systematic review and meta-analysis of published and unpublished randomised trials. Br J Psychiatry 2013; **203**:179–187.

39. Rothschild AJ. Selective serotonin reuptake inhibitor-induced sexual dysfunction: efficacy of a drug holiday. Am J Psychiatry 1995; **152**:1514–1516.

40. Serretti A et al. Treatment-emergent sexual dysfunction related to antidepressants: a meta-analysis. J Clin Psychopharmacol 2009; **29**:259–266.

41. Kennedy SH et al. A double-blind comparison of sexual functioning, antidepressant efficacy, and tolerability between agomelatine and venlafaxine XR. J Clin Psychopharmacol 2008; **28**:329–333.

42. Clayton AH et al. Bupropion extended release compared with escitalopram: effects on sexual functioning and antidepressant efficacy in 2 randomized, double-blind, placebo-controlled studies. J Clin Psychiatry 2006; **67**:736–746.

43. Clayton AH et al. Prevalence of sexual dysfunction among newer antidepressants. J Clin Psychiatry 2002; **63**:357–366.

44. Balon R et al. Survey of treatment practices for sexual dysfunction(s) associated with anti-depressants. J Sex Marital Ther 2008; **34**:353–365.

45. Ravindran LN et al. Combining mirtazapine and duloxetine in treatment-resistant depression improves outcomes and sexual function. J Clin Psychopharmacol 2008; **28**:107–108.

46. Ozmenler NK et al. Mirtazapine augmentation in depressed patients with sexual dysfunction due to selective serotonin reuptake inhibitors. Hum Psychopharmacol 2008; **23**:321–326.

47. Stryjer R et al. Trazodone for the treatment of sexual dysfunction induced by serotonin reuptake inhibitors: a preliminary open-label study. Clin Neuropharmacol 2009; **32**:82–84.

48. Clayton AH et al. Symptoms of sexual dysfunction in patients treated for major depressive disorder: a meta-analysis comparing selegiline transdermal system and placebo using a patient-rated scale. J Clin Psychiatry 2007; **68**:1860–1866.

49. Fava M et al. Efficacy and safety of sildenafil in men with serotonergic antidepressant-associated erectile dysfunction: results from a randomized, double-blind, placebo-controlled trial. J Clin Psychiatry 2006; **67**:240–246.

50. Nurnberg HG et al. Sildenafil treatment of women with antidepressant-associated sexual dysfunction: a randomized controlled trial. JAMA 2008; **300**:395–404.

51. Dording CM et al. A double-blind, randomized, pilot dose-finding study of maca root (L. meyenii) for the management of SSRI-induced sexual dysfunction. CNS Neurosci Ther 2008; **14**:182–191.

52. Modabbernia A et al. Effect of saffron on fluoxetine-induced sexual impairment in men: randomized double-blind placebo-controlled trial. Psychopharmacology (Berl) 2012; **223**:381–388.

53. Kashani L et al. Saffron for treatment of fluoxetine-induced sexual dysfunction in women: randomized double-blind placebo-controlled study. Hum Psychopharmacol 2013; **28**:54–60.

54. Taylor MJ et al. Strategies for managing sexual dysfunction induced by antidepressant medication. Cochrane Database Syst Rev 2013; **5**:CD003382.

Further reading

Williams VS et al. Prevalence and impact of antidepressant-associated sexual dysfunction in three European countries: replication in a cross-sectional patient survey. J Psychopharmacol 2010; **24**:489–496.

CHAPTER 4

SSRIs and bleeding

Serotonin is released from platelets in response to vascular injury and promotes vaso-constriction and morphological changes in platelets that lead to aggregation.[1] Serotonin alone is a relatively weak platelet aggregator. SSRIs inhibit the serotonin transporter which is responsible for the uptake of serotonin into platelets. It might thus be predicted that SSRIs will deplete platelet serotonin, leading to a reduced ability to form clots and a subsequent increase in the risk of bleeding. SSRIs also increase gastric acid secretion and therefore may be irritant to the gastric mucosa.[2] Use of SSRIs seems to increase the risk of peptic ulcer.[3]

Several database studies have found that patients who take SSRIs are at significantly increased risk of being admitted to hospital with an upper GI bleed compared with age-and-sex matched controls.[4-7] This association holds when age, gender and the effects of other drugs such as aspirin and NSAIDs are controlled for. Co-prescription of low-dose aspirin at least doubles the risk of GI bleeding associated with SSRIs alone and co-prescription of NSAIDs approximately quadruples risk.[8] Combined use of SSRIs and NSAIDs greatly increases the use of anti-acid drugs.[9] The elderly and those with a history of GI bleeding are at greatest risk.[6,7,10] The risk may be greatest with SSRIs that have a high affinity for the serotonin transporter.[5,11] Risk decreases to the same level as controls in past users of SSRIs, indicating that bleeding is likely to be associated with treatment itself rather than some inherent characteristic of the patients being treated.[5]

The excess risk of bleeding is not confined to upper GI bleeds. The risk of lower GI bleeds may also be increased[12] and an increased risk of uterine bleeding has also been reported.[13] SSRIs should be used cautiously in patients with cirrhosis or other risk factors for internal bleeding.[14]

Use of SSRIs in the perioperative period has been associated with a 20% increase in inpatient mortality (absolute risk 1:1000), although patient rather than drug factors could not be excluded as the cause.[15] One study found that patients prescribed SSRIs who underwent orthopaedic surgery had an almost four-fold risk of requiring a blood transfusion.[16] This equated to one additional patient requiring transfusion for every ten SSRI patients undergoing surgery and was double the risk of patients who were taking NSAIDs alone. It should be noted in this context that treatment with SSRIs has been associated with a 2.4-fold increase in the risk of hip fracture[17] and a two-fold increase of fracture in old age.[18] The combination of advanced age, SSRI treatment, orthopaedic surgery and NSAIDs clearly presents a very high risk. However, there does not seem to be an increased risk of bleeding in patients who undergo coronary artery bypass surgery.[19] Similarly, the risk of post-partum haemorrhage does not seem to be increased,[20] although a review of 13 studies found an increased odds ratio (1.21–4.14) of perioperative bleeding with SSRIs.[21] One study noted an increased risk of bleeding in women undergoing breast surgery[22] and the authors suggest withholding SSRIs for 2 weeks prior to such planned surgery. Others conclude that there is insufficient evidence to support routine discontinuation of SSRIs prior to surgery and call for RCTs to be conducted in this area of care.[23] Venlafaxine may have similar effects[21] but duloxetine may not affect bleeding risk.[24]

It is likely that SSRIs are responsible for an additional three episodes of bleeding in every 1000 patient-years of treatment over the normal background incidence[5,13] but this figure masks large variations in risk (see Table 4.21). For example, one in 85 patients with a history of GI bleed will have a further bleed attributable to treatment with a SSRI.[10] One database study suggests that gastroprotective drugs (proton pump inhibitors – PPIs) decrease the risk of GI bleeds associated with SSRIs (alone or in combination with NSAIDs) although not quite to control levels.[6]

Some studies have been prompted by the hypothesis that the increased risk of upper GI bleeds associated with SSRIs may be balanced by a decreased risk of embolic events. One database study failed to find a reduction in the risk of a first myocardial infarction in SSRI-treated patients compared with controls,[25] while another[26] found a reduction in the risk of being admitted to hospital with a first MI in smokers on SSRIs. The effect size in the second study was large: approximately one in ten hospitalisations were avoided in SSRI-treated patients.[26] This is similar to the effect size of other antiplatelet therapies such as aspirin.[27]

In patients who take warfarin, SSRIs increase the risk of a non-GI bleed 2–3-fold (similar to the effect size of NSAIDs) but do not seem to increase the risk of a GI bleed.[28,29] This does not seem to be associated with any effect on the INR, making it difficult to identify those at highest risk.[29] In keeping with these findings, SSRI use in anticoagulated patients being treated for acute coronary syndromes may decrease the risk of minor cardiac events at the expense of an increased risk of a bleed.[30]

Three large database studies have failed to find a reduction in the risk of an ischaemic stroke (or increase in the risk of haemorrhagic stroke) in SSRI users.[31–33] A single cohort study reported an increased risk of haemorrhagic stroke.[34] The absolute risk was small. A further nested case–control study showed an 11% increased odds of haemorrhagic stroke in people on SSRIs[35] (absolute risk 1:10,000 patient-years of treatment). Table 4.21 shows estimated relative odds/risk of bleeding events reported in more recent meta-analyses.

Table 4.21 Recent analyses of bleeding risk with SSRIs

Treatment	Upper GI bleed	Cerebral haemorrhage
SSRI[11]	OR 1.39	OR 1.39
SSRI[36]	–	RR 1.42
SSRI + oral anticoagulant[36]	–	RR 1.56 vs oral anticoagulant
SSRI[37]	OR 1.73	–
SSRI + NSAID[37]	OR 4.02	–
SSRI[38]	OR 1.66	–
SSRI[39]	OR 1.67	–
SSRI[40]	–	OR 1.32
SSRI[41]	OR 1.55	–
SSRI + warfarin[42]	–	OR 1.41 vs warfarin

GI, gastrointestinal; NSAID, non-steroidal anti-inflammatory drug; OR, odds ratio; RR, relative risk; SSRI, selective serotonin reuptake inhibitor.
Note: Absolute risk is important here in interpreting the clinical significance of these outcomes, but not all reviews give subject numbers. In the first listed review,[11] upper GI bleeding occurred in 3.7% of SSRI subjects and 2.5% of controls. The corresponding figures for intracranial bleeding were 3.5% and 2.3%. In the last listed review,[42] haemorrhage rates were 2.32/100 patient-years versus 1.35 per 100 patient-years.

CHAPTER 4

Summary

- SSRIs increase the risk of GI, cerebral and perioperative bleeding (those undergoing orthopaedic or breast surgery may be at greatest risk).
- Risk is increased still further in those also receiving aspirin, NSAIDs or oral anticoagulants.
- Try to avoid SSRIs in patients receiving NSAIDs, aspirin or oral anticoagulants or with history of cerebral or GI bleeds.
- If SSRI use cannot be avoided, monitor closely and prescribe gastroprotective proton pump inhibitors.

References

1. Skop BP et al. Potential vascular and bleeding complications of treatment with selective serotonin reuptake inhibitors. Psychosomatics 1996; 37:12–16.
2. Andrade C et al. Serotonin reuptake inhibitor antidepressants and abnormal bleeding: a review for clinicians and a reconsideration of mechanisms. J Clin Psychiatry 2010; 71:1565–1575.
3. Dall M et al. There is an association between selective serotonin reuptake inhibitor use and uncomplicated peptic ulcers: a population-based case-control study. Aliment Pharmacol Ther 2010; 32:1383–1391.
4. de Abajo FJ et al. Association between selective serotonin reuptake inhibitors and upper gastrointestinal bleeding: population based case-control study. BMJ 1999; 319:1106–1109.
5. Dalton SO et al. Use of selective serotonin reuptake inhibitors and risk of upper gastrointestinal tract bleeding: a population-based cohort study. Arch Intern Med 2003; 163:59–64.
6. de Abajo FJ et al. Risk of upper gastrointestinal tract bleeding associated with selective serotonin reuptake inhibitors and venlafaxine therapy: interaction with nonsteroidal anti-inflammatory drugs and effect of acid-suppressing agents. Arch Gen Psychiatry 2008; 65:795–803.
7. Lewis JD et al. Moderate and high affinity serotonin reuptake inhibitors increase the risk of upper gastrointestinal toxicity. Pharmacoepidemiol Drug Saf 2008; 17:328–335.
8. Paton C et al. SSRIs and gastrointestinal bleeding. BMJ 2005; 331:529–530.
9. de Jong JC et al. Combined use of SSRIs and NSAIDs increases the risk of gastrointestinal adverse effects. Br J Clin Pharmacol 2003; 55:591–595.
10. van Walraven C et al. Inhibition of serotonin reuptake by antidepressants and upper gastrointestinal bleeding in elderly patients: retrospective cohort study. BMJ 2001; 323:655–658.
11. Verdel BM et al. Use of serotonergic drugs and the risk of bleeding. Clin Pharmacol Ther 2011; 89:89–96.
12. Wessinger S et al. Increased use of selective serotonin reuptake inhibitors in patients admitted with gastrointestinal haemorrhage: a multicentre retrospective analysis. Aliment Pharmacol Ther 2006; 23:937–944.
13. Meijer WE et al. Association of risk of abnormal bleeding with degree of serotonin reuptake inhibition by antidepressants. Arch Intern Med 2004; 164:2367–2370.
14. Weinrieb RM et al. A critical review of selective serotonin reuptake inhibitor-associated bleeding: balancing the risk of treating hepatitis C-infected patients. J Clin Psychiatry 2003; 64:1502–1510.
15. Auerbach AD et al. Perioperative use of selective serotonin reuptake inhibitors and risks for adverse outcomes of surgery. JAMA Intern Med 2013; 173:1075–1081.
16. Movig KL et al. Relationship of serotonergic antidepressants and need for blood transfusion in orthopedic surgical patients. Arch Intern Med 2003; 163:2354–2358.
17. Liu B et al. Use of selective serotonin-reuptake inhibitors of tricyclic antidepressants and risk of hip fractures in elderly people. Lancet 1998; 351:1303–1307.
18. Richards JB et al. Effect of selective serotonin reuptake inhibitors on the risk of fracture. Arch Intern Med 2007; 167:188–194.
19. Andreasen JJ et al. Effect of selective serotonin reuptake inhibitors on requirement for allogeneic red blood cell transfusion following coronary artery bypass surgery. Am J Cardiovasc Drugs 2006; 6:243–250.
20. Salkeld E et al. The risk of postpartum hemorrhage with selective serotonin reuptake inhibitors and other antidepressants. J Clin Psychopharmacol 2008; 28:230–234.
21. Mahdanian AA et al. Serotonergic antidepressants and perioperative bleeding risk: a systematic review. Expert Opin Drug Saf 2014; 13:695–704.
22. Jeong BO et al. Use of serotonergic antidepressants and bleeding risk in patients undergoing surgery. Psychosomatics 2014; 55:213–220.
23. Mrkobrada M et al. Selective serotonin reuptake inhibitors and surgery: to hold or not to hold, that is the question: comment on 'Perioperative use of selective serotonin reuptake inhibitors and risks for adverse outcomes of surgery'. JAMA Intern Med 2013; 173:1082–1083.
24. Perahia DG et al. The risk of bleeding with duloxetine treatment in patients who use nonsteroidal anti-inflammatory drugs (NSAIDs): analysis of placebo-controlled trials and post-marketing adverse event reports. Drug Healthcare patient Saf 2013; 5:211–219.

25. Meier CR et al. Use of selective serotonin reuptake inhibitors and risk of developing first-time acute myocardial infarction. Br J Clin Pharmacol 2001; **52**:179–184.

26. Sauer WH et al. Selective serotonin reuptake inhibitors and myocardial infarction. Circulation 2001; **104**:1894–1898.

27. Antiplatelet Trialists' Collaboration. Collaborative overview of randomised trials of antiplatelet therapy – I: Prevention of death, myocardial infarction, and stroke by prolonged antiplatelet therapy in various categories of patients. BMJ 1994; **308**:81–106.

28. Schalekamp T et al. Increased bleeding risk with concurrent use of selective serotonin reuptake inhibitors and coumarins. Arch Intern Med 2008; **168**:180–185.

29. Wallerstedt SM et al. Risk of clinically relevant bleeding in warfarin-treated patients – influence of SSRI treatment. Pharmacoepidemiol Drug Saf 2009; **18**:412–416.

30. Ziegelstein RC et al. Selective serotonin reuptake inhibitor use by patients with acute coronary syndromes. Am J Med 2007; **120**:525–530.

31. Bak S et al. Selective serotonin reuptake inhibitors and the risk of stroke: a population-based case-control study. Stroke 2002; **33**:1465–1473.

32. Barbui C et al. Past use of selective serotonin reuptake inhibitors and the risk of cerebrovascular events in the elderly. Int Clin Psychopharmacol 2005; **20**:169–171.

33. Kharofa J et al. Selective serotonin reuptake inhibitors and risk of hemorrhagic stroke. Stroke 2007; **38**:3049–3051.

34. Smoller JW et al. Antidepressant use and risk of incident cardiovascular morbidity and mortality among postmenopausal women in the Women's Health Initiative study. Arch Intern Med 2009; **169**:2128–2139.

35. Douglas I et al. The use of antidepressants and the risk of haemorrhagic stroke: a nested case control study. Br J Clin Pharmacol 2011; **71**:116–120.

36. Hackam DG et al. Selective serotonin reuptake inhibitors and brain hemorrhage: a meta-analysis. Neurology 2012; **79**:1862–1865.

37. Oka Y et al. Meta-analysis of the risk of upper gastrointestinal hemorrhage with combination therapy of selective serotonin reuptake inhibitors and non-steroidal anti-inflammatory drugs. Biol Pharm Bull 2014; **37**:947–953.

38. Anglin R et al. Risk of upper gastrointestinal bleeding with selective serotonin reuptake inhibitors with or without concurrent nonsteroidal anti-inflammatory use: a systematic review and meta-analysis. Am J Gastroenterol 2014; **109**:811–819.

39. Wang YP et al. Short-term use of serotonin reuptake inhibitors and risk of upper gastrointestinal bleeding. Am J Psychiatry 2014; **171**:54–61.

40. Shin D et al. Use of selective serotonin reuptake inhibitors and risk of stroke: a systematic review and meta-analysis. J Neurol 2014; **261**:686–695.

41. Jiang HY et al. Use of selective serotonin reuptake inhibitors and risk of upper gastrointestinal bleeding: a systematic review and meta-analysis. Clin Gastroenterol Hepatol 2014; 30 June (epub ahead of print).

42. Quinn GR et al. Effect of selective serotonin reuptake inhibitors on bleeding risk in patients with atrial fibrillation taking warfarin. Am J Cardiol 2014; **114**:583–586.

CHAPTER 4

Antidepressants: relative adverse effects – a rough guide

Table 4.22 shows approximate relative severity of common adverse effects of antidepressants.

Table 4.22 Common adverse effects of antidepressants

Drug	Sedation	Hypotension	Cardiac conduction disturbance	Anticholinergic effects	Nausea/ vomiting	Sexual dysfunction
Tricyclics						
Amitriptyline	+++	+++	+++	+++	+	+++
Clomipramine	++	+++	+++	++	++	+++
Dosulepin	+++	+++	+++	++	+	+
Doxepin	+++	++	+++	+++	+	+
Imipramine	++	+++	+++	+++	+	+
Lofepramine	+	+	+	++	+	+
Nortriptyline	+	++	++	+	+	+
Trimipramine	+++	+++	++	++	+	+
Other antidepressants						
Agomelatine	+	–	–	–	–	–
Duloxetine	–	–	–	–	++	++
Mianserin	++	–	–	–	–	–
Mirtazapine	+++	+	–	+	+	–
Reboxetine	+	–	–	+	+	+
Trazodone	+++	+	+	+	+	+
Venlafaxine	–	–	+	–	+++	+++
Selective serotonin reuptake inhibitors (SSRIs)						
Citalopram	–	–	+	–	++	+++
Escitalopram	–	–	+	–	++	+++
Fluoxetine	–	–	–	–	++	+++
Fluvoxamine	+	–	–	–	+++	+++
Paroxetine	+	–	–	+	++	+++
Sertraline	–	–	–	–	++	+++
Vortioxetine*	–	+	–	–	++	++

Table 4.22 (Continued)

Drug	Sedation	Hypotension	Cardiac conduction disturbance	Anticholinergic effects	Nausea/ vomiting	Sexual dysfunction
Monoamine oxidase inhibitors (MAOIs)						
Isocarboxazid	+	++	+	++	+	+
Phenelzine	+	+	+	+	+	+
Tranylcypromine	−	+	+	+	+	+
Reversible inhibitor of monoamine oxidase A (RIMA)						
Moclobemide	−	−	−	−	+	+

Key: +++, high incidence/severity; ++, moderate; +, low; −, very low, none.
*Vortioxetine classed as an SSRI for convenience here – it has several other pharmacological effects.

Anxiety spectrum disorders

Anxiety is a normal emotion that is experienced by everyone at some time. Symptoms can be psychological, physical, or a mixture of both. Intervention is required when symptoms become disabling or reduce quality of life.

There are several disorders within the overall spectrum of anxiety disorders, each with its own characteristic symptoms. These are outlined briefly in Table 4.23. Anxiety disorders can occur on their own, be co-morbid with other psychiatric disorders (particularly depression), be a consequence of physical illness such as thyrotoxicosis or be drug induced (e.g. by caffeine). Co-morbidity with other psychiatric disorders is very common.

Anxiety spectrum disorders tend to be chronic and treatment is often only partially successful. Note that people with anxiety disorders may be particularly prone to adverse effects.[1] High initial doses of SSRIs in particular may be poorly tolerated.

Benzodiazepines

Benzodiazepines provide rapid symptomatic relief from acute anxiety states.[2] All guidelines and consensus statements recommend that this group of drugs should only be used to treat anxiety that is severe, disabling or subjecting the individual to extreme distress. Because of their potential to cause physical dependence and withdrawal symptoms, these drugs should be used at the lowest effective dose for the shortest period of time (maximum 4 weeks), while medium-/long-term treatment strategies are put in place, and with caution in patients with substance misuse. For the majority of patients, these recommendations are sensible and should be adhered to. A very small number of patients with severely disabling anxiety may benefit from long-term treatment with a benzodiazepine and these patients should not be denied treatment. Benzodiazepines are, however, known to be overprescribed in the long term for treatment of both anxiety[3] and depression,[4] usually in place of more appropriate treatment.

NICE recommends that benzodiazepines should not be used to treat panic disorder.[5] In other countries, alprazolam is widely used for this indication. Benzodiazepines should be used with care in post-traumatic stress disorder (PTSD).[6]

SSRIs/SNRIs

When used to treat **generalised anxiety disorder** (**GAD**), SSRIs should initially be prescribed at half the normal starting dose for the treatment of depression and the dose titrated upwards into the normal antidepressant dosage range as tolerated (initial worsening of anxiety may be seen when treatment is started[7]). The same advice applies to the use of venlafaxine and duloxetine. Response is usually seen within 6 weeks and continues to increase over time.[8] The optimal duration of treatment has not been determined but should be at least 1 year.[9,10] Effective treatment of GAD may prevent the development of major depression.[9] Fluoxetine is probably the most effective SSRI and sertraline the best tolerated.[11]

When used to treat **panic disorder**, the same starting dose and dosage titration as in GAD should be used. Doses of clomipramine,[12] citalopram[13] and sertraline[14] towards the bottom of the antidepressant range give the best balance between efficacy and side-effects, whereas higher doses of paroxetine (40 mg and above) may be required.[15] Higher doses of all drugs may be effective when standard doses have failed. Onset of action may be as long as 6 weeks. Women may respond better to SSRIs than men.[16] There is some evidence that augmentation with clonazepam leads to a more rapid response (but not a greater magnitude of response overall).[15] The optimal duration of treatment is unknown, but should be at least 8 months;[17] a large naturalistic study showed convincing evidence of benefit for at least 3 years.[18] Less than half are likely to remain well after medication is withdrawn.[19]

Lower starting doses are also required in **post-traumatic stress disorder (PTSD)**, although high doses (e.g. fluoxetine 60 mg) are often required for full effect. Response is usually seen within 8 weeks, but can take up to 12 weeks.[19] Treatment should be continued for at least 6 months and probably longer.[10,20,21]

Although the doses of SSRIs licensed for the treatment of **obsessive compulsive disorder (OCD)** are higher than those licensed for the treatment of depression (e.g. fluoxetine 60 mg, paroxetine 40–60 mg), lower (standard antidepressant) doses may be effective, particularly for maintenance treatment.[22] Initial response is usually slower to emerge than in depression (can take 10–12 weeks). Treatment should continue for at least 1 year.[10] The relapse rate in those who continue treatment for 2 years is half that of those who stop treatment after initial response (25–40% versus 80%).[23] In most people with OCD, the condition is persistent and symptom severity fluctuates over time.[24]

Body dysmorphic disorder (BDD) should be treated initially with CBT. If symptoms are moderate to severe, adding an SSRI may improve outcome.[25] Buspirone may usefully augment the SSRI.[25]

Standard antidepressant starting doses are well tolerated in **social phobia**,[26,27] and dosage titration may benefit some patients but is not always required. Response is usually seen within 8 weeks and treatment should be continued for at least a year and probably longer.[27] Note that NICE recommends CBT as first-line treatment for social anxiety.[28]

All patients treated with SSRIs should be monitored for the development of akathisia, increased anxiety and the emergence of suicidal ideation; the risk is thought to be greatest in those <30 years, those with co-morbid depression and those already known to be at higher risk of suicide.[25,29]

Selective serotonin reuptake inhibitors should not be stopped abruptly, as patients with anxiety spectrum disorders are particularly sensitive to discontinuation symptoms (see section on 'Antidepressant discontinuation symptoms' in this chapter). The dose should be reduced slowly as tolerated over several weeks to months.

Pregabalin

Pregabalin is licensed for the treatment of GAD. Several large RCTs have demonstrated its efficacy and tolerability and comparable speed of onset of action to a benzodiazepine.[30] The dose of pregabalin in GAD is initially 150 mg, increased gradually to maximum of 600 mg in 2–3 divided doses. Pregabalin should not be stopped abruptly as it may precipitate rebound anxiety and seizures.

CHAPTER 4

Psychological approaches

There is good evidence to support the efficacy of some psychological interventions in anxiety spectrum disorders.[10,31] Examples include exposure therapy in OCD and social phobia. Initial drug therapy may be required to help the patient become more receptive to psychological input. Some studies suggest that optimal outcome is achieved by combining psychological and drug therapies,[5] but negative studies also exist.[32,33]

A discussion of the evidence base for psychological interventions is outside the scope of these guidelines. Further information can be found at www.doh.gov.uk.[34] It is recognised that for many patients, psychological therapies are an appropriate first-line treatment, and indeed this is supported by NICE.[5]

Table 4.23 Characteristics and management of anxiety spectrum disorders

	Generalised anxiety disorder (GAD)[5-10,35-54]	Panic disorder[5,10,12,14,15,17,19,55-59]	Post-traumatic stress disorder (PTSD)[10,20,22,60-73]	Obsessive compulsive disorder (OCD)[10,23,74-87]	Social phobia[10,26,27,88-97]
Clinical presentation	■ Irrational worries ■ Motor tension ■ Hypervigilance ■ Somatic symptoms (e.g. hyperventilation, tachycardia and sweating) ■ GAD is often co-morbid with major depression, panic disorder or OCD	■ Sudden unpredictable episodes of severe anxiety usually 30–45 minutes in duration ■ Shortness of breath ■ Fear of suffocation/dying ■ Urgent desire to flee	■ History of a traumatic life event (as perceived by the sufferer) ■ Emotional numbness or detachment ■ Intrusive flashbacks or vivid dreams ■ Disabling fear of re-exposure, causing avoidance of perceived similar situations	■ Obsessional thinking (e.g. constantly thinking the door has been left unlocked) ■ Compulsive behaviour (e.g. constantly going back to check)	■ Extreme fear of social situations (e.g. eating in public or public speaking) ■ Fear of humiliation or embarrassment ■ Avoidant behaviour (e.g. never eating in restaurants) ■ Anxious anticipation (e.g. feeling sick on entering a restaurant)
Twelve-month prevalence[10]	1.7–3.4%	1.8%	1.1–2.9%	0.7%	2.3%
Emergency management	Benzodiazepines (normally for short-term use only: max. 2–4 weeks) although some are of the opinion that risks are overstated[98]	Benzodiazepines (have a rapid effect, although panic symptoms return quickly if the drug is withdrawn) NICE does *not* recommend benzodiazepines	Not usually appropriate	Not usually appropriate	Benzodiazepines (have a rapid effect and may be useful on a prn basis)
First-line drug treatment Treatment of anxiety may prevent the subsequent development of depression[9]	■ SSRIs (although may initially exacerbate symptoms. A lower starting dose is often required: fluoxetine and sertraline are preferred options) ■ Mirtazapine ■ Venlafaxine ■ Duloxetine ■ Pregabalin	■ SSRIs (therapeutic effect can be delayed and patients can experience an initial exacerbation of panic symptoms)	SSRIs	■ SSRIs ■ Clomipramine	■ SSRIs ■ Pregabalin ■ Gabapentin

Continued

Table 4.23 (Continued)

	Generalised anxiety disorder (GAD)[5–10,35–54]	Panic disorder[5,10,12,14,15,17,19,55–59]	Post-traumatic stress disorder (PTSD)[10,20,22,60–73]	Obsessive compulsive disorder (OCD)[10,23,74–87]	Social phobia[10,26,27,88–97]
Other treatments (less well tolerated, unlicensed or weaker evidence base)	■ Agomelatine ■ Buspirone (has a delayed onset of action) ■ Hydroxyzine ■ Quetiapine (as monotherapy; probably not effective as augmentation in treatment resistance[99]) ■ β-blockers (useful for somatic symptoms, particularly tachycardia) ■ Some TCAs (e.g. imipramine, clomipramine) ■ MAOIs	■ MAOIs ■ Mirtazapine ■ Some TCAs (e.g. imipramine, clomipramine) ■ Valproate ■ Venlafaxine	■ Antipsychotics (as augmentation) ■ Mirtazapine ■ MAOIs ■ Serotonergic TCAs ■ Venlafaxine ■ Duloxetine ■ Prazosin (as augmentation)	■ Antipsychotics as antidepressant augmentation; effect most marked when added to low-dose SSRIs ■ Clonazepam (benzodiazepines in general are mainly useful in reducing associated anxiety; only careful short-term use supported by NICE) ■ Citalopram augmentation of clomipramine ■ Mirtazapine augmentation of SSRI (supported by NICE) ■ Lamotrigine or topiramate augmentation of an SSRI (supported by the BAP[10])	■ Benzodiazepine augmentation of SSRI (modestly more effective than switching from an SSRI to venlafaxine) ■ Clonazepam (as augmentation) ■ Moclobemide ■ Olanzapine ■ Phenelzine ■ Propranolol (performance anxiety only) ■ Venlafaxine ■ Valproate
More experimental	■ Tiagabine ■ Vortioxetine (one positive and two negative studies) ■ Riluzole	■ Gabapentin ■ Inositol ■ Pindolol (as augmentation)	■ Carbamazepine ■ Clonidine ■ Lamotrigine ■ Phenytoin ■ Tiagabine ■ Valproate ■ IV ketamine	■ Duloxetine/venlafaxine (not recommended by NICE) ■ Buspirone ■ Clomipramine (IV pulse loading) ■ Anti-androgen treatment ■ Granisetron augmentation of an SSRI ■ Memantine ■ IV ketamine ■ N-acetylcysteine	■ Levetiracetam
Non-drug treatments See www.doh.org. uk (combined and NICE[5])	■ Reassurance ■ Anxiety management, including relaxation training drug and exposure therapy ■ CBT ■ Exercise	■ CBT ■ Anxiety management, including relaxation, training ■ Combined drug and psychological therapy not consistently better than pharmacological treatment alone	■ Debriefing should be available if desired ■ Counselling ■ Anxiety management ■ CBT, especially for avoidance behaviours or intrusive images ■ EMDR	■ Exposure therapy ■ Behavioural therapy ■ CBT ■ Combined drug and psychological therapy may be the most effective option ■ Surgery	■ CBT ■ Exposure therapy (combined drug and exposure therapy may be more effective)

BAP, British Association for Psychopharmacology; CBT, cognitive behavioural therapy; EMDR, eye movement desensitisation and reprocessing; IV, intravenous; MAOI, monoamine oxidase

Summary of NICE guidelines for the treatment of generalised anxiety disorder[5], panic disorder[5] and OCD[25]

- A 'stepped care' approach is recommended to help in choosing the most effective intervention.
- A comprehensive assessment is recommended that considers the degree of distress and functional impairment; the effect of any co-morbid mental illness, substance misuse or medical condition; and past response to treatment.
- Treat the primary disorder first.
- Psychological therapy is more effective than pharmacological therapy and should be used as first line where possible. Details of the types of therapy recommended and their duration can be found in the NICE guidelines.
- Pharmacological therapy is also effective. Most evidence supports the use of the SSRIs (sertraline as first line).
- Provide verbal and written information on the likely benefits and disadvantages of each mode of treatment.
- Consider combination therapy for complex anxiety disorders that are refractory to treatment.

Panic disorder

- Benzodiazepines should not be used.
- A SSRI should be used as first line. If SSRIs are contraindicated or there is no response, imipramine or clomipramine can be used.
- Self-help (based on CBT principles) should be encouraged.

Generalised anxiety disorder

- Benzodiazepines should not be used beyond 2–4 weeks.
- An SSRI should be used as first line.
- SNRIs and pregabalin are alternative choices.
- High-intensity psychological intervention and self-help (based on CBT principles) should be encouraged.

OCD (where there is moderate or severe functional impairment)

- Use an SSRI or intensive CBT.
- Combine the SSRI and CBT if response to single strategy is suboptimal.
- Use clomipramine if SSRIs fail.
- If response is still suboptimal, add an antipsychotic or combine clomipramine and citalopram.

References

1. Nash JR et al. Pharmacotherapy of anxiety. HandbExp Pharmacol 2005:**469-501**.
2. Martin JL et al. Benzodiazepines in generalized anxiety disorder: heterogeneity of outcomes based on a systematic review and meta-analysis of clinical trials. J Psychopharmacol 2007; **21**:774–782.
3. Benitez CI et al. Use of benzodiazepines and selective serotonin reuptake inhibitors in middle-aged and older adults with anxiety disorders: a longitudinal and prospective study. Am J Geriatr Psychiatry 2008; **16**:5–13.

4. Demyttenaere K et al. Clinical factors influencing the prescription of antidepressants and benzodiazepines: results from the European Study of the Epidemiology of Mental Disorders (ESEMeD). J Affect Disord 2008; 110:84–93.

5. National Institute for Health and Clinical Excellence. Generalised anxiety disorder and panic disorder (with or without agoraphobia) in adults. Clinical Guideline 113, 2011. http://guidance.nice.org.uk/CG113

6. Davidson JR. Use of benzodiazepines in social anxiety disorder, generalized anxiety disorder, and posttraumatic stress disorder. J Clin Psychiatry 2004; 65 Suppl 5:29–33.

7. Scott A et al. Antidepressant drugs in the treatment of anxiety disorders. Adv Psychiatr Treatment 2001; 7:275–282.

8. Ballenger JC. Remission rates in patients with anxiety disorders treated with paroxetine. J Clin Psychiatry 2004; 65:1696–1707.

9. Davidson JR et al. A psychopharmacological treatment algorithm for generalised anxiety disorder (GAD). J Psychopharmacol 2010; 24:3–26.

10. Baldwin DS et al. Evidence-based pharmacological treatment of anxiety disorders, post-traumatic stress disorder and obsessive-compulsive disorder: a revision of the 2005 guidelines from the British Association for Psychopharmacology. J Psychopharmacol 2014; 28:403–439.

11. Baldwin D et al. Efficacy of drug treatments for generalised anxiety disorder: systematic review and meta-analysis. BMJ 2011; 342:d1199.

12. Caillard V et al. Comparative effects of low and high doses of clomipramine and placebo in panic disorder: a double-blind controlled study. French University Antidepressant Group. Acta Psychiatr Scand 1999; 99:51–58.

13. Wade AG et al. The effect of citalopram in panic disorder. Br J Psychiatry 1997; 170:549–553.

14. Londborg PD et al. Sertraline in the treatment of panic disorder. A multi-site, double-blind, placebo-controlled, fixed-dose investigation. Br J Psychiatry 1998; 173:54–60.

15. Pollack MH et al. Combined paroxetine and clonazepam treatment strategies compared to paroxetine monotherapy for panic disorder. J Psychopharmacol 2003; 17:276–282.

16. Clayton AH et al. Sex differences in clinical presentation and response in panic disorder: pooled data from sertraline treatment studies. Arch Womens Ment Health 2006; 9:151–157.

17. Rickels K et al. Panic disorder: long-term pharmacotherapy and discontinuation. J Clin Psychopharmacol 1998; 18:12S–18S.

18. Choy Y et al. Three-year medication prophylaxis in panic disorder: to continue or discontinue? A naturalistic study. Compr Psychiatry 2007; 48:419–425.

19. Michelson D et al. Continuing treatment of panic disorder after acute response: randomised, placebo-controlled trial with fluoxetine. The Fluoxetine Panic Disorder Study Group. Br J Psychiatry 1999; 174:213–218.

20. Davidson J et al. Efficacy of sertraline in preventing relapse of posttraumatic stress disorder: results of a 28-week double-blind, placebo-controlled study. Am J Psychiatry 2001; 158:1974–1981.

21. Stein DJ et al. Pharmacotherapy for post traumatic stress disorder (PTSD). Cochrane Database Syst Rev 2006 Jan 25;(1):CD002795–

22. Martenyi F et al. Fluoxetine v. placebo in prevention of relapse in post-traumatic stress disorder. Br J Psychiatry 2002; 181:315–320.

23. Expert Consensus Panel for Obsessive-Compulsive Disorder. Treatment of obsessive-compulsive disorder. J Clin Psychiatry 1997; 58 Suppl 4: 2–72.

24. Catapano F et al. Obsessive-compulsive disorder: a 3-year prospective follow-up study of patients treated with serotonin reuptake inhibitors OCD follow-up study. J Psychiatr Res 2006; 40:502–510.

25. National Institute for Health and Clinical Excellence. Obsessive-compulsive disorder: core interventions in the treatment of obsessive-compulsive disorder and body dysmorphic disorder. Clinical Guideline 31, 2005. http://www.nice.org.uk

26. Blomhoff S et al. Randomised controlled general practice trial of sertraline, exposure therapy and combined treatment in generalised social phobia. Br J Psychiatry 2001; 179:23–30.

27. Hood SD et al. Psychopharmacological treatments: an overview. In: Crozier WR, ed. International Handbook of Social Anxiety Concepts, Research and Interventions Relating to the Self and Shyness. Oxford: John Wiley and Sons Ltd; 2001.

28. Mayo-Wilson E et al. Psychological and pharmacological interventions for social anxiety disorder in adults: a systematic review and network meta-analysis. Lancet Psychiatry 2014; 1:368–376.

29. National Institute for Health and Clinical Excellence. Depression in adults: the treatment and management of depression in adults. Clinical Guideline 90, 2009. http://www.nice.org.uk/Guidance/cg90

30. Pollack MH. Refractory generalized anxiety disorder. J Clin Psychiatry 2009; 70 Suppl 2:32–38.

31. Roberts NP et al. Early psychological interventions to treat acute traumatic stress symptoms. Cochrane Database Syst Rev 2010: 4:CD007944.

32. van Apeldoorn FJ et al. Is a combined therapy more effective than either CBT or SSRI alone? Results of a multicenter trial on panic disorder with or without agoraphobia. Acta Psychiatr Scand 2008; 117:260–270.

33. Marcus SM et al. A comparison of medication side effect reports by panic disorder patients with and without concomitant cognitive behavior therapy. Am J Psychiatry 2007; 164:273–275.

34. Department of Health. Treatment choice in psychological therapies and counselling: evidence based clinical practice guideline. http://www.dh.gov.uk/

35. Goodwin RD et al. Psychopharmacologic treatment of generalized anxiety disorder and the risk of major depression. Am J Psychiatry 2002; 159:1935–1937.

36. Allgulander C et al. Efficacy of sertraline in a 12-week trial for generalized anxiety disorder. Am J Psychiatry 2004; 161:1642–1649.

37. Lenox-Smith AJ et al. A double-blind, randomised, placebo controlled study of venlafaxine XL in patients with generalised anxiety disorder in primary care. Br J Gen Pract 2003; 53:772–777.

38. Rosenthal M. Tiagabine for the treatment of generalized anxiety disorder: a randomized, open-label, clinical trial with paroxetine as a positive control. J Clin Psychiatry 2003; 64:1245–1249.

39. Pande AC et al. Pregabalin in generalized anxiety disorder: a placebo-controlled trial. Am J Psychiatry 2003; 160:533–540.

CHAPTER 4

40. Mathew SJ et al. Open-label trial of riluzole in generalized anxiety disorder. Am J Psychiatry 2005; 162:2379–2381.

41. Schuurmans J et al. A randomized, controlled trial of the effectiveness of cognitive-behavioral therapy and sertraline versus a waitlist control group for anxiety disorders in older adults. Am J Geriatr Psychiatry 2006; 14:255–263.

42. Chessick CA et al. Azapirones for generalized anxiety disorder. Cochrane Database Syst Rev 2006; 3:CD006115.

43. Bakker A et al. SSRIs vs. TCAs in the treatment of panic disorder: a meta-analysis. Acta Psychiatr Scand 2002; 106:163–167.

44. Benjamin J et al. Double-blind, placebo-controlled, crossover trial of inositol treatment for panic disorder. Am J Psychiatry 1995; 152:1084–1086.

45. Otto MW et al. An effect-size analysis of the relative efficacy and tolerability of serotonin selective reuptake inhibitors for panic disorder. Am J Psychiatry 2001; 158:1989–1992.

46. Herring MP et al. The effect of exercise training on anxiety symptoms among patients: a systematic review. Arch Intern Med 2010; 170:321–331.

47. Lader M et al. A multicentre double-blind comparison of hydroxyzine, buspirone and placebo in patients with generalized anxiety disorder. Psychopharmacology (Berl) 1998; 139:402–406.

48. Montgomery S et al. Long-term treatment of anxiety disorders with pregabalin: a 1 year open-label study of safety and tolerability. Curr Med Res Opin 2013; 29:1223–1230.

49. Stein DJ et al. Agomelatine prevents relapse in generalized anxiety disorder: a 6-month randomized, double-blind, placebo-controlled discontinuation study. J Clin Psychiatry 2012; 73:1002–1008.

50. Stein DJ et al. Agomelatine in generalized anxiety disorder: an active comparator and placebo-controlled study. J Clin Psychiatry 2014; 75:362–368.

51. Mezhebovsky I et al. Double-blind, randomized study of extended release quetiapine fumarate (quetiapine XR) monotherapy in older patients with generalized anxiety disorder. Int J Geriatr Psychiatry 2013; 28:615–625.

52. Mahableshwarkar AR et al. A randomized, double-blind, fixed-dose study comparing the efficacy and tolerability of vortioxetine 2.5 and 10 mg in acute treatment of adults with generalized anxiety disorder. Hum Psychopharmacol 2014; 29:64–72.

53. Bidzan L et al. Vortioxetine (Lu AA21004) in generalized anxiety disorder: results of an 8-week, multinational, randomized, double-blind, placebo-controlled clinical trial. Eur Neuropsychopharmacol 2012; 22:847–857.

54. Rothschild AJ et al. Vortioxetine (Lu AA21004) 5 mg in generalized anxiety disorder: results of an 8-week randomized, double-blind, placebo-controlled clinical trial in the United States. Eur Neuropsychopharmacol 2012; 22:858–866.

55. Sheehan DV et al. Efficacy and tolerability of controlled-release paroxetine in the treatment of panic disorder. J Clin Psychiatry 2005; 66:34–40.

56. Bradwejn J et al. Venlafaxine extended-release capsules in panic disorder: flexible-dose, double-blind, placebo-controlled study. Br J Psychiatry 2005; 187:352–359.

57. Pollack M et al. A randomized controlled trial of venlafaxine ER and paroxetine in the treatment of outpatients with panic disorder. Psychopharmacology (Berl) 2007; 194:233–242.

58. Ferguson JM et al. Relapse prevention of panic disorder in adult outpatient responders to treatment with venlafaxine extended release. J Clin Psychiatry 2007; 68:58–68.

59. Buch S et al. Successful use of phenelzine in treatment-resistant panic disorder. J Clin Psychiatry 2007; 68:335–336.

60. Jakovljevic M et al. Olanzapine in the treatment-resistant, combat-related PTSD – a series of case reports. Acta Psychiatr Scand 2003; 107:394–396.

61. Otte C et al. Valproate monotherapy in the treatment of civilian patients with non-combat-related posttraumatic stress disorder: an open-label study. J Clin Psychopharmacol 2004; 24:106–108.

62. Davidson JR et al. Mirtazapine vs. placebo in posttraumatic stress disorder: a pilot trial. Biol Psychiatry 2003; 53:188–191.

63. Bremner DJ et al. Treatment of posttraumatic stress disorder with phenytoin: an open-label pilot study. J Clin Psychiatry 2004; 65:1559–1564.

64. Davidson J et al. Treatment of posttraumatic stress disorder with venlafaxine extended release: a 6-month randomized controlled trial. Arch Gen Psychiatry 2006; 63:1158–1165.

65. Raskind MA et al. A parallel group placebo controlled study of prazosin for trauma nightmares and sleep disturbance in combat veterans with post-traumatic stress disorder. Biol Psychiatry 2007; 61:928–934.

66. Padala PR et al. Risperidone monotherapy for post-traumatic stress disorder related to sexual assault and domestic abuse in women. Int Clin Psychopharmacol 2006; 21:275–280.

67. Connor KM et al. Fluoxetine in post-traumatic stress disorder. Randomised, double-blind study. Br J Psychiatry 1999; 175:17–22.

68. Taylor FB. Tiagabine for posttraumatic stress disorder: a case series of 7 women. J Clin Psychiatry 2003; 64:1421–1425.

69. Pivac N et al. Olanzapine versus fluphenazine in an open trial in patients with psychotic combat-related post-traumatic stress disorder. Psychopharmacology (Berl) 2004; 175:451–456.

70. Filteau MJ et al. Quetiapine reduces flashbacks in chronic posttraumatic stress disorder. Can J Psychiatry 2003; 48:282–283.

71. Watts BV et al. Meta-analysis of the efficacy of treatments for posttraumatic stress disorder. J Clin Psychiatry 2013; 74:e541–550.

72. Carey P et al. Olanzapine monotherapy in posttraumatic stress disorder: efficacy in a randomized, double-blind, placebo-controlled study. Hum Psychopharmacol 2012; 27:386–391.

73. Feder A et al. Efficacy of intravenous ketamine for treatment of chronic posttraumatic stress disorder: a randomized clinical trial. JAMA Psychiatry 2014; 71:681–688.

74. Dell'Osso B et al. Serotonin-norepinephrine reuptake inhibitors in the treatment of obsessive-compulsive disorder: a critical review. J Clin Psychiatry 2006; 67:600–610.

CHAPTER 4

75. Sousa MB et al. A randomized clinical trial of cognitive-behavioral group therapy and sertraline in the treatment of obsessive-compulsive disorder. J Clin Psychiatry 2006; 67:1133–1139.

76. Eriksson T. Anti-androgenic treatment of obsessive-compulsive disorder: an open-label clinical trial of the long-acting gonadotropin-releasing hormone analogue triptorelin. Int Clin Psychopharmacol 2007; 22:57–61.

77. Soomro GM et al. Selective serotonin re-uptake inhibitors (SSRIs) versus placebo for obsessive compulsive disorder (OCD). Cochrane Database Syst Rev 2008; 1:CD001765.

78. Skapinakis P et al. Antipsychotic augmentation of serotonergic antidepressants in treatment-resistant obsessive-compulsive disorder: a meta-analysis of the randomized controlled trials. Eur Neuropsychopharmacol 2007; 17:79–93.

79. Fineberg NA et al. Escitalopram prevents relapse of obsessive-compulsive disorder. Eur Neuropsychopharmacol 2007; 17:430–439.

80. Storch EA et al. Aripiprazole augmentation of incomplete treatment response in an adolescent male with obsessive-compulsive disorder. Depress Anxiety 2008; 25:172–174.

81. Denys D et al. Quetiapine addition in obsessive-compulsive disorder: is treatment outcome affected by type and dose of serotonin reuptake inhibitors? Biol Psychiatry 2007; 61:412–414.

82. Dold M et al. Antipsychotic augmentation of serotonin reuptake inhibitors in treatment-resistant obsessive-compulsive disorder: a meta-analysis of double-blind, randomized, placebo-controlled trials. Int J Neuropsychopharmacol 2013; 16:557–574.

83. Grant JE. Clinical practice: Obsessive-compulsive disorder. N Engl J Med 2014; 371:646–653.

84. Askari N et al. Granisetron adjunct to fluvoxamine for moderate to severe obsessive-compulsive disorder: a randomized, double-blind, placebo-controlled trial. CNS Drugs 2012; 26:883–892.

85. Ghaleiha A et al. Memantine add-on in moderate to severe obsessive-compulsive disorder: randomized double-blind placebo-controlled study. J Psychiatr Res 2013; 47:175–180.

86. Rodriguez CI et al. Randomized controlled crossover trial of ketamine in obsessive-compulsive disorder: proof-of-concept. Neuropsychopharmacology 2013; 38:2475–2483.

87. Afshar H et al. N-acetylcysteine add-on treatment in refractory obsessive-compulsive disorder: a randomized, double-blind, placebo-controlled trial. J Clin Psychopharmacol 2012; 32:797–803.

88. Simon NM et al. An open-label study of levetiracetam for the treatment of social anxiety disorder. J Clin Psychiatry 2004; 65:1219–1222.

89. Kinrys G et al. Valproic acid for the treatment of social anxiety disorder. Int Clin Psychopharmacol 2003; 18:169–172.

90. Mancini M et al. Use of duloxetine in patients with an anxiety disorder, or with comorbid anxiety and major depressive disorder: a review of the literature. Expert Opin Pharmacother 2010; 11:1167–1181.

91. Blanco C et al. A placebo-controlled trial of phenelzine, cognitive behavioral group therapy, and their combination for social anxiety disorder. Arch Gen Psychiatry 2010; 67:286–295.

92. Hansen RA et al. Efficacy and tolerability of second-generation antidepressants in social anxiety disorder. Int Clin Psychopharmacol 2008; 23:170–179.

93. Westenberg HG. Recent advances in understanding and treating social anxiety disorder. CNS Spectr 2009; 14:24–33.

94. Blanco C et al. Pharmacological treatment of social anxiety disorder: a meta-analysis. Depress Anxiety 2003; 18:29–40.

95. Stein MB et al. Efficacy of low and higher dose extended-release venlafaxine in generalized social anxiety disorder: a 6-month randomized controlled trial. Psychopharmacology (Berl) 2005; 177:280–288.

96. Aarre TF. Phenelzine efficacy in refractory social anxiety disorder: a case series. Nord J Psychiatry 2003; 57:313–315.

97. Pollack MH et al. A double-blind randomized controlled trial of augmentation and switch strategies for refractory social anxiety disorder. Am J Psychiatry 2014; 171:44–53.

98. Offidani E et al. Efficacy and tolerability of benzodiazepines versus antidepressants in anxiety disorders: a systematic review and meta-analysis. Psychother Psychosom 2013; 82:355–362.

99. Khan A et al. Extended-release quetiapine fumarate (quetiapine XR) as adjunctive therapy in patients with generalized anxiety disorder and a history of inadequate treatment response: a randomized, double-blind study. Ann Clin Psychiatry 2014; 26:3–18.

Benzodiazepines in the treatment of psychiatric disorders

Benzodiazepines are normally divided into two groups depending on their half-life: hypnotics (short half-life) or anxiolytics (long half-life). Although benzodiazepines have a place in the treatment of some forms of epilepsy and severe muscle spasm, and as premedicants in some surgical procedures, the vast majority of prescriptions are written for their hypnotic and anxiolytic effects. Benzodiazepines are also used for rapid tranquillisation (see section on 'Rapid tranquillisation' in Chapter 7) and, as adjuncts, in the treatment of depression and schizophrenia.

Benzodiazepines are commonly prescribed; a European study found that almost 10% of adults had taken a benzodiazepine over the course of a year.[1]

Anxiolytic effect

Benzodiazepines reduce pathological anxiety, agitation and tension. Although useful in the short-term management of generalised anxiety disorder,[2,3] either alone or to augment SSRIs, benzodiazepines are clearly addictive; many patients continue to take these drugs for years[4] with unknown benefits and many likely harms. Benzodiazepines may be less effective in the short term than hydroxyzine, an antihistamine that is not known to be addictive.[5] If a benzodiazepine is prescribed, this should not routinely be for longer than 1 month.

The National Institute for Health and Care Excellence recommends that benzodiazepines should not be routinely used in patients with generalised anxiety disorder except as a short-term measure during crisis.[6]

Repeat prescriptions should be avoided in those with major personality problems whose difficulties are unlikely ever to resolve. Benzodiazepines should also be avoided, if possible, in those with a history of substance misuse.

Hypnotic effect

Benzodiazepines inhibit REM sleep and a rebound increase is seen when they are discontinued. There is a debate over the significance of this property.[7]

Benzodiazepines are effective hypnotics, at least in the short term. RCTs support the effectiveness of Z-hypnotics over a period of at least 6 months[8,9] but it is unclear if this holds true for benzodiazepine hypnotics.

Physical causes (pain, dyspnoea, etc.) or substance misuse (most commonly high caffeine consumption) should always be excluded before a hypnotic drug is prescribed. A high proportion of hospitalised patients are prescribed hypnotics.[10] Care should be taken to avoid using hypnotics regularly or for long periods of time.

Be particularly careful to avoid routinely prescribing hypnotics on discharge from hospital, as this may result in iatrogenic dependence.

Use in depression

Benzodiazepines are not a treatment for major depressive illness. In the UK, the National Service Framework for Mental Health[11] at one time emphasised this point by including a requirement that GPs audit the ratio of benzodiazepines to antidepressants

CHAPTER 4

prescribed in their practice. NICE suggests that a benzodiazepine may be helpful for up to 2 weeks early in treatment, particularly in combination with an SSRI (to help with sleep and the management of SSRI-induced agitation).[6] Use beyond this timeframe is discouraged.

Use in psychosis

Benzodiazepines are commonly used for rapid tranquillisation, either alone[12,13] or in combination with an antipsychotic. However, a Cochrane review concludes that there is no convincing evidence that combining an antipsychotic and a benzodiazepine offers any advantage over the benzodiazepine alone.[14] A further Cochrane review concludes that there are no proven benefits of benzodiazepines in people with schizophrenia, outside short-term sedation.[15] A significant minority of patients with established psychotic illness fail to respond adequately to antipsychotics alone, and this can result in benzodiazepines being prescribed on a chronic basis.[16] There is limited evidence that some treatment-resistant patients may benefit from a combination of antipsychotics and benzodiazepines, either by showing a very marked antipsychotic response or by allowing the use of lower-dose antipsychotic regimens.

Side-effects

Headaches, confusion, ataxia, dysarthria, blurred vision, gastrointestinal disturbances, jaundice and paradoxical excitement are all possible side-effects. A high incidence of reversible psychiatric side-effects, specifically loss of memory and depression, led to the withdrawal of triazolam.[17] The use of benzodiazepines has been associated with at least a 50% increase in the risk of hip fracture in the elderly.[18,19] The risk is greatest in the first few days and after 1 month of continuous use. High doses are particularly problematic. This would seem to be a class effect (the risk is not reduced by using short half-life drugs). Benzodiazepines often cause anterograde amnesia[20] and can adversely affect driving performance.[21] They can also cause disinhibition; this seems to be more common with short-acting drugs.

Respiratory depression is rare with oral therapy but is possible when the IV route is used. A specific benzodiazepine antagonist, flumazenil, is available. Flumazenil has a much shorter half-life than diazepam, making close observation of the patient essential for several hours after administration.

Intravenous injections can be painful and lead to thrombophlebitis, because of the low water solubility of benzodiazepines, and therefore it is necessary to use solvents in the preparation of injectable forms. Diazepam is available in emulsion form (Diazemuls) to overcome these problems.

Drug interactions

Benzodiazepines do not induce microsomal enzymes and so do not frequently precipitate pharmacokinetic interactions with any other drugs. Most benzodiazepines are metabolised by CYP3A4, which is inhibited by erythromycin, several SSRIs and ketoconazole. It is theoretically possible that co-administration of these drugs will result in higher serum levels of benzodiazepines. Pharmacodynamic interactions (usually increased sedation) can occur. Benzodiazepines are associated with an important inter-action with methadone (see Chapter 5) and should be used with caution in patients prescribed clozapine (increased risk of cardiopulmonary depression).

References

1. Demyttenaere K et al. Clinical factors influencing the prescription of antidepressants and benzodiazepines: results from the European Study of the Epidemiology of Mental Disorders (ESEMeD). J Affect Disord 2008; 110:84–93.
2. Martin JL et al. Benzodiazepines in generalized anxiety disorder: heterogeneity of outcomes based on a systematic review and meta-analysis of clinical trials. J Psychopharmacol 2007; 21:774–782.
3. Davidson JR et al. A psychopharmacological treatment algorithm for generalised anxiety disorder (GAD). J Psychopharmacol 2010; 24:3–26.
4. Benitez CI et al. Use of benzodiazepines and selective serotonin reuptake inhibitors in middle-aged and older adults with anxiety disorders: a longitudinal and prospective study. Am J Geriatr Psychiatry 2008; 16:5–13.
5. Hidalgo RB et al. An effect-size analysis of pharmacologic treatments for generalized anxiety disorder. J Psychopharmacol 2007; 21:864–872.
6. National Institute for Health and Clinical Excellence. Generalised anxiety disorder and panic disorder (with or without agoraphobia) in adults. Clinical Guideline 113, 2011. http://www.nice.org.uk/
7. Vogel GW et al. Drug effects on REM sleep and on endogenous depression. Neurosci Biobehav Rev 1990; 14:49–63.
8. Krystal AD et al. Long-term efficacy and safety of zolpidem extended-release 12.5 mg, administered 3 to 7 nights per week for 24 weeks, in patients with chronic primary insomnia: a 6-month, randomized, double-blind, placebo-controlled, parallel-group, multicenter study. Sleep 2008; 31:79–90.
9. Krystal AD et al. Sustained efficacy of eszopiclone over 6 months of nightly treatment: results of a randomized, double-blind, placebo-controlled study in adults with chronic insomnia. Sleep 2003; 26:793–799.
10. Mahomed R et al. Prescribing hypnotics in a mental health trust: what consultants say and what they do. Pharm J 2002; 268:657–659.
11. Department of Health. *National Service Framework for Mental Health: Modern Standards and Service Models.* London: Department of Health; 1999.
12. TREC Collaborative Group. Rapid tranquillisation for agitated patients in emergency psychiatric rooms: a randomised trial of midazolam versus haloperidol plus promethazine. BMJ 2003; 327:708–713.
13. Alexander J et al. Rapid tranquillisation of violent or agitated patients in a psychiatric emergency setting. Pragmatic randomised trial of intramuscular lorazepam v. haloperidol plus promethazine. Br J Psychiatry 2004; 185:63–69.
14. Gillies D et al. Benzodiazepines for psychosis-induced aggression or agitation. Cochrane Database Syst Rev 2013; 9:CD003079.
15. Dold M et al. Benzodiazepines for schizophrenia. Cochrane Database Syst Rev 2012; 11:CD006391.
16. Paton C et al. Benzodiazepines in schizophrenia. Is there a trend towards long-term prescribing? Psychiatr Bull 2000; 24:113–115.
17. Anon. The sudden withdrawal of triazolam – reasons and consequences. Drug Ther Bull 1991; 29:89–90.
18. Wang PS et al. Hazardous benzodiazepine regimens in the elderly: effects of half-life, dosage, and duration on risk of hip fracture. Am J Psychiatry 2001; 158:892–898.
19. Cumming RG et al. Benzodiazepines and risk of hip fractures in older people: a review of the evidence. CNS Drugs 2003; 17:825–837.
20. Verwey B et al. Memory impairment in those who attempted suicide by benzodiazepine overdose. J Clin Psychiatry 2000; 61:456–459.
21. Barbone F et al. Association of road-traffic accidents with benzodiazepine use. Lancet 1998; 352:1331–1336.

Further reading

Chouinard G. Issues in the clinical use of benzodiazepines: potency, withdrawal, and rebound. J Clin Psychiatry 2004; 65 Suppl 5:7–12.

CHAPTER 4

Benzodiazepines: dependence and detoxification

Benzodiazepines are widely acknowledged to be addictive and withdrawal symptoms can occur after 4–6 weeks of continuous use (Box 4.1). At least a third of long-term users experience problems on dosage reduction or withdrawal.[1] Short-acting drugs such as lorazepam are associated with more problems on withdrawal than longer-acting drugs such as diazepam.[1,2] To avoid or reduce the severity of these problems, good practice dictates that benzodiazepines should not be prescribed as hypnotics or anxiolytics for longer than 4 weeks.[3,4] Intermittent use (i.e. not every day) may also help avoid dependence and tolerance.

Box 4.1 Problems on withdrawal from benzodiazepines[5]

Physical	Psychological
■ Stiffness	■ Anxiety/insomnia
■ Weakness	■ Nightmares
■ Gastrointestinal disturbance	■ Depersonalisation
■ Paraesthesia	■ Decreased memory and concentration
■ Flu-like symptoms	■ Delusions and hallucinations
■ Visual disturbances	■ Depression

In the majority, symptoms last no longer than a few weeks, although a minority experience disabling symptoms for much longer.[1] Minimal intervention strategies; for example simply sending the patient a letter advising them to stop taking benzodiazepine,[5] increases the odds of successfully stopping at least three-fold.[6,7] A cluster randomised trial supports the effectiveness of a face-to-face educational intervention.[8] Continuing support can be required (e.g. psychological therapies or self-help groups).

If clinically indicated and assuming the patient is in agreement, benzodiazepines should be withdrawn in line with the following considerations.

Confirming use

If benzodiazepines are not prescribed and patients are obtaining their own supply, use should be confirmed by urine screening (a negative urine screen in combination with an absence of benzodiazepine withdrawal rules out physical dependence). Very short-acting benzodiazepines may not give a positive urine screen despite daily use.

Tolerance test

This will be required if the patient has been obtaining illicit supplies. No benzodiazepines or alcohol should be consumed for 12 hours before the test. A test dose of 10 mg diazepam should be administered (20 mg if consumption of >50 mg daily is claimed or suspected) and the patient observed for 2–3 hours. If there are no signs of sedation, it is generally safe to prescribe the same dose as the test dose three times a day. Some patients may require much higher doses. Inpatient assessment may be desirable in these cases.

Switching to diazepam

Patients who take short- or intermediate-acting benzodiazepines should be offered an equivalent dose of diazepam (which has a long half-life and therefore provokes less severe withdrawal).[1] Note that Cochrane is lukewarm about this approach.[9] Approximate 'diazepam equivalent'[1] doses are shown in Table 4.24.

The half-lives of benzodiazepines vary greatly. The degree of sedation that they induce also varies, making it difficult to determine exact equivalents. Table 4.24 is an approximate guide only. Extra precautions apply in patients with hepatic dysfunction, as diazepam and other longer-acting drugs may accumulate to toxic levels. Diazepam substitution may not be appropriate in this group of patients.

Dosage reduction

Systematic reduction strategies are twice as likely to lead to abstinence than simply advising the patient to stop.[6] Although gradual withdrawal is more acceptable to patients than abrupt withdrawal,[9] note that there is no evidence to support the differential efficacy of different tapering schedules, be they fixed dose or symptom guided.[6] The following is a suggested taper schedule; some patients may tolerate more rapid reduction and others may require a slower taper.

- Reduce by 10 mg/day every 1–2 weeks, down to a daily dose of 50 mg.
- Reduce by 5 mg/day every 1–2 weeks, down to a daily dose of 30 mg.
- Reduce by 2 mg/day every 1–2 weeks, down to a daily dose of 20 mg.
- Reduce by 1 mg/day every 1–2 weeks until stopped.

Usually, no more than one week's supply (prescribe the exact number of tablets) should be issued at any one time.

Gradual dose reduction accompanied by psychological interventions (relaxation, CBT) is more likely to be successful than supervised dose reduction alone[10] or psychological interventions alone.[11]

CHAPTER 4

Table 4.24 Switching from benzodiazepines to diazepam: doses

Benzodiazepine	Approximate dose (mg) equivalent to 10 mg diazepam
Chlordiazepoxide	25 mg
Clonazepam	1–2 mg
Lorazepam	1 mg
Lormetazepam	1 mg
Nitrazepam	10 mg
Oxazepam	30 mg
Temazepam	20 mg

Anticipating problems[1,5,12]

Problematic withdrawal can be anticipated if previous attempts have been unsuccessful, the patient lacks social support, there is a history of alcohol/polydrug abuse or withdrawal seizures, the patient is elderly, or there is concomitant severe physical/psychiatric disorder or personality disorder. The acceptable rate of withdrawal may inevitably be slower in these patients. Some may never succeed. Risk–benefit analysis may conclude that maintenance treatment with benzodiazepines is appropriate, and there is support for a RCT examining the benefits and risks of this strategy.[13] Some patients may need interventions for underlying disorders masked by benzodiazepine dependence. If the patient is indifferent to withdrawal (i.e. is not motivated to stop), success is unlikely.

Too rapid withdrawal may be risky; a case report describes a fatal outcome.[14]

Adjunctive treatments

There is some evidence to support the use of antidepressant and mood-stabilising drugs as adjuncts during benzodiazepine withdrawal.[1,6,9,15–18] There is more limited evidence to support the use of pregabalin, even in patients who take very high daily doses of benzodiazepines.[19–21] People with insomnia may benefit from adjunctive treatment with melatonin and those with panic disorder may benefit from CBT during the taper period.[6]

References

1. Schweizer E et al. Benzodiazepine dependence and withdrawal: a review of the syndrome and its clinical management. Acta Psychiatr Scand 1998; 98 Suppl 393:95–101.
2. Uhlenhuth EH et al. International study of expert judgment on therapeutic use of benzodiazepines and other psychotherapeutic medications: IV. Therapeutic dose dependence and abuse liability of benzodiazepines in the long-term treatment of anxiety disorders. J Clin Psychopharmacol 1999; 19:23S–29S.
3. Joint Formulary Committee. BNF 67. London: Pharmaceutical Press; 2014. http://www.medicinescomplete.com/mc/bnf/current/
4. Medicines, CoSo. Benzodiazepines, dependence and withdrawal symptoms. Curr Probl 1988; 21:1–2.
5. Petursson H. The benzodiazepine withdrawal syndrome. Addiction 1994; 89:1455–1459.
6. Voshaar RCO et al. Strategies for discontinuing long-term benzodiazepine use: meta-analysis. Br J Psychiatry 2006; 189:213–220.
7. Salonoja M et al. One-time counselling decreases the use of benzodiazepines and related drugs among community-dwelling older persons. Age Ageing 2010; 39:313–319.
8. Tannenbaum C et al. Reduction of inappropriate benzodiazepine prescriptions among older adults through direct patient education: the EMPOWER cluster randomized trial. JAMA Intern Med 2014; DOI: 10.1001/jamainternmed.2014.949
9. Denis C et al. Pharmacological interventions for benzodiazepine mono-dependence management in outpatient settings. Cochrane Database Syst Rev 2006; 6:CD005194.
10. Parr JM et al. Effectiveness of current treatment approaches for benzodiazepine discontinuation: a meta-analysis. Addiction 2009; 104:13–24.
11. Gould RL et al. Interventions for reducing benzodiazepine use in older people: meta-analysis of randomised controlled trials. Br J Psychiatry 2014; 204:98–107.
12. Tyrer P. Risks of dependence on benzodiazepine drugs: the importance of patient selection. BMJ 1989; 298:102–105.
13. Tyrer, P. Benzodiazepine substitution for dependent patients-going with the flow. Addiction 2010; 105:1875–1876.
14. Lann MA et al. A fatal case of benzodiazepine withdrawal. Am J Forensic Med Pathol 2009; 30:177–179.
15. Rickels K et al. Imipramine and buspirone in treatment of patients with generalized anxiety disorder who are discontinuing long-term benzodiazepine therapy. Am J Psychiatry 2000; 157:1973–1979.
16. Tyrer P et al. A controlled trial of dothiepin and placebo in treating benzodiazepine withdrawal symptoms. Br J Psychiatry 1996; 168:457–461.
17. Schweizer E et al. Carbamazepine treatment in patients discontinuing long-term benzodiazepine therapy. Effects on withdrawal severity and outcome. Arch Gen Psychiatry 1991; 48:448–452.
18. Zitman FG et al. Chronic benzodiazepine use in general practice patients with depression: an evaluation of controlled treatment and taper-off: report on behalf of the Dutch Chronic Benzodiazepine Working Group. Br J Psychiatry 2001; 178:317–324.

19. Oulis P et al. Pregabalin in the discontinuation of long-term benzodiazepines' use. Hum Psychopharmacol 2008; **23**:337–340.
20. Oulis P et al. Pregabalin in the discontinuation of long-term benzodiazepine use: a case-series. Int Clin Psychopharmacol 2008; **23**:110–112.
21. Oulis P et al. Pregabalin in the treatment of alcohol and benzodiazepines dependence. CNS Neurosci Ther 2010; **16**:45–50.

Further reading

Ahmed M et al. A self-help handout for benzodiazepine discontinuation using cognitive behavioral therapy. Cogn Behav Pract 2008; **15**:317–324.
Heberlein A et al. Neuroendocrine pathways in benzodiazepine dependence: new targets for research and therapy. Hum Psychopharmacol 2008; **23**:171–181.

Benzodiazepines and disinhibition

Unexpected increases in aggressive or impulsive behaviour secondary to drug treatment are usually called disinhibitory or paradoxical reactions. These reactions may include acute excitement, hyperactivity, increased anxiety, vivid dreams, sexual disinhibition, hostility and rage. It is possible for a drug to have the potential to both decrease and increase aggressive behaviour. Examples of causative agents include amfetamines, methylphenidate, benzodiazepines and alcohol (note that all are potential drugs of misuse).

How common are disinhibitory reactions with benzodiazepines?

The incidence of disinhibitory reactions varies widely depending on the population studied (see section on 'Who is at risk?' below). For example, a meta-analysis of benzodiazepine RCTs that included many hundreds of patients with a wide range of diagnoses reported an incidence of less than 1% (similar to placebo);[2] a Norwegian study that reported on 415 cases of 'driving under the influence', in which flunitrazepam was the sole substance implicated, found that 6% of adverse effects could be described as due to disinhibitory reactions.[3] An RCT that recruited patients with panic disorder reported an incidence of 13%;[4] authors of case series (often reporting on use in high-risk patients) reported rates of 10–20%;[2] and an RCT that included patients with borderline personality disorder reported a rate of 58%.[5] Other hypnotics, particularly zolpidem, have also been linked to disinhibition associated with somnambulism, automatism and amnesia.[6–8]

Who is at risk?

Those who have learning disability, neurological disorder or central nervous system (CNS) degenerative disease,[9] are young (child or adolescent) or elderly,[9–11] or have a history of aggression/poor impulse control[5,12] are at increased risk of experiencing a disinhibitory reaction. The risk is further increased if the benzodiazepine is a high-potency drug, has a short half-life, is given in a high dose or is administered intravenously (giving rise to high and rapidly fluctuating plasma levels).[9,13–15] Some people may be genetically predisposed.[16] Combinations of risk factors are clearly important: long-acting benzodiazepines may cause disinhibition in high-risk populations such as children,[11] short-acting drugs are highly likely to cause disinhibition in personality disorder.

What is the mechanism?[13,17–19]

Various theories of the mechanism have been proposed: the anxiolytic and amnesic properties of benzodiazepines may lead to loss of the restraint that governs normal social behaviour, the sedative and amnesic properties of benzodiazepines may lead to a reduced ability to concentrate on the external social cues that guide appropriate behaviour, and the benzodiazepine-mediated increases in GABA neurotransmission may lead to a decrease in the restraining influence of the cortex, resulting in untrammelled excitement, anxiety and hostility.

Subjective reports

People who take benzodiazepines rate themselves as being more tolerant and friendly, but respond more to provocation, than placebo-treated patients.[20] People with impulse control problems who take benzodiazepines may self-report feelings of power and overwhelming self-esteem.[12] Psychology rating scales demonstrate increased suggestibility, failure to recognise anger in others and reduced ability to recognise social cues.

Clinical implications

Benzodiazepines are frequently used in rapid tranquillisation and the short-term management of disturbed behaviour. It is important to be aware of their propensity to cause disinhibitory reactions.

Paradoxical/disinhibitory/aggressive outbursts in the context of benzodiazepine use:

- are rare in the general population but more frequent in people with impulse control problems or CNS damage and in the very young or very old
- are most often associated with high doses of high-potency drugs that are administered parenterally
- usually occur in response to (very mild) provocation, the exact nature of which is not always obvious to others
- are recognised by others but often not by the sufferer, who often believes that he is friendly and tolerant.

Suspected paradoxical reactions should be clearly documented in the clinical notes. In extreme cases, flumazenil can be used to reverse the reaction. If the benzodiazepine was prescribed to control acute behavioural disturbance, future episodes should be managed with antipsychotic drugs[1] or other non-benzodiazepine sedatives.

References

1. Paton C. Benzodiazepines and disinhibition: a review. Psychiatr Bull 2002; **26**:460–462.
2. Dietch JT et al. Aggressive dyscontrol in patients treated with benzodiazepines. J Clin Psychiatry 1988; **49**:184–188.
3. Bramness JG et al. Flunitrazepam: psychomotor impairment, agitation and paradoxical reactions. Forensic Sci Int 2006; **159**:83–91.
4. O'Sullivan GH et al. Safety and side-effects of alprazolam. Controlled study in agoraphobia with panic disorder. Br J Psychiatry 1994; **165**:79–86.
5. Gardner DL et al. Alprazolam-induced dyscontrol in borderline personality disorder. Am J Psychiatry 1985; **142**:98–100.
6. Poceta JS. Zolpidem ingestion, automatisms, and sleep driving: a clinical and legal case series. J Clin Sleep Med 2011; **7**:632–638.
7. Pressman MR. Sleep driving: sleepwalking variant or misuse of z-drugs? Sleep Med Rev 2011; **15**:285–292.
8. Daley C et al. 'I did what?' Zolpidem and the courts. J Am Acad Psychiatry Law 2011; **39**:535–542.
9. Bond AJ. Drug-induced behavioural disinhibition incidence, mechanisms and therapeutic implications. CNS Drugs 1998; **9**:41–57.
10. Hawkridge SM et al. A risk-benefit assessment of pharmacotherapy for anxiety disorders in children and adolescents. Drug Saf 1998; **19**:283–297.
11. Kandemir H et al. Behavioral disinhibition, suicidal ideation, and self-mutilation related to clonazepam. J Child Adolesc Psychopharmacol 2008; **18**:409.
12. Daderman AM et al. Flunitrazepam (Rohypnol) abuse in combination with alcohol causes premeditated, grievous violence in male juvenile offenders. J Am Acad Psychiatry Law 1999; **27**:83–99.
13. van der Bijl P et al. Disinhibitory reactions to benzodiazepines: a review. J Oral Maxillofac Surg 1991; **49**:519–523.
14. McKenzie WS et al. Paradoxical reaction following administration of a benzodiazepine. J Oral Maxillofac Surg 2010; **68**:3034–3036.
15. Wilson KE et al. Complications associated with intravenous midazolam sedation in anxious dental patients. Prim Dent Care 2011; **18**:161–166.
16. Short TG et al. Paradoxical reactions to benzodiazepines – a genetically determined phenomenon? Anaesth Intensive Care 1987; **15**:330–331.

CHAPTER 4

17. Weisman AM et al. Effects of clorazepate, diazepam, and oxazepam on a laboratory measurement of aggression in men. Int Clin Psychopharmacol 1998; **13**:183–188.
18. Blair RJ et al. Selective impairment in the recognition of anger induced by diazepam. Psychopharmacology (Berl) 1999; **147**:335–338.
19. Wallace PS et al. Reduction of appeasement-related affect as a concomitant of diazepam-induced aggression: evidence for a link between aggression and the expression of self-conscious emotions. Aggress Behav 2009; **35**:203–212.
20. Bond AJ et al. Behavioural aggression in panic disorder after 8 weeks' treatment with alprazolam. J Affect Disord 1995; **35**:117–123.

Chapter 5

Children and adolescents

Principles of prescribing practice in childhood and adolescence[1]

- **Target symptoms, not diagnoses.** Diagnosis can be difficult in children and co-morbidity is very common. Treatment should target key symptoms. While a working diagnosis is beneficial to frame expectations and help communication with patients and parents, it should be kept in mind that it may take some time for the illness to evolve.
- **Technical aspects of paediatric prescribing.** The Medicines Act 1968 and European legislation make provision for doctors to use medicines in an 'off-label' or out-of-licence capacity or to use unlicensed medicines. However, individual prescribers are always responsible for ensuring that there is adequate information to support the quality, efficacy, safety and intended use of a drug before prescribing it. It is recognised that the informed use of unlicensed medicines, or of licensed medicines for unlicensed applications, ('off-label' use) is often necessary in paediatric practice.
  - Prescription writing: inclusion of age is a legal requirement in the case of prescription-only medicines for children under 12 years of age, but it is preferable to state the age for all prescriptions for children.
- **Begin with less, go slow and be prepared to end with more.** In out-patient care, dosage will usually commence lower in mg/kg per day terms than adults and finish higher in mg/kg per day terms, if titrated to a point of maximal response.
- **Multiple medications are often required in the severely ill.** Monotherapy is ideal. However, childhood-onset illness can be severe and may require treatment with psychosocial approaches in combination with more than one medication.[2]
- **Allow time for an adequate trial of treatment.** Children are generally more ill than their adult counterparts and will often require longer periods of treatment before responding. An adequate trial of treatment for those who have required in-patient care may well take 8 weeks for depression or schizophrenia.
- **Where possible, change one drug at a time.**

The Maudsley Prescribing Guidelines in Psychiatry, Twelfth Edition. David Taylor, Carol Paton and Shitij Kapur.
© 2015 David Taylor, Carol Paton and Shitij Kapur. Published 2015 by John Wiley & Sons, Ltd.

- **Monitor outcome in more than one setting.** For symptomatic treatments (such as stimulants for attention deficit hyperactivity disorder [ADHD]), bear in mind that the expression of problems may be different across settings (e.g. home and school); a dose titrated against parent reports may be too high for the daytime at school
- **Patient and family medication education is essential.** For some child and adolescent psychiatric patients the need for medication will be life-long. The first experiences with medications are therefore crucial to long-term outcomes and adherence.

References

1. Nunn K, Dey C. *The Clinician's Guide to Psychotropic Prescribing in Children and Adolescents.* Sydney: Glade Publishing; 2003.
2. Luk E, Reed E. Polypharmacy or Pharmacologically Rich? In: Nunn KP, Dey C, eds. *The Clinician's Guide to Psychotropic Prescribing in Children and Adolescents,* 2nd edn. Sydney: Glade Publishing; 2003, pp. 8–11.

Further reading

For detailed adverse effects of CNS drugs in children and adolescents, see:
Paediatric Formulary Committee. *BNF for Children* 2013–2014. London: Pharmaceutical Press; 2013.
Martin A, Scahill L, Charney DS, Leckman JF. *Pediatric Psychopharmacology: Principles and Practice.* New York: Oxford University Press; 2002.
Riddle MA et al. Introduction: Issues and viewpoints in pediatric psychopharmacology. Int Rev Psychiatry 2008; **20**:119–120.

Depression in children and adolescents

Psychological intervention

The National Institute for Health and Clinical Excellence (NICE) guidelines[1] recommend that psychological intervention should be considered as the first-line treatment for child and adolescent depression. Psycho-educational programmes, non-directive supportive therapy, group cognitive behavioural therapy (CBT) and self-help are indicated for mild-to-moderate depression. More specific and intensive psychological interventions including CBT, interpersonal psychotherapy and short-term family therapy are recommended for moderate-to-severe depression.[1] The NICE guideline recommends the introduction of medication in conjunction with psychological treatments if there is failure to respond to psychological treatment.[1] In the light of changing evidence this advice has recently been questioned with recommendations for the use of medication at a much earlier stage of treatment in cases of moderate-to-severe depression.[2]

Pharmacotherapy

The NICE guideline CG28[1] supports the use of selective serotonin reuptake inhibitors (SSRIs) but only in combination with psychological forms of therapy. Two US studies, Treatment of Adolescents with Depression Study (TADS)[3] and Treatment of Resistant Depression in Adolescence (TORDIA)[4] found that CBT confers benefit when used in combination with medication. A large UK study did not establish the benefits of combined therapy (fluoxetine plus CBT) and demonstrated that the use of fluoxetine on its own in addition to routine clinical care is effective in treating moderate-to-severe depression.[5,6] Whether CBT provides added value to treatment and outcomes remains a controversial area, but in view of the recent research it is recommended that medication is started at a much earlier stage in treatment, especially if the depression is severe.[2] Evidence[7] now supports the administration of fluoxetine for moderate-to-severe depression sooner than the 12 weeks currently recommended in the original NICE guideline.[2] The NICE Surveillance Group also suggests that the additional benefit of combining CBT and antidepressant treatment compared with the administration of antidepressants alone may not be as significant as previously thought.[2]

The more severe the depressive episode the more likely it is that medication, in combination with psychological treatment or on its own, will be efficacious in the early stages of treatment.[8,9] Good initial response is a sign of improved rates of recovery and outcomes.[3,4]

Fluoxetine is the first-line pharmacological treatment.[10] In the UK it is licensed for use for children and young people from 8–18 to treat moderate-to-severe major depression which is unresponsive to psychological therapy after 4–6 sessions. It is recommended that pharmacotherapy should be administered in combination with a concurrent psychological therapy.[1,10–13] Cochrane agree that fluoxetine is the drug of choice in this patient group.[8] A recent multiple-treatments meta-analysis[14] confirmed fluoxetine's superiority over CBT and other drugs, but concluded that sertraline and mirtazapine might offer the optimal balance of efficacy and tolerability.

CHAPTER 5

Fluoxetine and **escitalopram** are the only antidepressants approved by the US Food and Drug Administration (FDA) for adolescents and fluoxetine is the only FDA-approved medication for pre-pubertal children. Generally speaking, adolescents can be expected to respond better to antidepressants than younger children, particularly those under the age of 12.[15]

Studies in adults have shown that the elimination half-life of fluoxetine is 1–4 days and 7–15 days for its primary metabolite, norfluoxetine, making it a preferable SSRI for adolescents who are less likely to experience withdrawal effects when omitting a dose or stopping the medication abruptly.[16,17] Body weight influences fluoxetine concentrations and starting doses of medication have to be lowered in children. However, during treatment the half-lives of most antidepressants are much lower in children than in adolescents and higher doses may have to be administered in order to achieve adequate blood concentration and therapeutic effects.[15,17]

Fluoxetine should be started at a low dose of 10 mg daily[1] and increased weekly until a minimum effective dosage of 20 mg daily is achieved.[15] Patients and their parents/carers should be informed about the potential side-effects associated with SSRI treatment and know how to seek help in an emergency. Any pre-existing symptoms that might be interpreted as side-effects (e.g. agitation, anxiety, suicidality) should be noted.

Alternative SSRIs and other antidepressants

If there is no response to fluoxetine and pharmacotherapy is still considered to be the most favourable option, an alternative SSRI such as **sertraline** and **citalopram**[1] may be used cautiously by specialists. Evidence suggests some efficacy for sertraline[1,18,19] but one randomised controlled trial (RCT) showed it to be inferior to CBT.[20] Citalopram, also recommended by NICE,[1] may be less effective[10,21,22] and is probably more toxic in overdose.[23]

Escitalopram is the therapeutically active isomer of racemic citalopram.[24] It has been shown to be efficacious in two RCTs[25,26] and is approved by the FDA for use in 12–18 year olds.

Sertraline, citalopram and escitalopram are quickly metabolised by children and twice daily dosing should be considered.[27,28] Sertraline, citalopram and escitalopram should also be started at low doses and titrated weekly up to minimum effective doses; sertraline 50–100 mg; citalopram 20 mg and escitalopram 10 mg.[29]

Paroxetine is considered to be an unsuitable option.[1,10]

The placebo response rate is high in young people with depression.[8,29] On average drug and placebo response rates in children and adolescents differ by only 10%[12] and the benefits of active treatment are likely to be modest. It is estimated that 1 in 6–10 may benefit from the active treatment (although 60% or more show improvement).[1,12,30] There is some evidence to suggest dose increases can improve response.[31]

Tricyclic antidepressants (TCAs) are not effective in pre-pubertal children but may have marginal efficacy in adolescents.[12,32] Amitriptyline (up to 200 mg/day), imipramine (up to 300 mg/day) and nortriptyline have all been studied in RCTs. Note that due to more extensive metabolism, young people require higher mg/kg doses than adults. The side-effect burden associated with TCAs is considerable. Vertigo, orthostatic hypotension, tremor and dry mouth limit tolerability.[32] Tricyclics are also more cardiotoxic in young people than in adults. Baseline and on-treatment electrocardiograms (ECGs) should be performed. Co-prescribing with other drugs known to prolong the QTc interval should be avoided. There is no evidence that adolescents who fail to respond to SSRIs will respond to tricyclics.

There is little evidence for the use of mirtazapine[33] but it is sometimes used in clinical practice where sleep is a problem.

Omega-3 fatty acids may be effective in childhood depression but evidence is minimal.[34] St John's wort should be avoided because of the risk of interaction (see Chapter 7).

Severe depression that is life-threatening or unresponsive to other treatments may respond to electroconvulsive therapy (ECT).[35] ECT should not be used in children under 12.[1] The effects of ECT on the developing brain are unknown.

Safety of antidepressants

When prescribing SSRIs it is important that the dose is increased slowly to minimise the risk of treatment-emergent agitation and that patients are monitored closely for the development of treatment-emergent suicidal thoughts and acts. Patients should be seen at least weekly in the early stages of treatment. Side-effects linked to SSRIs include sedation, insomnia and gastrointestinal symptoms and, rarely, can induce bleeding, serotonin syndrome, activation and mania. More detailed reviews of these problems in adults can be found in Chapter 4.

There is evidence from meta-analyses of pooled trials that antidepressants increase the risk of suicidal behaviours in the short term although no completed suicides were reported in any of the trials.[3,30,36–42] The risk of spontaneously reported suicidal ideation and suicidal behaviour in adolescents treated with antidepressant medication is 1–3 out of every 100 children.[41] Conversely, some studies point to the risk of suicide associated with untreated depression.[43] Reduced prescribing of SSRIs in the USA[44] and The Netherlands[45] has been linked to an increase in the rate of suicide.

The TADS study, which compared CBT with fluoxetine, placebo and combined CBT and fluoxetine, showed that all treatment arms were effective in reducing suicidal ideation, but that the combined treatment of fluoxetine and CBT reduced the risk of suicidal events to the greatest extent.[3] Overall, the potential benefits of treatment with antidepressants outweigh the risks in relation to suicidal behaviours.

Starting and titrating the dose of SSRIs and alternative medication

The administration of all SSRIs should be monitored against the emergence of side-effects and the dose should be reduced if side-effects persist beyond one week. In this case the dose of the medication should be lowered to the highest tolerable dose. SSRI medication should be administered for a minimum of 4–6 weeks and if the child or young person fails to respond and remains symptomatic a dose increase should be considered. A switch to another medication should be made if there is insufficient improvement after approximately 10–12 weeks (switch earlier if there are *no* signs of improvement). Medication effectiveness should be initially monitored at weekly intervals and its effectiveness re-evaluated every 4–6 weeks.[28]

Duration of treatment and discontinuation of SSRIs

There is little evidence regarding optimum duration of treatment.[46] Adding CBT to fluoxetine during continuation treatment has shown sustained remission and lower rates of relapse in comparison to medication on its own.[47] To consolidate the response to the acute treatment and avoid relapse, treatment with fluoxetine should continue for at least 6 months and up to 12 months.[48,49] There is a significant reduction of the risk of relapse with a continuation of treatment for 6 months.[28,48]

At the end of treatment, the antidepressant dose should be tapered slowly to minimise discontinuation symptoms. Ideally this should be done over 6–12 weeks.[1,28] Because of fluoxetine's long duration of action it can probably be safely tapered over 2 weeks.

Refractory depression

There are no clear clinical guidelines for the management of treatment-resistant depression in adolescents[1,50] but there is evidence from the TORDIA published studies[4] that adolescents who failed to respond to treatment with one SSRI may improve when switched to another SSRI or venlafaxine when the pharmacotherapy was combined with concurrent CBT. A switch to an SSRI was just as efficacious as a switch to venlafaxine with less severe side-effects. Recent TORDIA results demonstrate that with continued treatment of depression among treatment-resistant adolescents approximately one third remit.[51] However, the venlafaxine group had more side-effects and there was an association with higher rates of suicidal events in those who entered the study with high suicidal ideation. Venlafaxine should be used with caution and under specialist guidance.[1,4,52] Note that a recent large study suggested no increased risk of suicidality for venlafaxine.[53]

Augmentation with a second medication has not been studied in RCTs in depressed children and adolescents who have either not responded to treatment or have only shown a partial improvement. Case studies and post hoc TORDIA studies have demonstrated some benefits from the addition of antipsychotics.[54–56]

Risk of bipolar disorder

Some young people, and especially children, will develop behavioural activation in response to the administration of SSRIs. It is estimated that 3–8% of young people prescribed SSRIs present with heightened mood, restlessness and silliness which is transitory in nature. This disinhibitory response to starting SSRI medication or being prescribed increasing doses of medication needs to be differentiated from hypomania or mania.[57] Early bipolar illness should be suspected when the presentation is one of severe depression, associated with psychosis or rapid mood shifts and the condition worsens on treatment with antidepressants. Early studies suggested that between 20% and 40% of children and young people presenting with depression will develop bipolar affective disorder (BAD)[58] when treated with antidepressants (the antidepressants acting so as to reveal the disorder, not cause it). In some studies in bipolar patients treatment with antidepressants is associated with new or worsening rapid cycling in as many as 23% of patients.[59] It seems that the younger the child, the greater the risk.[60] In the case of emergent mania early treatment with atypical antipsychotics and mood stabilisers should be considered.[61] More recently it has been advocated that cautiously administered SSRIs should not be withheld in cases of severe depression and BAD.[62] There is limited evidence from open label studies that lamotrigine is effective in treating depression in the context of BAD.[63,64] There is evidence from TORDIA that sub-syndromal manic symptoms at baseline and over time are predictors of poor outcome in adolescent depression.[65] Adult studies suggest that olanzapine, quetiapine and lurasidone are superior to antidepressants in bipolar depression (see Chapter 3).

Box 5.1 summarises the treatment of depression in children and adolescents.

Box 5.1 Summary of treatment of depression in children and adolescents	
First line	Fluoxetine + CBT
Second line	Escitalopram + CBT
Third line	Sertraline, citalopram (more toxic in overdose)
Fourth line	Venlafaxine (less well tolerated)
	Mirtazapine (where sedation required)
	Consider adding quetiapine/aripiprazole to SSRI treatment

References

1. National Institute for Health and Clinical Excellence. Depression in children and young people: identification and management in primary, community and secondary care. Clinical Guideline **28**, 2005. http://www.nice.org.uk
2. National Institute for Health and Care Excellence. Depression in children and young people: review decision - Oct 13. Clinical Guideline **28**, 2013. http://guidance.nice.org.uk/CG28/ReviewDecision/pdf/English
3. The TADS Team. The Treatment for Adolescents With Depression Study (TADS): long-term effectiveness and safety outcomes. Arch Gen Psychiatry 2007; **64**:1132–1143.
4. Brent D et al. Switching to another SSRI or to venlafaxine with or without cognitive behavioral therapy for adolescents with SSRI-resistant depression: The TORDIA Randomized Controlled Trial. JAMA 2008; **299**:901–913.
5. Goodyer I et al. Selective serotonin reuptake inhibitors (SSRIs) and routine specialist care with and without cognitive behaviour therapy in adolescents with major depression: randomised controlled trial. BMJ 2007; **335**:142.
6. Dubicka B, March J, Wilkinson P, Kelvin R, Vitiello B, Goodyer I. The treatment of adolescent major depression: A comparison of the ADAPT and TADS trials. In: Yule W, ed. *Depression in Childhood and Adolescence: The Way Forward*. London: Association for Child and Adolescent Mental Health; 2009.
7. Dubicka B et al. Combined treatment with cognitive-behavioural therapy in adolescent depression: meta-analysis. Br J Psychiatry 2010; **197**:433–440.
8. Hetrick SE et al. Newer generation antidepressants for depressive disorders in children and adolescents. Cochrane Database Syst Rev 2012; **11**:CD004851.
9. March J et al. Fluoxetine, cognitive-behavioral therapy, and their combination for adolescents with depression: Treatment for Adolescents With Depression Study (TADS) randomized controlled trial. JAMA 2004; **292**:807–820.
10. Medicines and Healthcare Products Regulatory Agency. Selective serotonin reuptake inhibitors (SSRIs): Overview of regulatory status and CSM advice relating to major depressive disorder (MDD) in children and adolescents including a summary of available safety and efficacy data. London: MHRA; 2005. http://www.mhra.gov.uk
11. Kratochvil CJ et al. Selective serotonin reuptake inhibitors in pediatric depression: is the balance between benefits and risks favorable? J Child Adolesc Psychopharmacol 2006; **16**:11–24.
12. Tsapakis EM et al. Efficacy of antidepressants in juvenile depression: meta-analysis. Br J Psychiatry 2008; **193**:10–17.
13. Whittington CJ et al. Selective serotonin reuptake inhibitors in childhood depression: systematic review of published versus unpublished data. Lancet 2004; **363**:1341–1345.

14. Ma D et al. Comparative efficacy, acceptability, and safety of medicinal, cognitive-behavioral therapy, and placebo treatments for acute major depressive disorder in children and adolescents: a multiple-treatments meta-analysis. Curr Med Res Opin 2014.

15. Sakolsky DJ et al. Antidepressant exposure as a predictor of clinical outcomes in the Treatment of Resistant Depression in Adolescents (TORDIA) study. J Clin Psychopharmacol 2011; 31:92–97.

16. Wilens TE et al. Fluoxetine pharmacokinetics in pediatric patients. J Clin Psychopharmacol 2002; 22:568–575.

17. Findling RL et al. The relevance of pharmacokinetic studies in designing efficacy trials in juvenile major depression. J Child Adolesc Psychopharmacol 2006; 16:131–145.

18. Donnelly CL et al. Sertraline in children and adolescents with major depressive disorder. J Am Acad Child Adolesc Psychiatry 2006; 45:1162–1170.

19. Rynn M et al. Long-term sertraline treatment of children and adolescents with major depressive disorder. J Child Adolesc Psychopharmacol 2006; 16:103–116.

20. Melvin GA et al. A comparison of cognitive-behavioral therapy, sertraline, and their combination for adolescent depression. J Am Acad Child Adolesc Psychiatry 2006; 45:1151–1161.

21. Wagner KD et al. A randomized, placebo-controlled trial of citalopram for the treatment of major depression in children and adolescents. Am J Psychiatry 2004; 161:1079–1083.

22. von Knorring AL et al. A randomized, double-blind, placebo-controlled study of citalopram in adolescents with major depressive disorder. J Clin Psychopharmacol 2006; 26:311–315.

23. Klein-Schwartz W et al. Comparison of citalopram and other selective serotonin reuptake inhibitor ingestions in children. Clin Toxicol (Phila) 2012; 50:418–423.

24. Hyttel J et al. The pharmacological effect of citalopram residues in the (S)-(+)-enantiomer. J Neural Transm Gen Sect 1992; 88:157–160.

25. Wagner KD et al. A double-blind, randomized, placebo-controlled trial of escitalopram in the treatment of pediatric depression. J Am Acad Child Adolesc Psychiatry 2006; 45:280–288.

26. Emslie GJ et al. Escitalopram in the treatment of adolescent depression: a randomized placebo-controlled multisite trial. J Am Acad Child Adolesc Psychiatry 2009; 48:721–729.

27. Axelson DA et al. Sertraline pharmacokinetics and dynamics in adolescents. J Am Acad Child Adolesc Psychiatry 2002; 41:1037–1044.

28. Sakolsky D et al. Developmentally informed pharmacotherapy for child and adolescent depressive disorders. Child Adolesc Psychiatr Clin N Am 2012; 21:313–25, viii.

29. Jureidini JN et al. Efficacy and safety of antidepressants for children and adolescents. BMJ 2004; 328:879–883.

30. Bridge JA et al. Clinical response and risk for reported suicidal ideation and suicide attempts in pediatric antidepressant treatment: a meta-analysis of randomized controlled trials. JAMA 2007; 297:1683–1696.

31. Heiligenstein JH et al. Fluoxetine 40-60 mg versus fluoxetine 20 mg in the treatment of children and adolescents with a less-than-complete response to nine-week treatment with fluoxetine 10-20 mg: a pilot study. J Child Adolesc Psychopharmacol 2006; 16:207–217.

32. Hazell P et al. Tricyclic drugs for depression in children and adolescents. Cochrane Database Syst Rev 2013; 6:CD002317.

33. Haapasalo-Pesu KM et al. Mirtazapine in the treatment of adolescents with major depression: an open-label, multicenter pilot study. J Child Adolesc Psychopharmacol 2004; 14:175–184.

34. Nemets H et al. Omega-3 treatment of childhood depression: a controlled, double-blind pilot study. Am J Psychiatry 2006; 163:1098–1100.

35. McKeough G. Electroconvulsive therapy. In: Nunn KP, Dey C, eds. *The Clinician's Guide to Psychotropic Prescribing in Children and Adolescents*. Sydney: Glade Publishing; 2003, pp. 358–365.

36. Martinez C et al. Antidepressant treatment and the risk of fatal and non-fatal self harm in first episode depression: nested case-control study. BMJ 2005; 330:389.

37. Kaizar EE et al. Do antidepressants cause suicidality in children? A Bayesian meta-analysis. Clin Trials 2006; 3:73–90.

38. Mosholder AD et al. Suicidal adverse events in pediatric randomized, controlled clinical trials of antidepressant drugs are associated with active drug treatment: a meta-analysis. J Child Adolesc Psychopharmacol 2006; 16:25–32.

39. Simon GE et al. Suicide risk during antidepressant treatment. Am J Psychiatry 2006; 163:41–47.

40. Olfson M et al. Antidepressant drug therapy and suicide in severely depressed children and adults: A case-control study. Arch Gen Psychiatry 2006; 63:865–872.

41. Hammad TA et al. Suicidality in pediatric patients treated with antidepressant drugs. Arch Gen Psychiatry 2006; 63:332–339.

42. Dubicka B et al. Suicidal behaviour in youths with depression treated with new-generation antidepressants: meta-analysis. Br J Psychiatry 2006; 189:393–398.

43. Gibbons RD et al. Relationship between antidepressants and suicide attempts: an analysis of the Veterans Health Administration data sets. Am J Psychiatry 2007; 164:1044–1049.

44. Libby AM et al. Decline in treatment of pediatric depression after FDA advisory on risk of suicidality with SSRIs. Am J Psychiatry 2007; 164:884–891.

45. Gibbons RD et al. Early evidence on the effects of regulators' suicidality warnings on SSRI prescriptions and suicide in children and adolescents. Am J Psychiatry 2007; 164:1356–1363.

46. Kennard BD et al. Relapse and recurrence in pediatric depression. Child Adolesc Psychiatr Clin N Am 2006; 15:1057–79, xi.

47. Kennard BD et al. Cognitive-behavioral therapy to prevent relapse in pediatric responders to pharmacotherapy for major depressive disorder. J Am Acad Child Adolesc Psychiatry 2008; 47:1395–1404.

48. Emslie GJ et al. Fluoxetine treatment for prevention of relapse of depression in children and adolescents: a double-blind, placebo-controlled study. J Am Acad Child Adolesc Psychiatry 2004; 43:1397–1405.

CHAPTER 5

49. Emslie GJ et al. Fluoxetine versus placebo in preventing relapse of major depression in children and adolescents. Am J Psychiatry 2008; **165**:459–467.

50. Birmaher B et al. Practice parameter for the assessment and treatment of children and adolescents with depressive disorders. J Am Acad Child Adolesc Psychiatry 2007; **46**:1503–1526.

51. Emslie GJ et al. Treatment of Resistant Depression in Adolescents (TORDIA): week 24 outcomes. Am J Psychiatry 2010; **167**:782–791.

52. Brent DA et al. Predictors of spontaneous and systematically assessed suicidal adverse events in the treatment of SSRI-resistant depression in adolescents (TORDIA) study. Am J Psychiatry 2009; **166**:418–426.

53. Cooper WO et al. Antidepressants and suicide attempts in children. Pediatrics 2014; **133**:204–210.

54. Vitiello B et al. Long-term outcome of adolescent depression initially resistant to selective serotonin reuptake inhibitor treatment: a follow-up study of the TORDIA sample. J Clin Psychiatry 2011; **72**:388–396.

55. Pathak S et al. Adjunctive quetiapine for treatment-resistant adolescent major depressive disorder: a case series. J Child Adolesc Psychopharmacol 2005; **15**:696–702.

56. Wagner KD et al. Out of the black box: treatment of resistant depression in adolescents and the antidepressant controversy. J Child Adolesc Psychopharmacol 2012; **22**:5–10.

57. Wilens TE et al. Disentangling disinhibition. J Am Acad Child Adolesc Psychiatry 1998; **37**:1225–1227.

58. Geller B et al. Rate and predictors of prepubertal bipolarity during follow-up of 6- to 12-year-old depressed children. J Am Acad Child Adolesc Psychiatry 1994; **33**:461–468.

59. Ghaemi SN et al. Diagnosing bipolar disorder and the effect of antidepressants: a naturalistic study. J Clin Psychiatry 2000; **61**:804–808.

60. Martin A et al. Age effects on antidepressant-induced manic conversion. Arch Pediatr Adolesc Med 2004; **158**:773–780.

61. Dubicka B et al. Pharmacological treatment of depression and bipolar disorder in children and adolescents. Adv Psychiatr Treat 2010; **16**:402–412.

62. Joseph MF et al. Antidepressant-coincident mania in children and adolescents treated with selective serotonin reuptake inhibitors. Future Neurol 2009; **4**:87–102.

63. Chang K et al. An open-label study of lamotrigine adjunct or monotherapy for the treatment of adolescents with bipolar depression. J Am Acad Child Adolesc Psychiatry 2006; **45**:298–304.

64. Pavuluri MN et al. Effectiveness of lamotrigine in maintaining symptom control in pediatric bipolar disorder. J Child Adolesc Psychopharmacol 2009; **19**:75–82.

65. Maalouf FT et al. Do sub-syndromal manic symptoms influence outcome in treatment resistant depression in adolescents? A latent class analysis from the TORDIA study. J Affect Disord 2012; **138**:86—95.

Bipolar illness in children and adolescents

Diagnostic issues

Bipolar affective disorder (BAD) in children has become an area of intense research interest and controversy in recent years.[1,2] While classical manic presentations fulfilling DSM-IV or ICD-10 criteria are well known to clinicians treating adolescents, they are rare in younger children.[3,4] Claims that mania in pre-puberty may present as chronic (non-episodic) irritability or with extremely short (few hours) episodes should be treated with great caution.[2] Short-lived episodes of exuberance are normative in children, while temper outbursts and mood lability can present in children with a wide range of other primary diagnoses (such as conduct, anxiety, depressive, and autism spectrum disorders).[5] A detailed developmental assessment should therefore be the basis of any treatment decisions.

Clinical guidance

Before prescribing

- Establish a clinical diagnosis informed by a structured instrument assessment if possible. Try to monitor symptom patterns prospectively with mood or sleep diaries. If in doubt, seek specialist advice early on.
- Explain the diagnosis to the patient and family and invest time and effort in psychoeducation. This is likely to improve adherence and there is evidence that it reduces relapse rates at least in adults.[6]
- Measure baseline symptoms of mania (e.g. Young Mania Rating Scale[7] [YMRS]), depression (e.g. Children's Depression Rating Scale[8] [CDRS]), and impairment (e.g. Clinical Global Impression - BAD version[9]). Use these to set a clear and realistic treatment goal.
- Measure baseline height, weight, blood pressure and baseline bloods (including fasting glucose, lipids and prolactin levels).

What to prescribe

- Either second-generation antipsychotics (SGA) or mood stabilisers (MS) may be used as first-line treatment for youth with BAD, according to existing guidelines.[10,11] Most of the evidence is for the treatment of acute episodes.
- SGAs seem to show greater short-term efficacy (effect size (ES) = 0.65 compared with placebo) than MS (ES = 0.20 compared with placebo) in youth, according to a recent meta-analysis.[12]
- SGA seem to produce significantly greater weight gain and somnolence in youth compared with adults.[12]
- Polycystic ovary syndrome and associated infertility are particular concerns when valproate is used in adolescent girls and NICE[11] recommends avoiding its use in women of child-bearing age. Beware of teratogenicity.

- Adherence to lithium and blood-level testing may be difficult in adolescents. Beware of teratogenicity.
- Combinations of SGAs with MS are common but NICE guidelines[11] should be noted.
- Overall, we recommend the use of SGAs as first line for the acute treatment of mania in children and adolescents (see Table 5.1, Table 5.2, Table 5.3), similar to recommendations in adults.

After prescribing

- Assess and measure symptoms on a regular basis to establish effectiveness.
- Monitor weight and height at each visit and repeat bloods at 3 months (then every 6 months). Offer advice on healthy lifestyle and exercise.
- The duration of most medication trials is between 3–5 weeks. This should guide decisions about how long to try a single drug in a patient. A complete absence of response at 1–2 weeks should prompt a switch to another SGA.
- If non-response, check compliance, measure levels (where possible), and consider increasing dose. Consider concurrent use of SGA and MS.
- Judicious extrapolation of the evidence from adults[13] is required because of the very limited evidence base in youth with BAD. This includes treatment duration and prophylaxis.[11,12]
- We recommend that a successful acute treatment of a mood episode should be continued as long-term prophylaxis.

Specific issues

- Bipolar depression is a common clinical challenge, the treatment of which has been understudied in youth. In adults, there is considerably better evidence about efficacious treatments (see section on 'Bipolar depression' in Chapter 3), such as quetiapine;[14,15] surprisingly, however, a small study in 32 adolescents,[16] followed by a larger RCT[17] (n = 193) failed to show effectiveness. This study had a high placebo response and this will need to be reviewed once the data have been published in an academic journal. Lurasidone was recently shown to be effective in bipolar depression in adults[18] with a benign metabolic profile, which makes it a good candidate for trials in youth. Note that lamotrigine has only modest, if any, effects in adult bipolar depression;[19] it has not been studied in RCTs in children and adolescents and is, therefore, not recommended. Antidepressants should be used with care and only in presence of an antimanic agent.[11] There is very little evidence for the benefit of antidepressants in bipolar depression in adults.[20] Due to the dearth of trials in youth, we would recommend careful extrapolation from adult studies and use of quetiapine in older adolescents as first-line treatment.
- The exact relationship between ADHD and BAD is still debated. Some evidence suggests that stimulants in children with ADHD and manic symptoms may be well tolerated[21] and that they may be safe and effective to use after mood stabilisation.[21] Caution and experience with prescribing these drugs are required.

CHAPTER 5

Table 5.1 Summary of RCT evidence on medication used in youth with bipolar mania

Medication	Comment
Lithium	One double-blind placebo-controlled randomised trial[23] showed *significant* reductions in substance use and clinical ratings after 6 weeks, in 25 adolescents with BAD and co-morbid substance abuse. In a double blind placebo-controlled discontinuation trial (n = 40) over 2 weeks, *no significant difference* in relapse rates were found between lithium and placebo[24]
	Lithium and divalproex *did not differ* in an 18-months maintenance trial in youths (n = 60) who initially stabilised on combination pharmacotherapy of lithium and divalproex[25]
Valproate	In an RCT (n = 150)[26] divalproex ER (titrated to clinical response or 80–125 mg/L) *did not lead to significant differences* in mean YMRS compared with placebo at 4 weeks
Oxcarbazepine	A double-blind placebo-controlled study (n = 116) *did not show significant differences* between placebo and oxcarbazepine (mean dose 15 mg/day) in reducing mania rating at 7 weeks[27]
Olanzapine	A double blind, placebo-controlled study (n = 161)[28] showed olanzapine (5–20 mg/day) to be *significantly more effective* than placebo in YMRS mean score reduction over a period of 3 weeks. Note the higher weight gain in the treatment group (weight gain was 3.7 kg for olanzapine versus 0.3 kg for placebo) and the associated significantly increased fasting glucose, total cholesterol, AST, ALT, and uric acid
Risperidone	A double blind, placebo-controlled study (n = 169) showed risperidone (at doses 0.5–2.5 or 3–6 mg) to be *significantly more effective* than placebo in YMRS mean score reduction in a 3-week follow up.[29] The lower dose seems to lead to same benefits at a lower risk of side-effects. Sleepiness and fatigue common in the treatment arms. Note, mean weight increase in treatment groups (0.7 kg versus 1.7 kg for the low and 1.4 kg for the high dose arm)
	In the Treatment of Early Age Mania (TEAM) study, *higher response rates* (and metabolic side-effects) occurred with risperidone (mean dose of 2.57 mg) versus lithium (mean level of 1.09 mmol/L) and divalproex sodium (mean level of 113.6 mg/L).[30] However, the results need to be interpreted with caution as the definition of mania was broad
Quetiapine	A double blind, placebo-controlled study (n = 277)[31] showed quetiapine (at doses of 400 mg/day or 600 mg/day) to be *significantly better* than placebo in reducing mean YMRS scores at 3 weeks. The most common side-effects included somnolence and sedation. Weight gain was 1.7 kg in the quetiapine group versus 0.4 kg for placebo
	Quetiapine is *effective* as an adjunct to valproate compared with valproate alone (n = 30, 6 weeks)[32] and was *equally effective* as valproate in a double blind trial (n = 50, 4 weeks)[33]
Aripiprazole	A double blind placebo controlled study[34,35] showed aripiprazole (at doses 10 mg/day or 30 mg/day) to be *significantly better* than placebo in reducing mean YMRS scores at both 4 weeks (n = 296)[34] and 30 weeks (n = 210)[35]. Note, the significantly higher incidence of extrapyramidal side-effects in the treatment groups (especially the higher dose). Weight gain was *significantly higher* in the treatment groups compared to placebo (3.0 kg versus 6.5 kg for the low and 6.6 kg for the high dose arm) at week 30 but not at week 4
Ziprasidone	A double blind, placebo-controlled trial (n = 237)[36] showed ziprasidone (at flexible doses 40–160 mg) to be *significantly more effective* than placebo in reducing mean YMRS scores at 4 weeks. Sedation and somnolence were the most common side-effects, while it demonstrated a neutral metabolic profile and no QTc prolongation
	Ziprasidone is not marketed in the UK and some other countries

ALT, alanine transaminase; AST, aspartate aminotransferase; BAD, bipolar affective disorder; ER, extended release; NICE, National Institute for Health and Clinical Excellence; RCT, randomised controlled trial; YMRS, Young Mania Rating Scale.

Table 5.2 Recommended first-line treatments for acute mania*

Drug	Dose
Aripiprazole	10 mg daily
Olanzapine	5–20 mg daily
Quetiapine	Up to 400 mg daily
Risperidone	0.5–2.5 mg daily

*Continue acutely effective dosing regimen as prophylaxis.

Table 5.3 Recommended first-line treatments for bipolar depression*

Drug	Dose
Lurasidone	18.5–111 (20–120) mg daily
Olanzapine	5–20 mg daily
Quetiapine	Up to 300 mg daily

*Continue acutely effective dosing regimen as prophylaxis.

- The DSM-5 has introduced the new category of Disruptive Mood Dysregulation Disorder (DMDD) to capture severely irritable children (who were commonly misdiagnosed as having BAD in parts of the USA). There is no established treatment for DMDD yet. Lithium is ineffective,[22] but SSRIs and psychological treatment options may be considered.[5]

Other treatments

There is evidence for adults and children that adjunct treatments including psycho-education, CBT and especially family-focused interventions, can enhance treatment and reduce depression relapse rates in bipolar disorder.[13]

References

1. Carlson GA et al. Phenomenology and diagnosis of bipolar disorder in children, adolescents, and adults: complexities and developmental issues. Dev Psychopathol 2006; 18:939–969.
2. Leibenluft E. Severe mood dysregulation, irritability, and the diagnostic boundaries of bipolar disorder in youths. Am J Psychiatry 2011; 168:129–142.
3. Costello EJ et al. The Great Smoky Mountains Study of Youth. Goals, design, methods, and the prevalence of DSM-III-R disorders. Arch Gen Psychiatry 1996; 53:1129–1136.
4. Stringaris A et al. Youth meeting symptom and impairment criteria for mania-like episodes lasting less than four days: an epidemiological enquiry. J Child Psychol Psychiatry 2010; 51:31–38.
5. Krieger FV et al. Bipolar disorder and disruptive mood dysregulation in children and adolescents: assessment, diagnosis and treatment. Evid Based Ment Health 2013; 16:93–94.

CHAPTER 5

6. Colom F et al. A randomized trial on the efficacy of group psychoeducation in the prophylaxis of recurrences in bipolar patients whose disease is in remission. Arch Gen Psychiatry 2003; **60**:402–407.

7. Young RC et al. A rating scale for mania: reliability, validity and sensitivity. Br J Psychiatry 1978; **133**:429–435.

8. Poznanski EO et al. Preliminary studies of the reliability and validity of the children's depression rating scale. J Am Acad Child Psychiatry 1984; **23**:191–197.

9. Spearing MK et al. Modification of the Clinical Global Impressions (CGI) Scale for use in bipolar illness (BP): the CGI-BP. Psychiatry Res 1997; **73**:159–171.

10. Kowatch RA et al. Treatment guidelines for children and adolescents with bipolar disorder. J Am Acad Child Adolesc Psychiatry 2005; **44**:213–235.

11. National Institute for Clinical Excellence. Bipolar disorder. The management of bipolar disorder in adults, children and adolescents, in primary and secondary care. Clinical Guideline 38, 2006. http://www.nice.org.uk

12. Correll CU et al. Antipsychotic and mood stabilizer efficacy and tolerability in pediatric and adult patients with bipolar I mania: a comparative analysis of acute, randomized, placebo-controlled trials. Bipolar Disord 2010; **12**:116–141.

13. Geddes JR et al. Treatment of bipolar disorder. Lancet 2013; **381**:1672–1682.

14. Calabrese JR et al. A randomized, double-blind, placebo-controlled trial of quetiapine in the treatment of bipolar I or II depression. Am J Psychiatry 2005; **162**:1351–1360.

15. Thase ME et al. Efficacy of quetiapine monotherapy in bipolar I and II depression: a double-blind, placebo-controlled study (the BOLDER II study). J Clin Psychopharmacol 2006; **26**:600–609.

16. Delbello MP et al. A double-blind, placebo-controlled pilot study of quetiapine for depressed adolescents with bipolar disorder. Bipolar Disord 2009; **11**:483–493.

17. AstraZeneca. An 8-week, multicenter, double-blind, randomized, parallel-group, placebo-controlled study of the efficacy and safety of quetiapine fumarate (SEROQUEL) extended-release in children and adolescent subjects with bipolar depression (Clinical Trial NCT00811473), 2012. http://clinicaltrials.gov/ct2/show/study/NCT00811473

18. Loebel A et al. Lurasidone monotherapy in the treatment of bipolar I depression: a randomized, double-blind, placebo-controlled study. Am J Psychiatry 2014; **171**:160–168.

19. Calabrese JR et al. Lamotrigine in the acute treatment of bipolar depression: results of five double-blind, placebo-controlled clinical trials. Bipolar Disord 2008; **10**:323–333.

20. Pacchiarotti I et al. The International Society for Bipolar Disorders (ISBD) task force report on antidepressant use in bipolar disorders. Am J Psychiatry 2013; **170**:1249–1262.

21. Goldsmith M et al. Antidepressants and psychostimulants in pediatric populations: is there an association with mania? Paediatr Drugs 2011; **13**:225–243.

22. Dickstein DP et al. Randomized double-blind placebo-controlled trial of lithium in youths with severe mood dysregulation. J Child Adolesc Psychopharmacol 2009; **19**:61–73.

23. Geller B et al. Double-blind and placebo-controlled study of lithium for adolescent bipolar disorders with secondary substance dependency. J Am Acad Child Adolesc Psychiatry 1998; **37**:171–178.

24. Kafantaris V et al. Lithium treatment of acute mania in adolescents: a placebo-controlled discontinuation study. J Am Acad Child Adolesc Psychiatry 2004; **43**:984–993.

25. Findling RL et al. Double-blind 18-month trial of lithium versus divalproex maintenance treatment in pediatric bipolar disorder. J Am Acad Child Adolesc Psychiatry 2005; **44**:409–417.

26. Wagner KD et al. A double-blind, randomized, placebo-controlled trial of divalproex extended-release in the treatment of bipolar disorder in children and adolescents. J Am Acad Child Adolesc Psychiatry 2009; **48**:519–532.

27. Wagner KD et al. A double-blind, randomized, placebo-controlled trial of oxcarbazepine in the treatment of bipolar disorder in children and adolescents. Am J Psychiatry 2006; **163**:1179–1186.

28. Tohen M et al. Olanzapine versus placebo in the treatment of adolescents with bipolar mania. Am J Psychiatry 2007; **164**:1547–1556.

29. Haas M et al. Risperidone for the treatment of acute mania in children and adolescents with bipolar disorder: a randomized, double-blind, placebo-controlled study. Bipolar Disord 2009; **11**:687–700.

30. Geller B et al. A randomized controlled trial of risperidone, lithium, or divalproex sodium for initial treatment of bipolar I disorder, manic or mixed phase, in children and adolescents. Arch Gen Psychiatry 2012; **69**:515–528.

31. Pathak S et al. Efficacy and safety of quetiapine in children and adolescents with mania associated with bipolar I disorder: a 3-week, double-blind, placebo-controlled trial. J Clin Psychiatry 2013; **74**:e100–e109.

32. Delbello MP et al. A double-blind, randomized, placebo-controlled study of quetiapine as adjunctive treatment for adolescent mania. J Am Acad Child Adolesc Psychiatry 2002; **41**:1216–1223.

33. Delbello MP et al. A double-blind randomized pilot study comparing quetiapine and divalproex for adolescent mania. J Am Acad Child Adolesc Psychiatry 2006; **45**:305–313.

34. Findling RL et al. Acute treatment of pediatric bipolar I disorder, manic or mixed episode, with aripiprazole: a randomized, double-blind, placebo-controlled study. J Clin Psychiatry 2009; **70**:1441–1451.

35. Findling RL et al. Aripiprazole for the treatment of pediatric bipolar I disorder: a 30-week, randomized, placebo-controlled study. Bipolar Disord 2013; **15**:138–149.

36. Findling RL et al. Ziprasidone in adolescents with schizophrenia: results from a placebo-controlled efficacy and long-term open-extension study. J Child Adolesc Psychopharmacol 2013; **23**:531–544.

Psychosis in children and adolescents

Schizophrenia is rare in children but the incidence increases rapidly in adolescence. Early-onset schizophrenia-spectrum (EOSS) disorder is often chronic and in the majority of cases requires long-term treatment with antipsychotic medication.[1]

There have been three major RCTs of first-generation antipsychotics (FGAs), all of them showing high rates of extrapyramidal side-effects (EPSs) and significant sedation.[1] Treatment-emergent dyskinesias can also be problematic.[2] First-generation antipsychotics should generally be avoided in children.

There have been a number of randomised controlled trials of second-generation antipsychotics in EOSS disorder.[3–8] Olanzapine, risperidone and aripiprazole have all been shown to be effective in the treatment of psychosis but there is no information to support the superiority of any one agent over another. There is also some evidence from uncontrolled trials for quetiapine[9–11] and for ziprasidone,[12] but concerns have been raised about the safety of ziprasidone.[13,14]

Children and adolescents are at greater risk than adults for side-effects such as extrapyramidal symptoms, raised prolactin, sedation, weight gain and metabolic effects.[15]

There is evidence that clozapine is effective in treatment-resistant psychosis in adolescents, although this population may be more prone to neutropenia and seizures than adults.[16–18]

Overall, algorithms for treating psychosis in young people are the same as those for adult patients (see Chapter 2). NICE[19] recommends oral antipsychotics in conjunction with family interventions and individual CBT. Doses should be at the lower end of the adult range if licensed for children and adolescents; below the lower range if not. See Box 5.2.

CHAPTER 5

Box 5.2 Summary of drug treatment of psychosis in children and adolescents

First choice	Allow patient to choose from: aripiprazole (to 10 mg), olanzapine (to 10 mg) risperidone (to 3 mg)
Second choice	Switch to alternative from list above*
Third choice	Clozapine

*Based on data obtained from the treatment of younger adults, olanzapine should be tried before moving to clozapine.[20]

References

1. Kumra S et al. Efficacy and tolerability of second-generation antipsychotics in children and adolescents with schizophrenia. Schizophr Bull 2008; **34**:60–71.

2. Connor DF et al. Neuroleptic-related dyskinesias in children and adolescents. J Clin Psychiatry 2001; **62**:967–974.

3. Sikich L et al. A pilot study of risperidone, olanzapine, and haloperidol in psychotic youth: a double-blind, randomized, 8-week trial. Neuropsychopharmacology 2004; **29**:133–145.

4. Findling RL et al. A multiple-center, randomized, double-blind, placebo-controlled study of oral aripiprazole for treatment of adolescents with schizophrenia. Am J Psychiatry 2008; **165**:1432–1441.

5. Haas M et al. A 6-week, randomized, double-blind, placebo-controlled study of the efficacy and safety of risperidone in adolescents with schizophrenia. J Child Adolesc Psychopharmacol 2009; 19:611–621.
6. Haas M et al. Efficacy, safety and tolerability of two dosing regimens in adolescent schizophrenia: double-blind study. Br J Psychiatry 2009; 194:158–164.
7. Sikich L et al. Double-blind comparison of first- and second-generation antipsychotics in early-onset schizophrenia and schizo-affective disorder: findings from the treatment of early-onset schizophrenia spectrum disorders (TEOSS) study. Am J Psychiatry 2008; 165:1420–1431.
8. Kryzhanovskaya L et al. Olanzapine versus placebo in adolescents with schizophrenia: a 6-week, randomized, double-blind, placebo-controlled trial. J Am Acad Child Adolesc Psychiatry 2009; 48:60–70.
9. McConville B et al. Long-term safety, tolerability, and clinical efficacy of quetiapine in adolescents: an open-label extension trial. J Child Adolesc Psychopharmacol 2003; 13:75–82.
10. Schimmelmann BG et al. A prospective 12-week study of quetiapine in adolescents with schizophrenia spectrum disorders. J Child Adolesc Psychopharmacol 2007; 17:768–778.
11. McConville BJ et al. Pharmacokinetics, tolerability, and clinical effectiveness of quetiapine fumarate: an open-label trial in adolescents with psychotic disorders. J Clin Psychiatry 2000; 61:252–260.
12. Patel NC et al. Experience with ziprasidone. J Am Acad Child Adolesc Psychiatry 2002; 41:495.
13. Scahill L et al. Sudden death in a patient with Tourette syndrome during a clinical trial of ziprasidone. J Psychopharmacol 2005; 19:205–206.
14. Blair J et al. Electrocardiographic changes in children and adolescents treated with ziprasidone: a prospective study. J Am Acad Child Adolesc Psychiatry 2005; 44:73–79.
15. Correll CU. Addressing adverse effects of antipsychotic treatment in young patients with schizophrenia. J Clin Psychiatry 2011; 72:e01.
16. Kumra S et al. Childhood-onset schizophrenia. A double-blind clozapine-haloperidol comparison. Arch Gen Psychiatry 1996; 53:1090–1097.
17. Shaw P et al. Childhood-onset schizophrenia: A double-blind, randomized clozapine-olanzapine comparison. Arch Gen Psychiatry 2006; 63:721–730.
18. Kumra S et al. Clozapine and "high-dose" olanzapine in refractory early-onset schizophrenia: a 12-week randomized and double-blind comparison. Biol Psychiatry 2008; 63:524–529.
19. National Institute for Health and Care Excellence. Psychosis and schizophrenia in children and young people: Recognition and management. Clinical Guideline 155, 2013. http://www.nice.org/
20. Agid O et al. An algorithm-based approach to first-episode schizophrenia: response rates over 3 prospective antipsychotic trials with a retrospective data analysis. J Clin Psychiatry 2011; 72:1439–1444.

Further reading

Masi G et al. Management of schizophrenia in children and adolescents: focus on pharmacotherapy. Drugs 2011; 71:179–208.

CHAPTER 5

Anxiety disorders in children and adolescents

Diagnostic issues

Fear and worry are common in children and they are part of normal development. At the same time, anxiety disorders often begin in childhood and adolescence[1] and they are the most common psychiatric disorders in this age group, with overall prevalence between 8% and 30% depending on the impairment cut-offs used.[2] Anxiety disorders may be even more common in children with neurodevelopment disorders.[3]

In children, the more obvious clinical presentation with distress and avoidance may be masked by prominent behavioural symptoms (e.g. irritability and angry outbursts linked to avoidance). Therefore, the assessment and treatment of anxiety disorders in children needs to be undertaken by clinicians who can discriminate normal, developmentally appropriate worries, fears and shyness from anxiety disorders that significantly impair a child's functioning, and who can appreciate developmental variations in the presentation of symptoms.

Clinical guidance

Anxiety symptoms in children and adolescents often improve with age, presumably in parallel to the development of the prefrontal cortex and, in particular, executive functions. However, anxiety disorders are distressing and impairing conditions that need to be treated promptly. Chronic stress mediators may have significant impact on brain development[4] and functional impairment linked to anxiety symptoms may prevent young people from accessing normative experiences that are critical for social, emotional, and cognitive development. Consistent with these detrimental effects, young people with anxiety disorders are, for example, three times more likely to have anxiety and depression in adult life compared to non-anxious youths.[5]

Guidelines for the treatment of anxiety disorders in children and adolescents have been made available in the UK and the US. NICE guidelines focus on the treatment of social anxiety disorder in children and adolescents, suggesting the use of cognitive behavioural therapy and cautioning against the routine use of pharmacological treatment for social anxiety in this age group.[6] Guidelines from the American Academy of Child and Adolescent Psychiatry (AACAP) cover the treatment of all non-obsessive compulsive disorder (OCD), non-post-traumatic stress disorder (PTSD) anxiety disorders[7]. AACAP guidelines suggest multimodal treatment including psycho-education, psychotherapy (e.g. a 12-session course of exposure-based CBT), and pharmacotherapy. Drug treatment is endorsed for moderate-to-severe anxiety symptoms, when impairment makes participation in psychotherapy difficult, or when psychotherapy leads to only partial response.

CHAPTER 5

Prescribing for anxiety disorders in children and adolescents

Before prescribing

- **Exclude other diagnoses.** Anxiety symptoms can be mimicked by a range of psychiatric disorders including depression (inattention, sleep problems), bipolar disorder (irritability, sleep problems, restlessness), oppositional-defiant disorder (irritability, oppositional behaviour), psychotic disorders (social withdrawal, restlessness), ADHD (inattention, restlessness), Asperger syndrome (social withdrawal, poor social skills, repetitive behaviours and routines), and learning disabilities. They may also be mimicked by a range of endocrine (hyperthyroidism, hypoglycaemia, pheochromocytoma), neurological (migraine, seizures, delirium, brain tumours), cardiovascular (cardiac arrhythmias), and respiratory (asthma) conditions and lead intoxication. Anxiety-like symptoms can be observed in response to several drugs and substances including anti-asthma medications, sympathomimetics, steroids, SSRIs, antipsychotics (akathisia), diet pills, cold medicines, caffeine and energy drinks.
- **Beware contraindications to SSRIs and potential interactions.**
- **Measure baseline severity.** Structured interviews including the Anxiety Disorders Interview Schedule (ADIS) and the Kiddie-Schedule for Affective Disorders and Schizophrenia (Kiddie-SADS). Questionnaires including the Revised Children's Anxiety and Depression Scale (RCADS), Screen for Child Anxiety and Related Emotional Disorders (SCARED), or the Multidimensional Anxiety Scale for Children (MASC). Measures of functional impairment including the Children's Global Assessment Scale (CGAS) and the Clinical Global Impression scales (CGI)
- **Obtain consent.** Discuss treatment with the young person and the family (e.g. name of medication, starting/estimated ending dose, titration timeline, possible side-effects and strategies to monitor/minimise them, strategies to monitor progress, interventions for treatment-resistant cases). Document consent in writing.

What to prescribe

- **SSRIs** are the medications of choice for the treatment of anxiety disorders in children and adolescents. A Cochrane systematic review[8] shows that there are seven short-term RCTs (<16 weeks; n treatment = 453, n control = 389) testing the efficacy of SSRIs (fluoxetine, fluvoxamine, paroxetine, sertraline) on changes in impairment for anxiety disorders in young people (CGI-I), with an overall relative risk of response of 2.38 [95% CI = 2.01–2.83] over placebo, number needed to treat (NNT) of 2–3, and no significant difference among SSRIs. The Childhood Anxiety Multimodal Study (CAMS) showed that monotherapy with sertraline (55% response) is as effective as CBT for anxiety (60% response) compared with placebo (24% response), and that combined therapy with sertraline and CBT is most likely to be successful (81% response).[9] Sertraline, fluoxetine and fluvoxamine have been approved by the US FDA for treatment of paediatric OCD, and fluoxetine and escitalopram have been approved for treatment of paediatric depression. In 2004, the US FDA issued a Black Box warning for concerns related to worsening of depression, agitation, and suicidal ideation linked to SSRIs. These concerns were based on a review of studies of adolescents with depression rather than young people with anxiety.

- **Venlafaxine** was tested in two short-term RCTs (n treatment = 295, n control = 311) with an overall relative risk of response of 1.46 [95% CI = 1.25–1.71] over placebo (which was significantly lower than the overall effect of SSRIs; see above). Because of the different pharmacodynamic actions, venlafaxine could be considered a second-line treatment when SSRIs are ineffective. The evidence base for this strategy in this group of patients is, however, non-existent.
- The efficacy and safety of **buspirone** and **mirtazapine** in young people with anxiety disorders is not known, although open-label studies[10,11] suggest that they might be effective in relieving anxiety symptoms.
- **Benzodiazepine** use is not supported by controlled trials in children,[12] and may lead to paradoxical disinhibition in some children. Nevertheless, benzodiazepine use is at times considered in clinical practice to 'potentiate' therapeutic effect during initial titration of SSRIs (or to mitigate adverse effects) and for rapid tranquillisation.

A summary of the medications and doses used in the treatment of anxiety disorders is shown in Table 5.4.

Table 5.4 Typical dosage of medications for treatment of anxiety disorders in children and adolescents

Medication	Starting dose (mg)	Dose range (mg)
SSRI		
Sertraline	12.5–25	25–200 od
Fluoxetine	5–10	10–60 od
Fluvoxamine	12.5–25	50–200 (bd if >50)
Paroxetine	5–10	10–40 od
Citalopram*	5–10	10–40 od
SNRI		
Venlafaxine ER	37.5	37.5–225 od
5-HT1A partial agonist		
Buspirone*	5 tds	15–60 od
Tetracyclic		
Mirtazapine*	7.5–15	7.5–30 at night
Benzodiazepine* (prn)		
Clonazepam	0.25–0.5	–
Lorazepam	0.5–1	–

Always check dose with latest formal guidance, e.g. *BNF for Children*.
*Treatments not supported by RCT evidence.
bd, *bis die* (twice a day); ER, extended release; od, *omni die* (once a day); prn, *pro re nata* (as required); SNRI, selective noradrenaline reuptake inhibitor; SSRI, selective serotonin reuptake inhibitor; tds, *ter die sumendus* (three times a day).

CHAPTER 5

After prescribing

- **Acute phase**
  - Start at low dose and titrate at regular (e.g. weekly) intervals.
  - Monitor response (e.g. RCADS, SCARED, MASC, CGAS, CGI-I) frequently and systematically.
  - Monitor side-effects. SSRIs are generally well tolerated during treatment for anxiety disorders in young people. However, side-effects including gastrointestinal symptoms (e.g. nausea, vomiting, dyspepsia, abdominal pain, diarrhoea, constipation), headache, increased motor activity, and insomnia may occur, often in mild and transient form.
  - Therapeutic effect should start after 3–6 weeks of treatment but maximum effect can take up to 12–16 weeks. It is important to communicate this to families.
  - If partial or non-response, consider accuracy of diagnosis, adequacy of medication trial, and compliance of patient.
  - To improve response, consider: adding CBT, changing medication (e.g. switch SSRIs, other classes), or combining medications (e.g. for co-morbidities, to treat side-effects, to potentiate action).
- **Maintenance phase**
  - Continue maintenance treatment for at least 1 year of stable improvement.
  - Monitor response and side-effects regularly.
- **Discontinuation phase**
  - Because of lack of information on long-term safety and possible improvement in symptoms with age and learning, consider discontinuing treatment after a period of stable improvement. A trial off-medication should be started at a period of low stress/demands. Discontinuation should also be considered if the medication is no longer working or the side-effects are too severe. Taper SSRIs slowly to minimise risk of withdrawal symptoms. Monitor closely for recurrence of symptoms/relapse and, if deterioration is noted, promptly restart medications.

Specific issues

Treatment of anxiety disorders in pre-school children must routinely focus on psychotherapy. In rare cases when a very young child has extreme ongoing symptoms and impairment, clinicians should reconsider diagnosis and case formulation, and reassess the adequacy of the psychotherapy trial. There are no RCTs of pharmacological interventions for anxiety in pre-school children but case reports suggest potential benefit of fluoxetine and buspirone.[13]

There has also been an interest in the role of pharmacological intervention to augment the effect of exposure therapy in PTSD.[14] An RCT showed that administration of d-cycloserine, a partial agonist of the N-methyl-D-aspartate (NMDA) receptor involved in fear learning and extinction, potentiates the therapeutic effect of psychotherapy in adults with social anxiety.[15] No study has tested this effect in young people.

References

1. Kessler RC et al. Lifetime prevalence and age-of-onset distributions of DSM-IV disorders in the National Comorbidity Survey Replication. Arch Gen Psychiatry 2005; **62**:593–602.

2. Merikangas KR et al. Lifetime prevalence of mental disorders in U.S. adolescents: results from the National Comorbidity Survey Replication – Adolescent Supplement (NCS-A). J Am Acad Child Adolesc Psychiatry 2010; **49**:980–989.

3. Simonoff E et al. Psychiatric disorders in children with autism spectrum disorders: prevalence, comorbidity, and associated factors in a population-derived sample. J Am Acad Child Adolesc Psychiatry 2008; **47**:921–929.

4. Danese A et al. Adverse childhood experiences, allostasis, allostatic load, and age-related disease. Physiol Behav 2012; **106**:29–39.

5. Pine DS et al. The risk for early-adulthood anxiety and depressive disorders in adolescents with anxiety and depressive disorders. Arch Gen Psychiatry 1998; **55**:56–64.

6. National Institute for Health and Care Excellence. Social anxiety disorder: recognition, assessment and treatment. Clinical Guideline **159**, 2013. http://www.nice.org.uk/

7. Connolly SD et al. Practice parameter for the assessment and treatment of children and adolescents with anxiety disorders. J Am Acad Child Adolesc Psychiatry 2007; **46**:267–283.

8. Ipser JC et al. Pharmacotherapy for anxiety disorders in children and adolescents. Cochrane Database Syst Rev 2009; CD005170.

9. Walkup JT et al. Cognitive behavioral therapy, sertraline, or a combination in childhood anxiety. N Engl J Med 2008; **359**:2753–2766.

10. Buitelaar JK et al. Buspirone in the management of anxiety and irritability in children with pervasive developmental disorders: results of an open-label study. J Clin Psychiatry 1998; **59**:56–59.

11. Mrakotsky C et al. Prospective open-label pilot trial of mirtazapine in children and adolescents with social phobia. J Anxiety Disord 2008; **22**:88–97.

12. Simeon JG et al. Clinical, cognitive, and neurophysiological effects of alprazolam in children and adolescents with overanxious and avoidant disorders. J Am Acad Child Adolesc Psychiatry 1992; **31**:29–33.

13. Gleason MM et al. Psychopharmacological treatment for very young children: contexts and guidelines. J Am Acad Child Adolesc Psychiatry 2007; **46**:1532–1572.

14. Parsons RG et al. Implications of memory modulation for post-traumatic stress and fear disorders. Nat Neurosci 2013; **16**:146–153.

15. Hofmann SG et al. Augmentation of exposure therapy with D-cycloserine for social anxiety disorder. Arch Gen Psychiatry 2006; **63**:298–304.

Obsessive compulsive disorder in children and adolescents

The treatment of obsessive compulsive disorder (OCD) in children follows the same principles as in adults (see Chapter 4). Cognitive behavioural therapy is effective in this patient group and is the treatment of first choice[1,2] although it may be combined with medication.[3]

Sertraline[4-6] (from 6 years of age) and **fluvoxamine** (from 8 years of age) are the SSRIs licensed in the UK for the treatment of OCD in young people. Studies spanning 20 years have established the efficacy of SSRIs in the paediatric population in placebo-controlled trials. Fluoxetine, fluvoxamine, paroxetine, citalopram, escitalopram and sertraline have all been shown to be efficacious and safe in young people with OCD. Clomipramine is a tricyclic with strong serotonin reuptake inhibition activity, which has been shown to be consistently superior to SSRIs[5] in the paediatric population (aged 6–18 years). Clomipramine therefore remains a useful drug for some individuals, although its side-effect profile (sedation, dry mouth, potential for cardiac side-effects) tend to limit its use in this age group. As a consequence SSRIs generally remain the recommended first choice medication for children and young people with OCD. All SSRIs appear to be equally effective, although they have different pharmacokinetics and side-effects.[5] A meta-analysis of 12 RCTs of pharmacotherapy against control, in young people (under 19 years of age) showed that medication is consistently significantly more effective than placebo, and that there is no evidence that there are any clinically relevant differences between SSRIs.[5]

Initiation of treatment with medication

Clomipramine and SSRIs show a similar slow and incremental effect on obsessions and compulsions from as early as 1–2 weeks after initiation and placebo-referenced improvements continue for at least 24 weeks. Symptoms of depression show improvements in parallel with the OCD. In some cases, the effects can take several weeks to appear. In addition, the earliest signs of improvement may be apparent to an informant before the patient. In some instances improvements may take some months to become apparent. In light of this response profile, it is important to inform patients and their families about this, in addition to not feeling rushed to change medication because of only modest initial changes in symptoms. The use of an observer-rated quantitative measure such as the Children's Yale-Brown Obsessive Compulsive Scale (CY-BOCS), may therefore be helpful to monitor progress in clinical settings. The British Association of Psychopharmacology suggest starting at the lowest dose known to be effective and waiting for up to 12 weeks before evaluating effectiveness.[7] Upward dosage titration is recommended if there is insufficient clinical response. In clinical practice, a balance has to be struck between tolerability and the rate of dosage increase in busy clinical services.

Prescribing SSRIs in children

In 2004, the British Medicines and Healthcare product and Regulatory Authority agency (MHRA) cautioned against the use of SSRIs in children and young people, due to a possible increased risk of suicidal ideation.[8] Subsequent reanalysis of SSRI use in depressed adolescents showed a modest two-fold rise in suicidal ideation or behaviours. There were no completed suicides in over 4400 children and adolescents. Careful re-analysis of treatment data highlights that SSRIs are clearly more efficacious in the OCD group of patients than they are in the treatment of moderate depressive episodes in children and young people. Investigators concluded that in the paediatric OCD group, the pooled risk for suicidal ideation and attempts was less than 1% across all studies. This of course is an important risk and should be explained and carefully monitored. Nonetheless, the naturalistic course of untreated OCD is that it tends not to spontaneously remit and has tremendous morbidity. Careful, judicious use of medication is therefore important in alleviating the considerable suffering caused by OCD in children and young people.

On occasion, medications (SSRIs) other than sertraline, fluvoxamine and clomipramine may be used as 'off-label' preparations with the appropriate and suitable caution. Indeed, NICE guidance[9] for the treatment of OCD recommends the use of SSRIs before use of clomipramine, due to the latter drug's greater propensity for side-effects and need for cardiac monitoring. Factors guiding the choice of other medications may include issues such as the presence of other disorders (fluoxetine for OCD with co-morbid depression); a good treatment response to a certain drug in other family members; the presence of other disorders, as well as cost and availability. Some children find tablets or capsules hard to swallow and there are no licensed OCD preparations available in liquid form, although 'off-label' efficacious alternatives would include fluoxetine and escitalopram.

NICE guidelines for the assessment and treatment of OCD

NICE published guidelines in 2005 on the evidence-based treatment options for OCD (and body dysmorphic disorder) for young people and adults. NICE recommends a 'stepped care' model, with increasing intensity of treatment according to clinical severity and complexity.[9] The assessment of the severity and impact of OCD can be aided by the use of the CY-BOCS questionnaire, both at baseline, and as a helpful monitoring tool.[10]

The summary treatment algorithm from the NICE guideline is shown in Figure 5.1.

CBT and medication in the treatment of childhood OCD

Medication has occasionally been used as initial treatment where there is no CBT available, or if the child is unable or unwilling to engage in CBT. Studies now show convincingly that CBT is superior to placebo and that that efforts should be made to try and ensure access to a suitably experienced CBT practitioner. On occasion, medication may be commenced before starting CBT, for instance in the context of significant co-morbid anxiety or depressed mood. Medication may also be indicated in those whose capacity to access CBT is limited by learning disabilities, although every attempt should be made to modify CBT protocols for such children.

The principle study that directly compared the efficacy of CBT, sertraline, and their combination, in children and adolescents, concluded that children with OCD should begin treatment with CBT alone or CBT plus an SSRI.[2]

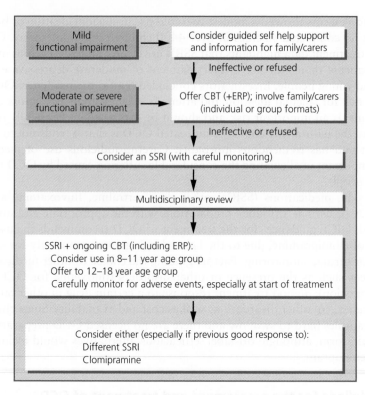

Figure 5.1 Treatment options for children and young people with OCD. CBT, cognitive behavioural therapy; ERP, exposure and response prevention; SSRI, selective serotonin reuptake inhibitor. Adapted from NICE guidance[9] and reproduced from Heyman et al.[11] with permission from BMJ Publishing Group Ltd.

Treatment of refractory OCD in children

Evidence from randomised trials suggests that up to three-quarters of medicated patients make an adequate response to treatment. Roughly one-quarter of children with OCD will therefore fail to respond to an initial SSRI, administered for at least 12 weeks at the maximum tolerated dose, in combination with an adequate trial of CBT and ERP. These children should be reassessed, clarifying compliance, and ensuring that co-morbidity is not being missed. These children should usually have additional trials of at least one other SSRI. Research suggests that approximately 40% respond to a second SSRI.[12] Following this, if the response is limited, a child should usually be referred to a specialist centre. Trials of clomipramine may be considered and/or augmentation with a low dose of risperidone.[11,13] Research hints at the fact that using a medication with a different method of action such as risperidone or clomipramine may benefit patients who have failed to respond to two adequate SSRI trials. There is evidence that antipsychotic augmentation, as an 'off-label' therapy, can benefit patients whose response to treatment has been inadequate despite at least 3 months of maximal tolerated SSRI. Unfortunately, only one-third of treatment-resistant adult cases showed a meaningful response to this augmentation strategy. The data would therefore suggest that caution should be exercised when augmenting treatment packages for OCD in children and young people. Often children whose OCD has been difficult to treat have co-morbidities such as autism spectrum disorder, ADHD, or tic disorders. The response to medication can be differentially affected by these co-morbidities. For instance, cases with tic disorders may benefit somewhat more from augmentation with second-generation antipsychotics. Careful clinical review and reformulation is important in OCD treatment resistance. The impact of co-morbidities and wider psychosocial factors need to be considered for their impact on the treatment response overall.

Neither ketamine[14] nor riluzole[15] are effective in refractory childhood OCD.

Duration of treatment and long-term follow-up

Untreated OCD tends to run a chronic course. A series of adult studies have shown that discontinuation of medication tends to result in symptomatic relapse. Some authors have suggested that those with co-morbidities are at the greatest risk of relapse. Given that studies frequently exclude cases with additional co-morbidities, it is likely that the relapse rates have been underestimated. NICE guidelines recommend that if a young person has responded to medication, treatment should continue for at least 6 months after remission. Clinical experience would suggest that when discontinuation of treatment is attempted it should be done slowly, cautiously and in a transparent manner with the patient and their family. Once again, the careful use of clinical outcome measures should be considered when stopping medication. The role of maintenance CBT and medication is under increasing scrutiny. Both appear to offer promise in maintaining gains made after initial treatment. It is important that throughout childhood, adolescence and into adult life, the individual with OCD should have access to health-care professionals, treatment opportunities and other support as needed, and NICE recommends that if relapse occurs, people with OCD should be seen as soon as possible rather than placed on a routine waiting list.

CHAPTER 5

References

1. O'Kearney RT et al. Behavioural and cognitive behavioural therapy for obsessive compulsive disorder in children and adolescents. Cochrane Database Syst Rev 2006; CD004856.
2. Freeman JB et al. Cognitive behavioral treatment for young children with obsessive-compulsive disorder. Biol Psychiatry 2007; 61:337–343.
3. Mancuso E et al. Treatment of pediatric obsessive-compulsive disorder: a review. J Child Adolesc Psychopharmacol 2010; 20:299–308.
4. The Pediatric OCD Treatment Study Team (POTS). Cognitive-behavior therapy, sertraline, and their combination for children and adolescents with obsessive-compulsive disorder: the Pediatric OCD Treatment Study (POTS) randomized controlled trial. JAMA 2004; 292:1969–1976.
5. Geller DA et al. Which SSRI? A meta-analysis of pharmacotherapy trials in pediatric obsessive-compulsive disorder. Am J Psychiatry 2003; 160:1919–1928.
6. March JS et al. Treatment benefit and the risk of suicidality in multicenter, randomized, controlled trials of sertraline in children and adolescents. J Child Adolesc Psychopharmacol 2006; 16:91–102.
7. Baldwin DS et al. Evidence-based pharmacological treatment of anxiety disorders, post-traumatic stress disorder and obsessive-compulsive disorder: A revision of the 2005 guidelines from the British Association for Psychopharmacology. J Psychopharmacol 2014; 28:403–439.
8. Medicines and Healthcare Products Regulatory Agency. Report of the CSM expert working group on the safety of selective serotonin reuptake inhibitor antidepressants. London: MHRA; 2004. http://www.mhra.gov.uk
9. National Institute for Health and Clinical Excellence. Obsessive-compulsive disorder: Core interventions in the treatment of obsessive-compulsive disorder and body dysmorphic disorder. Clinical Guideline 31, 2005. http://www.nice.org.uk.

10. Scahill L et al. Children's Yale-Brown Obsessive Compulsive Scale: reliability and validity. J Am Acad Child Adolesc Psychiatry 1997; 36:844–852.

11. Heyman I et al. Obsessive-compulsive disorder. BMJ 2006; 333:424–429.

12. Grados M et al. Pharmacotherapy in children and adolescents with obsessive-compulsive disorder. Child Adolesc Psychiatr Clin N Am 1999; 8:617–34, x.

13. Bloch MH et al. A systematic review: antipsychotic augmentation with treatment refractory obsessive-compulsive disorder. Mol Psychiatry 2006; 11:622–632.

14. Bloch MH et al. Effects of ketamine in treatment-refractory obsessive-compulsive disorder. Biol Psychiatry 2012; 72:964–970.

15. Grant PJ et al. 12-week, placebo-controlled trial of add-on riluzole in the treatment of childhood-onset obsessive-compulsive disorder. Neuropsychopharmacology 2014; 39:1453–1459.

Post-traumatic stress disorder in children and adolescents

Diagnostic issues

Traumatic events and post-traumatic stress disorder (PTSD) are common in young people. One in four children experiences traumatic events[1] and nearly 1 in 10 children develops PTSD[2] before the age of 18. The prevalence of PTSD in adolescents is 4% in males and 6% in females from the general population,[3] and could be as high as 30% in young people attending emergency departments. Furthermore, young people with significant PTSD symptoms, but sub-threshold criteria for diagnosis, may show similar impairment and distress to children and adolescents with a diagnosis of PTSD and thus require treatment.[4] Response to trauma may also involve other anxiety disorders, depression, self-harm, aggression, and substance abuse.

A diagnosis of PTSD is based on the triad of intrusive re-experiencing, avoidance of stimuli associated with the trauma, and hyper-arousal after trauma exposure. However, in children, re-experiencing may not be reported in the form of distressing visual flashbacks, but rather could be noted as compulsive repetition of aspects of trauma in play, drawings, or verbalisation, or as nightmares. Furthermore, certain types of avoidance (sense of a foreshortened future, inability to recall important aspects of the event) may not be detectable because of insufficient abilities with abstract cognition or verbal expression. In adolescents, PTSD symptoms are often associated with, and may be masked by, impulsive and aggressive behaviours.[5,6] Because of the varied clinical manifestations, the assessment and treatment of PTSD in children and adolescents needs to be undertaken by clinicians who can appreciate developmental variations in the presentation of symptoms.

Clinical guidance

Guidelines for treatment of PTSD in children and adolescents are available in the UK and the US. NICE guidelines advise that treatment should be 12-sessions of trauma-focused CBT for PTSD resulting from a single event (longer for chronic or recurrent events) and discourage routine prescription of medications.[7] Guidelines by the American Academy of Child and Adolescent Psychiatry (AACAP) recommend trauma-focused CBT as first-line treatment for young people with PTSD and use of pharmacotherapy if the child's symptom severity, lack of response, or co-morbidity suggest need for additional interventions.[8] The AACAP guidelines discuss SSRIs treatment, but also treatment with anti-adrenergic and second-generation antipsychotic medications.

Prescribing for anxiety disorders in young people

Before prescribing

- **Exclude other diagnoses.** (See section on 'Anxiety disorders in children and adolescents' earlier in this chapter.)
- **Beware contraindication to SSRIs and potential interactions.**

- **Measure baseline severity.** Structured interviews including the Anxiety Disorders Interview Schedule (ADIS) and the Kiddie-Schedule for Affective Disorders and Schizophrenia (Kiddie-SADS). Questionnaires, including the Child PTSD Symptom Scale (CPSS) and the UCLA Posttraumatic Stress Disorder Reaction Index. Measures of functional impairment including the Children's Global Assessment Scale (CGAS) and the Clinical Global Impression scales (CGI).
- **Obtain consent.** (See section on 'Anxiety disorders in children and adolescents' earlier in this chapter.)

What to prescribe

- **SSRIs** have shown only minimal evidence of clinical efficacy for the treatment of PTSD in children and adolescents, despite their efficacy in adults.[9] A small 12-week RCT of add-on sertraline (n = 11) to routine TF-CBT treatment showed only marginal benefit of pharmacological treatment over TF-CBT and placebo (n = 11), which was not statistically significant.[10] A larger 10-week RCT with flexibly dosed sertraline (n treated = 67; n placebo = 64) failed to detect a benefit over placebo.[11] A small (n = 8) open-label study suggests potential efficacy of citalopram.[12] It is possible that SSRIs may be more effective for the treatment of PTSD in young people in the presence of co-morbid major depressive episode, anxiety disorders, and OCD, although the evidence base for this is minimal.
- **Anti-adrenergic medications** have been studied for the treatment of PTSD in young people because of the evidence of noradrenergic hyperactivity in PTSD[13,14] and the suggestive evidence of efficacy in adults.[15] Clonidine is an α_2-adrenergic agonist that reduces norepinephrine release. Clonidine is used 'off-label' in several paediatric conditions and an open-label trial (n = 7) in children showed that clonidine can improve PTSD symptoms, in particular re-living symptoms.[16] Guanfacine is also an α_2-adrenergic agonist. A case study suggested that guanfacine can improve PTSD symptoms, again particularly re-living symptoms, in young people.[17] The most common side-effects of α_2-adrenergic agonist are dry mouth and dizziness. Blood pressure should be monitored regularly and discontinuation should be slow to avoid rebound hypertension. Prazosin is an α_1-adrenergic antagonist that reduces the post-synaptic effect of norepinephrine. Evidence in children and adolescents is limited to case reports which showed improvement of PTSD symptoms.[18] Prazosin should be titrated slowly (e.g. 1 mg/week) and blood pressure (risk of orthostatic hypotension) should be carefully monitored, particularly early in treatment. Propranolol is a β-antagonist that reduces the post-synaptic effect of norepinephrine. In a on-off-on study, propranolol was shown to improve PTSD in children and adolescents.[19] The most common side-effects include hypotension, bradycardia, dizziness, and bronchospasm. Blood pressure should be monitored regularly during titration.
- **Second-generation antipsychotics** have been studied for treatment of PTSD in children and adolescents based on the role of dopamine in various aspects of fear conditioning[20] and on the efficacy of risperidone, olanzapine, aripiprazole (either as monotherapy or as adjunctive to SSRI therapy) on PTSD in adults.[15,21] Evidence in children and adolescents is limited to case series and case studies with risperidone[22] and quetiapine,[23] which showed positive results.

Table 5.5 Typical dosage of medications for the treatment of PTSD in children and adolescents. These clinical guidelines are based on less than robust research evidence (e.g. case series) in children and adolescents and on extrapolation of data from adult trials

Medication	Starting dose (mg)	Dose range (mg)
SSRI		
Sertraline	12.5–25	50–200 od
Citalopram	5–10	10–40 od
Anti-Adrenergic		
Clonidine	0.05 nocte	0.1–0.2 nocte
Guanfacine	0.5 bd	1–3 nocte
Prazosin	1 nocte	2–4 nocte
Propranolol	10 tds	40–80/day
Second-generation antipsychotics		
Risperidone	0.5	0.5–1 od
Quetiapine	25–50	50–200 od (at night)

Always check dose against latest formal guidance, e.g. *BNF for Children*.
bd, *bis die* (twice a day); nocte, at night; od, *omni die* (once a day); tds, *ter die sumendus* (three times a day).

- **Mood stabilisers** have been studied for the treatment of PTSD in adults, generally adjunctively in combination with SSRIs, and have been found to be effective.[15] The literature in children and adolescents is limited to one open-label study (n = 28) with carbamazepine[24] and one open-label study (n = 12) with valproate semisodium[25] that showed positive results.

A summary of the medications and doses used in the treatment of PTSD is shown in Table 5.5.

After prescribing

- **Acute phase**
  - Start at low dose and titrate at regular (e.g. weekly) intervals.
  - Monitor response (e.g. CPSS, CGAS, CGI-I) frequently and systematically.
  - Monitor side-effects.
  - If partial or non-response, consider (1) accuracy of diagnosis, (2) adequacy of medication trial, and (3) compliance of patient.
- **Maintenance phase**
  - Monitor response and side-effects regularly.
- **Discontinuation phase**
  - Consider discontinuing treatment after a period of stable improvement.
  - A trial off medication should be started at a period of low stress/demands.

CHAPTER 5

- Discontinuation should also be considered if the medication is no longer working or the side-effects are too severe.
- Taper medications slowly to minimise risk of withdrawal symptoms.
- Monitor closely for recurrence of symptoms/relapse.

Specific issues

Treatment of PTSD in pre-school children must routinely focus on psychotherapy with either child–parent psychotherapy (CPP) or pre-school CBT. Pharmacological treatment of PTSD in pre-school children is not recommended.[26]

There has been an interest in preventive psychopharmacological interventions in the aftermath of trauma exposure, based on the findings that arousal and noradrenergic hyperactivity may promote consolidation of trauma memories.[27] After initial positive results with the use of propranolol,[28] subsequent larger studies and also studies in children and adolescents[29] failed to detect significant protective effects. Morphine has a similar ability to inhibit noradrenergic activity, and studies in children and adolescents[30] and adults[31] suggest that morphine use after trauma might be effective in preventing development of PTSD. These findings require replication and morphine should not be used to prevent PTSD in routine clinical practice.

There has also been an interest in the role of pharmacological intervention to augment the effect of exposure therapy in PTSD.[32] An RCT showed that administration of d-cycloserine, a partial agonist of the NMDA receptor involved in fear learning and extinction, potentiate the therapeutic effect of psychotherapy in adults with PTSD.[33] No study has tested this effect in children and adolescents.

References

1. Costello EJ et al. The prevalence of potentially traumatic events in childhood and adolescence. Trauma Stress 2002; 15:99–112.
2. Breslau N et al. Traumatic events and posttraumatic stress disorder in an urban population of young adults. Arch Gen Psychiatry 1991; 48:216–222.
3. Kilpatrick DG et al. Violence and risk of PTSD, major depression, substance abuse/dependence, and comorbidity: results from the National Survey of Adolescents. J Consult Clin Psychol 2003; 71:692–700.
4. Carrion VG et al. Toward an empirical definition of pediatric PTSD: the phenomenology of PTSD symptoms in youth. J Am Acad Child Adolesc Psychiatry 2002; 41:166–173.
5. Scheeringa MS et al. PTSD in children and adolescents: toward an empirically based algorithma. Depress Anxiety 2011; 28:770–782.
6. Meiser-Stedman R et al. The posttraumatic stress disorder diagnosis in preschool- and elementary school-age children exposed to motor vehicle accidents. Am J Psychiatry 2008; 165:1326–1337.
7. National Institute for Health and Clinical Excellence. Post-traumatic stress disorder (PTSD): The management of PTSD in adults and children in primary and secondary care. Clinical Guideline 26, 2005. http://www.nice.org.uk/guidance/CG26
8. Cohen JA et al. Practice parameter for the assessment and treatment of children and adolescents with posttraumatic stress disorder. J Am Acad Child Adolesc Psychiatry 2010; 49:414–430.
9. Stein DJ et al. Pharmacotherapy for post traumatic stress disorder (PTSD). Cochrane Database Syst Rev 2006; CD002795.
10. Cohen JA et al. A pilot randomized controlled trial of combined trauma-focused CBT and sertraline for childhood PTSD symptoms. J Am Acad Child Adolesc Psychiatry 2007; 46:811–819.
11. Robb AS et al. Sertraline treatment of children and adolescents with posttraumatic stress disorder: a double-blind, placebo-controlled trial. J Child Adolesc Psychopharmacol 2010; 20:463–471.
12. Seedat S et al. An open trial of citalopram in adolescents with post-traumatic stress disorder. Int Clin Psychopharmacol 2001; 16:21–25.
13. Geracioti TD, Jr. et al. CSF norepinephrine concentrations in posttraumatic stress disorder. Am J Psychiatry 2001; 158:1227–1230.
14. De B et al. Urinary catecholamine excretion in sexually abused girls. J Am Acad Child Adolesc Psychiatry 1994; 33:320–327.
15. Strawn JR et al. Psychopharmacologic treatment of posttraumatic stress disorder in children and adolescents: a review. J Clin Psychiatry 2010; 71:932–941.

CHAPTER 5

16. Harmon RJ et al. Clonidine for posttraumatic stress disorder in preschool children. J Am Acad Child Adolesc Psychiatry 1996; 35:1247–1249.

17. Horrigan JP. Guanfacine for PTSD nightmares. J Am Acad Child Adolesc Psychiatry 1996; 35:975–976.

18. Strawn JR et al. Prazosin treatment of an adolescent with posttraumatic stress disorder. J Child Adolesc Psychopharmacol 2009; 19:599–600.

19. Famularo R et al. Propranolol treatment for childhood posttraumatic stress disorder, acute type. A pilot study. Am J Dis Child 1988; 142:1244–1247.

20. Pezze MA et al. Mesolimbic dopaminergic pathways in fear conditioning. Prog Neurobiol 2004; 74:301–320.

21. Pae CU et al. The atypical antipsychotics olanzapine and risperidone in the treatment of posttraumatic stress disorder: a meta-analysis of randomized, double-blind, placebo-controlled clinical trials. Int Clin Psychopharmacol 2008; 23:1–8.

22. Keeshin BR et al. Risperidone treatment of an adolescent with severe posttraumatic stress disorder. Ann Pharmacother 2009; 43:1374.

23. Stathis S et al. A preliminary case series on the use of quetiapine for posttraumatic stress disorder in juveniles within a youth detention center. J Clin Psychopharmacol 2005; 25:539–544.

24. Looff D et al. Carbamazepine for PTSD. J Am Acad Child Adolesc Psychiatry 1995; 34:703–704.

25. Steiner H et al. Divalproex sodium for the treatment of PTSD and conduct disordered youth: a pilot randomized controlled clinical trial. Child Psychiatry Hum Dev 2007; 38:183–193.

26. Gleason MM et al. Psychopharmacological treatment for very young children: contexts and guidelines. J Am Acad Child Adolesc Psychiatry 2007; 46:1532–1572.

27. Cahill L et al. Beta-adrenergic activation and memory for emotional events. Nature 1994; 371:702–704.

28. Vaiva G et al. Immediate treatment with propranolol decreases posttraumatic stress disorder two months after trauma. Biol Psychiatry 2003; 54:947–949.

29. Nugent NR et al. The efficacy of early propranolol administration at reducing PTSD symptoms in pediatric injury patients: a pilot study. J Trauma Stress 2010; 23:282–287.

30. Saxe G et al. Relationship between acute morphine and the course of PTSD in children with burns. J Am Acad Child Adolesc Psychiatry 2001; 40:915–921.

31. Holbrook TL et al. Morphine use after combat injury in Iraq and post-traumatic stress disorder. N Engl J Med 2010; 362:110–117.

32. Parsons RG et al. Implications of memory modulation for post-traumatic stress and fear disorders. Nat Neurosci 2013; 16:146–153.

33. de Kleine RA et al. A randomized placebo-controlled trial of D-cycloserine to enhance exposure therapy for posttraumatic stress disorder. Biol Psychiatry 2012; 71:962–968.

Attention deficit hyperactivity disorder

ADHD in Children

- A diagnosis of attention deficit hyperactivity disorder (ADHD) should be made only after a comprehensive assessment by a specialist – usually, a child psychiatrist or a paediatrician with expertise in ADHD.[1] Appropriate psychological, psychosocial and behavioural interventions should be put in place. Drug treatments should be only a part of the overall treatment plan.
- The indication for drug treatment is the presence of impairment resulting from ADHD; in mild-to-moderate cases the first treatments are usually behaviour therapy and education; medication is indicated as first-line therapy only in severe cases (e.g. those diagnosed as hyperkinetic disorder), and as second-line when psychological approaches have not been successful within a reasonable time (e.g. 8 weeks) or are inappropriate.
- **Methylphenidate** is usually the first choice of drug when a drug is indicated. It is a central nervous stimulant with a large evidence base from trials. Adverse effects include insomnia, anorexia, raised blood pressure and growth deceleration, which can usually be managed by symptomatic management and/or dose reduction (see Box 5.3).
- **Dexamfetamine** is an alternative central nervous system (CNS) stimulant; effects and adverse reactions are broadly similar to methylphenidate, but there is much

---

Box 5.3 NICE guidance: summary of treatment for attention deficit hyperactivity disorder[19]

- Drug treatment should only be initiated by a specialist and only after comprehensive assessment of mental and physical health and social influences.
- For cases with moderate (or lesser) degrees of severity, psychological interventions are recommended as initial therapy, with medication subsequently if still required.
- For severe cases (i.e. those with pervasive impairment from their ADHD), medication will usually be the first-line treatment.
- Methylphenidate, dexamfetamine and atomoxetine are recommended within their licensed indications.
- Methylphenidate is usually first choice of medication, but decision should include consideration of:
  - co-morbid conditions (tics, Tourette's syndrome, epilepsy)
  - tolerability and adverse effects
  - convenience of dosing
  - potential for diversion
  - patient/parent preference.
- If using methylphenidate, consider modified-release preparations (convenience of single-day dosage, improving adherence, reducing stigma, acceptability to schools); or multiple doses of immediate-release (greater flexibility in controlling time-course of action, closer initial titration).
- Where more than one agent is considered suitable, the product with the lowest cost should be prescribed.
- Monitoring should include measurement of height and weight (with entry on growth charts) and recording of blood pressure and heart rate.

less evidence on efficacy and safety than exists for methylphenidate, and it plays a part in illegal drug taking. Both methylphenidate and dexamfetamine are Controlled Drugs; prescriptions should be written appropriately and for not more than 28 days.

- **Lisdexamfetamine** is a 'prodrug'; the dexamfetamine is complexed with the aminoacid lysine and in this form is inactive. It is gradually broken down (in red blood cells) so that dexamfetamine is gradually made available. It therefore has a similar practical role to extended-release preparations of methylphenidate; and, like them, is unlikely to be abused for recreational or dependency-driven purposes. Several randomised controlled trials have established it as superior to placebo in children[2,3] and adolescents.[4] Effect size from preliminary research appears to be at least as great as that of Oros-methylphenidate[3] and it seems to have a similar range of adverse effects.[5] Long-term data suggest that it can be considered as an alternative to extended-release methylphenidate.[6]

- **Atomoxetine**[7–10] is a suitable first-line alternative. It may be particularly useful for children who do not respond to stimulants or whose medication cannot be administered during the day. It may also be suitable where stimulant diversion is a problem or when 'dopaminergic' adverse effects (such as tics, anxiety and stereotypies) become problematic on stimulants. Parents should be warned of the possibilities of suicidal thinking and liver disease emerging and advised of the possible features that they might notice.

- Third-line drugs include **clonidine**[11] and **tricyclic antidepressants.**[12] Very few children should receive these drugs for ADHD alone. There is some evidence supporting the efficacy of **carbamazepine**[13] and **bupropion.** There is no evidence to support the use of **second-generation antipsychotics**[14] for ADHD symptoms, but risperidone may be helpful in reducing severe coexistent levels of aggression and agitation, especially in those with moderate learning disability.[15] **Modafanil** appears to be effective[16] but has not been compared with standard treatments and its safety is not established. **Guanfacine** is approved in the USA[17] but at present in the UK only for Phase 3 trials.

- Co-morbid psychiatric illness is common in ADHD children. Stimulants are often helpful overall[12] but are unlikely to be appropriate for children who have a psychotic illness and problems with substance misuse should be managed in their own right before considering ADHD treatment.[18]

- Once stimulant treatment has been established, it is appropriate for repeat prescriptions to be supplied through general practitioners.[19]

ADHD in adults

Adult ADHD is recognised by both ICD-10 and DSM-V, and NICE guidance regards the first-line treatment as medication, following the same principles as for drug treatment in children.

- At least 25% of ADHD children will still have symptoms at the age of 30. It is appropriate to **continue treatment started in childhood** in adults whose symptoms remain disabling.

CHAPTER 5

- A new diagnosis of ADHD in an adult should only be made after a comprehensive assessment, including information from other informants and where possible from adults who knew the patient as a child.
- The prevalence of substance misuse and antisocial personality disorder are high in adults whose ADHD was not recognised in childhood.[20] Methylphenidate can be effective in this population,[21] but caution is appropriate in prescribing and monitoring.
- **Methylphenidate** is usually the first choice of medication. **Atomoxetine** is also effective[22] and is the only medication licensed for use in adults – and then only when treatment was initiated before the age of 18 years. Monitoring for symptoms of liver dysfunction and suicidal thinking is advised.

References

1. National Institute for Health and Clinical Excellence. Methylphenidate, atomoxetine and dexamfetamine for attention deficit hyperactivity disorder (ADHD) in children and adolescents - guidance. Technology Appraisal 98, 2006. http://www.nice.org.uk
2. Biederman J et al. Lisdexamfetamine dimesylate and mixed amphetamine salts extended-release in children with ADHD: a double-blind, placebo-controlled, crossover analog classroom study. Biol Psychiatry 2007; 62:970–976.
3. Coghill D et al. European, randomized, phase 3 study of lisdexamfetamine dimesylate in children and adolescents with attention-deficit/hyperactivity disorder. Eur Neuropsychopharmacol 2013; 23:1208–1218.
4. Findling RL et al. Efficacy and safety of lisdexamfetamine dimesylate in adolescents with attention-deficit/hyperactivity disorder. J Am Acad Child Adolesc Psychiatry 2011; 50:395–405.
5. Heal DJ et al. Amphetamine, past and present–a pharmacological and clinical perspective. J Psychopharmacol 2013; 27:479–496.
6. Findling RL et al. Long-term effectiveness and safety of lisdexamfetamine dimesylate in school-aged children with attention-deficit/hyperactivity disorder. CNS Spectr 2008; 13:614–620.
7. Michelson D et al. Once-daily atomoxetine treatment for children and adolescents with attention deficit hyperactivity disorder: a randomized, placebo-controlled study. Am J Psychiatry 2002; 159:1896–1901.
8. Kratochvil CJ et al. Atomoxetine and methylphenidate treatment in children with ADHD: a prospective, randomized, open-label trial. J Am Acad Child Adolesc Psychiatry 2002; 41:776–784.
9. Weiss M et al. A randomized, placebo-controlled study of once-daily atomoxetine in the school setting in children with ADHD. J Am Acad Child Adolesc Psychiatry 2005; 44:647–655.
10. Kratochvil CJ et al. A Double-Blind, Placebo-Controlled Study of Atomoxetine in Young Children With ADHD. Pediatrics 2011; 127:e862–e868.
11. Connor DF et al. A meta-analysis of clonidine for symptoms of attention-deficit hyperactivity disorder. J Am Acad Child Adolesc Psychiatry 1999; 38:1551–1559.
12. Hazell P. Tricyclic antidepressants in children: is there a rationale for use? CNS Drugs 1996; 5:233–239.
13. Silva RR et al. Carbamazepine use in children and adolescents with features of attention-deficit hyperactivity disorder: a meta-analysis. J Am Acad Child Adolesc Psychiatry 1996; 35:352–358.
14. Einarson TR et al. Novel antipsychotics for patients with attention-deficit hyperactivity disorder: a systematic review. Ottawa: Canadian Coordinating Office for Health Technology Assessment (CCOHTA) 2001;Technology Report No 17.
15. Correia Filho AG et al. Comparison of risperidone and methylphenidate for reducing ADHD symptoms in children and adolescents with moderate mental retardation. J Am Acad Child Adolesc Psychiatry 2005; 44:748–755.
16. Biederman J et al. A comparison of once-daily and divided doses of modafinil in children with attention-deficit/hyperactivity disorder: a randomized, double-blind, and placebo-controlled study. J Clin Psychiatry 2006; 67:727–735.
17. Biederman J et al. A randomized, double-blind, placebo-controlled study of guanfacine extended release in children and adolescents with attention-deficit/hyperactivity disorder. Pediatrics 2008; 121:e73–e84.
18. Hutchins P, Hazell P, Nunn K. Attention deficit hyperactivity disorder (ADHD). In: Nunn KP, Dey C, eds. *The Clinician's Guide to Psychotropic Prescribing in Children and Adolescents*. Sydney: Glade Publishing; 2003, pp.162–171.
19. National Institute for Health and Clinical Excellence. Attention Deficit Hyperactivity Disorder: diagnosis and management of ADHD in children, young people and adults. Clinical Guideline 72, 2008. http://guidance.nice.org.uk.
20. Cosgrove PVF. Attention deficit hyperactivity disorder. Primary Care Psychiatry 1997; 3:101–114.
21. Spencer T et al. A double-blind, crossover comparison of methylphenidate and placebo in adults with childhood-onset attention-deficit hyperactivity disorder. Arch Gen Psychiatry 1995; 52:434–443.
22. Spencer T et al. Effectiveness and tolerability of atomoxetine in adults with attention deficit hyperactivity disorder. Am J Psychiatry 1998; 155:693–695.

Further reading

Kutcher S *et al*. International consensus statement on attention-deficit/hyperactivity disorder (ADHD) and disruptive behaviour disorders (DBDs): clinical implications and treatment practice suggestions. Eur Neuropsychopharmacol 2004;**14**:11–28.

Nutt DJ *et al*. Evidence-based guidelines for management of attention-deficit/hyperactivity disorder in adolescents in transition to adult services and in adults: recommendations from the British Association for Psychopharmacology. J Psychopharmacol 2007;**21**:10–41.

Taylor E et al. European clinical guidelines for hyperkinetic disorder – first upgrade. Eur Child Adolesc Psychiatry 2004;**13** Suppl 1:17–30.

Prescribing in attention deficit hyperactivity disorder

See Table 5.6 for prescribing in ADHD.

Table 5.6 Prescribing in attention deficit hyperactivity disorder

Medication	Onset and duration of action	Dose	Comment	Recommended monitoring
Methylphenidate immediate release (Ritalin, Equasym)[1,2]	Onset: 20–60 min Duration: 2–4 hours	Initially 5–10 mg daily titrated up to a maximum of 2 mg/kg/day in divided doses using weekly increments of 5–10 mg (maximum 100 mg)	Usually first-line treatment. Generally well tolerated[3] Controlled Drug	Blood pressure Pulse Height and weight Monitor for insomnia, mood and appetite change and the development of tics[4]
Methylphenidate sustained release (Concerta XL)[1,2,5–7] Also Equasym XL[8–9] Also Medikinet[10]	Concerta Onset: 30 min–2 hours Duration: 12 hours Equasym XL: Onset: 20–60 min Duration: 8 hours Onset: 20–60 min Duration up to 8 hours	Concerta: Initially 18 mg in the morning, titrated up to a maximum of 54 mg – or after review up to 108 mg in adults 18 mg Concerta = 15 mg Ritalin Equasym XL: Initially 10 mg increasing as necessary to 60 mg once daily (max 100 in adults) Dose as Equasym Capsules can be opened and sprinkled[11]	An afternoon dose of Ritalin may be required in some children to optimise treatment Controlled Drug Controlled Drug A larger fraction of the drug is available immediately than in other modified-release forms Controlled Drug	Discontinue if no benefits seen in 1 month
Dexamfetamine immediate release (Dexedrine)[3,12]	Onset: 20–60 min Duration: 3–6 hours	2.5–10 mg daily to start, titrated up to a maximum of 20 mg (occasionally 40 mg) in divided doses using weekly increments of 2.5 mg	Considered to be less well tolerated than methylphenidate[3] Controlled Drug	
Lisdexamfetamine (Elvanse)[13–15]	Onset: 20–60min Duration: 13+ hours	Initially 30mg in the morning, titrated up to a maximum of 70mg	Prodrug gradually hydrolysed to dexamfetamine Treat as Controlled Drug	As for methylphenidate Full long-term efficacy and safety data awaited
Atomoxetine[16,17]	Approximately 4–6 weeks (atomoxetine is a NA reuptake inhibitor)	When switching from a stimulant, continue stimulant for first 4 weeks of therapy For children <70 kg: start with 0.5mg/kg/day and increase after a minimum of 7 days to 1.2 mg/kg (single or divided doses) and increase up to 1.8 mg/kg/day if necessary For children >70 kg: start with 40 mg and increase after a minimum of 7 days to 80 mg	Efficacy may be a little lower than found for methylphenidate.[18] May be useful where stimulant diversion is a problem[19] Once-daily dosing convenient in schoolchildren Not a Controlled Drug	Pulse Blood pressure Height Weight

References

1. Wolraich ML et al. Pharmacokinetic considerations in the treatment of attention-deficit hyperactivity disorder with methylphenidate. CNS Drugs 2004; **18**:243–250.

2. Joint Formulary Committee. *BNF* 67 March-September 2014 (online). London: Pharmaceutical Press; 2014. http://www.medicinescomplete.com/mc/bnf/current/

3. Efron D et al. Side effects of methylphenidate and dexamphetamine in children with attention deficit hyperactivity disorder: a double-blind, crossover trial. Pediatrics 1997; **100**:662–666.

4. Gadow KD et al. Efficacy of methylphenidate for attention-deficit hyperactivity disorder in children with tic disorder. Arch Gen Psychiatry 1995; **52**:444–455.

5. Hoare P et al. 12-month efficacy and safety of OROS MPH in children and adolescents with attention-deficit/hyperactivity disorder switched from MPH. Eur Child Adolesc Psychiatry 2005; **14**:305–309.

6. Remschmidt H et al. Symptom control in children and adolescents with attention-deficit/hyperactivity disorder on switching from immediate-release MPH to OROS MPH Results of a 3-week open-label study. Eur Child Adolesc Psychiatry 2005; **14**:297–304.

7. Wolraich ML et al. Randomized, controlled trial of OROS methylphenidate once a day in children with attention-deficit/hyperactivity disorder. Pediatrics 2001; **108**:883–892.

8. Findling RL et al. Comparison of the clinical efficacy of twice-daily Ritalin and once-daily Equasym XL with placebo in children with Attention Deficit/Hyperactivity Disorder. Eur Child Adolesc Psychiatry 2006; **15**:450–459.

9. Anderson VR et al. Spotlight on Methylphenidate Controlled-Delivery Capsules (Equasymtrade markXL, Metadate CDtrade mark) in the treatment of children and adolescents with Attention-Deficit Hyperactivity Disorder. CNS Drugs 2007; **21**:173–175.

10. Haessler F et al. A pharmacokinetic study of two modified-release methylphenidate formulations under different food conditions in healthy volunteers. Int J Clin Pharmacol Ther 2008; **46**:466–476.

11. Fischer R et al. Bioequivalence of a methylphenidate hydrochloride extended-release preparation: comparison of an intact capsule and an opened capsule sprinkled on applesauce. Int J Clin Pharmacol Ther 2006; **44**:135–141.

12. Cyr M et al. Current drug therapy recommendations for the treatment of attention deficit hyperactivity disorder. Drugs 1998; **56**:215–223.

13. Biederman J et al. Lisdexamfetamine dimesylate and mixed amphetamine salts extended-release in children with ADHD: a double-blind, placebo-controlled, crossover analog classroom study. Biol Psychiatry 2007; **62**:970–976.

14. Coghill D et al. European, randomized, phase 3 study of lisdexamfetamine dimesylate in children and adolescents with attention-deficit/hyperactivity disorder. Eur Neuropsychopharmacol 2013; **23**:1208–1218.

15. Findling RL et al. Efficacy and safety of lisdexamfetamine dimesylate in adolescents with attention-deficit/hyperactivity disorder. J Am Acad Child Adolesc Psychiatry 2011; **50**:395–405.

16. Kelsey DK et al. Once-daily atomoxetine treatment for children with attention-deficit/hyperactivity disorder, including an assessment of evening and morning behavior: a double-blind, placebo-controlled trial. Pediatrics 2004; **114**:e1–e8.

17. Wernicke JF et al. Cardiovascular effects of atomoxetine in children, adolescents, and adults. Drug Saf 2003; **26**:729–740.

18. Kratochvil CJ et al. Atomoxetine and methylphenidate treatment in children with ADHD: a prospective, randomized, open-label trial. J Am Acad Child Adolesc Psychiatry 2002; **41**:776–784.

19. Heil SH et al. Comparison of the subjective, physiological, and psychomotor effects of atomoxetine and methylphenidate in light drug users. Drug Alcohol Depend 2002; **67**:149–156.

CHAPTER 5

Autism spectrum disorders

Autism spectrum disorders (ASD) are conditions characterised by core deficits in three areas of development (domains); language, social interaction and behaviour (stereotypies and/or restricted and unusual patterns of interests). The autism spectrum comprises autism, Asperger's syndrome and pervasive developmental disorders-not otherwise specified (PDD-NOS) and are categorised under pervasive developmental disorders (PDD) in ICD 10. Rett's syndrome and childhood disintegrative disorder are also categorised under PDD in the ICD, though they are aetiologically distinct, with different characteristics and outcomes from ASD. The focus of this section is on treatments for ASD.

Diagnosis of ASD is straightforward. There are a range of well validated instruments for history taking from parents/guardians and objective assessment of the individual in question. However, the heterogeneity of problems seen within ASD makes detailed clinical assessment essential. Often the greatest diagnostic difficulty occurs at the milder end of the spectrum. It is important to evaluate any co-morbid neurodevelopmental, medical and psychiatric disorders that may complicate the symptom profile. These include mental retardation, attention deficit hyperactivity disorder (ADHD), epilepsy, anxiety, obsessive-compulsive and mood disorders, sleep disturbance, self-harm, irritability and aggression towards others.

Pharmacotherapies are commonly used in individuals with ASD as adjuncts to psychological interventions and there are now several published reports describing controlled and open-label clinical trials. The bulk of the evidence to date is for the efficacy of risperidone, methylphenidate and some selective reuptake inhibitors in the treatment of problem behaviours or co-existing disorders in ASD. Preliminary controlled trials of sodium valproate, atomoxetine and aripiprazole are promising. There is a potential role for α_2-agonists, cholinergic agents, glutamatergic agents and oxytocin and these require further investigation.[1]

Currently there is no single medication for ASD that alleviates symptoms in all three domains. Targeting pharmacological interventions at problem behaviours and the level of impairment these cause, is essential. Such interventions should always be considered to be individual treatment trials. The efficacy and adverse effects associated with pharmacotherapy should be systematically monitored, bearing in mind that individuals with ASD often have impaired communication. Standardised behaviour ratings scales and adverse effect checklists are an essential tool in monitoring progress.[2] A very wide range of pharmacological interventions have been studied in autism (both allopathic and 'alternative') but few are well supported.[3]

Pharmacological treatment of core symptoms of ASD

Restricted repetitive behaviours and interests domain

Restricted repetitive behaviours and interests (RRBI) behaviours are distressing and disruptive to functioning and therefore an important treatment target to improve overall outcomes in ASD.[4] Behavioural therapies should be used as a first line but some behaviours can be difficult to manage. When these are severe, with significant impact on educational and social performance, and/or pose risks to others and/or self, then pharmacological treatment should be considered.

SSRIs have become the most the most widely prescribed medications to treat RRBIs in paediatric ASD populations. The evidence supporting the effectiveness of SSRIs in ameliorating these symptoms remains limited with the bulk of reports being from single case-studies and open-label trials with only a few RCTs published to date.[5-7] The SSRIs that have been studied include fluoxetine, fluvoxamine, sertraline, citalopram and escitalopram. While side-effects have generally been considered to be mild, increased activation and agitation occurred in some subjects. The current available literature reports inconsistent benefit from SSRIs and there remains uncertainty about the optimal dose regime, which may be lower than those used for treatment of depression in typically developing individuals.[8,9] The mean dose of fluoxetine has been approximately 10 mg per day, starting with 2.5 mg (see Box 5.5). Note that a recent Cochrane review found 'no evidence of effect of SSRIs in children and emerging evidence of harm'.[10]

Other potential pharmacological treatments include second-generation antipsychotics,[11] anticonvulsants[12] and the neuropeptide, oxytocin.[13] Research with respect to risperidone indicates that it is effective in reducing repetitive behaviours in children who have high levels of irritability or aggression.[14] Reductions in core repetitive behaviours have also been reported.[11,15,16]

Social and communication impairment domain

Currently, no drug has been consistently shown to improve the core social and communication impairments in ASD. Risperidone may have a secondary effect through improvement in irritability.[17] Glutamatergic drugs and oxytocin are currently the most promising.[18]

Pharmacological treatment of co-morbid problem behaviours in ASD

Inattention, over activity and impulsiveness in ASD (symptoms of ADHD)

Children with ASD have high rates of inattention, over activity and impulsiveness.[19] Adequate numbers of controlled trials of pharmacotherapy to treat these symptoms in children with ASD are lacking.[20] The largest controlled trial to date has been with methylphenidate and conducted by the Research Units on Paediatric Psychopharmacology (RUPP) Autism Network.[21,22] In a previous retrospective and prospective study of children with ASD, Santosh and colleagues[23] reported positive benefits of treatment with methylphenidate. In general, methylphenidate produces highly variable responses in children with ASD and ADHD symptoms. These responses range from a marked improvement with few side-effects through to poor response and/or problematic side-effects. Although there has recently been a slight shift in reporting positive effects of methylphenidate on ADHD symptoms in children with ASD, it is widely accepted that the efficacy in this group is limited and that adverse side-effects are more commonly reported compared to children with ADHD alone.[1,24,25] However, where ADHD

CHAPTER 5

symptoms are severe and/or disabling, it is reasonable to proceed with a treatment trial of methylphenidate. It is advisable to warn parents of the lower likelihood of response and the potential side-effects and to proceed with low initial does (~0.125 mg/kg three times daily) increasing with small increments. Treatment should be stopped immediately if behaviour deteriorates or there are unacceptable side-effects.

Atomoxetine is a noradrenergic reuptake inhibitor that has been licensed to treat ADHD. There is preliminary evidence from small open-label trials that it may be useful in children with ASD but large scale RCTs are awaited.[26] A recent review has suggested that atomoxetine is more effective in individuals with milder ASD symptoms.[27] Whilst the number of open label and RCTs is increasing, the evidence of benefit across the severity of ASD spectrum remains conflicting.[1]

There is some evidence from controlled studies for risperidone and α_2-agonists (clonidine and guanfacine) however there is little or no evidence in favour of SSRIs, venlafaxine benzodiazepines or anticonvulsant mood stabilisers.[28]

Irritability (aggression, self-injurious behaviour, tantrums)

Aggression to others and self is a common problem behaviour in ASD. Although behavioural and environment approaches are recommended as first-line treatments, more severe and dangerous behaviours usually necessitate pharmacological intervention.[29] Duration of recommended treatment is difficult to derive from published evidence but treatment appears to be beneficial for up to 6–12 months.[30] Efforts to reduce and possibly discontinue such treatment at the end of this period should be strongly considered.[29,30]

Second-generation antipsychotics are the first-line pharmacological treatment for children and adolescents with ASD and associated irritability.[30-32] The first licensed in children is risperidone.[33,34] Treatment of irritability in adults with ASD is reported in a placebo-controlled trial to respond in a similar way.[35] Though side-effects such as weight-gain, increased appetite and somnolence can be problematic,[36-39] an adverse impact on cognitive performance has not been found after up to 8 weeks of treatment.[40] See Box 5.4 for the Medicines and Healthcare Regulatory Agency (MHRA) recommended dosages for risperidone.

Aripiprazole is the other FDA-approved second-generation antipsychotic for use in children and adolescents with ASD.[41] A recent review and meta-analysis of short-term (8 weeks) aripiprazole in the treatment of irritability in ASD children aged 6–17 years[42] found there to be a significant reduction in irritability with a moderate effect size, when compared with placebo. A more recent Cochrane review[43] concludes that whilst aripiprazole may be beneficial in managing irritability, hyperactivity and stereotypies in children with ASD, it is not without side-effects which include weight gain, sedation, sialorrhoea and EPS. The usual recommended clinical dose for maintenance is between 5 and 15 mg daily.[30]

The effectiveness of other SGAs such as olanzapine and ziprasidone has not been tested in adequately powered RCTs. Available data suggest that mood stabilisers and anticonvulsants may not be as effective as SGAs for the treatment of irritability in ASD.[44] Limited data support the combination of risperidone and topiramate being better than risperidone alone.[1,45]

Sleep disturbance

Children with ASD have significant sleep problems[46] and there are a range of behavioural and pharmacological treatments available for this group. It is essential to understand the aetiology of the sleep problem before embarking on a course of treatment. Typical sleep problems in this group are sleep-onset insomnia, sleep-maintenance insomnia, and irregularities of the sleep–wake cycle, including early morning awakening. Abnormalities in the melatonin system have recently received much attention.[47]

Melatonin, has been shown in 17 studies to be beneficial in children with ASD.[48] More recent RCTs continue to show promising results, although larger RCTs are needed.[1,30] Doses range from 1 mg to 10 mg. Melatonin is usually very well tolerated. General seizures did not recur in children who were seizure free nor increase in those with epilepsy.[49] See section on 'Melatonin in the treatment of insomnia in children and adolescents' later in this chapter.

Risperidone may benefit sleep difficulties in those with extreme irritability. In the anxious or depressed child, antidepressants may be beneficial. Insomnia due to hyperarousal may benefit from clonidine or clonazepam.[50]

Pathologic aggression in children and adolescents with ASD

Children and adolescents with psychiatric illness, like adults, may display pathologic aggression (PA) that is destructive, severe, chronic, and unresponsive to psychosocial and psychopharmacological treatment of their underlying condition(s) and psychosocial interventions specifically targeting their aggression. For this subset of young people with persistent aggression, pharmacotherapy may be an appropriate treatment option to optimise their functioning. It is important to understand what drives the aggressive behaviour and to intervene appropriately. This topic is reviewed by Barzman and Findling.[51] In general, the use of pharmacological intervention for pathologic aggression should only be considered when (1) the underlying condition is adequately treated, (2) any current treatments are not contributing and (3) all other psychological and behavioural treatment options fail to ensure the safety and optimal functioning of the child or young person. With respect to co-morbid psychiatric illness, the most common primary diagnoses include bipolar disorders and psychotic illness. Learning disability is also common.

There is most evidence supporting the use of risperidone in aggressive behaviour.[52–54] There are fewer data for olanzapine, quetiapine, aripiprazole and clozapine. Risperidone can cause significant extrapyramidal side-effects in young people and like almost all SGAs can cause considerable weight gain, metabolic (hyperglycaemia) and hormonal (hyperprolactinaemia) imbalance. Weight gain is usually worse in children than in adults.[55] A more recent systematic review[56] highlights the importance of careful safety monitoring of SGAs used in children and adolescents and provides evidence based guidance on effectiveness and safety monitoring practice.

Controlled studies support the use of mood stabilisers such as lithium[57,58] and sodium valproate[59] as being effective in the treatment of persistent aggression in children and adolescents.

There are no controlled trials of pharmacological treatments in children younger than 5 years of age.

CHAPTER 5

Use of risperidone in children and adolescents

Box 5.4 MHRA guidance for risperidone prescribing in children and adolescents[60]

Risperidone is indicated for the treatment of autism in children (aged 5 and over) and adolescents. The dosage of risperidone should be individualised according to the response of the patient.

Doses of risperidone in paediatric patients with ASD (by total mg/day)

Weight categories	Days 1–3	Days 4–14+	Increments if dose increases are needed	Dose range
<20 kg	0.25 mg	0.5 mg	+0.25 mg at ≥2 week intervals	0.5 mg–1.5 mg
≥20 kg	0.5 mg	1.0 mg	+0.5 mg at ≥2 week intervals	1.0 mg–2.5 mg*

*Subjects weighing >45 kg may require higher doses: maximum dose studied was 3.5 mg/day.

For prescribers preferring to dose on a mg/kg/day basis the following guidance is provided.

Doses of risperidone in paediatric patients with ASD (by mg/kg/day)

Weight categories	Days 1–3	Days 4–14+	Increments if dose increases are needed	Dose range
All	0.01 mg/kg/day	0.02 mg/kg/day	+0.01 mg/kg/day at ≥2 week intervals	0.2 mg/kg/day –0.06 mg/kg/day

General considerations

- Risperidone can be administered once daily or twice daily.
- Patients experiencing somnolence may benefit from taking the whole daily dose at bedtime.
- Once sufficient clinical response has been achieved and maintained, consideration may be given to gradually lowering the dose to achieve the optimal balance of efficacy and safety.
- There is insufficient evidence from controlled trials to indicate how long treatment should continue.

Adverse effects

Weight gain, somnolence and hyperglycaemia require monitoring, and the long-term safety of risperidone in children and adolescents with ASD remains to be fully determined.

Fluoxetine in children and adolescents

When using fluoxetine to treat repetitive behaviours in ASD patients, doses much lower than those used to treat depression are normally required. It is advisable to use a liquid preparation and begin at the lowest possible dose, monitoring for side-effects. A suitable regime is outlined in Box 5.5.

Box 5.5 Use of fluoxetine in children and adolescents

Liquid fluoxetine: (as hydrochloride) 20 mg/5 mL
2.5 mg/day a day for 1 week; note that 2.5 mg = 0.625 mL which is difficult to measure accurately.

Follow with flexible titration schedule based on weight, tolerability, and side-effects up to a maximum dose of 0.8 mg/kg/day (0.3 mg/kg for week 2, 0.5 mg/kg/day for week 3, and 0.8 mg/kg/day subsequently). Reduction may be indicated if side-effects are problematic.

Adverse effects

- Monitor for emergent **suicidal** behaviour, self-harm and hostility, particularly at the beginning of treatment.
- Hyponatraemia is also possible – see section on 'Antidepressant-induced hyponatraemia' in Chapter 4.

References

1. Sung M et al. What's in the pipeline? Drugs in development for autism spectrum disorder. Neuropsychiatr Dis Treat 2014; **10**:371–381.
2. Greenhill LL. Assessment of safety in pediatric psychopharmacology. J Am Acad Child Adolesc Psychiatry 2003; **42**:625–626.
3. Rossignol DA. Novel and emerging treatments for autism spectrum disorders: a systematic review. Ann Clin Psychiatry 2009; **21**:213–236.
4. Leekam SR et al. Restricted and repetitive behaviors in autism spectrum disorders: a review of research in the last decade. Psychol Bull 2011; **137**:562–593.
5. McDougle CJ et al. A double-blind, placebo-controlled study of fluvoxamine in adults with autistic disorder. Arch Gen Psychiatry 1996; **53**:1001–1008.
6. Buchsbaum MS et al. Effect of fluoxetine on regional cerebral metabolism in autistic spectrum disorders: a pilot study. Int J Neuropsychopharmacol 2001; **4**:119–125.
7. Hollander E et al. A placebo controlled crossover trial of liquid fluoxetine on repetitive behaviors in childhood and adolescent autism. Neuropsychopharmacology 2005; **30**:582–589.
8. Aman MG et al. Medication patterns in patients with autism: temporal, regional, and demographic influences. J Child Adolesc Psychopharmacol 2005; **15**:116–126.
9. Soorya L et al. Psychopharmacologic interventions for repetitive behaviors in autism spectrum disorders. Child Adolesc Psychiatr Clin N Am 2008; **17**:753–771.
10. Williams K et al. Selective serotonin reuptake inhibitors (SSRIs) for autism spectrum disorders (ASD). Cochrane Database Syst Rev 2013; **8**: CD004677.
11. McDougle CJ et al. Risperidone for the core symptom domains of autism: results from the study by the autism network of the research units on pediatric psychopharmacology. Am J Psychiatry 2005; **162**:1142–1148.
12. Hollander E et al. A double-blind placebo-controlled pilot study of olanzapine in childhood/adolescent pervasive developmental disorder. J Child Adolesc Psychopharmacol 2006; **16**:541–548.
13. Hollander E et al. Oxytocin infusion reduces repetitive behaviors in adults with autistic and Asperger's disorders. Neuropsychopharmacology 2003; **28**:193–198.
14. McDougle CJ et al. A double-blind, placebo-controlled study of risperidone addition in serotonin reuptake inhibitor-refractory obsessive-compulsive disorder. Arch Gen Psychiatry 2000; **57**:794–801.
15. McCracken JT et al. Risperidone in children with autism and serious behavioral problems. N Engl J Med 2002; **347**:314–321.
16. Arnold LE et al. Parent-defined target symptoms respond to risperidone in RUPP autism study: customer approach to clinical trials. J Am Acad Child Adolesc Psychiatry 2003; **42**:1443–1450.
17. Canitano R et al. Risperidone in the treatment of behavioral disorders associated with autism in children and adolescents. Neuropsychiatr Dis Treat 2008; **4**:723–730.
18. Posey DJ et al. Developing drugs for core social and communication impairment in autism. Child Adolesc Psychiatr Clin N Am 2008; **17**:787–801.
19. Simonoff E et al. Psychiatric disorders in children with autism spectrum disorders: prevalence, comorbidity, and associated factors in a population-derived sample. J Am Acad Child Adolesc Psychiatry 2008; **47**:921–929.
20. Mahajan R et al. Clinical practice pathways for evaluation and medication choice for attention-deficit/hyperactivity disorder symptoms in autism spectrum disorders. Pediatrics 2012; **130** Suppl 2:S125–S138.
21. Research Units on Pediatric Psychopharmacology (RUPP) Autism Network. Randomized, controlled, crossover trial of methylphenidate in pervasive developmental disorders with hyperactivity. Arch Gen Psychiatry 2005; **62**:1266–1274.
22. Posey DJ et al. Positive effects of methylphenidate on inattention and hyperactivity in pervasive developmental disorders: an analysis of secondary measures. Biol Psychiatry 2007; **61**:538–544.
23. Santosh PJ et al. Impact of comorbid autism spectrum disorders on stimulant response in children with attention deficit hyperactivity disorder: a retrospective and prospective effectiveness study. Child Care Health Dev 2006; **32**:575–583.

CHAPTER 5

24. Siegel M et al. Psychotropic medications in children with autism spectrum disorders: a systematic review and synthesis for evidence-based practice. J Autism Dev Disord 2012; **42**:1592–1605.

25. Williamson ED et al. Psychotropic medications in autism: practical considerations for parents. J Autism Dev Disord 2012; **42**:1249–1255.

26. Arnold LE et al. Atomoxetine for hyperactivity in autism spectrum disorders: placebo-controlled crossover pilot trial. J Am Acad Child Adolesc Psychiatry 2006; **45**:1196–1205.

27. Ghanizadeh A. Atomoxetine for treating ADHD symptoms in autism: a systematic review. J Atten Disord 2013; **17**:635–640.

28. Aman MG et al. Treatment of inattention, overactivity, and impulsiveness in autism spectrum disorders. Child Adolesc Psychiatr Clin N Am 2008; **17**:713–38, vii.

29. National Institute for Health and Care Excellence. Autism: The management and support of children and young people on the autism spectrum. Clinical Guideline **170**, 2013. http://publications.nice.org.uk/autism-cg170

30. Kaplan G et al. Psychopharmacology of autism spectrum disorders. Pediatr Clin North Am 2012; **59**:175-87, xii.

31. McDougle CJ et al. Atypical antipsychotics in children and adolescents with autistic and other pervasive developmental disorders. J Clin Psychiatry 2008; **69** Suppl 4:15–20.

32. Parikh MS et al. Psychopharmacology of aggression in children and adolescents with autism: a critical review of efficacy and tolerability. J Child Adolesc Psychopharmacol 2008; **18**:157–178.

33. Jesner OS et al. Risperidone for autism spectrum disorder. Cochrane Database Syst Rev 2007; CD005040.

34. Scahill L et al. Risperidone approved for the treatment of serious behavioral problems in children with autism. J Child Adolesc Psychiatr Nurs 2007; **20**:188–190.

35. McDougle CJ et al. A double-blind, placebo-controlled study of risperidone in adults with autistic disorder and other pervasive developmental disorders. Arch Gen Psychiatry 1998; **55**:633–641.

36. Caccia S. Safety and pharmacokinetics of atypical antipsychotics in children and adolescents. Paediatr Drugs 2013; **15**:217–233.

37. Sharma A et al. Efficacy of risperidone in managing maladaptive behaviors for children with autistic spectrum disorder: a meta-analysis. J Pediatr Health Care 2012; **26**:291–299.

38. Kent JM et al. Risperidone dosing in children and adolescents with autistic disorder: a double-blind, placebo-controlled study. J Autism Dev Disord 2013; **43**:1773–1783.

39. Maayan L et al. Weight gain and metabolic risks associated with antipsychotic medications in children and adolescents. J Child Adolesc Psychopharmacol 2011; **21**:517–535.

40. Aman MG et al. Acute and long-term safety and tolerability of risperidone in children with autism. J Child Adolesc Psychopharmacol 2005; **15**:869–884.

41. Curran MP. Aripiprazole: in the treatment of irritability associated with autistic disorder in pediatric patients. Paediatr Drugs 2011; **13**:197–204.

42. Douglas-Hall P et al. Aripiprazole: a review of its use in the treatment of irritability associated with autistic disorder patients aged 6-17. Journal of Central Nervous System Diseases 2011; **3**:1–11.

43. Ching H et al. Aripiprazole for autism spectrum disorders (ASD). Cochrane Database Syst Rev 2012; **5**: CD009043.

44. Stigler KA et al. Pharmacotherapy of irritability in pervasive developmental disorders. Child Adolesc Psychiatr Clin N Am 2008; **17**:739–752.

45. Rezaei V et al. Double-blind, placebo-controlled trial of risperidone plus topiramate in children with autistic disorder. Prog Neuropsychopharmacol Biol Psychiatry 2010; **34**:1269–1272.

46. Krakowiak P et al. Sleep problems in children with autism spectrum disorders, developmental delays, and typical development: a population-based study. J Sleep Res 2008; **17**:197–206.

47. Sanchez-Barcelo EJ et al. Clinical uses of melatonin in pediatrics. Int J Pediatr 2011; **2011**:892624.

48. Doyen C et al. Melatonin in children with autistic spectrum disorders: recent and practical data. Eur Child Adolesc Psychiatry 2011; **20**:231–239.

49. Andersen IM et al. Melatonin for insomnia in children with autism spectrum disorders. J Child Neurol 2008; **23**:482–485.

50. Johnson KP et al. Sleep in children with autism spectrum disorders. Curr Treat Options Neurol 2008; **10**:350–359.

51. Barzman DH et al. Pharmacological treatment of pathologic aggression in children. Int Rev Psychiatry 2008; **20**:151–157.

52. Aman MG et al. Double-blind, placebo-controlled study of risperidone for the treatment of disruptive behaviors in children with subaverage intelligence. Am J Psychiatry 2002; **159**:1337–1346.

53. Snyder R et al. Effects of risperidone on conduct and disruptive behavior disorders in children with subaverage IQs. J Am Acad Child Adolesc Psychiatry 2002; **41**:1026–1036.

54. Reyes M et al. A randomized, double-blind, placebo-controlled study of risperidone maintenance treatment in children and adolescents with disruptive behavior disorders. Am J Psychiatry 2006; **163**:402–410.

55. De Hert M et al. Metabolic and endocrine adverse effects of second-generation antipsychotics in children and adolescents: A systematic review of randomized, placebo controlled trials and guidelines for clinical practice. Eur Psychiatry 2011; **26**:144–158.

56. Pringsheim T et al. Evidence-based recommendations for monitoring safety of second-generation antipsychotics in children and youth. Paediatr Child Health 2011; **16**:581–589.

57. Campbell M et al. Lithium in hospitalized aggressive children with conduct disorder: a double-blind and placebo-controlled study. J Am Acad Child Adolesc Psychiatry 1995; **34**:445–453.

58. Malone RP et al. A double-blind placebo-controlled study of lithium in hospitalized aggressive children and adolescents with conduct disorder. Arch Gen Psychiatry 2000; **57**:649–654.

59. Donovan SJ et al. Divalproex treatment for youth with explosive temper and mood lability: a double-blind, placebo-controlled crossover design. Am J Psychiatry 2000; **157**:818–820.

60. Medicines and Healthcare Products Regulatory Agency. Variation Assessment Form. London: MHRA; 2005. http://www.mhra.gov.uk/home/groups/pl-p/documents/websiteresources/con2025027.pdf

Tics and Tourette's syndrome

Transient tics occur in 5–20% of children. Tourette's syndrome (TS) occurs in about 1% of children and is defined by persistent motor and vocal tics. As many as 65% of individuals with TS will have no, or only very mild, tics in adult life. Tics wax and wane over time and are variably exacerbated by external factors such as stress, inactivity and fatigue, depending on the individual. Tics are about 2–3 times more common in boys than girls.[1]

Detection and treatment of co-morbidity

Co-morbid OCD, attention deficit hyperactivity disorder, depression, anxiety, and behavioural problems are more prevalent than would be expected by chance, and often cause the major impairment in people with tic disorders.[2] These co-morbid conditions are usually treated first before assessing the level of disability caused by the tics.[3]

Education and behavioural treatments

Most people with tics do not require pharmacological treatment; education for the individual with tics, their family and the people they interact with, especially schools, is crucial. Treatment aimed primarily at reducing tics is warranted if they cause distress to the patient or are functionally disabling. There has been a resurgence of interest in behavioural programs, and a recent randomised controlled trial of a comprehensive behavioural intervention achieved an effect-size of 0.68 which is comparable with the effect sizes achieved with medication for tics.[4] Habit reversal and exposure and response prevention are the behavioural treatments of choice.[5]

Pharmacological treatments

Studies of pharmacological interventions in TS are difficult to interpret for several reasons.

- There is a large inter-individual variation in tic frequency and severity. Small, randomised studies may include patients that are very different at baseline.
- The severity of tics in a given individual varies markedly over time, making it difficult to separate drug effect from natural variation.
- The bulk of the literature consists of case reports, case series, open studies and underpowered, randomised studies. Publication bias is also likely to be an issue.
- A high proportion of patients have co-morbid psychiatric illness. It can be difficult to disentangle any direct effect on tics from an effect on the co-morbid illness. This makes it difficult to interpret studies that report improvements in global functioning rather than specific reductions in tics.
- Large numbers of individuals attending clinics with TS appear to use complementary or alternative therapies and around 50% report benefit from these.[6]
- The placebo effect in clinical trials of tic disorders is not as large as previously thought.[7]

Most of the published literature concerns children and adolescents.

CHAPTER 5

Adrenergic α₂-agonists

Clonidine has been shown in open studies to reduce the severity and frequency of tics, but in one study this effect did not seem to be convincingly larger than the placebo.[8] Other studies have shown more substantial reductions in tics.[9-12] Guanfacine has been shown to lead to a 30% reduction in tic-rating-scale scores.[13] In the UK, only clonidine is readily available. Therapeutic doses of clonidine are in the order of 3–5 µg/kg, and the dose should be built up gradually. Main side-effects are sedation, postural hypotension and depression. Patients and their families should be informed not to stop clonidine suddenly because of the risk of rebound hypertension.

Antipsychotics

Adverse effects of antipsychotics may outweigh beneficial effects in the treatment of tics and so it is recommended that clonidine is tried first. Antipsychotics may however be more effective than clonidine in alleviating tics in some individuals.

A number of first-generation antipsychotics have been used in TS.[14] In a recent Cochrane review, pimozide demonstrated robust efficacy in a meta analysis of six trials.[15] In these trials, pimozide was compared with haloperidol (one trial), placebo (one trial), haloperidol and placebo (two trials) and risperidone (two trials) and was found to be more effective than placebo, as effective as risperidone and slightly less effective than haloperidol in reducing tics. It was associated with fewer adverse reactions compared with haloperidol but did not differ from risperidone in that respect. ECG monitoring is essential for pimozide and haloperidol. Haloperidol is often poorly tolerated. Given their side-effect profile, most authors recommend the use of second-generation rather than first-generation antipsychotics in the treatment of TS.[14]

Recent studies are suggestive that aripiprazole is an effective and well tolerated treatment of children with TS (and also tics[16]). A 10-week multicentre double-blind randomised placebo-controlled trial (n = 61) demonstrated the efficacy of aripiprazole in tic reduction in TS. Aripiprazole treatment was associated with significantly decreased serum prolactin concentration, increased mean body weight (by 1.6 kg), body mass index, and waist circumference.[17] Several case series are also in support of the use of aripiprazole.[18-21] A study evaluating the metabolic side-effects of aripiprazole (n = 25) and pimozide (n = 25) in TS over a 24-month period demonstrated that treatment was not associated with significant increase in body mass index. However, pimozide treatment was associated with increases in blood sugar which did not plateau from 12 to 24 months, aripiprazole treatment was associated with increased cholesterolaemia and both medications were associated with increased triglyceridaemia.[22]

Risperidone has, in addition to the studies mentioned above, also been shown to be more effective than placebo in a small (n = 34), randomised study.[23] Fatigue and increased appetite were problematic in the risperidone arm and a mean weight gain of 2.8 kg over 8 weeks was reported. A small double-blind crossover study suggested that olanzapine[24] may be more effective than pimozide. One small randomised, controlled trial found risperidone and clonidine to be equally effective.[25] Sulpiride has been shown to be effective and relatively well tolerated,[26] as has ziprasidone.[27] Open studies support the efficacy of quetiapine[28] and olanzapine.[29,30] One very small crossover study (n = 7) found no effect for clozapine.[31]

Overall, metabolic side-effects and weight gain are common with second-generation antipsychotics so benefit/risk ratios need careful discussion.[14]

Other drugs

A small, double-blind, placebo-controlled, crossover trial of **baclofen** was suggestive of beneficial effects in overall impairment rather than a specific effect on tics.[32] The numerical benefits shown in this study did not reach statistical significance. Similarly, a double-blind, placebo-controlled trial of **nicotine** augmentation of haloperidol found beneficial effects in overall impairment rather than a specific effect on tics.[33] These benefits persisted for several weeks after nicotine (in the form of patches) was withdrawn. Nicotine patches were associated with a high prevalence of nausea and vomiting (71% and 40% respectively). The authors suggest that *pro re nata* (prn)use may be appropriate. **Pergolide** (a D_1-D_2-D_3 agonist) given in low dose significantly reduced tics in a double-blind, placebo-controlled, crossover study in children and adolescents.[34] Side-effects included sedation, dizziness, nausea and irritability. Pergolide was also evaluated in a randomised trial in children and adolescents with chronic tics and TS, and showed significant tic reduction compared with placebo.[35] Flutamide, an antiandrogen, has been the subject of a small RCT in adults with TS. Modest, short-lived effects were seen in motor but not phonic tics.[36] A small randomised controlled trial has shown significant advantages for **metoclopramide** over placebo[37] and for **topiramate** over placebo.[38] A recent meta-analysis identified 14 randomised controlled trials (all from China) comparing topiramate with haloperidol or tiapride. It concluded that due to the overall low quality of the study designs, there is not enough evidence to support the routine use of topiramate in clinical practice.[39]

Case reports or case series describing positive effects for ondansetron,[40] clomifene,[41] tramadol,[42] ketanserin,[43] cyproterone,[44] levetiracetam[45] and cannabis[46] have been published. A recent Cochrane Review of cannabinoids concluded that there was little if any current evidence for efficacy.[47] Tetrabenazine may be useful as an add-on treatment.[48] Many other drugs have been reported to be effective in single case reports. Patients in these reports all had co-morbid psychiatric illness, making it difficult to determine the effect of these drugs on TS alone.

Botulinum toxin has been used to treat bothersome or painful focal motor tics, particularly those affecting neck muscles.[14]

There may be a sub-group of children who develop tics/and or OCD in association with streptococcal infection. This group has been given the acronym PANDAS (Paediatric Autoimmune Neuropsychiatric Disorder Associated with Streptococcus).[49] This is thought to be an autoimmune-mediated effect, and there have been trials of immunomodulatory therapy in these children. However, current clinical consensus is that tics or OCD should be treated in the usual way unless a child is part of a research trial. A normal course of antibiotic treatment should be given for any identified active infection (e.g. Strep sore throat) in a child who presents acutely with new onset tics and/or OCD.

References

1. Murphy TK et al. Practice parameter for the assessment and treatment of children and adolescents with tic disorders. J Am Acad Child Adolesc Psychiatry 2013; 52:1341–1359.
2. Cath DC et al. European clinical guidelines for Tourette syndrome and other tic disorders. Part I: assessment. Eur Child Adolesc Psychiatry 2011; 20:155–171.
3. Singer HS. Treatment of tics and tourette syndrome. Curr Treat Options Neurol 2010; 12:539–561.
4. Piacentini J et al. Behavior therapy for children with Tourette disorder: a randomized controlled trial. JAMA 2010; 303:1929–1937.
5. Verdellen C et al. European clinical guidelines for Tourette syndrome and other tic disorders. Part III: behavioural and psychosocial interventions. Eur Child Adolesc Psychiatry 2011; 20:197–207.
6. Kompoliti K et al. Complementary and alternative medicine use in Gilles de la Tourette syndrome. Mov Disord 2009; 24:2015–2019.
7. Cubo E et al. Impact of placebo assignment in clinical trials of tic disorders. Mov Disord 2013; 28:1288–1292.
8. Goetz CG et al. Clonidine and Gilles de la Tourette's syndrome: double-blind study using objective rating methods. Ann Neurol 1987; 21:307–310.
9. Leckman JF et al. Clonidine treatment of Gilles de la Tourette's syndrome. Arch Gen Psychiatry 1991; 48:324–328.
10. Tourette's Syndrome Study Group. Treatment of ADHD in children with tics: a randomized controlled trial. Neurology 2002; 58:527–536.
11. Du YS et al. Randomized double-blind multicentre placebo-controlled clinical trial of the clonidine adhesive patch for the treatment of tic disorders. Aust N Z J Psychiatry 2008; 42:807–813.
12. Hedderick EF et al. Double-blind, crossover study of clonidine and levetiracetam in Tourette syndrome. Pediatr Neurol 2009; 40:420–425.
13. Scahill L et al. A placebo-controlled study of guanfacine in the treatment of children with tic disorders and attention deficit hyperactivity disorder. Am J Psychiatry 2001; 158:1067–1074.
14. Roessner V et al. Pharmacological treatment of tic disorders and Tourette Syndrome. Neuropharmacology 2013; 68:143–149.
15. Pringsheim T et al. Pimozide for tics in Tourette's syndrome. Cochrane Database Syst Rev 2009; CD006996.
16. Yoo HK et al. An open-label study of the efficacy and tolerability of aripiprazole for children and adolescents with tic disorders. J Clin Psychiatry 2007; 68:1088–1093.
17. Yoo HK et al. A multicenter, randomized, double-blind, placebo-controlled study of aripiprazole in children and adolescents with Tourette's disorder. J Clin Psychiatry 2013; 74:e772–e780.
18. Davies L et al. A case series of patients with Tourette's syndrome in the United Kingdom treated with aripiprazole. Hum Psychopharmacol 2006; 21:447–453.
19. Seo WS et al. Aripiprazole treatment of children and adolescents with Tourette disorder or chronic tic disorder. J Child Adolesc Psychopharmacol 2008; 18:197–205.
20. Murphy TK et al. Open label aripiprazole in the treatment of youth with tic disorders. J Child Adolesc Psychopharmacol 2009; 19:441–447.
21. Wenzel C et al. Aripiprazole for the treatment of Tourette syndrome: a case series of 100 patients. J Clin Psychopharmacol 2012; 32:548–550.
22. Rizzo R et al. Metabolic effects of aripiprazole and pimozide in children with Tourette syndrome. Pediatr Neurol 2012; 47:419–422.
23. Scahill L et al. A placebo-controlled trial of risperidone in Tourette syndrome. Neurology 2003; 60:1130–1135.
24. Onofrj M et al. Olanzapine in severe Gilles de la Tourette syndrome: a 52-week double-blind cross-over study vs. low-dose pimozide. J Neurol 2000; 247:443–446.
25. Gaffney GR et al. Risperidone versus clonidine in the treatment of children and adolescents with Tourette's syndrome. J Am Acad Child Adolesc Psychiatry 2002; 41:330–336.
26. Robertson MM et al. Management of Gilles de la Tourette syndrome using sulpiride. Clin Neuropharmacol 1990; 13:229–235.
27. Sallee FR et al. Ziprasidone treatment of children and adolescents with Tourette's syndrome: a pilot study. J Am Acad Child Adolesc Psychiatry 2000; 39:292–299.
28. Mukaddes NM et al. Quetiapine treatment of children and adolescents with Tourette's disorder. J Child Adolesc Psychopharmacol 2003; 13:295–299.
29. Budman CL et al. An open-label study of the treatment efficacy of olanzapine for Tourette's disorder. J Clin Psychiatry 2001; 62:290–294.
30. McCracken JT et al. Effectiveness and tolerability of open label olanzapine in children and adolescents with Tourette syndrome. J Child Adolesc Psychopharmacol 2008; 18:501–508.
31. Caine ED et al. The trial use of clozapine for abnormal involuntary movement disorders. Am J Psychiatry 1979; 136:317–320.
32. Singer HS et al. Baclofen treatment in Tourette syndrome: a double-blind, placebo-controlled, crossover trial. Neurology 2001; 56:599–604.
33. Silver AA et al. Transdermal nicotine and haloperidol in Tourette's disorder: a double-blind placebo-controlled study. J Clin Psychiatry 2001; 62:707–714.
34. Gilbert DL et al. Tourette's syndrome improvement with pergolide in a randomized, double-blind, crossover trial. Neurology 2000; 54:1310–1315.
35. Gilbert DL et al. Tic reduction with pergolide in a randomized controlled trial in children. Neurology 2003; 60:606–611.
36. Peterson BS et al. A double-blind, placebo-controlled, crossover trial of an antiandrogen in the treatment of Tourette's syndrome. J Clin Psychopharmacol 1998; 18:324–331.
37. Nicolson R et al. A randomized, double-blind, placebo-controlled trial of metoclopramide for the treatment of Tourette's disorder. J Am Acad Child Adolesc Psychiatry 2005; 44:640–646.

38. Jankovic J et al. A randomised, double-blind, placebo-controlled study of topiramate in the treatment of Tourette syndrome. J Neurol Neurosurg Psychiatry 2010; **81**:70–73.

39. Yang CS et al. Topiramate for Tourette's syndrome in children: a meta-analysis. Pediatr Neurol 2013; **49**:344–350.

40. Toren P et al. Ondansetron treatment in patients with Tourette's syndrome. Int Clin Psychopharmacol 1999; **14**:373–376.

41. Sandyk R. Clomiphene citrate in Tourette's syndrome. Int J Neurosci 1988; **43**:103–106.

42. Shapira NA et al. Novel use of tramadol hydrochloride in the treatment of Tourette's syndrome. J Clin Psychiatry 1997; **58**:174–175.

43. Bonnier C et al. Ketanserin treatment of Tourette's syndrome in children. Am J Psychiatry 1999; **156**:1122–1123.

44. Izmir M et al. Cyproterone acetate treatment of Tourette's syndrome. Can J Psychiatry 1999; **44**:710–711.

45. Awaad Y et al. Use of levetiracetam to treat tics in children and adolescents with Tourette syndrome. Mov Disord 2005; **20**:714–718.

46. Sandyk R et al. Marijuana and Tourette's syndrome. J Clin Psychopharmacol 1988; **8**:444–445.

47. Curtis A et al. Cannabinoids for Tourette's Syndrome. Cochrane Database Syst Rev 2009; CD006565.

48. Porta M et al. Tourette's syndrome and role of tetrabenazine: review and personal experience. Clin Drug Invest 2008; **28**:443–459.

49. Martino D et al. The PANDAS subgroup of tic disorders and childhood-onset obsessive-compulsive disorder. J Psychosom Res 2009; **67**:547–557.

Melatonin in the treatment of insomnia in children and adolescents

Insomnia is a common symptom in childhood. Underlying causes may be behavioural (inappropriate sleep associations or bedtime resistance) physiological (delayed sleep phase syndrome) or related to underlying mood disorders (anxiety, depression and bipolar disorder). All forms of insomnia are more common in children with learning difficulties, autism, ADHD and sensory impairments (particularly visual). Although behavioural interventions should be the primary intervention and have a robust evidence base, exogenous melatonin is now the 'first-line' medication prescribed for childhood insomnia.[1]

Melatonin is a hormone that is produced by the pineal gland in a circadian manner. The evening rise in melatonin, enabled by darkness, precedes the onset of natural sleep by about 2 hours.[2] Melatonin is involved in the induction of sleep and in synchronisation of the circadian system.

There are a wide variety of unlicensed fast-release, slow-release and liquid preparations of melatonin. Many products rely on food-grade rather than pharmaceutical grade melatonin and some are very expensive. BioMelatonin is an immediate-release melatonin preparation of pharmaceutical grade which is soluble in water and so obviates the need for expensive liquid preparations. A prolonged release formulation of melatonin (Circadin) was licensed in the UK in April 2008 as a short-term treatment of insomnia in patients over 55 years of age. It has not been evaluated in children. Many children are unable to swallow tablets and use in this population will be 'off-label'. Despite these limitations the MHRA recommends prescription of this licensed formulation where possible.[3] Lack of any 'head to head' studies means that there are still no data on whether, or when, immediate or slow release melatonin preparations should be used. Sense would dictate that fast-release melatonin improves sleep latency whilst slow-release improves sleep time (and so a combined approach might be optimal). Nonetheless, there is very little evidence to support this and experience suggests that (1) Circadin can also effectively decrease sleep latency, and (2) sleep duration long term is only minimally altered by any form of melatonin. There are additionally a number of melatonin analogues already produced, or in development[4] although they are virtually never used in the paediatric population, with no evidence from equivalence studies of superiority over melatonin itself.

Efficacy

Two meta-analyses on the use of melatonin in sleep disorders have been published.[5,6] Both pooled data from studies in children and adults. The first considered melatonin in primary sleep disorders (not accompanied by any medical or psychiatric disorder likely to account for the sleep problem) and showed improvements in the time taken to fall asleep of 11.7 minutes across the group, but nearly 40 minutes if delayed sleep phase syndrome was the underlying cause. The study considering secondary sleep disorders in this heterogeneous group found no significant effect on sleep latency.

Since these meta-analyses, many smaller RCTs comparing melatonin with placebo in children have been published.[7-13] Studies have considered diverse groups including children with sleep phase delay, ADHD, autistic spectrum disorders, intellectual disability and epilepsy. Results are surprisingly consistent considering the different underlying disorders. Children in these studies fall asleep about 30 minutes quicker (26.9–34) and their total time asleep increases by a similar (19.8–48) amount of time. The effect size for sleep latency is much greater than for total sleep time confirming that melatonin is of most use for sleep initiation, rather than sleep maintenance. Importantly, over time a number of children who fall asleep earlier on melatonin will also start to wake up earlier on melatonin. The two largest randomised controlled studies to date considered the use of melatonin for children with ASD and neurodevelopmental delay.[14,15] Both employed a behavioural intervention, although with different designs. Together they demonstrated the value of a sleep behavioural intervention before melatonin treatment, and the value of continuing the behavioural intervention during melatonin administration. Both studies showed similar effectiveness of melatonin for sleep latency, but total sleep time was increased more in the study that used a combined slow/fast release preparation of melatonin.

Side-effects

Many of the children who have received melatonin in RCTs and published case series had developmental problems and/or sensory deficits. The scope for detecting subtle adverse effects in this population is limited. Screening for side-effects was not routine in all studies. Early reports included a very small case series cases where melatonin was been reported to worsen seizures[16] and exacerbate asthma[17,18] in the short term. Other reported side-effects include headache, depression, restlessness, confusion, nausea, tachycardia and pruritis.[19,20] In the more recent largest placebo-controlled studies to date involving children with learning difficulty, autism and epilepsy,[11,13,14] there were no excess adverse effects in the treatment group, and in particular seizures were not worsened.

Dose

The cut-off point between physiological and pharmacological doses in children is less than 500 µg. Physiological doses of melatonin may result in very high receptor occupancy. The doses used in RCTs and published case series vary hugely, between 500 µg and 5 mg being the most common, although much lower and higher doses have been used. The optimal dose is unknown and there is no evidence to support a direct relationship between dose and response.[21] In one large RCT 18% of children seemed to respond to a 500 µg dose but others seemed to require much higher doses (12 mg).[14] Increasing doses above 5 mg is likely to be utilising the sedative effects of melatonin, rather than its sleep-phase shifting properties. This might be necessary and still helpful for some children with severe and bilateral brain injury. The use of salivary melatonin measurements is likely to become important in identifying those children with the most delayed sleep phase (likely to have the best response to exogenous melatonin) and those children who are slow metabolisers of melatonin in whom serum levels accumulate during the daytime (particularly on higher doses) and eventually reduce efficiency.

See Figure 5.2 for a summary of recommendations for the use of melatonin.

CHAPTER 5

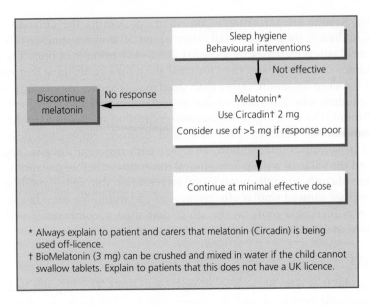

Figure 5.2 Melatonin – summary of recommendations.

References

1. Gringras P. When to use drugs to help sleep. Arch Dis Child 2008; **93**:976–981.
2. Macchi MM et al. Human pineal physiology and functional significance of melatonin. Front Neuroendocrinol 2004; **25**:177–195.
3. Medicines and Healthcare Products Regulatory Agency. Restrictions on the import of unlicensed Melatonin products following the grant of a marketing authorisation for Circadin® 2 mg tablets. London: MHRA; 2008. http://www.mhra.gov.uk
4. Arendt J et al. Melatonin and its agonists: an update. Br J Psychiatry 2008; **193**:267–269.
5. Buscemi N et al. The efficacy and safety of exogenous melatonin for primary sleep disorders. A meta-analysis. J Gen Intern Med 2005; **20**:1151–1158.
6. Buscemi N et al. Efficacy and safety of exogenous melatonin for secondary sleep disorders and sleep disorders accompanying sleep restriction: meta-analysis. BMJ 2006; **332**:385–393.
7. Van der Heijden KB et al. Effect of melatonin on sleep, behavior, and cognition in ADHD and chronic sleep-onset insomnia. J Am Acad Child Adolesc Psychiatry 2007; **46**:233–241.
8. Wasdell MB et al. A randomized, placebo-controlled trial of controlled release melatonin treatment of delayed sleep phase syndrome and impaired sleep maintenance in children with neurodevelopmental disabilities. J Pineal Res 2008; **44**:57–64.
9. Braam W et al. Melatonin treatment in individuals with intellectual disability and chronic insomnia: a randomized placebo-controlled study. J Intellect Disabil Res 2008; **52**:256–264.
10. Gupta M et al. Add-on melatonin improves sleep behavior in children with epilepsy: randomized, double-blind, placebo-controlled trial. J Child Neurol 2005; **20**:112–115.
11. Coppola G et al. Melatonin in wake-sleep disorders in children, adolescents and young adults with mental retardation with or without epilepsy: a double-blind, cross-over, placebo-controlled trial. Brain Dev 2004; **26**:373–376.
12. Weiss MD et al. Sleep hygiene and melatonin treatment for children and adolescents with ADHD and initial insomnia. J Am Acad Child Adolesc Psychiatry 2006; **45**:512–519.
13. Garstang J et al. Randomized controlled trial of melatonin for children with autistic spectrum disorders and sleep problems. Child Care Health Dev 2006; **32**:585–589.
14. Gringras P et al. Melatonin for sleep problems in children with neurodevelopmental disorders: randomised double masked placebo controlled trial. BMJ 2012; **345**:e6664.
15. Cortesi F et al. Controlled-release melatonin, singly and combined with cognitive behavioural therapy, for persistent insomnia in children with autism spectrum disorders: a randomized placebo-controlled trial. J Sleep Res 2012; **21**:700–709.
16. Sheldon SH. Pro-convulsant effects of oral melatonin in neurologically disabled children. Lancet 1998; **351**:1254.
17. Maestroni GJ. The immunoneuroendocrine role of melatonin. J Pineal Res 1993; **14**:1–10.
18. Sutherland ER et al. Elevated serum melatonin is associated with the nocturnal worsening of asthma. J Allergy Clin Immunol 2003; **112**:513–517.
19. Chase JE et al. Melatonin: therapeutic use in sleep disorders. Ann Pharmacother 1997; **31**:1218–1226.
20. Jan JE et al. Melatonin treatment of sleep-wake cycle disorders in children and adolescents. Dev Med Child Neurol 1999; **41**:491–500.
21. Sack RL et al. Sleep-promoting effects of melatonin: at what dose, in whom, under what conditions, and by what mechanisms? Sleep 1997; **20**:908–915.

Rapid tranquillisation in children and adolescents

As in adults, a comprehensive mental state assessment and appropriately implemented treatment plan along with staff skilled in the use of de-escalation techniques and appropriate placement of the patient are key to minimising the need for enforced parenteral medication.

Healthcare professionals undertaking rapid tranquillisation (RT) and/or restraint in children and adolescents should be trained and competent in undertaking these procedures in this population, and should be clear about the legal context for any restrictive practices they employ. Be particularly cautious when considering high-potency antipsychotic medication (such as haloperidol) especially in those who have not taken antipsychotic medication before, because of the increased risk of acute dystonic reactions in this age group.[1]

A wide dose range is given here for medication used in RT. Caution is required, especially for younger children, but in older adolescents consider the use of adult doses, especially in those who are not drug naïve and where doses in the lower end of the quoted dose range have proved ineffective.

Oral medication should always be offered (and repeated if necessary if the young person is willing to take it), before resorting to parenteral treatment (see Table 5.7). Monitoring after RT is the same as in adults (see section on 'Acutely disturbed or violent behaviour' in Chapter 7).

Table 5.7 Recommended drugs for rapid tranquillsation if the oral route is refused or has proven ineffective

Medication	Dose	Onset of action	Comment
Olanzapine IM[2,3]	2.5–10 mg	15–30 minutes	Possibly increased risk of respiratory depression when administered with benzodiazepines, particularly if alcohol has been consumed. Separate administration by at least one hour
Haloperidol IM[4]	<12 years: 0.025–0.075 mg/kg/dose (max 2.5 mg) IM Adolescents > 12 years can receive the adult dose (2.5–5 mg)	20–30 minutes	Must have parenteral anticholinergics present in case of laryngeal spasm (young people more vulnerable to severe dystonia) Adult data suggest co-administration of promethazine may reduce EPS risk[5] **ECG essential**
Lorazepam* IM[6,7]	<12 years: 0.5–1 mg >12 years: 0.5–2 mg	20–40 minutes	Slower onset of action than midazolam Flumazenil is the reversing agent for all benzodiazepines
Midazolam* IM, IV or buccal[7,8]	0.1–0.15 mg/kg (IM) Buccal midazolam 300 µg/kg or 6–10 years = 7.5 mg >10 years = 10 mg	10–20 minutes IM (1–3 minutes IV)	Quicker onset and shorter duration of action than lorazepam or diazepam IV administration should only be used (usually as a last resort) with extreme caution and where resuscitation facilities are available Shorter onset and duration of action than haloperidol When given as buccal liquid, onset of action is 15–30 minutes.[9] Some published data in mental health but only in adults.[10] Buccal liquid is unlicensed for this use
Diazepam* IV (not for IM administration)[11]	0.1 mg/kg/dose by slow IV injection. Max 40 mg total daily dose for <12 years and 60 mg for >12 years	1–3 minutes	Long half-life that does not correlate with length of sedation. Possibility of accumulation **Never give as IM injection**
Ziprasidone IM[12–15] (not UK)	10–20 mg	15–30 minutes IM	Apparently effective. QT prolongation is of concern in this patient group **ECG essential**
Aripiprazole IM[16,17]	9.75 mg	15–30 minutes	Evidence of effectiveness in adults but no data for children and adolescents
Promethazine IM	<12 years: 5–25 mg (max 50 mg/day) >12 years: 25–50 mg (max 100 mg/day)	Up to 60 minutes	An effective sedative, although has a slow onset of action. Useful if the cause of behavioural disturbance is unknown and there is concern about the use of antipsychotic medication in a child or young person

*Note that young people are particularly vulnerable to disinhibitory reactions with benzodiazepines.
ECG, electrocardiogram; EPS, extrapyramidal side-effects; IM, intramuscular; IV, intravenous.

References

1. National Institute for Health and Care Excellence. Psychosis and schizophrenia in children and young people: Recognition and management. Clinical Guideline **15**, 2013. http://www.nice.org/

2. Breier A et al. A double-blind, placebo-controlled dose-response comparison of intramuscular olanzapine and haloperidol in the treatment of acute agitation in schizophrenia. Arch Gen Psychiatry 2002; **59**:441–448.

3. Lindborg SR et al. Effects of intramuscular olanzapine vs. haloperidol and placebo on QTc intervals in acutely agitated patients. Psychiatry Res 2003; **119**:113–123.

4. Powney MJ et al. Haloperidol for psychosis-induced aggression or agitation (rapid tranquillisation). Cochrane Database Syst Rev 2012; **11**: CD009377.

5. TREC Collaborative Group. Rapid tranquillisation for agitated patients in emergency psychiatric rooms: a randomised trial of midazolam versus haloperidol plus promethazine. BMJ 2003; **327**:708–713.

6. Sorrentino A. Chemical restraints for the agitated, violent, or psychotic pediatric patient in the emergency department: controversies and recommendations. Curr Opin Pediatr 2004; **16**:201–205.

7. Nobay F et al. A prospective, double-blind, randomized trial of midazolam versus haloperidol versus lorazepam in the chemical restraint of violent and severely agitated patients. Acad Emerg Med 2004; **11**:744–749.

8. Kennedy RM et al. The "ouchless emergency department". Getting closer: advances in decreasing distress during painful procedures in the emergency department. Pediatr Clin North Am 1999; **46**:1215–1247.

9. Schwagmeier R et al. Midazolam pharmacokinetics following intravenous and buccal administration. Br J Clin Pharmacol 1998; **46**:203–206.

10. Taylor D et al. Buccal midazolam for agitation on psychiatric intensive care wards. Int J Psychiatry Clin Pract 2008; **12**:309–311.

11. Nunn K, Dey C. Medication Table. In: Nunn K, Dey C, eds. *The Clinician's Guide to Psychotropic Prescribing in Children and Adolescents.* Sydney: Glade Publishing; 2003, pp. 383–452.

12. Khan SS et al. A naturalistic evaluation of intramuscular ziprasidone versus intramuscular olanzapine for the management of acute agitation and aggression in children and adolescents. J Child Adolesc Psychopharmacol 2006; **16**:671–677.

13. Staller JA. Intramuscular ziprasidone in youth: a retrospective chart review. J Child Adolesc Psychopharmacol 2004; **14**:590–592.

14. Hazaray E et al. Intramuscular ziprasidone for acute agitation in adolescents. J Child Adolesc Psychopharmacol 2004; **14**:464–470.

15. Barzman DH et al. A retrospective chart review of intramuscular ziprasidone for agitation in children and adolescents on psychiatric units: prospective studies are needed. J Child Adolesc Psychopharmacol 2007; **17**:503–509.

16. Sanford M et al. Intramuscular aripiprazole: a review of its use in the management of agitation in schizophrenia and bipolar I disorder. CNS Drugs 2008; **22**:335–352.

17. National Institute for Health and Clinical Excellence. Aripiprazole for schizophrenia in people aged 15 to 17 years. Technology Appraisal **13**, 2011. http://guidance.nice.org.uk/TA213

Doses of commonly used psychotropic drugs in children and adolescents

See Table 5.8 for doses of commonly used psychotropic drugs in children and adolescents.

Table 5.8 Starting doses of commonly used psychotropic drugs in children and adolescents

Drug	Dose	Comment
Antipsychotics		
Aripiprazole	2 mg daily	Increase to 5–15 mg daily according to response
Clozapine	6.25–12.5 mg	Use plasma levels to determine maintenance dose
Haloperidol	0.5–1.0 mg daily	Little evidence for benefit of doses >4 mg a day in any condition
Olanzapine	2.5–5 mg	Use plasma levels to determine maintenance dose
Quetiapine	25 mg	Effective dose usually in the range 150–200 mg daily
Risperidone	0.25–2 mg	Adjust dose according to response and adverse effects
Antidepressants		
Amitriptyline	5–10 mg at night	Effective dose in neuropathic pain and nocturnal enuresis 10–50 mg at night
Escitalopram	5 mg	Effective dose 10–20 mg
Fluoxetine	5–10 mg/day	Adjust dose according to response and adverse effects
Sertraline	25–50 mg	Effective dose 50–100 mg, sometimes higher
Mood stabilisers		
Carbamazepine	5 mg/kg/day in divided doses	Use plasma levels to determine maintenance dose
Lithium	100–200 mg/day lithium carbonate	Use plasma levels to determine maintenance dose
Valproate	10–20 mg/kg/day in divided doses	Use plasma levels to determine maintenance dose

Suggested approximate oral starting doses (see primary literature for doses in individual indications). Lower dose in suggested range is for children weighing less than 25 kg.

Chapter 6

Substance misuse

Introduction

Mental and behavioural problems due to psychoactive substance use are common. The World Health Organization (WHO) in the International Classification of Diseases 10 (ICD-10)[1] identifies acute intoxication, harmful use, dependence syndrome, withdrawal state, withdrawal state with delirium, psychotic disorder, amnesic syndrome, residual and late onset psychotic disorder, other mental and behavioural disorders and unspecified mental and behavioural disorders as substance related disorders. A wide range of psychoactive substances may be problematic including alcohol, opioids, cannabinoids, sedatives, stimulants, hallucinogens, tobacco, volatile substances and so called 'legal highs'.

Substance misuse is commonly seen in people with severe mental illness (so-called dual diagnosis) and personality disorder. In many adult psychiatry settings, dual diagnosis is the norm rather than the exception. In contrast, substance misuse services are often commissioned and provided separately from psychiatric services. The model of care in most addiction services means that patients who are not motivated to engage will not be assertively treated and followed up. Dual diagnosis teams are not universally available resulting in sub-optimal treatment for substance misuse related problems for many patients with mental illness.

According to ICD-10, dependence syndrome is 'a cluster of physiological, behavioural, and cognitive phenomena in which the use of a substance or a class of substances takes on a much higher priority for a given individual than other behaviours that once had greater value'. A definite diagnosis of dependence should only be made if at least three of the following have been present togther in the last year:

- compulsion to take substance
- difficulties controlling substance-taking behaviour
- physiological withdrawal state
- evidence of tolerance

The Maudsley Prescribing Guidelines in Psychiatry, Twelfth Edition. David Taylor, Carol Paton and Shitij Kapur.

- neglect of alternative interests
- persistant use despite harm.

Substance use disorders should generally be treated with a combination of psychosocial and pharmacological interventions. This chapter will concentrate on pharmacological interventions for alcohol, opioids and nicotine use. Cocaine, other stimulants and benzodiazepine use will be discussed briefly. Note that various National Institute for Health and Care Excellence (NICE) Guidelines and Technology Appraisals (see relevant sections in this chapter), Department of Health Substance Misuse Guidelines,[2] and National Treatment Agency for Substance Misuse guidance[3] also provide a comprehensive overview of treatment approaches, as does the most recent British Association for Psychopharmacology consensus guideline.[4]

References

1. World Health Organisation. International Statistical Classification of Diseases and Related Health Problems. 10th revision version for 2007. Geneva: WHO; 2007. http://www.who.int/

2. Department of Health. Drug misuse and dependence. UK guidelines on clinical management. London: DH; 2007.

3. Day E. National Treatment Agency for Substance Misuse. Opiate detoxification in an inpatient setting. London: NTA, 2005. http://www.nta.nhs.uk/

4. Lingford-Hughes AR et al. Evidence-based guidelines for the pharmacological management of substance abuse, harmful use, addiction and comorbidity: recommendations from BAP. J Psychopharmacol 2012; 26:899–952.

CHAPTER 6

Alcohol dependence

What is a unit of alcohol?

One unit = 10 mL of ethanol or 1L of 1% alcohol. For example, 250 mL of wine that is 10% alcohol contains 2.5 units.

How much alcohol is too much?

NICE public health guideline on preventing harmful drinking cites the following weekly limits (in units):[2]

	Men	Women
Low risk (responsible drinking)	Up to 21	Up to 14
Increasing risk	22–50	15–35
High risk	>50	>35

The NICE guideline on the diagnosis, assessment and management of harmful drinking and alcohol dependence recommends that staff working in services providing care for problem drinkers should be competent in identifying and assessing harmful drinking and alcohol dependence.[1] The NICE public health guideline on reducing harmful drinking[2] recommends a session of brief structured advice based on FRAMES principles (Feedback, Responsibility, Advice, Menu, Empathy, Self-efficacy) as a useful intervention for everyone at increasing or high-risk of alcohol related problems.

Assessing alcohol use

Where consumption above recommended levels has been identified, a more detailed clinical assessment is required. This should include the following:

- history of alcohol use, including daily consumption and recent patterns of drinking
- history of previous episodes of alcohol withdrawal
- time of most recent drink
- history from family member or carer
- other drug (illicit and prescribed) use
- severity of dependence and of withdrawal symptoms
- co-existing medical and psychiatric problems
- physical examination including cognitive function
- breathalyser: absolute breath alcohol level and whether rising or falling (take at least 20 minutes after last drink to avoid falsely high readings from the mouth and 1 hour later)
- laboratory investigations: FBC, U&E, LFTs, INR, PT and urinary drug screen.

The following structured assessment tools are recommended.[1]

- The **Alcohol Use Disorders Identification Test (AUDIT)**[3] questionnaire, a 10-item questionnaire which is useful as a screening tool in those identified as being at increasing risk. Questions 1–3 address the quantity of alcohol consumed, 4–6 the signs and symptoms of dependence and 7–10 the behaviours and symptoms associated with harmful alcohol use. Each question is scored 0–4, giving a maximum total score of 40. A score of 8 or more is suggestive of hazardous or harmful alcohol use. Hazardous drinking = consumption of alcohol likely to cause harm. Harmful drinking = consumption already causing mental or physical health problems.
- The **Severity of Alcohol Dependence Questionnaire (SADQ)**[4] is a more detailed 20-item questionnaire with the score on each item ranging from 0–3, giving a maximum total score of 60.

Severity of alcohol dependence

Mild = SADQ score of 15 or less
Moderate = SADQ score 15–30
Severe = SADQ score >30

Alcohol withdrawal

In alcohol-dependent drinkers, the central nervous system has adjusted to the constant presence of alcohol in the body (neuro-adaptation). When the blood alcohol concentration (BAC) is suddenly lowered, the brain remains in a hyper-excited state, resulting in the withdrawal syndrome.

Self-limiting symptoms of withdrawal include tremor, sweating, nausea, retching, vomiting, tachycardia, agitation, headache, insomnia and malaise (essentially, a very bad hangover). Where large quantities of alcohol have been regularly consumed over a period of time (moderate-to-severe dependence), withdrawal can be associated with the development of seizures, Wernicke's encephalopathy and delirium tremens (DT), all of which are potentially life-threatening. See Table 6.1.

Table 6.1 Features of alcohol withdrawal

Manifestation of alcohol withdrawal	Usual timing of onset after the last drink	Other information
Somatic symptoms	3–12 hours	Symptoms peak at 24–48 hours, usual duration 5–14 days
Seizures*	12–18 hours	Adequate benzodiazepine cover reduces risk
Wernicke's encephalopathy*		Parenteral thiamine reduces risk
Delirium tremens*	3–4 days	Develops in 5% Mortality 10–20% if untreated

*Clinical presentation, prophylaxis and treatment are described below.

Pharmacologically assisted withdrawal (alcohol detoxification)

Alcohol withdrawal is associated with significant morbidity and mortality when improperly managed. Therefore all patients need general support and a proportion will need pharmacotherapy to modify the course of reversal of alcohol-induced neuro-adaptation.

Pharmacologically assisted withdrawal is likely to be needed when:

- regular consumption of >15 units/day
- AUDIT score >20.

Symptom scales can be helpful in determining whether the regimen prescribed is adequate, but not excessive with respect to managing symptoms. The Clinical Institute Withdrawal Assessment of Alcohol Scale, Revised (CIWA-Ar; see Figure 6.1)[5] and Short Alcohol Withdrawal Scale (SAWS; see Figure 6.2)[6] are both 10-item scales that can be completed in around 5 minutes. The CIWA-Ar is an objective scale and the SAWS is a self-complete tool. A CIWA-Ar score >15 or a SAWS score >12 should prompt assisted withdrawal.

Where assisted withdrawal is undertaken in the **community**, there should be someone at home (ideally 24 hours) who is able to monitor and supervise the withdrawal process. The treatment plan, including contingency plans, should be discussed with the patient and person who will be supporting them and shared with the GP. It is usually appropriate to arrange for medication to be picked up on a daily/alternate day basis and for the patient to be seen regularly during the assisted withdrawal process. Assisted withdrawal should stop if the patient resumes drinking. Outpatient-based programmes should include psychosocial support, such as motivational interviewing.

Most patients can be safely treated at home, however, **inpatient treatment is likely to be required in the following circumstances.**

- Regular consumption of >30 units/day.
- SADQ >30 (severe dependence).
- There is a history of seizures or DT.
- The patient is very young or elderly.
- There is current benzodiazepine use in combination with alcohol.
- Substances other than alcohol are also being misused/abused.
- There is co-morbid mental or physical illness, learning disability or cognitive impairment.
- The patient is pregnant.
- The patient is homeless or has no social support.
- There is a history of failed community detoxification(s).

Benzodiazepines are the treatment of choice for alcohol withdrawal. They exhibit cross-tolerance with alcohol and have anticonvulsant properties. Use is supported by NICE guidelines;[1,7] a Cochrane systematic review;[8] and the British Association for Psychopharmacology (BAP) guidelines.[9] **Parenteral thiamine**, and other vitamin replacement is an important adjunctive treatment for the prophylaxis and/or treatment of Wernicke–Korsakoff syndrome and other vitamin-related neuropsychiatric conditions.

Chlordiazepoxide is the benzodiazepine used for most patients in most centres as it is considered to have a relatively low dependence-forming potential. Some centres use

Patient:_____ Date: _____
Time: _____(24-h clock, midnight = 00:00)

Pulse or heart rate, taken for 1 min:_____
Blood pressure:_____

NAUSEA AND VOMITING – Ask 'Do you feel sick to your stomach? Have you vomited?' Observation.
0 no nausea and no vomiting
1 mild nausea with no vomiting
2
3
4 intermittent nausea with dry heaves
5
6
7 constant nausea, frequent dry heaves and vomiting

TACTILE DISTURBANCES – Ask 'Have you any itching, pins and needles sensations, any burning, any numbness, or do you feel bugs crawling on or under your skin?' Observation.
0 none
1 very mild itching, pins and needles, burning or numbness
2 mild itching, pins and needles, burning or numbness
3 moderate itching, pins and needles, burning or numbness
4 moderately severe hallucinations
5 severe hallucinations
6 extremely severe hallucinations
7 continuous hallucinations

TREMOR – Arms extended and fingers spread apart. Observation.
0 no tremor
1 not visible, but can be felt fingertip to fingertip
2
3
4 moderate, with patient's arms extended
5
6
7 severe, even with arms not extended

AUDITORY DISTURBANCES – Ask 'Are you more aware of sounds around you? Are they harsh? Do they frighten you? Are you hearing anything that is disturbing to you? Are you hearing things you know are not there?' Observation.
0 not present
1 very mild harshness or ability to frighten
2 mild harshness or ability to frighten
3 moderate harshness or ability to frighten
4 moderately severe hallucinations
5 severe hallucinations
6 extremely severe hallucinations
7 continuous hallucinations

PAROXYSMAL SWEATS – Observation.
0 no sweat visible
1 barely perceptible sweating, palms moist
2
3
4 beads of sweat obvious on forehead
5
6
7 drenching sweats

VISUAL DISTURBANCES – Ask 'Does the light appear to be too bright? Is its colour different? Does it hurt your eyes? Are you seeing anything that is disturbing to you? Are you seeing things you know are not there?' Observation.
0 not present
1 very mild sensitivity
2 mild sensitivity
3 moderate sensitivity
4 moderately severe hallucinations
5 severe hallucinations
6 extremely severe hallucinations
7 continuous hallucinations

ANXIETY – Ask 'Do you feel nervous?' Observation.
0 no anxiety, at ease
1 mildly anxious
2
3
4 moderately anxious, or guarded, so anxiety is inferred
5
6
7 equivalent to acute panic states as seen in severe delirium or acute schizophrenic reactions

HEADACHE, FULLNESS IN HEAD – Ask 'Does your head feel different? Does it feel like there is a band around your head?' Do not rate for dizziness or light-headedness. Otherwise, rate severity.
0 not present
1 very mild
2 mild
3 moderate
4 moderately severe
5 severe
6 very severe
7 extremely severe

AGITATION – Observation.
0 normal activity
1 somewhat more than normal activity
2
3
4 moderately fidgety and restless
5
6
7 paces back and forth during most of the interview, or constantly thrashes about

ORIENTATION AND CLOUDING OF SENSORIUM – Ask 'What day is this? Where are you? Who am I?'
0 oriented and can do serial additions
1 cannot do serial additions or is uncertain about date
2 disoriented for date by no more than 2 calendar days
3 disoriented for date by more than 2 calendar days
4 disoriented for place/or person

Scores
≤10 – mild withdrawal (does not need additional medication)
≤15 – moderate withdrawal
>15 – severe withdrawal

Total CIWA-Ar score _____
Rater's initials_____

Maximum possible score: 67

Figure 6.1 Clinical Institute Withdrawal Assessment of Alcohol Scale, Revised.[5] The CIWA-Ar is not copyrighted and may be reproduced freely.

	None (0)	Mild (1)	Moderate (2)	Severe (3)
Anxious				
Sleep disturbance				
Problems with memory				
Nausea				
Restless				
Tremor (shakes)				
Feeling confused				
Sweating				
Miserable				
Heart pounding				

Figure 6.2 Short Alcohol Withdrawal Scale (SAWS).[6] The SAWS is a self-completion questionnaire. SAWS is not copyrighted and may be reproduced freely. Symptoms cover the previous 24-hour period.

diazepam. Where hepatic impairment is clinically significant (that is, the patient is in liver failure), a short-acting benzodiazepine such as oxazepam or lorazepam is the treatment of choice.

There are three types of assisted withdrawal regimens; **fixed dose reduction** (the most common in non-specialist settings), **variable dose reduction** (usually results in less benzodiazepine being administered but best reserved for settings where staff have specialist skills in managing alcohol withdrawal), and finally **front-loading** (infrequently used).[1,9] Assisted withdrawal regimens should never be started if the blood alcohol concentration is very high or is still rising.

Fixed dose reduction regimen
Fixed dose regimens are recommended for use in community or non-specialist inpatient/ residential settings. Patients should be started on a dose of benzodiazepine, selected after an assessment of the severity of alcohol dependence (clinical history, number of units per drinking day and score on the SADQ). With respect to chlordiazepoxide, a

Table 6.2 Moderate alcohol dependence: example of a fixed dose chlordiazepoxide treatment regimen

Time	Dose	Total daily dose (mg)
Day 1	20 mg qds	80
Day 2	15 mg qds	60
Day 3	10 mg qds	40
Day 4	5 mg qds	20
Day 5	5 mg bd	10

bd, *bis die* (twice a day); qds, *quarter die sumendum* (four times a day).

general rule of thumb is that the starting dose can be estimated from current alcohol consumption. For example, if 20 units/day are being consumed, the starting dose should be 20 mg four times a day. The dose is then tapered to zero over 5–10 days. Alcohol withdrawal symptoms should be monitored using a validated instrument such as the CIWA-Ar[5] or SAWS.[6]

Mild alcohol dependence usually requires very small doses of chlordiazepoxide or else may be managed without medication.

For **moderate** alcohol dependence, a typical regime might be 10–20 mg chlordiazepoxide four times a day, reducing gradually over 5–7 days (see Table 6.2). Note that 5–7 days' treatment is adequate and longer treatment is rarely helpful or necessary. It is advisable to monitor withdrawal and BAC daily prior to providing the days medication. This may mean that community pharmacologically assisted alcohol withdrawals should start on a Monday to last 5 days.

Severe alcohol dependence will often require specialist/inpatient treatment. Intensive daily monitoring is advised for the first 2–3 days. This may require special arrangements over a weekend. Prescribing should not start if the patient is heavily intoxicated, and in such circumstances they should be advised to return when not intoxicated, at an early opportunity. The dose of benzodiazepine may need to be reduced over a 7–10 day period in this group (occasionally longer if dependence is very severe or there is a history of complications during previous detoxifications) (see Table 6.3).

Symptom-triggered regimen

This should be reserved for managing assisted withdrawal in specialist alcohol inpatient or residential settings. Regular monitoring (pulse, blood pressure [BP], temperature, level of consciousness, severity of withdrawal symptoms as determined using CIWA-Ar, SAWS or alternative validated measure) is required and medication is given only when withdrawal symptoms are observed. Symptom-triggered therapy is generally used in patients without a history of complications. A typical symptom-triggered regimen would be chlordiazepoxide 20–30 mg hourly as needed. Note that the total dose given each day would be expected to decrease from day 2 onwards. It is common for symptom-triggered treatment to last only 24–48 hours before switching to an individualised

Table 6.3 Severe alcohol dependence: example of a fixed dose chlordiazepoxide regimen

Time	Dose	Total daily dose (mg)
Day 1 (first 24 hours)	40 mg qds + 40 mg prn	200
Day 2	40 mg qds	160
Day 3	30 mg qds	120
Day 4	25 mg qds	100
Day 5	20 mg qds	80
Day 6	15 mg qds	60
Day 7	10 mg qds	40
Day 8	10 mg tds	30
Day 9	5 mg qds	20
Day 10	10 mg nocte	10

bd, *bis die* (twice a day); nocte, at night; prn, *pro re nata* (as required); qds, *quarter die sumendum* (four times a day); tds, *ter die sumendum* (three times a day).

fixed dose reducing schedule. Occasionally (e.g. in DT) the flexible regime may need to be prolonged beyond the first 24 hours.

Front-loading regimens

Front loading regimens involve giving an initial loading dose of medication, e.g. chlordiazepoxide 100 mg, followed by further doses of between 50 and 100 mg approximately every 4–6 hours until light sedation is achieved. The patient is monitored every 2 hours (or more frequently) with basic observations and a withdrawal scale. The long half-life of chlordiazepoxide ensures that withdrawal symptoms are alleviated. Front loading is contraindicated in advanced liver disease, chronic obstructive pulmonary disease or following a head injury. It should be reserved for use in well-monitored inpatient settings.

Whichever regimen is used, a CIWA-Ar score >15 or a SAWS score >12 during assisted withdrawal suggest that the regimen prescribed is inadequate and further intervention is required. If a patient suffers hallucinations or agitation, an increased dose of benzo-diazepine should be administered, according to clinical judgement.

Those with **liver cirrhosis and/or functional liver impairment** (see section on 'Hepatic impairment' in Chapter 7) should receive a shorter acting benzodiazepine such as oxazepam.[7] Some patients may need, and be able to tolerate, relatively high starting doses, e.g. 40 mg qds whereas others may only be able to tolerate lower doses. A withdrawal scale should be used as a marker of optimal dosing. It is important to note that the risk of alcohol withdrawal seizures may be higher with oxazepam although this is more of a clinical impression than proven fact. Oxazepam is also a useful option in patients with chronic respiratory disease (note that the majority of dependent drinkers are smokers). Chlordiazepoxide and oxazepam have broadly similar potencies (10 mg ≈ 10 mg)

Complications associated with alcohol withdrawal

Seizures

Alcohol withdrawal can precipitate seizures, but note that those who have a seizure for the first time during assisted withdrawal should be investigated to rule out organic disease or idiopathic epilepsy. A meta-analysis of trials assessing the efficacy of drugs preventing alcohol withdrawal seizures demonstrated that benzodiazepines, particularly long-acting preparations such as diazepam, significantly reduced seizures *de novo*;[10] longer-acting benzodiazepines are therefore recommended for medically assisted withdrawal in those with a previous history of seizures.[11] Some anticonvulsants are as effective as benzodiazepines in preventing seizures[10] and some units recommend carbamazepine loading in patients with untreated epilepsy, those with a history of more than two seizures during previous withdrawal episodes, or those who have experienced previous seizures despite adequate benzodiazepine loading. Note that phenytoin does not prevent alcohol-withdrawal seizures.[9] There is no need to continue an anticonvulsant long-term if it has been used to treat an alcohol-withdrawal related seizure.[9]

Hallucinations

Mild perceptual disturbances usually respond to chlordiazepoxide. However, those that do not can be treated with oral haloperidol.[12] Haloperidol may also be given intramuscularly or (very rarely) intravenously if necessary (but BP should be monitored for hypotension and electrocardiogram [ECG] for QT prolongation). Caution is needed because haloperidol can reduce the seizure threshold. It is also associated with acute dystonic reactions.

Delirium tremens

Delirium tremens is a toxic confusional state that occurs when alcohol withdrawal symptoms are severe. Risk factors include a long history of dependence or severe dependence, multiple previous admissions/assisted withdrawals, older age and a history of DT or alcohol-related seizures. DT is often associated with medical illness and are life-threatening. The classic triad of symptoms includes clouding of consciousness/confusion, vivid hallucinations affecting every sensory modality, and marked tremor. Clinical features also include paranoid delusions, agitation, sleeplessness and autonomic hyperactivity (tachycardia, hypertension, sweating and fever). Symptoms of DT typically peak between 72–96 hours after the last drink. Prodromal symptoms usually include night-time insomnia, restlessness, fear and confusion. Treatment of DT requires early diagnosis and prompt transfer to a general medical setting where intravenous diazepam can be given, medical disorders treated, fluids and electrolytes replaced, and thiamine and other vitamins administered intravenously.

Wernicke's encephalopathy

Wernicke's encephalopathy is a progressive neurological condition caused by thiamine deficiency. It can occur in any condition associated with poor nutrition; those who consume large quantities of alcohol tend to be malnourished secondary to a restricted diet and alcohol-related reduced absorption of thiamine.

Thiamine

Low-risk drinkers without neuropsychiatric complications and with an adequate diet should be offered oral thiamine: a minimum of 300 mg daily during assisted alcohol withdrawal and periods of continued alcohol intake.[9]

Thiamine is required to utilise glucose. A glucose load in a thiamine-deficient patient can precipitate Wernicke's encephalopathy.

It is advised that parenteral B-complex (Pabrinex) must be administered *before glucose is* administered in all patients presenting with altered mental status.

The 'classical' symptom triad of ophthalmoplegia, ataxia and confusion is rarely present in Wernicke's encephalopathy, and the syndrome is more common than is widely believed. A presumptive diagnosis of Wernicke's encephalopathy should therefore be made in any patient undergoing detoxification who experiences any of the following signs: ataxia, hypothermia, hypotension, confusion, ophthalmoplegia/nystagmus, memory disturbance and unconsciousness/coma. Any history of malnutrition, recent weight loss, vomiting or diarrhoea or peripheral neuropathy should also be noted.[13] Individuals at high risk of developing Wernicke's encephalopathy[7] include dependent drinkers in acute withdrawal who are malnourished or at risk of malnourishment or have decompensated liver disease and, in addition, attend the emergency department or are admitted to hospital with acute illness or injury, are homeless or are hospitalised for co-morbidity.

It is generally advised that patients undergoing inpatient detoxification should be given parenteral thiamine as **prophylaxis**[1,7,9,14,15] although there is insufficient evidence from randomised controlled trials (RCTs) as to the best dose, frequency or duration of use. Guidance is based on 'expert opinion'[9] and the standard advice is **one pair of Pabrinex IMHP daily** (containing thiamine 250 mg/dose) for 5 days, followed by oral thiamine and/or vitamin B compound for as long as needed (where diet is inadequate or alcohol consumption is resumed).[9] All inpatients should receive this regime as an absolute minimum.

Intramuscular (IM) thiamine preparations have a lower incidence of anaphylactic reactions than IV preparations, at 1 per 5 million pairs of ampoules of Pabrinex - far lower than many frequently used drugs that carry no special anaphylaxis warning. However, this risk has resulted in fears about using parenteral preparations and the inappropriate use of oral thiamine preparations (which do not offer adequate protection). Given the risks associated with Wernicke's encephalopathy, the benefit to risk ratio grossly favours parenteral thiamine.[9,14,16] Where parenteral thiamine is used, facilities for treating anaphylaxis should be available.[17–19]

If Wernicke's encephalopathy is suspected the patient should be transferred to a medical unit where intravenous thiamine can be administered. If untreated, Wernicke's encephalopathy progresses to Korsakoff's syndrome (permanent memory impairment, confabulation, confusion and personality changes).

Treatment for patients with suspected/established Wernicke's encephalopathy (acute medical ward) is at least 2 pairs of Pabrinex IVHP (i.e. 4 ampoules) three times daily for 3–5 days, followed by one pair of ampoules once daily for a further 3–5 days or longer[1,9] (until no further response is seen).

CHAPTER 6

Table 6.4 Alcohol withdrawal treatment interventions: summary

Severity	Supportive/ medical care	Pharmacotherapy for neuro-adaptation reversal	Thiamine supplementation	Setting
Mild CIWA-Ar ≤10	Moderate-to-high level supportive care, little, if any medical care required	Little to none required Simple remedies only (see below)	Oral likely to be sufficient if patient is well nourished	Home
Moderate CIWA-Ar ≤15	Moderate-to-high level supportive care, little medical care required	Little to none required Symptomatic treatment only	Pabrinex IMHP if the patient is malnourished followed by oral supplementation	Home or community team
Severe CIWA-Ar >15	High level supportive care plus medical monitoring	Symptomatic and substitution treatment (chlordiazepoxide) probably required	Pabrinex IMHP followed by oral supplementation	Community team or hospital
CIWA-Ar >10 plus co-morbid alcohol- related medical problems	High level supportive care plus specialist medical care	Symptomatic and substitution treatments usually required	Pabrinex IMHP followed by oral supplementation	Hospital

CIWA-Ar, Clinical Institute Withdrawal Assessment of Alcohol Scale, revised; IMHP, intramuscular high potency.

Table 6.5 Simple remedies for somatic complaints during assisted alcohol withdrawal

Symptom	Recommended treatment
Dehydration	Ensure adequate fluid intake in order to maintain hydration and electrolyte balance. Dehydration can precipitate life-threatening cardiac arrhythmia
Pain	Paracetamol
Nausea and vomiting	Metoclopramide 10 mg or prochlorperazine 5 mg 4–6 hourly
Diarrhoea	Diphenoxylate and atropine (Lomotil) or loperamide
Skin itching	Occurs commonly and not only in individuals with alcoholic liver disease: antihistamines

Alcohol withdrawal treatment interventions are summarised in Table 6.4.

Somatic complaints are common during assisted withdrawal. Some simple remedies are shown in Table 6.5.

Relapse prevention

There is no place for the continued use of benzodiazepines beyond treatment of the acute alcohol withdrawal syndrome. Acamprosate and supervised disulfiram are licensed for treatment of alcohol dependence in the UK and should be offered in combination with psychosocial treatment.[1] Treatment should be initiated by a specialist service. After 12 weeks, transfer of the prescribing to the GP may be appropriate, although specialist care may continue (shared care). Naltrexone is also recommended as an adjunct in the treatment of moderate and severe alcohol dependence.[1] As it does not have marketing authorisation for the treatment of alcohol dependence in the UK, informed consent should be sought and documented prior to commencing treatment.

Acamprosate

Acamprosate is a synthetic taurine analogue which acts as a functional glutamatergic NMDA antagonist and also increases GABA-ergic function. The 'number needed to treat' (NNT) for the maintenance of abstinence has been calculated as 9–11.[9] The treatment effect is most pronounced at 6 months, although it remains significant for up to 12 months.[1] Acamprosate should be initiated as soon as possible after abstinence has been achieved (the BAP consensus guidelines[9] recommend that acamprosate should be started 'during detoxification' because of its potential neuroprotective effect). NICE recommends that acamprosate should be continued for up to 6 months, with regular (monthly) supervision. The summary of product characteristics (SPC) recommends that it is given for one year.

Acamprosate is relatively well tolerated; side-effects include diarrhoea, abdominal pain, nausea, vomiting and pruritis.[1] It is contraindicated in severe renal or hepatic impairment, thus baseline liver and kidney function tests should be performed before commencing treatment. Acamprosate should be avoided in individuals who are pregnant or breast feeding. See Box 6.1.

Box 6.1 Acamprosate: NICE Clinical Guideline 115, 2011[1]

Acamprosate should be offered for relapse prevention in moderately to severely dependent drinkers, in combination with psychosocial treatment. It should be prescribed for up to 6 months, or longer for those who perceive benefit and wish to continue taking it. The dose is 1998 mg daily (666 mg three times per day) for individuals over 60 kg. For those under 60 kg, the dose is 1332 mg daily. Treatment should be stopped in those who continue to drink for 4–6 weeks after starting the drug.

Naltrexone

Opioid receptor blockade prevents increased dopaminergic activity after the consumption of alcohol, thus reducing its rewarding effects. Naltrexone, a non-selective opioid receptor antagonist significantly reduces relapse to heavy drinking but does not necessarily improve continuous abstinence rates.[1] Although early trials used a dose of 50 mg/day, more recent US studies have used 100 mg/day. In the UK the usual dose is 50 mg/day.

Naltrexone is well tolerated but side-effects include nausea (especially in the early stages of treatment), headache, abdominal pain, reduced appetite and tiredness. A comprehensive medical assessment should be carried out prior to commencing naltrexone, together with baseline renal and liver function tests. Naltrexone can be started when patients are still drinking or during medically-assisted withdrawal. There is no clear evidence as to the optimal duration of treatment but 6 months appears to be an appropriate period.[9] See Box 6.2.

Patients on naltrexone should not be given opioid agonist drugs for analgesia: non-opioid analgesics should be used instead. In the event that opioid analgesia is necessary, it can be instituted 48–72 hours after cessation of naltrexone. Hepatotoxicity has been described with high doses, so use should be avoided in acute liver failure.

Injectable naltrexone has been developed to improve poor compliance and side-effects are similar to those seen with the oral preparation.[20] NICE concluded that the initial evidence was encouraging but not enough to support routine use.

Box 6.2 Naltrexone: NICE Clinical Guideline 115, 2011[1]

Naltrexone (50 mg/day) should be offered for relapse prevention in moderately to severely dependent drinkers, in combination with psychosocial treatment. It should be prescribed for up to 6 months, or longer for those who perceive benefit and wish to continue taking it. Treatment should be stopped in those who continue to drink for 4–6 weeks after starting the drug or in those who feel unwell while taking it.

Nalmefene

Nalmefene is also an opioid antagonist. It effectively reduces heavy drinking days but does not promote abstinence.[21–23] There is limited and inconclusive evidence that it has a role in relapse prevention.

Disulfiram (Antabuse)

The evidence for disulfiram is weaker than for acamprosate and naltrexone.[1] NICE recommends its use 'as a second-line option for moderate-to-severe alcohol dependence for patients who are not suitable for acamprosate or naltrexone or have a specified preference for disulfiram and who **aim to stay abstinent from alcohol**'.[1] See Box 6.3. As with acamprosate and naltrexone it should be prescribed as part of a comprehensive treatment programme. 'Witnessing' (supervision) optimises compliance and contributes to effectiveness. Disulfiram inhibits aldehyde dehydrogenase, thus leading to acetaldehyde accumulation after drinking alcohol, which can cause extremely unpleasant physical effects. Continued drinking can lead to arrhythmias, hypotension and collapse. Despite being available for many years, the number of controlled clinical trials is limited.

Because of the known adverse effects of disulfiram the clinician must ensure that no alcohol has been consumed for at least 24 hours before commencing treatment. Contraindications to use include cardiac failure, coronary artery disease, hypertension, history of cerebrovascular disease, pregnancy and breast feeding, liver disease, peripheral neuropathy and severe mental illness. Urea and electrolytes and liver function tests should be carried out before starting disulfiram to rule out renal and liver impairment.

Doses as stated in the *BNF* are 800 mg for the first dose, reducing to 100–200mg daily for maintenance. It is sometimes given in higher doses. In co-morbid alcohol and

> **Box 6.3** Disulfiram: NICE Clinical Guideline 115, 2011[1]
>
> Disulfiram should be considered in combination with a psychological intervention for service users who wish to achieve abstinence, but for whom acamprosate or naltrexone are not suitable. Treatment should be started at least 24 hours after the last drink and should be overseen by a family member or carer. Monitoring is recommended every 2 weeks for the first 2 months, then monthly for the following 4 months. Medical monitoring should be continued at 6 monthly intervals after the first 6 months. Patients must not consume alcohol while taking disulfiram.

cocaine dependence doses of 500 mg daily have been given. Halitosis is a common side effect. If there is a sudden onset of jaundice (the rare complication of hepatotoxicity), the patient should stop the drug and seek urgent medical attention.

Baclofen

Baclofen is a GABA-β agonist that does not have a licence for use in alcohol dependence but is nevertheless used by some clinicians. It may have a role in reducing anxiety in severely dependent patients. It is well tolerated and can be given to alcohol dependent patients with liver cirrhosis. Studies have used a 10 mg tds dose, but a 20 mg tds dose may have superior outcomes.[24]

Anticonvulsants

Topiramate is not licensed for use in alcohol dependence, but has been show in RCTs to reduce the percentage of heavy drinking days and improve the harmful consequences of drinking, physical health and quality of life.[25] The dose is 25 mg daily, increasing to 300 mg daily. Its use is likely to be limited by its troublesome side-effect profile (parasthesiae, dizziness, taste perversion, anorexia and weight loss, difficulties with memory and concentration).

Gabapentin[26] and pregabalin[27] have been shown to have some efficacy in alcohol withdrawal and in reducing drinking, but the evidence is limited (although promising).

Pregnancy and alcohol use

Evidence indicates that alcohol consumption during pregnancy may cause harm to the foetus. NICE advises that women should not drink any alcohol at all during pregnancy.[28] If abstinence is not tolerable, NICE advises that alcohol should be avoided in the first 3 months of pregnancy, and consumption limited to '1–2 units once or twice a week' for the rest of the pregnancy.

For alcohol-dependent pregnant women who have withdrawal symptoms, pharmacological cover for detoxification should be offered, ideally in an inpatient setting. The timing of detoxification in relation to the trimester of pregnancy should be risk-assessed against continued alcohol consumption and risks to the foetus.[9] Chlordiazepoxide has been suggested as being unlikely to pose a substantial risk, however dose-dependent

CHAPTER 6

malformations have been observed.[9] The Regional Drugs and Therapeutics Centre Teratology Service[29] provides national advice for healthcare professionals and like to follow up on pregnancies that require alcohol detoxification. Please refer to the references below. Specialist advice should always be sought. (See also section on 'Pregnancy' in Chapter 7). No relapse prevention medication has been evaluated in pregnancy.[9]

Children and adolescents

Children and young people (10–17 years) should be assessed as outlined in the NICE Clinical Guideline 115, 2011.

The number of young people who are dependent and needing pharmacotherapy is likely to be small, but for those who are dependent there should be a lower threshold for admission to hospital. Doses of chlordiazepoxide for medically assisted withdrawal may need to be adjusted to lower levels, but the general principles of withdrawal management are the same as for adults. All young people should have a full health screen carried out routinely to allow identification of physical and mental health problems. The evidence base for acamprosate, naltrexone and disulfiram in 16–19 year olds is evolving.[9]

Older adults

There should be a lower threshold for inpatient medically-assisted alcohol withdrawal for older adults.[1] While benzodiazepines remain the treatment of choice, they may need to be prescribed in lower doses and in some situations shorter acting drugs may be preferred.[9] Older adults with alcohol use disorders should all have full routine health screens to identify physical and mental health problems. The evidence base for pharmacotherapy of alcohol use disorders in older people is limited.

Concurrent alcohol and drug use disorders

Where alcohol and drug use disorders are co-morbid, treat both conditions actively.[1]

Co-existing alcohol and benzodiazepine dependence

This is best managed with one benzodiazepine, either chlordiazepoxide or diazepam. The starting dose should take into account the requirements for medically-assisted alcohol withdrawal and the typical daily equivalent dose of the relevant benzodiazepine(s).[1] Inpatient treatment should be carried out over a 2–3 week period, possibly longer.[1]

Co-existing alcohol dependence and cocaine use

In co-morbid cocaine/alcohol dependence, naltrexone 150 mg/day resulted in reduced cocaine and alcohol use in men but not in women.[30]

Co-existing alcohol and opioid dependence

Both conditions should be treated, and attention paid to the increased mortality of individuals taking both drugs.

Co-morbid alcohol and nicotine dependence

Encourage individuals to stop smoking. Refer for smoking cessation in primary care and other settings. In in-patient settings offer nicotine patches/inhalator during assisted alcohol withdrawal.

Co-morbid mental health disorders

People with alcohol use disorders often present with other mental health disorders, particularly anxiety and depression. For most people these symptoms will diminish after 3–4 weeks of abstinence, so it is important to tackle the drinking problem as the first step in the treatment pathway. For some, the co-morbid disorder will have been the initial trigger to their drinking: for instance recurrent depressive disorder, bipolar affective disorder (BAD) and anxiety disorder (obsessive compulsive disorder [OCD]; social anxiety, post-traumatic stress disorder[PTSD]).

It may take time for the individual to admit to heavy drinking, so sympathetic history-taking skills and the use of questionnaires and blood tests will help to confirm any suspicions of an alcohol use disorder. Services for alcohol dependent individuals with co-morbidity are rarely integrated, so they may find themselves undergoing 'detox' on a general medical or psychiatric ward with subsequent referral to, and follow-up with, specialist addiction services for treatment of their alcohol problem and then referral to psychiatric services for treatment of their mental health problem(s). Some specialist addictions services within the NHS are able to offer psychological and pharmacological therapies for co-morbid mental health problem(s), but services contracted out to non-NHS agencies will not usually have this facility.

Depression

Depressive and anxiety symptoms occur commonly during alcohol withdrawal, but usually diminish by the third or fourth week of abstinence. Meta-analyses suggest that antidepressants with mixed pharmacology (the tricyclics imipramine or trimipramine) perform better than selective serotonin reuptake inhibitors (SSRIs; fluoxetine or sertraline) in reducing depressive symptoms in individuals with an alcohol use disorder, but the antidepressant effect is modest.[1,9] A greater antidepressant effect was seen if the diagnosis of depression was made after at least one week of abstinence, thus excluding those with affective symptoms caused by alcohol withdrawal. However, tricyclics are not recommended in clinical practice because of their potential for cardiotoxicity and toxicity in overdose. Preliminary research on newer drugs such as mirtazapine[31] or escitalopram[32] shows promise.

Relapse prevention medication should be considered in combination with antidepressants. Pettinati et al[33] have shown that the combination of sertraline (200 mg/day) with naltrexone (100 mg/day) had superior outcomes – improved drinking outcomes and better mood – than placebo and each drug alone.

Secondary analyses of acamprosate and naltrexone trials suggest that:

- acamprosate has an indirect modest beneficial effect on depression via increasing abstinence and
- in depressed alcohol dependent patients, the combination of naltrexone and an antidepressant is better than either drug alone[9]

Bipolar affective disorder

Bipolar patients tend to use alcohol to reduce symptoms of anxiety. Where there is co-morbidity it is important to treat the different phases as recommended in guidelines for bipolar disorder. It may be worth adding sodium valproate to lithium as two trials have shown that the combination was associated with better drinking outcomes than with lithium alone. However, the combination did not confer any extra benefit than lithium alone in improving mood (see BAP consensus 2012).[9] Note that, in those who continue to drink, electrolyte imbalance may precipitate lithium toxicity. Lithium is best avoided completely in binge drinkers.

Naltrexone should be offered, in the first instance, to help bipolar patients reduce their alcohol consumption.[9] If naltrexone is not effective then acamprosate should be offered. In the event that both naltrexone and acamprosate fail to promote abstinence, then disulfiram should be considered, and the risks made known to the patient.

Anxiety

Anxiety is commonly observed in alcohol dependent individuals during intoxication, withdrawal and in the early days of abstinence. Alcohol is typically used to self-medicate anxiety disorders, particularly social anxiety. In alcohol dependent individuals who experience anxiety it is often difficult to determine the extent to which the anxiety is a symptom of the alcohol use disorder or whether it is an independent disorder. Medically assisted withdrawal and supported abstinence for up to 8 weeks are required before a full assessment can be made. If a medically assisted withdrawal is not possible then treatment of the anxiety disorder should still be attempted, following guidelines for the respective anxiety disorder.

The use of benzodiazepines is controversial[9] because of the increased risk of benzodiazepine abuse and dependence. Benzodiazepines should only be considered following assessment in a specialist addiction service.

One meta-analysis suggests that buspirone is effective in reducing symptoms of anxiety, but not alcohol consumption.[9] Studies have also shown that paroxetine (up to 60 mg/day) was superior to placebo in reducing social anxiety in co-morbid patients: alcohol consumption was not affected.[9]

Either naltrexone or disulfiram, alone or combined, improved drinking outcomes compared with placebo in patients with PTSD and alcohol dependence. Both acamprosate and baclofen have shown benefit in reducing anxiety in *post hoc* analyses of alcohol dependence trials (see BAP consensus for references[9]). It is therefore important to ensure that these patients are enabled to become abstinent and are prescribed relapse prevention medication. Anxiety should then be treated according to the appropriate NICE guidelines.

Schizophrenia

Patients with schizophrenia who also have an alcohol use disorder should be assessed and alcohol specific relapse prevention treatment considered, either naltrexone or acamprosate. Antipsychotic medication should be optimised[9] and clozapine may be considered. However, there is insufficient evidence to recommend the use of any one antipsychotic medication over another.

References

1. National Institute for Health and Clinical Excellence. Alcohol use disorders: diagnosis, assessment and management of harmful drinking and alcohol dependence. Clinical Guideline 115, 2011. http://guidance.nice.org.uk/CG115

2. National Institute for Health and Clinical Excellence. Alcohol-use disorders: Preventing harmful drinking. Public Health Guideline 24, 2010. http://guidance.nice.org.uk/PH24

3. Babor T, Higgins-Biddle JC, Saunders JB, Monteiro MG. AUDIT: The Alcohol Use Disorders Identification Test Guidelines for Use in Primary Care, 2nd edn. Geneva: WHO, 2001. http://whqlibdoc.who.int/hq/2001/WHO_MSD_MSB_01.6a.pdf?ua=1.

4. Stockwell T et al. The severity of alcohol dependence questionnaire: its use, reliability and validity. Br J Addict 1983; **78**:145–155.

5. Sullivan JT et al. Assessment of alcohol withdrawal: the revised clinical institute withdrawal assessment for alcohol scale (CIWA-Ar). Br J Addict 1989; **84**:1353–1357.

6. Gossop M et al. A Short Alcohol Withdrawal Scale (SAWS): development and psychometric properties. Addict Biol 2002; **7**:37–43.

7. National Institute for Health and Clinical Excellence. Alcohol-use disorders: physical complications. Clinical Guideline 100, 2010. http://guidance.nice.org.uk/CG100

8. Amato L et al. Benzodiazepines for alcohol withdrawal. Cochrane Database Syst Rev 2010; CD005063.

9. Lingford-Hughes AR et al. Evidence-based guidelines for the pharmacological management of substance abuse, harmful use, addiction and comorbidity: recommendations from BAP. J Psychopharmacol 2012; **26**:899–952.

10. Minozzi S et al. Anticonvulsants for alcohol withdrawal. Cochrane Database Syst Rev 2010; CD005064.

11. Brathen G et al. EFNS guideline on the diagnosis and management of alcohol-related seizures: report of an EFNS task force. Eur J Neurol 2005; **12**:575–581.

12. Perry EC. Inpatient management of acute alcohol withdrawal syndrome. CNS Drugs 2014; **28**:401–410.

13. Thomson AD et al. Time to act on the inadequate management of Wernicke's encephalopathy in the UK. Alcohol Alcohol 2013; **48**:4–8.

14. Thomson AD et al. The Royal College of Physicians report on alcohol: guidelines for managing Wernicke's encephalopathy in the accident and emergency department. Alcohol Alcohol 2002; **37**:513–521.

15. Day E et al. Thiamine for prevention and treatment of Wernicke-Korsakoff Syndrome in people who abuse alcohol. Cochrane Database Syst Rev 2013; **7**:CD004033.

16. Thomson AD et al. The treatment of patients at risk of developing Wernicke's encephalopathy in the community. Alcohol Alcohol 2006; **41**:159–167.

17. Joint Formulary Committee. BNF 67 March-September 2014 (online). London: Pharmaceutical Press; 2014. http://www.medicinescomplete.com/mc/bnf/current/

18. Thomson AD et al. Parenteral thiamine and Wernicke's Encephalopathy: the balance of risks and perception of concern. Alcohol Alcohol 1997; **32**:207–209.

19. Committee on Safety of Medicine. Parentrovite and allergic reactions. Current Problems 1989; 24.

20. Krupitsky E et al. Injectable extended-release naltrexone (XR-NTX) for opioid dependence: long-term safety and effectiveness. Addiction 2013; **108**:1628–1637.

21. Karhuvaara S et al. Targeted nalmefene with simple medical management in the treatment of heavy drinkers: a randomized double-blind placebo-controlled multicenter study. Alcohol Clin Exp Res 2007; **31**:1179–1187.

22. Mason BJ et al. A double-blind, placebo-controlled study of oral nalmefene for alcohol dependence. Arch Gen Psychiatry 1999; **56**:719–724.

23. van den BW et al. Efficacy of as-needed nalmefene in alcohol-dependent patients with at least a high drinking risk level: results from a subgroup analysis of two randomized controlled 6-month studies. Alcohol Alcohol 2013; **48**:570–578.

24. Liu J et al. Baclofen for alcohol withdrawal. Cochrane Database Syst Rev 2013; **2**:CD008502.

25. Johnson BA et al. Topiramate for treating alcohol dependence: a randomized controlled trial. JAMA 2007; **298**:1641–1651.

26. Mason BJ et al. Gabapentin treatment for alcohol dependence: a randomized clinical trial. JAMA Intern Med 2014; **174**:70–77.

CHAPTER 6

27. Guglielmo R et al. Pregabalin for alcohol dependence: a critical review of the literature. Adv Ther 2012; **29**:947–957.

28. National Institute for Health and Clinical Excellence. Antenatal care: routine care for the healthy pregnant woman. Clinical Guideline 62, 2008. http://guidance.nice.org.uk/CG62.

29. Regional Drug and Therapeutics Centre. Regional Medicines Information Service, 2014. http://www.nyrdtc.nhs.uk/Services/teratology/teratology.html.

30. Pettinati HM et al. Gender differences with high-dose naltrexone in patients with co-occurring cocaine and alcohol dependence. J Subst Abuse Treat 2008; **34**:378–390.

31. Cornelius JR et al. Mirtazapine in comorbid major depression and alcohol dependence: An Open-Label Trial. J Dual Diagn 2012; **8**:200–204.

32. Han DH et al. Adjunctive aripiprazole therapy with escitalopram in patients with co-morbid major depressive disorder and alcohol dependence: clinical and neuroimaging evidence. J Psychopharmacol 2013; **27**:282–291.

33. Pettinati HM et al. A double-blind, placebo-controlled trial combining sertraline and naltrexone for treating co-occurring depression and alcohol dependence. Am J Psychiatry 2010; **167**:668–675.

Opioid misuse and dependence

Prescribing for opioid dependence

Important: Treatment of opioid dependence usually requires specialist intervention – generalists who do not have specialist experience should always contact substance misuse services before attempting to treat opioid dependence. It is strongly recommended that general adult psychiatrists *do not* initiate opioid substitute treatment unless directly advised by specialist services. **It cannot be over-emphasised that the use of methadone is readily fatal; opioid withdrawal is not.**

The treatment interventions used for opioid-dependent people in the UK range from low-intensity harm minimisation, such as needle exchange, through to substitution opioid maintenance therapy and high-intensity structured programmes, such as residential abstinence-based psychosocial treatment. Pharmacological treatments can be broadly categorised as maintenance, detoxification or abstinence[1] and should always be prescribed as part of a comprehensive care package.

Treatment aims

- To reduce or prevent withdrawal symptoms.
- To reduce or eliminate non-prescribed drug use.
- To stabilise drug intake and lifestyle.
- To reduce drug-related harm (particularly injecting behaviour).
- To engage and provide an opportunity to work with the patient.

Treatment

This will depend upon:

- what pharmacotherapies and/or other interventions are available
- patient's previous history of drug use and treatment
- patient's current drug use and circumstances
- location/service where treatment is initiated.

Most opioid substitute prescribing for people with mental health problems should be initiated by specialist addiction services. Community mental health teams should work collaboratively with addiction services following local care/referral pathways and joint working protocols. However, some people with mental health problems will be admitted to psychiatric services (e.g. due to mental health relapse) and general psychiatrists will need to take over, or initiate prescribing in the immediate term. Specialist support should be sought as soon as practicable.

The guidance here is generic, but where there are special considerations for psychiatric inpatient services these have been highlighted.

Principles of prescribing[2]

Use licensed medications for heroin-dependence treatment (methadone and buprenorphine).

- The prescriber should ensure that the patient is dependent on opioids and that the patient is given a safe initial dose with suitable supervision and review to minimise the risk of toxicity.
- Daily dispensing advised for at least the first 3 months of prescribing.
- Supervised consumption in the first 3 months usually or until stability achieved.

Evaluating opioid dependence

Before considering prescribing any substitute pharmacotherapy, care should be taken to ensure that the patient does have a diagnosis of opioid dependence as corroborated by the following points.

- A diagnosis of opioid dependence from history and examination of patient. Assessment should include details of what substances the person is taking, quantity, frequency, route of administration, duration at current level and date and time of last use.
- At least one positive recent urine or oral fluid drug screen for opioids (note that opioid-based medication such as co-codamol and codeine phosphate can also give a positive result on screening tests so it is important to get laboratory confirmation of actual opioids or use specific drug testing kits).
- Objective signs of opioid withdrawal (nausea, stomach cramps, muscular tension, muscle spasms/twitching, aches and pains, insomnia and the objective signs listed in Table 6.6).
- Recent sites of injection may also be present (depending on route of administration of opioid) but presence alone does not indicate dependence.

Table 6.6 Objective opioid withdrawal scale

Symptoms	Absent/normal	Mild-to-moderate	Severe
Lacrimation	Absent	Eyes watery	Eyes streaming/wiping eyes
Rhinorrhoea	Absent	Sniffing	Profuse secretion (wiping nose)
Agitation	Absent	Fidgeting	Can't remain seated
Perspiration	Absent	Clammy skin	Beads of sweat
Piloerection	Absent	Barely palpable hairs standing up	Readily palpable, visible
Pulse rate (bpm)	<80	>80 but <100	>100
Vomiting	Absent	Absent	Present
Shivering	Absent	Absent	Present
Yawning/10 min	<3	3–5	6 or more
Dilated pupils	Normal <4 mm	Dilated 4–6 mm	Widely dilated >6 mm

Untreated heroin withdrawal symptoms typically begin after 4–6 hours and reach their peak 32–72 hours after the last dose and symptoms will have subsided substantially after 5 days. Untreated methadone withdrawal typically reaches its peak between 4–6 days after last dose and symptoms do not substantially subside for 10–12 days.[2] Untreated buprenorphine withdrawal typically lasts for up to 10 days.

Specific opioid withdrawal scales are available, e.g. the Clinical Opiate Withdrawal Scale (COWS),[3] Objective Opiate Withdrawal Scale (OOWS)[4] and Short Opiate Withdrawal Scale (SOWS),[5] which can be used to help assess levels of dependence.

Induction and stabilisation of substitute prescribing

It is usually preferable to use a longer-acting opioid agonist or partial agonist (e.g. methadone or buprenorphine respectively) in opioid dependence, as it is generally easier to maintain stability.[2] However, patients with a less severe opioid dependency (e.g. history of using low doses of prescribed codeine or dihydrocodeine-containing preparations only) may in some cases be better managed by maintaining/detoxifying them using that preparation or equivalent.

Buprenorphine or methadone?

NICE guidance on the management of opioid dependence recommend oral methadone or buprenorphine as the pharmacotherapeutic options in opioid dependence.[1] The decision of which to use should be based on the client's preference; their past experience of maintenance with either methadone or buprenorphine; their long-term plans, including a preference for one or other as a detoxification regimen; and in the case of buprenorphine their ability to refrain from heroin use for long enough to avoid precipitated opioid withdrawal symptoms. These considerations are highlighted in Table 6.7; in cases where methadone and buprenorphine appear equally suitable, NICE guidance advises prescribing methadone as first choice.[1]

In rare cases, patients may be allergic to methadone or buprenorphine or to some of the constituents within the formulations.

Suboxone

With regards to the risk of diversion and subsequent injecting of buprenorphine, consideration may be given by the prescriber to a buprenorphine/naloxone preparation which theoretically may reduce the risk of diversion: the rationale is that as the presence of naloxone makes injecting the diverted drug less appealing due to the precipitation of opioid withdrawal symptoms. Extended treatment schedules (12 weeks) tend to be more effective than shorter detoxification regimes.[12] Suboxone is probably more effective in acute detoxification than clonidine.[13]

Dosing of this preparation is the same as for buprenorphine.

CHAPTER 6

Table 6.7 Choosing between buprenorphine and methadone

	Methadone	Buprenorphine
Withdrawal syndrome	Appears to be more marked – best for maintenance programmes	Appears to have a milder withdrawal syndrome than methadone and therefore may be preferred for detoxification programs[6,7]
Differences in side-effect profiles may effect patient preference	Methadone may be associated with QTc prolongation and torsade de pointes (see later in this section)	Buprenorphine is often perceived as less sedating then methadone
Chronic pain	Patients with chronic pain conditions that frequently require additional opioid analgesia may have difficulties being treated with buprenorphine because of the 'blockade' effect although in practice this does not appear to be a major problem	Buprenorphine appears to provide greater 'blockade' effects than doses of methadone <60 mg.[8-10] If a patient on buprenorphine requires treatment for acute pain, an additional opioid may be added titrated against response[11]
Effectiveness	Higher dose methadone maintenance treatment (>60 mg) appears more effective than buprenorphine. However there are no adequate trials of high dose buprenorphine (16–32 mg) compared with high dose methadone maintenance treatment[10]	Buprenorphine is less effective than methadone at retaining patients in treatment at the guidance dose ranges
Combining with other medications	Methadone levels may alter with drugs that inhibit/induce CYP3A4 such as erythromycin, several SSRIs, ribavirin and some anticonvulsants and HIV medications. This may make dose assessment difficult, if a person is not consistent in their use of these CYP3A4 inhibiting drugs	Buprenorphine is less affected by drug interactions and may be preferable for some patients
Pregnancy	Women who are pregnant or planning a pregnancy should consider methadone treatment	There is a risk of buprenorphine precipitated withdrawal or risk with awaiting spontaneous withdrawal prior to initiation of buprenorphine in pregnant women. However, if a patient already stable on buprenorphine becomes pregnant, a decision may be made to continue with that medication
Diversion	Patients at greater risk of diversion of medication (e.g. past history of this; treatment in a prison setting) may be better served with methadone treatment	Sublingual buprenorphine tablets can be more easily diverted with the risk of injecting tablets Available in combination with Naloxone (Suboxone) which may prevent diversion for injection
Transfer to buprenorphine		Methadone clients unable to reduce to doses of methadone <60 mg without becoming 'unstable' cannot easily be transferred to buprenorphine without going into withdrawal

HIV, human immune deficiency virus; SSRIs, selective serotonin reuptake inhibitors.

Methadone

Clinical effectiveness

Methadone, a long acting opioid agonist, has been shown to be an effective maintenance therapy intervention for the treatment of heroin dependence by retaining patients in treatment and decreasing heroin use more than non-opioid based replacement therapy.[14] In addition, higher doses of methadone (60 to 100 mg/day) have been shown to be more effective than lower dosages in retaining patients and in reducing illicit heroin and cocaine use during treatment.[15] Methadone is also effective at reducing withdrawal severity when used for detoxification from heroin, however there is a high relapse following termination of treatment.[16]

Prescribing information

Methadone is a Controlled Drug with a high dependency potential and a low lethal dose. The initial two weeks of treatment with methadone are associated with a substantially increased risk of overdose mortality.[2,16–19] It is important that appropriate assessment, titration of doses and monitoring is performed during this period.

There is also an increase in mortality immediately after completing treatment – one study found that risk of death increased eight-fold to nine-fold in the month immediately after the end of opiate substitution treatment.[17] There is also an increased risk of overdose immediately after leaving inpatient treatment.[18] Opiate substitution treatment was found to have a greater than 85% chance of reducing overall mortality among opiate users if the average duration approaches or exceeds 12 months.[17]

Prescribing should only commence if:

- opioid drugs are being taken on a regular basis (typically daily)
- there is convincing evidence of dependence including drug testing and objective evidence of withdrawal (see above)
- consumption of methadone can be supervised initially.

Supervised daily consumption is recommended for new prescriptions, for a minimum of 3 months.[2] If this is not possible, instalment prescriptions for daily dispensing and collection should be used. No more than one week's supply should be dispensed at one time, except in exceptional circumstances.[2]

Methadone should normally be prescribed as a 1 mg in 1 mL oral solution.[2] Tablets can potentially be crushed and inappropriately injected and therefore should not usually be prescribed.[2,19] However, there may be occasional circumstances in which tablets are prescribed, usually by experienced prescribing doctors in specialist services.

Important: All patients starting a methadone treatment programme must be informed of the risks of toxicity and overdose, and the necessity for safe storage of any take home medication.[2,20–22] Safe storage is vital, particularly if there are children in the household, as tragic deaths have occurred when children have ingested methadone. Prescribers should consider risks to children in all assessments and treatment plans of drug using patients.

Methadone dose: continuation for patients already being prescribed methadone

For patients who are *currently prescribed* methadone and who require the medication to be continued by a different doctor (for example if they are admitted to hospital) and if *all* the criteria listed below are met, then it is safe to prescribe the claimed dose.

- Dose confirmed in writing by the previous prescriber.
- Last consumption confirmed and supervised (e.g. pharmacy contacted) and has been regularly taking this dose including within the last 3 days (to ensure that tolerance has not been reduced).
- Previous prescriber has stopped prescribing and current prescription is completed or cancelled to date (to prevent a patient receiving a double dose).
- Patient is stable or 'comfortable' on dose (no signs of intoxication/withdrawal) and the patient is not presenting as intoxicated with other drugs and/or alcohol.
- No other contraindications or cautions are present.

Note: if there is any doubt about any of these conditions *do not* continue the prescription at the claimed dose.

Recommendations for prescribing methadone where recent use cannot be confirmed

If the patient has missed one or more doses within the last 3 days consider starting at a lower dose and titrating up in response to withdrawal symptoms.

If the person has not been supervised taking their methadone for 3 or more days they must be re-titrated (see below).

In determining the **starting dose** for patients using heroin or other opioids, not already on a prescription for methadone, consideration must be given to the potential for opioid toxicity, taking into account the following.

- Tolerance to opioids can be affected by a number of factors and significantly influences an individual's risk of toxicity.[23] Of particular importance in assessing this are the client's reported current quantity, frequency and route of administration; whilst being wary of possible over-reporting. A person's tolerance to methadone can be significantly reduced within 3 to 4 days of not using opioids, so caution must be exercised after this time, with careful re-titration from a starting dose.
- Use of other depressant drugs, e.g. alcohol, benzodiazepines and psychiatric medications increase risks of toxicity.
- Long half-life of methadone, as cumulative toxicity may develop.[24,25] For this reason a patient should be reviewed regularly for signs of intoxication and the dose must be omitted if there is any sign of drowsiness or other evidence of toxicity.
- Inappropriate dosing can result in fatal overdose, particularly in the first few days.[20,21,26,27] Deaths have occurred following the commencement of a daily dose of less than 30 mg methadone.[2]
- It is safer to start with a low dose that can subsequently be increased at intervals if this dose later proves to be insufficient.

Note: opioid withdrawal is *not* a life-threatening condition, opioid toxicity is.

Direct conversion tables for opioids and methadone should be viewed cautiously, as there are a number of factors influencing the values at any given time. It is much safer to titrate the dose against presenting withdrawal symptoms.

The Clinical Opioid Withdrawal Scale[3] or Short Opiate Withdrawal Scale[5] provide a systematic way of assessing withdrawals.

The **initial total** daily dose for most cases will be in the range of 10–30 mg methadone depending on the level of tolerance.[1,2] In an acute medical or psychiatric ward, starting doses of up to 20 mg daily are usually recommended, as patients in these settings are likely to be physically unwell in the former, or being treated with various other psychoactive drugs in the latter case. In inpatient settings it is recommended that the dose is divided, for example 10 mg twice daily, in case there is any sign of toxicity.

In specialist settings, an initial dose of up to 40 mg methadone may be prescribed by an experienced competent senior clinician for patients who are assessed as being heavily dependent and tolerant, but it is unwise to exceed this dose.[1,2] An additional dose of methadone can be given later the same day in cases where there is evidence of ongoing opioid withdrawal, but this should only be undertaken by experienced prescribers with the appropriate competencies.[1,2]

Note: onset of action should be evident within half an hour, with peak plasma levels being achieved after approximately two to four hours of dosing.

Recommendations for prescribing methadone by non-specialists in non-specialist areas (e.g. general psychiatric wards)

Day one – induction.

- The person must be exhibiting objective opioid withdrawal symptoms, as assessed on an opioid withdrawal scale, before any dose is prescribed.
- Give a dose of 5–10 mg of methadone mixture 1 mg/1 mL based on the severity of withdrawal. This should be given as a once only dose. Methadone will start to have an effect after 20–30 minutes with peak levels being reached at 4 hours.
- Continue to monitor for signs of withdrawal 2–4 hourly and give further doses as required – also observe for signs of intoxication.
- The initial daily dose (over 24 hours) will not usually be more than 30 mg.
- Consider prescribing naloxone as required, in case of overdose.

Day two – calculate the total dose given in the previous 24 hours, *but* divide and prescribe twice daily. It can then be withheld in case of over-sedation.

- Continue to monitor using an opioid withdrawal scale 4 hourly until symptoms have stabilised.
- Up to an additional 10 mg can be given in 24 hours if indicated (i.e. maximum of 40 mg).
- Liaise with the local specialist addiction service for ongoing advice and to develop a joint plan.

Ongoing prescribing.

- Once stability has been achieved continue to prescribe the required dose.

CHAPTER 6

In the acute inpatient setting it is usually advisable for the person to be maintained on a stable dose rather than commence detoxification.

Methadone stabilisation in the community

This applies to patients who have not been on a prescription in the previous 3 days or more.

This is usually undertaken in specialist services by those with appropriate competencies and after a full assessment with urine toxicology and clear evidence of opioid use and withdrawal.

- **First week.** Outpatients should attend daily for the first few days to enable assessment by the prescriber and any dose titration against withdrawal symptoms. Dose increases should not exceed 5–10 mg a day and not usually more than 30 mg in the first week above the initial starting dose.[1] Note that steady state plasma levels are only achieved approximately 5 days after the last dose increase. Once the patient has been stabilised on an adequate dose, methadone should be prescribed as a single regular daily dose. It should not be prescribed on a *pro re nata* basis or at variable dosage. It is good practice to supervise consumption for the first 3 months.
- **Subsequent period.** Subsequent increases of 5–10 mg methadone can continue after the first week, and there should be at least a few days between each successive increase.[2] It may take several weeks to reach the therapeutic daily dose of 60–120 mg.[2] Stabilisation is usually achieved within 6 weeks but may take longer. However, it is important to consider that some patients may require more rapid stabilisation. This would need to be balanced by a high level of supervision and observation thereby allowing the ability to increase doses more rapidly.

Methadone cautions

- **Intoxication.** Methadone should not be given to any patient showing signs of intoxication, especially due to alcohol or other depressant drugs (e.g. benzodiazepines).[23,28] Risk of fatal overdose is greatly enhanced when methadone is taken concomitantly with alcohol and other respiratory depressant drugs. Concurrent alcohol and illicit drug consumption must be borne in mind when considering subsequent prescribing of methadone due to the increased risk of overdose associated with polysubstance misuse.[21,26,28,29]
- **Severe hepatic/renal dysfunction.** Metabolism and elimination of methadone may be affected in which case the dose or dosing interval should be adjusted accordingly against clinical presentation. Because of extended plasma half-life, the interval between assessments during initial dosing may need to be extended.

Methadone overdose

In the event of methadone overdose, **naloxone** should be administered following the *BNF* guidelines. Naloxone can be given by intravenous, intramuscular or subcutaneous route. **The emergency services should always be called.** See Box 6.5 later in this section.

Dose: 0.4–2 mg repeated at intervals of 2–3 minutes to a maximum of 10 mg if respiratory function does not improve. If no response consider alternative causes for overdose.

Although the onset of action will be slower with the intramuscular route, this is the preferred route within the psychiatric setting or addiction service where the intravenous route may be difficult and actually take longer to administer.

In the medical setting a continuous intravenous infusion (2 mg/500 mL) at a rate adjusted according to response may be used.

Naloxone is short-acting and therefore the effect may reverse within 20 minutes to 1 hour, meaning that a patient can revert back into an overdose state. Therefore ongoing medical monitoring should be provided after naloxone administration and patients should be kept under observation in a suitable medical facility.

Analgesia for methadone-prescribed patients

Non-opioid analgesics should be used in preference (e.g. paracetamol, non-steroidal anti-inflammatory drugs [NSAIDs]) initially where appropriate. If opioid analgesia (e.g. codeine, dihydrocodeine, morphine) is indicated due to the type and severity of the pain, then this should be titrated accordingly for pain relief in line with usual analgesic protocols. There are specific considerations for patients receiving methadone, buprenorphine or naltrexone. In the case of patients prescribed methadone, if an opioid analgesic is appropriate, a non-methadone opioid may be co-prescribed, i.e. it is not necessary to 'rationalise' the patient's entire opioid requirements to one drug.[30] Titrating the methadone dose to provide analgesia may be used in certain circumstances but this should only be carried out by experienced specialists.

As outlined elsewhere in this chapter, patients taking buprenorphine or naltrexone may be relatively refractory to opioids prescribed for analgesia, although in practice if a patient on buprenorphine requires treatment for acute pain, an additional opioid may be added titrated against response.[11]

If naltrexone is stopped to allow for the prescribing of opioid analgesia, careful monitoring will be required because of the increased risk of both relapse and overdose.[17,30]

Patients with a history of substance misuse may also need acute pain management in hospital following surgery, trauma or other illness. The primary objectives during the period of acute pain are to manage the pain and avoid the consequences of withdrawal, so it is important to maintain sufficient background medication to achieve both. Liaison with both the inpatient pain team and the local addictions services, as well as collaborative discussion with the patient, are important. The patient may be known to the addictions services, who will be able to inform the treatment plan, assist in a reliable conversion from street drugs (if these are also being taken) to prescribed analgesics and help plan a smooth transition from acute pain intervention to ongoing management of the patient's substance misuse.[17] Further details can be found in a consensus document by the British Pain Society, Royal College of Psychiatrists, Royal College of GPs and The Advisory Council on the Misuse of Drugs.[30]

As advised in the consensus document, in palliative care, the principles of providing analgesia 'in substance misusers are fundamentally no different from those for other adult patients needing palliative care', although increased liaison with substance misuse

CHAPTER 6

services is essential. Those who are opioid dependent may receive maintenance therapy from a substance misuse service 'and this should be regarded as a separate prescription from that for analgesia when attending as a [pain clinic] outpatient', as also described in the context of chronic non-cancer pain above. During admission all medication would usually be received from the inpatient unit, but with 'a clear plan for separate follow-ups for substance misuse and symptom palliation … in place on discharge except during the terminal phase of an illness'.[30] Again, further details can be found in the consensus advice document.[30]

Methadone and risk of Torsades de Pointes/QT interval prolongation

It is possible that methadone either alone or combined with other QT prolonging agents may increase the likelihood of QT interval prolongation on the ECG, which is associated with Torsades de Pointes and can be fatal.[31–33]

Recommended ECG monitoring

In 2006, the Medicines and Healthcare product and Regulatory Authority (MHRA) recommended that patients with the following risk factors for QT interval prolongation are carefully monitored whilst taking methadone: heart or liver disease, electrolyte abnormalities, concomitant treatment with CYP3A4 inhibitors, or medicines with the potential to cause QT interval prolongation (e.g. some antipsychotics, erythromycin, amongst others). See Table 6.8. In addition, any patient requiring more than 100 mg of methadone per day should be closely monitored,[34] because of possible increased risk of QTc prolongation.[31] Thus, in individuals with such risk factors, e.g. those with known heart disease, and those being titrated up to doses of methadone exceeding 100 mg, should have a baseline ECG and subsequent ECG monitoring. The timeframe for the latter is not yet subject to a rigorous evidence base; annual checks in the absence of cardiac symptomatology would be a reasonable minimum frequency where there are

Table 6.8 Recommended ECG monitoring

	Borderline prolonged QTc	Action	Prolonged QTc	Action	Very prolonged QTc	Action
Females	≥470 ms	• Repeat ECG • Electrolytes • Try to modify QT risk factors • Regular ECG until normal	≥500 ms	• Repeat ECG • Electrolytes • Try to modify QT risk factors • Seek specialist help • Consider stopping methadone • Regular ECGs until normal	≥550 ms	• Urgent specialist referral • Repeat ECG • Electrolytes • Try to modify QT risk factors • Stop methadone
Males	≥450 ms					

risk factors as listed. It is also important to check the actions of any medications being prescribed with methadone for CYP3A4 inhibitory activity, to inform the risk-benefit analysis when commencing methadone.[35]

Buprenorphine appears to be associated with less QTc prolongation and therefore may be a safer alternative in this respect,[36] although there are few studies in this area at present; and there are many other factors to take into account when choosing an appropriate opioid substitute, as described earlier.

Remember that QT should be corrected for heart rate to produce a corrected QT (QTc) in milliseconds (ms). This is normally documented on the ECG recording. The ECG should be read by a professional with experience in reading ECGs. Brief guidelines as to actions to take are documented below. Always seek specialist advice where there is prolongation of the QT interval.

A recent review of ECG monitoring suggests that there is insufficient evidence for the efficacy of QTc screening strategies for preventing cardiac morbidity and mortality in methadone-maintained patients and there is concern that in some settings the procedures involved may be 'too demanding and too stressful' and may 'interfere with the availability of patients to undergo methadone maintenance and may expose patients to health consequences of untreated opioid addiction including increased mortality risk'.[37]

Patients on or about to start methadone in inpatient settings on both medical and psychiatric wards should always have an ECG, and patients on high doses or with other risk factors should if possible have ECGs when treated in the community, although consideration should be taken of the risks and benefits if a community patient refuses to attend for ECG monitoring.

Buprenorphine

Clinical effectiveness

Buprenorphine (Subutex) is a synthetic partial opioid agonist and with a low intrinsic activity and high affinity at μ opioid receptors. It is an effective treatment for use in maintenance treatment for heroin addiction, although not more effective than methadone at adequate dosages.[38] There is no significant difference between buprenorphine and methadone in terms of completion of detoxification treatment, but withdrawal symptoms may resolve more quickly with buprenorphine.[39]

Prescribing information

Buprenorphine is absorbed via the sublingual route which takes approximately 5–10 minutes to complete. It is effective in treating opioid dependence because:

- it alleviates/prevents opioid withdrawal and craving
- it reduces the effects of additional opioid use because of its high receptor affinity[8–10]
- it is long-acting allowing daily (or less frequent) dosing. The duration of action is related to the buprenorphine dose administered: low doses (e.g. 2 mg) exert effects for up to 12 hours; higher doses (e.g. 16–32 mg) exert effects for as long as 48–72 hours.

CHAPTER 6

Buprenorphine starting dose

The same principles as for methadone apply when starting treatment with buprenorphine. However, of particular interest with buprenorphine is the phenomenon of precipitated withdrawal. Patient education is an important factor in reducing the problems during induction.

Continuing an already established buprenorphine prescription

As for continuation of methadone prescribing, the following principles apply.

- Dose confirmed in writing by the previous prescriber.
- Last consumption confirmed and supervised (e.g. pharmacy contacted) and has been regularly taking this dose including within the last 3 days (to ensure that tolerance has not been reduced).
- Previous prescriber has stopped prescribing and current prescription is completed or cancelled to date (to prevent a patient receiving a double dose).
- Patient is stable or 'comfortable' on dose (no signs of intoxication/withdrawal) and the patient is not presenting as intoxicated with other drugs and/or alcohol.
- No other contraindications or cautions are present.

Starting buprenorphine

The first dose of buprenorphine should be administered when the patient is experiencing opioid withdrawal symptoms to reduce the risk of precipitated withdrawal. As with methadone, clear evidence of daily opioid use (including drug testing) and withdrawal symptoms are mandatory before commencing a prescription for buprenorphine. The initial dose recommendations are shown in Table 6.9.

No more than 8 mg buprenorphine should be given on the first day in a non-specialist setting. In some cases 8 mg may be sufficient, but this may be increased to 12–16 mg the following day if there is continuing evidence of withdrawal and no evidence of intoxication. The doses should be given in divided doses so that it can be reviewed promptly in the event of any intoxication. If there is concern that doses higher than 16 mg may be required specialist advice should be sought and only increased under advice from addiction specialists.

If patients are on other respiratory sedatives such as benzodiazepines, the lower doses should be used and the patient monitored for intoxication and respiratory depression.

Table 6.9 Recommended starting doses of buprenorphine in opioid withdrawal

Patient's condition	Dose of buprenorphine (mg)
Patient in withdrawal and no risk factors	8 mg
Patient not experiencing withdrawal and no risk factors	4 mg
Patient has concomitant risk factors (e.g. medical condition, polydrug misuse, low or uncertain severity of dependence, on other psychiatric medications.)	2–4 mg

Table 6.10 Factors affecting risk of precipitated withdrawal with buprenorphine

Factor	Discussion	Recommended strategy
Dose of methadone	More likely with doses of methadone above 30 mg Generally – the higher the dose the more severe the precipitated withdrawal[40]	Attempt transfer from doses of methadone <40 mg (preferably ≤30 mg) Transfer from >60 mg should not be attempted
Time between last methadone dose and first buprenorphine dose	Interval should be at least 24 hours. Increasing the interval reduces the incidence and severity of withdrawal[41,42]	Cease methadone and delay first dose until patient experiencing withdrawal from methadone
Dose of buprenorphine	Very low doses of buprenorphine (e.g. 2 mg) are generally inadequate to substitute for methadone High first doses of buprenorphine (e.g. 8 mg) are more likely to precipitate withdrawal	First dose should generally be 4 mg; review patient 2–3 hours later
Patient expectancy	Patients not prepared for precipitated withdrawal are more likely to become distressed and confused by the effect	Inform patients in advance Have contingency plan for severe symptoms
Use of other medications	Symptomatic medication (e.g. lofexidine) can be useful to relieve symptoms	Prescribe in accordance to management plan

Table 6.11 Recommended doses of buprenorphine for patients transferring from methadone (<40 mg (ideally ≤30 mg))

Last methadone dose	Day 1 initial buprenorphine dose	Day 2 buprenorphine dose
20–40 mg	4 mg	6–8 mg
10–20 mg	4 mg	4–8 mg
1–10 mg	2 mg	2–4 mg

CHAPTER 6

Transferring from methadone to buprenorphine

This should usually be under the supervision of a suitably experienced specialist prescriber. Patients transferring from methadone are at risk of experiencing precipitated withdrawal symptoms that may continue at a milder level for 1–2 weeks. Factors affecting precipitated withdrawal are listed in Table 6.10.

Transferring from methadone dose <40 mg (ideally ≤30 mg) to buprenorphine

Methadone should be ceased abruptly and the first dose of buprenorphine given at least 24 hours after the last methadone dose. The conversion rates shown in Table 6.11 at the start of treatment are recommended, but higher doses may be subsequently needed depending on clinical presentation.

Transferring from methadone 40–60 mg dose to buprenorphine

- The methadone dose should be reduced as far as possible without the patient becoming unstable or chaotic, and then abruptly stopped.
- The first buprenorphine dose should be delayed until the patient displays clear signs of withdrawal, generally 48–96 hours after the last dose of methadone. Symptomatic medication (lofexidine) may be useful to provide transitory relief.
- An initial dose of 2–4 mg should be given. The patient should then be reviewed 2–3 hours later.
- If withdrawal has been precipitated further symptomatic medication can be prescribed.
- If there has been no precipitation or worsening of withdrawal, an additional 2–4 mg of buprenorphine can be dispensed on the same day.
- The patient should be reviewed the following day at which point the dose should be increased to between 8–12 mg.

Transferring from methadone doses >60 mg to buprenorphine

Such transfers should not be attempted in an outpatient setting except in exceptional circumstances by an experienced practitioner. Usually patients would be partially detoxified from methadone and transferred to buprenorphine when the methadone was at or below 30 mg daily. However, if transfer from higher dose methadone to buprenorphine is required, a referral to an inpatient unit should be considered.

Transferring from other prescribed opioids to buprenorphine

There is little experience in transferring patients from other prescribed opioids (e.g. codeine, dihydrocodeine, morphine). Basic principles suggest that transferring from opioids with short half-lives should be similar to inducting heroin users; whereas transferring from opioids with longer half-lives will be similar to transferring from methadone.

Stabilisation dose of buprenorphine

Outpatients should attend regularly for the first few days to enable assessment by the prescriber and any dose titration. Dose increases should be made in increments of 2–4 mg at a time, daily if necessary, up to a maximum daily dose of 32 mg. Effective maintenance doses are usually in the range of 12–24 mg daily[43] and patients should generally be able to achieve maintenance levels within 1–2 weeks of starting buprenorphine.

Buphrenorphine less than daily dosing

Buprenorphine is licensed in the UK as a medication to be taken daily. International evidence and experience indicates that many clients can be comfortably maintained on one dose every 2–3 days.[81–84] This may be pertinent for patients in buprenorphine treatment who are considered unsuitable for take-away medication because of the risk of diversion.

The following conversion rate is recommended:

2-day buprenorphine dose = 2 × daily dose of buprenorphine (to a max 32 mg)
3-day buprenorphine dose = 3 × daily dose of buprenorphine (to a max 32 mg)

Note: in the event of patients being unable to stabilise comfortably on buprenorphine (often those transferring from methadone), the option of transferring to methadone should be available. Methadone can be commenced 24 hours after the last buprenorphine dose. Doses should be titrated according to clinical response, being mindful of the residual 'blockade' effect of buprenorphine which may last for several days.

Buprenorphine cautions

- **Liver function.** There is some evidence suggesting that high dose buprenorphine can cause changes in liver function in individuals with a history of liver disease.[48] Such patients should have liver funstion tests (LFTs) measured before commencing with follow-up investigations conducted 6–12 weeks after commencing buprenorphine. More frequent testing should be considered in patients of particular concern, e.g. severe liver disease. Elevated liver enzymes in the absence of clinically significant liver disease however does not necessarily contraindicate treatment with buprenorphine
- **Intoxication.** Buprenorphine should not be given to any patient showing signs of intoxication, especially due to alcohol or other depressant drugs (e.g. benzodiazepines). Buprenorphine in combination with other sedative drugs can result in respiratory depression, sedation, coma and death. Concurrent alcohol and illicit drug consumption must be borne in mind when considering subsequent prescribing of buprenorphine due to the increased risk of overdose associated with polysubstance misuse.

Overdose with buprenorphine

Buprenorphine as a single drug in overdose is generally regarded as safer than methadone and heroin because it causes less respiratory depression. However, in combination with other respiratory depressant drugs the effects may be harder to manage. Very high doses of naloxone (e.g. 10–15 mg) may be needed to reverse buprenorphine effects (although lower doses such as 0.8 to 2 mg may be sufficient), hence ventilator support is often required in cases where buprenorphine is contributing to respiratory depression (e.g. in polydrug overdose). **The emergency services should always be called.** See Box 6.5 later in this section.

Analgesia for buprenorphine-prescribed patients

Non-opioid analgesics should be used in preference (e.g. paracetamol, NSAIDs). Buprenorphine reduces or blocks the effect of full opioid agonists complicating their use as analgesics in patients on buprenorphine. If adequate pain control cannot be achieved then it may be necessary to transfer the patient to a stable methadone dose so that an opioid analgesic can be effectively used for pain control (see notes on analgesia for methadone-prescribed patients earlier in this chapter).

Suboxone

With regards to the risk of diversion and subsequent injecting of buprenorphine, consideration may be given by the prescriber to a buprenorphine/naloxone preparation which theoretically may reduce the risk of diversion. The different sublingual and parenteral potency profiles of buprenorphine and naloxone is key: if used sublingually the naloxone will have negligible effects. However, if the combined preparation is injected, the naloxone will have a substantial effect and can attenuate the effects of the buprenorphine in the short-term and is also likely to precipitate withdrawal in opioid dependent individuals on full opioid agonists.[49]

Alternative oral preparations

Oral methadone and buprenorphine should continue to be the mainstay of treatment;[2] other oral options such as slow release oral morphine (SROM) preparations and dihydrocodeine are not licensed in the UK for the treatment of opiate dependence.[2]

However, a specialised clinician may in very exceptional circumstances prescribe oral dihydrocodeine as maintenance therapy, where clients are unable to tolerate methadone or buprenorphine, or in other exceptional circumstances; taking into account the difficulties associated with its short half-life, supervision requirements, and diversion potential.[2]

Slow release oral morphine preparations have been shown elsewhere in Europe to be useful as maintenance therapy in those failing to tolerate methadone; again only for prescribing by specialised clinicians.[2] A recent review of studies on slow release oral morphine suggested that there was insufficient evidence to assess the effectiveness of this treatment.[50]

Injectable opioid maintenance prescribing

With regard to the prescribing of injectable opioids, a small number of patients in the UK continue to receive these under the former 'British system',[2] and a further minority are being treated in trial clinics in the UK,[51] modelled on the recent Swiss and Dutch injectable opioid maintenance clinics. The trials in Europe have shown promising results, and the UK results have also shown favourable outcomes. Meanwhile, injectable opioid treatment is not currently available in all specialist services in the UK.[2] Notably, a Home Office licence is required to prescribe diamorphine for addictions treatment, and specialist levels of competence are required to prescribe injectable substitute opioids.[2]

At present, clients should only be considered for injectable opioid prescribing in combination with psychosocial interventions, as part of a wider package of care, as an option in cases where the individual has not responded adequately to oral opioid substitution treatment, and in an area where it can be supported by locally commissioned and provided mechanisms for supervised consumption.[2,51] Patients are generally seen for supervised injecting in a specialist facility twice a day.

Opioid detoxification and reduction regimes

Opioid maintenance can be continued from the short term to almost indefinitely, depending on clinical need. Some patients are keen to detoxify after short periods of stability and other patients may decide to detoxify after medium- to long-term periods of stability on maintenance prescriptions. All detoxification programmes should be part of a care programme. Given the risk of serious fatal overdose post detoxification, services providing such treatment should educate the patient about these risks and supply and train them with naloxone and overdose training for emergency use.[1,52,53]

Regarding the length of detoxification, the NICE guidelines state 'dose reduction can take place over anything from a few days to several months, with a higher initial stabilisation dose taking longer to taper', and indicate that 'up to 3 months is typical for methadone reduction, while buprenorphine reductions are typically carried out over 14 days to a few weeks'.[54] In practice, detoxification in the community may extend over a longer period, if this facilitates the client's comfort during the process, compliance with the care-plan, continued abstinence from illicit use during detoxification, and subsequent abstinence following detoxification.

Detoxification in an inpatient setting, the NICE guidelines indicate, may take place over a shorter time than in the community (suggesting 14–21 days for methadone and 7–14 days for buprenorphine) 'as the supportive environment helps a service user to tolerate emerging withdrawal symptoms'.[55] As in the community, stabilisation on the dose of a substitute opioid is first achieved, followed by gradual dose reduction; with additive medications judiciously prescribed for withdrawal symptoms if and as needed.

Detoxification carries a recognised risk of relapse and indeed fatal overdose. Therefore, if a patient is being detoxified there needs to be adequate aftercare in place, such as a rehabilitation programme and community support. For patients having emergency psychiatric or medical admissions, detoxification is not usually indicated unless with the support of specialist services and aftercare arrangements are in place.

Opioid withdrawal in a community setting

Methadone

Following a period of stabilisation with methadone, or a longer period of maintenance, the patient and prescriber may agree a reduction programme as part of a care plan to reduce the daily methadone dose. The usual reduction would be by 5–10 mg weekly or fortnightly, although there can be much variation in the reduction and speed of reduction. In the community setting, patient preference is the most important variable in terms of dose reduction and rate of reduction. The detoxification programme should be reviewed regularly and remain flexible to adjustments and changes, such as relapse to illicit drug use or patient anxieties about speed of reduction. Factors such as an increase in heroin or other drug use or worsening of the patient's physical, psychological or social well-being, may warrant a temporary increase, or stabilisation of the dose or a slowing-down of the reduction rate. Towards the end of the detoxification the dose reduction may be slower 1–2 mg per week. Recent studies show that length of stability on maintenance treatment and prolonged reduction schedules (up to a year) substantially improve the chances of achieving abstinence.[56]

Buprenorphine

The same principles as for methadone apply when planning a buprenorphine detoxification regime. Dose reduction should be gradual to minimise withdrawal discomfort. A suggested reduction regime is shown in Table 6.12.

CHAPTER 6

Table 6.12 Recommended dose reduction schedule for buprenorphine

Daily buprenorphine dose	Reduction rate
Above 16 mg	4 mg every 1–2 weeks
8–16 mg	2–4 mg every 1–2 weeks
2–8 mg	2 mg per week or fortnight
Below 2 mg	Reduce by 0.4–0.8 mg per week

Opioid withdrawal in a specialist addiction inpatient setting

Methadone

Patients should have a starting dose assessment of methadone, over 48 hours by a specialist inpatient team. The dose may then be reduced following a linear regime over up to 4 weeks.[54]

Buprenorphine

Buprenorphine can be used effectively for short-term inpatient detoxifications following the same principles as for methadone.

Lofexidine

Lofexidine, an α_2-adrenergic agonist, can counteract the adrenergic hyperactivity associated with opioid withdrawal[57] (demonstrated by characteristic signs and symptoms, such as tachycardia, sweating, runny nose, hair standing on end, shivering, and goose bumps). Thus, it is licensed for the management of symptoms of opioid withdrawal,[54] although additional short term adjunctive medications may be needed, such as loperamide for diarrhoea.[2] Detoxification using lofexidine is much faster than with methadone or buprenorphine, typically lasting 5–7 days, and up to a maximum of 10 days. The usual regimen commences at 800 μg daily, rising to 2.4 mg in split doses, which is then reduced over subsequent days.[22] Side-effects may include a dry mouth, drowsiness, and clinically significant hypotension and bardycardia;[2] the latter two in particular must therefore be monitored during lofexidine prescribing. Lofexidine should be used with caution in patients with cardiovascular disease or being treated with medications associated with QT prolongation.

Although lofexidine is not useful for detoxification of those with substantial opioid dependence,[2] there are certain circumstances in which this regimen may have a role: in cases where the client has made an informed and clinically appropriate decision not to use methadone or buprenorphine for detoxification; where they have made a similarly informed and clinically appropriate decision to detoxify within a short time period; and where there is only mild or uncertain opioid dependence (including young people).[54] Treatment also enables early initiation onto naltrexone.

Relapse prevention – psychosocial interventions

Psychosocial and behavioural therapies play an important role in the treatment of drug misuse. By helping people develop skills to resist drug misuse and cope with associated problems, they form an important adjunct to pharmacological treatments.[2]

These include brief interventions, such as exploring ambivalence about drug use and possible treatment, with the aim of increasing motivation to change behaviour; providing information about self-help groups (e.g. Narcotics Anonymous); behavioural couples therapy; family therapy, community reinforcement approach and other psychosocial therapies.[2] One particular form of therapy is Contingency Management, considered by NICE[55] as having a strong evidence base from a growing body of work in the US. The principle of this therapy is to provide structured external incentives focused on changing specific behaviours. For example, low monetary value vouchers may be provided in a structured setting contingent on each presentation of a drug-negative test until stability is achieved. Vouchers of higher monetary value (e.g. £10) should be considered to encourage harm reduction on a one-off basis or over a limited duration for managing physical health problems, such as concordance with, or completion of:

- hepatitis B/C and HIV testing
- hepatitis B immunisation
- tuberculosis testing.[55]

'The emphasis on reinforcing positive behaviours is consistent with current knowledge about the underlying neuropsychology of many people who misuse drugs and is more likely to be effective than penalising negative behaviours. There is good evidence that contingency management increases the likelihood of positive behaviours and is cost effective'.[55] Further details are beyond the scope of this text and the interested reader is therefore referred to the 2007 NICE guidelines on psychosocial interventions in drug misuse.

The 2011 review comments on the 2007 NICE guidelines, although not leading to a current updating of the guidelines,[58] highlighted that the 2007 guidelines did not sufficiently emphasise the importance, from world-wide experience of psychosocial interventions outside the realms of double-blind trials, such as the 12-step programme, which also has an important role to play in relapse prevention and recovery- 'the experience of the millions who have recovered through a 12-step programme'.[59]

Naltrexone in relapse prevention

Evidence for the effectiveness of naltrexone as a treatment for relapse prevention in opioid misusers has been inconclusive.[60] However, for those who preferred an abstinence programme, are fully informed of the potential adverse effects and benefits of treatment, are highly motivated to remain on treatment, and have a partner supporting concordance, naltrexone treatment has been found by NICE to be a cost-effective treatment strategy in aiding abstinence from opioid misuse.[61] The naltrexone implant, not currently licensed in the UK, may also have a role to play in reducing opioid use in a motivated population of patients[62] following further research.

Close monitoring is particularly important when naltrexone treatment is initiated because of the higher risk of fatal overdose at this time. Discontinuation of naltrexone may also be associated with an increase in inadvertent overdose from illicit opioids. Thus, supervision of naltrexone administration, and careful choice of who is prescribed it (those who are abstinence-focused and motivated) is very important. Moreover, people taking naltrexone often experience adverse effects of unease (dysphoria), depression and insomnia, which can lead to relapse to illicit opioid use while on naltrexone treatment, or failure to continue on treatment. The dysphoria may be caused by either withdrawal from illicit drugs or by the naltrexone treatment itself, emphasising the importance of prescribing naltrexone as part of a care programme that includes psychosocial therapy and general support.[61]

Initiating naltrexone treatment

Naltrexone has the propensity to cause a severe withdrawal reaction in patients who are either currently taking opioid drugs or who were previously taking opioid drugs and there has not been a sufficient 'wash-out' period prior to administering naltrexone.

The minimum recommended interval between stopping the opioid and starting naltrexone depends on the opioid used, duration of use and the amount taken as a last dose. Opioid agonists with long half-lives such as methadone will require a wash-out period of up to 10 days, whereas shorter acting opioids such as heroin may only require up to 7 days.

Experience with buprenorphine indicates that a wash-out period of up to 7 days is sufficient (final buprenorphine dose >2 mg; duration of use >2 weeks) and in some cases naltrexone may be started within 2–3 days of a patient stopping (final buprenorphine dose <2 mg; duration of use <2 weeks).

A test dose of naloxone (0.2–0.8 mg), which has a much shorter half-life than naltrexone, may be given to the patient as an intramuscular (IM) dose prior to starting naltrexone treatment. Any withdrawal symptoms precipitated will be of shorter duration than if precipitated by naltrexone.

Patients *must* be advised of the risk of withdrawal prior to giving the dose. It is worth thoroughly questioning the patient as to whether they have taken any opioid containing preparation unknowingly (e.g. over-the-counter analgesic). See Box 6.4.

Box 6.4 Important points regarding prescribing naltrexone

- Ensure the client is fully informed of the increased risk of fatal opioid overdose.
- Following detoxification and any period of abstinence, an individual's tolerance to opioids will decrease markedly. At such a time, using opioids puts the individual at greatly increased risk of overdose.
- Discontinuation of naltrexone may also be associated with an increase in inadvertent overdose from illicit opioids, emphasising the need for close monitoring and support of the client at this time.

Dose of naltrexone

An initial dose of 25 mg naltrexone should be administered after a suitable opioid-free interval (and naloxone challenge if appropriate). The patient should be monitored for 4 hours after the first dose, for symptoms of opioid withdrawal. Symptomatic medication for withdrawal (lofexidine) should be available for use, if necessary, on the first day of naltrexone dosing (withdrawal symptoms may last up to 4–8 hours). Once the patient has tolerated this low naltrexone dose, subsequent doses can be increased to 50 mg daily as a maintenance dose.

Naltrexone is contraindicated in patients with hepatic dysfunction and liver function tests should be monitored during treatment.

Pregnancy and opioid use

Substitute prescribing can occur at any time in pregnancy and carries a lower risk than continuing illicit use.[2]

Women can present with opioid dependency at any stage in pregnancy and stabilisation on substitute methadone is the treatment of choice at any stage in pregnancy. Detoxification in the first trimester is contraindicated due to the risk of spontaneous abortion and in the third trimester it is associated with preterm delivery. If detoxification is requested, this is most safely achieved in the second trimester but should only be supervised by specialists with the appropriate competencies and with careful monitoring for any evidence of instability. Enforcing detoxification is contraindicated as it is likely to deter some clients from seeking help, and the majority will then return to opioid use at some point during their pregnancy;[63] fluctuating opioid concentrations in the maternal blood from intermittent use of illicit opioids may then lead to foetal withdrawal or overdose.[64,65] Given the value of a comprehensive care package, pregnant women attending treatment usually have better general health than those using drugs who are not in treatment, even if the former continue to also use illicit drugs.[2] The emphasis must therefore be on early engagement in treatment,[2] and, methadone maintenance treatment during pregnancy, in the context of a multidisciplinary team (including obstetricians, neonatologists, and addictions specialists) and detailed holistic package of care, (including comprehensive psychosocial input);[63] this is currently regarded as the gold standard.[64,65]

The majority of neonates born to methadone-maintained mothers will, however, require treatment for neonatal abstinence syndrome (NAS).[64] NAS is characterised by a variety of signs and symptoms relating to the autonomic nervous system, gastrointestinal tract and respiratory system;[64] with methadone it usually commences after 48 hours.[66] In the case of any mother using drugs or in opioid substitution treatment, it is important to have access to skilled neonatal paediatric care, to monitor the neonate and treat as required.

Specialist advice should be obtained before initiating opioid substitution treatment or detoxification, particularly with regards to management and treatment plan during pregnancy. Maternal metabolism of methadone may increase towards the third trimester of pregnancy. At this time an increased methadone dose may be required or occasionally split dosing on the medication to prevent withdrawal.

Limited controlled data are available on the treatment of opioid dependence in pregnancy,[63,65,67] and particularly the use of buprenorphine in pregnancy.[63,68]

A review of the evidence suggests that there were no significant differences between methadone, buprenorphine and slow release oral morphine in pregnancy.[67] However, the buprenorphine cases recorded to date suggest that buprenorphine, compared with methadone, may lead to a less severe abstinence syndrome in the neonate,[54] while methadone may be related to better treatment retention.[67]

It is useful to anticipate potential problems for women prescribed opioids during pregnancy with regard to opioid pain relief: such women should be managed in specialist antenatal clinics due to the increased associated risks. Antenatal assessment by anaesthetists may be recommended with regard to anticipating any anaesthetic risks, any analgesic requirements and problems with venous access.

Pregnancy and breast feeding – methadone

Although the newborn may experience a withdrawal syndrome, as described, there is no evidence of an increase in congenital defects with methadone.

Methadone is considered compatible with breast feeding, although other risk factors such as HIV, hepatitis C, use of benzodiazepines, cocaine and other drugs need to be considered and may mean that breast feeding is contraindicated. The NICE guidelines[2] recommend that breast feeding should still be encouraged, but that with regards to methadone and breast feeding 'the dose is kept as low as possible while maintaining stability, and the infant monitored to avoid sedation'.

Pregnancy and breast feeding – buprenorphine

Currently buprenorphine is not licensed as an opioid substitute treatment during pregnancy or breast feeding although there is increasing experience of the use of this drug in pregnancy. More evidence is available on the safety of methadone, which for that reason makes it the preferred choice. However, women well maintained on buprenorphine prior to pregnancy may remain on buprenorphine following full informed consent and advice that safety of buprenorphine in pregnancy has not been fully established.[2] All such decisions should be made by experienced prescribers and fully documented.

Opioids overdose

The recommended procedure in the event of an opioids overdose is shown in Box 6.5.

'Take-home' naloxone

Research trials have assessed the impact of providing take-home naloxone and overdose-management training to opioid-using patients.[52,53] With overdose-management training, opiate users can be trained to execute appropriate actions to assist the successful reversal of potentially fatal opiate overdose.[69] Some services are providing one dose of take-home naloxone (400 μg) in combination opioid overdose-management training (as above) to opioid-using clients in treatment, and wider provision may reduce opioid-related deaths further.[69]

Box 6.5 Opioid overdose and use of naloxone

All addictions services and psychiatric units should have naloxone available.

ALWAYS CALL THE EMERGENCY SERVICES

1. Call 999
2. Check airways and breathing
3. Administer IM naloxone; repeat dose if needed
4. Stay with the client and await the ambulance

Opioid overdose with heroin or other opioids can be recognised by:

- Pin-point pupils.
- Respiratory depression (<8 breaths per minute).
- Cold to touch/blue lips.
- Unconsciousness.

Actions to be taken on discovering an opioid overdose:

- Check area safe, then try to rouse overdose victim.
- If unrousable – call for help/ambulance.
- Check airway and breathing
  - if not breathing, give 2 rescue breaths (optional)
  - if breathing – place in recovery position.
- Administer 0.4 mg Naloxone IM.
- Repeat this dose if there is no response after 5–10 minutes.
- Consider use of high flow oxygen (where available).
- Await emergency team/ambulance.
- Patient to have medical monitoring for several hours after naloxone as the effects of naloxone are short acting (between 30 minutes to one hour) and the effects of an opioid overdose may re-emerge. Patients may need additional doses of naloxone.

NICE guidelines related to substance abuse

The National Institute of Health and Care Excellence has issued various guidelines related to substance misuse. These are summarised in Boxes 6.6–6.10.

Box 6.6 NICE guidance: methadone and buprenorphine for the management of opioid dependence[1]

- Methadone and buprenorphine (oral formulations), using flexible dosing regimens, are recommended as options for maintenance therapy in the management of opioid dependence.
- The decision about which drug to use should be made on a case-by-case basis, taking into account a number of factors, including the person's history of opioid dependence, their commitment to a particular long-term management strategy, and an estimate of the risks and benefits of each treatment made by the responsible clinician in consultation with the person. If both drugs are equally suitable, methadone should be prescribed as the first choice.
- Methadone and buprenorphine should be administered daily, under supervision, for at least the first 3 months. Supervision should be relaxed only when the patient's compliance is assured. Both drugs should be given as part of a programme of supportive care.

Box 6.7 Naltrexone for the management of opioid dependence[61]

- Naltrexone is recommended as a treatment option in detoxified formerly opioid-dependent people who are highly motivated to remain in an abstinence programme.
- Naltrexone should only be administered under adequate supervision to people who have been fully informed of the potential adverse effects of treatment. It should be given as part of a programme of supportive care.
- The effectiveness of naltrexone in preventing opioid misuse in people being treated should be reviewed regularly. Discontinuation of naltrexone treatment should be considered if there is evidence of such misuse.

Box 6.8 Drug misuse: psychological interventions[55]

Brief interventions
- Opportunistic brief interventions focused on motivation should be offered to people in limited contact with drug services (e.g. those attending a needle and syringe exchange).
- These interventions should aim to increase motivation to change behaviour, and provide non-judgemental feedback.

Self help
- Provide people who misuse drugs with information about self-help groups, e.g. Narcotics Anonymous and Cocaine Anonymous.

Contingency management
- Introduce contingency management to reduce illicit drug use and/or promote engagement with services for people receiving methadone maintenance treatment.

Box 6.9 Drug misuse: opioid detoxification[54]

- Detoxification should be an available option for those who have expressed an informed choice to become abstinent.
- Give detailed information about detoxification and the associated risks, including the loss of opioid tolerance following detoxification, the ensuing increased risk of overdose and death from illicit drug use; and the importance of continued support to maintain abstinence and reduce the risk of adverse outcomes.
- Methadone or buprenorphine should be offered as the first-line treatment in opioid detoxification.
- Ultra-rapid detoxification under general anaesthesia or heavy sedation (where the airway needs to be supported) must not be offered. This is because of the risk of serious adverse events, including death.
- Offer a community-based programme to all service users considering opioid detoxification. Exceptions to this may include service users who:
  - have not benefited from previous formal community-based detoxification
  - need care because of significant co-morbid physical or mental health problems
  - require complex polydrug detoxification, e.g. concurrent detoxification from alcohol or benzodiazepines and who are experiencing significant social problems that will limit the benefit of community-based detoxification.
- Residential detoxification should be considered for people who have significant co-morbid physical or mental health problems, or who require concurrent detoxification from opioids and benzodiazepines or sequential detoxification from opioids and alcohol, and for people who would benefit significantly from a residential rehabilitation programme during and after detoxification.
- Inpatient detoxification should be considered for people who need a high level of medical and/or nursing support because of significant and severe co-morbid physical or mental health problems, or who need concurrent detoxification from alcohol or other drugs that requires a high level of medical and nursing expertise.

Box 6.10 Psychosis with coexisting substance misuse[70]

- Consider seeking specialist advice and initiating joint working arrangements with specialist substance misuse services for adults and young people with psychosis being treated by community mental health teams and known to be dependent on opioids.
- Adult community mental health teams or CAMHS should continue to provide coordination and treatment for the psychosis within joint working arrangements.
- If a person with psychosis and coexisting substance misuse requires planned detoxification from drugs this should take place in an inpatient setting.
- When developing a treatment plan:
  - tailor the plan and the sequencing of treatments to the person
  - take account of the relative severity of both conditions and different times and the person's social and treatment context and the person's readiness to change.
- Offer evidence-based treatment (see NICE Clinical Guideline 51 and 52).
- When prescribing medication:
  - take into account the level and type of substance misuse, especially alcohol
  - warn about potential interaction between substances of misuse and prescribed medications
  - discuss problems and potential dangers of using non-prescribed substances and alcohol to counteract the effects or side-effects of prescribed medication.

Inpatient mental health services
- Ensure that planned detoxification from drugs is undertaken only:
  - with the involvement and advice of substance misuse services
  - in an inpatient setting, preferably in specialist detoxification units, or designated detoxification beds within inpatient mental health services
  - as part of an overall treatment plan.

References

1. National Institute for Health and Clinical Excellence. Methadone and buprenorphine for the management of opioid dependence. Technology Appraisal **114**, 2007. http://www.nice.org.uk
2. Department of Health. Drug misuse and dependence. UK guidelines on clinical management. London: DH; 2007.
3. Wesson DR et al. The Clinical Opiate Withdrawal Scale (COWS). J Psychoactive Drugs 2003; **35**:253–259.
4. Handelsman L et al. Two new rating scales for opiate withdrawal. Am J Drug Alcohol Abuse 1987; **13**:293–308.
5. Gossop M. The development of a Short Opiate Withdrawal Scale (SOWS). Addict Behav 1990; **15**:487–490.
6. Seifert J et al. Detoxification of opiate addicts with multiple drug abuse: a comparison of buprenorphine vs. methadone. Pharmacopsychiatry 2002; **35**:159–164.
7. Jasinski DR et al. Human pharmacology and abuse potential of the analgesic buprenorphine: a potential agent for treating narcotic addiction. Arch Gen Psychiatry 1978; **35**:501–516.
8. Bickel WK et al. Buprenorphine: dose-related blockade of opioid challenge effects in opioid dependent humans. J Pharmacol Exp Ther 1988; **247**:47–53.
9. Walsh SL et al. Acute administration of buprenorphine in humans: partial agonist and blockade effects. J Pharmacol Exp Ther 1995; **274**:361–372.
10. Comer SD et al. Buprenorphine sublingual tablets: effects on IV heroin self-administration by humans. Psychopharmacology 2001; **154**:28–37.
11. Alford DP et al. Acute pain management for patients receiving maintenance methadone or buprenorphine therapy. Ann Intern Med 2006; **144**:127–134.
12. Woody GE et al. Extended vs short-term buprenorphine-naloxone for treatment of opioid-addicted youth: a randomized trial. JAMA 2008; **300**:2003–2011.
13. Ziedonis DM et al. Predictors of outcome for short-term medically supervised opioid withdrawal during a randomized, multicenter trial of buprenorphine-naloxone and clonidine in the NIDA clinical trials network drug and alcohol dependence. Drug Alcohol Depend 2009; **99**:28–36.
14. Mattick RP et al. Buprenorphine maintenance versus placebo or methadone maintenance for opioid dependence. Cochrane Database Syst Rev 2014; **2**: CD002207.
15. Faggiano F et al. Methadone maintenance at different dosages for opioid dependence. Cochrane Database Syst Rev 2003; CD002208.
16. Amato L et al. Methadone at tapered doses for the management of opioid withdrawal. Cochrane Database Syst Rev 2013; **2**: CD003409.
17. Cornish R et al. Risk of death during and after opiate substitution treatment in primary care: prospective observational study in UK General Practice Research Database. BMJ 2010; **341**:c5475.

18. Strang J et al. Loss of tolerance and overdose mortality after inpatient opiate detoxification: follow up study. BMJ 2003; **326**:959–960.

19. Department of Health Task Force to Review Services for Drug Misusers. Report of an independent review of drug treatment services in England. London: DH; 1996. http://www.dh.gov.uk/.

20. Caplehorn JR. Deaths in the first two weeks of maintenance treatment in NSW in 1994: identifying cases of iatrogenic methadone toxicity. Drug Alcohol Rev 1998; **17**:9–17.

21. Zador D et al. Deaths in methadone maintenance treatment in New South Wales, Australia 1990–1995. Addiction 2000; **95**:77–84.

22. Hall W. Reducing the toll of opioid overdose deaths in Australia. Drug Alcohol Rev 1999; **18**:213–220.

23. White JM et al. Mechanisms of fatal opioid overdose. Addiction 1999; **94**:961–972.

24. Wolff K et al. The pharmacokinetics of methadone in healthy subjects and opiate users. Br J Clin Pharmacol 1997; **44**:325–334.

25. Rostami-Hodjegan A et al. Population pharmacokinetics of methadone in opiate users: characterization of time-dependent changes. Br J Clin Pharmacol 1999; **48**:43–52.

26. Harding-Pink D. Methadone: one person's maintenance dose is another's poison. Lancet 1993; **341**:665–666.

27. Drummer OH et al. Methadone toxicity causing death in ten subjects starting on a methadone maintenance program. Am J Forensic Med Pathol 1992; **13**:346–350.

28. Farrell M et al. Suicide and overdose among opiate addicts. Addiction 1996; **91**:321–323.

29. Neale J. Methadone, methadone treatment and non-fatal overdose. Drug Alcohol Depend 2000; **58**:117–124.

30. The British Pain Society, Royal College of Psychiatrists, Royal College of General Practitioners, Advisory Council on the Misuse of Drugs. Pain and substance misuse: improving the patient experience. A consensus statement prepared by The British Pain Society in collaboration with The Royal College of Psychiatrists, The Royal College of General Practitionersand The Advisory Council on the Misuse of Drugs. London: BPS; 2007. http://www.britishpainsociety.org/book_drug_misuse_main.pdf.

31. Krantz MJ et al. Torsade de pointes associated with very-high-dose methadone. Ann Intern Med 2002; **137**:501–504.

32. Kornick CA et al. QTc interval prolongation associated with intravenous methadone. Pain 2003; **105**:499–506.

33. Martell BA et al. The impact of methadone induction on cardiac conduction in opiate users. Ann Intern Med 2003; **139**:154–155.

34. Medicines and Healthcare Products Regulatory Agency. Risk of QT interval prolongation with methadone. Current Problems in Pharmacovigilance 2006; **31**:6.

35. Cruciani RA. Methadone: to ECG or not to ECG...That is still the question. J Pain Symptom Manage 2008; **36**:545–552.

36. Wedam EF et al. QT-interval effects of methadone, levomethadyl, and buprenorphine in a randomized trial. Arch Intern Med 2007; **167**:2469–2475.

37. Pani PP et al. QTc interval screening for cardiac risk in methadone treatment of opioid dependence. Cochrane Database Syst Rev 2013; **6**: CD008939.

38. Mattick RP et al. Buprenorphine maintenance versus placebo or methadone maintenance for opioid dependence. Cochrane Database Syst Rev 2008; CD002207.

39. Gowing L et al. Buprenorphine for the management of opioid withdrawal. Cochrane Database Syst Rev 2009; CD002025.

40. Walsh SL et al. Effects of buprenorphine and methadone in methadone-maintained subjects. Psychopharmacology 1995; **119**:268–276.

41. Strain EC et al. Acute effects of buprenorphine, hydromorphone and naloxone in methadone-maintained volunteers. J Pharmacol Exp Ther 1992; **261**:985–993.

42. Strain EC et al. Buprenorphine effects in methadone-maintained volunteers: effects at two hours after methadone. J Pharmacol Exp Ther 1995; **272**:628–638.

43. Ling W et al. Buprenorphine maintenance treatment of opiate dependence: a multicenter, randomized clinical trial. Addiction 1998; **93**:475–486.

44. Amass L et al. Alternate-day buprenorphine dosing is preferred to daily dosing by opioid-dependent humans. Psychopharmacology 1998; **136**:217–225.

45. Amass L et al. Alternate-day dosing during buprenorphine treatment of opioid dependence. Life Sci 1994; **54**:1215–1228.

46. Johnson RE et al. Buprenorphine treatment of opioid dependence: clinical trial of daily versus alternate-day dosing. Drug Alcohol Depend 1995; **40**:27–35.

47. Eissenberg T et al. Controlled opioid withdrawal evaluation during 72 h dose omission in buprenorphine-maintained patients. Drug Alcohol Depend 1997; **45**:81–91.

48. Berson A et al. Hepatitis after intravenous buprenorphine misuse in heroin addicts. J Hepatol 2001; **34**:346–350.

49. Stoller KB et al. Effects of buprenorphine/naloxone in opioid-dependent humans. Psychopharmacology (Berl) 2001; **154**:230–242.

50. Ferri M et al. Slow-release oral morphine as maintenance therapy for opioid dependence. Cochrane Database Syst Rev 2013; **6**: CD009879.

51. Strang J et al. Supervised injectable heroin or injectable optimised methadone versus optimised oral methadone as treatment for chronic heroin addicts in England after persistent failure in orthodox treatment (RIOTT): a randomised trial. Lancet 2010; **375**:1885–1895.

52. Baca CT et al. Take-home naloxone to reduce heroin death. Addiction 2005; **100**:1823–1831.

53. Strang J et al. Emergency naloxone for heroin overdose. BMJ 2006; **333**:614–615.

54. National Institute for Health and Clinical Excellence. Drug misuse: opioid detoxification. Clinical Guideline 52, 2007.

55. National Institute for Health and Clinical Excellence. Drug misuse: psychosocial interventions. Clinical Guideline 51, 2007. http://www.nice.org.uk/

56. Nosyk B et al. Defining dosing pattern characteristics of successful tapers following methadone maintenance treatment: results from a population-based retrospective cohort study. Addiction 2012; **107**:1621–1629.

57. Yu E et al. A Phase 3 placebo-controlled, double-blind, multi-site trial of the alpha-2-adrenergic agonist, lofexidine, for opioid withdrawal. Drug Alcohol Depend 2008; **97**:158–168.

CHAPTER 6

58. National Institute for Health and Clinical Excellence. Drug misuse: psychosocial interventions - review decision on Clinical Guideline 51, 2011. http://www.nice.org.uk/nicemedia/live/11812/53564/53564.pdf

59. National Institute for Health and Clinical Excellence. Drug misuse: psychosocial interventions - Guideline Review Consultation Comments Table on Clinical Guideline 51, 24 January 2011 -7 February 2011. http://www.nice.org.uk/nicemedia/live/11812/53565/53565.doc

60. Minozzi S et al. Oral naltrexone maintenance treatment for opioid dependence. Cochrane Database Syst Rev 2011; 4: CD001333.

61. National Institute for Health and Clinical Excellence. Naltrexone for the management of opioid dependence. Technology Apprasial 115, 2007. http://www.nice.org.uk

62. Kunoe N et al. Naltrexone implants after in-patient treatment for opioid dependence: randomised controlled trial. Br J Psychiatry 2009; 194:541–546.

63. Winklbaur B et al. Treating pregnant women dependent on opioids is not the same as treating pregnancy and opioid dependence: a knowledge synthesis for better treatment for women and neonates. Addiction 2008; 103:1429–1440.

64. Finnegan LP. Neonatal Abstinence Syndrome. In: Hoekelman RA, Friedman SB, Nelson N, Seidel HM, eds. *Primary Pediatric Care*. St Louis: Mosby; 1992. 1367–1378.

65. Winklbaur B et al. Opioid dependence and pregnancy. Curr Opin Psychiatry 2008; 21:255–259.

66. Fischer G et al. Methadone versus buprenorphine in pregnant addicts: a double-blind, double-dummy comparison study. Addiction 2006; 101:275–281.

67. Minozzi S et al. Maintenance agonist treatments for opiate-dependent pregnant women. Cochrane Database Syst Rev 2013; 12: CD006318.

68. Kayemba-Kay's S et al. Buprenorphine withdrawal syndrome in newborns: a report of 13 cases. Addiction 2003; 98:1599–1604.

69. Strang J et al. Overdose training and take-home naloxone for opiate users: prospective cohort study of impact on knowledge and attitudes and subsequent management of overdoses. Addiction 2008; 103:1648–1657.

70. National Institute for Health and Clinical Excellence. Psychosis with coexisting substance misuse. Clinical Guideline 120, 2011. http://guidance.nice.org.uk/CG120

Nicotine and smoking cessation

Smoking remains the Western world's major preventable cause of early death. Reductions in smoking behaviour have a major positive impact on numerous health outcomes.

NICE guidance on smoking cessation

Harmful effects from nicotine dependence are generally related to the harm caused by smoking cigarettes and therefore the primary goal of treatment is complete cessation of smoking. The three main treatments licensed in the UK for smoking cessation are nicotine replacement (all formulations are available over the counter), the antidepressant bupropion prolonged-release and varenicline tartrate. Nicotine replacement therapy (NRT) has been investigated in a large number of well conducted RCTs, and varenicline and bupropion in a smaller number of such trials. NICE have developed tobacco treatment guidance[1-3] relating to planned abrupt cessation of tobacco which is the optimal approach, gradual smoking reduction prior to cessation (a form of harm reduction) for those unable or unwilling to stop smoking completely, and managing temporary abstinence when smokers are unable to smoke, ie. due to smoking restrictions such as during an inpatient stay.

For smoking cessation NICE make the following recommendations.

- NRT, varenicline and bupropion are recommended for those who want to stop smoking.
- NRT, varenicline and bupropion should only be prescribed as part of an 'abstinent-contingent treatment' model in which smokers make a committment to stop smoking on a particular date and medication is only continued if the user remains abstinent from smoking at follow-ups. To increase cost-efficacy, the total treatment course is dispensed in divided prescriptions. NRT should initially be prescribed to last for 2 weeks after the stopping date and varenicline and bupropion for 3–4 weeks after the stop date. Subsequent prescriptions should be given if the smoker is making good progress at their quit attempt.
- Varenicline and bupropion should not be used in the under 18 s, pregnant and breast-feeding women.
- Explain the risks and benefits of using NRT to young people aged from 12 to 17, pregnant or breast-feeding women, and people who have unstable cardiovascular disorders. To maximise the benefits of NRT, people in these groups should also be strongly encouraged to use behavioural support in their quit attempt.
- Varenicline or bupropion may be offered to people with unstable cardiovascular disorders, subject to clinical judgement.
- NHS-funded smoking cessation treatments should not usually be offered within 6 months of an unsuccessful attempt at smoking cessation with either NRT, varenicline or bupropion, unless there are external circumstances which lead to relapse.
- Do not offer NRT, varenicline or buproprion in any combination.
- Consider offering a combination of nicotine patches and an acute form of NRT (such as gum, inhalator, lozenge or nasal/mouth spray) to people who show a high level of dependence on nicotine or who have found single forms of NRT inadequate in the past.

- Factors to consider when deciding which of the three treatments to initate include:
  - motivation to stop
  - availability of counselling
  - previous experience with smoking cessation aids
  - contraindications to use and the potential for adverse events
  - personal preference of smoker.

More recently, in recognition of the fact that not all smokers are able or willing to stop smoking, or abstain from nicotine completely, NICE have recommended smokers to use one or more licensed nicotine-containing products while still smoking and for as long as needed to prevent relapse. Healthcare staff are encouraged to raise awareness of this new strategy among smokers. For those forced into temporary tobacco abstinence by smoking restrictions NICE also advises using such products to alleviate nicotine withdrawal symptoms.[3]

Another development has been a focus on tackling smoking cessation in people with mental health conditions. NICE, the Royal College of Physicians and the Royal College of Psychiatrists have all recently called for radical changes in the prioritisation, service provision and prevention of tobacco related deaths and disability in people with mental health disorders.[2,4] Widely held misconceptions that such smokers are not motivated to stop, are unable to do so if they try, or that their mental health might deteriorate as a result of quitting, are not supported by the data. In fact there is evidence that smoking cessation is associated with reduced depression, anxiety, stress, and improved positive mood and quality of life compared to continuing to smoke in those with and without psychiatric disorders.[5]

NICE has also made recommendations on brief interventions and referral to NHS smoking cessation services some of which are outlined below.[6]

- Everyone who smokes should be advised to stop.
- All smokers should be asked how interested they are in stopping.
- Healthcare workers (including GPs and hospital doctors) should offer referral to smoking cessation services and if the person does not want to attend these services, can initiate pharmacotherapy as per NICE guidelines if sufficiently experienced.

Nicotine replacement therapy (NRT)

Clinical effectiveness

A Cochrane review of 117 RCTs of NRT against placebo or non-NRT for smoking cessation[7] concluded that all six commercially available forms of NRT are effective. NRT increases the odds of quitting by approximately 1.5- to 2-fold regardless of clinical setting. NRT significantly reduces the severity of nicotine withdrawal symptoms and urge to smoke and should be given as per recommended doses in the *BNF* and outlined below. The dosages may vary according to the degree of nicotine dependence as indicated by markers such as daily cigarette consumption, latency to first cigarette in the morning, and severity of withdrawal symptoms on previous quit attempts. There was a tendency for nicotine inhaler and nasal spray to be more effective than gums, lozenges or patches.

In order to widen access of NRT in at-risk patient groups, the MHRA state that NRT may be used by:

- **Adolescents aged 12 to 18**, but as there are limited data on the safety and efficacy, duration should be restricted to 12 weeks. Treatment should only be continued longer than 12 weeks on the advice of a healthcare professional.

- **Pregnant women** – ideally they should stop smoking without using NRT but, if this is not possible, NRT may be recommended to assist a stopping attempt as it is considered that the risk to the foetus of continued smoking by the mother outweighs any potential adverse effects of NRT. The decision to use NRT should be made following a risk-benefit assessment as early in pregnancy as possible. The aim should be to discontinue NRT use after 2–3 months. Intermittent (oral) forms of NRT are preferable during pregnancy although a patch may be appropriate if nausea and/or vomiting are a problem. If patches are used, they should be removed before going to bed at night. Generally clinicians are advised to use only 16-hour patches with pregnant women as then the onus is not on the woman to remember to remove the patch. If she forgets to take 16-hour one off there is no further nicotine delivery.

- **Breast-feeding women** – NRT can be used by women who are breast feeding. The amount of nicotine the infant is exposed to from breast milk is relatively small and less hazardous than the second-hand smoke they would otherwise be exposed to if the mother continued to smoke. If possible, patches should be avoided. NRT products taken intermittently (oral forms) are preferred as their use can be adjusted to allow the maximum time between their administration and feeding of the baby, to minimise the amount of nicotine in the milk.

- **Patients with cardiovascular disease** – dependent smokers with a myocardial infarction (MI), severe dysrhythmia or recent cerebrovascular accident (CVA) who are in hospital, should be encouraged to stop smoking with non-pharmacological interventions. If this fails NRT may be considered, but as data on safety in these patient groups are limited, initiation of NRT should only be done under medical supervision. For patients with stable cardiovascular disease, NRT is a lesser risk than continuing to smoke.

- **Patients with diabetes** – nicotine releases catecholamines, which can affect carbohydrate metabolism. Diabetic patients should be advised to monitor their blood sugar levels more closely than usual when starting NRT.

- **Patients with renal or hepatic impairment** – NRT should be used with caution in patients with moderate to severe hepatic impairment and/or severe renal impairment, as the clearance of nicotine or its metabolites may be decreased, with the potential for increased adverse effects.

- **Patients taking other drugs** – drug interactions may occur as a *result of stopping smoking* rather from NRT per se. The only interaction that is possibly directly attributable to NRT is with adenosine (adverse haemodynamic effects).

Preparations and dose

All NRTs, when used to make an abrupt attempt to stop smoking, should be used for about 8–12 weeks but may be continued beyond this time if needed to prevent relapse. They can also be used in combination if required, usually the patch plus a faster-acting oral or nasal NRT for relief of situational urges to smoke. Cochrane report an odds ratio of 1.34 for combination NRT versus patch alone for long term abstinence.[7] Unless given adequate behavioural support in combination with NRT, and enough information about how these products work, smokers tend not to use sufficient NRT for relief of withdrawal and do not use it for long enough to prevent relapse. Even the fastest acting NRTs (nasal and mouth spray) deliver nicotine much more slowly than inhaled tobacco smoke and so do not give the same subjective satisfaction.

- Sublingual tablet (2 mg): recommended dose of one tablet per hour or, for heavy smokers (smoking more than 20 cigarettes per day), two tablets per hour maximum 40 × 2 mg daily.
- Gum (2 mg or 4 mg, variety of flavours, chewed slowly when urge to smoke occurs) up to maximum of 15 pieces daily. Gum needs to be rested against the gums or buccal mucosa for absorption to occur. There is some evidence of reduced efficacy for the 2 mg preparation.[7]
- Patch: two different types are available (24 hour or 16 hour). There is no difference in efficacy. Both types come in three strengths to allow gradual weaning.
  - 16 hour patches deliver nicotine over a 16 hour period and are removed at bedtime (dose 25 mg, 15 mg, 10 mg)
  - 24 hour patches are worn throughout the night and taken off and replaced in the morning (21 mg, 14 mg, 7 mg).
- Nasal spray (each metered spray delivers 0.5 mg nicotine. A dose = 1 spray to each nostril, up to maximum of 2 doses per hour or 32 doses per day). Most suitable for highly dependent smokers.
- Inhalator (15 mg/cartridge) used with a plastic mouthpiece. Dose initially up to 6 cartridges per day – puffed for 20 minutes every hour.
- Lozenge (1 mg, 2 mg and 4 mg) up to maximum of 15 per day. Again, as with gum, needs to be used correctly. Patients should be advised not to suck the lozenge, rest between gum and cheek or put under the tongue.
- Nicotine oromucal spray (1 mg): Apply 1–2 sprays into the mouth every 30 minutes, for 8 weeks, then reduce use by 50% over 2–4 weeks and down to 0 within another 2 weeks.
- Orodispersable nicotine mouth strips (2.5 mg): One strip every 1–2 hours for 6 weeks, then one every 2–4 hours for 3 weeks reducing to one every 4–8 hours for 3 weeks. Minimum of 9 to maximum of 15 strips a day. Suitable for less nicotine dependent smokers.

E-cigarettes

In the past two or three years the number of people switching partly or wholly to e-cigarettes has massively increased. Smoking e-cigarettes ('vaping') is essentially unsupervised NRT. The advantage is a fast delivery of nicotine which mimics tobacco smoking. Disadvantages include the normalisation of smoking in a different form and the possibility that carcinogens may still be present in the tobacco-derived nicotine solutions. Many smokers find delivery from some e-cigarettes to be unsatisfactory, and so equipment which allows the user to alter the nicotine delivery may be preferred.

Side-effects

Mainly mild local irritant effects such as skin irritation, hiccups, stinging in the mouth/throat/nose depending on formulation. These usually disappear with continued use as tolerance develops rapidly.

Bupropion (amfebutamone)

Clinical effectiveness

Bupropion (Zyban) is an atypical antidepressant with dopaminergic and noradrenergic actions, and has been advocated by NICE for smoking cessation. A systematic review of 65 RCTs of bupropion revealed a near doubling of smoking cessation as compared to the placebo control (where NRT is not used).[8] Trials show it significantly reduces the severity of nicotine withdrawal symptoms and urges to smoke and in some patients will make smoking less pleasurable and rewarding.

There is a risk of about 1 in 1000 of seizures associated with bupropion use and therefore this must be considered before initiation of treatment.

Bupropion is contraindicated in patients with a history of seizures, eating disorders, a CNS tumour, bipolar disorder, pregnancy, breast feeding or those experiencing acute benzodiazepine or alcohol withdrawal. As many drugs reduce seizure threshold, including other antidepressants, a risk-benefit assessment must be made in such cases and if bupropion is prescribed it should be at half dose.

Side-effects

Insomnia, dry mouth, headache (common ~30%). Seizure, hypersensitivity reaction or rash (rare ~0.1%).

Start 1–2 weeks before the planned 'quit date' at 150 mg daily for 6 days, then 150 mg twice daily for a maximum of 7–9 weeks. The dose will need to be reduced in the elderly or in those experiencing side-effects. Not recommended for those <18 years old.

Varenicline (Champix)

Varenicline tartrate is a partial agonist binding with high affinity to the $\alpha_4\beta_2$ nicotinic acetylcholine receptor. Two large scale randomised placebo-controlled trials comparing it directly with bupropion suggest it is nearly 80% more effective.[9,10] The Cochrane review gives a number needed to treat (NNT) of 10 for varenicline to achieve an additional successful 6–12 month quitter compared with placebo, compared with an NNT of 20 for bupropion and 10 for single NRT.[11] Varenicline is also more effective than 24 hour NRT.[12] Like NRT and bupropion, varenicline significantly reduces nicotine withdrawal symptoms, but there is also evidence it makes smoking less rewarding so may help prevent 'slips' develop into full relapse.

Dose

Days 1–3: 0.5 mg once daily
Days 4–7: 0.5 mg twice daily
Day 8–end of week 12: 1.0 mg twice daily

Smokers should be advised to set a 'quit date' between days 8–14 but can delay quitting for up to 35 days. For patients who have successfully stopped smoking at the end of 12 weeks, an additional course of 12 weeks treatment at 1 mg twice daily may be considered. The only contraindication is hypersensitivity to the drug or excipients. There are no known drug interactions.

Warnings and precautions

Smoking cessation, with or without pharmacotherapy, has been associated with exacerbation of underlying psychiatric illness (e.g. depression). It should not be used in the under 18s, pregnant or breast-feeding women, or in those with end stage renal disease. Those with severe renal impairment may require a dosage reduction.

Side-effects

The main side effect is nausea (30%). Depression and suicidality have also been reported[13] during post-marketing surveillance and care should be taken to monitor patients for any signs of agitation, mood changes or suicidal thoughts.[14]

Extra considerations for those with a psychiatric diagnosis

People with mental health problems who smoke tend to be more highly nicotine-dependent than the general population of smokers and may find withdrawal intolerable,[15] a factor which predicts lower success rates with smoking cessation interventions. The relationship between tobacco use and different psychiatric disorders has been extensively reviewed.[4,15] Clinicians should also be aware of the possible emergence of depression in patients who attempt to stop smoking. Switching to e-cigarettes (wholly or partly) might be considered desirable in many patients.

Bupropion has been shown to be effective in people with schizophrenia particularly when combined with NRT.[16] Benefits of bupropion treatment must be weighed against the risk of seizures – see section on 'Bupropion' on the previous page. Noradrenergic antidepressants such as nortriptyline[8,17] and venlafaxine[18] may also be effective smoking cessation treatments in those with schizophrenia, but SSRIs are not.

Varenicline is the most effective smoking cessation treatment but may also be associated with higher risks than NRT. There is MHRA advice about suicidal behaviour and varenicline which can be found in the *BNF*; 'Patients should be advised to discontinue treatment and seek prompt medical advice if they develop agitation, depressed mood or suicidal thoughts. Patients with a history of psychiatric illness should be monitored closely while taking varenicline. If you have a history of depression, you may be more likely to experience common side-effects of varenicline and/or the symptoms of nicotine withdrawal, i.e. tension/agitation, irritability/anger, confusion and depression'.[19] Recent published research has provided some reassuring findings and to date no causal association between varenicline and neuropsychiatric adverse effects has been found.[20-22]

Effects of stopping smoking on other drugs

Stopping smoking may alter the pharmacokinetics or pharmacodynamics of other drugs, including several used in psychiatry, for which dosage adjustment may be necessary irrespective of which or whether any stop smoking medication is being used (examples include alprazolam, theophylline, chlorpromazine, diazepam, warfarin, insulin, clomipramine, clozapine, desipramine, doxepin, fluphenazine, haloperidol, imipramine and oxazepam). Stopping smoking is not thought to alter blood levels of chlordiazepoxide, ethanol, lorazepam or midazolam. These interactions are caused by the components in the smoke (polycyclic aromatic hydrocarbons) and not the nicotine. It is unclear if quitting affects blood levels of amitriptyline and nortriptyline. Smoking cessation usually results in an increase of plasma levels of CYP1A2 substrates (smoking induces CYP1A2). See section 'Smoking and psychotropic drugs' in Chapter 8.

References

1. National Institute for Health and Clinical Excellence. Smoking cessation services in primary care, pharmacies, local authorities and workplaces, particularly for manual working groups, pregnant women and hard to reach communities. Public Health Guidance 10, 2008. http://www.nice.org.uk/PH010
2. National Institute for Health and Care Excellence. Smoking cessation - acute, maternity and mental health services. Public Health Guidance 48, 2013. http://guidance.nice.org.uk/PH48
3. National Institute for Health and Care Excellence. Tobacco harm reduction. Public Health Guidance 45, 2013. http://guidance.nice.org.uk/PH45
4. Royal College of Physicians, Royal College of Psychiatrists. Smoking and mental health: A joint report by the Royal College of Physicians and the Royal College of Psychiatrists. London: RCP; 2013. http://www.rcplondon.ac.uk/publications/smoking-and-mental-health.
5. Taylor G et al. Change in mental health after smoking cessation: systematic review and meta-analysis. BMJ 2014; **348**:g1151.
6. National Institute for Health and Clinical Excellence. Brief interventions and referral for smoking cessation in primary care and other settings. Public Health Intervention Guidance 1, 2006. http://www.nice.org.uk/
7. Stead LF et al. Nicotine replacement therapy for smoking cessation. Cochrane Database Syst Rev 2012; **11**:CD000146.
8. Hughes JR et al. Antidepressants for smoking cessation. Cochrane Database Syst Rev 2014; **1**:CD000031.
9. Gonzales D et al. Varenicline, an alpha4beta2 nicotinic acetylcholine receptor partial agonist, vs sustained-release bupropion and placebo for smoking cessation: a randomized controlled trial. JAMA 2006; **296**:47–55.
10. Jorenby DE et al. Efficacy of varenicline, an alpha4beta2 nicotinic acetylcholine receptor partial agonist, vs placebo or sustained-release bupropion for smoking cessation: a randomized controlled trial. JAMA 2006; **296**:56–63.
11. Cahill K et al. Nicotine receptor partial agonists for smoking cessation. Cochrane Database Syst Rev 2012; **4**:CD006103.
12. Aubin HJ et al. Varenicline versus transdermal nicotine patch for smoking cessation: results from a randomised open-label trial. Thorax 2008; **63**:717–724.
13. McIntyre RS. Varenicline and suicidality: a new era in medication safety surveillance. Expert Opin Drug Saf 2008; **7**:511–514.
14. Medicines and Healthcare Products Regulatory Agency. Varenicline: adverse psychiatric reactions including depression. Drug Safety Update 2008; **2**:2–3.
15. Ziedonis D et al. Tobacco use and cessation in psychiatric disorders: National Institute of Mental Health report. Nicotine Tob Res 2008; **10**:1691–1715.
16. Tsoi DT et al. Interventions for smoking cessation and reduction in individuals with schizophrenia. Cochrane Database Syst Rev 2013; **2**:CD007253.
17. Wagena EJ et al. Should nortriptyline be used as a first-line aid to help smokers quit? Results from a systematic review and meta-analysis. Addiction 2005; **100**:317–326.
18. Cinciripini PM et al. Combined effects of venlafaxine, nicotine replacement, and brief counseling on smoking cessation. Exp Clin Psychopharmacol 2005; **13**:282–292.
19. McClure JB et al. Mood, side-effects and smoking outcomes among persons with and without probable lifetime depression taking varenicline. J Gen Intern Med 2009; **24**:563–569.
20. Anthenelli RM et al. Effects of varenicline on smoking cessation in adults with stably treated current or past major depression: a randomized trial. Ann Intern Med 2013; **159**:390–400.
21. Thomas KH et al. Smoking cessation treatment and risk of depression, suicide, and self harm in the Clinical Practice Research Datalink: prospective cohort study. BMJ 2013; **347**:f5704.
22. Gibbons RD et al. Varenicline, smoking cessation, and neuropsychiatric adverse events. Am J Psychiatry 2013; **170**:1460–1467.

Pharmacological treatment of dependence on stimulants

The most commonly misused stimulants are cocaine (as hydrochloride or free base), amfetamine sulfate and methamfetamine hydrochloride. These drugs are usually insufflated (snorted) (e.g. cocaine HCL; amfetamine SO_4), smoked (cocaine base) or injected. There are no effective pharmacotherapies for the treatment of stimulant dependence. A wide variety of pharmacological agents have been assessed and found lacking,[1] although research is ongoing.[2] Effective medications are available for some psychiatric complications of stimulant use. For example, antidepressants have a role in treating major depressive disorder associated with stimulant use[3] as do antipsychotics for amfetamine psychosis.[4] However, neither class of drug is efficacious in treating stimulant dependence itself.[5–7]

The recommended treatment for dependence on stimulants is psychosocial; in particular contingency management,[8] although benefit has also been shown for cognitive behavioural and relapse prevention approaches.[9]

Cocaine

Detoxification

There are no currently used evidence-based pharmacological treatments for the management of cocaine withdrawal. Symptoms of withdrawal include depressed mood, agitation and insomnia.[10] These are usually self limiting. It should be noted that given cocaine's short half-life and the binge nature of cocaine use, many patients essentially detoxify themselves regularly with no pharmacological therapy. Symptomatic relief such as the short-term use of hypnotics may be helpful in some but these agents may be diverted for illicit use or become agents of dependence themselves.[3]

Substitution treatment

There is little evidence for substitution therapy for the treatment of cocaine misuse and it should not be prescribed.[3]

Ongoing research

There is inconclusive evidence that some agents may increase rates of abstinence. These include drugs that increase extracellular dopamine by stimulating dopamine release (dexamfetamine),[11,12] inhibiting dopamine reuptake (bupropion and modafinil),[11–14] or inhibiting dopamine metabolism (disulfiram).[15] The anticonvulsant vigabatrin has shown some efficacy in both increasing abstinence and retention in treatment.[16] Most of these medications have substantial side-effects and all have uncertain long-term outcomes. Hence they remain subjects for further research rather than clinical treatment options.

Vaccination

Anti-addiction vaccines may offer an alternative pharmacological approach. Vaccinated individuals produce antibodies which bind to drug molecules inhibiting their passage across the blood–brain barrier and reducing their subjective effects.[17] The first

CHAPTER 6

placebo-controlled RCT of a cocaine vaccine (administered as 5 injections over 12 weeks) in opioid and cocaine dependent patients showed a significant decrease in cocaine use in patients who attained effective serum anticocaine antibody levels.[18] However, only 38% of vaccinated patients attained such levels and this occurred slowly such that the decrease in cocaine use only became significant between weeks 9 and 16 and then rapidly dropped off. It remains to be seen how far these issues can be addressed and whether anti-addiction vaccines will have a role in the treatment of cocaine and other drug dependence in the future.

Amfetamines

A wide variety of amfetamines are misused including 'street' amfetamine, methamfetamine and pharmaceutical dexamfetamine. Any drug in this class is likely to have misuse potential. As with cocaine there is no evidence base for pharmacological treatment of withdrawal,[3,4,7] although the number of agents that have been investigated is limited.[4,7] A recent systematic review of dexamfetamine, bupropion, methylphenidate and modafinil as replacement therapies found no reduction in amfetamine use or craving and no increase in sustained abstinence.[19] Future research may change this outcome in view of the small sample sizes and paucity of studies available for review. Naltrexone has shown promise in initial trials by attenuating the subjective effects of dexamfetamine[20] and reducing amfetamine use in dependent individuals.[21]

Detoxification

Treatment should focus on symptomatic relief, although many symptoms of amfetamine withdrawal (low mood, listlessness, fatigue, etc.) are short-lived and may not be amenable to pharmacological treatment. Insomnia can be treated with short courses of hypnotics.

Maintenance

Dexamfetamine maintenance should not be initiated. There is no good evidence for this practice.[3] There are, however, patients that have been prescribed dexamfetamine as a maintenance treatment for drug dependence for many years. Ideally, such patients should be gradually detoxified over several months. For some, though, the consequences of enforced detoxification may be worse than continuing to prescribe dexamfetamine. In these cases the best decision may be to continue to prescribe. A decision to continue prescribing dexamfetamine should only be made by an addiction specialist.[3]

Polysubstance abuse

In those that are dependent on opioids and cocaine, the provision of effective substitution therapy for treatment of the opioid dependence with either methadone or buprenorphine can lead to a reduction in cocaine use.[3]

References

1. de Lima MS et al. Pharmacological treatment of cocaine dependence: a systematic review. Addiction 2002; **97**:931–949.
2. Haile CN et al. Pharmacotherapy for stimulant-related disorders. Curr Psychiatry Rep 2013; **15**:415.
3. Department of Health. Drug misuse and dependence. UK guidelines on clinical management. London: DH; 2007.
4. Shoptaw SJ et al. Treatment for amphetamine withdrawal. Cochrane Database Syst Rev 2009;CD003021.
5. Amato L et al. Antipsychotic medications for cocaine dependence. Cochrane Database Syst Rev 2007;CD006306.
6. Pani PP et al. Antidepressants for cocaine dependence and problematic cocaine use. Cochrane Database Syst Rev 2011;CD002950.
7. Srisurapanont M et al. Treatment for amphetamine dependence and abuse. Cochrane Database Syst Rev 2001;CD003022.
8. National Institute for Health and Clinical Excellence. Drug misuse: psychosocial interventions. Clinical Guideline 51, 2007. http://www.nice.org.uk/.
9. Dutra L et al. A meta-analytic review of psychosocial interventions for substance use disorders. Am J Psychiatry 2008; **165**:179–187.
10. Rounsaville BJ. Treatment of cocaine dependence and depression. Biol Psychiatry 2004; **56**:803–809.
11. Castells X et al. Efficacy of psychostimulant drugs for cocaine dependence. Cochrane Database Syst Rev 2010;CD007380.
12. Perez-Mana C et al. Efficacy of indirect dopamine agonists for psychostimulant dependence: a systematic review and meta-analysis of randomized controlled trials. J Subst Abuse Treat 2011; **40**:109–122.
13. Anderson AL et al. Modafinil for the treatment of cocaine dependence. Drug Alcohol Depend 2009; **104**:133–139.
14. Martinez-Raga J et al. Modafinil: a useful medication for cocaine addiction? Review of the evidence from neuropharmacological, experimental and clinical studies. Curr Drug Abuse Rev 2008; **1**:213–221.
15. Pani PP et al. Disulfiram for the treatment of cocaine dependence. Cochrane Database Syst Rev 2010;CD007024.
16. Brodie JD et al. Randomized, double-blind, placebo-controlled trial of vigabatrin for the treatment of cocaine dependence in Mexican parolees. Am J Psychiatry 2009; **166**:1269–1277.
17. Shen XY et al. Vaccines against drug abuse. Clin Pharmacol Ther 2012; **91**:60–70.
18. Martell BA et al. Cocaine vaccine for the treatment of cocaine dependence in methadone-maintained patients: a randomized, double-blind, placebo-controlled efficacy trial. Arch Gen Psychiatry 2009; **66**:1116–1123.
19. Perez-Mana C et al. Efficacy of psychostimulant drugs for amphetamine abuse or dependence. Cochrane Database Syst Rev 2013; **9**:CD009695.
20. Jayaram-Lindstrom N et al. Naltrexone attenuates the subjective effects of amphetamine in patients with amphetamine dependence. Neuropsychopharmacology 2008; **33**:1856–1863.
21. Jayaram-Lindstrom N et al. Naltrexone for the treatment of amphetamine dependence: a randomized, placebo-controlled trial. Am J Psychiatry 2008; **165**:1442–1448.

Benzodiazepine misuse (see section in Chapter 4)

Benzodiazepine prescribing increased during the 1970s, mainly because of their improved safety profile relative to barbiturates. However, it was soon noted that benzodiazepines have a high potential for causing dependence. Prescriptions originally started for other disorders may be continued long-term and develop into dependence. This is particularly common in elderly patients and those with anxiety spectrum disorders or depression.

A Cochrane review evaluated the evidence for pharmacological interventions for benzodiazepine mono-dependence and concluded that a gradual reduction of benzodiazepine dose (by about an eighth of the dose per fortnight) was preferable to an abrupt discontinuation[1] (see section on 'Benzodiazepines' in Chapter 4 for suggested regimens). A more recent review confirmed that withdrawal over a period of less than 6 months is appropriate for most patients.[2] A meta-analysis supports the effectiveness of multi-faceted prescribing interventions (usually including psychological interventions/support) in reducing benzodiazepine use in older patients[3] and a recent RCT has demonstrated that a simple educational approach based on self-efficacy theory resulted in almost a quarter of long-term elderly benzodiazepine users engaging voluntarily in reducing and discontinuing use.[4]

A large number of patients presenting to addictions services may be using illicit benzodiazepines on top of their primary substance of abuse. Although some services provide prescriptions for benzodiazepines, there is no evidence that substitute prescribing of benzodiazepines reduces benzodiazepine misuse. If benzodiazepines are prescribed, this should ideally be for a short-term, time-limited (2–3 weeks) prescription and with a view to detoxification.

If patients have been prescribed benzodiazepines for a substantial period of time, it may be preferable to convert to equivalents of diazepam as this is longer acting and so less likely to be associated with withdrawal symptoms between doses. Benzodiazepine dependence as part of polysubstance dependence should also be treated by a gradual withdrawal of the medication. Benzodiazepines prescribed at greater than 30 mg diazepam equivalent per day may cause harm[5] and so this should be avoided if at all possible. Psychosocial interventions including contingency management have had some success at reducing benzodiazepine use.

Pregnancy and benzodiazepine misuse

Benzodiazepines are not major human teratogens but should ideally be gradually discontinued before a planned pregnancy. If a woman is prescribed benzodiazepines and found to be pregnant, the prescription should be gradually withdrawn over as short a time as possible, being mindful of the risk of withdrawal seizures and the potential consequences for the pregnant woman and foetus. A risk benefit analysis should be undertaken and specialist advice sought (see section on 'Pregnancy' in Chapter 7).

References

1. Denis C et al. Pharmacological interventions for benzodiazepine mono-dependence management in outpatient settings. Cochrane Database Syst Rev 2006;CD005194.
2. Lader M et al. Withdrawing benzodiazepines in primary care. CNS Drugs 2009; 23:19–34.
3. Gould RL et al. Interventions for reducing benzodiazepine use in older people: meta-analysis of randomised controlled trials. Br J Psychiatry 2014; 204:98–107.
4. Tannenbaum C et al. Reduction of Inappropriate Benzodiazepine Prescriptions Among Older Adults Through Direct Patient Education: The EMPOWER Cluster Randomized Trial. JAMA Intern Med 2014.
5. Department of Health. Drug misuse and dependence. UK guidelines on clinical management. London: DH; 2007.

GBL and GHB dependence

GBL (γ-butaryl-lactone, a pro-drug of GHB) and GHB (γ-hydroxybutyrate) use is uncommon, but medically important because in dependent users withdrawal can proceed rapidly to agitated delirium with paranoia and muscle rigidity so severe that it can occasionally cause rhabdomyolysis and acute renal failure. Doctors in emergency departments and psychiatric admission wards need to be able to recognise and manage acute withdrawal.

GBL and GHB reduce anxiety and produce disinhibition and sedation, primarily through actions at the gamma-aminobutyric acid (GABA)-β receptor. These drugs are used for socialising and facilitating sex, and sometimes for sleep. The drugs have a narrow therapeutic index and overdose is not uncommon. Dependence on these drugs is quite rare, but in dependent users withdrawal has a rapid onset and can produce severe delirium and muscle rigidity.[1,2] Fatalities associated with withdrawal have been reported.[3]

The GBL withdrawal syndrome[1,2,4]

Dependent users take GBL 'round the clock' (every 3–4 hours or more frequently). Onset of withdrawal is usually 3–4 hours after the last dose of GBL and is characterised by anxiety, sweating, fine tremor and resting tachycardia. Untreated, this can proceed to delirium, often with psychotic features (visual and tactile hallucinations, paranoia), followed by severe tremors and muscle rigidity. Muscle rigidity may be so severe as to produce fever, and rhabdomyolysis and acute renal failure have been observed. The requirement for medication eases over 4–6 days, although there are case reports of more prolonged withdrawal.

The principle of managing withdrawal is to treat early and prevent the development of delirium and other complications, as once established, delirium can be difficult to control. Early treatment with high doses of benzodiazepines are required, and baclofen (a GABA-β agonist) has been included in management to reduce the risk of muscle rigidity.[5] See Box 6.11. Existing withdrawal scales are unlikely to be helpful.

Box 6.11 Acute GBL and GHB withdrawal management

- Initiate treatment with diazepam, 20 mg, once early withdrawal symptoms are observed. Diazepam can be repeated at 2-hourly intervals until symptoms are controlled; most cases of GBL withdrawal require 60–80 mg diazepam in the first 24 hours. Baclofen, 10–20 mg every eight hours should also be given. If the patient becomes drowsy, withhold diazepam and review diagnosis. If after a total dose of diazepam greater than 100 mg in the first 24 hours is not controlling symptoms, medical consultation is recommended. One to one nursing care may assist in managing severe cases.
- Further, smaller doses of diazepam, titrated against response, may be required on day 2 and 3 of withdrawal.
- Baclofen can be continued for the first 3 days.

Management of elective GBL withdrawal

In such patients, withdrawal should be medically supervised. After withdrawal, persisting anxiety and insomnia are common, and there is a high risk of relapse. Before initiating elective withdrawal management, a plan should be in place to monitor and support patients for 4 weeks to minimise risk of relapse. Patients with good social support who live in proximity to where treatment is to be delivered can be managed on an ambulatory basis, other patients should be managed in an inpatient setting.

Community detoxification

- Ambulatory detoxification should only be attempted if there is someone at home who is able to monitor and supervise the withdrawal process and there is the option available of transferring the patient to an inpatient unit if symptoms are not well-controlled.
- Discuss treatment plan with the patient and person who will be supporting them. It is helpful to write this out and keep a copy in notes.
- On day one of planned ambulatory detoxification, the patient is asked to attend having used no GBL for 2 hours and advised to dispose of their remaining supplies of GBL. They will need to stay at the clinic for 4 hours on day one. They must be advised that they cannot drive motor vehicles during withdrawal and should be advised not to drink alcohol during withdrawal.
- Initiate treatment once signs and symptoms develop – pulse >90, sweaty palms, fine tremor, and/or anxiety – administer diazepam 20 mg, repeat after 2 hours, at which time also administer baclofen 10 mg. Monitor hourly for anxiety/sedation.
- Once 6 hours have passed since last GBL usage and the patient has had at least 40 mg diazepam and 10 mg baclofen, they may be dispensed a further 40 mg diazepam and 30 mg baclofen and then seen on the following two days.
- At each daily review, adjust medication. Diazepam is seldom needed beyond 5 days.

Inpatient treatment

Patients lacking social support are more safely managed in inpatient settings. Pharmacological management is as for ambulatory withdrawal – early initiation of high dose benzodiazepines, titrated against response. In both situations, it is advisable to have flumazenil available.

References

1. Bell J et al. Gamma-butyrolactone (GBL) dependence and withdrawal. Addiction 2011; **106**:442–447.
2. McDonough M et al. Clinical features and management of gamma-hydroxybutyrate (GHB) withdrawal: a review. Drug Alcohol Depend 2004; **75**:3–9.
3. Zvosec DL et al. Case series of 226 gamma-hydroxybutyrate-associated deaths: lethal toxicity and trauma. Am J Emerg Med 2011; **29**:319–332.
4. Wojtowicz JM et al. Withdrawal from gamma-hydroxybutyrate, 1,4-butanediol and gamma-butyrolactone: a case report and systematic review. CJEM 2008; **10**:69–74.
5. LeTourneau JL et al. Baclofen and gamma-hydroxybutyrate withdrawal. Neurocrit Care 2008; **8**:430–433.

Drugs of misuse: a summary

One in twelve adults use illicit drugs in any one year,[1] and at least a third of those with mental illness can be classified as having a 'dual diagnosis'.[2,3] There is now compelling evidence that cannabis use increases the risk of psychosis.[4,5] It is therefore important to be aware of the main mental state changes associated with drugs of abuse. Note also that substance misuse in fully compliant patients with schizophrenia increases relapse rate to the levels seen in those who are non-compliant[6] (that is, substance misuse negates the benefits of antipsychotic treatment). Urine-testing for illicit drugs is routine on many psychiatric wards. It is important to be aware of the duration of detection of drugs in urine and of other commonly used substances and drugs that can give a false-positive result. Some false positives are unexpected and so not readily predictable, for example amisulpride can give a false positive for buprenorphine.[7] False positive results are most likely with point of care testing kits. If a positive result has implications for a patient's liberty, and the patient denies use of substances, a second sample should be sent to the laboratory. Table 6.13 summarises the physical and mental changes associated with various drugs, withdrawal from those drugs and general results for urine testing.

Table 6.13 Drugs of misuse: effects, withdrawal and testing

Drug	Physical signs/ symptoms of intoxication	Most common mental state changes[8]	Withdrawal symptoms	Duration of withdrawal	Duration of detection in the urine[9]	Other substances which give a positive result[10]
Amfetamine-type stimulants[11]	Tachycardia Increased BP Anorexia Tremor Restlessness	Visual/tactile/ olfactory auditory hallucinations Paranoia Elation	Fatigue Hunger Depression Irritability Craving Social withdrawal	Peaks 7–34 hours Lasts maximum of 5 days	Depends on half-life, mostly 48–72 hours	Cough and decongestant preparations Bupropion Chloroquine Chlorpromazine Promethazine Ranitidine Selegiline Large quantities of tyramine Tranylcypromine Trazodone
GHB/GBL	Drowsiness Coma Disinhibition	Sociability Confidence	Tremor Tachycardia Paranoia Delirium Psychosis Visual/ tactile/ olfactory/ auditory hallucinations	3–4 days	Difficult to detect Not routinely screened for	
Benzodiazepines	Sedation Disinhibition	Relaxation Visual hallucinations Disorientation Sleep disturbance	Anxiety Insomnia Delirium Seizures; Visual/tactile/ olfactory auditory hallucinations Psychosis;	Usually short-lived but may last weeks to months	Up to 28 days: depending on half-life of drug taken	Nefopam Sertraline Zopiclone
Cannabis[12,13]	Tachycardia Lack of co-ordination Red eyes Postural hypotension	Elation Psychosis Perceptual distortions Disturbance of memory/ judgement Two-fold increase in risk of developing schizophrenia[14]	Restlessness Irritability Insomnia Anxiety[15]	Uncertain Probably less than 1 month[12] (longer in heavy users)	Single use: 3 days; chronic heavy use: up to 21 days	Passive 'smoking' of cannabis Efavirenz
Cocaine	Tachycardia/ tachypnoea Increased BP/ headache Respiratory depression Chest pain	Euphoria Paranoid psychosis Panic attacks/ anxiety Insomnia/ excitement	Fatigue Hunger Depression Irritability Craving Social withdrawal	12–18 hours	Up to 96 hours	Food/tea containing coco leaves Codeine Ephedrine/ pseudoephedrine

(Continued)

Table 6.13 (*Continued*)

Drug	Physical signs/ symptoms of intoxication	Most common mental state changes[8]	Withdrawal symptoms	Duration of withdrawal	Duration of detection in the urine[9]	Other substances which give a positive result[10]
Heroin	Pinpoint pupils Clammy skin Respiratory depression	Drowsiness Euphoria Hallucinations	Dilated pupils Nausea Diarrhoea Generalised pains Gooseflesh Runny nose/ eyes;	Peaks after 36–72 hours	Up to 72 hours	Diphenoxylate Naltrexone Opiate analgesics Food/tea containing poppy seed
Methadone	Pinpoint pupils Respiratory depression Pulmonary oedema	As above	As above but milder and longer lasting	Peaks after 4–6 days; can last 6 weeks	Up to 7 days with chronic use	

References

1. UK National Statistics. Drug Misuse: Findings from the 2012 to 2013 Crime Survey for England and Wales. https://www.gov.uk/government/uploads/system/uploads/attachment_data/file/225122/Drugs_Misuse201213.pdf.
2. Menezes PR et al. Drug and alcohol problems among individuals with severe mental illness in south London. Br J Psychiatry 1996; 168:612–619.
3. Phillips P. et al. Drug and alcohol misuse among in-patients with psychotic illnesses in three inner-London psychiatric units. Psychiatr Bull 2003; 27:217–220.
4. Sara GE et al. The impact of cannabis and stimulant disorders on diagnostic stability in psychosis. J Clin Psychiatry 2014; 75:349–356.
5. Di FM et al. High-potency cannabis and the risk of psychosis. Br J Psychiatry 2009; 195:488–491.
6. Hunt GE et al. Medication compliance and comorbid substance abuse in schizophrenia: impact on community survival 4 years after a relapse. Schizophr Res 2002; 54:253–264.
7. Couchman L et al. Amisulpride and sulpiride interfere in the C&DIA DAU buprenorphine test. Ann Clin Psychiatry 2008; 45 Suppl 1.
8. Truven Health Analytics. Micromedex 2.0. http://www.micromedex.com/ . 2013.
9. Substance Abuse and Mental Health Services Administration (US). Substance abuse: clinical issues in intensive outpatient treatment. Treatment Improvement Protocol (TIP) Series, No. 47. http://store.samhsa.gov/product/TIP-47-Substance-Abuse-Clinical-Issues-in-Intensive-Outpatient-Treatment/SMA13-4182. 2006.
10. Brahm NC et al. Commonly prescribed medications and potential false-positive urine drug screens. Am J Health Syst Pharm 2010; 67:1344–1350.
11. Shoptaw SJ et al. Treatment for amphetamine psychosis. Cochrane Database Syst Rev 2009;CD003026.
12. Johns A. Psychiatric effects of cannabis. Br J Psychiatry 2001; 178:116–122.
13. Hall W et al. Long-term cannabis use and mental health. Br J Psychiatry 1997; 171:107–108.
14. Arseneault L et al. Causal association between cannabis and psychosis: examination of the evidence. Br J Psychiatry 2004; 184:110–117.
15. Budney AJ et al. Review of the validity and significance of cannabis withdrawal syndrome. Am J Psychiatry 2004; 161:1967–1977.

Interactions between 'street drugs' and prescribed psychotropic drugs

There are some significant interactions between 'street drugs' and drugs that are prescribed for the treatment of mental illness. Information comes from case reports or theoretical assumptions, rarely from systematic investigation. A summary can be found in Table 6.14, but remember that the evidence base is poor. Always be cautious.

In all patients who misuse street drugs:

- Infection with hepatitis B and C is common. The associated liver damage may lead to a reduced ability to metabolise other drugs and increased sensitivity to adverse effects.
- Infection with HIV is common.[1,2] Antiretroviral drugs are involved in pharmacokinetic interactions with a number of prescribed drugs. For example, ritonavir can decrease the metabolism of Ecstasy and precipitate toxicity, and a number of antiretrovirals can increase or decrease methadone metabolism;[3] see section on 'HIV' in Chapter 7 for a summary.
- Prescribed drugs may be used in the same way as illicit drugs (i.e. erratically and not as intended). Large quantities of prescribed drugs should not be given to outpatients.
- Additive or synergistic effects of respiratory depressants may play a contributory role in deaths from overdose with methadone or other opioid agonists.[4] Caution is needed in prescribing sedative medicines such as benzodiazepines.

Acute behavioural disturbance

Acute intoxication with street drugs may result in behavioural disturbance. Non-drug management is preferable. If at all possible a urine drug screen should be performed to determine the drugs that have been taken before prescribing any psychotropic. A physical examination should be done if possible (BP, TPR and ECG).

If intervention with a psychotropic is unavoidable, promethazine 50 mg *or* olanzapine 10 mg po/IM are probably the safest options. Temperature, pulse, respiration and blood pressure *must* be monitored afterwards. Benzodiazepines are commonly misused with other street drugs and so standard doses may be ineffective in tolerant users. Interactions are also possible (see Table 6.14). Try to avoid the use of benzodiazepines: they are unlikely to be effective at standard clinical doses.

Table 6.14 Interactions between 'street drugs' and psychotropics

	Cannabis	Heroin/methadone[5]	Cocaine Amfetamines, Ecstasy, MDA, 6-APD	Alcohol
General considerations	▪ Usually smoked in cigarettes (induces CYP1A2) ▪ Can be sedative ▪ Dose-related tachycardia	▪ Can produce sedation/respiratory depression ▪ QTc prolongation also reported with methadone (see section on 'Methadone' in this chapter)	▪ Stimulants (cocaine can be sedative in higher doses) ▪ Arrhythmia possible ▪ Cerebral/cardiac ischaemia with cocaine – may be fatal ▪ Hyperthermia/dehydration with ecstasy[6]	▪ Sedative ▪ Liver damage possible
Older antipsychotics	▪ Antipsychotics reduce the psychotropic effects of almost all drugs of abuse by blocking dopamine receptors (dopamine is the neurotransmitter responsible for 'reward') ▪ Patients prescribed antipsychotics may increase their consumption of illicit substances to compensate ▪ Patients who have taken ecstasy may be more prone to EPS ▪ Cardiotoxic or very sedative antipsychotics are best avoided, at least initially. Sulpiride is a reasonably safe first choice			
Atypicals	▪ Risk of additive sedation ▪ Cannabis can reduce plasma levels of olanzapine and clozapine via induction of CYP1A2[7] ▪ Clozapine might reduce cannabis and alcohol consumption[8]	▪ Risk of additive sedation ▪ Case report of methadone withdrawal being precipitated by risperidone[9] ▪ Isolated report of quetiapine increasing methadone levels, especially in those with slowed CYP2D6 hepatic metabolism[10]	▪ Antipsychotics may reduce craving and cocaine-induced euphoria[11–15] ▪ Olanzapine may worsen cocaine dependency[16] ▪ Clozapine may increase cocaine levels but diminish subjective response[17]	▪ Increased risk of hypotension with olanzapine (and possibly other α-blockers)
Antidepressants	Tachycardia has been reported (monitor pulse and take care with TCAs[18])	▪ Avoid very sedative antidepressants ▪ Some SSRIs can increase methadone plasma levels[19] (citalopram is SSRI of choice but note the small risk of additive QTc prolongation) ▪ Case report of serotonin syndrome occurring when sertraline prescribed with methadone for a palliative care patient[20]	▪ Avoid TCAs (arrhythmia risk) ▪ MAOIs contraindicated (hypertension) ▪ SSRI antidepressants are generally ineffective at attenuating withdrawal effects from cocaine[21] ▪ Risk of SSRIs increasing cocaine levels, especially fluoxetine[22] ▪ Concomitant use of SSRIs, cocaine or other stimulants (especially MDA and 6-APD) could precipitate a serotonin syndrome[23] ▪ SSRIs may enhance subjective reaction to cocaine[24]	▪ Avoid very sedative antidepressants ▪ Avoid antidepressants that are toxic in OD ▪ Impaired psychomotor skills (not SSRIs)

(Continued)

Table 6.14 (Continued)

	Cannabis	Heroin/methadone[5]	Cocaine Amfetamines, Ecstasy, MDA, 6-APD	Alcohol
Anticholinergics	■ Misuse is likely. Try to avoid if at all possible (by using a second-generation drug if an antipsychotic is required) ■ Can cause hallucinations, elation and cognitive impairment			
Lithium	■ Very toxic if taken erratically ■ Always consider the effects of dehydration (particularly problematic with alcohol or ecstasy)			
Carbamazepine/ valproate		■ Carbamazepine (CBZ) decreases methadone levels[25] (danger if CBZ stopped suddenly) ■ Valproate seems less likely to interact	■ Carbamazapine induces CYP3A4, which leads to increased formation of norcocaine (hepatotoxic and more cardiotoxic than cocaine)[26]	■ Monitor LFTs
Benzodiazepines (Always remember that benzodiazepines are liable to misuse)	Monitor level of sedation	■ Oversedation (and respiratory depression possible) ■ Concomitant use can lead to accidental overdose ■ Possible pharmacokinetic interaction (increased methadone levels)	■ Oversedation (if high doses of cocaine have been taken) ■ Widely used after cocaine intoxication ■ Future misuse possible detoxification	■ Oversedation (and respiratory depression) possible ■ Widely used in alcohol detoxification

6-APB, 6-(2-aminopropyl)benzofuran or 1-benzofuran-6-ylpropan-2-amine; CBZ, carbamazepine; LFT, liver function test; MAOI, monoamine oxidase inhibitor; MDA, 3,4-methylenedioxyamfetamine; OD, overdose; SSRI, selective serotonin reuptake inhibitor; TCA, tricyclic antidepressant.

References

1. Vocci FJ et al. Medication development for addictive disorders: the state of the science. Am J Psychiatry 2005; **162**:1432–1440.
2. Tsuang J et al. Pharmacological treatment of patients with schizophrenia and substance abuse disorders. Addict Disord Treat 2005; **4**:127–137.
3. Gruber VA et al. Methadone, buprenorphine, and street drug interactions with antiretroviral medications. Curr HIV /AIDS Rep 2010; **7**:152–160.
4. National Institute for Health and Clinical Excellence. Drug misuse: opioid detoxification. Clinical Guideline 52, 2007.
5. Department of Health. Drug misuse and dependence. UK guidelines on clinical management. London: DH; 2007.
6. Gowing LR et al. The health effects of ecstasy: a literature review. Drug Alcohol Rev 2002; **21**:53–63.
7. Zullino DF et al. Tobacco and cannabis smoking cessation can lead to intoxication with clozapine or olanzapine. Int Clin Psychopharmacol 2002; **17**:141–143.
8. Green AI et al. Alcohol and cannabis use in schizophrenia: effects of clozapine vs. risperidone. Schizophr Res 2003; **60**:81–85.
9. Wines JD, Jr. et al. Opioid withdrawal during risperidone treatment. J Clin Psychopharmacol 1999; **19**:265–267.
10. Uehlinger C et al. Increased (R)-methadone plasma concentrations by quetiapine in cytochrome P450s and ABCB1 genotyped patients. J Clin Psychopharmacol 2007; **27**:273–278.
11. Poling J et al. Risperidone for substance dependent psychotic patients. Addict Disord Treat 2005; **4**:1–3.
12. Albanese MJ et al. Risperidone in cocaine-dependent patients with comorbid psychiatric disorders. J Psychiatr Pract 2006; **12**:306–311.
13. Sattar SP et al. Potential benefits of quetiapine in the treatment of substance dependence disorders. J Psychiatry Neurosci 2004; **29**:452–457.
14. Grabowski J et al. Risperidone for the treatment of cocaine dependence: randomized, double-blind trial. J Clin Psychopharmacol 2000; **20**:305–310.
15. Kishi T et al. Antipsychotics for cocaine or psychostimulant dependence: systematic review and meta-analysis of randomized, placebo-controlled trials. J Clin Psychiatry 2013; **74**:e1169–e1180.
16. Kampman KM et al. A pilot trial of olanzapine for the treatment of cocaine dependence. Drug Alcohol Depend 2003; **70**:265–273.
17. Farren CK et al. Significant interaction between clozapine and cocaine in cocaine addicts. Drug Alcohol Depend 2000; **59**:153–163.
18. Benowitz NL et al. Effects of delta-9-tetrahydrocannabinol on drug distribution and metabolism. Antipyrine, pentobarbital, and ethanol. Clin Pharmacol Ther 1977; **22**:259–268.
19. Hemeryck A et al. Selective serotonin reuptake inhibitors and cytochrome P-450 mediated drug-drug interactions: an update. Curr Drug Metab 2002; **3**:13–37.
20. Bush E et al. A case of serotonin syndrome and mutism associated with methadone. J Palliat Med 2006; **9**:1257-1259.
21. Pani PP et al. Antidepressants for cocaine dependence and problematic cocaine use. Cochrane Database Syst Rev 2011;CD002950.
22. Fletcher PJ et al. Fluoxetine, but not sertraline or citalopram, potentiates the locomotor stimulant effect of cocaine: possible pharmacokinetic effects. Psychopharmacology (Berl) 2004; **174**:406–413.
23. Silins E et al. Qualitative review of serotonin syndrome, ecstasy (MDMA) and the use of other serotonergic substances: hierarchy of risk. Aust N Z J Psychiatry 2007; **41**:649–655.
24. Soto PL et al. Citalopram enhances cocaine's subjective effects in rats. Behav Pharmacol 2009; **20**:759–762.
25. Miller BL et al. Neuropsychiatric Effects of Cocaine: SPECT Measurements. In: Paredes A, Gorelick DA, eds. Cocaine: Physiological and Physiopathological Effects. 1 ed. New York: Haworth Press; 1993. 47–58.
26. Roldan CJ, Habal R. Toxicity, cocaine. http://www.emedicine.com/ . 2004.

Further reading

Hunt GE et al. Psychosocial interventions for people with both severe mental illness and substance misuse. Cochrane Database Syst Rev 2013; **10**:CD001088

Chapter 7

Use of psychotropic drugs in special patient groups

The elderly

General principles of prescribing in the elderly

The pharmacokinetics and pharmacodynamics of most drugs are altered to an important extent in the elderly. These changes in drug handling and action must be taken into account if treatment is to be effective and adverse effects minimised. The elderly often have a number of concurrent illnesses and may require treatment with several drugs. This leads to a greater chance of problems arising because of drug interactions and to a higher rate of drug-induced problems in general.[1] It is reasonable to assume that all drugs are more likely to cause adverse effects in the elderly than in younger patients.

How drugs affect the ageing body (altered pharmacodynamics)

As we age, control over reflex actions such as blood pressure and temperature regulation is reduced. Receptors may become more sensitive. This results in an increased incidence and severity of side-effects. For example, drugs that decrease gut motility are more likely to cause constipation (e.g. anticholinergics and opioids) and drugs that affect blood pressure are more likely to cause falls (e.g. tricyclic antidepressants [TCAs] and diuretics). The elderly are more sensitive to the effects of benzodiazepines than younger adults. Therapeutic response can also be delayed; the elderly may take longer to respond to antidepressants than younger adults.[2]

The elderly may be more prone to develop serious side-effects from some drugs such as agranulocytosis[3] and neutropenia[4] with clozapine, stroke with antipsychotic drugs[5] and bleeding with selective serotonin reuptake inhibitors (SSRIs).

The Maudsley Prescribing Guidelines in Psychiatry, Twelfth Edition. David Taylor, Carol Paton and Shitij Kapur.
© 2015 David Taylor, Carol Paton and Shitij Kapur. Published 2015 by John Wiley & Sons, Ltd.

How ageing affects drug therapy (altered pharmacokinetics)[6]

Absorption

Gut motility decreases with age, as does secretion of gastric acid. This leads to drugs being absorbed more slowly, resulting in a slower onset of action. The same *amount* of drug is absorbed as in a younger adult, but rate of absorption is slower.

Distribution

The elderly have more body fat, less body water and less albumin than younger adults. This leads to an increased volume of distribution and a longer duration of action for some fat-soluble drugs (e.g. diazepam), higher concentrations of some drugs at the site of action (e.g. digoxin) and a reduction in the amount of drug bound to albumin (increased amounts of active 'free drug', e.g. warfarin, phenytoin).

Metabolism

The majority of drugs are hepatically metabolised. Liver size is reduced in the elderly, but in the absence of hepatic disease or significantly reduced hepatic blood flow, there is no significant reduction in metabolic capacity. The magnitude of pharmacokinetic interactions is unlikely to be altered but the pharmacodynamic consequences of these interactions may be amplified.

Excretion

Renal function declines with age: 35% of function is lost by the age of 65 years and 50% by the age of 80.

More function is lost if there are concurrent medical problems such as heart disease, diabetes or hypertension. Measurement of serum creatinine or urea can be misleading in the elderly because muscle mass is reduced, so less creatinine is produced. It is particularly important that estimated glomerular filtration rate (eGFR)[7] is used as a measure of renal function in this age group. It is best to assume that all elderly patients have at most two-thirds of normal renal function.

Most drugs are eventually (after metabolism) excreted by the kidney. A few do not undergo biotransformation first. Lithium and sulpiride are important examples. Drugs primarily excreted via the kidney will accumulate in the elderly, leading to toxicity and side-effects. Dosage reduction is likely to be required (see section on 'Renal impairment' in this chapter).

Drug interactions

Some drugs have a narrow therapeutic index (a small increase in dose can cause toxicity and a small reduction in dose can cause a loss of therapeutic action). The most commonly prescribed ones are: digoxin, warfarin, theophylline, phenytoin and lithium. Changes in the way these drugs are handled in the elderly and the greater chance of interaction with other drugs mean that toxicity and therapeutic failure are more likely. These drugs can be used safely but extra care must be taken and blood concentrations should be measured where possible. See Box 7.1.

Some drugs inhibit or induce hepatic metabolising enzymes. Important examples include some SSRIs, erythromycin and carbamazepine. This may lead to the metabolism of another drug being altered. Many drug interactions occur through this mechanism.

Box 7.1 Reducing drug-related risk in the elderly

Adherence to the following principles will reduce drug-related morbidity and mortality.
- Use drugs only when absolutely necessary.
- Avoid, if possible, drugs that block α_1-adrenoceptors, have anticholinergic side-effects, are very sedative, have a long half-life or are potent inhibitors of hepatic metabolising enzymes.
- Start with a low dose and increase slowly but do not undertreat. Some drugs still require the full adult dose.
- Try not to treat the side-effects of one drug with another drug. Find a better-tolerated alternative.
- Keep therapy simple; that is, once daily administration whenever possible.

Details of individual interactions and their consequences can be found in Appendix 1 of the *BNF*.[8] Most can be predicted by a sound knowledge of pharmacology.

Administering medicines in foodstuffs[9–11]

Sometimes patients may refuse treatment with medicines, even when such treatment is thought to be in their best interests. Where the patient has a mental illness or has capacity, the Mental Health Act should be used, but if the patient lacks capacity, this option may not be desirable. Medicines should never be administered covertly to elderly patients with dementia without a full discussion with the multi-disciplinary team (MDT) and the patient's relatives. The outcome of this discussion should be clearly documented in the patient's clinical notes. Medicine should be administered covertly only if the clear and express purpose is to reduce suffering for the patient. For further information, see section on 'Covert administration of medicines within food and drink' in Chapter 8.

For advice on dosing of psychotropics in the elderly, see Table 7.1.

References

1. Royal College of Physicians. Medication for older people. Summary and recommendations of a report of a working party. J R Coll Physicians Lond 1997; **31**:254–257.
2. Baldwin R et al. Management of depression in later life. Adv Psychiatr Treat 2004; **10**:131–139.
3. Munro J et al. Active monitoring of 12,760 clozapine recipients in the UK and Ireland. Beyond pharmacovigilance. Br J Psychiatry 1999; **175**:576–580.
4. O'Connor DW et al. The safety and tolerability of clozapine in aged patients: a retrospective clinical file review. World J Biol Psychiatry 2010; **11**:788–791.
5. Douglas IJ et al. Exposure to antipsychotics and risk of stroke: self controlled case series study. BMJ 2008; **337**:a1227.
6. Mayersohn M. Special pharmacokinetic considerations in the elderly. In: Evans WE, Schentag JJ, Jusko WJ, eds. *Applied Pharmacokinetics Principles of Therapeutic Drug Monitoring*. Spokane, WA: Applied Therapeutics Inc; 1986. pp. 229–293.
7. Morriss R et al. Lithium and eGFR: a new routinely available tool for the prevention of chronic kidney disease. Br J Psychiatry 2008; **193**:93–95.
8. Joint Formulary Committee. BNF 67 March-September 2014 (online). London: Pharmaceutical Press; 2014. http://www.medicinescomplete.com/mc/bnf/current/
9. Royal College of Psychiatrists. College Statement on Covert Administration of Medicines. Psychiatr Bull 2004; **28**:385–386.
10. Haw C et al. Administration of medicines in food and drink: a study of older inpatients with severe mental illness. Int Psychogeriatr 2010; **22**:409–416.
11. Haw C et al. Covert administration of medication to older adults: a review of the literature and published studies. J Psychiatr Ment Health Nurs 2010; **17**:761–768.

Further reading

National Service Framework for Older People. London: Department of Health; 2001.

CHAPTER 7

Table 7.1 A guide to medication doses of commonly used psychotropics in older adults

Drug	Specific indication/additional notes	Starting dose	Usual maintenance dose	Maximum dose in elderly
Antidepressants				
Agomelatine	Depression Monitor LFTs Data suggest agomelatine is not effective in patients >75 years	25 mg nocte	25–50 mg daily	50 mg nocte
Citalopram	Depression/anxiety disorder	10 mg mane	10–20 mg mane	20 mg mane
Clomipramine	Depression/phobic and obsessional states	10 mg nocte (dose increases should be cautious)	30–75 mg daily[1] should be reached after about 10 days	75 mg daily*
Desvenlafaxine	No formal recommendations are available for dosing in older adults[2]			
Duloxetine	Depression/anxiety disorder	30 mg daily*	60 mg daily	120 mg daily* (caution as limited data in elderly for this dose)
Escitalopram	Depression/anxiety disorder	5 mg mane	5–10 mg mane	10 mg mane
Fluoxetine	Depression/anxiety disorder Caution as long half-life and inhibitor of several CYP enzymes	20 mg mane	20 mg mane	40 mg mane usually (but 60 mg can be used)
Lofepramine	Depression	35 mg nocte*	70 mg nocte*	140 mg nocte or in divided doses* (occasionally 210 mg nocte required)
Mirtazapine	Depression	7.5 mg nocte or usually 15 mg nocte*	15–30mg nocte	45 mg nocte
Sertraline	Depression/anxiety disorder	25–50 mg mane (25 mg can be increased to 50 mg mane after 1 week)	50–100 mg mane*	100 mg (occasionally up to 150 mg mane)*

Drug	Specific indication/additional notes	Starting dose	Usual maintenance dose	Maximum dose in elderly
Trazodone	Depression	50 mg bd	100–200 mg daily*	300 mg daily[4]
	Agitation in dementia Avoid single doses >100 mg	25 mg bd*	25–100 mg daily*	200 mg daily* (in divided doses)
Venlafaxine	Depression/anxiety disorder Monitor BP on initiation	37.5 mg mane (increased to 75 mg [ER] mane after 1 week)*	75–150 mg (ER) mane*	150 mg daily (occasionally 225 mg daily necessary)*
Vortioxetine	Major depressive disorder	5–10 mg daily[5]	5–20 mg daily[5]	20 mg daily[5]
Drug	**Specific indication/additional notes**	**Starting dose**	**Usual maintenance dose**	**Maximum dose in elderly**
Antipsychotics				
Amisulpride	Chronic schizophrenia	50 mg daily*	100–200 mg daily*	400 mg daily[6] (caution >200 mg daily)*
	Late life psychosis	25–50mg daily*	50–100 mg daily* (increase in 25 mg steps)	200 mg daily[7] (caution >100 mg daily)*
	Agitation/psychosis in dementia Caution QTc prolongation	25 mg nocte[8]	25–50mg daily[8]	50 mg daily[8]
Aripiprazole	Schizophrenia, mania (oral)	5 mg mane*	5–15 mg daily*	20 mg mane*
	Control of agitation (IM injection)	5.25 mg*	5.25–9.75 mg*	15 mg daily* (combined oral + IM)
Clozapine	Schizophrenia	6.25–12.5 mg daily[9,10] increased by no more than 6.25–12.5 mg once or twice a week[9]	50–100 mg daily[9,10]	100 mg daily[9,10]
	Parkinson's related psychosis	6.25 mg daily[11]	25–37.5 mg daily[11]	50 mg daily[11]
Iloperidone	No formal recommendations are available for dosing in older adults			
Lurasidone	No formal recommendations are available for dosing in older adults In elderly patients (65 to 85years) lurasidone concentrations were similar to those in young subjects. It is unknown whether dose adjustment is necessary on the basis of age alone (but dose reduction required in moderate and severe renal impairment- see product information)[12]			

(Continued)

Table 7.1 (*Continued*)

Drug	Specific indication/additional notes	Starting dose	Usual maintenance dose	Maximum dose in elderly
Olanzapine	Schizophrenia	2.5 mg nocte*	5–10 mg daily*	15 mg nocte[10]
	Agitation/psychosis in dementia	2.5 mg nocte*	2.5–10 mg daily*	10 mg nocte* (optimal dose is 5 mg daily)[10]
Quetiapine	Schizophrenia	12.5–25 mg daily[10]	75–125 mg daily[9]	200–300 mg daily[10]
	Agitation/psychosis in dementia	12.5–25 mg daily*	50–100 mg daily*	100–300 mg daily[10]
Risperidone	Psychosis	0.5 mg bd (0.25–0.5 mg daily in some cases)[10]	1.0–2.5 mg daily[9]	4 mg daily
	Late onset psychosis	0.5 mg daily*	1 mg daily*	2 mg daily* (optimal dose is 1 mg daily)
	Agitation/psychosis in dementia	0.25 mg daily* or bd	0.5 mg bd	2 mg daily (optimal dose is 1 mg daily)[10]
Haloperidol	Psychosis	0.25–0.5 mg daily[9]	1.0–3.5 mg daily[9]	Caution >3.5 mg – assess tolerability and ECG Max 10 mg/day (oral) Max 5 mg/day (IM)
	Agitation Avoid in older adults (except in delirium) owing to risk of QTc prolongation	0.25–0.5mg daily*	0.5–1.5 mg daily or bd	

Drug	Specific indication/additional notes	Starting dose	Usual maintenance dose	Maximum dose in elderly
Long-acting conventional antipsychotic drugs				
Flupentixol decanoate (Depixol)		Test dose: 5–10 mg	After at least 7 days of test dose: 10–20mg every 2–4 weeks* Dose increased gradually according to response and tolerability in steps of 5–10 mg every 2 weeks*	40 mg every 2 weeks* (extend frequency to every 3–4 weeks if EPS develop) (occasionally up to 50 or 60 mg every 2 weeks* may be used if tolerated)

Drug			
Fluphenazine decanoate	Caution – high risk of EPS	Test dose 6.25 mg	After 4–7 days of test dose: 12.5–25mg every 2–4 weeks Dose increased gradually according to response and tolerability in steps of 12.5 mg every 2–4 weeks*	50 mg every 4 weeks*
Haloperidol decanoate	Risk of EPS and QTc prolongation	(No test dose) 12.5–25 mg every 4 weeks	12.5–25 mg every 4 weeks	50 mg every 4 weeks*
Pipotiazine palmitate		Test dose: 5–10 mg (or 12.5 mg*)	After 4–7 days of test dose: 12.5–25 mg every 2–4 weeks (initially can be every 2 weeks to achieve steady state quickly) then 25–50 mg every 4 weeks*	50 mg every 4 weeks*
Zuclopenthixol decanoate (Clopixol)		Test dose: 25–50 mg	After at least 7 days of test dose: 50–200 mg every 2–4 weeks*	200 mg every 2 weeks*

Long-acting atypical antipsychotic drugs

Drug			
Aripiprazole Long-acting injection	No formal recommendations are available for dosing in older adults However, no detectable effect of age on pharmacokinetics[13]		
Paliperidone palmitate	Dose based on renal function- Because elderly patients may have diminished renal function, they are dosed as in mild renal impairment even if tests show normal renal function*	Loading doses: Day 1: 100 mg Day 8: 75 mg (lower loading doses may be appropriate in some)*	25–100 mg monthly*	100 mg monthly*
Risperidone Long-acting injection	Monitor renal function	25 mg every 2 weeks	25 mg every 2 weeks	25 mg every 2 weeks Consider 37.5mg every 2 weeks in patients treated with oral risperidone doses >4 mg/day[14]

(Continued)

Table 7.1 (Continued)

Drug	Specific indication/additional notes	Starting dose	Usual maintenance dose	Maximum dose in elderly
Mood stabilisers				
Carbamazepine	Bipolar disorder Caution – drug interactions Check LFTs, FBC and U&Es Consider checking plasma levels	50 mg bd or 100 mg bd*	200–400 mg/day*	600–800 mg/day*
Lamotrigine	Bipolar disorder (titration as in young adults) Check for interactions and make appropriate dose alterations (see *BNF*)	25 mg daily (monotherapy) 25 mg on alternate days (if with valproate) 50 mg daily (if with carbamazepine)	Increase by 25 mg steps every 14 days Increase by 25 mg steps every 14 days Increase by 50 mg steps every 14 days	200 mg/day* 100 mg/day* 100 mg bd*
Lithium carbonate M/R	Bipolar disorder Mania/depression Caution – drug interactions Check renal and thyroid function and regularly monitor plasma levels	100–200 mg nocte*	200–600 mg daily*	600–1200 mg daily (aim for plasma levels 0.4–0.8 mmol/L in elderly)[15]
Sodium valproate	Bipolar disorder Check LFTs and consider checking plasma levels	Sodium valproate: 100 mg–200 mg bd* Semi-sodium valproate: 250 mg daily or bd*	Sodium valproate: 200–400 mg bd* Semi-sodium valproate: 500 mg –1g daily*	Sodium valproate: 400 mg bd* Semi-sodium valproate: 1g daily*
	Agitation in dementia (not licensed and not recommended) Check response, tolerability and plasma levels for guide	Sodium valproate: 50 mg bd (liquid) or 100 mg bd*	Sodium valproate: 100–200 mg bd*	Sodium valproate: 200 mg bd*
Anxiolytics/hypnotics				
Clonazepam	Agitation	0.5 mg daily	1–2 mg/day*	4 mg/day*
Diazepam	Agitation	1 mg tds		6 mg/day*

Lorazepam	PRN only- avoid regular use due to short half-life and risk of dependence	0.5 mg daily	0.5–2 mg daily*	2 mg/day
Melatonin	Insomnia- short term use (up to 13 weeks)	2 mg (modified release) once daily (1–2 hours before bedtime)		
Pregabalin	Generalised anxiety disorder Dose adjustment based on renal function (see product information)[16]	Usually 25 mg bd (increase by 25 mg bd weekly) Up to 75 mg bd (if healthy and normal renal function)	Usually 150 mg daily* Up to 150 mg bd (if healthy and normal renal function)	150–300 mg/day*
Zolpidem	Insomnia (short term use – up to 4 weeks)	5 mg nocte	5 mg nocte	5 mg nocte
Zopiclone	Insomnia (short term use – up to 4 weeks)	3.75 mg nocte	3.75–7.5 mg nocte	7.5 mg nocte

*There is no information available in the literature for these drug doses in elderly patients – the doses stated are a guide only. Where there are no data, the maximum doses are conservative and may be exceeded if the drug is well tolerated and following clinician's assessment.

All doses are from the *British National Formulary* (66th edition 2013) unless otherwise indicated.

bd, *bis die* (twice a day); BP, blood pressure; CYP, cytochrome P450; EPS, extrapyramidal side-effects; ER, extended release; FBC, full blood count; IM, intramuscular; LFTs, liver function tests; mane, morning; nocte, at night; prn, *pro re nata* (as required); tds, *ter die sumendum* (three times a day); U&Es, urea and electrolytes.

CHAPTER 7

References

1. Novartis Pharmaceuticals UK Ltd. Summary of Product Characteristics. Anafranil 75mg SR Tablets. 2014. http://www.medicines.org.uk/emc/medicine/1267
2. Physicians' Desk Reference. Drug Summary - Desvenlafaxine. 2014. http://www.pdr.net/drug-summary/pristiq?druglabelid=625
3. Eli Lilly and Company Limited. Summary of Product Characteristics. Cymbalta 30mg hard gastro-resistant capsules, Cymbalta 60mg hard gastro-resistant capsules. 2013. http://www.medicines.org.uk/
4. Zentiva. Summary of Product Characteristics. Molipaxin 100mg Capsules. 2013. http://www.medicines.org.uk/
5. Physicians' Desk Reference. Drug Summary - Vortioxetine. 2014. http://www.pdr.net/drug-summary/brintellix?druglabelid=3348
6. Muller MJ et al. Amisulpride doses and plasma levels in different age groups of patients with schizophrenia or schizoaffective disorder. J Psychopharmacol 2009; **23**:278–286.
7. Psarros C et al. Amisulpride for the treatment of very-late-onset schizophrenia-like psychosis. Int J Geriatr Psychiatry 2009; **24**:518–522.
8. Clark-Papasavas C et al. Towards a therapeutic window of D2/3 occupancy for treatment of psychosis in Alzheimer's disease, with [F]fallypride positron emission tomography. Int J Geriatr Psychiatry 2014; Epub ahead of print.
9. Jeste DV et al. Conventional vs. newer antipsychotics in elderly patients. Am J Geriatr Psychiatry 1999; **7**:70–76.
10. Karim S et al. Treatment of psychosis in elderly people. Adv Psychiatr Treat 2005; **11**:286–296.
11. The Parkinson Study Group. Low-dose clozapine for the treatment of drug-induced psychosis in Parkinson's Disease. N Engl J Med 1999; **340**:757–763.
12. Physicians' Desk Reference. Drug Summary - Lurasidone Hydrochloride. 2014. http://www.pdr.net/drug-summary/latuda?druglabelid=553
13. Otsuka Pharmaceuticals (UK) Ltd. Summary of Product Characteristics. ABILIFY MAINTENA 400 mg powder and solvent for prolonged-release suspension for injection. 2014. https://www.medicines.org.uk/
14. Janssen-Cilag Ltd. Risperdal Consta 25, 37.5 and 50 mg powder and solvent for prolonged-release suspension for intramuscular injection. 2013. http://www.medicines.org.uk/
15. Sanofi. Summary of Product Characteristics. Priadel 200mg prolonged release tablets. 2013. http://www.medicines.org.uk
16. Pfizer Limited. Summary of Product Characteristics. Lyrica Capsules. 2014. http://www.medicines.org.uk/

Dementia

Dementia is a progressive, degenerative, neurological syndrome affecting around 5% of those aged over 65 years, rising to 20% in the over 80s. This age-related disorder is characterised by cognitive decline, impaired memory and thinking, and a gradual loss of skills needed to carry out activities of daily living. Often, other mental functions may also be affected, including changes in mood, personality and social behaviour.[1]

The various types of dementia are classified according to the different disease processes affecting the brain. The most common cause of dementia is Alzheimer's disease, accounting for around 60% of all cases. Vascular dementia and dementia with Lewy bodies (DLB) are responsible for most other cases. Alzheimer's disease and vascular dementia may co-exist and are often difficult to separate clinically. Dementia is also encountered in about 30% to 70% of patients with Parkinson's disease[1] (see section on 'Parkinson's disease' in this chapter).

Alzheimer's disease

Mechanism of action of cognitive enhancers used in Alzheimer's disease

Acetylcholinesterase (AChE) inhibitors

The cholinergic hypothesis of Alzheimer's disease is predicated on the observation that the cognitive deterioration associated with the disease results from progressive loss of cholinergic neurones and decreasing levels of acetylcholine (ACh) in the brain.[2] Both acetylcholinesterase (AChE) and butyrylcholinesterase (BuChE) have been found to play an important role in the degradation of ACh.[3]

Three inhibitors of AChE are currently licensed in the UK for the treatment of mild to moderate dementia in Alzheimer's disease: donepezil, rivastigmine and galantamine. In addition, rivastigmine is licensed in the treatment of mild-to-moderate dementia associated with Parkinson's disease. Cholinesterase inhibitors differ in pharmacological action: donepezil selectively inhibits AChE, rivastigmine affects both AChE and BuChE and galantamine selectively inhibits AChE and also has nicotinic receptor agonist properties.[4] To date, these differences have not been shown to result in differences in efficacy or tolerability. See Table 7.2 for comparison of AChE inhibitors.

Memantine

Memantine is licensed in the UK for the treatment of moderate-to-severe dementia in Alzheimer's disease. It acts as an antagonist at N-methyl-D-aspartate (NMDA) glutamate receptors. See Table 7.2.

Efficacy of drugs used in dementia

All three AChE-inhibitors seem to have broadly similar clinical effects, as measured with the Mini Mental State Examination (MMSE), a 30-point basic evaluation of cognitive function, and the Alzheimer's Disease Assessment Scale-cognitive subscale (ADAS-cog), a 70-point evaluation largely of cognitive dysfunction. Estimates of the number needed to treat (NNT) (improvement of >4 points ADAS-cog) range from 4 to 12.[14]

Cochrane reviews for all three AChE-Is have been carried out, both collectively as a group and individually for each drug. In the review for all AChE-Is, which included

CHAPTER 7

Table 7.2 Characteristics of cognitive enhancers[5-13]

Characteristic	Donepezil (Aricept®) (Pfizer, Eisai)	Rivastigmine (Exelon®) (Novartis)	Galantamine (Reminyl®) (Shire/Janssen-Cilag)	Memantine (Exiba®) (Lundbeck)
Primary mechanism	AChE-I (selective + reversible)	AChE-I (pseudo-irreversible)	AChE-I (selective + reversible)	NMDA receptor antagonist
Other mechanism	None	BuChE-I	Nicotine modulator	5-HT$_3$ receptor antagonist
Starting dose	5 mg daily	1.5 mg bd (oral) (or 4.6 mg/24 hours patch)	4 mg bd (or 8 mg ER daily)	5 mg daily
Usual treatment dose (max. dose)	10 mg daily	6 mg bd (oral) or 9.5 mg /24 hours patch	12 mg bd (or 24 mg ER daily)	20 mg daily or (10 mg bd)
Recommended minimum interval between dose increases	4 weeks (increase by 5 mg daily)	2 weeks for oral (increase by 1.5 mg twice a day) 4 weeks for patch (increase to 9.5 mg/ 24 hours) (can consider increase to 13.3 mg/24 hours after 6 months if tolerated and meaningful cognitive/ functional decline occurs on 9.5 mg/24 hours)	4 weeks (increase by 4 mg twice a day or 8 mg ER daily)	1 week (increase by 5 mg daily)
Adverse effects[5-12]	Diarrhoea* Nausea* Headache* Common cold Anorexia Hallucinations Agitation Aggressive behaviour Abnormal dreams and nightmares Syncope Dizziness Insomnia Vomiting Abdominal disturbance Rash Pruritis Muscle cramps Urinary incontinence Fatigue Pain	Anorexia* Dizziness* Nausea* Vomiting* Diarrhoea* Agitation Confusion Anxiety Headache Somnolence Tremor Abdominal pain and dyspepsia Sweating Fatigue and asthenia, Malaise Weight loss	Nausea* Vomiting* Decreased appetite Anorexia Hallucinations Depression Syncope Dizziness Tremor Headache Somnolence Lethargy Bradycardia Hypertension Abdominal pain and discomfort Diarrhoea Dyspepsia Sweating Muscle spasms Fatigue and asthenia Malaise Weight loss Fall	Drug hypersensitivity Somnolence Dizziness Balance disorders Hypertension Dyspnoea Constipation Elevated liver function test Headache

Table 7.2 *(Continued)*

Characteristic	Donepezil (Aricept®) (Pfizer, Eisai)	Rivastigmine (Exelon®) (Novartis)	Galantamine (Reminyl®) (Shire/Janssen-Cilag)	Memantine (Exiba®) (Lundbeck)
Half life (hours)	~70	~1 (oral) 3.4 (patch)	7–8 (tablets/oral solution) 8–10 (ER capsules)	60–100
Metabolism	CYP 3A4 CYP 2D6 (minor)	Non-hepatic	CYP 3A4 CYP 2D6	Primarily non-hepatic
Drug–drug interactions	Yes (see Table 7.3)	Interactions unlikely	Yes (see Table 7.3)	Yes (see Table 7.3)
Effect of food on absorption	None	Delays rate and extent of absorption	Delays rate but not extent of absorption	None
Cost of preparations[13] (for 1-month treatment at usual i.e. max. dose)	Tablets: £1.60 Orodispersible tablets: £12.00	Capsules:£33.24 Oral solution (2 mg/mL): £126.71 Patches (Exelon®) 4.6 mg, 9.5 mg and 13.3 mg: £77.97	Tablets: £74.10 Capsules MR: £79.80 Oral solution (Reminyl®) (4 mg/mL): £201.60	Tablets: £28.85 Oral solution (10 mg/mL): £67.12 NB: Bottles supplied with a dosing pump dispensing 5 mg in 0.5 mL per actuation
Relative cost	$	$$	$$$	$$
Patent status	Generic available	Generic available (but not patches)	Generic available (branded oral solution cheaper than generic)	Generic available

*very common: ≥1/10 and common: ≥1/100.
AChE-I, acetylcholinesterase inhibitor; bd, *bis die* (twice a day); BuChE-I, butyrylcholinesterase inhibitor; CYP, cytochrome P450; ER, extended release; 5-HT3, 5-hydroxytryptamine (serotonin); MR, modified release; NMDA, N-methyl-D-aspartate.

10 randomised controlled trials (RCTs), results demonstrated that treatment over 6 months produced improvements in cognitive function, of, on average, –2.7 points (95% CI –3.0 to –2.3, p < 0.00001) on the ADAS-cog scale. Benefits were also noted on measures of Activities of Daily Living (ADL) and behaviour, although none of these treatment effects was large. Despite the slight variations in the mode of action of the three drugs, there is no evidence of any differences between them with respect to efficacy.[15]

A review of the Technology Appraisal for AChE-Is and memantine concluded that the evidence of additional clinical effectiveness continues to suggest clinical benefit from AChE-Is in alleviating the symptoms of Alzheimer's disease, although there is considerable debate about the magnitude of effect. There is also some evidence that AChE-Is have an impact on controlling disease progression. Although there is also new evidence for the effectiveness of memantine, it remains less robust than the evidence supporting AChE-Is.[16]

Donepezil

Pivotal trials of donepezil[17–19] suggest an advantage over placebo of 2.5–3.1 points on the ADAS-cog scale. Results from the donepezil Cochrane review suggested statistically significant improvements for both 5 mg and 10 mg/day at 24 weeks compared with placebo on the ADAS-cog scale with a 2.01 point and a 2.80 point reduction, respectively.[20] A long-term placebo-controlled trial of donepezil in 565 patients with mild-to-moderate Alzheimer's disease found a small but significant benefit on cognition compared with placebo. This was reflected in a 0.8 point difference in the MMSE score (95% CI 0.5–1.2; p < 0.0001).[21] The size of the effect is similar to other trials.

Rivastigmine

Studies for rivastigmine[22,23] suggest an advantage of 2.6–4.9 points on the ADAS-cog scale over placebo. In the Cochrane review, high dose rivastigmine (6–12 mg daily) was associated with a 2 point improvement in cognitive function on the ADAS-cog score compared with placebo and a 2.2 point improvement in ADL at 26 weeks. At lower doses (4 mg daily or lower) differences were in the same direction but were only statistically significant for cognitive function.[15] **Rivastigmine transdermal patch** (9.5 mg/24 hours) has been shown to be as effective as the highest doses of capsules but with a superior tolerability profile in a 6-month double-blind, placebo-controlled RCT.[24]

Galantamine

Studies with galantamine[25–27] suggest an advantage over placebo of 2.9–3.9 on the ADAS-cog scale. The galantamine Cochrane review reported that treatment with the drug led to a significantly greater proportion of subjects with improved or unchanged global scale rating at all doses except for 8 mg/day. Point estimate of effect was lower for 8 mg/day but similar for 16–36 mg/day. Treatment effect for 24 mg/day over 6 months was 3.1 point reduction in ADAS-cog.[28] Data from two trials of galantamine in mild cognitive impairment suggest marginal clinical benefit but a yet unexplained excess in death rate.[28] Galantamine has been shown to be effective (albeit marginally so) in severe Alzheimer's disease in subjects with MMSE scores of 5–12 points.[29]

Memantine

A number needed to treat analysis of memantine found it to have an NNT (improvement) of 3–8.[30] The efficacy of memantine is evaluated using the ADAS-cog subscale to evaluate cognitive abilities in mild to moderate Alzheimer's disease and the Severe Impairment Battery (SIB) to evaluate cognitive functions in moderate to severe Alzheimer's disease. The SIB is a 40-item test with scores ranging from 0 to 100, higher scores reflecting higher levels of cognitive ability.[31] Trials in moderate-to-severe dementia found that memantine showed significant benefits on both scales.[32] A Cochrane review of memantine concluded that it had a small beneficial effect at 6 months in moderate-to-severe Alzheimer's disease. Statistically significant effects were detected on cognition, ADL and behaviour.[33]

Early data suggested memantine was effective in mild-to-moderate Alzheimer's disease with an advantage over placebo of 1.9 points on ADAS-cog.[34] Pooled data from unpublished studies in the Cochrane review in mild-to-moderate Alzheimer's disease indicated a marginal benefit at 6 months on cognition which was barely detectable clinically (0.99 points on ADAS-cog) but no effect on behaviour, ADL or observed case analysis of cognition.[33] A meta-analysis however found no significant differences between memantine and placebo on any outcome for patients with mild Alzheimer's disease either within any individual trial or when data were combined (ADAS-cog

–0.17; p = 0.82). For patients with moderate Alzheimer's disease, there were no significant differences between memantine and placebo on the ADAS-cog in any individual trial, although there was a significant effect when the three trials were statistically combined (–1.33; p = 0.006).[35]

Since these systematic reviews, a large multicentre study[36] of community-dwelling patients with moderate or severe Alzheimer's disease investigated the long-term effects of donepezil over 12 months compared with stopping donepezil after 3 months, switching to memantine or combining donepezil with memantine. Continued treatment with donepezil was associated with continued cognitive benefits and patients with a MMSE score as low as 3 were still benefiting from treatment. This suggests that patients should continue treatment with AChE-Is for as long as possible and there should not be a cut-off MMSE score where treatment is stopped automatically.

A meta-analysis evaluating the efficacy of the three AChE-Is and memantine in relation to the severity of Alzheimer's disease found that the efficacy of all drugs except memantine was independent of dementia severity in all domains. The effect of memantine on functional impairment was better in patients with more severe Alzheimer's disease. Results demonstrated that patients in differing stages of Alzheimer's disease retain the ability to respond to treatment with AChE-Is and memantine. Medication effects are therefore substantially independent from disease severity and patients with a wide range of severities can benefit from drug therapy. This suggests that the severity of a patient's illness should not preclude treatment with these drugs.[37]

Quantifying the effects of drugs in dementia

All the above results need to be interpreted with caution because of differences in the populations included in the different studies, especially as so few head-to-head studies have been published. Alzheimer's disease is usually characterised by inexorable cognitive decline, which is generally well quantified by tests such as ADAS-cog and MMSE. The average annual rate of decline in untreated patients ranges between 6 to 12 points on the ADAS-cog (and the annual increase in ADAS-cog in patients with untreated moderate Alzheimer's disease has been estimated to be as much as 9 to 11 points per year). A 4-point change in the ADAS-cog score is considered clinically meaningful.[38] It is, however, difficult to accurately predict treatment effect in individual patients. Acetylcholinesterase inhibitors, on average, have a modest symptomatic effect on cognition.

Switching between drugs used in dementia

The benefits of treatment with AChE-Is are rapidly lost when drug administration is interrupted[39] and may not be fully regained when drug treatment is reinitiated.[40] Poor tolerability with one agent does not rule out good tolerability with another.[41] Two cases of discontinuation syndrome upon stopping donepezil have been published[42] suggesting that a gradual withdrawal should be carried out where possible. However, a study comparing abrupt versus stepwise switching from donepezil to memantine found no clinically relevant differences in adverse effects despite patients in the abrupt group experiencing more frequent adverse effects than the stepwise discontinuation group (46% versus 32% respectively).[43] See section on 'Tolerability', below, for switching to a rivastigmine patch.

Following a systematic review of the literature,[44] a practical approach to switching between AChE-Is has been proposed: in the case of intolerance, switching to another agent should be done only after complete resolution of side-effects following discontinuation of the initial agent. In the case of lack of efficacy, switching can be done overnight, with a quicker titration scheme thereafter. Switching to another AChE-I is not recommended in individuals who show loss of benefit several years after initiation of therapy.

Other effects

AChE inhibitors may also affect non-cognitive aspects of Alzheimer's disease and other dementias. Several studies have investigated their safety and efficacy in managing the non-cognitive symptoms of dementia. For more information about the management of these symptoms, see section on 'Management of non-cognitive symptoms of dementia' in this chapter.

Dosing

Different titration schedules do, to some extent, differentiate AChE-Is (see Table 7.2 for dosing information). Donepezil has been perhaps the easiest to use and is given once daily. Both rivastigmine and galantamine have prolonged titration schedules and used to be given twice a day. These factors may be important to prescribers, patients and carers. This was demonstrated in a retrospective analysis of the patterns of use of AChE-Is, where it was shown that donepezil was significantly more likely to be prescribed at an effective dose than either rivastigmine or galantamine.[45] Galantamine, however, is now usually given once daily as the controlled-release formulation and rivastigmine is now available as a patch. Memantine once-daily dosing has been found to be similar in safety and tolerability as twice-daily dosing and may be more practical.[46]

Tolerability

Drug tolerability may differ between AChE-Is, but, again, in the absence of sufficient direct comparisons, it is difficult to draw definitive conclusions. Overall tolerability can be broadly evaluated by reference to the numbers withdrawing from clinical trials. Withdrawal rates in trials of donepezil[17,18] ranged from 4% to 16% (placebo 1–7%). With rivastigmine[22,23], rates ranged from 7% to 29% (placebo 7%) and with galantamine[25-27] from 7% to 23% (placebo 7–9%). These figures relate to withdrawals specifically associated with adverse effects. The number needed to harm (NNH) has been reported to be 12.[14] A study of the French pharmacovigilance database identified age, the use of antipsychotic drugs, antihypertensives, and drugs targeting the alimentary tract and metabolism, as factors associated with serious reactions to AChE-Is.[47]

Tolerability seems to be affected by speed of titration and, perhaps less clearly, by dose. Most adverse effects occurred in trials during titration, and slower titration schedules are recommended in clinical use. This may mean that these drugs are equally well tolerated in practice.

Rivastigmine patch may offer convenience and a superior tolerability profile to rivastigmine capsules.[24] Data from three trials found that rivastigmine patch was better tolerated than the capsules with fewer gastrointestinal adverse effects and discontinuations due to these adverse effects.[48] Data support recommendations for patients on high doses of rivastigmine capsules (>6 mg/day) to switch directly to the 9.5 mg/24-hours patch, while those on lower doses (≤6 mg/day) should start on 4.6 mg/hour patch for 4 weeks before increasing to the 9.5 mg/hour patch. This latter switch is also recommended for patients switching from other oral cholinesterase inhibitors to the rivastigmine patch (with a 1 week washout period in patients sensitive to adverse effects or who have very low body weight or a history of bradycardia).[49] A new strength for rivastigmine patches (13.3 mg/24 hours) has recently been approved. It is possible to consider increasing the dose to 13.3 mg/24 hours after 6 months on 9.5 mg/24 hours if tolerated and meaningful cognitive or functional decline occurs. A 48-week RCT found the higher strength patch to significantly reduce deterioration in instrumental activities of daily living (IADL) compared with the 9.5 mg/24-hours patch and was well tolerated.[50]

Memantine appears to be well tolerated[51,52] and the only conditions associated with warnings include hepatic impairment and epilepsy/seizures.[53]

Adverse effects

When adverse effects occur with **AChE-Is**, they are largely predictable: excess cholinergic stimulation can lead to nausea, vomiting, dizziness, insomnia and diarrhoea.[54] Such effects are most likely to occur at the start of therapy or when the dose is increased. They are dose-related and tend to be transient. Urinary incontinence has also been reported.[55] There appear to be no important differences between drugs in respect to type or frequency of adverse events, although clinical trials do suggest a relatively lower frequency of adverse events for donepezil. This may simply be a reflection of the aggressive titration schedules used in trials of other drugs. Gastrointestinal effects appeared to be more common with oral rivastigmine in clinical trials than with other cholinesterase inhibitors, however slower titration, ensuring oral rivastigmine is taken with food or using the patch, reduces the risk of gastrointestinal effects.

In view of their pharmacological action, AChE-Is may have vagotonic effects on heart rate (i.e. bradycardia). The potential for this action may be of particular importance in patients with 'sick sinus syndrome' or other supraventricular cardiac conduction disturbances, such as sinoatrial or atrioventricular block.[5–11]

Concerns over the potential cardiac adverse effects associated with AChE-Is were raised following findings from controlled trials of galantamine in mild cognitive impairment (MCI) in which increased mortality was associated with galantamine compared with placebo (1.5% versus 0.5% respectively).[56] Although no specific cause of death was predominant, half the deaths reported were due to cardiovascular disorders. As a result, the FDA issued a warning restricting galantamine in patients with MCI. The relevance in Alzheimer's disease remains unclear.[57] A Cochrane review of pooled data from RCTs of the AChE-Is revealed that there was a significantly higher incidence of syncope amongst the AChE-I groups compared with the placebo groups (3.43 versus 1.87%, p=0.02). A population-based study using a case-time-control design examined health records for 1.4 million older adults in Ontario and found that treatment with AChE-Is was associated with doubling the risk of hospitalisation for bradycardia. (The drugs were resumed at discharge in over half the cases suggesting that cardiovascular toxicity of AChE-Is is underappreciated by clinicians.)[58] It seems that patients with DLB are more susceptible to the bradyarrhythmic adverse effects of these drugs owing to the autonomic insufficiency associated with the disease.[59] A similar study found hospital visits for syncope were also more frequent in people receiving AChE-Is than in controls: 31.5 versus 18.6 events per 1000 person-years (adjusted HR 1.76; 95% CI, 1.57–1.98).[60]

The manufacturers of all three agents therefore advise that the drugs should be used with caution in patients with cardiovascular disease or in those taking concurrent medicines that reduce heart rate, e.g. digoxin or beta-blockers. Although a pre-treatment mandatory electrocardiogram (ECG) has been suggested,[57] a review of published evidence showed that the incidence of cardiovascular side-effects is low and that serious adverse effects are rare. In addition, the value of pre-treatment screening and routine ECGs is questionable and is not currently routinely recommended by the National Institute of Health and Care Excellence (NICE). However, in patients with a history of cardiovascular disease, or who are prescribed concomitant negative chronotropic drugs with AChE-Is, an ECG may be advised.

A study of 204 elderly patients with Alzheimer's disease had their ECG and blood pressure assessed before and after starting AChE-I therapy. It was noted that none of the AChE-Is was associated with increased negative chronotropic, arrythmogenic or hypotensive effects and therefore a preferred drug could not be established with regards to vagotonic effects.[61] Similarly, a Danish retrospective cohort study[62] found no substantial differences in the risk of myocardial infarction (MI) or heart failure between participants on donepezil and those using the other AChE-Is. Memantine was in fact associated with greatest risk of all-cause mortality, although sicker individuals were selected for memantine therapy. A Swedish cohort study[63] found that AChE-Is were associated with a 35% reduced risk of MI or death in patients with Alzheimer's disese. These associations were stronger with increasing doses of AChE-Is. RCTs are required in order to confirm findings from this observational study.

An analysis of pooled data for **memantine** revealed that the most frequently reported adverse effects in placebo-controlled trials included agitation (7.5% memantine versus 12% placebo), falls (6.8% versus 7.1%), dizziness (6.3% versus 5.7%), accidental injury (6.0% versus 7.2%), influenza-like symptoms (6.0% versus 5.8%), headache (5.2% versus 3.7%) and diarrhoea (5.0% versus 5.6%).[64]

An analysis of the French pharmacovigilance database compared adverse effects reported with **donepezil** with **memantine**. The most frequent adverse drug reactions with donepezil alone and memantine alone were respectively: bradycardia (10% versus 7%), weakness (5% versus 6%) and convulsions (4% versus 3%). Although it is well known that donepezil is often associated with bradycardia, and memantine associated with seizures, this analysis suggests that memantine can also induce bradycardia and donepezil can also induce seizures; thus highlighting the care required when treating patients with dementia who have a history of bradycardia or epilepsy.[65]

Interactions

Potential for interaction may also differentiate currently available cholinesterase inhibitors. Donepezil[66] and galantamine[67] are metabolised by cytochromes 2D6 and 3A4 and so drug levels may be altered by other drugs affecting the function of these enzymes.

Cholinesterase inhibitors themselves may also interfere with the metabolism of other drugs, although this is perhaps a theoretical consideration. Rivastigmine has almost no potential for interaction since it is metabolised at the site of action and does not affect hepatic cytochromes. A prospective pharmacodynamic analysis of potential drug interactions between rivastigmine and other medications (22 different therapeutic classes) commonly prescribed in the elderly population compared adverse effects odds ratios between rivastigmine and placebo. Rivastigmine did not reveal any significant pattern of increase in adverse effects that would indicate a drug interaction compared with placebo.[68]

Rivastigmine appears to be least likely to cause problematic drug interactions, a factor that may be important in an elderly population subject to polypharmacy (see Table 7.3).

Analysis of the French pharmacovigilance database found that the majority of reported drug interactions concerning AChE-Is were found to be pharmacodynamic in nature and most frequently involved the combination of AChE-I and bradycardic drugs (beta-blockers, digoxin, amiodarone, calcium channel antagonists). Almost a third of these interactions resulted in cardiovascular adverse drug reactions (ADRs) such as bradycardia, atrioventricular block and arterial hypotension. The second most frequent drug interaction reported was the combination of AChE-I with anticholinergic drugs leading to pharmacological antagonism.[69]

The pharmacodynamics, pharmacokinetic and pharmacogenetic aspects of drugs used in dementia have recently been summarised in a comprehensive review.[70]

Combination treatment

The benefits of adding memantine to AChE-Is are not clear but the combination appears to be well tolerated[71,72] and may even result in a decreased incidence of gastrointestinal adverse effects compared with monotherapy with an AChE-I.[73] Studies investigating the benefits of combining AChE-Is with memantine have found conflicting results. Long-term observational controlled studies have shown that combination therapy is associated with better cognitive outcomes and greater delays in time to nursing home admission compared with monotherapy or no treatment.[74]. Whilst a recent review[75] found that combination treatment in moderate-to-severe Alzheimer's disease produces consistent benefits that appear to increase over time and that are beyond AChE-Is therapy alone, a meta-analysis[76] concluded that despite significant changes found in favour of the combination, it was unclear if these were clinically significant. Similarly, a large multicentre study[36] concluded that the efficacy of donepezil and of memantine did not differ significantly in the presence or absence of the other and that there were no significant benefits for the combination over donepezil alone. Studies have confirmed that there are no pharmacokinetic or pharmacodynamic interactions between AChE-Is and memantine.[77,78]

NICE recommendations

NICE guidance on dementia[1], which has been amended to incorporate the updated NICE technology appraisal of drugs for Alzheimer's disease, was published in March 2011[81] and is due to be reviewed in 2015. See Box 7.2.

CHAPTER 7

Table 7.3 Drug–drug interactions[6–11,79,80]

Drug	Metabolism	Plasma levels increased by	Plasma levels decreased by	Pharmacodynamic interactions
Donepezil (Aricept®)	Substrate at 3A4 and 2D6	**Ketoconazole Itraconazole Erythromycin Quinidine Fluoxetine**	**Rifampicin Phenytoin Carbamazepine Alcohol**	Antagonistic with **anticholinergic drugs** Potential for synergistic activity with **cholinomimetics** such as **neuro-muscular blocking agents** (e.g. **succinylcholine**), **cholinergic agonists** and **peripherally acting cholinesterase inhibitors**, e.g. **neostigmine** **Beta-blockers, amiodarone** or **calcium channel blockers** may have additive effects on cardiac conduction
Rivastigmine (Exelon®)	Non-hepatic metabolism	Metabolic interactions appear unlikely Rivastigmine may inhibit the butyryl-cholinesterase-mediated metabolism of other substances, e.g. **cocaine**		Antagonistic effects with **anticholinergic** drugs and additive effects with **cholinomimetic** drugs, **succinylcholine-type muscle relaxants, cholinergic agonists**, e.g. **bethanecol, or peripherally acting cholinesterase inhibitors**, e.g. **neostigmine** Synergistic effects on cardiac conduction with **beta-blockers, amiodarone** and **calcium channel blockers**
Galantamine (Reminyl®)	Substrate at 3A4 and 2D6	**Ketoconazole Erythromycin Ritonavir Quinidine Paroxetine Fluoxetine Fluvoxamine Amitriptyline**	None known	Antagonistic effects with **anticholinergic** drugs and additive effects with **cholinomimetics, succinylcholine-type muscle relaxants, cholinergic agonists** and **peripherally acting cholinesterase inhibitors, e.g. neostigmine** Possible interaction with agents that significantly reduce heart rate, e.g. **digoxin, beta-blockers, certain calcium-channel blockers** and **amiodarone** Caution with agents that can cause torsades de pointes (manufacturers recommend ECG in such cases)

Table 7.3 (*Continued*)

Drug	Metabolism	Plasma levels increased by	Plasma levels decreased by	Pharmacodynamic interactions
Memantine (Exiba®)	Primarily non-hepatic metabolism Renally eliminated	**Cimetidine** **Ranitidine** **Procainamide** **Quinidine** **Quinine** **Nicotine** Isolated cases of INR increases reported with concomitant warfarin (close monitoring of prothrombin time or INR advisable). Drugs that alkalinize urine (pH ~8) may reduce renal elimination of memantine, e.g. **carbonic anhydrase inhibitors, sodium bicarbonate**	None known Possibility of reduced serum level of **hydrochlorothiazide** when co administered with memantine	Effects of **L-dopa, dopaminergic agonists** and **anticholinergics** may be enhanced Effects of **barbiturates** and **neuroleptics** may be reduced Avoid concomitant use with **amantadine, ketamine** and **dextromethorphan** -risk of pharmacotoxic psychosis. One published case report on possible risk for **phenytoin** and memantine combination Dosage adjustment may be necessary for **antispasmodic agents, dantrolene** or **baclofen** when administered with memantine

Note: this list is not exhaustive - caution with other drugs that are also inhibitors or enhancers of CYP 3A4 and 2D6 enzymes.

ECG, electrocardiogram; INR, international normalised ratio.

Box 7.2 Summary of NICE guidance for the treatment of Alzheimer's disease[1,81]

- The three acetylcholinesterase inhibitors (AChE-Is) donepezil, galantamine and rivastigmine are recommended for managing mild-to-moderate Alzheimer's disease.
- Memantine is recommended for managing moderate Alzheimer's disease for people who are intolerant of, or have a contraindication to, AChE-Is, or for managing severe Alzheimer's disease.
- Carers' view on the patient's condition should be sought at baseline and follow-up.
- Patients who continue on the drug should be reviewed regularly using cognitive, global, functional and behavioural assessment. Treatment should be reviewed by an appropriate specialist team, unless there are locally agreed protocols for shared care.
- Therapy with AChE-I should be initiated with a drug with the lowest acquisition cost (taking into account required daily dose and the price per dose once shared care has started). An alternative may be considered on the basis of adverse effects profile, expectations about adherence, medical co-morbidity, possibility of drug interactions and dosing profiles.
- When assessing the severity of Alzheimer's disease and the need for treatment, healthcare professionals should not rely solely on cognition scores in circumstances in which it would be inappropriate to do so, and should take into account any physical, sensory or learning disabilities, or communication difficulties that could affect the results. Any adjustments considered appropriate should be made.

Other treatments

Ginkgo biloba

A Cochrane review found that although *Ginkgo biloba* appears to be safe with no excess side-effects compared with placebo, there was no convincing evidence that it is efficacious for dementia and cognitive impairment. Many of the trials were too small and used unsatisfactory methods and publication bias could not be excluded. The review concluded that ginkgo's clinical benefit in dementia or cognitive impairment is somewhat inconsistent and unconvincing.[82] A randomised, double-blind trial, which compared *Ginkgo biloba*, donepezil, or both combined, found no statistically significant or clinically relevant differences between the three groups with respect to efficacy. In addition, they noted that combined treatment adverse effects were less frequent than with donepezil alone.[83] Several reports have noted that ginkgo may increase the risk of bleeding.[84] The drug is widely used in Germany but less so elsewhere.

Vitamin E

A Cochrane review of vitamin E for Alzheimer's disease and mild cognitive impairment (MCI) examined two studies meeting the inclusion criteria. The authors' conclusions were that there is no evidence of efficacy of vitamin E in prevention or treatment of people with Alzheimer's disease or MCI and that further research is required in order to identify its role in this area.[85] A more recent RCT[86] compared the effects of vitamin E (alpha tocopherol) 2000 IU/day, memantine 20 mg/day, the combination or placebo in 613 patients with mild-to-moderate Alzheimer's disease. Findings showed that alpha tocopherol resulted in slower functional decline than placebo. However, there were no significant differences between memantine alone or memantine plus alpha tocopherol groups. Due to limitations of this trial, further evidence is needed to support these findings.

Folic acid

A placebo-controlled pilot RCT of 1 mg folic acid supplementation of AChE-Is over 6 months in 57 patients with Alzheimer's disease showed significant benefit in combined IADL and social behaviour scores (folate + 1.50 (SD 5.32) versus placebo −2.29 (SD 6.16) (p = 0.03) but no change in MMSE scores.[87] Another RCT examining the efficacy of **multivitamins and folic acid** as an adjunctive to AChE-Is over 26 weeks in 89 patients with Alzheimer's disease found no statistically significant benefits between the two groups on cognition or ADL function.[88] A Cochrane review found no evidence that **folic acid** with or without **vitamin B$_{12}$** improves cognitive function of unselected elderly people with or without dementia. However, long term supplementation may benefit cognitive function of healthy older people with high homocysteine levels.[89]

Elevated homocysteine, decreased folate and low vitamin B$_{12}$ serum levels are associated with poor cognitive function, cognitive decline and dementia. A systematic and critical review of the literature did not provide any clear evidence that supplementation with vitamin B$_{12}$ and/or folate improves cognition or dementia even though it might normalise homocysteine levels.[90] A small RCT found that vitamin B, which lowers homocysteine levels, appeared to slow cognitive and clinical decline in people with MCI, in particular those with elevated homocysteine levels, however further trials are needed to establish whether reducing homocysteine levels will slow or prevent conversion from MCI to dementia.[91]

Omega-3

Omega-3 supplementation in mild-to-moderate Alzheimer's disease has been evaluated in 174 patients in a placebo-controlled RCT but there were no significant overall effects on neuropsychiatric symptoms, on activities of daily living or on caregiver's burden, although some possible positive effects were seen on depressive symptoms (assessed by Montgomery-Asberg Depression Rating Scale [MADRS]) and agitation symptoms (assessed by neuropsychiatric inventory [NPI]).[92]

Ginseng

A prospective open-label study of ginseng in Alzheimer's disease measured cognitive performance in 97 patients randomly assigned ginseng or placebo for 12 weeks and then 12 weeks after the ginseng had been discontinued. After ginseng treatment, the cognitive subscales of ADAS and MMSE score began to show improvement continued up to 12 weeks (p = 0.029 and p = 0.009 versus baseline respectively) but scores declined to levels of the control group following discontinuation of ginseng.[93]

Dimebon

Dimebon, a non-selective antihistamine previously approved in Russia but later discontinued for commercial reasons, has been assessed for safety, tolerability and efficacy in the treatment of patients with mild-to-moderate Alzheimer's disease. It acts as a weak inhibitor of butyrylcholinesterase and acetylcholinesterase, weakly blocks the NMDA-receptor signalling pathway and inhibits the mitochondrial permeability transition pore opening.[94] A meta-analysis found that dimebon generally presented a good safety profile and was well tolerated. Heterogeneous results were noted between trials, however, and it failed to exert a significant beneficial effect (although it tended to improve cognitive scores).[95]

Hirudin

Natural hirudin, isolated from salivary gland of medicinal leech, is a direct thrombin inhibitor and has been used for many years in China. It does not share the usual limitations of other anticoagulant drugs like heparin, such as the potential to cause bleeding and variable anticoagulant effects. Since thrombosis and ischaemia are the primary vascular risk factors, improvement of cerebral blood flow may be helpful in the treatment and rehabilitation of patients with Alzheimer's disease. A 20-week open label RCT of 84 patients receiving donepezil or donepezil plus hirudin (3 g/day) found that patients on the combination showed significant decrease in ADAS-cog scores and significant increase in ADL scores compared with donepezil alone. However, haemorrhage and hypersensitivity reactions were more common in the combination group compared with donepezil group (11.9% and 7.1% versus 2.4% and 2.4% respectively).[96]

Huperzine A

Huperzine A, a novel alkaloid isolated from the Chinese herb *Huperzia serrata*, is a potent, highly selective, reversible AChE-I used for treating Alzheimer's disease since 1994 in China and available as a nutraceutical in the US. A recent meta-analysis found that huperzine A 300–500 μg daily for 8–24 weeks in Alzheimer's disease led to significant improvements in MMSE (mean change 3.5157; p < 0.05) and ADL with effect size shown to increase over treatment time. Most adverse effects were cholinergic in nature and no serious adverse effects occurred.[97] A Cochrane review of huperzine A in vascular dementia, however, found no convincing evidence for its value in vascular dementia.[98] Similarly, a Cochrane review of huperzine A for mild cognitive impairment concluded that the current evidence is insufficient for this indication as no eligible trials were identified.[99]

Saffron

There is increasing evidence to suggest possible efficacy of *Crocus sativus* (saffron) in the management of Alzheimer's disease. In a 16-week placebo-controlled RCT, saffron produced a significantly better outcome on cognitive function than placebo and there were no significant differences between the two groups in terms of observed adverse events.[100] A 22-week double-blind study included 55 patients randomly assigned to saffron capsules 15 mg bd or donepezil 5 mg bd. Results found no significant differences between the two groups in terms of efficacy or adverse effects, although vomiting occurred significantly more frequently in the donepezil group.[101]

Cerebrolysin

Cerebrolysin is a parenterally administered, porcine brain-derived peptide preparation that has pharmacodynamic properties similar to those of endogenous neurotrophic factors. Cerebrolysin was superior to placebo in improving global outcome measures and cognitive ability in several RCTs of up to 28 weeks in patients with Alzheimer's disease. In addition, a large RCT comparing cerebrolysin, donepezil or combination therapy showed beneficial effects on global measures and cognition for all three treatment groups compared with baseline. Although not as extensively studied in vascular dementia, cerebrolysin has also showed beneficial effects on global measures and cognition in this patient group. Cerebrolysin was generally well tolerated in trials with dizziness being the most frequently reported adverse event.[102]

Statins

In Alzheimer's disease, amyloid protein is deposited in the form of extracellular plaques and studies have determined that amyloid protein generation is cholesterol-dependent. Hypercholesterolaemia has also been implicated in the pathogenesis of vascular dementia. Due to the role of statins in cholesterol reduction, they have been explored as a means to treat dementia. A Cochrane review, however, found that there is still insufficient evidence to recommend statins for the treatment of dementia. Analysis from the studies available, indicate that they have no benefit on the outcome measures ADAS-Cog or MMSE.[103]

Cocoa

Sixty older people were studied in a clinical trial of neurovascular coupling and cognition in response to 30 days of cocoa consumption. Two cups of cocoa daily for 30 days resulted in higher neurovascular coupling (NVC) and individuals with higher NVC had better cognitive function and greater cerebral white matter structural integrity.[104]

Souvenaid

Souvenaid is a medical food for the dietary management of early Alzheimer's disease. The mix of nutrients in this drink is suggested to have a beneficial effect on cognitive function; however health claims for medical foods are not checked by government agencies. Souvenaid has been investigated in three clinical trials. The first trial showed that Souvenaid produced a significant improvement in delayed verbal recall, but not in other psychological tests.[105] The second and largest trial showed no effect on any outcome.[106] A third trial showed no significant effect at 12 or 24 weeks, but a significant difference in the 24-week time course of the composite memory score.[107] However, none of these outcomes was clearly specified as a primary outcome at trial registration. There is currently therefore no convincing proof that Souvenaid benefits cognitive function. Further regulated and robust efficacy data are required.

Three new drugs have failed to improve clinical outcomes in phase III trials for Alzheimer's disease. These include: Semagacestat, a γ-secretase inhibitor,[108] solanezumab, a humanised monoclonal antibody that binds soluble forms of amyloid and promotes its clearance from the brain[109] and bapineuzumab, a humanised anti-amyloid-β monoclonal antibody.[110]

Vascular dementia (VaD)

Vascular dementia has been reported to comprise 10–50% of dementia cases and is the second most common type of dementia after Alzheimer's disease. It is caused by ischaemic damage to the brain and is associated with cognitive impairment and behavioural disturbances. The management options are currently very limited and focus on controlling the underlying risk factors for cerebrovascular disease.[111]

None of the currently available drugs is formally licensed in the UK for vascular dementia. The management of vascular dementia has been summarised.[112,113] Unlike the situation with stroke, there is no conclusive evidence that treatment of hyperlipidemia with statins, or treatment of blood clotting abnormalities with acetylsalicylic acid, do have an effect on vascular dementia incidence or disease progression.[114] Similarly, a Cochrane review found that there were no studies supporting the role of statins in the treatment of VaD.[103] There is however growing evidence for donepezil,[115,116] rivastigmine,[117,118] galantamine[119–121] and memantine.[122,123] The largest clinical trial of donepezil in vascular dementia found small but significant improvement on the vascular ADAS-cog subscale but no difference was seen on the Clinician's Interview-Based Impression of Change (CIBIC-Plus)[124]. These results are consistent with prior trials suggesting that donepezil may have a greater impact on cognitive rather than global outcomes in vascular dementia. The Cochrane review for donepezil in vascular cognitive impairment however found evidence to support its benefit in improving cognition function, clinical global impression and activities of daily living after 6 months treatment.[116] In the Cochrane review for galantamine for vascular cognitive impairment,[15,125] there were limited data suggesting some advantage over placebo in areas of cognition and global clinical state. However, authors thought more studies were needed to confirm these results. Trials of galantamine reported high rates of gastrointestinal side effects. The Cochrane review for rivastigmine in vascular cognitive impairment found some evidence of benefit, however the conclusion was based on one large study and side effects with rivastigmine lead to withdrawal in a significant proportion of patient.[103,126] Furthermore, a meta-analysis of RCTs found that cholinesterase inhibitors and memantine produce small benefits in cognition of uncertain clinical significance and concluded that data were insufficient to support widespread use of these agents in vascular dementia.[111]

Note that it is impossible to diagnose with certainty vascular or Alzheimer's dementia and much dementia has mixed causation. This might explain why certain AChE-Is do not always provide consistent results in probable vascular dementia and the data indicating efficacy in cognitive outcomes was derived from older patients, who were therefore likely to have concomitant Alzheimer's disease pathology.[127]

Dementia with Lewy bodies

It has been suggested that dementia with Lewy bodies (DLB) may account for 15–25% of cases of dementia (although autopsy suggests much lower rates). Characteristic symptoms are dementia with fluctuation of cognitive ability, early and persistent visual hallucinations and spontaneous motor features of parkinsonism. Falls, syncope, transient disturbances of consciousness, neuroleptic sensitivity and hallucinations in other modalities are also common.[128]

A Cochrane review for AChE-Is in DLB and Parkinson's disease dementia and cognitive impairment found evidence supporting their use in Parkinson's disease but no statistically significant improvement was observed in patients with DLB and that further trials were necessary to clarify their effects in this patient group.[129] A comparative analysis of cholinesterase inhibitors in DLB, which included open label trials as well as the placebo-controlled randomized trial of rivastigmine, found that, so far, there is no compelling evidence that one AChE-I is better that the other in DLB.[130] Despite certain reports of patients with DLB worsening or responding adversely when exposed to memantine,[131] a recent RCT of memantine (funded by the manufacturer) found it to be mildly beneficial in terms of global clinical status and behavioural symptoms in patients with DLB.[132]

Mild cognitive impairment (MCI)

Mild cognitive impairment is hypothesised to represent a pre-clinical stage of dementia but forms a heterogeneous group with variable prognosis. A Cochrane review assessing the safety and efficacy of AChE-Is in MCI found there was very little evidence that they affect progression to dementia or cognitive test scores. This weak evidence was countered by the increased risk of adverse effects, particularly gastrointestinal effects, meaning that AChE-Is could not be recommended in MCI.[133] A recent systematic review[134] found that there was no replicated evidence that any intervention was effective for MCI including AChE-Is and the non-steroidal anti-inflammatory drug (NSAID) rofecoxib.

Summary of clinical practice guidance with anti-dementia drugs from BAP

A revised consensus statement from the British Association of Psychopharmacology (BAP)[135] states that: AChE-Is are effective in mild-to-moderate Alzheimer's disease and memantine in moderate-to-severe Alzheimer's disease. Other drugs including statins, anti-inflammatory drugs, vitamin E and ginkgo cannot be recommended either for the treatment

Table 7.4 Summary of recommendations

	First choice	Second choice
Alzheimer's disease	AChE-Is	Memantine
Vascular dementia	None	None
Mixed dementia	AChE-Is	Memantine
Dementia with Lewy bodies	AChE-Is	Memantine
Mild cognitive impairment	None	None
Dementia with Parkinson's disease	AChE-Is	None

or prevention of Alzheimer's disease. Neither AChE-Is nor memantine are effective in MCI. AChE-Is are not effective in frontotemporal dementia and may cause agitation. AChE-Is may be used for people with DLB (can produce cognitive improvements) and Parkinson's disease dementia, especially for neuropsychiatric symptoms. There is no clear evidence that any intervention can prevent or delay the onset of dementia. See Table 7.4.

References

1. National Institute for Health and Clinical Excellence. Dementia. Supporting people with dementia and their carers in health and social care. Clincial Guideline 42, 2011. Updated March 2011. http://www.nice.org.uk/nicemedia/live/10998/30318/30318.pdf
2. Francis PT et al. The cholinergic hypothesis of Alzheimer's disease: a review of progress. J Neurol Neurosurg Psychiatry 1999; **66**:137–147.
3. Mesulam M et al. Widely spread butyrylcholinesterase can hydrolyze acetylcholine in the normal and Alzheimer brain. Neurobiol Dis 2002; **9**:88–93.
4. Weinstock M. Selectivity of cholinesterase inhibition: clinical implications for the treatment of alzheimer's disease. CNS Drugs 1999; **12**:307–323.
5. Joint Formulary Committee. *BNF* 67 March-September 2014 (online). London: Pharmaceutical Press; 2014. http://www.medicinescomplete.com/mc/bnf/current/
6. Eisai Ltd. Summary of Product Characteristics. Aricept Tablets. 2013. https://www.medicines.org.uk/
7. Novartis Pharmaceuticals UK Limited, Novar. Summary of Product Characteristics. Exelon 4.6 mg/24 h, 9.5 mg/24 h, 13.3 mg/24 h transdermal patch. 2013. https://www.medicines.org.uk/
8. Novartis Pharmaceuticals UK Limited. Summary of Product Characteristics. Exelon. 2013. https://www.medicines.org.uk
9. Shire Pharmaceuticals Limited. Summary of Product Characteristics. Reminyl XL 8 mg, 16 mg and 24 mg prolonged release capsules. 2013. https://www.medicines.org.uk/
10. Shire Pharmaceuticals Limited. Summary of Product Characteristics. Reminyl Oral Solution. 2013. https://www.medicines.org.uk/
11. Shire Pharmaceuticals Limited. Summary of Product Characteristics. Reminyl Tablets. 2013. https://www.medicines.org.uk
12. Lundbeck Limited. Summary of Product Characteristics. Ebixa 5 mg/pump actuation oral solution, 20 mg and 10 mg Tablets and Treatment Initiation Pack. 2013. https://www.medicines.org.uk/
13. NHS Prescription Services. Drug Tariff - May 2014. 2014. http://www.ppa.org.uk/ppa/edt_intro.htm
14. Lanctot KL et al. Efficacy and safety of cholinesterase inhibitors in Alzheimer's disease: a meta-analysis. CMAJ 2003; **169**:557–564.
15. Birks J. Cholinesterase inhibitors for Alzheimer's disease. Cochrane Database Syst Rev 2006; CD005593.
16. Bond M et al. The effectiveness and cost-effectiveness of donepezil, galantamine, rivastigmine and memantine for the treatment of Alzheimer's disease (review of Technology Appraisal No. 111): a systematic review and economic model. Health Technol Assess 2012; **16**:1–470.
17. Rogers SL et al. Donepezil improves cognition and global function in Alzheimer disease: a 15-week, double-blind, placebo-controlled study. Donepezil Study Group. Arch Intern Med 1998; **158**:1021–1031.
18. Rogers SL et al. A 24-week, double-blind, placebo-controlled trial of donepezil in patients with Alzheimer's disease. Donepezil Study Group. Neurology 1998; **50**:136–145.
19. Rogers SL et al. Long-term efficacy and safety of donepezil in the treatment of Alzheimer's disease: final analysis of a US multicentre open-label study. Eur Neuropsychopharmacol 2000; **10**:195–203.
20. Birks J et al. Donepezil for dementia due to Alzheimer's disease. Cochrane Database Syst Rev 2006; CD001190.
21. AD2000 Collaborative Group. Long-term donepezil treatment in 565 patients with Alzheimer's disease (AD2000): randomised double-blind trial. Lancet 2004; **363**:2105–2115.

22. Corey-Bloom J et al. A randomized trial evaluating the efficacy and safety of ENA 713 (rivastigmine tartrate), a new acetylcholinesterase inhibitor, in patients with mild to moderately severe Alzheimer's disease. Int J Geriatr Psychopharmacol 1998; 1:55–64.

23. Rosler M et al. Efficacy and safety of rivastigmine in patients with Alzheimer's disease: international randomised controlled trial. BMJ 1999; 318:633–638.

24. Winblad B et al. A six-month double-blind, randomized, placebo-controlled study of a transdermal patch in Alzheimer's disease--rivastigmine patch versus capsule. Int J Geriatr Psychiatry 2007; 22:456–467.

25. Tariot PN et al. A 5-month, randomized, placebo-controlled trial of galantamine in AD. The Galantamine USA-10 Study Group. Neurology 2000; 54:2269–2276.

26. Raskind MA et al. Galantamine in AD: A 6-month randomized, placebo-controlled trial with a 6-month extension. The Galantamine USA-1 Study Group. Neurology 2000; 54:2261–2268.

27. Wilcock GK et al. Efficacy and safety of galantamine in patients with mild to moderate Alzheimer's disease: multicentre randomised controlled trial. Galantamine International-1 Study Group. BMJ 2000; 321:1445–1449.

28. Loy C et al. Galantamine for Alzheimer's disease and mild cognitive impairment. Cochrane Database Syst Rev 2006;CD001747.

29. Burns A et al. Safety and efficacy of galantamine (Reminyl) in severe Alzheimer's disease (the SERAD study): a randomised, placebo-controlled, double-blind trial. The Lancet Neurology 2009; 8:39–47.

30. Livingston G et al. The place of memantine in the treatment of Alzheimer's disease: a number needed to treat analysis. Int J Geriatr Psychiatry 2004; 19:919–925.

31. Schmitt FA et al. The severe impairment battery: concurrent validity and the assessment of longitudinal change in Alzheimer's disease. The Alzheimer's Disease Cooperative Study. Alzheimer Dis Assoc Disord 1997; 11 Suppl 2:S51–S56.

32. Mecocci P et al. Effects of memantine on cognition in patients with moderate to severe Alzheimer's disease: post-hoc analyses of ADAS-cog and SIB total and single-item scores from six randomized, double-blind, placebo-controlled studies. Int J Geriatr Psychiatry 2009; 24:532–538.

33. McShane R et al. Memantine for dementia. Cochrane Database Syst Rev 2006; CD003154.

34. Peskind ER et al. Memantine Treatment in Mild to Moderate Alzheimer Disease: A 24-Week Randomized, Controlled Trial. Am J Geriatr Psychiatry 2006; 14:704–715.

35. Schneider LS et al. Lack of evidence for the efficacy of memantine in mild Alzheimer Disease. Arch Neurol 2011; 68:991–998.

36. Howard R et al. Donepezil and memantine for moderate-to-severe Alzheimer's disease. N Engl J Med 2012; 366:893–903.

37. Di Santo SG et al. A meta-analysis of the efficacy of donepezil, rivastigmine, galantamine, and memantine in relation to severity of Alzheimer's disease. J Alzheimers Dis 2013; 35:349–361.

38. Stern RG et al. A longitudinal study of Alzheimer's disease: measurement, rate, and predictors of cognitive deterioration. Am J Psychiatry 1994; 151:390–396.

39. Burns A et al. Efficacy and safety of donepezil over 3 years: an open-label, multicentre study in patients with Alzheimer's disease. Int J Geriatr Psychiatry 2007; 22:806–812.

40. Doody RS et al. Open-label, multicenter, phase 3 extension study of the safety and efficacy of donepezil in patients with Alzheimer disease. Arch Neurol 2001; 58:427–433.

41. Farlow MR et al. Effective pharmacologic management of Alzheimer's disease. Am J Med 2007; 120:388–397.

42. Singh S et al. Discontinuation syndrome following donepezil cessation. Int J Geriatr Psychiatry 2003; 18:282–284.

43. Waldemar G et al. Tolerability of switching from donepezil to memantine treatment in patients with moderate to severe Alzheimer's disease. Int J Geriatr Psychiatry 2008; 23:979–981.

44. Massoud F et al. Switching cholinesterase inhibitors in older adults with dementia. Int Psychogeriatr 2011; 23:372–378.

45. Dybicz SB et al. Patterns of cholinesterase-inhibitor use in the nursing home setting: a retrospective analysis. Am J Geriatr Pharmacother 2006; 4:154–160.

46. Jones RW et al. Safety and tolerability of once-daily versus twice-daily memantine: a randomised, double-blind study in moderate to severe Alzheimer's disease. Int J Geriatr Psychiatry 2007; 22:258–262.

47. Pariente A et al. Factors associated with serious adverse reactions to cholinesterase inhibitors: a study of spontaneous reporting. CNS Drugs 2010; 24:55–63.

48. Sadowsky CH et al. Safety and tolerability of rivastigmine transdermal patch compared with rivastigmine capsules in patients switched from donepezil: data from three clinical trials. Int J Clin Pract 2010; 64:188–193.

49. Sadowsky C et al. Switching from oral cholinesterase inhibitors to the rivastigmine transdermal patch. CNS Neurosci Ther 2010; 16:51–60.

50. Cummings J et al. Randomized, double-blind, parallel-group, 48-week study for efficacy and safety of a higher-dose rivastigmine patch (15 vs. 10 cm(2)) in Alzheimer's disease. Dement Geriatr Cogn Disord 2012; 33:341–353.

51. Parsons CG et al. Memantine is a clinically well tolerated N-methyl-D-aspartate (NMDA) receptor antagonist--a review of preclinical data. Neuropharmacology 1999; 38:735–767.

52. Reisberg B et al. Memantine in moderate-to-severe Alzheimer's disease. N Engl J Med 2003; 348:1333–1341.

53. Jones RW. A review comparing the safety and tolerability of memantine with the acetylcholinesterase inhibitors. Int J Geriatr Psychiatry 2010; 25:547–553.

54. Dunn NR et al. Adverse effects associated with the use of donepezil in general practice in England. J Psychopharmacol 2000; 14:406–408.

55. Hashimoto M et al. Urinary incontinence: an unrecognised adverse effect with donepezil. Lancet 2000; 356:568.

56. FDA Alert for Healthcare Professionals. Galantamine hydrobromide (marketed as Razadyne, formerly Reminyl). 2005. http://www.fda.gov/

57. Malone DM et al. Cholinesterase inhibitors and cardiovascular disease: a survey of old age psychiatrists' practice. Age Ageing 2007; 36:331–333.

58. Park-Wyllie LY et al. Cholinesterase inhibitors and hospitalization for bradycardia: a population-based study. PLoS Med 2009; 6:e1000157.

59. Rosenbloom MH et al. Donepezil-associated bradyarrhythmia in a patient with dementia with Lewy bodies (DLB). Alzheimer Dis Assoc Disord 2010; 24:209–211.

60. Gill SS et al. Syncope and its consequences in patients with dementia receiving cholinesterase inhibitors: a population-based cohort study. Arch Intern Med 2009; 169:867–873.

61. Isik AT et al. Which cholinesterase inhibitor is the safest for the heart in elderly patients with Alzheimer's disease? Am J Alzheimers Dis Other Demen 2012; 27:171–174.

62. Fosbol EL et al. Comparative cardiovascular safety of dementia medications: a cross-national study. J Am Geriatr Soc 2012; 60:2283–2289.

63. Nordstrom P et al. The use of cholinesterase inhibitors and the risk of myocardial infarction and death: a nationwide cohort study in subjects with Alzheimer's disease. Eur Heart J 2013; 34:2585–2591.

64. Farlow MR et al. Memantine for the treatment of Alzheimer's disease: tolerability and safety data from clinical trials. Drug Saf 2008; 31:577–585.

65. Babai S et al. Comparison of adverse drug reactions with donepezil versus memantine: analysis of the French Pharmacovigilance Database. Therapie 2010; 65:255–259.

66. Dooley M et al. Donepezil: a review of its use in Alzheimer's disease. Drugs Aging 2000; 16:199–226.

67. Scott LJ et al. Galantamine: a review of its use in Alzheimer's disease. Drugs 2000; 60:1095–1122.

68. Grossberg GT et al. Lack of adverse pharmacodynamic drug interactions with rivastigmine and twenty-two classes of medications. Int J Geriatr Psychiatry 2000; 15:242–247.

69. Tavassoli N et al. Drug interactions with cholinesterase inhibitors: an analysis of the French pharmacovigilance database and a comparison of two national drug formularies (Vidal, British National Formulary). Drug Saf 2007; 30:1063–1071.

70. Noetzli M et al. Pharmacodynamic, pharmacokinetic and pharmacogenetic aspects of drugs used in the treatment of Alzheimer's disease. Clin Pharmacokinet 2013; 52:225–241.

71. Tariot PN et al. Memantine treatment in patients with moderate to severe Alzheimer disease already receiving donepezil: a randomized controlled trial. JAMA 2004; 291:317–324.

72. Hartmann S et al. Tolerability of memantine in combination with cholinesterase inhibitors in dementia therapy. Int Clin Psychopharmacol 2003; 18:81–85.

73. Olin JT et al. Safety and tolerability of rivastigmine capsule with memantine in patients with probable Alzheimer's disease: a 26-week, open-label, prospective trial (Study ENA713B US32). Int J Geriatr Psychiatry 2010; 25:419–426.

74. Rountree SD et al. Effectiveness of antidementia drugs in delaying Alzheimer's disease progression. Alzheimers Dement 2013; 9:338–345.

75. Gauthier S et al. Benefits of combined cholinesterase inhibitor and memantine treatment in moderate-severe Alzheimer's disease. Alzheimers Dement 2013; 9:326–331.

76. Muayqil T et al. Systematic review and meta-analysis of combination therapy with cholinesterase inhibitors and memantine in Alzheimer's disease and other dementias. Dement Geriatr Cogn Dis Extra 2012; 2:546–572.

77. Periclou AP et al. Lack of pharmacokinetic or pharmacodynamic interaction between memantine and donepezil. Ann Pharmacother 2004; 38:1389–1394.

78. Grossberg GT et al. Rationale for combination therapy with galantamine and memantine in Alzheimer's disease. J Clin Pharmacol 2006; 46:17S–26S.

79. Stockley's Drug Interactions. London: Pharamceutical Press; 2014. https://www.medicinescomplete.com/

80. Truven Health Analytics. Micromedex 2.0. 2013. https://www.medicinescomplete.com/

81. National Institute for Health and Clinical Excellence. Donepezil, galantamine, rivastigmine and memantine for the treatment of Alzheimer's disease. TA 217, 2011. http://www.nice.org.uk/guidance/index.jsp?action=byID&o=13419

82. Birks J et al. Ginkgo biloba for cognitive impairment and dementia. Cochrane Database Syst Rev 2009; CD003120.

83. Yancheva S et al. Ginkgo biloba extract EGb 761(R), donepezil or both combined in the treatment of Alzheimer's disease with neuropsychiatric features: a randomised, double-blind, exploratory trial. Aging Ment Health 2009; 13:183–190.

84. Bent S et al. Spontaneous bleeding associated with ginkgo biloba: a case report and systematic review of the literature: a case report and systematic review of the literature. J Gen Intern Med 2005; 20:657–661.

85. Issac MG et al. Vitamin E for Alzheimer's disease and mild cognitive impairment (review). Cochrane Database Syst Rev 2008; CD002854.

86. Dysken MW et al. Effect of vitamin E and memantine on functional decline in Alzheimer disease: the TEAM-AD VA cooperative randomized trial. JAMA 2014; 311:33–44.

87. Connelly PJ et al. A randomised double-blind placebo-controlled trial of folic acid supplementation of cholinesterase inhibitors in Alzheimer's disease. Int J Geriatr Psychiatry 2008; 23:155–160.

88. Sun Y et al. Efficacy of multivitamin supplementation containing vitamins B6 and B12 and folic acid as adjunctive treatment with a cholinesterase inhibitor in Alzheimer's disease: a 26-week, randomized, double-blind, placebo-controlled study in Taiwanese patients. Clin Ther 2007; 29:2204–2214.

89. Malouf R et al. Folic acid with or without vitamin B12 for the prevention and treatment of healthy elderly and demented people. Cochrane Database Syst Rev 2008; CD004514.

90. Vogel T et al. Homocysteine, vitamin B12, folate and cognitive functions: a systematic and critical review of the literature. Int J Clin Pract 2009; 63:1061–1067.

91. de Jager CA et al. Cognitive and clinical outcomes of homocysteine-lowering B-vitamin treatment in mild cognitive impairment: a randomized controlled trial. Int J Geriatr Psychiatry 2012; 27:592–600.

CHAPTER 7

92. Freund-Levi Y et al. Omega-3 supplementation in mild to moderate Alzheimer's disease: effects on neuropsychiatric symptoms. Int J Geriatr Psychiatry 2008; 23:161–169.

93. Lee ST et al. Panax ginseng enhances cognitive performance in Alzheimer disease. Alzheimer Dis Assoc Disord 2008; 22:222–226.

94. Doody RS et al. Effect of dimebon on cognition, activities of daily living, behaviour, and global function in patients with mild-to-moderate Alzheimer's disease: a randomised, double-blind, placebo-controlled study. Lancet 2008; 372:207–215.

95. Cano-Cuenca N et al. Evidence for the efficacy of latrepirdine (Dimebon) treatment for improvement of cognitive function: a meta-analysis. J Alzheimers Dis 2014; 38:155–164.

96. Li DQ et al. Donepezil combined with natural hirudin improves the clinical symptoms of patients with mild-to-moderate Alzheimer's disease: a 20-week open-label pilot study. Int J Med Sci 2012; 9:248–255.

97. Wang BS et al. Efficacy and safety of natural acetylcholinesterase inhibitor huperzine A in the treatment of Alzheimer's disease: an updated meta-analysis. J Neural Transm 2009; 116:457–465.

98. Hao Z et al. Huperzine A for vascular dementia. Cochrane Database Syst Rev 2009; CD007365.

99. Yue J et al. Huperzine A for mild cognitive impairment. Cochrane Database Syst Rev 2012; 12: CD008827.

100. Akhondzadeh S et al. Saffron in the treatment of patients with mild to moderate Alzheimer's disease: a 16-week, randomized and placebo-controlled trial. J Clin Pharm Ther 2010; 35:581–588.

101. Akhondzadeh S et al. A 22-week, multicenter, randomized, double-blind controlled trial of Crocus sativus in the treatment of mild-to-moderate Alzheimer's disease. Psychopharmacology (Berl) 2010; 207:637–643.

102. Plosker GL et al. Spotlight on cerebrolysin in dementia. CNS Drugs 2010; 24:263–266.

103. McGuinness B et al. Cochrane review on 'Statins for the treatment of dementia'. Int J Geriatr Psychiatry 2013; 28:119–126.

104. Sorond FA et al. Neurovascular coupling, cerebral white matter integrity, and response to cocoa in older people. Neurology 2013; 81:904–909.

105. Scheltens P et al. Efficacy of a medical food in mild Alzheimer's disease: A randomized, controlled trial. Alzheimers Dement 2010; 6:1–10.

106. Shah RC et al. The S-Connect study: results from a randomized, controlled trial of Souvenaid in mild-to-moderate Alzheimer's disease. Alzheimers Res Ther 2013; 5:59.

107. Scheltens P et al. Efficacy of Souvenaid in mild Alzheimer's disease: results from a randomized, controlled trial. J Alzheimers Dis 2012; 31:225–236.

108. Doody RS et al. A phase 3 trial of semagacestat for treatment of Alzheimer's disease. N Engl J Med 2013; 369:341–350.

109. Doody RS et al. Phase 3 trials of solanezumab for mild-to-moderate Alzheimer's disease. N Engl J Med 2014; 370:311–321.

110. Salloway S et al. Two phase 3 trials of bapineuzumab in mild-to-moderate Alzheimer's disease. N Engl J Med 2014; 370:322–333.

111. Kavirajan H et al. Efficacy and adverse effects of cholinesterase inhibitors and memantine in vascular dementia: a meta-analysis of randomised controlled trials. Lancet Neurol 2007; 6:782–792.

112. Bocti C et al. Management of dementia with a cerebrovascular component. Alzheimer's and Dementia 2007; 3:398–403.

113. Demaerschalk BM et al. Treatment of vascular dementia and vascular cognitive impairment. Neurologist 2007; 13:37–41.

114. Baskys A et al. Pharmacological prevention and treatment of vascular dementia: approaches and perspectives. Exp Gerontol 2012; 47:887–891.

115. Roman GC et al. Donepezil in vascular dementia: combined analysis of two large-scale clinical trials. Dement Geriatr Cogn Disord 2005; 20:338–344.

116. Malouf R et al. Donepezil for vascular cognitive impairment. Cochrane Database Syst Rev 2004; CD004395.

117. Moretti R et al. Rivastigmine superior to aspirin plus nimodipine in subcortical vascular dementia: an open, 16-month, comparative study. Int J Clin Pract 2004; 58:346–353.

118. Moretti R et al. Rivastigmine in subcortical vascular dementia: a randomized, controlled, open 12-month study in 208 patients. Am J Alzheimers Dis Other Demen 2003; 18:265–272.

119. Small G et al. Galantamine in the treatment of cognitive decline in patients with vascular dementia or Alzheimer's disease with cerebrovascular disease. CNS Drugs 2003; 17:905–914.

120. Kurz AF et al. Long-term safety and cognitive effects of galantamine in the treatment of probable vascular dementia or Alzheimer's disease with cerebrovascular disease. Eur J Neurol 2003; 10:633–640.

121. Erkinjuntti T et al. Efficacy of galantamine in probable vascular dementia and Alzheimer's disease combined with cerebrovascular disease: a randomised trial. Lancet 2002; 359:1283–1290.

122. Wilcock G et al. A double-blind, placebo-controlled multicentre study of memantine in mild to moderate vascular dementia (MMM500). Int Clin Psychopharmacol 2002; 17:297–305.

123. Orgogozo JM et al. Efficacy and safety of memantine in patients with mild to moderate vascular dementia: a randomized, placebo-controlled trial (MMM 300). Stroke 2002; 33:1834–1839.

124. Roman GC et al. Randomized, placebo-controlled, clinical trial of donepezil in vascular dementia: differential effects by hippocampal size. Stroke 2010; 41:1213–1221.

125. Craig D et al. Galantamine for vascular cognitive impairment. Cochrane Database Syst Rev 2006; CD004746.

126. Birks J et al. Rivastigmine for vascular cognitive impairment. Cochrane Database Syst Rev 2013; 5: CD004744.

127. Wang J et al. Cholinergic deficiency involved in vascular dementia: possible mechanism and strategy of treatment. Acta Pharmacol Sin 2009; 30:879–888.

128. Wild R et al. Cholinesterase inhibitors for dementia with Lewy bodies. Cochrane Database Syst Rev 2003; CD003672.

129. Rolinski M et al. Cholinesterase inhibitors for dementia with Lewy bodies, Parkinson's disease dementia and cognitive impairment in Parkinson's disease. Cochrane Database Syst Rev 2012; 3: CD006504.

130. Bhasin M et al. Cholinesterase inhibitors in dementia with Lewy bodies: a comparative analysis. Int J Geriatr Psychiatry 2007; 22:890–895.

131. Sabbagh MN et al. The use of memantine in dementia with Lewy bodies. J Alzheimers Dis 2005; 7:285–289.

132. Emre M et al. Memantine for patients with Parkinson's disease dementia or dementia with Lewy bodies: a randomised, double-blind, placebo-controlled trial. Lancet Neurol 2010; 9:969–977.

133. Russ TC et al. Cholinesterase inhibitors for mild cognitive impairment. Cochrane Database Syst Rev 2012; 9: CD009132.

134. Cooper C et al. Treatment for mild cognitive impairment: systematic review. Br J Psychiatry 2013; 203:255–264.

135. O'Brien JT et al. Clinical practice with anti-dementia drugs: a revised (second) consensus statement from the British Association for Psychopharmacology. J Psychopharmacol 2011; 25:997–1019.

Safer prescribing of physical health medicines in dementia

People with dementia are more susceptible to cognitive side-effects of drugs. Drugs may affect cognition through their action on cholinergic, histaminergic or opioid neurotransmitter pathways or through more complex actions. Medications prescribed for physical disorders may also interact with cognitive-enhancing medication.

Anticholinergic drugs

Anticholinergic drugs reduce the efficacy of acetylcholinesterase inhibitors and so concomitant use should be avoided.[1,2] Anticholinergic drugs also cause sedation, cognitive impairment, delirium[3] and falls.[4] These effects may be worse in older patients with dementia.[5] Table 7.5 summarises the anticholinergic potency of drugs commonly used in physical health conditions.[6] Combining several drugs with anticholinergic activity increases the anticholinergic cognitive burden (ACB) for an individual. One study showed that a high ACB total score was associated with a greater decline in MMSE score and a higher mortality.[7] It is good practice to keep the ACB to a minimum in older people, especially if they have cognitive impairment.

Where possible, drugs with an equivalent therapeutic effect, but a mode of action which does not affect the cholinergic system, should be used. If this is not possible, the prescription of a drug with low anticholinergic activity or high specificity to the site of action (and thus minimal central activity) should be encouraged. Anticholinergic drugs that do not cross the blood–brain barrier have less profound effects on cognitive function.[8]

Anticholinergic drugs used in urinary incontinence

Oxybutynin easily penetrates the central nervous system (CNS) and has consistently been associated with deterioration in cognitive function. Although studies of tolterodine found no adverse CNS effects,[9] case reports have described adverse effects including memory loss, hallucinations and delirium.[10–12] In contrast, darifenacin, an M_3 selective receptor antagonist, has been investigated in healthy elderly subjects for its effects on cognitive function and was noted to have no significant effects on cognitive tests compared with placebo;[13,14] although studies in dementia are lacking. Solifenacin has been shown to cause impairment of working memory[15] although it was investigated in stroke patients and was found not to affect their short term cognitive performance.[16] A study looking at the use of trospium with galantamine in patients with Alzheimer's disease

CHAPTER 7

Table 7.5 Anticholinergic potency for some physical health drugs commonly used in elderly patients

Drugs with unknown anticholinergic effect	Drugs with improbable or no anticholinergic action		Low effect anticholinergic drugs *Caution*	High effect anticholinergic drugs *Avoid*
	A to K	L to Z		
Colchicine	Allopurinol	Lansoprazole	Amantadine	Atropine
Digoxin	Amlodipine	Levodopa	Baclofen	Benzatropine
Furosemide	Amoxicillin	Lisinopril	Bromocriptine	Chlorphenamine
Metoclopramide	Ampicillin	Losartan	Carbamazepine	Clemastine
	Aspirin	Metformin	Cetirizine	Cyproheptadine
	Atenolol	Methotrexate	Cimetidine	Flavoxate
	Atorvastatin	Metoprolol	Codeine	Hydroxyzine
	Azathioprine	Naratriptan	Disopyramide	Hyoscine
	Benazapril	Nifedipine	Domperidone	Ipratropium
	Betaxolol	Omeprazole	Entacapone	Orphenadrine
	Bisacodyl	Pantoprazole	Fentanyl	Oxybutynin
	Captopril	Paracetamol	Fexofenadine	Procyclidine
	Carbidopa	Phenobarbital	Hydrocodone	Promethazine
	Cefalexin (+other cephalosporins)	Phenytoin	Ketorolac	Propantheline
		Pioglitazone	Loperamide	Tolterodine
	Celecoxib	Piperacillin	Loratadine	Tizanidine
	Ciclosporin	Piroxicam	Meperidine	Trihexyphenidyl
	Clindamycin	Prednisolone	Methadone	(benzhexol)
	Clopidogrel	Propranolol	Methocarbamol	
	Cortisone	Pseudoephedrine	Morphine	
	Cycloserine	Rabeprazole	Oxcarbazepine	
	Dexamethasone	Ropinirole	Oxycodone	
	Dextromethorphan	Rosiglitazone	Prochlorperazine	
	Dicycloverine	Salmeterol	Ranitidine	
	Diltiazem	Selegiline	Theophylline	
	Dipyridamole	Senna	Tramadol	
	Duloxetine	Simvastatin		
	Enalapril	Spironolactone		
	Famotidine	Sumatriptan		
	Fluticasone	Tamoxifen		
	Gemfibrozil	Terbutaline		
	Glipizide	Timolol		
	Glyceryl trinitrate (GTN)	Topiramate		
	Gentamicin	Trandolapril		
	Guaifenesin	Triamcinolone		
	Hydralazine	Triamterene		
	Hydrochlorothiazide	Trimethoprim		
	Hydrocortisone	Valproate		
	Ibuprofen	Verapamil		
	Insulin	Vancomycin		
	Isosorbide mononitrate	Warfarin		
	Ketoprofen	Zolmitriptan		

Note: This list is not exhaustive and includes drugs used for physical health conditions only (i.e. not psychotropic drugs).
Adapted from Bishara D et al.[20] with permission.

found no significant change in cognitive function.[17] There are no *in vivo* studies investigating whether or not fesoterodine causes cognitive impairment but *in vitro* evaluation found that its active metabolite 5-hydroxy-methyl-tolterodine (5-HMT) had one of the highest detectable serum anticholinergic activities and therefore it has potential to induce central anticholinergic adverse effects. However, anticholinergic activity measured in serum does not necessarily reflect brain concentrations[18] and theoretically, fesoterodine has a very low ability to cross the blood–brain barrier.[15]

All tertiary amine drugs, i.e. oxybutynin, tolterodine, fesoterodine and darifenacin are metabolised by cytochrome P450 (CYP450) enzymes. Increasing age or co-administration of drugs that inhibit these enzymes (e.g. erythromycin, fluoxetine) can lead to higher serum levels and therefore increased adverse effects. The metabolism of trospium is unknown, although metabolism via CYP450 system does not occur, meaning that pharmacokinetic drug interactions are unlikely with this drug.[9]

See Table 7.6 for a summary of the physiochemical properties of anticholinergic drugs used in urinary incontinence.

Alpha-blockers for urinary retention

Alpha-blockers such as tamsulosin, alfuzosin and prazosin are reported to cause drowsiness, dizziness and depression.[21] There is no published literature reporting their effects on cognition and alpha-blockers do not feature on any anticholinergic cognitive burden list.

Drugs used in gastrointestinal disorders

- **Loperamide:** although loperamide may have some anticholinergic activity, there are no data to suggest that it can worsen cognitive function in patients with dementia. It may add to the anticholinergic cognitive burden if used in conjunction with other anticholinergic drugs, however.
- **Laxatives:** there is no evidence to suggest that laxatives have any negative impact on cognitive function. In fact since constipation can lead to behavioural and psychological symptoms of dementia (BPSD), treating it can improve these symptoms in many cases.
- **Antiemetics**
  - **Cyclizine** is a first-generation histamine antagonist and can impair cognitive and psychomotor performance (see section on 'Antihistamines' in this section).[22]
  - **Metoclopramide** has little anticholinergic action, but the D_2 receptor antagonism of both metoclopramide and prochlorperazine can produce movement disorders and so these drugs must be used with great caution in people with dementia.
  - **Domperidone** is a dopamine D_2 receptor antagonist that does not usually cross the blood–brain barrier. However, since blood–brain barrier alterations can occur in dementia, CNS penetration of domperidone and resulting adverse effects can occur.[23] Recent reports have highlighted a small increased risk of serious cardiac adverse effects with domperidone, especially in older people. The maximum dose has been reduced to 30 mg/day and the maximum treatment duration should not exceed one week. Domperidone is now contraindicated in

CHAPTER 7

Table 7.6 Physiochemical properties of anticholinergic drugs in urinary incontinence[15,19]

Drug	Muscarinic receptor (M₃:M₁ affinity ratio)	Polarity	Lipophilicity	Molecular weight (kDa)	P-gp substrate	Theoretical ability to cross blood–brain barrier	Effect on cognition
Darifenacin	Mainly M$_3$ (9.3:1)	Neutral	High	507.5 (relatively large)	Yes	High (but bladder selective and P-gp substrate)	–
Fesoterodine	Non-selective	Neutral	Very low	411.6	Yes	Very low	No data yet
Oxybutynin	Non-selective	Neutral	Moderate	357 (relatively small)	No	Moderate/ high	+++
Solifenacin	Mainly M$_3$ (2.5:1)	Neutral	Moderate	480.6	No	Moderate	–/+
Tolterodine	Non-selective	Neutral	Low	475.6	No	Low	+
Trospium chloride	Non-selective	Positively charged	Not lipophilic	428	Yes	Almost none	–

P-gp, P-glycoprotein.

–, no reports of adverse effects on cognition; +, some adverse effects on cognition reported; +++, consistent reports of adverse effects on cognition.

Adapted from Bishara D et al.[20] with permission.

CHAPTER 7

those with underlying cardiac conditions or severe hepatic impairment and in patients receiving other medications known to prolong QT interval or potent CYP3A4 inhibitors.[24]

- **Serotonin 5HT$_3$ receptor antagonists**, used for treating chemotherapy-induced nausea and vomiting do not have adverse effects on cognition, and may have some cognitive enhancing action.[25] These drugs carry cardiovascular warnings and should be used cautiously in patients with cardiac co-morbidities or taking concomitant arrhythmogenic drugs or drugs known to prolong QT interval. Granisetron allows for once daily administration, which is preferable in elderly patients with memory problems or swallowing difficulties. Granisetron is metabolised exclusively via a single CYP family (CYP3A4) and thus has lower propensity for drug interactions.[26] All 5HT$_3$ antagonists cause constipation.
- **Antispasmodics**
  - **Hyoscine hydrobromide** (scopolamine) is a centrally acting anticholinergic which is lipophilic and penetrates the blood–brain barrier easily. It impairs memory, speed of processing and attention. Older patients suffer these symptoms at lower doses and are more vulnerable to confusion and hallucinations.[27] People with Alzheimer's disease have experienced clinically significant cognitive impairment at lower doses compared with healthy, aged-matched controls.[5] The effect that hyoscine has on cognition is so significant that it is used in trials to produce memory deficits similar to those seen in dementia (the scopolamine challenge test).[28]
  - **Hyoscine butylbromide** (Buscopan) exerts topical spasmolytic action on smooth muscle of the GI tract. Hyoscine butylbromide does not enter the CNS, therefore anticholinergic adverse effects at the CNS are extremely rare.[29]
  - **Alverine, mebeverine** and **peppermint oil** are relaxants of intestinal smooth muscle and do not appear to have an effect on cognition.

Bronchodilators

- **Beta-agonists:** in patients with co-existing Parkinson's disease or essential tremor, tremor induced by beta-agonists may result in misdiagnosis and over-treatment of Parkinson's disease.[30] Tremor is a common adverse effect of cholinesterase inhibitors so caution should be exercised when used with beta-agonists.
- **Anticholinergic bronchodilators:** inhaled anticholinergic drugs have few systemic side effects compared with oral medication.[30] A randomised, double blind placebo controlled comparison of ipratropium and theophylline treatment was unable to detect a negative effect with either drug on the psychometric test performance of elderly patients. This suggests that treatment with inhaled ipratropium is not associated with significant cognitive impairment in older people.[31]
- **Theophylline:** as with cholinesterase inhibitors, nausea and vomiting are common adverse effects of theophylline. Neurological effects such as headaches, anxiety, behavioural disturbances, depression and seizures can occur in 50% of patients on theophylline. Although seizures are rare, they are significantly more likely in older people than younger people. Theophylline does not cause significant cognitive impairment.[31]

CHAPTER 7

Hypersalivation

Oral anticholinergic agents used for hypersalivation (e.g. hyoscine hydrobromide) should be avoided in the elderly because of the risk of cognitive impairment, delirium and constipation (see section on 'Anticholinergic drugs' in this section). Pirenzepine is a relatively selective M_1 and M_4 muscarinic receptor antagonist which does not cross the blood–brain barrier and therefore has little CNS penetration.[32]

Atropine solution given sublingually or used as a mouthwash is sometimes used to manage hypersalivation. There are no data available for the extent of penetration through the blood–brain barrier when atropine is administered by this route.

Myasthenia gravis

Unlike acetylcholinesterase inhibitors used in Alzheimer's disease (donepezil, rivastigmine and galantamine), those used in myasthenia gravis (pyridostigmine, neostigmine) act peripherally and do not cross the blood–brain barrier (so as to minimise unwanted central effects).[33] It is possible that combining peripheral and central acetylcholinesterase inhibitors may add to the cholinomimetic adverse effect burden (e.g. nausea, vomiting diarrhoea, abdominal cramps and increased salivation). Memantine may be an alternative to cholinesterase inhibitors in cases where the combined cholinomimetic effects of drugs used for myasthenia gravis and Alzheimer's disease are not tolerated.

Analgesics

NSAIDs and paracetamol

Paracetamol is a safe drug and there is no evidence that it causes cognitive impairment other than in overdose when it may cause delirium.[34] There is some evidence that chronic use of aspirin can cause confusional states.[35] Case reports implicate non-steroidal anti-inflammatory drugs (NSAIDs) in causing delirium and psychosis[36] although clinical trials have not demonstrated significant adverse effects on cognition with naproxen[37] or indomethacin.[38] NSAIDs are difficult to use in older people due to their cardiovascular risk and risk of gastrointestinal bleeding.[39] It is good practice to prescribe gastroprotection with these drugs. Although there is little evidence for their efficacy and safety in dementia, consideration should be given to the use of topical NSAIDs (if clinically appropriate), to reduce GI risk.

Opiates

Sedation is a potential problem with all opiates.[40] Delirium induced by opioids may be associated with agitation, hallucinations or delusions.[40] Pethidine is associated with a high risk of cognitive impairment, as its metabolites have anticholinergic properties, and accumulate rapidly if renal function is impaired.[41] Codeine may increase the risk of falls, and both tramadol and codeine have a high risk of drug–drug interactions, as well as considerable variation in response and adverse effects.[42] Fentanyl patches, useful as they can be in chronic pain and palliative care, should not be used to initiate opioid analgesia in frail older people[43] because of their long duration of action even after the patch is removed, making the treatment of side-effects more difficult.[42] Morphine is a very effective analgesic but is likely to cause cognitive problems and other adverse effects in elderly patients.[44] Oxycodone has a short half-life, few drug–drug interactions, and more predictable dose–response relationships than other opiates. It is therefore, theoretically at least, a good candidate for oral analgesia in dementia.[42] Buprenorphine transdermal patches probably have fewer side effects than many other opiates.

Antihistamines

First-generation H_1 antihistamines include chlorphenamine, hydroxyzine, cyclizine and promethazine. They are non-selective, have anticholinergic activity and readily penetrate the blood–brain barrier, which can lead to unwanted cognitive side-effects. They can impair cognitive and psychomotor performance and can trigger seizures, dyskinesia, dystonia and hallucinations. The second-generation H_1 antihistamines (such as loratadine, cetirizine and fexofenadine) penetrate poorly into the CNS and are considerably less likely to cause these adverse effects. Moreover, they lack any anticholinergic effects.[22]

Statins

A recent Cochrane systematic review assessed the clinical efficacy and tolerability of statins in the treatment of dementia[45] and showed that there was no significant benefit from statins in terms of cognitive function, but equally no evidence that statins were detrimental to cognition. Earlier case reports had highlighted subjective complaints of memory loss associated with the use of statins.[46] This tended to occur in the first two months after starting the drug, and was most commonly associated with simvastatin. In the event of a patient experiencing cognitive problems on simvastatin it may be worth first stopping the drug, and if the complaint resolves, try atorvastatin or pravastatin instead, as these drugs are less likely to cross the blood–brain barrier.

Antihypertensives

Mid-life hypertension has negative effects on cognition and increases the risk of a person developing dementia.[47] A recent systematic review found that treatment reduced the risk of all-cause dementia by 9% in comparison with the control group.[48] Antihypertensive treatment, regardless of drug class, had a positive effect on global cognition and on all cognitive functions except language. Angiotensin II receptor blockers (ARBs) were more effective than beta-blockers, diuretics, and angiotensin-converting enzyme inhibitors in improving scores of cognition.

Other cardiac drugs

Digoxin has been associated with acute confusional states at therapeutic drug concentrations.[49] It has also been reported to cause nightmares.[50] However, one study showed the treatment of cardiac failure with digoxin improved cognitive performance in 25% of patients treated (and in 23% of the patients treated who did not have cardiac failure).[51] There are some case reports of amiodarone being associated with delirium.[52,53]

Table 7.7 Recommended drugs and drugs to avoid in dementia

Condition	Drug class or drug name	Drugs to avoid in dementia	Recommended drugs in dementia
Allergic conditions	Antihistamines	Chlorphenamine Promethazine Hydroxyzine Cyproheptadine Cyclizine (and other first-generation antihistamines)	Cetirizine Loratadine Fexofenadine (and other second-generation antihistamines)
Asthma/COPD	Bronchodilators		Beta-agonists Inhaled anticholinergics (have not been reported to affect cognition) Theophylline
Constipation	Laxatives	No evidence to suggest that laxatives have any negative impact on cognitive function Constipation itself may worsen cognition	
Diarrhoea	Loperamide	Low-potency anticholinergic Not known to have effects on cognitive function, however may add to the anticholinergic cognitive burden if used in combination with other anticholinergics	
Hyperlipidaemia	Statins		All are safe but atorvastatin and pravastatin less likely to cross blood–brain barrier
Hypersalivation	Anticholinergics	Hyoscine hydrobromide	Pirenzepine Atropine (sublingually)
Hypertension	Antihypertensives	Beta-blockers (avoidance may not always be possible)	Calcium channel blockers, angiotensin converting enzyme inhibitors, and angiotensin receptor blockers may all improve cognitive function
Infections	Antibiotics	Delirium reported most commonly with quinolone and macrolide antibiotics But given the importance of treating infections, the most appropriate antibiotic for the infections should be used	
Myasthenia gravis	Peripheral acetylcholinesterase inhibitors, e.g. neostigmine and pyridostigmine	May add to the cholinergic adverse effects of central acetylcholinesterase inhibitors (e.g. donepezil, etc.) in patients with dementia, i.e. increased risk of nausea, vomiting, etc.	
Nausea/vomiting	Antiemetics	Cyclizine Metoclopramide Prochlorperazine	Domperidone (see text for restrictions) Serotonin $5HT_3$ receptor antagonists
Other gastrointestinal conditions	Antispasmodics	Atropine sulphate Dicycloverine hydrochloride	Alverine Mebeverine Peppermint oil Hyoscine-n-butylbromide Propantheline bromide

Table 7.7 (Continued)

Condition	Drug class or drug name	Drugs to avoid in dementia	Recommended drugs in dementia
Pain	Analgesics	Pethidine Pentazocine Dextropropoxyphene Codeine Tramadol Methadone	Paracetamol Oxycodone Buprenorphine Topical NSAIDs (where appropriate)
		Fentanyl patches (caution in opioid naïve patients) Morphine (may be indicated in treatment resistant pain or palliative care; use cautiously due to associated cognitive and other adverse effects)	
Urinary frequency	Anticholinergic drugs used in overactive bladder	Oxybutynin Tolterodine	Darifenacin Trospium Solifenacin (use if others not available; some reports of cognitive adverse effects)
		Data for fesoterodine are still lacking; it is non-selective, has high central anticholinergic activity but theoretically has very low ability to cross the blood–brain barrier	
Urinary retention	Alpha-blockers	Not known to have effects on cognitive function	

COPD, chronic obstructive pulmonary disease; NSAIDs, non-steroidal anti-inflammatory drugs.
Adapted from Bishara D et al.[20] with permission.

H$_2$ antagonists and proton pump inhibitors

Although histamine-2 (H$_2$) receptor antagonists (e.g. cimetidine, ranitidine) are not used widely now, it is not uncommon to see patients with dementia who have been prescribed these drugs for several years. Central nervous system reactions to these drugs have been reviewed.[54] Neurotoxicity in the form of delirium, sometimes with agitation and hallucinations, generally occurred in the first two weeks of therapy and resolved within three days of stopping the drug. The estimated incidence of these reactions was 0.2% or less in outpatients, but much higher in hospitalised patients, particularly in patients with hepatic and liver failure.[55] So if someone with dementia is stable on a H$_2$ antagonist, there is no reason to stop it. Proton pump inhibitors appear less likely to cause cognitive problems.

Antibiotics

Many antibiotics have been associated rarely with delirium but there is no consistent pattern of them causing cognitive impairment. Given the importance of treating infection in dementia the most appropriate antibiotic for the infection being treated should be used. The evidence might suggest that if there is a choice between either a quinolone or macrolide antibiotic with another class of antibiotic, the other class might be the preferred for someone with dementia given the possible risk of these two classes of drugs triggering cognitive disorders. Antituberculous therapy, particularly isoniazid, has attracted some case reports of adverse psychiatric reactions.[56]

Table 7.7 summarises those drugs that are recommended for use in dementia and the drugs to avoid.

CHAPTER 7

References

1. Sink KM et al. Dual use of bladder anticholinergics and cholinesterase inhibitors: long-term functional and cognitive outcomes. J Am Geriatr Soc 2008; **56**:847–853.
2. Lu CJ et al. Chronic exposure to anticholinergic medications adversely affects the course of Alzheimer disease. Am J Geriatr Psychiatry 2003; **11**:458–461.
3. Modi A et al. Concomitant use of anticholinergics with acetylcholinesterase inhibitors in Medicaid recipients with dementia and residing in nursing homes. J Am Geriatr Soc 2009; **57**:1238–1244.
4. Aizenberg D et al. Anticholinergic burden and the risk of falls among elderly psychiatric inpatients: a 4-year case-control study. Int Psychogeriatr 2002; **14**:307–310.
5. Sunderland T et al. Anticholinergic sensitivity in patients with dementia of the Alzheimer type and age-matched controls. A dose-response study. Arch Gen Psychiatry 1987; **44**:418–426.
6. Duran CE et al. Systematic review of anticholinergic risk scales in older adults. Eur J Clin Pharmacol 2013; **69**:1485–1496.
7. Fox C et al. Anticholinergic medication use and cognitive impairment in the older population: the medical research council cognitive function and ageing study. J Am Geriatr Soc 2011; **59**:1477–1483.
8. Wagg A. The cognitive burden of anticholinergics in the elderly - implications for the treatment of overactive bladder. Eur Uro Rev 2012; **7**:42–49.
9. Pagoria D et al. Antimuscarinic drugs: review of the cognitive impact when used to treat overactive bladder in elderly patients. Curr Urol Rep 2011; **12**:351–357.
10. Womack KB et al. Tolterodine and memory: dry but forgetful. Arch Neurol 2003; **60**:771–773.
11. Tsao JW et al. Transient memory impairment and hallucinations associated with tolterodine use. N Engl J Med 2003; **349**:2274–2275.
12. Edwards KR et al. Risk of delirium with concomitant use of tolterodine and acetylcholinesterase inhibitors. J Am Geriatr Soc 2002; **50**:1165–1166.
13. Kay G et al. Differential effects of the antimuscarinic agents darifenacin and oxybutynin ER on memory in older subjects. Eur Urol 2006; **50**:317–326.
14. Lipton RB et al. Assessment of cognitive function of the elderly population: effects of darifenacin. J Urol 2005; **173**:493–498.
15. Chancellor MB et al. Blood-brain barrier permeation and efflux exclusion of anticholinergics used in the treatment of overactive bladder. Drugs Aging 2012; **29**:259–273.
16. Park JW. The Effect of Solifenacin on Cognitive Function following Stroke. Dement Geriatr Cogn Dis Extra 2013; **3**:143–147.
17. Isik AT et al. Trospium and cognition in patients with late onset Alzheimer disease. J Nutr Health Aging 2009; **13**:672–676.
18. Jakobsen SM et al. Evaluation of brain anticholinergic activities of urinary spasmolytic drugs using a high-throughput radio receptor bioassay. J Am Geriatr Soc 2011; **59**:501–505.
19. Kay GG et al. Preserving cognitive function for patients with overactive bladder: evidence for a differential effect with darifenacin. Int J Clin Pract 2008; **62**:1792–1800.
20. Bishara D et al. Safe prescribing of physical health medication in patients with dementia. Int J Geriatr Psychiatry 2014; in press.
21. Joint Formulary Committee. *BNF* 67 March-September 2014 (online). London: Pharmaceutical Press; 2014. http://www.medicinescomplete.com/mc/bnf/current/
22. Mahdy AM et al. Histamine and antihistamines. Anaesthesia and Intensive Care Medicine 2011; **12**:324–329.
23. Roy-Desruisseaux J et al. Domperidone-induced tardive dyskinesia and withdrawal psychosis in an elderly woman with dementia. Ann Pharmacother 2011; **45**:e51.
24. Medicines and Healthcare Products Regulatory Agency. Domperidone: risks of cardiac side effects - indication restricted to nausea and vomiting, new contraindications, and reduced dose and duration of use. 2014. http://www.mhra.gov.uk/Safetyinformation/DrugSafetyUpdate/CON418518
25. Bentley KR et al. Therapeutic Potential of Serotonin 5-HT3 Antagonists in neuropsychiatric disorders. CNS Drugs 1995; **3**:363–392.
26. Gridelli C. Same old story? Do we need to modify our supportive care treatment of elderly cancer patients? Focus on antiemetics. Drugs Aging 2004; **21**:825–832.
27. Flicker C et al. Hypersensitivity to scopolamine in the elderly. Psychopharmacology (Berl) 1992; **107**:437–441.
28. Ebert U et al. Scopolamine model of dementia: electroencephalogram findings and cognitive performance. Eur J Clin Invest 1998; **28**:944–949.
29. Boehringer Ingelheim Limited. Buscopan Tablets. 2013. https://www.medicines.org.uk/
30. Gupta P et al. Potential adverse effects of bronchodilators in the treatment of airways obstruction in older people: recommendations for prescribing. Drugs Aging 2008; **25**:415–443.
31. Ramsdell JW et al. Effects of theophylline and ipratropium on cognition in elderly patients with chronic obstructive pulmonary disease. Ann Allergy Asthma Immunol 1996; **76**:335–340.
32. Fritze J et al. Pirenzepine for clozapine-induced hypersalivation. Lancet 1995; **346**:1034.
33. Pohanka M. Acetylcholinesterase inhibitors: a patent review 2. Expert Opin Ther Pat 2012; **22**:871–886.
34. Gray SL et al. Drug-induced cognition disorders in the elderly: incidence, prevention and management. Drug Saf 1999; **21**:101–122.
35. Bailey RB et al. Chronic salicylate intoxication. A common cause of morbidity in the elderly. J Am Geriatr Soc 1989; **37**:556–561.
36. Hoppmann RA et al. Central nervous system side effects of nonsteroidal anti-inflammatory drugs. Aseptic meningitis, psychosis, and cognitive dysfunction. Arch Intern Med 1991; **151**:1309–1313.
37. Wysenbeek AJ et al. Assessment of cognitive function in elderly patients treated with naproxen. A prospective study. Clin Exp Rheumatol 1988; **6**:399–400.

38. Bruce-Jones PN et al. Indomethacin and cognitive function in healthy elderly volunteers. Br J Clin Pharmacol 1994; **38**:45–51.

39. Barber JB et al. Treatment of chronic non-malignant pain in the elderly: safety considerations. Drug Saf 2009; **32**:457–474.

40. Ripamonti C et al. CNS Adverse Effects of Opioids in Cancer Patients. CNS Drugs 1997; **8**:21–37.

41. Alagiakrishnan K et al. An approach to drug induced delirium in the elderly. Postgrad Med J 2004; **80**:388–393.

42. McLachlan AJ et al. Clinical pharmacology of analgesic medicines in older people: impact of frailty and cognitive impairment. Br J Clin Pharmacol 2011; **71**:351–364.

43. Dosa DM et al. Frequency of long-acting opioid analgesic initiation in opioid-naive nursing home residents. J Pain Symptom Manage 2009; **38**:515–521.

44. Tannenbaum C et al. A systematic review of amnestic and non-amnestic mild cognitive impairment induced by anticholinergic, antihistamine, GABAergic and opioid drugs. Drugs Aging 2012; **29**:639–658.

45. McGuinness B et al. Cochrane review on 'Statins for the treatment of dementia'. Int J Geriatr Psychiatry 2013; **28**:119–126.

46. Wagstaff LR et al. Statin-associated memory loss: analysis of 60 case reports and review of the literature. Pharmacotherapy 2003; **23**:871–880.

47. Qiu C et al. The age-dependent relation of blood pressure to cognitive function and dementia. Lancet Neurol 2005; **4**:487–499.

48. Levi MN et al. Antihypertensive classes, cognitive decline and incidence of dementia: a network meta-analysis. J Hypertens 2013; **31**:1073–1082.

49. Eisendrath SJ et al. Toxic neuropsychiatric effects of digoxin at therapeutic serum concentrations. Am J Psychiatry 1987; **144**:506–507.

50. Brezis M et al. Nightmares from digoxin. Ann Intern Med 1980; **93**:639–640.

51. Laudisio A et al. Digoxin and cognitive performance in patients with heart failure: a cohort, pharmacoepidemiological survey. Drugs Aging 2009; **26**:103–112.

52. Athwal H et al. Amiodarone-induced delirium. Am J Geriatr Psychiatry 2003; **11**:696–697.

53. Foley KT et al. Separate episodes of delirium associated with levetiracetam and amiodarone treatment in an elderly woman. Am J Geriatr Pharmacother 2010; **8**:170–174.

54. Cantu TG et al. Central nervous system reactions to histamine-2 receptor blockers. Ann Intern Med 1991; **114**:1027–1034.

55. Vial T et al. Side effects of ranitidine. Drug Saf 1991; **6**:94–117.

56. Kass JS et al. Nervous system effects of antituberculosis therapy. CNS Drugs 2010; **24**:655–667.

Management of non-cognitive symptoms of dementia

The non-cognitive or neuropsychiatric symptoms of dementia can include: psychosis, agitation and mood disorder[1] and can affect more than 90% of patients to varying degrees.[2] More specifically, they often present as delusions, hallucinations, agitation, aggression, wandering, abnormal vocalisations and disinhibition (often of a sexual nature). The number, type and severity of these symptoms vary amongst patients and the fact that several types occur simultaneously in individuals, makes it difficult to target specific ones therapeutically. The safe and effective management of these symptoms is the subject of a longstanding debate because treatment is not well informed by properly conducted studies[3] and many available agents have been linked to serious adverse effects.

Analgesics

It has been suggested that pain in patients with impaired language and abstract thinking may manifest as agitation and therefore treatment of undiagnosed pain may contribute to the overall prevention and management of agitation.[4] An RCT investigating the effects of a stepwise protocol of treatment with analgesics in patients with moderate-to-severe dementia and agitation noted significant improvement in agitation, overall neuropsychiatric symptoms and pain. The majority of patients in the study received only paracetamol (acetaminophen).

Recommendation: the assessment and effective treatment of pain is important. Even in people without overt pain, a trial of paracetamol is worthwhile.

Non-drug measures

A variety of non-pharmacological methods[5] have been developed and some are reasonably well supported by cogent research.[6-8] Behavioural management techniques, and caregiver psycho-education, centred on individual patient's behaviour are generally successful and the effects can last for months.[7] Music therapy[9] and some types of sensory stimulation are useful during the sessions but have no longer-term effects.[7,10] Snoezelen (specially designed rooms with soothing and stimulating environment) have shown some short term benefits in the past,[11] however, a recent Cochrane Summary found that two new trials did not show any significant effects on behaviour, interactions, and mood of people with dementia.[12] A number of different complementary therapies[13] have been used in dementia including massage, reflexology, administration of herbal medicines and aromatherapy. Aromatherapy[14,15] is the fastest growing of these therapies, with extracts from lavender and *Melissa officinalis* (lemon balm) most commonly used.[5] While some positive results from controlled trials have shown significant reduction in agitation,[16] when assessed using a rigorous blinded RCT, there was no evidence that *Melissa* aromatherapy is superior to placebo or donepezil.[17] Overall, the evidence base remains sparse and the side effect profile relatively unexplored.[18] A systematic review of aromatherapy use in non-cognitive symptoms of dementia identified adverse effects including vomiting, dizziness, abdominal pain and wheezing when essential oils were taken orally and diarrhoea, allergic skin reactions, drowsiness and serious unspecified adverse events when administered topically or by inhalation.[15] Given concerns over almost all drug therapies, non-pharmacological measures should always be considered first.

Recommendation: evidence-based, non-drug measures are first-line treatments.

Antipsychotics in non-cognitive symptoms of dementia

First-generation antipsychotics (FGAs) have been widely used for decades in behavioural disturbance associated with dementia. They are probably effective[19] but, because of extrapyramidal and other adverse effects, are less well tolerated[20,21] than second-generation antipsychotics (SGAs). SGAs have been shown to be comparable in efficacy to FGAs for behavioural symptoms of dementia,[22-24] with one study finding risperidone to be superior to haloperidol.[25] SGAs were once widely recommended in dementia-related behaviour disturbance[26] but their use is now highly controversial.[27,28] There are three reasons for this: effect size is small,[29-32] tolerability is poor[32-34] and there is a tentative association with increased mortality.[35]

Various reviews and trials support the efficacy of olanzapine,[22,36] risperidone,[37-41] quetiapine,[24,42-44] aripiprazole[45-47] and amisulpride.[48,49] One study comparing olanzapine with risperidone[31] and one comparing quetiapine with risperidone[50] found no significant differences between treatment groups. However, more recent data outlined below have led to risperidone (licensed) followed by olanzapine (unlicensed) being the treatments of choice in managing psychosis or aggression in dementia. One study found clozapine to be beneficial in treatment resistant agitation associated with dementia.[51]

The most compelling data come from the CATIE-AD trial. This study[52] showed very minor effectiveness advantages for olanzapine and risperidone (but not for quetiapine) over placebo in terms of time to discontinuation, but all drugs were poorly tolerated because of sedation, confusion and extrapyramidal side-effects (the last of these not a problem with quetiapine). Similarly, in a second report[53] greater improvement was noted with olanzapine or risperidone on certain neuropsychiatric rating scales compared with placebo (but not with quetiapine). A Cochrane review[54] of atypical antipsychotics for aggression and psychosis in Alzheimer's disease found that evidence suggests that risperidone and olanzapine are useful in reducing aggression and risperidone reduces psychosis. However, the authors concluded that because of modest efficacy and significant increase in adverse effects, neither risperidone nor olanzapine should be routinely used to treat patients with dementia unless there is severe distress or a serious risk of physical harm to those living or working with the patient.

Increased mortality with antipsychotics in dementia

Following analysis of published and unpublished data in 2004, initial warnings were issued in the UK and USA regarding increased mortality in patients with dementia using certain SGAs (mainly risperidone and olanzapine).[55-57] These warnings have been extended to include all SGAs as well as conventional antipsychotics[57,58] in view of more recent data. The inclusion of a warning about a possible risk of cerebrovascular accidents (CVAs) has now been added to product labelling for all FGAs and SGAs.

Several published analyses support these warnings,[35,59] confirming an association between SGAs and stroke.[60,61] The magnitude of increased mortality with FGAs has been shown to be similar[62-64] to that with SGAs and possibly even greater.[65-69] Some studies suggested that the risk of CVAs in elderly users of antipsychotics may not be cumulative.[70,71] The risk was found to be elevated especially during the first weeks of treatment but then decreased over time, returning to base level after 3 months. In contrast, a long-term study (24–54 months) deduced that mortality was progressively increased over time for antipsychotic-treated (risperidone and FGAs) patients compared with those receiving placebo.[72] At present this is not a widely held view.

Whether the risk of mortality differs from one antipsychotic to another has recently been investigated in two separate studies. The first study[73] found that among nursing home residents prescribed antipsychotics, when compared with risperidone, haloperidol users had an increased risk of mortality whereas quetiapine users had a decreased risk. No clinically meaningful differences were observed for the other drugs investigated: olanzapine, aripiprazole and ziprasidone. The effects were strongest shortly after the start of treatment and remained after adjustment for dose. There was a dose–response relation for all drugs except quetiapine.[73] The second study[74] confirmed these findings. This study included elderly patients with dementia and also assessed risk of mortality with valproic acid. Haloperidol was associated with the highest rates of mortality, followed by risperidone, olanzapine, valproic acid and then quetiapine. One study[70] suggests affinity for M_1 and α_2-receptors predicts effects on stroke.

Several mechanisms have been postulated for the underlying causes of CVAs with antipsychotics.[75] Orthostatic hypotension may aggravate the deficit in cerebral

CHAPTER 7

perfusion in an individual with cerebrovascular insufficiency or atherosclerosis thus causing a CVA. Tachycardia may similarly decrease cerebral perfusion or dislodge a thrombus in a patient with atrial fibrillation (see section on 'Atrial fibrillation' in this chapter). Following an episode of orthostatic hypotension, there could be a rebound excess of catecholamines with vasoconstriction thus aggravating cerebral insufficiency. In addition, hyperprolactinaemia could in theory accelerate atherosclerosis and sedation might cause dehydration and haemoconcentration, each of which are possible mechanisms for increased risk of cerebrovascular events.[75]

A review of the literature on the safety of antipsychotics in elderly patients with dementia found that overall, atypical and typical antipsychotics were associated with similar increased risk for all-cause mortality and cerebrovascular events. Patients being treated with typical agents have an increased risk of cardiac arrhythmias and extrapyramidal symptoms relative to atypical users. Conversely, users of atypical antipsychotics are exposed to an increased risk of venous thromboembolism and aspiration pneumonia. Despite metabolic effects having consistently been documented in studies with atypical antipsychotics, this effect tends to be attenuated with advancing age and in elderly patients with dementia.[76]

Both typical[77] and atypical antipsychotics[78] may also hasten cognitive decline in dementia, although there is some evidence to refute this.[50,79,80]

Recommendation: use of risperidone (licensed for persistent aggression in Alzheimer's disease) and olanzapine may be justified in some cases. Effect is modest at best.

Clinical information for antipsychotic use in dementia

Risperidone is the only drug licensed in the UK for the management of non-cognitive symptoms associated with dementia and is therefore the agent of choice. It is specifically indicated for short term treatment (up to 6 weeks) of persistent aggression in patients with moderate-to-severe Alzheimer's disease unresponsive to non-pharmacological approaches and when there is a risk of harm to self or others.[81] Risperidone is licensed up to 1 mg twice a day[82], although optimal dose in dementia has been found to be 500 μg twice a day (1 mg daily).[83]

Monitoring recommendations are as follows.

- Baseline ECG, weight, pulse and BP, fasting blood glucose, HbA1c, blood lipid profile and prolactin levels. Routine bloods also include U&Es, LFTs and FBC.
- Pulse, BP and above tests should be repeated at 3 months, at 1 year and then annually (more frequently for in-patients).
- The ECG should be repeated at between 4 weeks and 3 months and then annually (or when clinically indicated)
- Weights should be recorded monthly for the first 3 months, then at 1 year and then annually provided weight is stable.
- Very ill or physically frail patients may need more frequent physical health monitoring than this.
- Review of the antipsychotic drug needs to be done at 4–6 weeks (may be earlier for in-patients), then at 3 months and then every 6 months if physically stable and there are no adverse effects.

Alternative antipsychotic drugs may be used (off-licence) if risperidone is contraindicated or not tolerated. Olanzapine has some positive efficacy data for reducing aggression in dementia,[54] work is underway investigating the efficacy and tolerability of amisulpride in dementia,[84] and quetiapine (although not as effective as risperidone and olanzapine) may be considered in patients with Parkinson's disease, or Lewy body dementia (at very small doses) because of its low propensity for causing movement disorders.

Other pharmacological agents in non-cognitive symptoms of dementia

Cognitive enhancers

Donepezil,[85,86] rivastigmine[87–90] and galantamine[91–93] may afford some benefit in reducing behavioural disturbance in dementia. Their effect seems apparent only after several weeks of treatment.[94] However, the evidence is somewhat inconsistent and a study of donepezil in agitation associated with dementia found no apparent benefit compared with placebo.[95] Rivastigmine has shown positive results for neuropsychiatric symptoms associated with vascular[87] and Lewy body dementia.[87,96] A meta-analysis investigating the impact of acetylcholinesterase inhibitors (AChE-Is) on non-cognitive symptoms of dementia found a statistically significant reduction in symptoms among patients with Alzheimer's disease, however the clinical relevance of this effect remained unclear.[97] A systematic review of RCTs concluded that cholinesterase inhibitors have, at best, a modest impact on non-cognitive symptoms of dementia. However, in the absence of alternative safe and effective pharmacological options, a trial of a cholinesterase inhibitor is an appropriate pharmacological strategy for the management of behavioural disturbances in Alzheimer's disease.[98]

NICE guidance suggests considering a cholinesterase inhibitor only for:[99,100]

- people with Lewy body dementia who have non-cognitive symptoms causing significant distress or leading to behaviour that challenges
- people with mild, moderate or severe Alzheimer's disease who have non-cognitive symptoms and/or behaviour that challenges causing significant distress or potential harm to the individual if:
    - a non-pharmacological approach is inappropriate or has been ineffective, and
    - antipsychotic drugs are inappropriate or have been ineffective.

Growing evidence for memantine also suggests benefits for neuropsychiatric symptoms associated with Alzheimer's disease.[101–103] A Cochrane review[104] of memantine found that slightly fewer patients with moderate-to-severe Alzheimer's disease taking memantine develop agitation, but one study[105] found no effect for memantine in established agitation. The review also suggested that memantine may have a small beneficial effect on behaviour in mild-to-moderate vascular dementia but this was not supported by clinical global measures.[104] Despite apparently positive findings in studies (often manufacturer-sponsored) the use of cognitive enhancing agents for behavioural disturbance remains controversial.

Recommendation: use of AChE-Is or memantine can be justified in situations described above. Effect is modest at best.

Benzodiazepines

Benzodiazepines[106,107] are widely used but their use is poorly supported. Benzodiazepines have been associated with cognitive decline[106] and may contribute to increased frequency of falls and hip fractures[107,108] in the elderly population.

Recommendation: avoid.

Antidepressants

Substantial evidence suggests that depression can be considered both a cause and consequence of Alzheimer's disease. Depression is considered causative because it is a risk factor for Alzheimer's disease. In fact, the prevalence rate of depression and Alzheimer's disease co-morbidity is estimated to be 30–50%.[109] Two potential mechanisms by which antidepressants affect cognition in depression have been postulated: a direct effect caused by the pharmacological action of the drugs on specific neurotransmitters and a secondary effect caused by improvement of depression.[110]

Despite reports of a possible modest advantage over placebo, SSRIs have shown doubtful efficacy in non-cognitive symptoms of dementia in the past.[111,112] One review however, contradicted previous findings and indicated that antidepressants (mainly SSRIs) not only showed efficacy in treating non-cognitive symptoms, but were also well tolerated.[113] The authors noted that the most common antidepressants used in dementia were sertraline followed by citalopram and trazodone. Some of the clinical evidence demonstrating the beneficial effects of SSRIs in patients with Alzheimer's disease either alone or in combination with cholinesterase inhibitors have been summarised in recent papers.[109,114] The Citalopram for Agitation in AD Study (CitAD) found that the addition of citalopram titrated up to 30 mg/day significantly reduced agitation and caregivers' distress compared with placebo in 186 patients who were receiving psychosocial intervention. This is perhaps of academic interest only, as the maximum dose of citalopram in this group of patients is 20 mg a day because of the drug's effect on cardiac QT interval.[115]

Findings suggest that in patients with Alzheimer's disease treated with cholinesterase inhibitors, SSRIs may exert some degree of protection against the negative effects of depression on cognition. To date, literature analysis does not clarify if the combined effect of SSRIs and AChE-Is is synergistic, additive or independent.[110] In addition, it is still unclear whether SSRIs have beneficial effects on cognition in patients with Alzheimer's disease who are not actively manifesting mood or behavioural problems.[114]

Trazodone[116,117] is sometimes used for non-cognitive symptoms although evidence is limited. It has been found to reduce irritability and cause a slight reduction in agitation, most probably by means of its sedative effects.[116,117] A Cochrane review of trazodone for agitation in dementia[116] however found insufficient evidence from RCTs to support its use in dementia.

A second, more recent Cochrane review investigating the efficacy and safety of antidepressants for agitation and psychosis in dementia has also been published.[118] The authors concluded that there are currently relatively few studies available but there is some evidence to support the use of certain antidepressants for agitation and psychosis in dementia. The SSRIs sertraline and citalopram were associated with a reduction in symptoms of agitation when compared with placebo in two studies. Both SSRIs and trazodone appear to be tolerated reasonably well when compared with placebo, typical antipsychotics and atypical antipsychotics. Future studies involving more subjects are required however to determine the effectiveness and safety of SSRIs, trazodone, or other antidepressants in managing these symptoms.

A Cochrane review investigating whether antidepressants are clinically effective and acceptable for the treatment of patients with depression in the context of dementia concluded that antidepressants are not necessarily ineffective in dementia but rather there is not much evidence to support their efficacy and therefore they should be used with caution.[119] Furthermore, a large, independent, parallel group RCT found no difference in depression scores when comparing placebo, sertraline or mirtazapine in patients with dementia suggesting that first line treatment for depression in Alzheimer's disease should be reconsidered.[120]

Tricyclic antidepressants are best avoided in patients with dementia. They can cause falls, possibly via orthostatic hypotension, and increase confusion because of their anticholinergic adverse effects.[121]

Recommendation: use of SSRIs may be justified in some cases. Effect is modest at best. Supporting evidence is weak.

Mood stabilisers/anticonvulsants

Randomised controlled trials of mood stabilisers in non-cognitive symptoms of dementia have been completed for oxcarbazepine[122] carbamazepine[123] and valproate.[124] Gabapentin, lamotrigine and topiramate have also been used.[125] Of the mood stabilisers, carbamazepine has the most robust evidence of efficacy in non-cognitive symptoms.[126] However, its serious adverse effects (especially Stevens-Johnson syndrome) and its potential for drug interactions somewhat limit its use. One RCT of valproate, which included an open-label extension, found valproate to be ineffective in controlling symptoms. Seven of the thirty-nine patients enrolled died during the 12-week extension phase study period, although the deaths could not be attributed to the drug.[127] A study investigating the optimal dose of valproic acid in dementia found that whilst serum levels between 40 and 60 µg/L and relatively low doses (7–12 mg/kg per day) are associated with improvements in agitation in some patients, similar levels produced no significant improvements in others and led to substantial side-effects.[128] A Cochrane review of valproate for the treatment of agitation in dementia found no evidence of efficacy but advocated the need for further research into its use in dementia.[129] Valproate does not delay emergence of agitation in dementia.[130] Literature reviews of anticonvulsants in non-cognitive symptoms of dementia found that valproate, oxcarbazepine and lithium showed low or no evidence of efficacy and that more RCTs are needed to strengthen the evidence for gabapentin, topiramate and lamotrigine.[126] Although clearly beneficial in some patients, anticonvulsant mood stabilisers cannot be recommended for routine use in the treatment of the neuropsychiatric symptoms in dementia at present.[125]

Recommendation: limited evidence to support use. Use may be justified where other treatments are contraindicated or ineffective. Valproate best avoided.

CHAPTER 7

Miscellaneous agents

There is growing evidence for the effects of *Ginkgo biloba* on neuropsychiatric symptoms of dementia especially for apathy, anxiety, depression and irritability.[131] A once daily dose of 240 mg was safe and effective in patients with mild-to-moderate dementia.[132]

Summary

The evidence base available to guide treatment in this area is insufficient to allow specific recommendations on appropriate management and drug choice. The basic approach is to try non-drug measures and analgesia before resorting to the use of psychotropics. Whichever drug is chosen, the following approach should be noted.

- Exclude physical illness potentially precipitating non-cognitive symptoms of dementia, e.g. constipation, infection, pain.
- Target the symptoms requiring treatment.
- Consider non-pharmacological methods.
- Carry out a risk–benefit analysis tailored to individual patient needs when selecting a drug.
- Make evidence-based decisions when choosing a drug.
- Discuss treatment options and explain the risks to patient (if they have capacity) and family/carers.
- Titrate drug from a low starting dose and maintain the lowest dose possible for the shortest period necessary.
- Review appropriateness of treatment regularly so that the ineffective drug is not continued unnecessarily.
- Monitor for adverse effects.
- Document clearly treatment choices and discussions with patient, family or carers.

References

1. Aalten P et al. Behavioral problems in dementia: a factor analysis of the neuropsychiatric inventory. Dement Geriatr Cogn Disord 2003; 15:99–105.
2. Steinberg M et al. Point and 5-year period prevalence of neuropsychiatric symptoms in dementia: the Cache County Study. Int J Geriatr Psychiatry 2008; 23:170–177.
3. Salzman C et al. Elderly patients with dementia-related symptoms of severe agitation and aggression: consensus statement on treatment options, clinical trials methodology, and policy. J Clin Psychiatry 2008; 69:889–898.
4. Husebo BS et al. Efficacy of treating pain to reduce behavioural disturbances in residents of nursing homes with dementia: cluster randomised clinical trial. BMJ 2011; 343:d4065.
5. Douglas S et al. Non-pharmacological interventions in dementia. Adv Psychiatr Treat 2004; 10:171–177.
6. Ayalon L et al. Effectiveness of nonpharmacological interventions for the management of neuropsychiatric symptoms in patients with dementia: a systematic review. Arch Intern Med 2006; 166:2182–2188.
7. Livingston G et al. Systematic review of psychological approaches to the management of neuropsychiatric symptoms of dementia. Am J Psychiatry 2005; 162:1996–2021.
8. Robinson L et al. Effectiveness and acceptability of non-pharmacological interventions to reduce wandering in dementia: a systematic review. Int J Geriatr Psychiatry 2007; 22:9–22.
9. Raglio A et al. Efficacy of music therapy in the treatment of behavioral and psychiatric symptoms of dementia. Alzheimer Dis Assoc Disord 2008; 22:158–162.
10. Chaudhury H et al. The role of physical environment in supporting person-centered dining in long-term care: a review of the literature. Am J Alzheimers Dis Other Demen 2013; 28:491–500.
11. Chung JC et al. Snoezelen for dementia. Cochrane Database Syst Rev 2002; CD003152.

12. Chung JCC, Lay CKY. Cochrane Summary - No evidence of the efficacy of snoezelen or multi-sensory stimulation programmes for people withdementia.2009.http://summaries.cochrane.org/CD003152/no-evidence-of-the-efficacy-of-snoezelen-or-multi-sensory-stimulation-programmes-for-people-with-dementia

13. McCarney R et al. Homeopathy for dementia. Cochrane Database Syst Rev 2003; CD003803.

14. Thorgrimsen L et al. Aroma therapy for dementia. Cochrane Database Syst Rev 2003; CD003150.

15. Fung JK et al. A systematic review of the use of aromatherapy in treatment of behavioral problems in dementia. Geriatr Gerontol Int 2012; 12:372–382.

16. Ballard CG et al. Aromatherapy as a safe and effective treatment for the management of agitation in severe dementia: the results of a double-blind, placebo-controlled trial with Melissa. J Clin Psychiatry 2002; 63:553–558.

17. Burns A et al. A double-blind placebo-controlled randomized trial of Melissa officinalis oil and donepezil for the treatment of agitation in Alzheimer's disease. Dement Geriatr Cogn Disord 2011; 31:158–164.

18. Nguyen QA et al. The use of aromatherapy to treat behavioural problems in dementia. Int J Geriatr Psychiatry 2008; 23:337–346.

19. Devanand DP et al. A randomized, placebo-controlled dose-comparison trial of haloperidol for psychosis and disruptive behaviors in Alzheimer's disease. Am J Psychiatry 1998; 155:1512–1520.

20. Chan WC et al. A double-blind randomised comparison of risperidone and haloperidol in the treatment of behavioural and psychological symptoms in Chinese dementia patients. Int J Geriatr Psychiatry 2001; 16:1156–1162.

21. Tariot PN et al. Quetiapine treatment of psychosis associated with dementia: a double-blind, randomized, placebo-controlled clinical trial. Am J Geriatr Psychiatry 2006; 14:767–776.

22. Verhey FR et al. Olanzapine versus haloperidol in the treatment of agitation in elderly patients with dementia: results of a randomized controlled double-blind trial. Dement Geriatr Cogn Disord 2006; 21:1–8.

23. De Deyn PP et al. A randomized trial of risperidone, placebo, and haloperidol for behavioral symptoms of dementia. Neurology 1999; 53:946–955.

24. Savaskan E et al. Treatment of behavioural, cognitive and circadian rest-activity cycle disturbances in Alzheimer's disease: haloperidol vs. quetiapine. Int J Neuropsychopharmacol 2006; 9:507–516.

25. Suh GH et al. Comparative efficacy of risperidone versus haloperidol on behavioural and psychological symptoms of dementia. Int J Geriatr Psychiatry 2006; 21:654–660.

26. Lee PE et al. Atypical antipsychotic drugs in the treatment of behavioural and psychological symptoms of dementia: systematic review. BMJ 2004; 329:75.

27. Jeste DV et al. Atypical antipsychotics in elderly patients with dementia or schizophrenia: review of recent literature. Harv Rev Psychiatry 2005; 13:340–351.

28. Jeste DV et al. ACNP White Paper: update on use of antipsychotic drugs in elderly persons with dementia. Neuropsychopharmacology 2008; 33:957–970.

29. Aupperle P. Management of aggression, agitation, and psychosis in dementia: focus on atypical antipsychotics. Am J Alzheimers Dis Other Demen 2006; 21:101–108.

30. Yury CA et al. Meta-analysis of the effectiveness of atypical antipsychotics for the treatment of behavioural problems in persons with dementia. Psychother Psychosom 2007; 76:213–218.

31. Deberdt WG et al. Comparison of olanzapine and risperidone in the treatment of psychosis and associated behavioral disturbances in patients with dementia. Am J Geriatr Psychiatry 2005; 13:722–730.

32. Schneider LS et al. Efficacy and adverse effects of atypical antipsychotics for dementia: meta-analysis of randomized, placebo-controlled trials. Am J Geriatr Psychiatry 2006; 14:191–210.

33. Anon. How safe are antipsychotics in dementia? Drug Ther Bull 2007; 45:81–86.

34. Rosack J. Side-effect risk often tempers antipsychotic use for dementia. Psychiatr News 2006; 41:1–a.

35. Schneider LS et al. Risk of death with atypical antipsychotic drug treatment for dementia: meta-analysis of randomized placebo-controlled trials. JAMA 2005; 294:1934–1943.

36. Street JS et al. Olanzapine treatment of psychotic and behavioral symptoms in patients with Alzheimer disease in nursing care facilities: a double-blind, randomized, placebo-controlled trial. The HGEU Study Group. Arch Gen Psychiatry 2000; 57:968–976.

37. Bhana N et al. Risperidone: a review of its use in the management of the behavioural and psychological symptoms of dementia. Drugs Aging 2000; 16:451–471.

38. Katz I et al. The efficacy and safety of risperidone in the treatment of psychosis of Alzheimer's disease and mixed dementia: a meta-analysis of 4 placebo-controlled clinical trials. Int J Geriatr Psychiatry 2007; 22:475–484.

39. Onor ML et al. Clinical experience with risperidone in the treatment of behavioral and psychological symptoms of dementia. Prog Neuropsychopharmacol Biol Psychiatry 2007; 31:205–209.

40. Rabinowitz J et al. Treating behavioral and psychological symptoms in patients with psychosis of Alzheimer's disease using risperidone. Int Psychogeriatr 2007; 19:227–240.

41. Kurz A et al. Effects of risperidone on behavioral and psychological symptoms associated with dementia in clinical practice. Int Psychogeriatr 2005; 17:605–616.

42. McManus DQ et al. Quetiapine, a novel antipsychotic: experience in elderly patients with psychotic disorders. Seroquel Trial 48 Study Group. J Clin Psychiatry 1999; 60:292–298.

43. Onor ML et al. Efficacy and tolerability of quetiapine in the treatment of behavioral and psychological symptoms of dementia. Am J Alzheimers Dis Other Demen 2006; 21:448–453.

44. Zhong KX et al. Quetiapine to treat agitation in dementia: a randomized, double-blind, placebo-controlled study. Curr Alzheimer Res 2007; 4:81–93.

CHAPTER 7

45. Laks J et al. Use of aripiprazole for psychosis and agitation in dementia. Int Psychogeriatr 2006; **18**:335–340.

46. De Deyn P et al. Aripiprazole for the treatment of psychosis in patients with Alzheimer's disease: a randomized, placebo-controlled study. J Clin Psychopharmacol 2005; **25**:463–467.

47. Mintzer JE et al. Aripiprazole for the treatment of psychoses in institutionalized patients with Alzheimer dementia: a multicenter, randomized, double-blind, placebo-controlled assessment of three fixed doses. Am J Geriatr Psychiatry 2007; **15**:918–931.

48. Mauri M et al. Amisulpride in the treatment of behavioural disturbances among patients with moderate to severe Alzheimer's disease. Acta Neurol Scand 2006; **114**:97–101.

49. Lim HK et al. Amisulpride versus risperidone treatment for behavioral and psychological symptoms in patients with dementia of the Alzheimer type: a randomized, open, prospective study. Neuropsychobiology 2006; **54**:247–251.

50. Rainer M et al. Quetiapine versus risperidone in elderly patients with behavioural and psychological symptoms of dementia: efficacy, safety and cognitive function. Eur Psychiatry 2007; **22**:395–403.

51. Lee HB et al. Clozapine for treatment-resistant agitation in dementia. J Geriatr Psychiatry Neurol 2007; **20**:178–182.

52. Schneider LS et al. Effectiveness of atypical antipsychotic drugs in patients with Alzheimer's disease. N Engl J Med 2006; **355**:1525–1538.

53. Sultzer DL et al. Clinical symptom responses to atypical antipsychotic medications in Alzheimer's disease: phase 1 outcomes from the CATIE-AD effectiveness trial. Am J Psych 2008; **165**:844–854.

54. Ballard C et al. Atypical antipsychotics for aggression and psychosis in Alzheimer's disease (review). Cochrane Database Syst Rev 2006; DOI: 10.1002/14651858.CD003476.

55. Pharmacovigilance Working Party. Antipsychotics and cerebrovascular accident. SPC wording for antipsychotics. 2005. http://www.mhra.gov.uk

56. Duff G. Atypical antipsychotic drugs and stroke - Committee on Safety of Medicines. 2004. http://www.mhra.gov.uk/home/groups/pl-p/documents/websiteresources/con019488.pdf

57. FDA. Information on Conventional Antipsychotics - FDA Alert [6/16/2008]. 2008. http://www.fda.gov/

58. European Medicines Agency. CHMP Assessment Report on conventional antipsychotics. 2008. http://www.emea.europa.eu

59. Kryzhanovskaya LA et al. A review of treatment-emergent adverse events during olanzapine clinical trials in elderly patients with dementia. J Clin Psychiatry 2006; **67**:933–945.

60. Herrmann N et al. Do atypical antipsychotics cause stroke? CNS Drugs 2005; **19**:91–103.

61. Douglas IJ et al. Exposure to antipsychotics and risk of stroke: self controlled case series study. BMJ 2008; **337**:a1227.

62. Kales HC et al. Mortality risk in patients with dementia treated with antipsychotics versus other psychiatric medications. Am J Psychiatry 2007; **164**:1568–1576.

63. Herrmann N et al. Atypical antipsychotics and risk of cerebrovascular accidents. Am J Psychiatry 2004; **161**:1113–1115.

64. Trifiro G et al. All-cause mortality associated with atypical and typical antipsychotics in demented outpatients. Pharmacoepidemiol Drug Saf 2007; **16**:538–544.

65. Nasrallah HA et al. Lower mortality in geriatric patients receiving risperidone and olanzapine versus haloperidol: preliminary analysis of retrospective data. Am J Geriatr Psychiatry 2004; **12**:437–439.

66. Gill SS et al. Antipsychotic drug use and mortality in older adults with dementia. Ann Intern Med 2007; **146**:775–786.

67. Sacchetti E et al. Risk of stroke with typical and atypical anti-psychotics: a retrospective cohort study including unexposed subjects. J Psychopharmacol 2008; **22**:39–46.

68. Wang PS et al. Risk of death in elderly users of conventional vs. atypical antipsychotic medications. N Engl J Med 2005; **353**:2335–2341.

69. Hollis J et al. Antipsychotic medication dispensing and risk of death in veterans and war widows 65 years and older. Am J Geriatr Psychiatry 2007; **15**:932–941.

70. Wu CS et al. Association of stroke with the receptor-binding profiles of antipsychotics-a case-crossover study. Biol Psychiatry 2013; **73**:414–421.

71. Kleijer BC et al. Risk of cerebrovascular events in elderly users of antipsychotics. J Psychopharmacol 2008.

72. Ballard C et al. The dementia antipsychotic withdrawal trial (DART-AD): long-term follow-up of a randomised placebo-controlled trial. Lancet Neurol 2009; **8**:151–157.

73. Huybrechts KF et al. Differential risk of death in older residents in nursing homes prescribed specific antipsychotic drugs: population based cohort study. BMJ 2012; **344**:e977.

74. Kales HC et al. Risk of mortality among individual antipsychotics in patients with dementia. Am J Psychiatry 2012; **169**:71–79.

75. Smith DA et al. Association between risperidone treatment and cerebrovascular adverse events: examining the evidence and postulating hypotheses for an underlying mechanism. J Am Med Dir Assoc 2004; **5**:129–132.

76. Trifiro G et al. Use of antipsychotics in elderly patients with dementia: do atypical and conventional agents have a similar safety profile? Pharmacol Res 2009; **59**:1–12.

77. McShane R et al. Do neuroleptic drugs hasten cognitive decline in dementia? Prospective study with necropsy follow up. BMJ 1997; **314**:266–270.

78. Ballard C et al. Quetiapine and rivastigmine and cognitive decline in Alzheimer's disease: randomised double blind placebo controlled trial. BMJ 2005; **330**:874.

79. Livingston G et al. Antipsychotics and cognitive decline in Alzheimer's disease: the LASER-Alzheimer's disease longitudinal study. J Neurol Neurosurg Psychiatry 2007; **78**:25–29.

80. Paleacu D et al. Quetiapine treatment for behavioural and psychological symptoms of dementia in Alzheimer's disease patients: a 6-week, double-blind, placebo-controlled study. Int J Geriatr Psychiatry 2008; **23**:393–400.

81. Janssen-Cilag Ltd. Risperdal Tablets, Liquid & Quicklet. 2013. https://www.medicines.org.uk/

82. Joint Formulary Committee. *BNF* 67 March-September 2014 (online). London: Pharmaceutical Press; 2014. http://www.medicinescomplete.com/mc/bnf/current/

83. Katz IR et al. Comparison of risperidone and placebo for psychosis and behavioral disturbances associated with dementia: a randomized, double-blind trial. Risperidone Study Group. J Clin Psychiatry 1999; **60**:107–115.

84. UK Clinical Research Network. Optimisation of amisulpride prescribing in older people. 2014. http://public.ukcrn.org.uk/search/StudyDetail.aspx?StudyID=12780

85. Terao T et al. Can donepezil be considered a mild antipsychotic in dementia treatment? A report of donepezil use in 6 patients. J Clin Psychiatry 2003; **64**:1392–1393.

86. Weiner MF et al. Effects of donepezil on emotional/behavioral symptoms in Alzheimer's disease patients. J Clin Psychiatry 2000; **61**:487–492.

87. Figiel G et al. A systematic review of the effectiveness of rivastigmine for the treatment of behavioral disturbances in dementia and other neurological disorders. Curr Med Res Opin 2008; **24**:157–166.

88. Finkel SI. Effects of rivastigmine on behavioral and psychological symptoms of dementia in Alzheimer's disease. Clin Ther 2004; **26**:980–990.

89. Rosler M et al. Effects of two-year treatment with the cholinesterase inhibitor rivastigmine on behavioural symptoms in Alzheimer's disease. Behav Neurol 1998; **11**:211–216.

90. Cummings JL et al. Effects of rivastigmine treatment on the neuropsychiatric and behavioral disturbances of nursing home residents with moderate to severe probable Alzheimer's disease: a 26-week, multicenter, open-label study. Am J Geriatr Pharmacother 2005; **3**:137–148.

91. Cummings JL et al. Reduction of behavioral disturbances and caregiver distress by galantamine in patients with Alzheimer's disease. Am J Psychiatry 2004; **161**:532–538.

92. Herrmann N et al. Galantamine treatment of problematic behavior in Alzheimer disease: post-hoc analysis of pooled data from three large trials. Am J Geriatr Psychiatry 2005; **13**:527–534.

93. Tangwongchai S et al. Galantamine for the treatment of BPSD in Thai patients with possible Alzheimer's disease with or without cerebrovascular disease. Am J Alzheimers Dis Other Demen 2008; **23**:593–601.

94. Barak Y et al. Donepezil for the treatment of behavioral disturbances in Alzheimer's disease: a 6-month open trial. Arch Gerontol Geriatr 2001; **33**:237–241.

95. Howard RJ et al. Donepezil for the treatment of agitation in Alzheimer's disease. N Engl J Med 2007; **357**:1382–1392.

96. McKeith I et al. Efficacy of rivastigmine in dementia with Lewy bodies: a randomised, double-blind, placebo-controlled international study. Lancet 2000; **356**:2031–2036.

97. Campbell N et al. Impact of cholinesterase inhibitors on behavioral and psychological symptoms of Alzheimer's disease: a meta-analysis. Clin Interv Aging 2008; **3**:719–728.

98. Rodda J et al. Are cholinesterase inhibitors effective in the management of the behavioral and psychological symptoms of dementia in Alzheimer's disease? A systematic review of randomized, placebo-controlled trials of donepezil, rivastigmine and galantamine. Int Psychogeriatr 2009; **21**:813–824.

99. National Institute for Health and Clinical Excellence. Donepezil, galantamine, rivastigmine and memantine for the treatment of Alzheimer's disease. TA 217, 2011. http://www.nice.org.uk/guidance/index.jsp?action=byID&o=13419

100. National Institute for Health and Clinical Excellence. Dementia. Supporting people with dementia and their carers in health and social care. Clincial Guideline 42, 2011. Updated March 2011. http://www.nice.org.uk/nicemedia/live/10998/30318/30318.pdf

101. Cummings JL et al. Behavioral effects of memantine in Alzheimer disease patients receiving donepezil treatment. Neurology 2006; **67**:57–63.

102. Wilcock GK et al. Memantine for agitation/aggression and psychosis in moderately severe to severe Alzheimer's disease: a pooled analysis of 3 studies. J Clin Psychiatry 2008; **69**:341–348.

103. Gauthier S et al. Improvement in behavioural symptoms in patients with moderate to severe Alzheimer's disease by memantine: a pooled data analysis. Int J Geriatr Psychiatry 2007; **23**:537–545.

104. McShane R et al. Memantine for dementia. Cochrane Database Syst Rev 2006;CD003154.

105. Fox C et al. Efficacy of memantine for agitation in Alzheimer's dementia: a randomised double-blind placebo controlled trial. PLoS One 2012; **7**:e35185.

106. Verdoux H et al. Is benzodiazepine use a risk factor for cognitive decline and dementia? A literature review of epidemiological studies. Psychol Med 2005; **35**:307–315.

107. Lagnaoui R et al. Benzodiazepine utilization patterns in Alzheimer's disease patients. Pharmacoepidemiol Drug Saf 2003; **12**:511–515.

108. Chang CM et al. Benzodiazepine and risk of hip fractures in older people: a nested case-control study in Taiwan. Am J Geriatr Psychiatry 2008; **16**:686–692.

109. Aboukhatwa M et al. Antidepressants are a rational complementary therapy for the treatment of Alzheimer's disease. Mol Neurodegener 2010; **5**:10.

110. Rozzini L et al. Efficacy of SSRIs on cognition of Alzheimer's disease patients treated with cholinesterase inhibitors. Int Psychogeriatr 2010; **22**:114–119.

111. Deakin JB et al. Paroxetine does not improve symptoms and impairs cognition in frontotemporal dementia: a double-blind randomized controlled trial. Psychopharmacology 2004; **172**:400–408.

112. Finkel SI et al. A randomized, placebo-controlled study of the efficacy and safety of sertraline in the treatment of the behavioral manifestations of Alzheimer's disease in outpatients treated with donepezil. Int J Geriatr Psychiatry 2004; **19**:9–18.

CHAPTER 7

113. Henry G et al. Efficacy and tolerability of antidepressants in the treatment of behavioral and psychological symptoms of dementia, a literature review of evidence. Am J Alzheimers Dis Other Demen 2011; 26:169–183.

114. Chow TW et al. Potential cognitive enhancing and disease modification effects of SSRIs for Alzheimer's disease. Neuropsychiatr Dis Treat 2007; 3:627–636.

115. Porsteinsson AP et al. Effect of citalopram on agitation in Alzheimer disease: the CitAD randomized clinical trial. JAMA 2014; 311:682–691.

116. Martinon-Torres G et al. Trazodone for agitation in dementia. Cochrane Database Syst Rev 2004; CD004990.

117. Lopez-Pousa S et al. Trazodone for Alzheimer's disease: a naturalistic follow-up study. Arch Gerontol Geriatr 2008; 47:207–215.

118. Seitz DP et al. Antidepressants for agitation and psychosis in dementia. Cochrane Database Syst Rev 2011; 2: CD008191.

119. Bains J et al. The efficacy of antidepressants in the treatment of depression in dementia. Cochrane Database Syst Rev 2002; CD003944.

120. Banerjee S et al. Sertraline or mirtazapine for depression in dementia (HTA-SADD): a randomised, multicentre, double-blind, placebo-controlled trial. Lancet 2011; 378:403–411.

121. Ballard C et al. Management of neuropsychiatric symptoms in people with dementia. CNS Drugs 2010; 24:729–739.

122. Sommer OH et al. Effect of oxcarbazepine in the treatment of agitation and aggression in severe dementia. Dement Geriatr Cogn Disord 2009; 27:155–163.

123. Tariot PN et al. Efficacy and tolerability of carbamazepine for agitation and aggression in dementia. Am J Psychiatry 1998; 155:54–61.

124. Lonergan E et al. Valproate preparations for agitation in dementia. Cochrane Database Syst Rev 2009; CD003945.

125. Konovalov S et al. Anticonvulsants for the treatment of behavioral and psychological symptoms of dementia: a literature review. Int Psychogeriatr 2008; 20:293–308.

126. Yeh YC et al. Mood stabilizers for the treatment of behavioral and psychological symptoms of dementia: an update review. Kaohsiung J Med Sci 2012; 28:185–193.

127. Sival RC et al. Sodium valproate in aggressive behaviour in dementia: a twelve-week open label follow-up study. Int J Geriatr Psychiatry 2004; 19:305–312.

128. Dolder CR et al. Valproic acid in dementia: does an optimal dose exist? J Pharm Pract 2012; 25:142–150.

129. Lonergan E et al. Valproate preparations for agitation in dementia. Cochrane Database Syst Rev 2009; CD003945.

130. Tariot PN et al. Chronic divalproex sodium to attenuate agitation and clinical progression of Alzheimer disease. Arch Gen Psychiatry 2011; 68:853–861.

131. Scripnikov A et al. Effects of Ginkgo biloba extract EGb 761 on neuropsychiatric symptoms of dementia: findings from a randomised controlled trial. Wien Med Wochenschr 2007; 157:295–300.

132. Bachinskaya N et al. Alleviating neuropsychiatric symptoms in dementia: the effects of Ginkgo biloba extract EGb 761. Findings from a randomized controlled trial. Neuropsychiatr Dis Treat 2011; 7:209–215.

Parkinson's disease

Parkinson's disease is a progressive, degenerative neurological disorder characterised by resting tremor, cogwheel rigidity, bradykinesia and postural instability. The prevalence of co-morbid psychiatric disorders is high. Approximately 25% will suffer from major depression at some point during the course of their illness, a further 25% from milder forms of depression, 25% from anxiety spectrum disorders, 25% from psychosis and up to 80% will develop dementia.[1-3] While depression and anxiety can occur at any time, psychosis, dementia and delirium are more prevalent in the later stages of the illness. Close co-operation between the psychiatrist and neurologist is required to optimise treatment for this group of patients.

Depression in Parkinson's disease

Depression in Parkinson's disease predicts greater cognitive decline, deterioration in functioning and progression of motor symptoms;[4] possibly reflecting more advanced and widespread neurodegeneration involving multiple neurotransmitter pathways.[5] Depression may also occur after the withdrawal of dopamine agonists.[6] Pre-existing dementia is an established risk factor for the development of depression. Recommendations for the treatment of depression in Parkinson's disease are shown in Box 7.3.

Box 7.3 Recommendations for the treatment of depression in Parkinson's disease

Step	Intervention
1	Exclude/treat organic causes such as hypothyroidism (the prevalence of which is relatively high in Parkinson's disease[4]).
2	**SSRIs** are considered to be first-line treatment although the effect size is modest.[7-9] Some patients may experience a worsening of motor symptoms although the absolute risk is low.[10,11] Care must be taken when combining SSRIs with selegiline, as the risk of serotonin syndrome is increased.[4] The **SNRIs** venlafaxine[12] and duloxetine[13] also appear to have some effect although venlafaxine may modestly worsen motor symptoms.[12] **TCAs** are generally poorly tolerated because of their anticholinergic (can worsen cognitive problems; constipation) and alpha-blocking effects (can worsen symptoms of autonomic dysfunction). Note though that several meta-analyses[8,9] have reported that low dose TCAs to be more effective than SSRIs,[14-16] although low dose amitriptyline and sertraline seem to be equally effective.[17] Atomoxetine is not effective.[18] **CBT** should always be considered.[19]
3	Consider augmentation with dopamine agonists/releasers such as pramiprexole.[20] Note though that these drugs increase the risk of impulse control disorders.[21,22] They have also been associated with the development of psychosis.[23]
4	Consider **ECT**. Depression and motor symptoms generally respond well[4] but the risk of inducing delirium is high,[24] particularly in patients with pre-existing cognitive impairment.
5	Follow the algorithm for treatment-resistant depression (see section on 'Treatment of refractory depression' in Chapter 4) from this point. Be aware of the increased propensity for adverse effects and drug interactions in this patient group.

CBT, cognitive behavioural therapy; ECT, electroconvulsive therapy; SNRI, selective noradrenaline reuptake inhibitor; SSRI, selective serotonin reuptake inhibitor; TCA, tricyclic antidepressants.

CHAPTER 7

Psychosis in Parkinson's disease

Psychosis in Parkinson's disease is often characterised by visual hallucinations.[25] Auditory hallucinations and delusions occur far less frequently,[26] and usually in younger patients.[27] Psychosis and dementia frequently co-exist. Having one predicts the development of the other.[28] Sleep disorders are also an established risk factor for the development of psychosis.[29]

Abnormalities in dopamine, serotonin and acetylcholine neurotransmission have all been implicated, but the exact aetiology of Parkinson's disease psychosis is poorly understood. In the majority of patients, psychotic symptoms are thought to be secondary to dopaminergic medication rather than part of Parkinson's disease itself; psychosis secondary to medication may be determined at least in part through polymorphisms

---

Box 7.4 Recommendations for the treatment of psychosis in Parkinson's disease

Step	Intervention
1	Exclude organic causes (delirium).
2	Optimise the environment to maximise orientation and minimise problems due to poor caregiver–patient interactions.
3	If the patient has insight and hallucinations are infrequent and not troubling, do not treat.
4	Consider reducing or stopping anticholinergics and dopamine agonists. Monitor for signs of motor deterioration. Be prepared to restart/increase the dose of these drugs again to achieve the best balance between psychosis and mobility.
5	Try an atypical antipsychotic. The efficacy of clozapine (see point 7) is supported by placebo-controlled randomised controlled trials.[25] In contrast, there are several negative placebo-controlled trials each for quetiapine and olanzapine.[25] Low dose quetiapine is the best tolerated, although extrapyramidal side-effects and stereotypical movements can occur. It is probably reasonable to try quetiapine before clozapine but the success rate may be low. Olanzapine, ziprasidone and aripiprazole are likely to all have greater adverse effects on motor function than quetiapine, although one small trial[32] supports the safe use of ziprasidone. Risperidone and typical antipsychotics should be avoided completely. Severe rebound psychosis has been described when antipsychotic drugs (quetiapine or clozapine) are discontinued. Note that all antipsychotics may be even less effective in managing psychotic symptoms in patients with dementia, and such patients may be more prone to developing motor and cognitive side effects.[33] Antipsychotics have been associated with an increased risk of vascular events in the elderly. See section on 'Antipsychotics and non-cognitive symptoms of dementia' in this chapter.
6	Consider a **cholinesterase inhibitor**, particularly if the patient has co-morbid dementia.[25,34] Cholinesterase inhibitors may also reduce the risk of falls.[35]
7	Try **clozapine**. Start at 6.25 mg – usual dose 25 mg–35 mg/day.[25,32] Usually safe but neuroleptic malignant syndrome has been reported.[36] Monitor as for clozapine in schizophrenia. The elderly are more prone to develop serious blood dyscrasia. A case of aplastic anaemia has been reported.[37]
8	Consider **ECT**.[38] Psychotic and motor symptoms usually respond well[39] but the risk of inducing delirium is high,[24] particularly in patients with pre-existing cognitive impairment.

ECT, electroconvulsive therapy.

of the angiotensin-converting enzyme (ACE) gene.[30] From the limited data available, anticholinergics and dopamine agonists seem to be associated with a higher risk of inducing psychosis than levodopa or catechol-O-methyltransferase (COMT) inhibitors.[26,31] Psychosis is a major contributor to caregiver distress and a risk factor for institutionalisation and early death.[28]

Recommendations for the treatment of psychosis in Parkinson's disease are shown in Box 7.4. In addition to the studies described, there is one failed RCT of pimavanserin, a $5HT_{2a}$ inverse agonist[40] and one demonstrating useful activity.[41] Pimavanserin remains unlicensed.

Dementia in Parkinson's disease

Cholinesterase inhibitors have been shown to improve cognition, delusions and hallucinations in patients with Lewy body dementia (which has some similarities to Parkinson's disease). Motor function may deteriorate.[42,43] Improvements in cognitive functioning are modest.[44,45] A Cochrane review and recent large RCTs[45–47] conclude that there is evidence that cholinesterase inhibitors lead to improvements in global functioning, cognition, behavioural disturbance and activities of daily living in Parkinson's disease. Again, motor function may deteriorate.[47,48] Evidence for memantine is mixed.[49,50]

Most patients with Parkinson's disease use complementary therapies, some of which may be modestly beneficial. See Zesiewicz et al.[40] Caffeine may offer a protective effect against the development of Parkinson's disease and also modestly improve motor function in established disease.[51]

References

1. Hely MA et al. The Sydney multicenter study of Parkinson's disease: the inevitability of dementia at 20 years. Mov Disord 2008; 23:837–844.
2. Riedel O et al. Frequency of dementia, depression, and other neuropsychiatric symptoms in 1,449 outpatients with Parkinson's disease. J Neurol 2010; 257:1073–1082.
3. Reijnders JS et al. A systematic review of prevalence studies of depression in Parkinson's disease. Mov Disord 2008; 23:183–189.
4. McDonald WM et al. Prevalence, etiology, and treatment of depression in Parkinson's disease. Biol Psychiatry 2003; 54:363–375.
5. Palhagen SE et al. Depressive illness in Parkinson's disease--indication of a more advanced and widespread neurodegenerative process? Acta Neurol Scand 2008; 117:295–304.
6. Rabinak CA et al. Dopamine agonist withdrawal syndrome in Parkinson disease. Arch Neurol 2010; 67:58–63.
7. Rocha FL et al. Antidepressants for depression in Parkinson's disease: systematic review and meta-analysis. J Psychopharmacol 2013; 27:417–423.
8. Liu J et al. Comparative efficacy and acceptability of antidepressants in Parkinson's disease: a network meta-analysis. PLoS One 2013; 8:e76651.
9. Troeung L et al. A meta-analysis of randomised placebo-controlled treatment trials for depression and anxiety in Parkinson's disease. PLoS One 2013; 8:e79510.
10. Gony M et al. Risk of serious extrapyramidal symptoms in patients with Parkinson's disease receiving antidepressant drugs: a pharmacoepidemiologic study comparing serotonin reuptake inhibitors and other antidepressant drugs. Clin Neuropharmacol 2003; 26:142–145.
11. Kulisevsky J et al. Motor changes during sertraline treatment in depressed patients with Parkinson's disease. Eur J Neurol 2008; 15:953–959.
12. Richard IH et al. A randomized, double-blind, placebo-controlled trial of antidepressants in Parkinson disease. Neurology 2012; 78:1229–1236.
13. Bonuccelli U et al. A non-comparative assessment of tolerability and efficacy of duloxetine in the treatment of depressed patients with Parkinson's disease. Expert Opin Pharmacother 2012; 13:2269–2280.
14. Serrano-Duenas M. A comparison between low doses of amitriptyline and low doses of fluoxetine used in the control of depression in patients suffering from Parkinson's disease (Spanish). Rev Neurol 2002; 35:1010–1014.
15. Menza M et al. A controlled trial of antidepressants in patients with Parkinson disease and depression. Neurology 2009; 72:886–892.
16. Devos D et al. Comparison of desipramine and citalopram treatments for depression in Parkinson's disease: a double-blind, randomized, placebo-controlled study. Mov Disord 2008; 23:850–857.

17. Antonini A et al. Randomized study of sertraline and low-dose amitriptyline in patients with Parkinson's disease and depression: effect on quality of life. Mov Disord 2006; 21:1119–1122.

18. Weintraub D et al. Atomoxetine for depression and other neuropsychiatric symptoms in Parkinson disease. Neurology 2010; 75:448–455.

19. Dobkin RD et al. Cognitive-behavioral therapy for depression in Parkinson's disease: a randomized, controlled trial. Am J Psychiatry 2011; 168:1066–1074.

20. Barone P et al. Pramipexole versus sertraline in the treatment of depression in Parkinson's disease: a national multicenter parallel-group randomized study. J Neurol 2006; 253:601–607.

21. Antonini A et al. A reassessment of risks and benefits of dopamine agonists in Parkinson's disease. Lancet Neurol 2009; 8:929–937.

22. Weintraub D et al. Impulse control disorders in Parkinson disease: a cross-sectional study of 3090 patients. Arch Neurol 2010; 67:589–595.

23. Li CT et al. Pramipexole-induced psychosis in Parkinson's disease. Psychiatry Clin Neurosci 2008; 62:245.

24. Figiel GS et al. ECT-induced delirium in depressed patients with Parkinson's disease. J Neuropsychiatry Clin Neurosci 1991; 3:405–411.

25. Friedman JH. Parkinson's disease psychosis 2010: a review article. Parkinsonism Relat Disord 2010; 16:553–560.

26. Ismail MS et al. A reality test: How well do we understand psychosis in Parkinson's disease? J Neuropsychiatry Clin Neurosci 2004; 16:8–18.

27. Kiziltan G et al. Relationship between age and subtypes of psychotic symptoms in Parkinson's disease. J Neurol 2007; 254:448–452.

28. Factor SA et al. Longitudinal outcome of Parkinson's disease patients with psychosis. Neurology 2003; 60:1756–1761.

29. Reich SG et al. Ten most commonly asked questions about the psychiatric aspects of Parkinson's disease. Neurologist 2003; 9:50–56.

30. Lin JJ et al. Genetic polymorphism of the angiotensin converting enzyme and L-dopa-induced adverse effects in Parkinson's disease. J Neurol Sci 2007; 252:130–134.

31. Ives NJ et al. Dopamine agonist therapy in early Parkinson's disease: a systematic review of randomised controlled trials. Mov Disord 2004; 19 Suppl 9.

32. Pintor L et al. Ziprasidone versus clozapine in the treatment of psychotic symptoms in Parkinson disease: a randomized open clinical trial. Clin Neuropharmacol 2012; 35:61–66.

33. Prohorov T et al. The effect of quetiapine in psychotic Parkinsonian patients with and without dementia. An open-labeled study utilizing a structured interview. J Neurol 2006; 253:171–175.

34. Marti M et al. Dementia in Parkinson's disease. J Neurol 2007; 254 Suppl 1:41–48.

35. Chung KA et al. Effects of a central cholinesterase inhibitor on reducing falls in Parkinson disease. Neurology 2010; 75:1263–1269.

36. Mesquita J et al. Fatal neuroleptic malignant syndrome induced by clozapine in Parkinson's psychosis. J Neuropsychiatry Clin Neurosci 2014; 26:E34.

37. Ziegenbein M et al. Clozapine-induced aplastic anemia in a patient with Parkinson's disease. Can J Psychiatry 2003; 48:352.

38. Factor SA et al. Combined clozapine and electroconvulsive therapy for the treatment of drug-induced psychosis in Parkinson's disease. J Neuropsychiatry Clin Neurosci 1995; 7:304–307.

39. Martin BA. ECT for Parkinson's? CMAJ 2003; 168:1391–1392.

40. Zesiewicz TA et al. Potential influences of complementary therapy on motor and non-motor complications in Parkinson's disease. CNS Drugs 2009; 23:817–835.

41. Cummings J et al. Pimavanserin for patients with Parkinson's disease psychosis: a randomised, placebo-controlled phase 3 trial. Lancet 2014; 383:533–540.

42. Richard IH et al. Rivastigmine-induced worsening of motor function and mood in a patient with Parkinson's disease. Mov Disord 2001; 16:33–34.

43. McKeith I et al. Efficacy of rivastigmine in dementia with Lewy bodies: a randomised, double-blind, placebo-controlled international study. Lancet 2000; 356:2031–2036.

44. Emre M et al. Rivastigmine for dementia associated with Parkinson's disease. N Engl J Med 2004; 351:2509–2518.

45. Aarsland D et al. Donepezil for cognitive impairment in Parkinson's disease: a randomised controlled study. J Neurol Neurosurg Psychiatry 2002; 72:708–712.

46. Rolinski M et al. Cholinesterase inhibitors for dementia with Lewy bodies, Parkinson's disease dementia and cognitive impairment in Parkinson's disease. Cochrane Database Syst Rev 2012; 3: CD006504.

47. Dubois B et al. Donepezil in Parkinson's disease dementia: a randomized, double-blind efficacy and safety study. Mov Disord 2012; 27:1230–1238.

48. Connolly BS et al. Pharmacological treatment of Parkinson disease: a review. JAMA 2014; 311:1670–1683.

49. Emre M et al. Memantine for patients with Parkinson's disease dementia or dementia with Lewy bodies: a randomised, double-blind, placebo-controlled trial. Lancet Neurol 2010; 9:969–977.

50. Seppi K et al. The Movement Disorder Society Evidence-Based Medicine Review Update: Treatments for the non-motor symptoms of Parkinson's disease. Mov Disord 2011; 26 Suppl 3:S42–S80.

51. Postuma RB et al. Caffeine for treatment of Parkinson disease: a randomized controlled trial. Neurology 2012; 79:651–658.

Further reading

Goldman JG et al. Treatment of psychosis and dementia in Parkinson's disease. Curr Treat Options Neurol 2014; 16:281.

Multiple sclerosis

Multiple sclerosis (MS) is a common cause of neurological disability affecting approximately 85,000 people in the UK with the onset usually between 20–50 years of age. Individuals with MS experience a variety of psychiatric/neurological disorders such as depression, anxiety, pathological laughter and crying (PLC) (pseudobulbar affect, PBA), mania and euphoria, psychosis/bipolar disorder, fatigue and cognitive impairment. Psychiatric disorders result from the psychological impact of MS diagnosis and prognosis, perceived lack of social support or unhelpful coping styles,[1] increased stress,[2] iatrogenic effects of treatments commonly used with MS,[3] or damage to neuronal pathways.[3] According to some studies, shorter duration of illness confers a greater risk of depression.

Depression

In people with MS, depression is common with a point prevalence of 14–27%[4,5] and lifetime prevalence of up to 50%.[5] Suicide rates are 2–7.5 times higher than the general population.[6] Depression is often associated with fatigue and pain, though the relationship direction is unclear. Overlapping symptoms of depression, PBA and MS can complicate diagnosis and so co-operation between neurologists and psychiatrists is essential to ensure optimal treatment for individuals with MS.

The role of interferon-beta in the aetiology of MS depression is unclear, but it is now thought that depression occurs no more frequently in people treated with interferon-beta.[7,8] Standard care for initiation of interferon-beta should include assessment for depression and, for those with a past history of depressive illness, prophylactic treatment with an antidepressant.[3] Recommendations for the treatment of depression in MS are shown in Box 7.5.

Anxiety

Anxiety affects many people with MS, with a point prevalence of up to 50%[25] and lifetime incidence of 35–37%[26]. Elevated rates in comparison with the general population are seen for generalized anxiety disorder, panic disorder, obsessive compulsive disorder[26] and social anxiety. Anxiety appears linked to perceived lack of support, increased pain, fatigue, sleep disturbance, depression, alcohol misuse, and suicidal ideas. There are no published trials for the treatment of anxiety in MS, but SSRIs can be used and, in non-responsive cases, venlafaxine might be an option.

Benzodiazepines may be used for acute and severe anxiety of less than 4 weeks duration but should not be prescribed in the long term. Buspirone and beta-blockers could also be considered although there is unproven efficacy in MS. Pregabalin is also licensed for anxiety and may be useful in this population group. People with MS may also respond to CBT. Generally treatment is as for non-MS anxiety disorders (see section on 'Anxiety spectrum disorders' in Chapter 4)

Pseudobulbar affect (PBA)

Up to 10% of individuals with MS experience PLC. It is more common in the advanced stages of the disease and is associated with cognitive impairment.[26] There have been a few open label trials recommending the use of small doses of TCAs, e.g.

Box 7.5 Recommendations for the treatment of depression in MS

Step	Intervention
1	Screen for depression with PHQ-9 HADS/BDI[9]/CES-D.[10] Exclude and treat any organic causes. Consider iatrogenic effects of medications as potential cause of depression. Ensure there is no past history of mania or bipolar disorder. People with mild depression could be considered for CBT[11] or self-help.[12]
2	SSRIs should be first line treatment[3,10,13] because of their relatively benign side- effect profile. Sertraline was as effective as CBT in one trial,[14] but paroxetine was found to be no more effective than placebo in another study.[15] Because of reduced tolerability of side-effects in this patient group, medications should be titrated from an initial half dose. Many MS patients are prescribed low dose TCAs for pain/bladder disturbance and so SSRIs should be used with caution and patients should be observed for serotonin syndrome. For those with co-morbid pain, consideration should be given to treating with an SNRI such as duloxetine or venlafaxine.[16] One RCT of desipramine showed it was more effective than placebo but tricyclics are often poorly tolerated.[17] Cochrane is not convinced by the studies cited here,[18] but there is no reason to suppose that antidepressants are any less effective in depression associated with physical illness.[19] CBT is the most appropriate psychological intervention with best efficacy in comparison to supportive therapy or usual care, and should be used in conjunction with medication for those who are moderately-severely depressed.[13,14,20] Mindfulness training may also help.[21]
3	If SSRIs are not tolerated, or there is no response, there are limited data that moclobemide is effective and well tolerated.[23,23] There are no published trials on venlafaxine, duloxetine and mirtazapine but these are used widely.
4	ECT could be considered for people who are actively suicidal or severely depressed and at high risk, but it may trigger an exacerbation of MS symptoms, although some studies suggest that no neurological disturbance occurs.[24]

BDI, Beck Depression Inventory; CBT, cognitive behavioural therapy; HADS, Hospital Anxiety and Depression Scale; CES-D, Centre for Epidemiological Studies Depression Scale; MS, multiple sclerosis; PHQ-9, Patient Health Questionnaire-9; RCT, randomised controlled trial; SNRI, serotonin noradrenaline reuptake inhibitor; SSRI, selective serotonin reuptake inhibitor; TCA, tricyclic antidepressant.

---

amitriptyline, or SSRIs, e.g. fluoxetine[27,28] in MS. Citalopram[29] or sertraline[30] have been investigated in people with post-stroke PLC and shown reasonable efficacy and rapid response. The combination of dextromethorphan and quinidine (Nuedexta) is effective.[31]

Mania/euphoria/bipolar disorder

Incidence of bipolar disorder can be as high as 13% in the MS population[2] compared with 1–6% in the general population. Mania can be induced by drugs such as steroids or baclofen.[32]

Anecdotal evidence suggests that patients presenting with mania/bipolar disorder should be treated with mood stabilisers such as sodium valproate as these are better tolerated than lithium.[33]

Lithium can cause diuresis and thus lead to increased difficulties with tolerance. Mania accompanied by psychosis could be treated with low dose atypical antipsychotics such as risperidone, olanzapine,[2] ziprasidone.[34] Patients requiring psychiatric treatment for steroid-induced mania with psychosis have been known to respond well to olanzapine;[35] further case reports suggest risperidone is also useful. There have been no trials in this area.

Psychosis

Psychosis occurs in 1.1% of the MS population and compared with other psychiatric disorders is relatively uncommon.[34] There have been few published trials, but risperidone or clozapine have been recommended because of their low risk of extra pyramidal symptoms.[32] On this basis, olanzapine, aripiprazole and quetiapine might also, in theory at least, be possible options.

Psychosis may rarely be the presentation of an MS relapse in which case steroids may be beneficial but would need to be given under close supervision. Note also the small risk of psychotic reactions in patients receiving cannabinnoids for MS.[36]

Cognitive impairment

Cognitive impairment occurs in at least 40–65% of people with MS. Some of the effects of medications commonly prescribed can worsen cognition, e.g. tizanidine, diazepam, gabapentin.[37] Although there are no published trials, evidence from clinical case studies suggests that the treatment of sleep difficulties, depression and fatigue can enhance cognitive function.[37] There have been two small, underpowered trials with donepezil for people with mild-to-moderate cognitive impairment showing moderate efficacy.[442,443] A larger study found no effect.[40] Similarly, data supporting the use of memantine are weak.[41] Overall, no symptomatic treatment has proven efficacy and disease modifying agents offer greater promise.[42]

Fatigue

Fatigue is a common symptom in MS with up to 80% of people with MS affected.[43] The aetiology of fatigue is unclear but there have been suggestions that disruption of neuronal networks,[44] depression or psychological reactions,[32] sleep disturbances or medication may play a role in its development. Pharmacological and non-pharmacological strategies[43] should be used in a treatment strategy.

Non-pharmacological strategies include reviewing history for any possible contributing factors, assessment and treatment of underlying depression if present, medication, pacing activities and appropriate exercise. One trial suggests that CBT reduces fatigue scores.[45]

Pharmacological strategies include the use of amantadine[46] or modafinil. NICE guidelines suggest no medicine should be used routinely but that amantadine could have a small benefit.[47] A Cochrane review of amantadine in people with MS suggests that the quality and outcomes of the amantadine trials are inconsistent and therefore efficacy remains unclear.[46] In the only study published since then,[48] amantadine outperformed placebo on some measures of fatigue. Modafinil has mixed results in clinical trials. Early studies[49,50] showed statistically significant improvements in fatigue, but these studies were subject to some bias. A later randomized placebo-controlled double blind study[51] found no improvement in fatigue compared with placebo. The most recent study[52] showed distinct advantages for modafinil over placebo. Despite doubts over its efficacy modafinil is widely used in MS.[53]

Other pharmacological agents recommended for use in MS fatigue include: pemoline or aspirin. A double blind crossover study of aspirin compared with placebo favoured aspirin but further studies are required.[54] Data relating to ginseng are mixed.[55,56]

References

1. Ron MA. Do neurologists provide adequate care for depression in patients with multiple sclerosis? Nat Clin Pract Neurol 2006; 2:534–535.

2. Patten SB et al. Biopsychosocial correlates of lifetime major depression in a multiple sclerosis population. Mult Scler 2000; 6:115–120.

3. Servis ME. Psychiatric comorbidity in parkinson's disease, multiple sclerosis, and seizure disorder. Continuum 2006; 12:72–86.

4. Gottberg K et al. A population-based study of depressive symptoms in multiple sclerosis in Stockholm county: association with functioning and sense of coherence. J Neurol Neurosurg Psychiatry 2007; 78:60–65.

5. Patten SB et al. Major depression in multiple sclerosis: a population-based perspective. Neurology 2003; 61:1524–1527.

6. Sadovnick AD et al. Cause of death in patients attending multiple sclerosis clinics. Neurology 1991; 41:1193–1196.

7. Zephir H et al. Multiple sclerosis and depression: influence of interferon beta therapy. Mult Scler 2003; 9:284–288.

8. Patten SB et al. Anti-depressant use in association with interferon and glatiramer acetate treatment in multiple sclerosis. Mult Scler 2008; 14:406–411.

9. Moran PJ et al. The validity of Beck Depression Inventory and Hamilton Rating Scale for Depression items in the assessment of depression among patients with multiple sclerosis. J Behav Med 2005; 28:35–41.

10. Pandya R et al. Predictive value of the CES-D in detecting depression among candidates for disease-modifying multiple sclerosis treatment. Psychosomatics 2005; 46:131–134.

11. Minden SL et al. Evidence-based guideline: assessment and management of psychiatric disorders in individuals with MS: report of the Guideline Development Subcommittee of the American Academy of Neurology. Neurology 2014; 82:174–181.

12. Rickards H. Depression in neurological disorders: Parkinson's disease, multiple sclerosis, and stroke. J Neurol Neurosurg Psychiatry 2005; 76 Suppl 1:i48–i52.

13. Siegert RJ et al. Depression in multiple sclerosis: a review. J Neurol Neurosurg Psychiatry 2005; 76:469–475.

14. Mohr DC et al. Comparative outcomes for individual cognitive-behavior therapy, supportive-expressive group psychotherapy, and sertraline for the treatment of depression in multiple sclerosis. J Consult Clin Psychol 2001; 69:942–949.

15. Ehde DM et al. Efficacy of paroxetine in treating major depressive disorder in persons with multiple sclerosis. Gen Hosp Psychiatry 2008; 30:40–48.

16. Hilty DM et al. Psychopharmacology for neurologists: principles, algorithms, and other resources. Continuum 2006; 12:33–46.

17. Barak Y et al. Treatment of depression in patients with multiple sclerosis. Neurologist 1998; 4:99–104.

18. Koch MW et al. Pharmacologic treatment of depression in multiple sclerosis. Cochrane Database Syst Rev 2011; 2: CD007295.

19. Taylor D et al. Pharmacological interventions for people with depression and chronic physical health problems: systematic review and meta-analyses of safety and efficacy. The British Journal of Psychiatry 2011; 198:179–188.

20. Larcombe NA et al. An evaluation of cognitive-behaviour therapy for depression in patients with multiple sclerosis. Br J Psychiatry 1984; 145:366–371.

21. man P et al. MS quality of life, depression, and fatigue improve after mindfulness training: a randomized trial. Neurology 2010; 75:1141–1149.

22. Schiffer RB et al. Antidepressant pharmacotherapy of depression associated with multiple sclerosis. Am J Psychiatry 1990; 147:1493–1497.

23. Barak Y et al. Moclobemide treatment in multiple sclerosis patients with comorbid depression: an open-label safety trial. J Neuropsychiatry Clin Neurosci 1999; 11:271–273.

24. Rasmussen KG et al. Electroconvulsive therapy in patients with multiple sclerosis. J ECT 2007; 23:179–180.

25. Jones KH et al. A large-scale study of anxiety and depression in people with Multiple Sclerosis: a survey via the web portal of the UK MS Register. PLoS One 2012; 7:e41910.

26. Korostil M et al. Anxiety disorders and their clinical correlates in multiple sclerosis patients. Mult Scler 2007; 13:67–72.

27. Feinstein A et al. The effects of anxiety on psychiatric morbidity in patients with multiple sclerosis. Mult Scler 1999; 5:323–326.

28. Feinstein A et al. Prevalence and neurobehavioral correlates of pathological laughing and crying in multiple sclerosis. Arch Neurol 1997; 54:1116–1121.

29. Andersen G et al. Citalopram for post-stroke pathological crying. Lancet 1993; 342:837–839.

30. Burns A et al. Sertraline in stroke-associated lability of mood. Int J Geriatr Psychiatry 1999; 14:681–685.

31. Pioro EP et al. Dextromethorphan plus ultra low-dose quinidine reduces pseudobulbar affect. Ann Neurol 2010; 68:693–702.

32. Jefferies K. The neuropsychiatry of multiple sclerosis. Adv Psychiatr Treat 2006; 12:214–220.

33. Stip E et al. Valproate in the treatment of mood disorder due to multiple sclerosis. Can J Psychiatry 1995; 40:219–220.

34. Davids E et al. Antipsychotic treatment of psychosis associated with multiple sclerosis. Prog Neuropsychopharmacol Biol Psychiatry 2004; 28:743–744.

35. Budur K et al. Olanzapine for corticosteroid-induced mood disorders. Psychosomatics 2003; **44**:353.

36. Aragona M et al. Psychopathological and cognitive effects of therapeutic cannabinoids in multiple sclerosis: a double-blind, placebo controlled, crossover study. Clin Neuropharmacol 2009; **32**:41–47.

37. Pierson SH et al. Treatment of cognitive impairment in multiple sclerosis. Behav Neurol 2006; **17**:53–67.

38. Krupp LB et al. Donepezil improved memory in multiple sclerosis in a randomized clinical trial. Neurology 2004; **63**:1579–1585.

39. Greene YM et al. A 12-week, open trial of donepezil hydrochloride in patients with multiple sclerosis and associated cognitive impairments. J Clin Psychopharmacol 2000; **20**:350–356.

40. Krupp LB et al. Multicenter randomized clinical trial of donepezil for memory impairment in multiple sclerosis. Neurology 2011; **76**:1500–1507.

41. Lovera JF et al. Memantine for cognitive impairment in multiple sclerosis: a randomized placebo-controlled trial. Mult Scler 2010; **16**:715–723.

42. Patti F. Treatment of cognitive impairment in patients with multiple sclerosis. Expert Opin Investig Drugs 2012; **21**:1679–1699.

43. Bakshi R. Fatigue associated with multiple sclerosis: diagnosis, impact and management. Mult Scler 2003; **9**:219–227.

44. Sepulcre J et al. Fatigue in multiple sclerosis is associated with the disruption of frontal and parietal pathways. Mult Scler 2009; **15**:337–344.

45. van KK et al. A randomized controlled trial of cognitive behavior therapy for multiple sclerosis fatigue. Psychosom Med 2008; **70**:205–213.

46. Pucci E et al. Amantadine for fatigue in multiple sclerosis. Cochrane Database Syst Rev 2007; CD002818.

47. National Institute for Health and Clinical Excellence. Management of multiple sclerosis in primary and secondary care. Clinical Guideline 8, 2003. http://www.nice.org.uk/

48. Ashtari F et al. Does amantadine have favourable effects on fatigue in Persian patients suffering from multiple sclerosis? Neurol Neurochir Pol 2009; **43**:428–432.

49. Rammohan KW et al. Efficacy and safety of modafinil (Provigil) for the treatment of fatigue in multiple sclerosis: a two centre phase 2 study. J Neurol Neurosurg Psychiatry 2002; **72**:179–183.

50. Zifko UA et al. Modafinil in treatment of fatigue in multiple sclerosis. Results of an open-label study. J Neurol 2002; **249**:983–987.

51. Stankoff B et al. Modafinil for fatigue in MS: A randomized placebo-controlled double-blind study. Neurology 2005; **64**:1139–1143.

52. Lange R et al. Modafinil effects in multiple sclerosis patients with fatigue. J Neurol 2009; **256**:645–650.

53. Davies M et al. Safety profile of modafinil across a range of prescribing indications, including off-label use, in a primary care setting in England: results of a modified prescription-event monitoring study. Drug Saf 2013; **36**:237–246.

54. Wingerchuk DM et al. A randomized controlled crossover trial of aspirin for fatigue in multiple sclerosis. Neurology 2005; **64**:1267–1269.

55. Kim E et al. American ginseng does not improve fatigue in multiple sclerosis: a single center randomized double-blind placebo-controlled crossover pilot study. Mult Scler 2011; **17**:1523–1526.

56. Etemadifar M et al. Ginseng in the treatment of fatigue in multiple sclerosis: a randomized, placebo-controlled, double-blind pilot study. Int J Neurosci 2013; **123**:480–486.

CHAPTER 7

Huntington's disease

Huntington's disease is a genetic condition involving slow progressive degeneration of neurones in the basal ganglia and cerebral cortex. Prevalence is estimated to be 12.4/100,000 population in Western societies.[1] Neurones are damaged when the mutated Huntingtin protein gradually aggregates and interferes with normal metabolism and functioning. The mechanism is poorly understood[2] making it difficult to develop drugs that slow or stop progression. Therefore, only symptomatic treatment is used in an attempt to improve quality of life. Choreiform movements occur in approximately 90% of patients and between 23% and 73% develop depression or psychosis during the course of their illness.[3] Anxiety, apathy, obsessions, compulsions, impulsivity, irritability and aggression can all be problematic.[4] Dementia is inevitable.

There is very little primary literature to guide practice in this area. A summary can be found in Table 7.8. Clinicians who treat patients with Huntington's disease are

Table 7.8 Recommendations for the treatment of symptoms in Huntington's disease

Symptoms	Treatment
Choreiform movements	Note that these are often more distressing for carers and healthcare professionals than they are for the patient and it should not be assumed that intervention is always in the patient's best interests
	■ Discontinue dopaminergic drugs such as piracetam and cabergoline.[5] Consider the contribution of psychotropic drugs with dopaminergic effects such as aripiprazole and venlafaxine or bupropion
	■ The use of tetrabenazine is supported by RCTs.[6–8] Up to 80% of patients experience dose-limiting symptoms[9] such as depression, anxiety and insomnia, but a pre-existing diagnosis of depression is not an absolute contraindication to treatment.[9] Studies suggest that clinical benefits can be observed rapidly and a multiple daily dosing regimen (e.g. tds) may be needed[10]
	■ A small dose of a conventional antipsychotic such as haloperidol, fluphenazine,[11] or sulpiride[9] is established clinical practice[12]
	■ Findings with second-generation antipsychotics are mixed. Two open studies of olanzapine 5 mg were negative[13,14] but a third using 30 mg showed improved motor function.[15] Case reports support the use of risperidone both at low[16] and higher dose.[17,18] Quetiapine[19] and aripiprazole[20] may also be effective. There is a small positive RCT of pridopidine (a dopamine partial agonist)[21]
	■ A small, open-label study suggested levetiracetam may be effective in reducing chorea. Side-effects included somnolence and dyskinesias[22]
	■ A large, double-blind trial found no benefit with riluzole in symptomatic effects or neuroprotection[23]
	■ The results of several small studies suggest that amantadine may help chorea at a dose of >400 mg/day. Improvements are modest and transient and unlikely to be clinically useful.[24] Possible side-effects include agitation, confusion and sleep disturbances[9]
	■ Valproic acid does not seem to be effective in treating chorea.[9] However, cortical myoclonus, a rare, but potentially disabling feature of adult Huntington's disease, was shown in several case reports to improve with valproic acid[9,25]
	■ Positive and negative data also exists for lamotrigine in the treatment of motor and mood symptoms in Huntington's disease[9,26]
	■ A small RCT found nabilone to be more effective than placebo in the treatment of motor symptoms, cognition and behaviour[27]

Table 7.8 (*Continued*)

Symptoms	Treatment
Hypokinetic rigidity	■ Treatment is similar to that of Parkinson's disease although response is often suboptimal. Anticholinergics and dopamine agonists are sometimes used. Note the potential for such drugs to exacerbate choreiform movements and precipitate psychosis ■ Muscle relaxants, such as diazepam can also be effective in treating rigidity and are usually well tolerated,[5] although aspiration secondary to sedation is a potential risk
Psychosis	There are no RCTs to guide choice. Treatment is empirical. Note that antipsychotic drugs may exacerbate any underlying movement disorder ■ Some evidence supports the efficacy of conventional antipsychotics, particularly haloperidol, when the Huntington's disease is mild to moderate.[12] As Huntington's disease progresses, typicals tend to be poorly tolerated because of dystonia and parkinsonism[12] ■ Case reports support the efficacy of risperidone,[17,18,28] quetiapine[29] and amisulpride[30] although extrapyramidal side-effects can be problematic with all of these drugs. A positive case report also exists for aripiprazole[31]
Depression	There are no RCTs to guide choice. Note that the suicide rate in patients with Huntington's disease is 4–6 times higher than in the background population[12] ■ An open study supports the efficacy of venlafaxine, although adverse effects can be problematic[32] ■ Case reports support the efficacy of a wide range of antidepressants but TCAs are poorly tolerated (sedation, falls and anticholinergic-induced cognitive impairment) and MAOIs can worsen choreiform movements. SSRIs are preferred[33,34] ■ Reviews state that lithium is best avoided; clinical experience suggests that response is likely to be poor and that toxic effects may be particularly problematic.[12] There is no primary literature ■ ECT seems to be relatively well tolerated in patients with Huntington's disease [12]
Dementia	Positive and negative case reports exist for the use of cholinesterase inhibitors in patients with Huntington's disease ■ Based on available evidence, the treatment of Huntington's disease with acetylcholinesterase inhibitors does not significantly alter cognitive decline, and has little impact on daily functionality of patients with Huntington's disease. Therefore these drugs have no specific indication in the treatment of this disease[9] ■ One small sample study concluded that donepezil was not an effective treatment for Huntington's disease[35] ■ However, a two year follow-up of rivastigmine treatment showed positive results in slowing motor deterioration and possibly reducing cognitive impairment[36] ■ Positive case reports also exist for memantine in preventing the progression of cognitive symptoms[37] ■ A large (n = 403) RCT found no benefit for latrepirdine (an experimental drug that stabilises mitochondrial membranes and function) with respect to improving cognition or global function[38]

ECT, electroconvulsive therapy; MAOI, monoamine oxidase inhibitor; RCT, randomised controlled trial; SSRI, selective serotonin reuptake inhibitor; TCA, tricyclic antidepressant; tds, *ter die sumendus* (three times a day).

encouraged to publish reports of both positive and negative outcomes to increase the primary literature base.

Table 7.8 represents a review of the literature rather than a guide to treatment. Readers are directed to the reports cited here for details of dosage regimens and further information about tolerability.

References

1. Spinney L. Uncovering the true prevalence of Huntington's disease. Lancet Neurol 2010; 9:760–761.
2. American Psychiatric Association. *Diagnostic and Statistical Manual of Mental Disorders*, 5th edn (DSM-5). Arlington, VA: American Psychiatric Association; 2013.
3. Petrikis P et al. Treatment of Huntington's disease with galantamine. Int Clin Psychopharmacol 2004; 19:49–50.
4. Scher LM et al. How to target psychiatric symptoms of Huntington's disease. Current Psychiatry 2012; 11:34–38.
5. Bonelli RM et al. Huntington's disease: present treatments and future therapeutic modalities. Int Clin Psychopharmacol 2004; 19:51–62.
6. McLellan DL et al. A double-blind trial of tetrabenazine, thiopropazate, and placebo in patients with chorea. Lancet 1974; 1:104–107.
7. Jankovic J. Treatment of hyperkinetic movement disorders with tetrabenazine: a double-blind crossover study. Ann Neurol 1982; 11:41–47.
8. Mestre T et al. Therapeutic interventions for symptomatic treatment in Huntington's disease. Cochrane Database Syst Rev 2009; CD006456.
9. Adam OR et al. Symptomatic treatment of Huntington disease. Neurotherapeutics 2008; 5:181–197.
10. Kenney C et al. Short-term effects of tetrabenazine on chorea associated with Huntington's disease. Mov Disord 2007; 22:10–13.
11. Bonelli RM et al. Pharmacological management of Huntington's disease: an evidence-based review. Curr Pharm Des 2006; 12:2701–2720.
12. Rosenblatt A et al. Neuropsychiatry of Huntington's disease and other basal ganglia disorders. Psychosomatics 2000; 41:24–30.
13. Squitieri F et al. Short-term effects of olanzapine in Huntington disease. Neuropsychiatry Neuropsychol Behav Neurol 2001; 14:69–72.
14. Paleacu D et al. Olanzapine in Huntington's disease. Acta Neurol Scand 2002; 105:441–444.
15. Bonelli RM et al. High-dose olanzapine in Huntington's disease. Int Clin Psychopharmacol 2002; 17:91–93.
16. Erdemoglu AK et al. Risperidone in chorea and psychosis of Huntington's disease. Eur J Neurol 2002; 9:182–183.
17. Dallocchio C et al. Effectiveness of risperidone in Huntington chorea patients. J Clin Psychopharmacol 1999; 19:101–103.
18. Duff K et al. Risperidone and the treatment of psychiatric, motor, and cognitive symptoms in Huntington's disease. Ann Clin Psychiatry 2008; 20:1–3.
19. Bonelli RM et al. Quetiapine in Huntington's disease: a first case report. J Neurol 2002; 249:1114–1115.
20. Brusa L et al. Treatment of the symptoms of Huntington's disease: preliminary results comparing aripiprazole and tetrabenazine. Mov Disord 2009; 24:126–129.
21. Lundin A et al. Efficacy and safety of the dopaminergic stabilizer Pridopidine (ACR16) in patients with Huntington's disease. Clin Neuropharmacol 2010; 33:260–264.
22. Zesiewicz TA et al. Open-label pilot study of levetiracetam (Keppra) for the treatment of chorea in Huntington's disease. Mov Disord 2006; 21:1998–2001.
23. Landwehrmeyer GB et al. Riluzole in Huntington's disease: a 3-year, randomized controlled study. Ann Neurol 2007; 62:262–272.
24. Reilmann R. Pharmacological treatment of chorea in Huntington's disease-good clinical practice versus evidence-based guideline. Mov Disord 2013; 28:1030–1033.
25. Saft C et al. Dose-dependent improvement of myoclonic hyperkinesia due to Valproic acid in eight Huntington's Disease patients: a case series. BMC Neurol 2006; 6:11.
26. Shen YC. Lamotrigine in motor and mood symptoms of Huntington's disease. World J Biol Psychiatry 2008; 9:147–149.
27. Curtis A et al. A pilot study using nabilone for symptomatic treatment in Huntington's disease. Mov Disord 2009; 24:2254–2259.
28. Madhusoodanan S et al. Use of risperidone in psychosis associated with Huntington's disease. Am J Geriatr Psychiatry 1998; 6:347–349.
29. Seitz DP et al. Quetiapine in the management of psychosis secondary to huntington's disease: a case report. Can J Psychiatry 2004; 49:413.
30. Saft C et al. Amisulpride in Huntington's disease. Psychiatr Prax 2005; 32:363–366.
31. Lin WC et al. Aripiprazole effects on psychosis and chorea in a patient with Huntington's disease. Am J Psychiatry 2008; 165:1207–1208.
32. Holl AK et al. Combating depression in Huntington's disease: effective antidepressive treatment with venlafaxine XR. Int Clin Psychopharmacol 2010; 25:46–50.
33. De Marchi N et al. Fluoxetine in the treatment of Huntington's disease. Psychopharmacology 2001; 153:264–266.
34. Rosenblatt A et al. *A Physician's Guide to the Management of Huntington's Disease*, 2nd edn. New York: Huntington's Disease Society of America; 1999.
35. Cubo E et al. Effect of donepezil on motor and cognitive function in Huntington disease. Neurology 2006; 67:1268–1271.
36. de TM et al. Two years' follow-up of rivastigmine treatment in Huntington disease. Clin Neuropharmacol 2007; 30:43–46.
37. Cankurtaran ES et al. Clinical experience with risperidone and memantine in the treatment of Huntington's disease. J Natl Med Assoc 2006; 98:1353–1355.
38. HORIZON Investigators of the Huntington Study Group and European Huntington's Disease Network. A randomized, double-blind, placebo-controlled study of latrepirdine in patients with mild to moderate Huntington disease. JAMA Neurol 2013; 70:25–33.

Further reading

Armstrong MJ et al. Evidence-based guideline: pharmacologic treatment of chorea in Huntington disease: report of the guideline development subcommittee of the American Academy of Neurology. Neurology 2012; 79:597–603.
Tyagi SN et al. Symptomatic Treatment and Management of Huntington's Disease: An Overview. Global J Pharmacol 2010; 4:6–12.

Pregnancy

A 'normal' outcome to pregnancy can never be guaranteed. The spontaneous abortion rate in confirmed early pregnancy is 10–20% and the risk of spontaneous major malformation is 2–3% (approximately 1 in 40 pregnancies).[1]

Lifestyle factors have an important influence on pregnancy outcome. It is well established that smoking cigarettes, eating a poor diet and drinking alcohol during pregnancy can have adverse consequences for the foetus. Moderate maternal caffeine consumption has been associated with low birth weight,[2] and pre-pregnancy obesity increases the risk of neural tube defects; (obese women seem to require higher doses of folate supplementation than women who have a BMI in the healthy range[3]).

In addition, psychiatric illness during pregnancy is an independent risk factor for congenital malformations and perinatal mortality.[4] Affective illness increases the risk of pre-term delivery.[5,6] Note that pre-term delivery is associated with an increased risk of depression, bipolar disorder and schizophrenia spectrum disorders in adult life.[7]

Drugs account for a very small proportion of abnormalities (approximately 5% of the total). Potential risks of drugs include major malformation (first-trimester exposure), neonatal toxicity (third-trimester exposure), longer-term neurobehavioural effects and increased risk of physical health problems in adult life.

The safety of psychotropics in pregnancy cannot be clearly established because robust, prospective trials are obviously unethical. Individual decisions on psychotropic use in pregnancy are therefore based on database studies that have many limitations (e.g. failure to control for the effects of illness and other medication, multiple statistical tests increasing the risk of Type 2 error and exposure status based on pharmacy data), limited prospective data from teratology information centres, and published case reports which are known to be biased towards adverse outcomes. At worst there may be no human data at all, only animal data from early preclinical studies. With new drugs early reports of adverse outcomes may or may not be replicated and a 'best guess' assessment must be made of the risks and benefits associated with withdrawal or continuation of drug treatment. Even with established drugs, data related to long-term outcomes are rare. Pregnancy does not protect against mental illness and may even elevate overall risk. The patient's view of risks and benefits will have paramount importance. This section provides a brief summary of the relevant issues and evidence to date.

General principles of prescribing in pregnancy

Box 7.6 outlines the general principles of prescribing in pregnancy.

What to include in discussions with pregnant women[13]

Discussions should include the following.

- The woman's ability to cope with untreated illness/sub-threshold symptoms.
- The potential impact of an untreated mental disorder on the foetus or infant.
- The risks from stopping medication abruptly.
- Severity of previous episodes, response to treatment and the woman's preference.

Box 7.6 General principles of prescribing in pregnancy

In all women of child bearing potential
- Always discuss the possibility of pregnancy; half of all pregnancies are unplanned.[8]
- Avoid using drugs that are contraindicated during pregnancy in women of reproductive age, (especially valproate and carbamazepine). If these drugs are prescribed, women should be made fully aware of their teratogenic properties even if not planning pregnancy. Consider prescribing folate. Valproate should be reserved for post-menopausal women only. Its use in younger women should be treatment of last resort.

If mental illness is newly diagnosed in a pregnant woman
- Try to avoid all drugs in the first trimester (when major organs are being formed) unless benefits outweigh risks.
- If non-drug treatments are not effective/appropriate, use an established drug at the lowest effective dose.

If a woman taking psychotopic drugs is planning a pregnancy
- Consideration should be given to discontinuing treatment if the woman is well and at low risk of relapse.
- Discontinuation of treatment for women with severe mental illness and at a high risk of relapse is unwise, but consideration should be given to switching to a low risk drug. Be aware that switching drugs may increase the risk of relapse.

If a woman taking psychotropic medication discovers that she is pregnant
- Abrupt discontinuation of treatment post-conception for women with severe mental illness and at a high risk of relapse is unwise; relapse may ultimately be more harmful to the mother and child than continued, effective drug therapy.
- Consider remaining with current (effective) medication rather than switching, to minimise the number of drugs to which the foetus is exposed.

If the patient smokes (smoking is more common in pregnant women with psychiatric illness)[9]
- Always encourage switching to nicotine replacement therapy; smoking has numerous adverse outcomes, nicotine replacement therapy (NRT) does not.[10] Referral to smoking cessation services is very desirable.

In all pregnant women
- Ensure that the parents are as involved as possible in all decisions.
- Use the lowest effective dose.
- Use the drug with the lowest known risk to mother and foetus.
- Prescribe as few drugs as possible both simultaneously and in sequence.
- Be prepared to adjust doses as pregnancy progresses and drug handling is altered. Dose increases are frequently required in the third trimester[11] when blood volume expands by around 30%. Plasma level monitoring is helpful, where available. Note that hepatic enzyme activity changes markedly during pregnancy; CYP2D6 activity is increased by almost 50% by the end of pregnancy while the activity of CYP1A2 is reduced by up to 70%.[12]
- Consider referral to specialist perinatal services.
- Ensure adequate foetal screening.
- Be aware of potential problems with individual drugs around the time of delivery.
- Inform the obstetric team of psychotropic use and possible complications.
- Monitor the neonate for withdrawal effects after birth.
- Document all decisions.

- The background risk of foetal malformations for pregnant women without a mental disorder.
- The increased risk of harm associated with drug treatments during pregnancy, and the post-natal period, including the risk in overdose (and acknowledge uncertainty surrounding risks).
- The possibility that stopping a drug with known teratogenic risk after pregnancy is confirmed may not remove the risk of malformations.

Where possible, written material should be provided to explain the risks (preferably individualised). Absolute and relative risks should be discussed. Risks should be described using natural frequencies rather than percentages (for example, 1 in 10 rather than 10%) and common denominators (for example, 1 in 100 and 25 in 100, rather than 1 in 100 and 1 in 4).

Psychosis during pregnancy and post-partum

- Pregnancy does not protect against relapse.
- Psychiatric illness during pregnancy predicts post-partum psychosis.[14]
- The risk of perinatal psychosis is 0.1–0.25% in the general population, but is about 50% in women with a history of bipolar disorder.
- During the month after childbirth there is a 20-fold increase (to 30–50%) in the relative risk of psychosis.
- The risk of recurrent post-partum psychosis is 50–90%.
- The mental health of the mother in the perinatal period influences foetal well-being, obstetric outcome and child development.

The risks of not treating psychosis include:

- harm to the mother through poor self-care or judgement, lack of obstetric care or impulsive acts
- harm to the foetus or neonate (ranging from neglect to infanticide).

It has long been established that people with schizophrenia are more likely to have minor physical anomalies than the general population. Some of these anomalies may be apparent at birth, while others are more subtle and may not be obvious until later in life. This background risk complicates assessment of the effects of antipsychotic drugs. (Psychiatric illness itself during pregnancy is an independent risk factor for congenital malformations and perinatal mortality.)

Treatment with antipsychotics

Older, **first-generation antipsychotics** are generally considered to have minimal risk of teratogenicity,[15,16] although data are less than convincing, as might be expected.

- Most data originate from studies that included primarily women with hyperemesis gravidarum (a condition associated with an increased risk of congenital malformations) treated with low doses of phenothiazines. The modest increase in risk identified in some of these studies, along with no clear clustering of congenital abnormalities suggest that the condition being treated may be responsible rather than drug treatment.

- There may be an association between haloperidol and limb defects, but if real, the risk is likely to be extremely low.
- A recent prospective study that included 284 women who took an FGA (mostly haloperidol, promethazine or flupentixol) during pregnancy concluded that pre-term birth and low birth weight were more common with FGAs than SGAs (or no antipsychotic exposure).[17] In total, 20% of neonates exposed to an FGA in the last week of gestation experienced early somnolence and jitteriness. The rate of major malformations, at 5%, was double that of controls (no antipsychotic exposure) but there was no clustering of abnormalities.
- Neonatal dyskinesia has been reported with FGAs.[18]
- Neonatal jaundice has been reported with phenothiazines.[15]

It remains uncertain whether FGAs are entirely without risk to the foetus or to later development.[15,16] However, this continued uncertainty and the wide use of these drugs over several decades suggest that any risk is small – an assumption borne out by most studies.[19]

Second-generation antipsychotics are unlikely to be major teratogens but are associated with some problems.

- There are most data for olanzapine which has been associated with both lower birth weight and increased risk of intensive care admission,[20] a large head circumference[21] and with macrosomia;[22] the last of these is consistent with the reported increase in the risk of gestational diabetes.[15,21,23,24] Olanzapine seems to be relatively safe with respect to congenital malformations; the prevalence being consistent with population norms in a study that reported on 610 prospectively followed pregnancies.[25] Olanzapine has however been associated with a range of problems including hip dysplasia,[26] meningocele, ankyloblepharon,[27] and neural tube defects;[15] (an effect that could be related to pre-pregnancy obesity rather than drug exposure[2]). Importantly there is no clustering of congenital malformations. Further, a recent prospective study that included 561 women who took an SGA (mostly olanzapine, quetiapine, clozapine, risperidone or aripiprazole) during pregnancy concluded that SGA exposure was associated with increased birth weight, a modestly increased risk of cardiac septal defects (possibly due to screening bias or co-exposure to SSRIs), and, as with FGAs, withdrawal effects in 15% neonates.[17]
- The risk of gestational diabetes may be increased with all SGAs.[21]
- The use of clozapine appears to present no increased risk of malformation, although gestational diabetes and neonatal seizures may be more likely to occur.[23] There is a single case report of maternal overdose resulting in foetal death[15] and there are theoretical concerns about the risk of agranulocytosis in the foetus/neonate.[15] NICE has, in the past, recommended that pregnant women should be switched from clozapine to another antipsychotic.[13] However, for almost all women who are prescribed clozapine, a switch to a different antipsychotic will result in relapse. On the balance of evidence available, clozapine should usually be continued.
- A small prospective case control study reported that babies who were exposed to antipsychotics *in utero*, had delayed cognitive, motor and social-emotional

development at 2 and 6 months old but not at 12 months.[28] The clinical significance of this finding, if any, is unclear.

Overall, these data do not allow an assessment of relative risks associated with different agents and certainly do not confirm absolutely the safety of any particular drug. At least two studies have suggested a small increased risk of malformation,[17,20] and one study a higher risk of caesarean section in people receiving antipsychotics.[20] As with other drugs, decisions must be based on the latest available information and an individualised assessment of probable risks and benefits. If possible, specialist advice should be sought, and primary reference sources consulted. Box 7.7 summarises the recommendations for the treatment of psychosis in pregnancy.

Box 7.7 Recommendations for the treatment of psychosis in pregnancy

- Patients with a history of psychosis who are maintained on antipsychotic medication should be advised to discuss a planned pregnancy as early as possible.
- Be aware that drug-induced hyperprolactinaemia may prevent pregnancy. Consider switching to alternative drug.
- Such patients, particularly if they have suffered repeated relapses, are best maintained on antipsychotics during and after pregnancy. This may minimise foetal exposure by avoiding the need for higher doses, and/or multiple drugs should relapse occur.
- There is most experience with **chlorpromazine** (constipation and sedation can be a problem), **trifluoperazine, haloperidol, olanzapine, quetiapine** and **clozapine** (gestational diabetes may be a problem with all SGAs). If the patient is established on another antipsychotic, the most up-to-date advice should always be obtained; a change in treatment may not be necessary or wise.
- NICE recommends avoiding depot preparations and anticholinergic drugs in pregnancy.
- A few authorities recommend discontinuation of antipsychotics 5–10 days before anticipated delivery to minimise the chances of neonatal effects. This may, however, put mother and infant at risk and needs to be considered carefully. Antipsychotic discontinuation symptoms can occur in the neonate (e.g. crying, agitation, increased suckling). This is thought to be a class effect.[29] When antipsychotics are taken in pregnancy it is recommended that the woman gives birth in a unit that has access to paediatric intensive care facilities.[17] Some centres used mixed (breast/bottle) feeding to minimise withdrawal symptoms.

Depression during pregnancy and post-partum[30–32]

- Approximately 10% of pregnant women develop a depressive illness and a further 16% a self-limiting depressive reaction. Much post-partum depression begins before birth.
- Risk may be at least partially genetically determined.
- There is a significant increase in new psychiatric episodes in the first 3 months after delivery. At least 80% are mood disorders, primarily depression.
- Women who have had a previous episode of depressive illness (post-partum or not) are at higher risk of further episodes during pregnancy and post-partum. The risk is highest in women with bipolar illness.
- It is unclear if depression increases the risk of spontaneous abortion, having a low birth weight or small for gestational age baby, or of pre-term delivery.[33,34] The mental health of the mother influences foetal well-being, obstetric outcome and child development.

The risks of not treating depression include:

- harm to the mother through poor self-care, lack of obstetric care or self-harm
- harm to the foetus or neonate (ranging from neglect to infanticide).

Treatment with antidepressants

The use of antidepressants during pregnancy is common; in the Netherlands, up to 2% of women are prescribed antidepressants during the first trimester,[35] and in the US around 10% of women are prescribed antidepressants at some point during their pregnancy,[33,36] and this rate is increasing.[37] The majority of prescriptions are for SSRIs. In the UK, the large majority of women who are prescribed antidepressants, stop taking them in very early pregnancy (<6 weeks gestation),[38] most likely because of concerns about teratogenicity. A large Danish study has also noted that pregnant women are considerably less likely to be prescribed antidepressants than women who are not pregnant.[39] **Relapse rates are high** in those with a history of depression who discontinue medication. One study found that 68% of women who were well on antidepressant treatment and stopped during pregnancy relapsed, compared with 26% who continued antidepressants.[30] Some data suggest that antidepressants may increase the risk of spontaneous abortion (but note that confounding factors were not controlled for).[33,40] SSRIs do not increase the risk of stillbirth or neonatal mortality.[41,42] Antidepressants may increase the risk of pre-term delivery, respiratory distress in the neonate, a low Apgar score at birth and admission to a special care baby unit.[33,43-48] Note though that most studies are observational and do not control for maternal depression. Limited data suggest that when this is done, antidepressants pose no additional risk, at least with respect to pre-term birth.[49] While **it is reasonably certain that commonly used antidepressants are not major teratogens,**[50] some antidepressants have been associated with specific congenital malformations, many of which are rare. Most of these potential associations remain unreplicated.[33] There are conflicting data on the issue of the influence of duration of antidepressant use.[51,52] The effects on early growth and neuro-development are poorly studied; the limited data that do exist are reassuring.[47,53,54] One small study reported abnormal general movements in neonates exposed to SSRIs *in utero*.[55] A small increase in the risk of childhood autism has also been suggested.[56,57]

Women who take antidepressants during pregnancy may be at increased risk of developing **hypertension** (NNH 83),[58] **pre-eclampsia** (NNH 40)[59] and **post-partum haemorrhage** (NNH 80). It has been suggested that SSRIs may cause the last of these by reducing serotonin-mediated uterine contraction as well as interfering with hemostasis.[60] A subsequent smaller study did not confirm this association; possibly because it was underpowered to do so.[61]

Tricyclic antidepressants

- Foetal exposure to TCAs (via umbilicus and amniotic fluid) is high.[62,63]
- TCAs have been widely used throughout pregnancy without apparent detriment to the foetus[50,64,65] and have for many years been agents of choice in pregnancy.
- A weak association between clomipramine use and cardiovascular defects cannot be excluded[66] and the European SPC for Anafranil states: 'Neonates whose mothers had taken tricyclic antidepressants until delivery have developed dyspnoea, lethargy, colic,

irritability, hypotension or hypertension, tremor or spasms, during the first few hours or days. Studies in animals have shown reproductive toxicity. Anafranil is not recommended during pregnancy and in women of childbearing potential not using contraception.'

- Limited data suggest *in utero* exposure to TCAs has no effects on later development.[67,68]
- Some authorities recommend the use of nortriptyline and desipramine (not available in the UK) because these drugs are less anticholinergic and hypotensive than amitriptyline and imipramine (respectively, their tertiary amine parent molecules).
- TCA use during pregnancy increases the risk of pre-term delivery.[64,65,69]
- Use of TCAs in the third trimester is well known to produce neonatal withdrawal effects; agitation, irritability, seizures, respiratory distress and endocrine and metabolic disturbances.[64] These are usually mild and self-limiting.
- Little is known of the developmental effects of prenatal exposure to TCAs, although one small study detected no adverse consequences.[67]

SSRIs
- Sertraline appears to result in the least placental exposure.[70]
- SSRIs appear not to be major teratogens,[50,52,64,71] with most data supporting the safety of fluoxetine.[67,72–75] Note though that one study revealed a slight overall increase in rate of malformation with SSRIs.[76] Database and case control studies have reported an association between SSRIs and anencephaly, craniosynostosis, omphalocele, and persistent pulmonary hypertension of the newborn.[77,78] These associations have not been replicated.
- Paroxetine has been specifically associated with cardiac malformations[79,80] particularly after high dose (>25 mg/day), first trimester exposure.[81] However, some studies have failed to replicate this finding for paroxetine,[64,82] and have implicated other SSRIs.[83,84] Other studies have found no association between any SSRI and an increased risk of cardiac septal defects.[78,85,86] Note that one database study reported that foetal alcohol disorders were 10 times more common in those exposed to SSRIs *in utero* than controls,[87] and that alcohol use during pregnancy is associated with an increased risk of cardiac defects in the foetus.[66]
- SSRIs have also been associated with decreased gestational age[88] (usually a few days which is of questionable clinical significance[49]), spontaneous abortion[89] and decreased birth weight (mean 175 g).[72,73,90] It is possible that these effects are primarily associated with maternal depression rather than specifically with antidepressant treatment.[49] The longer the duration of *in utero* exposure, the greater the chance of low birth weight and respiratory distress.[51] Three groups of symptoms are seen in neonates exposed to antidepressants in late pregnancy; those associated with serotonergic toxicity, those associated with antidepressant discontinuation symptoms and those related to early birth.[91] Third-trimester exposure to sertraline has been associated with reduced early APGAR scores.[72] Third-trimester use of paroxetine may give rise to neonatal complications, presumably related to abrupt withdrawal.[92,93] Other SSRIs have similar, possibly less severe effects.[93,94] Body temperature instability, poor feeding, respiratory distress, cardiac rhythm disturbance, lethargy, muscle tone anomalies, jitteriness, jerky movements and seizures have been reported.[66]

CHAPTER 7

- Data relating to neurodevelopmental outcome of foetal exposure to SSRIs suggest that these drugs are safe, although data are less than conclusive.[67,68,95,96] Depression itself may have more obvious adverse effects on development.[67]
- When taken in late pregnancy, SSRIs may increase the risk of persistent pulmonary hypertension of the newborn (NNH 300). Note this increased risk is compared with population norms, not women with depression, in whom the risk is unquantified.[97]

Other antidepressants
- No specific risks were identified with duloxetine in a study that prospectively followed 233 women through pregnancy and delivery.[98]
- Rather more scarce data suggest the absence of teratogenic potential with **moclobemide**[99]and **reboxetine**.[100] **Venlafaxine** may be associated with cardiac defects, anencephaly and cleft palate[101] and neonatal withdrawal may occur.[73,102,103] Second trimester exposure to venlafaxine has been associated with babies being born small for gestational age.[45] None of these drugs can be specifically recommended. Similarly, **trazodone, bupropion** (amfebutamone) and **mirtazapine** cannot be recommended because there are few data supporting their safety.[73,104,105] Data suggest that both bupropion and mirtazapine are not associated with malformations but, like SSRIs, may be linked to an increased rate of spontaneous abortion.[106,107] Bupropion exposure *in utero* has been associated with an increased risk of attention deficit hyperactivity disorder (ADHD) in young children.[108,109]
  - **Monoamine oxidase inhibitors** (MAOIs) should be avoided in pregnancy because of a suspected increased risk of congenital malformation and because of the risk of hypertensive crisis.[110]
- There is no evidence to suggest that **ECT** causes harm to either the mother or foetus during pregnancy[111] although general anaesthesia is, of course, not without risks. In resistant depression, NICE recommend that ECT is used before/instead of drug combinations.
- **Omega-3 fatty acids** may also be a treatment option[112] although efficacy and safety data are scant.

Box 7.8 summarises the recommendations for the treatment of depression in pregnancy.

Bipolar illness during pregnancy and post-partum

- The risk of relapse during pregnancy if mood stabilising medication is discontinued is high; one study found that bipolar women who were euthymic at conception and discontinued mood stabilisers were twice as likely to relapse and spent five times as long in relapse ill than women who continued mood stabilisers.[113]
- The risk of relapse after delivery is hugely increased: up to eight-fold in the first month post-partum.
- The mental health of the mother influences foetal well-being, obstetric outcome and child development.
- Women with bipolar illness are 50% more likely than controls to have their labour induced or a caesarean delivery, a pre-term delivery, and a neonate that is small for gestational age; the neonate is also more likely to have hypoglycaemia and microcephaly.[6] These associations hold true in both treated and untreated women.

Box 7.8 Recommendations for the treatment of depression in pregnancy

- Patients who are already receiving antidepressants and are at high risk of relapse are best maintained on antidepressants during and after pregnancy.
- Those who develop a moderate or severe depressive illness during pregnancy should be treated with antidepressant drugs.
- There is most experience with **amitriptyline, imipramine** (constipation and sedation can be a problem with both; withdrawal symptoms may occur) **sertraline** (low infant exposure) and **fluoxetine** (increased chance of earlier delivery and reduced birth weight). If the patient is established on another antidepressant, always obtain the most up-to-date advice. Experience with other drugs is growing and a change in treatment may not be necessary or wise. **Paroxetine may be less safe than other SSRIs.**
- Screen for alcohol use and be vigilant for the development of hypertension and pre-eclampsia. Women who take SSRIs may be at increased risk of post-partum haemorrhage.
- When taken in late pregnancy, SSRIs may increase the risk of persistent pulmonary hypertension of the newborn.
- The neonate may experience discontinuation symptoms such as agitation and irritability, or even respiratory distress and convulsions (with SSRIs). The risk is assumed to be particularly high with short half-life drugs such as paroxetine and venlafaxine. Continuing to breast feed and then 'weaning' by switching to mixed (breast/bottle) feeding may help reduce the severity of reactions.

- Bipolar illness itself does not seem to significantly increase the malformation rate; any such association is with mood stabilising drugs.[6]

The risks of not stabilising mood include:

- harm to the mother through poor self-care, lack of obstetric care or self-harm
- harm to the foetus or neonate (ranging from neglect to infanticide).

Treatment with mood stabilisers

- **Lithium** completely equilibrates across the placenta.[114]
- Although the overall risk of major malformations in infants exposed *in utero* has probably been overestimated, lithium should be avoided in pregnancy if possible. Slow discontinuation before conception is the preferred course of action[23,115] because abrupt discontinuation is suspected of worsening the risk of relapse. The relapse rate post-partum may be as high as 70% in women who discontinued lithium before conception.[116] If discontinuation is unsuccessful during pregnancy – restart and continue.
- Lithium use during pregnancy has a well-known association with the cardiac malformation Ebstein's anomaly (relative risk is 10–20 times more than control, but the absolute risk is low at 1:1000).[117] The period of maximum risk to the foetus is 2–6 weeks after conception,[118] before many women know that they are pregnant. The risk of atrial and ventricular septal defects may also be increased.[20] A recent review suggests the exact nature and incidence of congenital malformation is 'uncertain'.[119]
- If lithium is continued during pregnancy, high-resolution ultrasound and echocardiography should be performed at 6 and 18 weeks of gestation.

- In the third trimester, the use of lithium may be problematic because of changing pharmacokinetics: an increasing dose of lithium is required to maintain the lithium level during pregnancy as total body water increases, but the requirements return abruptly to pre-pregnancy levels immediately after delivery.[120] Lithium plasma levels should be monitored every month during pregnancy and immediately after birth. Women taking lithium should deliver in hospital where fluid balance can be monitored and maintained.
- Neonatal goitre, hypotonia, lethargy and cardiac arrhythmia can occur.

Most data relating to **carbamazepine, valproate** and **lamotrigine** come from studies in epilepsy, a condition associated with increased neonatal malformation. These data may not be precisely relevant to use in mental illness.

- Both carbamazepine and valproate have a clear causal link with increased risk of a variety of foetal abnormalities, particularly spina bifida.[121] Both drugs should be avoided, if possible, and an antipsychotic prescribed instead. Valproate confers a higher risk than carbamazapine[122,123] and should not be used in women of child-bearing age except where all other treatment has failed. Although 1 in 20 women of child-bearing age who are in long term contact with mental health services are prescribed mood stabilising drugs, awareness of the teratogenic potential of these drugs amongst psychiatrists is low.[121]
- Valproate monotherapy has also been associated with an increased relative risk of atrial septal defects, cleft palate, hypospadias, polydactyly and craniosynostosis, although absolute risks are low.[124] Valproate is also associated with a reduced head circumference in the neonate.[125]
- Where continued use of valproate or carbamazepine is deemed essential, low-dose monotherapy is strongly recommended, as the teratogenic effect is probably dose-related.[126,127] NICE recommends that the dose of valproate should be limited to 1000 mg a day. The dose of carbamazepine is also best limited to 1000 mg a day.[128,129]
- Vulnerability to valproate-induced neural tube defects may be genetically determined via genes that code for folate metabolism/handling.[130]
- Ideally, all patients should take folic acid (5 mg daily) for at least a month before conception (this may reduce the risk of neonatal neural tube defects). Note, however, that some authorities recommend a lower dose,[131] presumably because of a risk of twin births.[132] Note that there is no evidence that folate protects against anticonvulsant-induced neural tube defects if given during pregnancy,[128] but may do so if given prior to conception (the neural tube is essentially formed by the eighth week of pregnancy[133] before many women realise they are pregnant). However, folate supplementation may be beneficial with regard to early neurodevelopment and so should always be offered.[128]
- Use of carbamazepine in the third trimester may necessitate maternal vitamin K.
- There is growing evidence that lamotrigine is safer in pregnancy than carbamazepine or valproate across a range of outcomes.[128,129,134] Clearance of lamotrigine seems to increase radically during pregnancy[135] and then reduces post-partum.[136] NICE suggest that lamotrigine should not be routinely prescribed in pregnancy.

Box 7.9 summarises the recommendations for the treatment of bipolar disorder in pregnancy.

> **Box 7.9** Recommendations for the treatment of bipolar disorder in pregnancy
>
> - For women who have had a long period without relapse, the possibility of switching to a safer drug (antipsychotic) or withdrawing treatment completely before conception and for at least the first trimester should be considered.
> - The risk of relapse both pre- and post-partum is very high if medication is discontinued abruptly.
> - Women with severe illness or who are known to relapse quickly after discontinuation of a mood stabiliser should be advised to continue their medication following discussion of the risks.
> - No mood stabiliser is clearly safe. Women prescribed lithium should undergo level two ultrasound of the foetus at 6 and 18 weeks' gestation to screen for Ebstein's anomaly. Those prescribed valproate or carbamazepine (both teratogenic) should receive prophylactic folic acid to reduce the incidence of neural tube defects, and receive appropriate antenatal screening tests.
> - If carbamazepine is used, prophylactic vitamin K should be administered to the mother and neonate after delivery.
> - Valproate (the most teratogenic) and combinations of mood stabilisers should be avoided.
> - NICE recommends the use of mood-stabilising antipsychotics as a preferable alternative to continuation with a mood stabiliser.
> - In acute mania in pregnancy use an antipsychotic and if ineffective consider ECT.
> - In bipolar depression during pregnancy use CBT for moderate depression and an SSRI for more severe depression. Olanzapine plus fluoxetine may also be used.

Epilepsy during pregnancy and post-partum

- In pregnant women with epilepsy, there is an increased risk of maternal complications such as severe morning sickness, eclampsia, vaginal bleeding and premature labour. Women should get as much sleep and rest as possible and comply with medication (if prescribed) in order to minimise the risk of seizures.
- The risk of having a child with minor malformations may be increased regardless of treatment with anticonvulsants.

The risks of not treating epilepsy include:

- the increased risk of accidents resulting in foetal injury if seizures are inadequately controlled. Post-partum, the mother may be less able to look after herself and her child
- tonic-clonic seizures during pregnancy can lead to foetal lactic acidosis and hypoxia,[125] the long term consequences of which include neurodevelopmental delay and poor school performance[129]
- the risk of seizures during delivery is 1–2%, potentially worsening maternal and neonatal mortality. Overall, 5% maternal deaths are in women with epilepsy.[125]

Treatment with anticonvulsant drugs

It is established that treatment with anticonvulsant drugs increases the risk of having a child with major congenital malformation to two- to three-fold that seen in the general population. Congenital heart defects (1.8%) and facial clefts (1.7%) are the most common congenital malformations.

Both carbamazepine and valproate are associated with a hugely increased incidence of spina bifida at 0.5–1% and 1–2%, respectively. The risk of other neural tube defects is also increased. In women with epilepsy, the risk of foetal malformations with

> **Box 7.10** Recommendations for the treatment of epilepsy in pregnancy
>
> - For women who have been seizure free for a long period, the possibility of withdrawing treatment before conception, and for at least the first trimester, should be considered.
> - No anticonvulsant is clearly safer. Valproate should be avoided if possible. Women prescribed valproate or carbamazepine should receive prophylactic folic acid, ideally starting prior to conception. Prophylactic vitamin K should be administered to the mother and neonate after delivery.
> - Valproate and combinations of anticonvulsants should be avoided if possible
> - All women with epilepsy should have a full discussion with their neurologist to quantify the risks and benefits of continuing anticonvulsant drugs during pregnancy.

carbamazepine is 2.6%;[128] with lamotrigine 2.3%;[128] and with valproate 7.2%,[137] possibly even higher.[123,127–129] Higher doses (particularly doses of valproate exceeding 1000 mg/day) and anticonvulsant polypharmacy are particularly problematic.[127–129,138] The risks of malformation with carbamazepine and lamotrigine are also probably dose related with risk increasing sharply above daily doses of 1000 mg and 400 mg respectively.[128] It should be noted that these data are derived from databases (they are essentially observational) and it is therefore possible that women prescribed higher doses had more difficult to control seizures which may independently affect outcomes.

It is of note that women prescribed anticonvulsant medication who have given birth to a child with congenital abnormalities, have a 10-fold increased risk of their subsequent child also having abnormalities if they continue to take the same treatment (particularly if this treatment is valproate), suggesting a genetically determined vulnerability.[139] Interestingly, the nature of abnormalities is not consistent across pregnancies.

Cognitive deficits have been reported in older children who have been exposed to valproate *in utero*,[109,125] as have both childhood autism and autistic spectrum disorder.[140] Those exposed to carbamazepine may not be similarly disadvantaged.[141]

Barbiturates (rarely used in the management of epilepsy) are major teratogens, being particularly associated with cardiac malformations.[125] Growing, but still limited, data do not raise any particular concerns over the teratogenic potential of oxcarbazepine, topiramate, gabapentin or levetiracetam.[134]

Pharmacokinetics change during pregnancy, and there is marked inter-individual variation.[142] Dosage adjustment may be required to keep the patient seizure-free.[143] Serum levels usually return to pre-pregnancy levels within a month of delivery often much more rapidly. Doses may need to be reduced at this point.

Best practice guidelines recommend that a woman should receive the lowest possible dose of a single anticonvulsant. Box 7.10 summarises the recommendations for the treatment of epilepsy in pregnancy.

Anxiety disorders and insomnia: sedatives

Anxiety disorders and insomnia are commonly seen in pregnancy.[144] Preferred treatments are CBT and sleep-hygiene measures respectively.

- First-trimester exposure to **benzodiazepines** has been associated with an increased risk of oral clefts in newborns,[145] although two subsequent studies have failed to confirm this association.[146,147]

- Benzodiazepines have been associated with pylorostenosis and alimentary tract atresia.[146] A large Swedish cohort study (n = 1,406 women who took a benzodiazepine during pregnancy) did not confirm these associations, nor suggest others.[147] Note that data on elective terminations were not available.
- There is an association between benzodiazepine use in pregnancy, low birth weight and pre-term delivery.[43,46]
- Third-trimester use is commonly associated with neonatal difficulties (floppy baby syndrome).[148]
- **Promethazine** has been used in hyperemesis gravidarum and appears not to be teratogenic, although data are limited.
- NICE recommends the use of low dose chlorpromazine or amitriptyline.

Rapid tranquillisation

There is almost no published information on the use of rapid tranquillisation in pregnant women. The acute use of short-acting benzodiazepines such as lorazepam and of the sedative antihistamine promethazine is unlikely to be harmful. Presumably, the use

Table 7.9 Recommendations* for the use of psychotropic drugs in pregnancy
Minimise the number of drugs the foetus is exposed to.

Psychotropic group	Recommendations
Antidepressants	**Nortriptyline** **Amitriptyline** **Imipramine** **Sertraline**
Antipsychotics	No clear evidence that any antipsychotic is a major teratogen Consider using/continuing drug mother has previously responded to rather than switching prior to/during pregnancy Most experience with **chlorpromazine, trifluoperazine, haloperidol, olanzapine** Experience growing with **risperidone, quetiapine and aripiprazole** Screen for adverse metabolic effects Arrange for the woman to give birth in a unit with access to neonatal intensive care facilities
Mood stabilisers	Consider using an **antipsychotic** as a mood stabiliser rather than an anticonvulsant drug **Lamotrigine** is also an option (bipolar depression only) Avoid other **anticonvulsants** unless risks and consequences of relapse outweigh the known risk of teratogenesis Women of childbearing potential taking carbamazepine or valproate should receive prophylactic **folic acid** Avoid valproate and combinations where possible
Sedatives	**Non drug measures are preferred** **Benzodiazepines** are probably not teratogenic but are best avoided in late pregnancy **Promethazine** is widely used but supporting safety data are scarce

*It cannot be overstated that treatment needs to be individualised for each patient. This summary box is not intended to suggest that all patients should be switched to a recommended drug. For each patient, take into account their current prescription, response to treatment, history of response to other treatments and the risks known to apply in pregnancy (both for current treatment and for switching).

of either drug will be problematic immediately before birth. NICE also recommends the use of an antipsychotic but do not specify a particular drug.[13] Note that antipsychotics are not generally recommended as a first line treatment for managing acute behavioural disturbance (see section on 'Acutely disturbed and violent behaviour' in this chapter)

Attention deficit hyperactivity disorder

Limited data suggest that methylphenidate is not a major teratogen.[149]

Table 7.9 summarises the recommendations for the use of psychotropic drugs in pregnancy.

References

1. McElhatton PR. Pregnancy: (2) General principles of drug use in pregnancy. Pharm J 2003; **270**:232–234.
2. CARE Study Group. Maternal caffeine intake during pregnancy and risk of fetal growth restriction: a large prospective observational study. BMJ 2008; **337**:a2332.
3. Rasmussen SA et al. Maternal obesity and risk of neural tube defects: a metaanalysis. Am J Obstet Gynecol 2008; **198**:611–619.
4. Schneid-Kofman N et al. Psychiatric illness and adverse pregnancy outcome. Int J Gynaecol Obstet 2008; **101**:53–56.
5. MacCabe JH et al. Adverse pregnancy outcomes in mothers with affective psychosis. Bipolar Disord 2007; **9**:305–309.
6. Boden R et al. Risks of adverse pregnancy and birth outcomes in women treated or not treated with mood stabilisers for bipolar disorder: population based cohort study. BMJ 2012; **345**:e7085.
7. Nosarti C et al. Preterm birth and psychiatric disorders in young adult life. Arch Gen Psychiatry 2012; **69**:E1–E8.
8. de La Rochebrochard E et al. Children born after unplanned pregnancies and cognitive development at 3 years: social differentials in the United Kingdom Millennium Cohort. Am J Epidemiol 2013; **178**:910–920.
9. Goodwin RD et al. Mental disorders and nicotine dependence among pregnant women in the United States. Obstet Gynecol 2007; **109**:875–883.
10. Tobacco Advisory group of the Royal College of Physicians. Harm reduction in nicotine addiction. Helping people who can't quit. 2007. http://www.rcplondon.ac.uk/.
11. Sit DK et al. Changes in antidepressant metabolism and dosing across pregnancy and early postpartum. J Clin Psychiatry 2008; **69**:652–658.
12. Ter Horst PG et al. Pharmacological aspects of neonatal antidepressant withdrawal. Obstet Gynecol Surv 2008; **63**:267–279.
13. National Institute for Health and Clinical Excellence. Antenatal and postnatal mental health. Clinical management and service guidance. Clinical Guideline 45, 2007. http://www.nice.org.uk/
14. Harlow BL et al. Incidence of hospitalization for postpartum psychotic and bipolar episodes in women with and without prior prepregnancy or prenatal psychiatric hospitalizations. Arch Gen Psychiatry 2007; **64**:42–48.
15. Gentile S. Antipsychotic therapy during early and late pregnancy. A systematic review. Schizophr Bull 2010; **36**:518–544.
16. Diav-Citrin O et al. Safety of haloperidol and penfluridol in pregnancy: a multicenter, prospective, controlled study. J Clin Psychiatry 2005; **66**:317–322.
17. Habermann F et al. Atypical antipsychotic drugs and pregnancy outcome: a prospective, cohort study. J Clin Psychopharmacol 2013; **33**:453–462.
18. Collins KO et al. Maternal haloperidol therapy associated with dyskinesia in a newborn. Am J Health Syst Pharm 2003; **60**:2253–2255.
19. Trixler M et al. Use of antipsychotics in the management of schizophrenia during pregnancy. Drugs 2005; **65**:1193–1206.
20. Reis M et al. Maternal use of antipsychotics in early pregnancy and delivery outcome. J Clin Psychopharmacol 2008; **28**:279–288.
21. Boden R et al. Antipsychotics during pregnancy: relation to fetal and maternal metabolic effects. Arch Gen Psychiatry 2012; **69**:715–721.
22. Newham JJ et al. Birth weight of infants after maternal exposure to typical and atypical antipsychotics: prospective comparison study. Br J Psychiatry 2008; **192**:333–337.
23. Ernst CL et al. The reproductive safety profile of mood stabilizers, atypical antipsychotics, and broad-spectrum psychotropics. J Clin Psychiatry 2002; **63 Suppl** 4:42–55.
24. McKenna K et al. Pregnancy outcome of women using atypical antipsychotic drugs: a prospective comparative study. J Clin Psychiatry 2005; **66**:444–449.
25. Brunner E et al. Olanzapine in pregnancy and breastfeeding: a review of data from global safety surveillance. BMC Pharmacol Toxicol 2013; **14**:38.
26. Spyropoulou AC et al. Hip dysplasia following a case of olanzapine exposed pregnancy: a questionable association. Arch Womens Ment Health 2006; **9**:219–222.
27. Arora M et al. Meningocele and ankyloblepharon following in utero exposure to olanzapine. Eur Psychiatry 2006; **21**:345–346.

28. Peng M et al. Effects of prenatal exposure to atypical antipsychotics on postnatal development and growth of infants: a case-controlled, prospective study. Psychopharmacology (Berl) 2013; 228:577–584.

29. European Medicines Agency. Antipsychotics - Risk of extrapyramidal effects and withdrawal symptoms in newborns after exposure during pregnancy. Pharmacovigilance Working Party, July 2011 plenary meeting. Issue 1107. 2011. http://www.ema.europa.eu/docs/en_GB/document_library/Report/2011/07/WC500109581.pdf

30. Cohen LS et al. Relapse of major depression during pregnancy in women who maintain or discontinue antidepressant treatment. JAMA 2006; 295:499–507.

31. Munk-Olsen T et al. New parents and mental disorders: a population-based register study. JAMA 2006; 296:2582–2589.

32. Mahon PB et al. Genome-wide linkage and follow-up association study of postpartum mood symptoms. Am J Psychiatry 2009; 166:1229–1237.

33. Yonkers KA et al. The management of depression during pregnancy: a report from the American Psychiatric Association and the American College of Obstetricians and Gynecologists. Gen Hosp Psychiatry 2009; 31:403–413.

34. Engelstad HJ et al. Perinatal outcomes of pregnancies complicated by maternal depression with or without selective serotonin reuptake inhibitor therapy. Neonatology 2014; 105:149–154.

35. Ververs T et al. Prevalence and patterns of antidepressant drug use during pregnancy. Eur J Clin Pharmacol 2006; 62:863–870.

36. Andrade SE et al. Use of antidepressant medications during pregnancy: a multisite study. Am J Obstet Gynecol 2008; 198:194–195.

37. Alwan S et al. Patterns of Antidepressant Medication Use Among Pregnant Women in a United States Population. J Clin Pharmacol 2010; 51:264–270.

38. Petersen I et al. Pregnancy as a major determinant for discontinuation of antidepressants: an analysis of data from The Health Improvement Network. J Clin Psychiatry 2011; 72:979–985.

39. Munk-Olsen T et al. Prevalence of antidepressant use and contacts with psychiatrists and psychologists in pregnant and postpartum women. Acta Psychiatr Scand 2012; 125:318–324.

40. Nakhai-Pour HR et al. Use of antidepressants during pregnancy and the risk of spontaneous abortion. CMAJ 2010; 182:1031–1037.

41. Jimenez-Solem E et al. SSRI use during pregnancy and risk of stillbirth and neonatal mortality. Am J Psychiatry 2013; 170:299–304.

42. Stephansson O et al. Selective serotonin reuptake inhibitors during pregnancy and risk of stillbirth and infant mortality. JAMA 2013; 309:48–54.

43. Calderon-Margalit R et al. Risk of preterm delivery and other adverse perinatal outcomes in relation to maternal use of psychotropic medications during pregnancy. Am J Obstet Gynecol 2009; 201:579–8.

44. Lund N et al. Selective serotonin reuptake inhibitor exposure in utero and pregnancy outcomes. Arch Pediatr Adolesc Med 2009; 163:949–954.

45. Ramos E et al. Association between antidepressant use during pregnancy and infants born small for gestational age. Can J Psychiatry 2010; 55:643–652.

46. Jensen HM et al. Maternal depression, antidepressant use in pregnancy and Apgar scores in infants. Br J Psychiatry 2013; 202:347–351.

47. Wisner KL et al. Does fetal exposure to SSRIs or maternal depression impact infant growth? Am J Psychiatry 2013; 170:485–493.

48. Leibovitch L et al. Short-term neonatal outcome among term infants after in utero exposure to serotonin reuptake inhibitors. Neonatology 2013; 104:65–70.

49. Andrade C. Antenatal exposure to selective serotonin reuptake inhibitors and duration of gestation. J Clin Psychiatry 2013; 74:e633–e635.

50. Ban L et al. Maternal depression, antidepressant prescriptions, and congenital anomaly risk in offspring: a population-based cohort study. BJOG 2014; Epub ahead of print.

51. Oberlander TF et al. Effects of timing and duration of gestational exposure to serotonin reuptake inhibitor antidepressants: population-based study. Br J Psychiatry 2008; 192:338–343.

52. Ramos E et al. Duration of antidepressant use during pregnancy and risk of major congenital malformations. Br J Psychiatry 2008; 192:344–350.

53. Nulman I et al. Neurodevelopment of children following prenatal exposure to venlafaxine, selective serotonin reuptake inhibitors, or untreated maternal depression. Am J Psychiatry 2012; 169:1165–1174.

54. Suri R et al. A prospective, naturalistic, blinded study of early neurobehavioral outcomes for infants following prenatal antidepressant exposure. J Clin Psychiatry 2011; 72:1002–1007.

55. de Vries NK et al. Early neurological outcome of young infants exposed to selective serotonin reuptake inhibitors during pregnancy: results from the observational SMOK study. PLoS One 2013; 8:e64654.

56. Hviid A et al. Use of selective serotonin reuptake inhibitors during pregnancy and risk of autism. N Engl J Med 2013; 369:2406–2415.

57. Rai D et al. Parental depression, maternal antidepressant use during pregnancy, and risk of autism spectrum disorders: population based case-control study. BMJ 2013; 346:f2059.

58. De Vera MA et al. Antidepressant use during pregnancy and the risk of pregnancy-induced hypertension. Br J Clin Pharmacol 2012; 74:362–369.

59. Palmsten K et al. Antidepressant use and risk for preeclampsia. Epidemiology 2013; 24:682–691.

60. Palmsten K et al. Use of antidepressants near delivery and risk of postpartum hemorrhage: cohort study of low income women in the United States. BMJ 2013; 347:f4877.

61. Lupattelli A et al. Risk of vaginal bleeding and postpartum hemorrhage after use of antidepressants in pregnancy: a study from the Norwegian Mother and Child Cohort Study. J Clin Psychopharmacol 2014; 34:143–148.

62. Loughhead AM et al. Placental passage of tricyclic antidepressants. Biol Psychiatry 2006; 59:287–290.

63. Loughhead AM et al. Antidepressants in amniotic fluid: another route of fetal exposure. Am J Psychiatry 2006; 163:145–147.

64. Davis RL et al. Risks of congenital malformations and perinatal events among infants exposed to antidepressant medications during pregnancy. Pharmacoepidemiol Drug Saf 2007; **16**:1086–1094.

65. Kallen B. Neonate characteristics after maternal use of antidepressants in late pregnancy. Arch Pediatr Adolesc Med 2004; **158**:312–316.

66. Gentile S. Tricyclic antidepressants in pregnancy and puerperium. Expert Opin Drug Saf 2014; **13**:207–225.

67. Nulman I et al. Child development following exposure to tricyclic antidepressants or fluoxetine throughout fetal life: a prospective, controlled study. Am J Psychiatry 2002; **159**:1889–1895.

68. Nulman I et al. Neurodevelopment of children exposed in utero to antidepressant drugs. N Engl J Med 1997; **336**:258–262.

69. Maschi S et al. Neonatal outcome following pregnancy exposure to antidepressants: a prospective controlled cohort study. BJOG 2008; **115**:283–289.

70. Hendrick V et al. Placental passage of antidepressant medications. Am J Psychiatry 2003; **160**:993–996.

71. Gentile S. Selective serotonin reuptake inhibitor exposure during early pregnancy and the risk of birth defects. Acta Psychiatr Scand 2011; **123**:266–275.

72. Hallberg P et al. The use of selective serotonin reuptake inhibitors during pregnancy and breast-feeding: a review and clinical aspects. J Clin Psychopharmacol 2005; **25**:59–73.

73. Gentile S. The safety of newer antidepressants in pregnancy and breastfeeding. Drug Saf 2005; **28**:137–152.

74. Kallen BA et al. Maternal use of selective serotonin re-uptake inhibitors in early pregnancy and infant congenital malformations. Birth Defects Res A Clin Mol Teratol 2007; **79**:301–308.

75. Einarson TR et al. Newer antidepressants in pregnancy and rates of major malformations: a meta-analysis of prospective comparative studies. Pharmacoepidemiol Drug Saf 2005; **14**:823–827.

76. Wogelius P et al. Maternal use of selective serotonin reuptake inhibitors and risk of congenital malformations. Epidemiology 2006; **17**:701–704.

77. Chambers CD et al. Selective serotonin-reuptake inhibitors and risk of persistent pulmonary hypertension of the newborn. N Engl J Med 2006; **354**:579–587.

78. Alwan S et al. Use of selective serotonin-reuptake inhibitors in pregnancy and the risk of birth defects. N Engl J Med 2007; **356**:2684–2692.

79. Thormahlen GM. Paroxetine use during pregnancy: is it safe? Ann Pharmacother 2006; **40**:1834–1837.

80. Myles N et al. Systematic meta-analysis of individual selective serotonin reuptake inhibitor medications and congenital malformations. Aust N Z J Psychiatry 2013; **47**:1002–1012.

81. Berard A et al. First trimester exposure to paroxetine and risk of cardiac malformations in infants: the importance of dosage. Birth Defects Res B Dev Reprod Toxicol 2007; **80**:18–27.

82. Einarson A et al. Evaluation of the risk of congenital cardiovascular defects associated with use of paroxetine during pregnancy. Am J Psychiatry 2008; **165**:749–752.

83. Diav-Citrin O et al. Paroxetine and fluoxetine in pregnancy: a prospective, multicentre, controlled, observational study. Br J Clin Pharmacol 2008; **66**:695–705.

84. Louik C et al. First-trimester use of selective serotonin-reuptake inhibitors and the risk of birth defects. N Engl J Med 2007; **356**:2675–2683.

85. Margulis AV et al. Use of selective serotonin reuptake inhibitors in pregnancy and cardiac malformations: a propensity-score matched cohort in CPRD. Pharmacoepidemiol Drug Saf 2013; **22**:942–951.

86. Riggin L et al. The fetal safety of fluoxetine: a systematic review and meta-analysis. J Obstet Gynaecol Can 2013; **35**:362–369.

87. Malm H et al. Selective serotonin reuptake inhibitors and risk for major congenital anomalies. Obstet Gynecol 2011; **118**:111–120.

88. Ross LE et al. Selected pregnancy and delivery outcomes after exposure to antidepressant medication: a systematic review and meta-analysis. JAMA Psychiatry 2013; **70**:436–443.

89. Hemels ME et al. Antidepressant use during pregnancy and the rates of spontaneous abortions: a meta-analysis. Ann Pharmacother 2005; **39**:803–809.

90. Oberlander TF et al. Neonatal outcomes after prenatal exposure to selective serotonin reuptake inhibitor antidepressants and maternal depression using population-based linked health data. Arch Gen Psychiatry 2006; **63**:898–906.

91. Boucher N et al. A new look at the neonate's clinical presentation after in utero exposure to antidepressants in late pregnancy. J Clin Psychopharmacol 2008; **28**:334–339.

92. Haddad PM et al. Neonatal symptoms following maternal paroxetine treatment: serotonin toxicity or paroxetine discontinuation syndrome? J Psychopharmacol 2005; **19**:554–557.

93. Sanz EJ et al. Selective serotonin reuptake inhibitors in pregnant women and neonatal withdrawal syndrome: a database analysis. Lancet 2005; **365**:482–487.

94. Koren G. Discontinuation syndrome following late pregnancy exposure to antidepressants. Arch Pediatr Adolesc Med 2004; **158**:307–308.

95. Gentile S. SSRIs in pregnancy and lactation: emphasis on neurodevelopmental outcome. CNS Drugs 2005; **19**:623–633.

96. Casper RC et al. Follow-up of children of depressed mothers exposed or not exposed to antidepressant drugs during pregnancy. J Pediatr 2003; **142**:402–408.

97. Grigoriadis S et al. Prenatal exposure to antidepressants and persistent pulmonary hypertension of the newborn: systematic review and meta-analysis. BMJ 2014; **348**:f6932.

98. Hoog SL et al. Duloxetine and pregnancy outcomes: safety surveillance findings. Int J Med Sci 2013; **10**:413–419.

99. Rybakowski JK. Moclobemide in pregnancy. Pharmacopsychiatry 2001; **34**:82–83.

100. Pharmacia Ltd. Erdronax: Use on pregnancy, renally and hepatically impaired patients. Personal Communication. 2003.

101. Polen KN et al. Association between reported venlafaxine use in early pregnancy and birth defects, national birth defects prevention study, 1997-2007. Birth Defects Res A Clin Mol Teratol 2013; **97**:28–35.

102. Einarson A et al. Pregnancy outcome following gestational exposure to venlafaxine: a multicenter prospective controlled study. Am J Psychiatry 2001; **158**:1728–1730.

103. Ferreira E et al. Effects of selective serotonin reuptake inhibitors and venlafaxine during pregnancy in term and preterm neonates. Pediatrics 2007; **119**:52–59.

104. Einarson A et al. A multicentre prospective controlled study to determine the safety of trazodone and nefazodone use during pregnancy. Can J Psychiatry 2003; **48**:106–110.

105. Rohde A et al. Mirtazapine (Remergil) for treatment resistant hyperemesis gravidarum: rescue of a twin pregnancy. Arch Gynecol Obstet 2003; **268**:219–221.

106. Djulus J et al. Exposure to mirtazapine during pregnancy: a prospective, comparative study of birth outcomes. J Clin Psychiatry 2006; **67**:1280–1284.

107. Cole JA et al. Bupropion in pregnancy and the prevalence of congenital malformations. Pharmacoepidemiol Drug Saf 2007; **16**:474–484.

108. Figueroa R. Use of antidepressants during pregnancy and risk of attention-deficit/hyperactivity disorder in the offspring. J Dev Behav Pediatr 2010; **31**:641–648.

109. Forsberg L et al. School performance at age 16 in children exposed to antiepileptic drugs in utero-A population-based study. Epilepsia 2010; **52**:364–369.

110. Hendrick V et al. Management of major depression during pregnancy. Am J Psychiatry 2002; **159**:1667–1673.

111. Miller LJ. Use of electroconvulsive therapy during pregnancy. Hosp Community Psychiatry 1994; **45**:444–450.

112. Freeman MP et al. An open trial of Omega-3 fatty acids for depression in pregnancy. Acta Neuropsychiatr 2006; **18**:21–24.

113. Viguera AC et al. Risk of recurrence in women with bipolar disorder during pregnancy: prospective study of mood stabilizer discontinuation. Am J Psychiatry 2007; **164**:1817–1824.

114. Newport DJ et al. Lithium placental passage and obstetrical outcome: implications for clinical management during late pregnancy. Am J Psychiatry 2005; **162**:2162–2170.

115. Dodd S et al. The pharmacology of bipolar disorder during pregnancy and breastfeeding. Expert Opin Drug Saf 2004; **3**:221–229.

116. Viguera AC et al. Risk of recurrence of bipolar disorder in pregnant and nonpregnant women after discontinuing lithium maintenance. Am J Psychiatry 2000; **157**:179–184.

117. Cohen LS et al. A reevaluation of risk of in utero exposure to lithium. JAMA 1994; **271**:146–150.

118. Yonkers KA et al. Lithium during pregnancy: drug effects and therapeutic implications. CNS Drugs 1998; **4**:269.

119. McKnight RF et al. Lithium toxicity profile: a systematic review and meta-analysis. Lancet 2012; **379**:721–728.

120. Blake LD et al. Lithium toxicity and the parturient: case report and literature review. Int J Obstet Anesth 2008; **17**:164–169.

121. James L et al. Informing patients of the teratogenic potential of mood stabilising drugs; a case notes review of the practice of psychiatrists. J Psychopharmacol 2007; **21**:815–819.

122. Wide K et al. Major malformations in infants exposed to antiepileptic drugs in utero, with emphasis on carbamazepine and valproic acid: a nation-wide, population-based register study. Acta Paediatr 2004; **93**:174–176.

123. Wyszynski DF et al. Increased rate of major malformations in offspring exposed to valproate during pregnancy. Neurology 2005; **64**:961–965.

124. Jentink J et al. Valproic acid monotherapy in pregnancy and major congenital malformations. N Engl J Med 2010; **362**:2185–2193.

125. Tomson T et al. Teratogenic effects of antiepileptic drugs. Lancet Neurol 2012; **11**:803–813.

126. Vajda FJ et al. Critical relationship between sodium valproate dose and human teratogenicity: results of the Australian register of anti-epileptic drugs in pregnancy. J Clin Neurosci 2004; **11**:854–858.

127. Vajda FJ et al. Maternal valproate dosage and foetal malformations. Acta Neurol Scand 2005; **112**:137–143.

128. Campbell E et al. Malformation risks of antiepileptic drug monotherapies in pregnancy: updated results from the UK and Ireland Epilepsy and Pregnancy Registers. J Neurol Neurosurg Psychiatry 2014; Epub ahead of print.

129. Tomson T et al. Dose-dependent risk of malformations with antiepileptic drugs: an analysis of data from the EURAP epilepsy and pregnancy registry. Lancet Neurol 2011; **10**:609–617.

130. Duncan S. Teratogenesis of sodium valproate. Curr Opin Neurol 2007; **20**:175–180.

131. Yonkers KA et al. Management of bipolar disorder during pregnancy and the postpartum period. Am J Psychiatry 2004; **161**:608–620.

132. Czeizel AE. Folic acid and the prevention of neural-tube defects. N Engl J Med 2004; **350**:2209–2211.

133. Bestwick JP et al. Prevention of neural tube defects: a cross-sectional study of the uptake of folic acid supplementation in nearly half a million women. PLoS One 2014; **9**:e89354.

134. Molgaard-Nielsen D et al. Newer-generation antiepileptic drugs and the risk of major birth defects. JAMA 2011; **305**:1996–2002.

135. de Haan GJ et al. Gestation-induced changes in lamotrigine pharmacokinetics: a monotherapy study. Neurology 2004; **63**:571–573.

136. Clark CT et al. Lamotrigine dosing for pregnant patients with bipolar disorder. Am J Psychiatry 2013; **170**:1240–1247.

137. National Institute for Health and Clinical Excellence. The epilepsies: the diagnosis and management of the epilepsies in adults and children in primary and secondary care. Clinical Guideline 137, 2012. http://guidance.nice.org.uk/CG137

138. Vajda FJ et al. The Australian Register of Antiepileptic Drugs in Pregnancy: the first 1002 pregnancies. Aust N Z J Obstet Gynaecol 2007; **47**:468–474.

139. Vajda FJ et al. Teratogenesis in repeated pregnancies in antiepileptic drug-treated women. Epilepsia 2013; **54**:181–186.

140. Christensen J et al. Prenatal valproate exposure and risk of autism spectrum disorders and childhood autism. JAMA 2013; **309**:1696–1703.

CHAPTER 7

141. Gaily E et al. Normal intelligence in children with prenatal exposure to carbamazepine. Neurology 2004; 62:28–32.

142. Brodtkorb E et al. Seizure control and pharmacokinetics of antiepileptic drugs in pregnant women with epilepsy. Seizure 2008; 17:160–165.

143. Adab N. Therapeutic monitoring of antiepileptic drugs during pregnancy and in the postpartum period: is it useful? CNS Drugs 2006; 20:791–800.

144. Ross LE et al. Anxiety disorders during pregnancy and the postpartum period: A systematic review. J Clin Psychiatry 2006; 67:1285–1298.

145. Dolovich LR et al. Benzodiazepine use in pregnancy and major malformations or oral cleft: meta-analysis of cohort and case-control studies. BMJ 1998; 317:839–843.

146. Wikner BN et al. Use of benzodiazepines and benzodiazepine receptor agonists during pregnancy: neonatal outcome and congenital malformations. Pharmacoepidemiol Drug Saf 2007; 16:1203–1210.

147. Reis M et al. Combined use of selective serotonin reuptake inhibitors and sedatives/hypnotics during pregnancy: risk of relatively severe congenital malformations or cardiac defects. A register study. BMJ Open 2013; 3:e002166.

148. McElhatton PR. The effects of benzodiazepine use during pregnancy and lactation. Reprod Toxicol 1994; 8:461–475.

149. Pottegard A et al. First-trimester exposure to methylphenidate: a population-based cohort study. J Clin Psychiatry 2014; 75:e88–e93.

Further reading

National Institute for Health and Care Excellence. Antenatal and postnatal mental health: clinical management and service guidance. Clinical Guideline 192, 2014. https://www.nice.org.uk/guidance/cg192

Paton C. Prescribing in pregnancy. Br J Psychiatry 2008; 192:321–322.

Ruchkin V et al. SSRIs and the developing brain. Lancet 2005; 365:451–453.

Sanz EJ et al. Selective serotonin reuptake inhibitors in pregnant women and neonatal withdrawal syndrome: a database analysis. Lancet 2005; 365:482–487.

Other sources of information

National Teratology Information Service. http://www.hpa.org.uk/

Breastfeeding

Data on the safety of psychotropic medication in breastfeeding are largely derived from small studies or case reports and case series. Reported infant and neonatal outcomes in most cases are limited to short term acute adverse effects. Long-term safety cannot therefore be guaranteed for the psychotropics reviewed here. The information presented must be interpreted with caution with respect to the limited data from which it is derived and the need for such information to be regularly updated.

Infant exposure

All psychotropics are excreted in breast milk, to varying degrees. The most direct measure of infant exposure is, of course, infant plasma levels, but these data are often not available. Instead, many cases report drug concentrations in breast milk and maternal plasma. These data can be used to estimate the daily infant dose (by assuming a milk intake of 150 mL/kg/day). The infant weight-adjusted dose when expressed as a proportion of the maternal weight-adjusted dose is known as the relative infant dose (RID). Drugs with a RID below 10% are widely regarded as safe in breastfeeding.

$$RID = infant\ dose\,(mg/kg/day)/maternal\ dose\,(mg/kg/day)$$

Where measured, infant plasma levels below 10% of average maternal plasma levels have been proposed as safe in breastfeeding.[1]

The RIDs, where available from the literature, are given in Tables 7.11–7.14. The RID should be used as a guide only, as values are estimates and vary widely in the literature for individual drugs.

General principles of prescribing psychotropics in breastfeeding

- In each case, the benefits of breastfeeding to the mother and infant must be weighed against the risk of drug exposure in the infant.
- The infants should be monitored for any specific adverse effects of the drugs as well as for feeding patterns and growth and development.
- Neonates and infants do not have the same capacity for drug clearance as adults. In addition, premature infants and infants with renal, hepatic, cardiac or neurological impairment are at a greater risk from exposure to drugs.
- It is usually inappropriate to withhold treatment to allow breastfeeding where there is a high risk of relapse. Treatment of maternal illness is the highest priority.
- Where a mother has taken a particular psychotropic drug during pregnancy and until delivery, continuation with the drug while breastfeeding may be appropriate as this may minimise withdrawal symptoms in the infant. However, it is important to note that certain drugs may persist in infant plasma after delivery, leading to high levels in the early post-natal stage during breastfeeding.
- Half-lives of the drugs should be considered: drugs with a long half-life can accumulate in breast milk and infant serum.
- Infant plasma levels should be monitored if toxicity is suspected.
- Women receiving sedating medication should be strongly advised not to sleep with the baby in bed with them.

Wherever possible:

- use the lowest effective dose
- avoid polypharmacy
- time dosing to avoid feeding at peak plasma/milk levels or express milk to give later (this may be impractical in small infants feeding every 2–3 hours).

Table 7.10 summarises the recommendations for drug use in breastfeeding. Further information is provided in Tables 7.11–7.14.

Table 7.10 Summary of recommendations

Drug group	Recommended drugs
Antidepressants	**Sertraline** (others may be used, e.g. paroxetine, nortriptyline, imipramine, see Table 7.11)
Antipsychotics	**Olanzapine** (others may be used, see Table 7.12)
Mood stabilisers	Often best to switch to **mood-stabilising antipsychotic** (see Table 7.13) **Valproate** can be used but only where there is adequate protection against pregnancy (breastfeeding itself is not adequate protection). Beware risk of hepatotoxicity in breastfed infants
Sedatives	**Lorazepam** for anxiety and sleep (see Table 7.14)

Antidepressants in breast-feeding

Manufacturers' advice on drugs in breastfeeding is available in the Summary of Product Characteristics or European Public Assessment Report for individual drugs. Table 7.11 does not include or repeat this advice, but instead uses primary reference sources.

Table 7.11 Antidepressants in breastfeeding

Drug	Comment	Estimated daily infant dose as proportion of maternal dose (RID)
Agomelatine[11,91]	Peak breast milk levels were seen 1–2 hours post dose in a mother taking 25mg agomelatine. The drug was undetectable 4 hours post dose. Effects in the neonate were not reported.	Not available
Bupropion[11,21,82–87]	Reported infant serum levels range from low to undetectable. Bupropion has been detected in the urine of 1 infant. No adverse effects were noted in four infants (in three separate case reports) exposed to bupropion in breast milk. Infant effects were not assessed in the other cases. There is one report of a seizure in a 6-month-old infant exposed to bupropion in breast milk. Neither breast milk nor infant serum levels were determined in this case.	0.2–2%
Citalopram[1,2,11,13–22]	Reported infant serum levels are variable, ranging from undetectable or low to >10% of maternal serum levels. Recorded levels are higher than those for fluvoxamine, sertraline, paroxetine and escitalopram, but lower than for fluoxetine. Breast milk peak levels have been observed 3–9 hours after maternal dose. There is one case report of uneasy sleep in an infant exposed to citalopram while breastfeeding which resolved on halving the mother's dose. Irregular breathing, sleep disorder, hypo- and hypertonia were observed up to 3 weeks after delivery in another breastfeeding infant exposed to citalopram *in utero*. The symptoms were attributed to withdrawal syndrome from citalopram despite the mother continuing citalopram post-partum. In a study of 31 exposed infants, one case each of colic, decreased feeding, and irritability/restlessness was reported. Normal growth and development were noted in a 6-month old infant whose mother took a combination of ziprasidone and citalopram whilst breastfeeding (and during pregnancy). In a study of 78 breastfeeding infants of mothers taking an SSRI or venlafaxine no difference in weight was noted at 6 months when compared with the 'normative' weight. In one study, normal neurodevelopment was observed, up to the age of 1-year, in all 11 infants exposed to citalopram *in utero* and through breast milk. One of the children, at 1-year, was unable to walk. However, the neurological status of this child was deemed normal 6 months later.	3–10.9%
Duloxetine[11,21,88–90]	In a study of six nursing women breast-milk concentrations of duloxetine were found to be low. Neither infant serum levels nor infant effects were assessed. In two separate case reports infant serum levels of duloxetine were found to be low. In addition, no short-term adverse effects were noted in the infants.	<1%

(Continued)

Table 7.11 (*Continued*)

Drug	Comment	Estimated daily infant dose as proportion of maternal dose (RID)
Escitalopram[11,21,23–28]	Reported infant serum levels are low or undetectable. Adverse effects were not seen in two separate case reports. In a study of eight women breast milk peak levels of escitalopram were observed 2–11 hours post maternal dose. No adverse effects were noted in the infants. There is one case of necrotising enterocolitis (necessitating intensive care admission and intravenous antibiotic treatment) in a 5-day old infant exposed to escitalopram *in utero* and through breast milk. The infant's symptoms on admission were lethargy, decreased oral intake and blood in the stools.	3–8.3%
Fluoxetine[1,2,11,21,22,36–46]	Reported infant serum levels are variable and higher than those for paroxetine, fluvoxamine, sertraline, citalopram and escitalopram. In a pooled analysis of antidepressant levels fluoxetine produced the highest proportion of infant levels above 10% of the average maternal levels. Peak breast milk levels have been observed approximately 8 hours post maternal dose. Adverse effects have not been reported for the majority of fluoxetine-exposed infants. Reported adverse effects include colic, excessive crying, decreased sleep, diarrhoea and vomiting, somnolence, decreased feeding, hypotonia, moaning, grunting, hyperactivity. Seizure activity at 3 weeks, 4 months and then 5 months was reported in an infant whose mother was taking a combination of fluoxetine and carbamazepine. A retrospective study found the growth curves of breastfed infants of mothers taking fluoxetine to be significantly below those of infants receiving breast milk free of fluoxetine. However, in another study of 78 breastfeeding infants of mothers taking an SSRI or venlafaxine no difference in weight was noted at 6 months when compared with the 'normative' weight. Neurological developments and weight gain were found to be normal in 11 infants exposed to fluoxetine during pregnancy and lactation. No developmental abnormalities were noted in another four infants exposed to fluoxetine during breastfeeding. In a study of eleven infants exposed to fluoxetine whilst breastfeeding, a drop in platelet serotonin was noted in one of the infants.	1.6–14.6%
Fluvoxamine[1,2,11,21,22,36–46]	Reported infant serum levels vary from undetectable to up to half the maternal serum level. No infant adverse effects have been reported. Peak drug levels in breast milk have been observed 4 hours after maternal dose.	1–2%
Monoamine oxidase inhibitors (MAOIs)	No published data could found.	
Mianserin[11,76]	Adverse effects were not seen in two infants studied.	

Table 7.11 (*Continued*)

Drug	Comment	Estimated daily infant dose as proportion of maternal dose (RID)
Mirtazapine[1,2,11,21,22,36-46]	Reported infant serum levels range from undetectable to low. Psychomotor development in one infant after 6 weeks of exposure was found to be normal. No adverse effects were noted in any of the eight infants in a study of exposure to mirtazapine in breast milk. In addition, developmental milestones were being achieved by all infants at the time of the study. However, the weights for three of the infants were observed to be between the 10th to 25th percentiles. All three were noted to also have a low birth weight. There is one case of higher mirtazapine serum levels in a breastfeeding infant than have been previously reported. The authors explain this by suggesting that there may be a large difference in mirtazapine elimination rates between individual infants. In this same infant the mother reported a greater weight gain and uninterrupted night-time sleep compared with her other children.	0.5–4.4%
Moclobemide[1,2,11,21,22,36-46]	Reported infant serum levels appear to be low. No adverse effects were detected in these infants. Peak drug levels in breast milk were seen at 3 hours. The manufacturers of moclobemide advise that its use in breastfeeding can be considered if the benefits outweigh the risk to the child.	3.4%
Paroxetine[1,2,11,21,22,36-46]	Reported infant serum levels vary from low to undetectable. Adverse effects have not been reported for the majority of paroxetine-exposed infants. However, vomiting and irritability were reported in a breastfeeding baby of 18 months. The symptoms were attributed to severe hyponatraemia in the infant. The maternal paroxetine dose was 40 mg. Paroxetine levels were not determined in the breast milk or infant serum. In a study of 78 breastfeeding infants of mothers taking an SSRI or venlafaxine no difference in weight was noted at 6 months when compared with the 'normative' weight. Breastfed infants of 27 women taking paroxetine reached the usual developmental milestones at 3, 6 and 12 months, similar to a control group. The manufacturers of paroxetine advise that its use in breastfeeding can be considered.	0.5–2.8%
Reboxetine[11,21,65]	Reported infant serum levels range from low to undetectable and no adverse effects were noted in four infants. In addition, normal developmental milestones were reached by three of the infants. The fourth had developmental problems thought not to be related to maternal reboxetine therapy. Breast milk peak levels were observed 1–9 hours after maternal dose. The manufacturers of reboxetine advise that its use in breastfeeding can be considered if the benefits outweigh the risk to the child.	1–3%

(*Continued*)

CHAPTER 7

Table 7.11 (*Continued*)

Drug	Comment	Estimated daily infant dose as proportion of maternal dose (RID)
Sertraline[11,21,22,40,51,56–64]	Reported infant serum levels appear to be low and in some cases undetectable. Peak drug levels in breast milk have been observed 7–10 hours after the maternal dose. There is one report of an unusually high infant serum level (half maternal serum level). The infant was reported to be 'clinically thriving'. Adverse effects have not been observed in the majority of nursing infants. A drop in platelet serotonin levels was *not* seen in a study of 14 breastfeeding infants of mothers taking sertraline. Serotonergic overstimulation, associated with exposure through breast milk, has been reported in one pre-term infant. Reported symptoms included hyperthermia, shivering, myoclonus and tremor, irritability, decreased suckling reflex and reactivity, tremor and high pitched crying. The symptoms ceased on discontinuation of breastfeeding. The neonate was exposed to sertraline *in utero*. In a study of 78 breastfeeding infants of mothers taking an SSRI or venlafaxine no difference in weight was noted at 6 months when compared with the 'normative' weight. Withdrawal symptoms (agitation, restlessness, insomnia and an enhanced startle reaction) developed in a breastfed neonate, after abrupt withdrawal of maternal sertraline. The neonate was exposed to sertraline *in utero*. The manufacturers of sertraline advise against its use in breastfeeding, but NICE state that breast milk levels of sertraline are relatively lower (than what, it is not clear) and so tacitly recommends the use of sertraline.[12]	0.5–3%
Trazodone[11,81]	Trazodone is excreted into breast milk in small quantities, based on assessments after a single maternal dose.	2.8%
Tricyclic antidepressants (TCAs)[1–11]	Reported infant serum levels range from undetectable to low. Adverse effects have not been reported in infants exposed to amitriptyline, nortriptyline, clomipramine, imipramine, dothiepin (dosulepin) and desipramine. There are two case reports of doxepin exposure during breastfeeding leading to adverse effects in the infant. In one, an 8-week-old infant experienced respiratory depression, which resolved 24 hours after stopping nursing. In the other, poor suckling, muscle hypotonia and drowsiness were observed in a newborn, again resolving 24 hours after removing doxepin exposure. A study of 15 children did not show a negative outcome on cognitive development in children 3 to 5 years post-partum, following breast milk exposure to dothiepin. NICE states that imipramine, nortriptyline are present in breast milk 'at relatively low levels'.[12] Thus these drugs are at least tacitly recommended by NICE. However, nortriptyline is formally contraindicated in breastfeeding mothers. Data on TCAs not mentioned in this section were not available and their use can therefore not be recommended unless used during pregnancy.	Nortriptyline, Amitriptyline, Clomipramine } = 1–3%

Table 7.11 (*Continued*)

Drug	Comment	Estimated daily infant dose as proportion of maternal dose (RID)
Venlafaxine.[11,21,22,40,51,66–73]	Reported infant serum levels appear to be higher than those seen with fluvoxamine, sertraline and paroxetine. No adverse effects have been reported. Symptoms of lethargy, jitteriness, rapid breathing, poor suckling and dehydration seen two days after delivery of an infant exposed to venlafaxine *in utero*, subsided over a week on exposure to venlafaxine via breast milk. It was suggested in this case that breastfeeding may have helped manage the withdrawal symptoms experienced post-partum. In a study of 13 infants the highest levels of venlafaxine (and desvenlafaxine) were noted 8 hours after maternal dose. Concentrations in breast milk were found to be higher for desvenlafaxine than venlafaxine. An infant exposed to a combination of venlafaxine and amisulpride from the age of 2 months was found to be healthy during a clinical assessment at 5 months. No health issues were observed and the infant was found to have a Denver developmental age consistent with its chronological age. In a study of 78 breastfeeding infants of mothers taking an SSRI or venlafaxine no difference in weight was noted at 6 months when compared with the 'normative' weight. 'Typical' development (measured using the Bayley Scale of Infant Development) was observed in two infants exposed to a combination of venlafaxine and quetaipine whilst breastfeeding. In one of the cases the mother was also taking trazodone.	6–9%
Vortioxetine	No data available.	Not available

Table 7.12 Antipsychotics in breastfeeding

Drug	Comment	Estimated daily infant dose as proportion of maternal dose (RID)
Amisulpride[11,69,103]	In two separate cases, amisulpride concentrations in breast milk were found to be high. Infant serum levels were not directly measured in either case. However, the estimated relative infant dose was calculated in one case to be above the accepted safe level and in the other within the safe limit. The doses of amisulpride in the above cases were 400 mg and 250 mg, respectively. No acute adverse effects or health issues were observed in either infant. The Denver developmental age was consistent, for both infants, with the chronological age. In one of the cases the mother was also taking venlafaxine. Breastfeeding is contraindicated by the manufacturers of amisulpride.	10.7%
Aripiprazole[11,104–107]	A 3-month old infant was found to be growing 'normally' after exposure to aripiprazole in breast milk and *in utero*. No further infant data were available. Aripiprazole was undetectable in the three breast milk specimens analysed in this case. A plasma level of 7.6 ng/ml (approximately 4% of maternal plasma concentration) was recorded 6 days after delivery in a breastfed infant exposed to aripiprazole *in utero*. The authors proposed that a proportion of the drug detected may be due to placental transfer of aripiprazole. Adverse effects were not noted in the neonate. There is one case of a woman's failure to lactate after being treated with aripiprazole during pregnancy.	0.9%
Asenapine	No data available.	Not available
Butyrophenones[2,3,11,40,92–94]	Reported breast milk concentrations are variable. Normal development was noted in one infant. However, delayed development was noted in three infants exposed to a combination of haloperidol and chlorpromazine in breast milk. Data on butyrophenones not mentioned in this section were not available.	Haloperidol = 0.2–12%
Clozapine[2,3,11,40,93,108,109]	In a study of four infants exposed to clozapine in breast milk, sedation was noted in one and another developed agranulocytosis, which resolved on stopping clozapine. No adverse effects were noted in the other two. Decreased sucking reflex, irritability, seizures and cardiovascular instability have also been reported in nursing infants exposed to clozapine. A high breast milk clozapine level (2–3 times maternal plasma level) was reported in one case. The infant was not breastfed. There is one case report of delayed speech acquisition in an infant who was exposed to clozapine during breastfeeding. The infant was also exposed to clozapine *in utero*. Because of the risk of neutropenia and seizures, it is advisable to avoid breastfeeding while on clozapine until more data become available.	1.4%

Table 7.12 (*Continued*)

Drug	Comment	Estimated daily infant dose as proportion of maternal dose (RID)
Lurasidone	No data available.	Not available
Olanzapine[2,11,40,110–117]	Reported infant serum levels range from undetectable to low. There is one case of an infant developing jaundice and sedation on exposure to olanzapine during breastfeeding. This continued on cessation of breastfeeding. This infant was exposed to olanzapine *in utero* and had cardiomegaly. In another, no adverse effects were noted. No adverse effects were reported in four of seven breastfed infants of mothers taking olanzapine. Of the rest, one was not assessed, one had a lower developmental age than chronological age (but the mother had also been taking additional psychotropic medication), and drowsiness was noted in another, which resolved on halving the maternal dose. The median maximum concentration in the milk was found at around 5 hours after maternal ingestion. In one breastfeeding infant, olanzapine serum levels decreased over the course of 5 months. The authors' explanation for this is that the infant's capacity to metabolise olanzapine 'developed rapidly' around the age of 4 months. No increase in the rate of adverse outcomes (at the age of 1–2 years) was noted in a study comparing 37 infants exposed to olanzapine whilst breastfeeding with non-exposed infants. However, speech delay was noted in one olanzapine-exposed infant and motor developmental delay in another. 'Failure to gain weight' was reported in the case of two infants. Other reported adverse effects include somnolence, irritability, tremor and insomnia in infants exposed to olanzapine whilst breastfeeding.	1.0–1.6%
Paliperidone	No specific data available. See data for risperidone.	Not available
Phenothiazines[2,3,11,92–94]	Most of the data relate to chlorpromazine. There is a wide variation in the breast milk concentrations quoted. Similarly, infant serum levels vary greatly. Lethargy was reported in one infant whose mother was taking chlorpromazine while breastfeeding. In another case, however, an infant exposed to much higher levels showed no signs of lethargy. There is a report of delayed development in three infants exposed to a combination of chlorpromazine and haloperidol while breastfeeding. In the one case of perphenazine exposure and two cases of trifluoperazine exposure, no adverse effects were noted in the infants. Data on phenothiazines not mentioned in this section were not available.	Chlorpromazine=0.3%

CHAPTER 7

Table 7.12 (Continued)

Drug	Comment	Estimated daily infant dose as proportion of maternal dose (RID)
Quetiapine[11,70,118–126]	Peak breast milk concentrations have been reported one hour after maternal dose (using IR dosage form). Adverse effects were not noted in infants in three separate case reports. One of these infants was exposed to a combination of quetiapine and paroxetine. In addition, no adverse effects were noted in an infant exposed to a combination of quetiapine and fluvoxamine whilst breastfeeding. The baby reached developmental milestones. In a separate small study of quetiapine augmentation of maternal antidepressant therapy, two out of six babies showed mild developmental delays not thought to be related to quetiapine treatment. The doses in this study ranged from 25–400 mg/day. Quetiapine was undetected in milk samples from four of mothers, all of whom were taking a dose below 100 mg. There is one reported case of an infant 'sleeping more than expected' whilst exposed to quetiapine, mirtazapine and a benzodiazepine in breast milk. The drowsiness is thought to be a result of exposure to the benzodiazepine.	0.09–0.1%
Risperidone[11,127–131]	Reported breast milk concentrations of risperidone are higher than for olanzapine and quetiapine. No adverse effects were noted in the reported cases. In two cases where development was assessed, no abnormalities were observed.	Risperidone = 2.8–9.1% 9-hydoxyrisperidone = 3.46–4.7% (based on breast milk concentrations of lactating women taking risperidone)
Sertindole	No published data could be found.	
Sulpiride[11,98–102]	There are a number of small studies in which sulpiride has been shown to improve lactation in nursing mothers. Relative infant dose estimations are high. No adverse effects were noted in the nursing infants.	2.7–20.7%
Thioxanthenes[2,11,94–97]	There are two cases of infant exposure to flupentixol and seven to zuclopentixol. No adverse effects or developmental abnormalities were noted in the infant exposed infant exposed to flupentixol. The clinical status of the other infant was not reported. No adverse effects were reported in the cases of zuclopentixol exposure.	Zuclopentixol = 0.4–0.9%
Ziprasidone[11,20,94,132]	In one case, where breast-milk concentrations were measured, levels were found to be undetectable or low. Infant effects were not determined in this case. In another case, normal growth and development were noted in a 6-month old infant whose mother took a combination of ziprasidone and citalopram whilst breastfeeding (and during pregnancy). Ziprasidone plasma levels in breast milk were not determined in this case.	0.07–1.2%
Iloperidone	No data available.	Not available

Table 7.13 Mood stabilisers in breastfeeding

Drug	Comment	Estimated daily infant dose as proportion of maternal dose (RID)
Carbamazepine[2,11,133–142]	Reported infant serum levels are generally low although higher levels of up 4.8 μg/mL have been reported. Adverse effects have been reported in a number of infants exposed to carbamazepine during breastfeeding. These include one case of cholestatic hepatitis, and one of transient hepatic dysfunction with hyperbilirubinaemia and elevated gamma-glutamyl transferase (GGT). The adverse effects in the first case resolved after discontinuation of breastfeeding and the second resolved despite continued feeding. Other adverse effects reported include seizure-like activity, drowsiness, irritability and high-pitched crying in one infant whose mother was on multiple agents, hyperexcitability in two infants, poor suckling in one and poor feeding in another three. In contrast, in a number of infants, no adverse effects were noted. A prospective study of children of women with epilepsy found that breastfeeding whilst taking an anticonvulsant was not associated with adverse development of infants at ages 6 to 36 months. The study assessed outcomes in children exposed to anticonvulsants *in utero* who were subsequently breastfed compared with those who were not. A study of 199 infants exposed to anticonvulsant medications (carbamazepine, valproate, phenytoin, lamotrigine) during breastfeeding failed to show a difference in IQ between breastfed and non-breastfed infants at the age of 3 years. The infants were exposed to anticonvulsant medications *in utero*. The manufacturers of carbamazepine advise that breastfeeding can be considered if the benefits outweigh the risk to the child. The infant must be observed for possible adverse reactions.	1.1–7.3%
Lamotrigine[11,136,141,143–152]	Lamotrigine is excreted in breast milk. Infant serum levels range between 18% and 50% of maternal serum levels. No adverse effects were noted in 30 nursing infants exposed to lamotrigine. In particular none of the infants developed a rash. In addition, no change in the hepatic and electrolyte profiles was noted in 10 of the infants for whom clinical laboratory data were available. However, thrombocytosis was noted in seven infants. A case of a severe cyanotic episode (preceded by mild episodes of apnoea) requiring resuscitation has been reported in a 16-day old infant exposed to lamotrigine *in utero* and through breast milk. Neonatal serum concentration was in the upper therapeutic range. The mother was taking a high dose (850 mg/day). A prospective study of children of women with epilepsy found that breastfeeding whilst taking an anticonvulsant was not associated with adverse development of infants at ages 6 to 36 months. The study assessed outcomes in children exposed to anticonvulsants *in utero* who were subsequently breastfed compared with those who were not. Three infants exposed to lamotrigine *in utero* and through breast milk were reported to be showing 'normal growth and development' at 15 to 18 months of age. All three developed a rash 3 and 4 months post-partum. In one case the rash was attributed to eczema, and to soy allergy in another. The third case resolved spontaneously.	9.2–18.3%

(Continued)

Table 7.13 (*Continued*)

Drug	Comment	Estimated daily infant dose as proportion of maternal dose (RID)
	Because of the theoretical risk of life-threatening rashes, it is advisable to avoid lamotrigine while breastfeeding until more data on its effects become available. A study of 199 infants exposed to anticonvulsant medications (carbamazepine, valproate, phenytoin, lamotrigine) during breastfeeding failed to show a difference in IQ between breastfed and non-breastfed infants at the age of 3 years. The infants were exposed to anticonvulsant medications *in utero*.	12–30.1%
Lithium[11,133,135,153–156]	Infant serum levels range from 10% to 50% of maternal serum concentrations. In a study of 10 infants, growth and developmental delays were not reported by any of the mothers. In the same study an elevated thyroid stimulating hormone (TSH) was seen in one case (following exposure *in utero*), an increased urea in a further two and a raised creatinine in another. Adverse effects have been reported in infants exposed to lithium while breastfeeding. One infant developed cyanosis, lethargy, hypothermia, hypotonia and a heart murmur, all of which resolved within 3 days of stopping breastfeeding. The infant was exposed to lithium *in utero*. Non-specific signs of toxicity have been reported in others. Early feeding problems have been reported in two infants exposed to lithium *in utero* and through breast milk. There are also reports of no adverse effects in some infants exposed to lithium while breastfeeding. Opinions on the use of lithium while breastfeeding vary from absolute contraindication to mother's informed choice. Conditions which may alter the infant's electrolyte balance and state of hydration must be borne in mind. If it is used, the infant must be carefully monitored for signs of toxicity. Breastfeeding is contraindicated by the manufacturers of lithium. NICE recommends that lithium should not routinely be prescribed for women who are breastfeeding.	
Valproate[2,11,133–136,141,157,158]	Valproate is excreted into breast milk. Reported infant serum levels are low. Thrombocytopenia and anaemia were reported in a 3-month-old infant exposed to valproate *in utero* and while breastfeeding. This reversed on stopping breastfeeding. A study of 199 infants exposed to anticonvulsant medications (carbamazepine, valproate, phenytoin, lamotrigine) during breastfeeding failed to show a difference in IQ between breastfed and non-breastfed infants at the age of 3 years. The infants were exposed to anticonvulsant medications *in utero*. A prospective study of children of women with epilepsy found that breastfeeding whilst taking an anticonvulsant was not associated with adverse development of infants at ages 6 to 36 months. The study assessed outcomes in children exposed to anticonvulsants *in utero* who were subsequently breastfed compared with those who were not. The manufacturers of valproate state that there appears to be no contraindication to its use in breastfeeding. However, hepatotoxicity due to valproate is much more likely in the young so there is a theoretical and important risk in breastfed infants.	1.4–1.7%

Table 7.14 Sedatives in breastfeeding

Drug	Comment	
Benzodiazepines[2,11,40,159–166]	Diazepam can accumulate in breast milk and in infant serum. Reported adverse effects include sedation, lethargy, weight loss and mild jaundice. No adverse effects have been reported in others. Lorazepam, temazepam and clonazepam are excreted in breast milk in small amounts. Apart from one case report of persistent apnoea in one infant exposed to clonazepam *in utero* and during breastfeeding, no adverse effects were reported. Restlessness has been reported in one infant and mild drowsiness in another whose mothers were taking alprazolam during breastfeeding. In a telephone survey of 124 women taking benzodiazepines two mothers reported central nervous system (CNS) depression in their breastfeeding neonates. One of the children was exposed to benzodiazepines *in utero*. Benzodiazepines with a long half-life, such as diazepam should be avoided in breastfeeding. Any infant exposed to benzodiazepines in breast milk should be monitored for CNS depression and apnoea.	Not available
Promethazine	No published data could be found. The manufacturers of promethazine issue no specific advice on its use in breastfeeding.	Not available
Zopiclone, zolpidem and zaleplon[11,167–169]	All three are excreted into breast milk in small amounts. No adverse effects were noted in exposed infants. Zolpidem was detected in the breast milk of five lactating women for up to 4 hours after a 20 mg dose. Zaleplon peak breast milk levels were found 1 hour after the dose and breast milk concentrations were approximately 50% of plasma concentrations.	Zaleplon = 1.5% Zopiclone = 1.5% Zolpidem = 4.7–19.1%

References

1. Weissman AM et al. Pooled analysis of antidepressant levels in lactating mothers, breast milk, and nursing infants. Am J Psychiatry 2004; **161**:1066–1078.
2. Burt VK et al. The use of psychotropic medications during breast-feeding. Am J Psychiatry 2001; **158**:1001–1009.
3. Yoshida K et al. Psychotropic drugs in mothers' milk: a comprehensive review of assay methods, pharmacokinetics and of safety of breast-feeding. J Psychopharmacol 1999; **13**:64–80.
4. Misri S et al. Benefits and risks to mother and infant of drug treatment for postnatal depression. Drug Saf 2002; **25**:903–911.
5. Yoshida K et al. Investigation of pharmacokinetics and of possible adverse effects in infants exposed to tricyclic antidepressants in breast-milk. J Affect Disord 1997; **43**:225–237.
6. Frey OR et al. Adverse effects in a newborn infant breast-fed by a mother treated with doxepin. Ann Pharmacother 1999; **33**:690–693.
7. Ilett KF et al. The excretion of dothiepin and its primary metabolites in breast milk. Br J Clin Pharmacol 1992; **33**:635–639.
8. Kemp J et al. Excretion of doxepin and N-desmethyldoxepin in human milk. Br J Clin Pharmacol 1985; **20**:497–499.
9. Buist A et al. Effect of exposure to dothiepin and northiaden in breast milk on child development. Br J Psychiatry 1995; **167**:370–373.
10. Khachman D et al. Clomipramine in breast milk: a case study (article in French). Journal de Pharmacie Clinique 2007; **28**:33–38.
11. Hale TW. *Medications and Mothers' Milk*, 15th edn. Texas, USA: Hale Publishing; 2012.
12. National Institute for Health and Clinical Excellence. Antenatal and postnatal mental health. Clinical management and service guidance (reissued April 2007). http://www.nice.org.uk/
13. Lee A et al. Frequency of infant adverse events that are associated with citalopram use during breast-feeding. Am J Obstet Gynecol 2004; **190**:218–221.
14. Heikkinen T et al. Citalopram in pregnancy and lactation. Clin Pharmacol Ther 2002; **72**:184–191.

15. Jensen PN et al. Citalopram and desmethylcitalopram concentrations in breast milk and in serum of mother and infant. Ther Drug Monit 1997; **19**:236–239.

16. Spigset O et al. Excretion of citalopram in breast milk. Br J Clin Pharmacol 1997; **44**:295–298.

17. Rampono J et al. Citalopram and demethylcitalopram in human milk; distribution, excretion and effects in breast fed infants. Br J Clin Pharmacol 2000; **50**:263–268.

18. Schmidt K et al. Citalopram and breast-feeding: serum concentration and side effects in the infant. Biol Psychiatry 2000; **47**:164–165.

19. Franssen EJ et al. Citalopram serum and milk levels in mother and infant during lactation. Ther Drug Monit 2006; **28**:2–4.

20. Werremeyer A. Ziprasidone and citalopram use in pregnancy and lactation in a woman with psychotic depression. Am J Psychiatry 2009; **166**:1298.

21. Berle JO et al. Antidepressant use during breastfeeding. Curr Womens Health Rev 2011; **7**:28–34.

22. Hendrick V et al. Weight gain in breastfed infants of mothers taking antidepressant medications. J Clin Psychiatry 2003; **64**:410–412.

23. Gentile S. Escitalopram late in pregnancy and while breast-feeding (Letter). Ann Pharmacother 2006; **40**:1696–1697.

24. Castberg I et al. Excretion of escitalopram in breast milk. J Clin Psychopharmacol 2006; **26**:536–538.

25. Rampono J et al. Transfer of escitalopram and its metabolite demethylescitalopram into breastmilk. Br J Clin Pharmacol 2006; **62**:316–322.

26. Potts AL et al. Necrotizing enterocolitis associated with in utero and breast milk exposure to the selective serotonin reuptake inhibitor, escitalopram. J Perinatol 2007; **27**:120–122.

27. Ilett KF et al. Estimation of infant dose and assessment of breastfeeding safety for escitalopram use in postnatal depression. Ther Drug Monit 2005; **27**:248.

28. Bellantuono C et al. The safety of escitalopram during pregnancy and breastfeeding: a comprehensive review. Hum Psychopharmacol 2012; **27**:534–539.

29. Hendrick V et al. Use of sertraline, paroxetine and fluvoxamine by nursing women. Br J Psychiatry 2001; **179**:163–166.

30. Piontek CM et al. Serum fluvoxamine levels in breastfed infants. J Clin Psychiatry 2001; **62**:111–113.

31. Yoshida K et al. Fluvoxamine in breast-milk and infant development. Br J Clin Pharmacol 1997; **44**:210–211.

32. Hagg S et al. Excretion of fluvoxamine into breast milk. Br J Clin Pharmacol 2000; **49**:286–288.

33. Arnold LM et al. Fluvoxamine concentrations in breast milk and in maternal and infant sera. J Clin Psychopharmacol 2000; **20**:491–492.

34. Kristensen JH et al. The amount of fluvoxamine in milk is unlikely to be a cause of adverse effects in breastfed infants. J Hum Lact 2002; **18**:139–143.

35. Wright S et al. Excretion of fluvoxamine in breast milk. Br J Clin Pharmacol 1991; **31**:209.

36. Yoshida K et al. Fluoxetine in breast-milk and developmental outcome of breast-fed infants. Br J Psychiatry 1998; **172**:175–178.

37. Lester BM et al. Possible association between fluoxetine hydrochloride and colic in an infant. J Am Acad Child Adolesc Psychiatry 1993; **32**:1253–1255.

38. Hendrick V et al. Fluoxetine and norfluoxetine concentrations in nursing infants and breast milk. Biol Psychiatry 2001; **50**:775–782.

39. Hale TW et al. Fluoxetine toxicity in a breastfed infant. Clin Pediatr 2001; **40**:681–684.

40. Malone K et al. Antidepressants, antipsychotics, benzodiazepines, and the breastfeeding dyad. Perspect Psychiatr Care 2004; **40**:73–85.

41. Heikkinen T et al. Pharmacokinetics of fluoxetine and norfluoxetine in pregnancy and lactation. Clin Pharmacol Ther 2003; **73**:330–337.

42. Epperson CN et al. Maternal fluoxetine treatment in the postpartum period: effects on platelet serotonin and plasma drug levels in breast-feeding mother-infant pairs. Pediatrics 2003; **112**:e425.

43. Taddio A et al. Excretion of fluoxetine and its metabolite, norfluoxetine, in human breast milk. J Clin Pharmacol 1996; **36**:42–47.

44. Brent NB et al. Fluoxetine and carbamazepine concentrations in a nursing mother/infant pair. Clin Pediatr (Phila) 1998; **37**:41–44.

45. Kristensen JH et al. Distribution and excretion of fluoxetine and norfluoxetine in human milk. Br J Clin Pharmacol 1999; **48**:521–527.

46. Burch KJ et al. Fluoxetine/norfluoxetine concentrations in human milk. Pediatrics 1992; **89**:676–677.

47. Begg EJ et al. Paroxetine in human milk. Br J Clin Pharmacol 1999; **48**:142–147.

48. Stowe ZN et al. Paroxetine in human breast milk and nursing infants. Am J Psychiatry 2000; **157**:185–189.

49. Misri S et al. Paroxetine levels in postpartum depressed women, breast milk, and infant serum. J Clin Psychiatry 2000; **61**:828–832.

50. Ohman R et al. Excretion of paroxetine into breast milk. J Clin Psychiatry 1999; **60**:519–523.

51. Berle JO et al. Breastfeeding during maternal antidepressant treatment with serotonin reuptake inhibitors: infant exposure, clinical symptoms, and cytochrome p450 genotypes. J Clin Psychiatry 2004; **65**:1228–1234.

52. Merlob P et al. Paroxetine during breast-feeding: infant weight gain and maternal adherence to counsel. Eur J Pediatr 2004; **163**:135–139.

53. Abdul Aziz A et al. Severe paroxetine induced hyponatremia in a breast fed infant. J Bahrain Med Soc 2004; **16**:195–198.

54. Hendrick V et al. Paroxetine use during breast-feeding. J Clin Psychopharmacol 2000; **20**:587–589.

55. Spigset O et al. Paroxetine level in breast milk. J Clin Psychiatry 1996; **57**:39.

56. Llewellyn A et al. Psychotropic medications in lactation. J Clin Psychiatry 1998; **59 Suppl** 2:41–52.

57. Mammen OK et al. Sertraline and norsertraline levels in three breastfed infants. J Clin Psychiatry 1997; **58**:100–103.

58. Altshuler LL et al. Breastfeeding and sertraline: a 24-hour analysis. J Clin Psychiatry 1995; **56**:243–245.

59. Dodd S et al. Sertraline analysis in the plasma of breast-fed infants. Aust N Z J Psychiatry 2001; **35**:545–546.

60. Dodd S et al. Sertraline in paired blood plasma and breast-milk samples from nursing mothers. Hum Psychopharmacol 2000; **15**:161–264.

61. Epperson N et al. Maternal sertraline treatment and serotonin transport in breast-feeding mother-infant pairs. Am J Psychiatry 2001; **158**:1631–1637.

62. Stowe ZN et al. The pharmacokinetics of sertraline excretion into human breast milk: determinants of infant serum concentrations. J Clin Psychiatry 2003; **64**:73–80.

63. Muller MJ et al. Serotonergic overstimulation in a preterm infant after sertraline intake via breastmilk. Breastfeed Med 2013; **8**:327–329.

64. Wisner KL et al. Serum sertraline and N-desmethylsertraline levels in breast-feeding mother-infant pairs. Am J Psychiatry 1998; 155:690–692.

65. Hackett LP et al. Transfer of reboxetine into breastmilk, its plasma concentrations and lack of adverse effects in the breastfed infant. Eur J Clin Pharmacol 2006; 62:633–638.

66. Koren G et al. Can venlafaxine in breast milk attenuate the norepinephrine and serotonin reuptake neonatal withdrawal syndrome. J Obstet Gynaecol Can 2006; 28:299–302.

67. Ilett KF et al. Distribution of venlafaxine and its O-desmethyl metabolite in human milk and their effects in breastfed infants. Br J Clin Pharmacol 2002; 53:17–22.

68. Newport DJ et al. Venlafaxine in human breast milk and nursing infant plasma: determination of exposure. J Clin Psychiatry 2009; 70:1304–1310.

69. Ilett KF et al. Assessment of infant dose through milk in a lactating woman taking amisulpride and desvenlafaxine for treatment-resistant depression. Ther Drug Monit 2010; 32:704–707.

70. Misri S et al. Quetiapine augmentation in lactation: a series of case reports. J Clin Psychopharmacol 2006; 26:508–511.

71. Hendrick V et al. Venlafaxine and breast-feeding. Am J Psychiatry 2001; 158:2089–2090.

72. Rampono J et al. Estimation of desvenlafaxine transfer into milk and infant exposure during its use in lactating women with postnatal depression. Arch Womens Ment Health 2011; 14:49–53.

73. Ilett KF et al. Distribution and excretion of venlafaxine and O-desmethylvenlafaxine in human milk. Br J Clin Pharmacol 1998; 45:459–462.

74. Buist A et al. Plasma and human milk concentrations of moclobemide in nursing mothers. Hum Psychopharmacol 1998; 13:579–582.

75. Pons G et al. Moclobemide excretion in human breast milk. Br J Clin Pharmacol 1990; 29:27–31.

76. Buist A et al. Mianserin in breast milk (Letter). Br J Clin Pharmacol 1993; 36:133–134.

77. Aichhorn W et al. Mirtazapine and breast-feeding. Am J Psychiatry 2004; 161:2325.

78. Klier CM et al. Mirtazapine and breastfeeding: maternal and infant plasma levels. Am J Psychiatry 2007; 164:348–349.

79. Kristensen JH et al. Transfer of the antidepressant mirtazapine into breast milk. Br J Clin Pharmacol 2007; 63:322–327.

80. Tonn P et al. High mirtazapine plasma levels in infant after breast feeding: case report and review of the literature. J Clin Psychopharmacol 2009; 29:191–192.

81. Verbeeck RK et al. Excretion of trazodone in breast milk. Br J Clin Pharmacol 1986; 22:367–370.

82. Briggs GG et al. Excretion of bupropion in breast milk. Ann Pharmacother 1993; 27:431–433.

83. Chaudron LH et al. Bupropion and breastfeeding: a case of a possible infant seizure. J Clin Psychiatry 2004; 65:881–882.

84. Nonacs RM et al. Bupropion SR for the treatment of postpartum depression: a pilot study. Int J Neuropsychopharmacol 2005; 8:445–449.

85. Haas JS et al. Bupropion in breast milk: an exposure assessment for potential treatment to prevent post-partum tobacco use. Tob Control 2004; 13:52–56.

86. Baab SW et al. Serum bupropion levels in 2 breastfeeding mother-infant pairs. J Clin Psychiatry 2002; 63:910–911.

87. Davis MF et al. Bupropion levels in breast milk for 4 mother-infant pairs: more answers to lingering questions. J Clin Psychiatry 2009; 70:297–298.

88. Boyce PM et al. Duloxetine transfer across the placenta during pregnancy and into milk during lactation. Arch Womens Ment Health 2011; 14:169–172.

89. Briggs GG et al. Use of duloxetine in pregnancy and lactation. Ann Pharmacother 2009; 43:1898–1902.

90. Lobo ED et al. Pharmacokinetics of duloxetine in breast milk and plasma of healthy postpartum women. Clin Pharmacokinet 2008; 47:103–109.

91. Schmidt FM et al. Agomelatine in breast milk. Int J Neuropsychopharmacol 2013; 16:497–499.

92. Yoshida K et al. Breast-feeding and psychotropic drugs. Int Rev Psychiatry 1996; 8:117–124.

93. Patton SW et al. Antipsychotic medication during pregnancy and lactation in women with schizophrenia: evaluating the risk. Can J Psychiatry 2002; 47:959–965.

94. Klinger G et al. Antipsychotic drugs and breastfeeding. Pediatr Endocrinol Rev 2013; 10:308–317.

95. Matheson I et al. Milk concentrations of flupenthixol, nortriptyline and zuclopenthixol and between-breast differences in two patients. Eur J Clin Pharmacol 1988; 35:217–220.

96. Kirk L et al. Concentrations of Cis(Z)-flupentixol in maternal serum, amniotic fluid, umbilical cord serum, and milk. Psychopharmacology 1980; 72:107–108.

97. aes-Jorgensen T et al. Zuclopenthixol levels in serum and breast milk. Psychopharmacology (Berl) 1986; 90:417–418.

98. Ylikorkala O et al. Treatment of inadequate lactation with oral sulpiride and buccal oxytocin. Obstet Gynecol 1984; 63:57–60.

99. Aono T et al. Augmentation of puerperal lactation by oral administration of sulpiride. J Clin Endocrinol Metab 1970; 48:478–482.

100. Ylikorkala O et al. Sulpiride improves inadequate lactation. Br Med J 1982; 285:249–251.

101. Aono T et al. Effect of sulpiride on poor puerperal lactation. Am J Obstet Gynecol 1982; 143:927–932.

102. Polatti F. Sulpiride isomers and milk secretion in puerperium. Clin Exp Obstet Gynecol 1982; 9:144–147.

103. Teoh S et al. Estimation of rac-amisulpride transfer into milk and of infant dose via milk during its use in a lactating woman with bipolar disorder and schizophrenia. Breastfeed Med 2010; 6:85–88.

104. Schlotterbeck P et al. Aripiprazole in human milk. Int J Neuropsychopharmacol 2007; 10:433.

105. Lutz UC et al. Aripiprazole in pregnancy and lactation: a case report. J Clin Psychopharmacol 2010; 30:204–205.

106. Watanabe N et al. Perinatal use of aripiprazole: a case report. J Clin Psychopharmacol 2011; 31:377–379.

107. Mendhekar DN et al. Aripiprazole use in a pregnant schizoaffective woman. Bipolar Disord 2006; 8:299–300.

CHAPTER 7

108. Mendhekar DN. Possible delayed speech acquisition with clozapine therapy during pregnancy and lactation. J Neuropsychiatry Clin Neurosci 2007; **19**:196–197.

109. Barnas C et al. Clozapine concentrations in maternal and fetal plasma, amniotic fluid, and breast milk. Am J Psychiatry 1994; **151**:945.

110. Goldstein DJ et al. Olanzapine-exposed pregnancies and lactation: early experience. J Clin Psychopharmacol 2000; **20**:399–403.

111. Croke S et al. Olanzapine excretion in human breast milk: estimation of infant exposure. Int J Neuropsychopharmacol 2002; **5**:243–247.

112. Gardiner SJ et al. Transfer of olanzapine into breast milk, calculation of infant drug dose, and effect on breast-fed infants. Am J Psychiatry 2003; **160**:1428–1431.

113. Ambresin G et al. Olanzapine excretion into breast milk: a case report. J Clin Psychopharmacol 2004; **24**:93–95.

114. Lutz UC et al. Olanzapine treatment during breast feeding: a case report. Ther Drug Monit 2008; **30**:399–401.

115. Whitworth A et al. Olanzapine and breast-feeding: changes of plasma concentrations of olanzapine in a breast-fed infant over a period of 5 months. J Psychopharmacol 2010; **24**:121–123.

116. Eli Lilly and Company Limited. Personal Correspondence - Olanzapine - Use in Pregnant or Nursing Women. 2011.

117. Gilad O et al. Outcome of infants exposed to olanzapine during breastfeeding. Breastfeed Med 2010; **6**:55–58.

118. Lee A et al. Excretion of quetiapine in breast milk. Am J Psychiatry 2004; **161**:1715–1716.

119. Gentile S. Quetiapine-fluvoxamine combination during pregnancy and while breastfeeding (Letter). Arch Womens Ment Health 2006; **9**:158–159.

120. Seppala J. Quetiapine (Seroquel) is effective and well tolerated in the treatment of psychotic depression during breast feeding. Eur Neuropsychopharmacol 2004; S245.

121. Kruninger U et al. Pregnancy and lactation under treatment with quetiapine. Psychiatr Prax 2007; **34 Suppl** 1:S75–S76.

122. Ritz S. Quetiapine monotherapy in post-partum onset bipolar disorder with a mixed affective state. Eur Neuropsychopharmacol 2005; **15 Suppl** 3–:S407.

123. Rampono J et al. Quetiapine and breast feeding. Ann Pharmacother 2007; **41**:711–714.

124. Tanoshima R et al. Quetiapine in human breast milk – population PK analysis of milk levels and simulated infant exposure. J Popul Ther Clin Pharmacol 2012; **19**:e259–e298.

125. Yazdani-Brojeni P et al. Quetiapine in human milk and simulation-based assessment of infant exposure. Clinical Pharmacology & Therapeutics 2010; **87 Suppl** 1:S3–S4.

126. Var L et al. Management of postpartum manic episode without cessation of breastfeeding: A longitudinal follow up of drug excretion into breast milk. Eur Neuropsychopharmacol 2013; **23 Suppl** 2:S382.

127. Hill RC et al. Risperidone distribution and excretion into human milk: case report and estimated infant exposure during breast-feeding. J Clin Psychopharmacol 2000; **20**:285–286.

128. Aichhorn W et al. Risperidone and breast-feeding. J Psychopharmacol 2005; **19**:211–213.

129. Ilett KF et al. Transfer of risperidone and 9-hydroxyrisperidone into human milk. Ann Pharmacother 2004; **38**:273–276.

130. Ratnayake T et al. No complications with risperidone treatment before and throughout pregnancy and during the nursing period. J Clin Psychiatry 2002; **63**:76–77.

131. Weggelaar NM et al. A case report of risperidone distribution and excretion into human milk: how to give good advice if you have not enough data available. J Clin Psychopharmacol 2011; **31**:129–131.

132. Schlotterbeck P et al. Low concentration of ziprasidone in human milk: a case report. Int J Neuropsychopharmacol 2009; **12**:437–438.

133. Chaudron LH et al. Mood stabilizers during breastfeeding: a review. J Clin Psychiatry 2000; **61**:79–90.

134. Wisner KL et al. Serum levels of valproate and carbamazepine in breastfeeding mother-infant pairs. J Clin Psychopharmacol 1998; **18**:167–169.

135. Ernst CL et al. The reproductive safety profile of mood stabilizers, atypical antipsychotics, and broad-spectrum psychotropics. J Clin Psychiatry 2002; **63 Suppl** 4:42–55.

136. Meador KJ et al. Effects of breastfeeding in children of women taking antiepileptic drugs. Neurology 2010; **75**:1954–1960.

137. Zhao M et al. [A case report of monitoring on carbamazepine in breast feeding woman]. Beijing Da Xue Xue Bao 2010; **42**:602–603.

138. Froescher W et al. Carbamazepine levels in breast milk. Ther Drug Monit 1984; **6**:266–271.

139. Frey B et al. Transient cholestatic hepatitis in a neonate associated with carbamazepine exposure during pregnancy and breast-feeding. Eur J Pediatr 1990; **150**:136–138.

140. Merlob P et al. Transient hepatic dysfunction in an infant of an epileptic mother treated with carbamazepine during pregnancy and breast-feeding. Ann Pharmacother 1992; **26**:1563–1565.

141. Veiby G et al. Early child development and exposure to antiepileptic drugs prenatally and through breastfeeding: a prospective cohort study on children of women with epilepsy. JAMA Neurology 2013; **70**:1367–1374.

142. Pynnonen S et al. Letter: Carbamazepine and mother's milk. Lancet 1975; **2**:563.

143. Ohman I et al. Lamotrigine in pregnancy: pharmacokinetics during delivery, in the neonate, and during lactation. Epilepsia 2000; **41**:709–713.

144. Liporace J et al. Concerns regarding lamotrigine and breast-feeding. Epilepsy Behav 2004; **5**:102–105.

145. Gentile S. Lamotrigine in pregnancy and lactation (Letter). Arch Womens Ment Health 2005; **8**:57–58.

146. Page-Sharp M et al. Transfer of lamotrigine into breast milk (Letter). Ann Pharmacother 2006; **40**:1470–1471.

147. Rambeck B et al. Concentrations of lamotrigine in a mother on lamotrigine treatment and her newborn child. Eur J Clin Pharmacol 1997; **51**:481–484.

148. Tomson T et al. Lamotrigine in pregnancy and lactation: a case report. Epilepsia 1997; **38**:1039–1041.

149. Newport DJ et al. Lamotrigine in breast milk and nursing infants: determination of exposure. Pediatrics 2008; **122**:e223–e231.

150. Fotopoulou C et al. Prospectively assessed changes in lamotrigine-concentration in women with epilepsy during pregnancy, lactation and the neonatal period. Epilepsy Res 2009; **85**:60–64.

151. Nordmo E et al. Severe apnea in an infant exposed to lamotrigine in breast milk. Ann Pharmacother 2009; **43**:1893–1897.

152. Wakil L et al. Neonatal outcomes with the use of lamotrigine for bipolar disorder in pregnancy and breastfeeding: a case series and review of the literature. Psychopharmacol Bull 2009; **42**:91–98.

153. Moretti ME et al. Monitoring lithium in breast milk: an individualized approach for breast-feeding mothers. Ther Drug Monit 2003; **25**:364–366.

154. Viguera AC et al. Lithium in breast milk and nursing infants: clinical implications. Am J Psychiatry 2007; **164**:342–345.

155. Bogen DL et al. Three cases of lithium exposure and exclusive breastfeeding. Arch Womens Ment Health 2012; **15**:69–72.

156. Tunnessen WW, Jr. et al. Toxic effects of lithium in newborn infants: a commentary. J Pediatr 1972; **81**:804–807.

157. Piontek CM et al. Serum valproate levels in 6 breastfeeding mother-infant pairs. J Clin Psychiatry 2000; **61**:170–172.

158. Bjornsson E. Hepatotoxicity associated with antiepileptic drugs. Acta Neurol Scand 2008; **118**:281–290.

159. Malone K et al. Antidepressants, antipsychotics, benzodiazepines, and the breastfeeding dyad. Perspect Psychiatr Care 2004; **40**:73–85.

160. Hagg S et al. Anticonvulsant use during lactation. Drug Saf 2000; **22**:425–440.

161. Iqbal MM et al. Effects of commonly used benzodiazepines on the fetus, the neonate, and the nursing infant. Psychiatr Serv 2002; **53**:39–49.

162. Buist A et al. Breastfeeding and the use of psychotropic medication: a review. J Affect Disord 1990; **19**:197–206.

163. Fisher JB et al. Neonatal apnea associated with maternal clonazepam therapy: a case report. Obstet Gynecol 1985; **66**:34S–35S.

164. Davanzo R et al. Benzodiazepine e allattamento materno. Medico e Bambino 2008; **27**:109–114.

165. Kelly LE et al. Neonatal benzodiazepines exposure during breastfeeding. J Pediatr 2012; **161**:448–451.

166. Birnbaum CS et al. Serum concentrations of antidepressants and benzodiazepines in nursing infants: A case series. Pediatrics 1999; **104**:e11.

167. Darwish M et al. Rapid disappearance of zaleplon from breast milk after oral administration to lactating women. J Clin Pharmacol 1999; **39**:670–674.

168. Pons G et al. Excretion of psychoactive drugs into breast milk. Pharmacokinetic principles and recommendations. Clin Pharmacokinet 1994; **27**:270–289.

169. Matheson I et al. The excretion of zopiclone into breast milk. Br J Clin Pharmacol 1990; **30**:267–271.

Further reading

Field T. Breastfeeding and antidepressants. Infant Behav Dev 2008; **31**:481–487.

Gentile S et al. SSRIs during breastfeeding: spotlight on milk-to-plasma ratio. Arch Womens Ment Health 2007; **10**:39–51.

Gentile S. Infant safety with antipsychotic therapy in breast-feeding: a systematic review. J Clin Psychiatry 2008; **69**:666–673.

National Institute for Health and Care Excellence. Antenatal and postnatal mental health: clinical management and service guidance. Clinical Guideline 192, 2014. https://www.nice.org.uk/guidance/cg192

CHAPTER 7

Renal impairment

Using drugs in patients with renal impairment needs careful consideration. This is because some drugs are nephrotoxic and also because pharmacokinetics (absorption, distribution, metabolism, excretion) of drugs are altered in renal impairment. Essentially, **patients with renal impairment have a reduced capacity to excrete drugs** and their metabolites.

General principles of prescribing in renal impairment

- **Estimate the excretory capacity of the kidney** by calculating the glomerular filtration rate (GFR). GFR can be directly measured by collection of urine over 24 hours, isotope determination or estimated in *adults* in one of two ways;[1] that is creatinine clearance (CrCl) using the Cockroft and Gault equation or estimated GFR (eGFR) using the modification of diet in renal disease (MDRD) below.

Cockroft and Gault equation*

$$CrCl(mL/min) = \frac{F(140 - age\ (in\ years)) \times ideal\ body\ weight(kg))}{Serum\ creatinine(\mu mol/L)}$$

F = 1.23 (men) and 1.04 (women)
Ideal body weight should be used for patients at extremes of body weight or else the calculation is inaccurate
    For men, ideal body weight (kg) = 50 kg + 2.3 kg per inch over 5 feet
    For women, ideal body weight (kg) = 45.5 kg + 2.3 kg per inch over 5 feet

*This equation is not accurate if plasma creatinine is unstable, in pregnant women, children or in diseases causing production of abnormal amounts of creatinine and has only been validated in Caucasian patients. Creatinine clearance is less representative of GFR in severe renal failure.

When calculating drug doses use estimated CrCl from the Cockroft and Gault equation. Do not use MDRD formula for dose calculation because most current dose recommendations are based on the creatinine clearance estimations from Cockroft and Gault.

Modification of diet in renal disease (MDRD) formula

This gives an estimated GFR (eGFR) for a 1.73 m² body surface area. If the body surface area is > or < than 1.73 m² then eGFR becomes less accurate and representative (use correction below). Adjustments are made for female gender and Black ethnicity. Many pathology departments report eGFR.
    Actual GFR can be calculated as follows:

Actual GFR = (eGFR × BSA/1.73)

$$BSA = body\ surface\ area = \sqrt{\frac{Height(cm) \times Weight(kg)}{3600}}$$

Use Cockroft and Gault for drug dose calculation.

Classify the stage of renal impairment as below:

Stage	Description
1	GFR > 90 mL/min/1.73 m² with other evidence of chronic kidney damage*
2	Mild impairment; GFR 60–89 mL/min/1.73 m² with other evidence of kidney damage*
3	Moderate impairment, GFR 30–59 mL/min/1.73 m²
4	Severe impairment, GFR 15–29 mL/min/1.73 m²
5	Established renal failure, GFR <15 mL/min/1.73 m² or on dialysis

*Other evidence of chronic kidney damage is one or more of the following; persistent microalbuminuria; persistent proteinuria; persistent haematuria; structural kidney abnormalities; biopsy-proven chronic glomerulonephritis.

- **Elderly patients (>65 years) are assumed to have mild renal impairment.** Their serum creatinine may not be raised because they have a smaller muscle mass.
- **Avoid drugs that are nephrotoxic** (e.g. lithium) in moderate or severe renal failure.
- **Chose a drug that is safer to use in renal impairment** (see Tables 7.16–7.20 below).
- **Be cautious when using drugs that are extensively renally cleared** (e.g. sulpiride, amisulpride, lithium).
- **Start at a low dose and increase slowly** because, in renal impairment, the half-life of a drug and the time for it to reach steady state are often prolonged. Plasma level monitoring may be useful for some drugs.
- **Avoid long acting drugs** (e.g. depot preparations). Their dose and frequency cannot be easily adjusted should renal function change.
- **Prescribe as few drugs as possible.** Patients with renal failure take many medications requiring regular review. Interactions and side effects can be avoided if fewer drugs are used.
- **Monitor patient for adverse effects.** Patients with renal impairment are more likely to experience side effects and they may take longer to develop than in healthy patients. Adverse effects such as sedation, confusion and postural hypotension can be more common.
- **Be cautious when using drugs with anticholinergic effects,** since they may cause urinary retention.
- There are **few clinical studies** of the use of psychotropic drugs in people with renal impairment. Advice about drug use in renal impairment is often based on knowledge of the drug's pharmacokinetics in healthy patients.
- **The effect of renal replacement therapies (e.g. dialysis) on drugs is difficult to predict.** Dosing advice is available from tables and data on each drug's volume of distribution and protein binding affinity. Seek specialist advice.
- **Avoid drugs known to prolong QTc interval.** In established renal failure electrolyte changes are common so probably best to avoid antipsychotics with the greatest risk of QTc prolongation (see section on 'QT prolongation' in Chapter 2).
- **Monitor weight carefully.** Weight gain predisposes to diabetes which can cause rhabdomyolysis[2] and renal failure. Psychotropic medications commonly cause weight gain.
- **Be vigilant for serotonin syndrome with antidepressants, dystonias and neuroleptic malignant syndrome (NMS) with antipsychotics.** The resulting rhabdomyolysis can cause

renal failure and there are case reports of rhabdomyolysis occurring with antipsychotics without other symptoms of NMS.[3-5]

- **Depression is common in chronic kidney disease** but evidence on effectiveness of antidepressants in this condition is lacking.[6]

Table 7.15 summarises the recommendations for psychotropic drug use in renal impairment. Further information is given in Tables 7.16–7.20.

Table 7.15 Recommendations for the use of psychotropics in renal impairment

Drug group	Recommended drugs
Antipsychotics	No agent clearly preferred to another, however: ■ avoid sulpiride and amisulpride ■ avoid highly anticholinergic agents because they may cause urinary retention ■ first-generation antipsychotic – suggest **haloperidol** 2–6 mg a day ■ second-generation antipsychotic – suggest **olanzapine** 5 mg a day
Antidepressants	No agent clearly preferred to another, however: ■ **citalopram (care QTc prolonging effects)** and **sertraline** are suggested as reasonable choices
Mood stabilisers	No agent clearly preferred to another, however: ■ avoid lithium if possible ■ suggest start one the following at a low dose and increase slowly, monitor for adverse effects: **valproate**, **carbamazepine** or **lamotrigine**
Anxiolytics and hypnotics	No agent clearly preferred to another, however: ■ excessive sedation is more likely to occur in patients with renal impairment, so monitor all patients carefully ■ **lorazepam** and **zopiclone** are suggested as reasonable choices
Anti-dementia drugs	No agent clearly preferred to another, however: **rivastigmine** is a reasonable choice

Table 7.16 Antipsychotics in renal impairment

Drug	Comments
Amisulpride[7–10]	Primarily renally excreted. 50% excreted unchanged in urine. Limited experience in renal disease. Manufacturer states no data with doses of >50 mg but recommends following dosing: 50% of dose if GFR 30-60 mL/min; 33% of dose if GFR is 10–30 mL/min; no recommendations for GFR <10 mL/min so **best avoided in established renal failure**
Aripiprazole[7,8,10–13]	Less than 1% of unchanged aripiprazole renally excreted. Manufacturer states no dose adjustment required in renal failure as pharmacokinetics are similar in healthy and severely renally diseased patients. There is one case report of safe use of oral aripiprazole 5 mg in an 83-year-old man having haemodialysis. Avoid depot formulation – no current experience
Asenapine[8,14]	Manufacturer states no dose adjustment required for patients with renal impairment but no experience with use if GFR < 15 mL/min. A 5 mg single dose study in renal impairment suggests that no dose adjustment is needed
Chlorpromazine[7,8,10,15,16]	Less than 1% excreted unchanged in urine. Manufacturer advises avoiding in renal dysfunction. Dosing: GFR 10–50 mL/min, dose as in normal renal function; GFR <10 mL/min, start with a small dose because of an increased risk of anticholinergic, sedative and hypotensive side effects. Monitor carefully
Clozapine[8,10,17–20]	Only trace amounts of unchanged clozapine excreted in urine; however there are rare case reports of interstitial nephritis and acute renal failure. Nocturnal enuresis and urinary retention are common side-effects. Contraindicated by manufacturer in severe renal disease. Anticholinergic, sedative and hypotensive side effects occur more frequently in patients with renal disease. Dosing: GFR 10–50 mL/min as in normal renal function but with caution; GFR <10 mL/min start with a low dose and titrate slowly (based on renal expert opinion). Levels are useful to guide dosing. May cause and aggravate diabetes, a common cause of renal disease
Flupentixol[7,8,10]	Negligible renal excretion of unchanged flupentixol. Dosing: GFR 10–50 mL/min dose as in normal renal function; GFR < 10 mL/min start with one-quarter to one-half of normal dose and titrate slowly. May cause hypotension and sedation in renal impairment and can accumulate. Manufacturer recommends caution in renal failure. Avoid depot preparations in renal impairment
Fluphenazine[8,10]	Little information available; manufacturer cautions in renal impairment and contraindicates in renal failure. Dosing: GFR 10–50 mL/min dose as in normal renal function; GFR <10 mL/min start with a low dose and titrate slowly. Avoid depot preparations in renal impairment
Haloperidol[4,7,8,10,21,22]	Less than 1% excreted unchanged in the urine. Manufacturer advises caution in renal failure. Dosing: GFR 10–50 mL/min, dose as in normal renal function; GFR <10 mL/min start with a lower dose as can accumulate with repeated dosing. A case report of haloperidol use in renal failure suggests starting at a low dose and increasing slowly. Has been used to treat uraemia associated nausea in renal failure. Avoid depot preparations in renal impairment
Lurasidone[23]	9% excreted unchanged in the urine. Manufacturer recommends dose adjustment if GFR <30 mL/min to 50 mL/min patients (starting dose is 20 mg/day, maximum 80 mg/day). Renal failure has been reported rarely
Olanzapine[3,7,8,10,22,24]	57% of olanzapine is excreted mainly as metabolites (7% excreted unchanged) in urine. Dosing: GFR < 50 mL/min initially 5 mg daily and titrate as necessary. Avoid long acting preparations in renal impairment unless the oral dose is well tolerated and effective. Manufacturer recommends a lower long acting injection starting dose of 150 mg 4-weekly in patients with renal impairment. May cause and aggravate diabetes, a common cause of renal disease. Hypothermia has been reported when used in renal failure

(Continued)

Table 7.16 (*Continued*)

Drug	Comments
Paliperidone[7,8,10]	Paliperidone is also a metabolite of risperidone. 59% excreted unchanged in urine. Dosing: GFR 30–80 mL/min, 3 mg daily and increase according to response to maximum of 6 mg daily; GFR 10–30 mL/min, 3 mg alternate days increasing to 3 mg daily according to response. Use with caution as clearance is reduced by 71% in severe kidney disease. Manufacturer contraindicates oral if GFR < 10 mL/min due to lack of experience and depot preparation if GFR <50 mL/min (reduced loading doses if GFR ≥ 50 to <80 mL/min)
Pimozide[7,8,10]	Less than 1% of pimozide is excreted unchanged in the urine; dose reductions not usually needed in renal impairment. Dosing: GFR 10–50 mL/min, dose as in normal renal function; GFR <10 mL/min start at a low dose and increase according to response. Manufacturer cautions in renal failure
Pipotiazine[8]	Little information available; contraindicated in renal failure by manufacturer. Avoid depot preparations in renal impairment
Quetiapine[7,8,10,25,26]	Less than 5% of quetiapine excreted unchanged in the urine. Plasma clearance reduced by an average of 25% in patients with a GFR <30 mL/min. In patients with GFR of <10 to 50 mL/min start at 25 mg/day and increase in daily increments of 25–50 mg to an effective dose. Two separate case reports one of thrombotic thrombocytopenic purpura and another of non-NMS rhabdomyolyisis both resulting in acute renal failure with quetiapine have been published
Risperidone[7,8,10,22,27–29]	Clearance of risperidone and the active metabolite of risperidone is reduced by 60% in patients with moderate to severe renal disease. Dosing : GFR <50 mL/min 0.5 mg twice daily for at least 1 week then increasing by 0.5 mg twice daily to 1–2 mg bd. The manufacturer advises caution when using risperidone in renal impairment. The long-acting injection should only be used after titration with oral risperidone as described above. If 2 mg orally is tolerated, 25 mg intramuscularly every 2 weeks can be administered. However there is a case report of successful use of risperidone long-acting injection at a dose of 50 mg 2- weekly in a patient on haemodialysis. Another describes the successful use of risperidone in a child with steroid-induced psychosis and nephrotic syndrome
Sulpiride[2,7,8,10,30]	Almost totally renally excreted, with 95% excreted in urine and faeces as unchanged sulpiride. Dosing regimen: GFR 30–60 mL/min, give 70% of normal dose; GFR 10–30 mL/min give 50% of normal dose; GFR <10 mL/min give 34% of normal dose. There is a case report of renal failure with sulpiride due to diabetic coma and rhabdomyolyisis. **Probably best avoided in renal impairment**
Trifluoperazine[10]	Less than 1% excreted unchanged in the urine. Dose GFR <10–50 mL/min as for normal renal function - start with a low dose. Very limited data
Ziprasidone[7,22,31,32]	<1% is renally excreted unchanged. No dose adjustment needed for GFR >10 mL/min but care needed with using the injection as it contains a renally eliminated excipient (cyclodextrin sodium)
Zuclopentixol[7,8,10]	10–20% of unchanged drug and metabolites excreted unchanged in urine. Manufacturer cautions use in renal disease as can accumulate. Dosing: 10–50 mL/min dose as in normal renal function; GFR <10 mL/min start with 50% of the dose and titrate slowly. Avoid both depot preparations (acetate and decanoate) in renal impairment

GFR, glomerular filtration rate.

Table 7.17 Antidepressants in renal impairment[6]

Drug	Comments
Agomelatine[8]	Negligible renal excretion of unchanged agomelatine. No data on use in renal disease. Manufacturer says pharmacokinetics unchanged in small study of 25 mg dose in severe renal impairment but cautions use in moderate or severe renal disease
Amitriptyline[7,8,10,16,22,33–35]	<2% excreted unchanged in urine; no dose adjustment needed in renal failure. Dose as in normal renal function but start at a low dose and increase slowly. Monitor patient for urinary retention, confusion, sedation and postural hypotension. Has been used to treat pain in those with renal disease. Plasma level and ECG monitoring may be useful
Bupropion[7,8,10,16,22,36,37] (amfebutamone)	0.5% excreted unchanged in the urine. Dosing: GFR <50 mL/min, 150 mg once daily. A single dose study in haemodialysis patients (stage 5 disease) recommended a dose of 150 mg every 3 days. Metabolites may accumulate in renal impairment and clearance is reduced. Elevated levels increase risk of seizures
Citalopram[7,8,10,22,38–43]	<13% of citalopram is excreted unchanged in the urine. Single-dose studies in mild and moderate renal impairment show no change in the pharmacokinetics of citalopram. Dosing is as for normal renal function; however, use with caution if GFR <10 mL/min due to reduced clearance. The manufacturer does not advise use if GFR <20 mL/min. Renal failure has been reported with citalopram overdose. Citalopram can treat depression in chronic renal failure and improve quality of life. A case report of hyponatraemia has been reported in a renal transplant patient on citalopram
Clomipramine[7,8,10,16,44]	2% of unchanged clomipramine is excreted in the urine. Dosing: GFR 20–50 mL/min, dose as for normal renal function; GFR <20 mL/min, effects unknown, start at a low dose and monitor patient for urinary retention, confusion, sedation and postural hypotension as accumulation can occur. There is a case report of clomipramine-induced interstitial nephritis and reversible acute renal failure
Desvenlafaxine[6,7,45,46]	45% of desvenlafaxine is excreted unchanged in the urine. Dosing advice is conflicting. Manufacturer recommends: GFR 30 to 50 mL/min, 50 mg per day; GFR <30 mL/min, 50 mg every other day. However other authors[6] recommend 25 mg per day in all stages of renal impairment. Half-life is prolonged and desvenlafaxine accumulates as GFR decreases. Urinary retention, delay when starting to pass urine and proteinuria have been reported as adverse effects
Dosulepin[7,10,47] (dothiepin)	56% of mainly active metabolites renally excreted. They have a long half-life and may accumulate, resulting in excessive sedation. Dosing: GFR 20–50 mL/min, dose as for normal renal function; GFR <20 mL/min, start with a small dose and titrate to response. Monitor patient for urinary retention, confusion, sedation and postural hypotension
Doxepin[7,8,10,16]	<1% excreted unchanged in urine. Dose as in normal renal function but monitor patient for urinary retention, confusion, sedation and postural hypotension. Manufacturer advises using with caution. Haemolytic anaemia with renal failure has been reported with doxepin
Duloxetine[7,10,48,49]	<1% excreted unchanged in urine. Manufacturer states no dose adjustment is necessary for GFR >30 mL/min; however, starting at a low dose and increasing slowly is advised. Duloxetine is contraindicated in patients with a GFR <30 mL/min as it can accumulate in chronic kidney disease. Licensed to treat diabetic neuropathic pain and stress incontinence in women. Diabetes is a common cause of renal impairment. A case report of acute renal failure with duloxetine has been reported

(Continued)

Table 7.17 (Continued)

Drug	Comments
Escitalopram[7,10,50–52]	8% excreted unchanged in urine. The manufacturer states dosage adjustment is not necessary in patients with mild or moderate renal impairment but caution is advised if GFR < 30 mL/min so start with a low dose and increase slowly. A case report of reversible renal tubular defects and another of renal failure have been reported with escitalopram. One study says effective versus placebo in end stage renal disease
Fluvoxamine[7,10,16,22]	2% is excreted unchanged in urine. Little information on its use in renal impairment. Manufacturer cautions in renal impairment. Dosing: GFR 10–50 mL/min dose as for normal renal function; GFR < 10 mL/min dose as for normal renal function but start on a low dose and titrate slowly
Fluoxetine[7,8,10,16,22,53–56]	2.5–5% of fluoxetine and 10% of the active metabolite norfluoxetine are excreted unchanged in the urine. Dosing: GFR 20–50 mL/min dose as normal renal function; GFR <20 mL/min use a low dose or on alternate days and increase according to response. Plasma levels after 2 months treatment with 20 mg (in patients on dialysis with GFR < 10 mL/min) are similar to those with normal renal function. Efficacy studies of fluoxetine in depression and renal disease are conflicting. One small placebo controlled study of fluoxetine in patients on chronic dialysis found no significant differences in depression scores between the two groups after 8 weeks of treatment. Another found fluoxetine effective
Imipramine[7,8,10,16,33]	<5% excreted unchanged in the urine. No specific dose adjustment necessary in renal impairment (GFR <10–50 mL/min). Monitor patient for urinary retention, confusion, sedation and postural hypotension. Renal impairment with imipramine has been reported and manufacturer advises caution in severe renal impairment. Renal damage reported rarely
Lofepramine[7,8,10,57]	There is little information about the use of lofepramine in renal impairment. Less than 5% is excreted unchanged in the urine. Dosing: GFR 10–50 mL/min dose as in normal renal function; GFR < 10 mL/min start with a small dose and titrate slowly. Manufacturer contraindicates in severe renal impairment
Mirtazapine[7,8,10,58]	75% excreted unchanged or as metabolites in the urine. Clearance is reduced by 30% in patients with a GFR of 11–39 mL/min and by 50% in patients with a GFR <10 mL/min. Dosing advice: GFR 10–50 mL/min dose as for normal renal function; GFR <10 mL/min start at a low dose and monitor closely. Mirtazapine has been used to treat puritis caused by renal failure and is associated with kidney calculus formation
Moclobemide[7,8,10,59,60]	<1% of parent drug excreted unchanged in the urine. However, an active metabolite was found to be raised in patients with renal impairment but was not thought to affect dosing. The manufacturer advises that dose adjustments are not required in renal impairment. Dosing: GFR <10–50 mL/min dose as in normal renal function
Nortriptyline[7,10,16,22,33,61]	<5% excreted unchanged in urine. If GFR 10–50 mL/min, dose as in normal renal function; if GFR <10 mL/min start at a low dose. Plasma level monitoring recommended at doses of >100 mg/day, as plasma concentrations of active metabolites are raised in renal impairment. Worsening of GFR in elderly patients has also been reported. Plasma level monitoring can be useful

Table 7.17 (*Continued*)

Drug	Comments
Paroxetine[7,8,10,16,62–65]	Less than 2% of oral dose is excreted unchanged in the urine. Single-dose studies show increased plasma concentrations of paroxetine when GFR <30 mL/min. Dosing advice differs: GFR 30–50 mL/min dose as normal renal function; GFR <10–30 mL/min start at 10 mg/day (other source says start at 20 mg) and increase dose according to response. Paroxetine 10 mg daily and psychotherapy have been used sucessfully to treat depression in patients on chronic haemodialysis. Rarely associated with Fanconi syndrome and acute renal failure
Phenelzine[7,10]	Approximately 1% excreted unchanged in the urine. No dose adjustment required in renal failure
Reboxetine[7,8,10,66,67]	Approximately 10% of unchanged drug is excreted unchanged in the urine. Dosing: GFR <20 mL/min, 2 mg twice daily, adjusting dose according to response. Half-life is prolonged as renal function decreases
Vortioxetine[68]	Negligible amounts are excreted unchanged in urine. Manufacturer advises that no dose adjustment is needed in renal impairment and end stage disease
Sertraline[7,8,10,16,69–72]	<0.2% of unchanged sertraline excreted in urine. Pharmacokinetics in renal impairment are unchanged in single dose studies but no published data on multiple dosing. Dosing is as for normal renal function. Sertraline has been used to treat dialysis-associated hypotension and uraemic pruritis; however acute renal failure has been reported so it should be used with caution. An RCT of sertraline in kidney disease is ongoing. Has been associated with serotonin syndrome when used in patents on haemodialysis
Trazodone[7,8,10,73]	<5% excreted unchanged in urine but care needed as approximately 70% of active metabolite also excreted. Dosing: GFR 20–50 mL/min, dose as normal renal function; GFR 10–20 mL/min, dose as normal renal function but start with small dose and increase gradually; GFR <10 mL/min, start with small doses and increase gradually
Trimipramine[7,10,16,33,74,75]	No dose reduction required in renal impairment; however, elevated urea, acute renal failure and interstitial nephritis have been reported. As with all tricyclic antidepressants, monitor patient for urinary retention, confusion, sedation and postural hypotension as patients with renal impairment are at increased risk of having these side-effects
Venlafaxine[7,8,16,76–78]	1–10% is excreted unchanged in the urine (30% as the active metabolite). Clearance is decreased and half-life prolonged in renal impairment. Dosing advice differs: GFR 30–50 mL/min, dose as in normal renal function or reduce by 50%; GFR 10–30 mL/min reduce dose by 50% and give tablets once daily; GFR <10 mL/min, reduce dose by 50% and give once daily however manufacturer advises avoiding use in these patients. Avoid using the ER preparation if GFR < 30 mL/min. Rhabdomyolyisis and renal failure have been reported rarely with venlafaxine. Has been used to treat peripheral diabetic neuropathy in haemodialysis patients. High doses may cause hypertension

ECG, electrocardiogram; ER, extended release; GFR, glomerular filtration rate; RCT, randomised controlled trial.

Table 7.18 Mood stabilisers in renal impairment

Drug	Comments
Carbamazepine[7,8,10,79–86]	2–3% of the dose is excreted unchanged in urine. Dose reduction not necessary in renal disease, although cases of renal failure, tubular necrosis and tubulointerstitial nephritis have been reported rarely and metabolites may accumulate. Can cause Stevens-Johnson syndrome and toxic epidermal necrolysis which may result in acute renal failure
Lamotrigine[7,8,10,87–90]	<10% of lamotrigine is excreted unchanged in the urine. Single-dose studies in renal failure show pharmacokinetics are little affected: however, inactive metabolites can accumulate (effects unknown) and half-life can be prolonged. Renal failure and interstitial nephritis have also been reported. Dosing: GFR <10–50 mL/min, use cautiously, start with a low dose, increase slowly and monitor closely. One source suggests in GFR < 10 mL/min use 100 mg every other day
Lithium[7,8,10,16,91,92]	Lithium is nephrotoxic and contraindicated in severe renal impairment; 95% is excreted unchanged in the urine. Long-term treatment may result in impaired renal function ('creatinine creep'), permanent changes in kidney histology, nephrogenic diabetes insipidus, nephrotic syndrome and both reversible and irreversible kidney damage. If lithium is used in renal impairment, toxicity is more likely. The manufacturer contraindicates lithium in renal impairment. Dosing: GFR 10–50 mL/min, avoid or reduce dose (50–75% of normal dose) and monitor levels; GFR <10 mL/min, avoid if possible, however if used it is essential to reduce dose (25–50% of normal dose). Renal damage is more likely with chronic toxicity than acute
Valproate[7,8,10,93–99]	Approximately 2% excreted unchanged. Dose adjustment usually not required in renal impairment; however, free valproate levels may be increased. Renal impairment, interstitial nephritis, Fanconi syndrome, renal tubular acidosis and renal failure have been reported. Dose as in normal renal function, however, in severe impairment (GFR < 10 mL/min) it may be necessary to alter doses according to free (unbound) valproate levels

GFR, glomerular filtration rate.

Table 7.19 Anxiolytics and hypnotics in renal impairment

Drug	Comments
Buspirone[7,8,10,16]	Less than 1% is excreted unchanged; however, active metabolite is renally excreted. Dosing advice contradictory, suggest: GFR 10–50 mL/min dose as normal; GFR <10 mL/min avoid if possible due to accumulation of active metabolites;if essential, reduce dose by 25–50% if patient is anuric. Manufacturer contraindicates in severe renal impairment
Clomethiazole[7,8,10,100] (chlormethiazole)	0.1–5% of unchanged drug excreted unchanged in urine. Dose as in normal renal function but monitor for excessive sedation. Manufacturer recommends caution in renal disease
Chlordiazepoxide[8,10,16]	1–2%% excreted unchanged but chlordiazepoxide has a long-acting active metabolite that can accumulate. Dosing: GFR 10–50 mL/min, dose as normal renal function; GFR< 10 mL/min, reduce dose by 50%. Monitor for excessive sedation. Manufacturer cautions in chronic renal disease
Clonazepam[7,8,10,101]	<0.5% of clonazepam excreted unchanged in urine. Dose adjustment not required in impaired renal function; however with long-term administration, active metabolites may accumulate so start at a low doses and increase according to response. Monitor for excessive sedation. Has been used for insomnia in patients on haemodialysis
Diazepam[7,10,16,102]	Less than 0.5% is excreted unchanged. Dosing: GFR 20–50 mL/min, dose as in normal renal function; GFR <20 mL/min, use small doses and titrate to response. Long-acting, active metabolites accumulate in renal impairment; monitor patients for excessive sedation and encephalopathy. One case of interstitial nephritis with diazepam has been reported in a patient with chronic renal failure
Eszopiclone[103]	Less than 10% excreted unchanged in the urine. No dose adjustment is needed in renal impairment
Lorazepam[7,8,10,16,104–109]	<1% excreted unchanged in urine. Dose as in normal renal function but carefully according to response as some may need lower doses. Monitor for excessive sedation. Impaired elimination reported in two patients with severe renal impairment and also reports of propylene glycol in lorazepam injection causing renal impairment and acute tubular necrosis. However, lorazepam injection has been successfully used to treat catatonia in two patients with renal failure
Nitrazepam[8,10]	Less than 5% excreted unchanged in the urine. Dosing GFR 10–50 mL/min as per normal renal function; GFR <10 mL/min start with small dose and increase slowly. Manufacturer advises reducing dose in renal impairment. Monitor patient for sedation
Oxazepam[7,10,16,110]	Less than 1% excreted unchanged in the urine. Dose adjustment needed in severe renal impairment. Oxazepam may take longer to reach steady state in patients with renal impairment. Dosing: GFR 10–50 mL/min, dose as in normal renal function; GFR <10 mL/min, start at a low dose and increase according to response. Monitor for excessive sedation
Promethazine[7,8,10,16,111]	Dose reduction usually not necessary; however, promethazine has a long half-life so monitor for excessive sedative effects in patients with renal impairment. Manufacturer advises caution in renal impairment. There is a case report of interstitial nephritis in a patient who was a poor metaboliser of promethazine

(Continued)

Table 7.19 (Continued)

Drug	Comments
Temazepam[7,8,10,16]	<2% excreted unchanged in urine. In renal impairment the inactive metabolite can accumulate. Monitor for excessive sedative effects. Dosing: GFR 20–50 mL/min, dose as normal renal function; GFR <20 mL/min, dose as in normal renal function but start with 5 mg
Zaleplon[7,8,112,113]	In renal impairment inactive metabolites accumulate. No dose adjustment appears to be necessary in patients with a GFR >20 mL/min. Zaleplon is not recommended if GFR <20 mL/min, however, it has been used in patients on haemodialysis
Zolpidem[7,8,10,101,112]	Clearance moderately reduced in renal impairment. No dose adjustment required in renal impairment. Zolpidem 1 mg has been used to treat insomnia in patients on haemodialysis
Zopiclone[7,8,10,114,115]	Less than 5% excreted unchanged in urine. Manufacturer states no accumulation of zopiclone in renal impairment but suggests starting at 3.75 mg. Dosing: GFR <10 mL/min, start with lower dose. Interstitial nephritis reported rarely

GFR, glomerular filtration rate.

Table 7.20 Anti-dementia drugs in renal impairment

Drug	Comments
Donepezil[8,10,116–118]	17% excreted unchanged in urine. Dosing is as in normal renal function for GFR < 10–50 mL/min. Manufacturer states that clearance not affected by renal impairment. Single dose studies find similar pharmacokinetics in moderate and severe renal impairment compared with healthy controls. Has been used at a dose of 3 mg/day in an elderly patient with Alzheimer's dementia on dialysis
Galantamine[8,10]	18–22% is excreted unchanged in urine. Dose as in normal renal function for GFR 10–50 mL/min and at GFR < 10 mL/min start at a low dose and increase slowly. Manufacturer contraindicates use in GFR <10 mL/min. Plasma levels may be increased in patients with moderate and severe renal impairment
Memantine[7,8,119]	Manufacturers recommend a 10 mg dose if GFR 5–29 mL/min; 10 mg daily for 7 days then increased to 20 mg daily if tolerated for GFR > 30–49 mL/min. Renal tubular acidosis, severe urinary tract infections and alkalisation of urine (e.g. by drastic dietary changes) can increase plasma levels of memantine. Acute renal failure has been reported
Rivastigmine[8,10]	0% excreted unchanged in urine. Dosing advice for GFR <50 mL/min start at a low dose and gradually increase

GFR, glomerular filtration rate.

References

1. Devaney A et al. Chronic kidney disease — new approaches to classification. Hosp Pharm 2006; **13**:406–410.
2. Toprak O et al. New-onset type II diabetes mellitus, hyperosmolar non-ketotic coma, rhabdomyolysis and acute renal failure in a patient treated with sulpiride. Nephrol Dial Transplant 2005; **20**:662–663.
3. Baumgart U et al. Olanzapine-induced acute rhabdomyolysis-a case report. Pharmacopsychiatry 2005; **38**:36–37.
4. Marsh SJ et al. Rhabdomyolysis and acute renal failure during high-dose haloperidol therapy. Ren Fail 1995; **17**:475–478.
5. Smith RP et al. Quetiapine overdose and severe rhabdomyolysis. J Clin Psychopharmacol 2004; **24**:343.

6. Nagler EV et al. Antidepressants for depression in stage 3-5 chronic kidney disease: a systematic review of pharmacokinetics, efficacy and safety with recommendations by European Renal Best Practice (ERBP). Nephrol Dial Transplant 2012; 27:3736–3745.

7. Truven Health Analytics. Micromedex 2.0, 2013. http://www.micromedex.com/

8. Datapharm Communications Ltd. Electronic Medicines Compendium, 2014. http://www.medicines.org.uk/emc/

9. Noble S et al. Amisulpride: a review of its clinical potential in dysthymia. CNS Drugs 1999; 12:471–483.

10. Ashley C et al. *The Renal Drug Handbook*, 3rd edn. Oxford: Radcliffe Publishing Ltd; 2009.

11. Aragona M. Tolerability and efficacy of aripiprazole in a case of psychotic anorexia nervosa comorbid with epilepsy and chronic renal failure. Eat Weight Disord 2007; 12:e54–e57.

12. Mallikaarjun S et al. Effects of hepatic or renal impairment on the pharmacokinetics of aripiprazole. Clin Pharmacokinet 2008; 47:533–542.

13. Tzeng NS et al. Delusional parasitosis in a patient with brain atrophy and renal failure treated with aripiprazole: case report. Prog Neuropsychopharmacol Biol Psychiatry 2010; 34:1148–1149.

14. Peeters P et al. Asenapine pharmacokinetics in hepatic and renal impairment. Clin Pharmacokinet 2011; 50:471–481.

15. Fabre J et al. Influence of renal insufficiency on the excretion of chloroquine, phenobarbital, phenothiazines and methacycline. Helv Med Acta 1967; 33:307–316.

16. Aronoff GR et al. *Drug Prescribing in Renal Failure: Dosing Guidelines for Adults and Children*, 5th edn. Philadelphia: American College of Physicians; 2007.

17. Fraser D et al. An unexpected and serious complication of treatment with the atypical antipsychotic drug clozapine. Clin Nephrol 2000; 54:78–80.

18. Au AF et al. Clozapine-induced acute interstitial nephritis. Am J Psychiatry 2004; 161:1501.

19. Elias TJ et al. Clozapine-induced acute interstitial nephritis. Lancet 1999; 354:1180–1181.

20. Siddiqui BK et al. Simultaneous allergic interstitial nephritis and cardiomyopathy in a patient on clozapine. NDT Plus 2008; 1:55–56.

21. Lobeck F et al. Haloperidol concentrations in an elderly patient with moderate chronic renal failure. J Geriatr Drug Ther 1986; 1:91–97.

22. Cohen LM et al. Update on psychotropic medication use in renal disease. Psychosomatics 2004; 45:34–48.

23. Sunovion Pharmaceuticals Inc. Highlights of Prescribing Information: LATUDA (lurasidone hydrochloride) tablets, 2013. http://www.latuda.com/LatudaPrescribingInformation.pdf

24. Kansagra A et al. Prolonged hypothermia due to olanzapine in the setting of renal failure: a case report and review of the literature. Ther Adv Psychopharmacol 2013; 3:335–339.

25. Thyrum PT et al. Single-dose pharmacokinetics of quetiapine in subjects with renal or hepatic impairment. Prog Neuropsychopharmacol Biol Psychiatry 2000; 24:521–533.

26. Huynh M et al. Thrombotic thrombocytopenic purpura associated with quetiapine. Ann Pharmacother 2005; 39:1346–1348.

27. Snoeck E et al. Influence of age, renal and liver impairment on the pharmacokinetics of risperidone in man. Psychopharmacology 1995; 122:223–229.

28. Herguner S et al. Steroid-induced psychosis in an adolescent: treatment and prophylaxis with risperidone. Turk J Pediatr 2006; 48:244–247.

29. Batalla A et al. Antipsychotic treatment in a patient with schizophrenia undergoing hemodialysis. J Clin Psychopharmacol 2010; 30:92–94.

30. Bressolle F et al. Pharmacokinetics of sulpiride after intravenous administration in patients with impaired renal function. Clin Pharmacokinet 1989; 17:367–373.

31. Aweeka F et al. The pharmacokinetics of ziprasidone in subjects with normal and impaired renal function. Br J Clin Pharmacol 2000; 49:27S–33S.

32. Pfizer. Highlights of Prescribing Information: GEODON (ziprasidone HCl) capsules; GEODON (ziprasidone mesylate) injection for intramuscular use, 2013. http://labeling.pfizer.com/ShowLabeling.aspx?id=584

33. Lieberman JA et al. Tricyclic antidepressant and metabolite levels in chronic renal failure. Clin Pharmacol Ther 1985; 37:301–307.

34. Mitas JA et al. Diabetic neuropathic pain: control by amitriptyline and fluphenazine in renal insufficiency. South Med J 1983; 76:462–3, 467.

35. Murphy EJ. Acute pain management pharmacology for the patient with concurrent renal or hepatic disease. Anaesth Intensive Care 2005; 33:311–322.

36. Turpeinen M et al. Effect of renal impairment on the pharmacokinetics of bupropion and its metabolites. Br J Clin Pharmacol 2007; 64:165–173.

37. Worrall SP et al. Pharmacokinetics of bupropion and its metabolites in haemodialysis patients who smoke. A single dose study. Nephron Clin Pract 2004; 97:c83–c89.

38. Joffe P et al. Single-dose pharmacokinetics of citalopram in patients with moderate renal insufficiency or hepatic cirrhosis compared with healthy subjects. Eur J Clin Pharmacol 1998; 54:237–242.

39. Kalender B et al. Antidepressant treatment increases quality of life in patients with chronic renal failure. Ren Fail 2007; 29:817–822.

40. Kelly CA et al. Adult respiratory distress syndrome and renal failure associated with citalopram overdose. Hum Exp Toxicol 2003; 22:103–105.

41. Spigset O et al. Citalopram pharmacokinetics in patients with chronic renal failure and the effect of haemodialysis. Eur J Clin Pharmacol 2000; 56:699–703.

42. Hosseini SH et al. Citalopram versus psychological training for depression and anxiety symptoms in hemodialysis patients. Iran J Kidney Dis 2012; 6:446–451.

43. Sran H et al. Confusion after starting citalopram in a renal transplant patient. BMJ Case Rep 2013; 2013.

44. Onishi A et al. Reversible acute renal failure associated with clomipramine-induced interstitial nephritis. Clin Exp Nephrol 2007; 11:241–243.

45. Pfizer. Highlights of Prescribing Information: PRISTIQR (desvenlafaxine) Extended-Release Tablets, 2013. http://labeling.pfizer.com/showlabeling.aspx?id=497

46. Nichols AI et al. The pharmacokinetics and safety of desvenlafaxine in subjects with chronic renal impairment. Int J Clin Pharmacol Ther 2011; 49:3–13.

47. Rees JA. Clinical interpretation of pharmacokinetic data on dothiepin hydrochloride (Dosulepin, Prothiaden). J Int Med Res 1981; 9:98–102.

48. Lobo ED et al. Effects of varying degrees of renal impairment on the pharmacokinetics of duloxetine: analysis of a single-dose phase I study and pooled steady-state data from phase II/III trials. Clin Pharmacokinet 2010; 49:311–321.

49. Ho NV, Setters B. *Duloxetine-Induced Multi-System Organ Failure: A Case Report.* 2011. Poster presented at American Geriatrics Society Annual Meeting, May 11-15, 2011: National Harbor, Maryland.

50. Miriyala K et al. Renal failure in a depressed adolescent on escitalopram. J Child Adolesc Psychopharmacol 2008; 18:405–408.

51. Adiga GU et al. Renal tubular defects from antidepressant use in an older adult: An uncommon but reversible adverse drug effect. Clin Drug Invest 2006; 26:607–610.

52. Yazici AE et al. Efficacy and Tolerability of Escitalopram in Depressed Patients with end Stage Renal Disease: an Open Placebo-controlled Study. Bull Clin Psychopharmacol 2012; 22:23–30.

53. Bergstrom RF et al. The effects of renal and hepatic disease on the pharmacokinetics, renal tolerance, and risk-benefit profile of fluoxetine. Int Clin Psychopharmacol 1993; 8:261–266.

54. Blumenfield M et al. Fluoxetine in depressed patients on dialysis. Int J Psychiatry Med 1997; 27:71–80.

55. Levy NB et al. Fluoxetine in depressed patients with renal failure and in depressed patients with normal kidney function. Gen Hosp Psychiatry 1996; 18:8–13.

56. Rabindranath KS et al. Physical measures for treating depression in dialysis patients. Cochrane Database Syst Rev 2005; CD004541.

57. Lancaster SG et al. Lofepramine. A review of its pharmacodynamic and pharmacokinetic properties, and therapeutic efficacy in depressive illness. Drugs 1989; 37:123–140.

58. Davis MP et al. Mirtazapine for pruritus. J Pain Symptom Manage 2003; 25:288–291.

59. Schoerlin MP et al. Disposition kinetics of moclobemide, a new MAO-A inhibitor, in subjects with impaired renal function. J Clin Pharmacol 1990; 30:272–284.

60. Stoeckel K et al. Absorption and disposition of moclobemide in patients with advanced age or reduced liver or kidney function. Acta Psychiatr Scand Suppl 1990; 360:94–97.

61. Pollock BG et al. Metabolic and physiologic consequences of nortriptyline treatment in the elderly. Psychopharmacol Bull 1994; 30:145–150.

62. Doyle GD et al. The pharmacokinetics of paroxetine in renal impairment. Acta Psychiatr Scand Suppl 1989; 350:89–90.

63. Ishii T et al. A rare case of combined syndrome of inappropriate antidiuretic hormone secretion and Fanconi syndrome in an elderly woman. Am J Kidney Dis 2006; 48:155–158.

64. Kaye CM et al. A review of the metabolism and pharmacokinetics of paroxetine in man. Acta Psychiatr Scand Suppl 1989; 350:60–75.

65. Koo JR et al. Treatment of depression and effect of antidepression treatment on nutritional status in chronic hemodialysis patients. Am J Med Sci 2005; 329:1–5.

66. Coulomb F et al. Pharmacokinetics of single-dose reboxetine in volunteers with renal insufficiency. J Clin Pharmacol 2000; 40:482–487.

67. Dostert P et al. Review of the pharmacokinetics and metabolism of reboxetine, a selective noradrenaline reuptake inhibitor. Eur Neuropsychopharmacol 1997; 7 Suppl 1:S23–S35.

68. Takeda Pharmaceuticals America Inc. Highlights of Prescribing Information: BRINTELLIX (vortioxetine) tablets, 2013. http://www.takeda.us/products/default.aspx

69. Brewster UC et al. Addition of sertraline to other therapies to reduce dialysis-associated hypotension. Nephrology (Carlton) 2003; 8:296–301.

70. Chan KY et al. Use of sertraline for antihistamine-refractory uremic pruritus in renal palliative care patients. J Palliat Med 2013; 16:966–970.

71. Chander WP et al. Serotonin syndrome in maintenance haemodialysis patients following sertraline treatment for depression. J Indian Med Assoc 2011; 109:36–37.

72. Jain N et al. Rationale and design of the Chronic Kidney Disease Antidepressant Sertraline Trial (CAST). Contemp Clin Trials 2013; 34:136–144.

73. Catanese B et al. A comparative study of trazodone serum concentrations in patients with normal or impaired renal function. Boll Chim Farm 1978; 117:424–427.

74. Leighton JD et al. Trimipramine-induced acute renal failure (Letter). N Z Med J 1986; 99:248.

75. Simpson GM et al. A preliminary study of trimipramine in chronic schizophrenia. Curr Ther Res Clin Exp 1966; 99:248.

76. Troy SM et al. The effect of renal disease on the disposition of venlafaxine. Clin Pharmacol Ther 1994; 56:14–21.

77. Guldiken S et al. Complete relief of pain in acute painful diabetic neuropathy of rapid glycaemic control (insulin neuritis) with venlafaxine HCL. Diabetes Nutr Metab 2004; 17:247–249.

78. Pascale P et al. Severe rhabdomyolysis following venlafaxine overdose. Ther Drug Monit 2005; 27:562–564.

79. Hegarty J et al. Carbamazepine-induced acute granulomatous interstitial nephritis. Clin Nephrol 2002; 57:310–313.

80. Hogg RJ et al. Carbamazepine-induced acute tubulointerstitial nephritis. J Pediatr 1981; 98:830–832.

81. Imai H et al. Carbamazepine-induced granulomatous necrotizing angiitis with acute renal failure. Nephron 1989; 51:405–408.

82. Jubert P et al. Carbamazepine-induced acute renal failure. Nephron 1994; 66:121.

83. Nicholls DP et al. Acute renal failure from carbamazepine (Letter). Br Med J 1972; 4:490.

84. Tutor-Crespo MJ et al. Relative proportions of serum carbamazepine and its pharmacologically active 10,11-epoxy derivative: effect of polytherapy and renal insufficiency. Ups J Med Sci 2008; 113:171–180.

85. Verrotti A et al. Renal tubular function in patients receiving anticonvulsant therapy: a long-term study. Epilepsia 2000; 41:1432–1435.

86. Hung CC et al. Acute renal failure and its risk factors in Stevens-Johnson syndrome and toxic epidermal necrolysis. Am J Nephrol 2009; 29:633–638.

87. Fervenza FC et al. Acute granulomatous interstitial nephritis and colitis in anticonvulsant hypersensitivity syndrome associated with lamotrigine treatment. Am J Kidney Dis 2000; 36:1034–1040.

88. Fillastre JP et al. Pharmacokinetics of lamotrigine in patients with renal impairment: influence of haemodialysis. Drugs Exp Clin Res 1993; 19:25–32.

89. Schaub JE et al. Multisystem adverse reaction to lamotrigine. Lancet 1994; 344:481.

90. Wootton R et al. Comparison of the pharmacokinetics of lamotrigine in patients with chronic renal failure and healthy volunteers. Br J Clin Pharmacol 1997; 43:23–27.

91. Gitlin M. Lithium and the kidney: an updated review. Drug Saf 1999; 20:231–243.

92. Lepkifker E et al. Renal insufficiency in long-term lithium treatment. J Clin Psychiatry 2004; 65:850–856.

93. Smith GC et al. Anticonvulsants as a cause of Fanconi syndrome. Nephrol Dial Transplant 1995; 10:543–545.

94. Fukuda Y et al. Immunologically mediated chronic tubulo-interstitial nephritis caused by valproate therapy. Nephron 1996; 72:328–329.

95. Watanabe T et al. Secondary renal Fanconi syndrome caused by valproate therapy. Pediatr Nephrol 2005; 20:814–817.

96. Zaki EL et al. Renal injury from valproic acid: case report and literature review. Pediatr Neurol 2002; 27:318–319.

97. Tanaka H et al. Distal type of renal tubular acidosis after anti-epileptic therapy in a girl with infantile spasms. Clin Exp Nephrol 1999; 3:311–313.

98. Knorr M et al. Fanconi syndrome caused by antiepileptic therapy with valproic acid. Epilepsia 2004; 45:868–871.

99. Rahman MH et al. Acute hemolysis with acute renal failure in a patient with valproic acid poisoning treated with charcoal hemoperfusion. Hemodial Int 2006; 10:256–259.

100. Pentikainen PJ et al. Pharmacokinetics of chlormethiazole in healthy volunteers and patients with cirrhosis of the liver. Eur J Clin Pharmacol 1980; 17:275–284.

101. Dashti-Khavidaki S et al. Comparing effects of clonazepam and zolpidem on sleep quality of patients on maintenance hemodialysis. Iran J Kidney Dis 2011; 5:404–409.

102. Sadjadi SA et al. Allergic interstitial nephritis due to diazepam. Arch Intern Med 1987; 147:579.

103. Sunovion Pharmaceuticals Inc. Highlights of Prescribing Information: Lunesta (eszopiclone) tablets, 2012. http://www.lunesta.com/pdf/PostedApprovedLabelingText.pdf

104. Huang CE et al. Intramuscular lorazepam in catatonia in patients with acute renal failure: a report of two cases. Chang Gung Med J 2010; 33:106–109.

105. Reynolds HN et al. Hyperlactatemia, increased osmolar gap, and renal dysfunction during continuous lorazepam infusion. Crit Care Med 2000; 28:1631–1634.

106. Verbeeck RK et al. Impaired elimination of lorazepam following subchronic administration in two patients with renal failure. Br J Clin Pharmacol 1981; 12:749–751.

107. Yaucher NE et al. Propylene glycol-associated renal toxicity from lorazepam infusion. Pharmacotherapy 2003; 23:1094–1099.

108. Zar T et al. Acute kidney injury, hyperosmolality and metabolic acidosis associated with lorazepam. Nat Clin Pract Nephrol 2007; 3:515–520.

109. Hayman M et al. Acute tubular necrosis associated with propylene glycol from concomitant administration of intravenous lorazepam and trimethoprim-sulfamethoxazole. Pharmacotherapy 2003; 23:1190–1194.

110. Murray TG et al. Renal disease, age, and oxazepam kinetics. Clin Pharmacol Ther 1981; 30:805–809.

111. Leung N et al. Acute kidney injury in patients with inactive cytochrome P450 polymorphisms. Ren Fail 2009; 31:749–752.

112. Drover DR. Comparative pharmacokinetics and pharmacodynamics of short-acting hypnosedatives: zaleplon, zolpidem and zopiclone. Clin Pharmacokinet 2004; 43:227–238.

113. Sabbatini M et al. Zaleplon improves sleep quality in maintenance hemodialysis patients. Nephron Clin Pract 2003; 94:c99–103.

114. Goa KL et al. Zopiclone. A review of its pharmacodynamic and pharmacokinetic properties and therapeutic efficacy as an hypnotic. Drugs 1986; 32:48–65.

115. Hussain N et al. Zopiclone-induced acute interstitial nephritis. Am J Kidney Dis 2003; 41:E17.

116. Suwata J et al. New acetylcholinesterase inhibitor (donepezil) treatment for Alzheimer's disease in a chronic dialysis patient. Nephron 2002; 91:330–332.

117. Nagy CF et al. Steady-state pharmacokinetics and safety of donepezil HCl in subjects with moderately impaired renal function. Br J Clin Pharmacol 2004; 58 Suppl 1:18–24.

118. Tiseo PJ et al. An evaluation of the pharmacokinetics of donepezil HCl in patients with moderately to severely impaired renal function. Br J Clin Pharmacol 1998; 46 Suppl 1:56–60.

119. Periclou A et al. Pharmacokinetic study of memantine in healthy and renally impaired subjects. Clin Pharmacol Ther 2006; 79:134–143.

Hepatic impairment

Patients with hepatic impairment may have the following characteristics.

- **Reduced capacity to metabolise** biological waste products, dietary proteins and foreign substances such as drugs. Clinical consequences include hepatic encephalopathy and increased dose-related side-effects from drugs.
- **Reduced ability to synthesise** plasma proteins and vitamin K-dependent clotting factors. Clinical consequences include hypoalbuminaemia, leading in extreme cases to ascites. Increased toxicity from highly protein-bound drugs should be anticipated. There is also an increased risk of bleeding from GI irritant drugs and perhaps with SSRIs.
- **Reduced hepatic blood flow.** Clinical consequences include oesophageal varices and elevated plasma levels of drugs subject to first pass metabolism.

General principles of prescribing in hepatic impairment

Liver function tests (LFTs) are a poor marker of hepatic metabolising capacity, as the hepatic reserve is large. Note that many patients with chronic liver disease are asymptomatic or have fluctuating clinical symptoms. Always consider the clinical presentation rather than adhere to rigid rules involving LFTs.

There are few clinical studies relating to the use of psychotropic drugs in people with hepatic disease. The following principles should be adhered to:

- Prescribe as **few drugs** as possible.
- Use **lower starting doses,** particularly of drugs that are highly protein bound. TCAs, SSRIs (except citalopram), trazodone and antipsychotics may have increased free plasma levels, at least initially. This will not be reflected in measured (total) plasma levels. Use lower doses of drugs known to be subject to extensive first pass metabolism. Examples include TCAs and haloperidol.
- Be **cautious with drugs that are extensively hepatically metabolised** (most psychotropic drugs). Lower doses may be required. Exceptions are sulpiride, amisulpride, lithium and gabapentin, which all undergo no or minimal hepatic metabolism.
- **Leave longer intervals between dosage increases.** Remember that the half-life of most drugs is prolonged in hepatic impairment, so it will take longer for plasma levels to reach steady state.
- If albumin is reduced, consider the implications for drugs that are **highly protein bound,** and **if ascites is present consider the increased volume of distribution for water soluble drugs.**
- Avoid medicines with a **long-half life** or those that need to be metabolised to render them active (**pro-drugs**).
- Always **monitor carefully for side-effects,** which may be delayed.
- **Avoid drugs that are very sedative** because of the risk of precipitating hepatic encephalopathy.
- **Avoid drugs that are very constipating** because of the risk of precipitating hepatic encephalopathy.
- **Avoid drugs that are known to be hepatotoxic** in their own right (e.g. MAOIs, chlorpromazine).

- **Choose a low-risk drug** (see Tables 7.22–7.25) and **monitor LFTs** weekly, at least initially. If LFTs deteriorate after a new drug is introduced, consider switching to another drug.

These rules should always be observed in severe liver disease (low albumin, increased clotting time, ascites, jaundice, encephalopathy, etc.). The information above, and on the following pages, should be interpreted in the context of the patient's clinical presentation. Table 7.21 summarises the recommendations for psychotropic drug use in hepatic impairment. Further information is given in Tables 7.22–7.25.

Antipsychotics in hepatic impairment

One third of patients who are prescribed antipsychotic medication have at least one abnormal LFT and in 4% at least one LFT is elevated three times above the upper limit of normal. Transaminases are most often affected and this generally occurs within 1–6 weeks of treatment initiation. Only rarely does clinically significant hepatic damage result.[1]

Antidepressants in hepatic impairment

Of those treated with antidepressants, 0.5–3% develop asymptomatic mild elevation of hepatic transaminases. Onset is normally between several days and six months of treatment initiation and the elderly are more vulnerable. Frank clinically significant liver damage, however, is rare, mostly idiosyncratic (unpredictable and not related to dose). Cross toxicity within class has been described.[23]

Drug-induced hepatic damage

Hy's rule, defined as the occurrence of ALT > 3 times the upper limit of normal combined with serum bilirubin > 2 times the upper limit of normal is recommended by the FDA to assess the hepatotoxicity of new drugs.[55]

Table 7.21 Recommendations for the use of psychotropics in hepatic impairment

Drug group	Recommended drugs
Antipsychotics	**Haloperidol**: low dose *or* **Sulpiride/amisulpride**: no dosage reduction required if renal function is normal **Paliperidone:** if depot required
Antidepressants	**Imipramine**: start with 25 mg/day and titrate slowly (weekly at most) if required *or* **Paroxetine** or **citalopram**: start at 10 mg if severe hepatic impairment. Titrate slowly (if required) as above
Mood stabilisers	**Lithium**: use plasma levels to guide dosage. Care needed if ascites status changes
Sedatives	**Lorazepam, oxazepam, temazepam**: as short half-life with no active metabolites. Use low doses with caution, as sedative drugs can precipitate hepatic encephalopathy **Zopiclone**: 3.75 mg with care in moderate hepatic impairment

CHAPTER 7

Table 7.22 Antipsychotics in hepatic impairment

Drug	Comments
Amisulpride[2,3]	Predominantly renally excreted, so dosage reduction should not be necessary as long as renal function is normal *but* there are no clinical studies in people with hepatic impairment and little clinical experience. Caution required
Aripiprazole[2]	Extensively hepatically metabolised. Limited data that hepatic impairment has minimal effect on pharmacokinetics. SPC states no dosage reduction required in mild-moderate hepatic impairment, but caution required in severe impairment. Limited clinical experience. Caution required. Small number of reports of hepatotoxicity; increased LFTs, hepatitis and jaundice
Asenapine[2]	Hepatically metabolised. SPC recommends avoid in severe hepatic disease
Clozapine[2–6]	Very sedative and constipating. Contraindicated in active liver disease associated with nausea, anorexia or jaundice, progressive liver disease or hepatic failure. In less severe disease, start with 12.5 mg and increase slowly, using plasma levels to gauge metabolising capacity and guide dosage adjustment. Transient elevations in AST, ALT and GGT to over twice the normal range occur in over 10% of physically healthy people. Clozapine-induced hepatitis, jaundice, cholestasis and liver failure have been reported. If jaundice develops, clozapine should be discontinued
Flupentixol/ zuclopenthixol[2,3,7,8]	Both are extensively hepatically metabolised. Small, transient elevations in transaminases have been reported in some patients treated with zuclopenthixol. No other literature reports of use or harm. Both drugs have been in use for many years. Depot preparations are best avoided, as altered pharmacokinetics will make dosage adjustment difficult and side-effects from dosage accumulation more likely
Haloperidol[2,9]	Drug of choice in clinical practice and no problems reported although UK SPC states 'caution in liver disease'. Isolated reports of cholestatic hepatitis
Iloperidone[10]	Hepatically metabolised. Reduce dose in moderate hepatic impairment and avoid completely in severe hepatic impairment
Lurasidone[11]	Hepatically metabolised. SPC recommends starting dose of 20 mg in hepatic impairment and maximum dose of 40 mg/day in severe hepatic impairment
Olanzapine[2–4,12]	Although extensively hepatically metabolised, the pharmacokinetics of olanzapine seem to change little in severe hepatic impairment. It is sedative and anticholinergic (can cause constipation) so caution is advised. Start with 5 mg/day and consider using plasma levels to guide dosage (aim for 20–40 µg/L). Dose-related, transient, asymptomatic elevations in ALT and AST reported in physically healthy adults. People with liver disease may be at increased risk. Rare cases of hepatitis in the literature
Paliperidone[13]	Mainly excreted unchanged by the kidneys so no dosage adjustment required. However, no data are available with respect to severe hepatic impairment and clinical experience is limited. Caution required
Phenothiazines[2,3,14–16]	All cause sedation and constipation. Associated with cholestasis and some reports of fulminant hepatic cirrhosis. Best avoided completely in hepatic impairment. Chlorpromazine is particularly hepatotoxic
Quetiapine[2,17–20]	Extensively hepatically metabolised but short half-life. Clearance reduced by a mean of 30% in hepatic impairment so small dosage adjustments may be required. Can cause sedation and constipation. Little clinical experience in hepatic impairment so caution recommended. One case of fatal hepatic failure and another of hepatocellular damage reported in the literature

Table 7.22 (Continued)

Drug	Comments
Risperidone[2-4]	Extensively hepatically metabolised and highly protein bound. Manufacturers recommend a reduced starting dose, slower dose titration and a maximum dose of 4 mg in hepatic impairment. Transient, asymptomatic elevations in LFTs, cholestatic hepatitis and rare cases of hepatic failure have been reported. Steatohepatitis may arise as a result of weight gain. Clinical experience limited in hepatic impairment so caution recommended
Sulpiride[2,3,21,22]	Almost completely renally excreted with a low potential to cause sedation or constipation. Dosage reduction should not be required. Some clinical experience in hepatic impairment with few problems. Fairly old established drug. Isolated case reports of cholestatic jaundice and primary biliary cirrhosis. SPC states contraindicated in severe hepatic disease

ALT, alanine aminotransferase; AST, aspartate aminotransferase; GGT, gamma-glutamyl transferase; LFT, liver function test; SPC, summary of product characteristics.

Table 7.23 Antidepressants in hepatic impairment

Drug	Comments
Agomelatine[23-25]	Liver injury including hepatic failure reported. Best avoided in established liver disease. SPC recommends LFTs at baseline, 3, 6, 12, 24 weeks and thereafter where clinically indicated
Duloxetine[2,3,26,27]	Hepatically metabolised. Clearance markedly reduced even in mild impairment. Reports of hepatocellular injury and, less commonly, jaundice. Isolated case report of fulminant hepatic failure. Limited experience. Best avoided
Fluoxetine[2,3,28-32]	Extensively hepatically metabolised with a long half-life. Kinetic studies demonstrate accumulation in compensated cirrhosis. Although dosage reduction (of at least 50%) or alternate day dosing could be used, it would take many weeks to reach steady-state serum levels, making fluoxetine complex to use. Asymptomatic increases in LFTs found in 0.5% of healthy adults. Rare cases of hepatitis reported
MAOIs[2,3,33,34]	People with hepatic impairment reported to be more sensitive to the side-effects of MAOIs. MAOIs are also more hepatotoxic than other antidepressants, so best avoided completely
Mirtazapine[2,3,35]	Hepatically metabolised and sedative. 50% dose reduction recommended based on kinetic data, but clinical experience limited. Mild, asymptomatic increases in LFTs seen in healthy adults (ALT > 3 times the upper limit of normal in 2%). Few cases of cholestatic and hepatocellular damage reported. Best avoided
Moclobemide[2,3,36,37]	Clinical experience limited but probably safer than the irreversible MAOIs. 50% reduction in dose advised by manufacturers. Rare cases of hepatotoxicity reported. Caution advised
Other SSRIs[2,3,32,38-49]	All are hepatically metabolised and accumulate on chronic dosing. Dosage reduction may be required. Sertraline has been found to be both safe and effective in a placebo controlled RCT of the management of cholestatic pruritus. Raised LFTs and rare cases of hepatitis, including chronic active hepatitis, have been reported with paroxetine. Sertraline and fluvoxamine have also been associated with hepatitis. Citalopram and escitalopram have minimal effects on hepatic enzymes and may be the SSRI of choice although clinical experience is limited and occasional hepatotoxicity has been reported. Paroxetine is used by some specialised liver units with few apparent problems
Reboxetine[2,3,50]	50% reduction in starting dose recommended. Clinical experience limited. Does not seem to be associated with hepatotoxicity. Caution advised

(Continued)

Table 7.23 (Continued)

Drug	Comments
Tricyclics[2,3,51]	All are hepatically metabolised, highly protein bound and will accumulate. They vary in their propensity to cause sedation and constipation. All are associated with raised LFTs and rare cases of hepatitis. There is most clinical experience with imipramine. Sedative TCAs such as trimipramine, dothiepin (dosulepin) and amitriptyline are best avoided. Lofepramine is possibly the most hepatotoxic and should be avoided completely
Venlafaxine/ desvenlafaxine[2,3,52–54]	Dosage reduction of 50% advised in moderate hepatic impairment. Little clinical experience. Rare cases of cholestatic hepatitis reported. Caution advised

ALT, alanine aminotransferase; LFT, liver function test; MAOI, monoamine oxidase inhibitor; RCT, randomised controlled trial; SPC, summary of product characteristics; SSRI, selective serotonin reuptake inhibitor; TCA, tricyclic antidepressants.

Table 7.24 Mood stabilisers in hepatic impairment[945,946,998]

Drug	Comments
Carbamazepine[55]	Extensively hepatically metabolised and potent inducer of CYP450 enzymes. Contraindicated in acute liver disease. In chronic stable disease, caution advised. Reduce starting dose by 50%, and titrate up slowly, using plasma levels to guide dosage. Stop if LFTs deteriorate. Associated with hepatitis, cholangitis, cholestatic and hepatocellular jaundice, and hepatic failure (rare). Adverse hepatic effects are most common in the first month of treatment. Hepatocellular damage is often associated with a poor outcome. Vulnerability to carbamazepine-induced hepatic damage may be genetically determined
Lamotrigine	Manufacturers recommend 50% reduction in initial dose, dose escalation and maintenance dose in moderate hepatic impairment and 75% in severe hepatic impairment. Discontinue if lamotrigine-induced rash (which can be serious). Extreme caution advised, particularly if co-prescribed with valproate. Elevated LFTs and hepatitis reported
Lithium[56,57]	Not metabolised so dosage reduction not required as long as renal function is normal. Use serum levels to guide dosage and monitor more frequently if ascites status changes (volume of distribution will change). One case of ascites and one of hyperbilirubinaemia reported over many decades of lithium use worldwide
Valproate[58]	Highly protein bound and hepatically metabolised. Dosage reduction with close monitoring of LFTs in moderate hepatic impairment. Use plasma levels (free levels if possible) to guide dosage. Caution advised. Contraindicated in severe and/or active hepatic impairment; impairment of usual metabolic pathway can lead to generation of hepatotoxic metabolites via alternative pathway. Associated with elevated LFTs and serious hepatotoxicity including fulminant hepatic failure. Mitochondrial disease, learning disability, polypharmacy, metabolic disorders and underlying hepatic disease may be risk factors. Particularly hepatotoxic in very young children. The greatest risk is in the first 3 months of treatment.

LFT, liver function test.

Table 7.25 Stimulants in hepatic impairment[59]

Drug	Comments
Atomoxetine	Rare reports of liver toxicity, manifested by elevated hepatic enzymes, and raised bilirubin with jaundice. SPC states 'discontinue in patients with jaundice or laboratory evidence of liver injury, and do not restart'
Methylphenidate	Rare reports of liver dysfunction and hypersensitivity reactions. Limited clinical experience. Caution advised

SPC, summary of product characteristics.

Hepatic toxicity

Drug induced hepatic damage can be due to:

- direct dose-related hepatotoxicity (Type 1 ADR). A small number of drugs fall into this category e.g. paracetamol, alcohol
- hypersensitivity reactions (Type 2 ADR). These can present with rash, fever and eosinophilia. Almost all drugs have been associated with cases of heptatoxicity; frequency varies.

Almost any type of liver damage can occur, ranging from mild transient asymptomatic increases in LFTs to fulminant hepatic failure. See Tables 7.22–7.25 for details of the hepatotoxic potential of individual drugs.

Risk factors for drug-induced hepatotoxicity include:[60]

- increasing age
- female gender
- alcohol consumption
- co-prescription of enzyme inducing drugs
- genetic predisposition
- obesity
- pre-existing liver disease (small effect).

When interpreting LFTs, remember that:[61]

- 12% of the healthy adult population have one LFT outside (above or below) the normal reference range
- up to 10% of patients with clinically significant hepatic disease have normal LFTs
- individual LFTs lack specificity for the liver, but >1 abnormal test greatly increases the likelihood of liver pathology
- the absolute values of LFTs are a poor indicator of disease severity.

When monitoring LFTs:

- ideally LFTs should be measured before treatment starts so that 'baseline' values are available
- LFT elevations of <2 times the upper limit of the normal reference range are rarely clinically significant
- most drug related LFT elevations occur early in treatment (first month) and are transient. They may indicate adaptation of the liver to the drug rather than damage per se. Transient LFT elevations may also occur during periods of weight gain[62]

- if LFTs are persistently elevated >3 fold, continuing to rise or accompanied by clinical symptoms, the suspected drugs should be withdrawn
- when tracking change, >20% change in liver enzymes is required to exclude biological or analytical variation.

References

1. Marwick KF et al. Antipsychotics and abnormal liver function tests: systematic review. Clin Neuropharmacol 2012; **35**:244–253.
2. Datapharm Communications Ltd. Electronic Medicines Compendium, 2014. https://www.medicines.org.uk/emc/
3. Truven Health Analytics. Micromedex 2.0, 2014. http://micromedex.com/
4. Atasoy N et al. A review of liver function tests during treatment with atypical antipsychotic drugs: a chart review study. Prog Neuropsychopharmacol Biol Psychiatry 2007; **31**:1255–1260.
5. Brown CA et al. Clozapine toxicity and hepatitis. J Clin Psychopharmacol 2013; **33**:570–571.
6. Tucker P. Liver toxicity with clozapine. Aust N Z J Psychiatry 2013; **47**:975–976.
7. Amdisen A et al. Zuclopenthixol acetate in viscoleo - a new drug formulation. An open Nordic multicentre study of zuclopenthixol acetate in Viscoleo in patients with acute psychoses including mania and exacerbation of chronic psychoses. Acta Psychiatr Scand 1987; **75**:99–107.
8. Wistedt B et al. Zuclopenthixol decanoate and haloperidol decanoate in chronic schizophrenia: a double-blind multicentre study. Acta Psychiatr Scand 1991; **84**:14–21.
9. Ozcanli T et al. Severe liver enzyme elevations after three years of olanzapine treatment: a case report and review of olanzapine associated hepatotoxicity. Prog Neuropsychopharmacol Biol Psychiatry 2006; **30**:1163–1166.
10. Novartis Pharmaceuticals Corporation. Highlights of Prescribing Information. FANAPT® (iloperidone) tablets, 2014. http://www.pharma. us.novartis.com/product/pi/pdf/fanapt.pdf
11. Sunovion Pharmaceuticals Inc. Highlights of Prescribing Information: LATUDA (lurasidone hydrochloride) tablets, 2013. http://www.latuda. com/LatudaPrescribingInformation.pdf
12. Dominguez-Jimenez JL et al. Liver toxicity due to olanzapine. Rev Esp Enferm Dig 2012; **104**:617–618.
13. Vermeir M et al. Absorption, metabolism, and excretion of paliperidone, a new monoaminergic antagonist, in humans. Drug Metab Dispos 2008; **36**:769–779.
14. Regal RE et al. Phenothiazine-induced cholestatic jaundice. Clin Pharm 1987; **6**:787–794.
15. Zimmerman HJ et al. Drug-induced cholestasis. Med Toxicol 1987; **2**:112–160.
16. de Abajo FJ et al. Acute and clinically relevant drug-induced liver injury: a population based case-control study. Br J Clin Pharmacol 2004; **58**:71–80.
17. Thyrum PT et al. Single-dose pharmacokinetics of quetiapine in subjects with renal or hepatic impairment. Prog Neuropsychopharmacol Biol Psychiatry 2000; **24**:521–533.
18. Nemeroff CB et al. Quetiapine: preclinical studies, pharmacokinetics, drug interactions, and dosing. J Clin Psychiatry 2002; **63 Suppl** 13:5–11.
19. El Hajj I et al. Subfulminant liver failure associated with quetiapine. Eur J Gastroenterol Hepatol 2004; **16**:1415–1418.
20. Lin CH et al. Quetiapine-induced hepatocellular damage. Psychosomatics 2012; **53**:601–602.
21. Melzer E et al. Severe cholestatic jaundice due to sulpiride. Isr J Med Sci 1987; **23**:1259–1260.
22. Ohmoto K et al. Symptomatic primary biliary cirrhosis triggered by administration of sulpiride. Am J Gastroenterol 1999; **94**:3660–3661.
23. Voican CS et al. Antidepressant-induced liver injury: a review for clinicians. Am J Psychiatry 2014; **171**:404–415.
24. Dolder CR et al. Agomelatine treatment of major depressive disorder. The Annals of Pharmacotherapy 2008; **42**:1822–1831.
25. Stuhec M. Agomelatine-induced hepatotoxicity. Wien Klin Wochenschr 2013; **125**:225–226.
26. Hanje AJ et al. Case report: fulminant hepatic failure involving duloxetine hydrochloride. Clin Gastroenterol Hepatol 2006; **4**:912–917.
27. Vuppalanchi R et al. Duloxetine hepatotoxicity: a case-series from the drug-induced liver injury network. Aliment Pharmacol Ther 2010; **32**:1174–1183.
28. Schenker S et al. Fluoxetine disposition and elimination in cirrhosis. Clin Pharmacol Ther 1988; **44**:353–359.
29. Cai Q et al. Acute hepatitis due to fluoxetine therapy. Mayo Clin Proc 1999; **74**:692–694.
30. Friedenberg FK et al. Hepatitis secondary to fluoxetine treatment. Am J Psychiatry 1996; **153**:580.
31. Johnston DE et al. Chronic hepatitis related to use of fluoxetine. Am J Gastroenterol 1997; **92**:1225–1226.
32. Hale AS. New antidepressants: use in high-risk patients. J Clin Psychiatry 1993; **54 Suppl**:61–70.
33. Gomez-Gil E et al. Phenelzine-induced fulminant hepatic failure. Ann Intern Med 1996; **124**:692–693.
34. Bonkovsky HL et al. Severe liver injury due to phenelzine with unique hepatic deposition of extracellular material. Am J Med 1986; **80**:689–692.
35. Kang SG et al. Mirtazapine-induced hepatocellular-type liver injury. Ann Pharmacother 2011; **45**:825–826.
36. Stoeckel K et al. Absorption and disposition of moclobemide in patients with advanced age or reduced liver or kidney function. Acta Psychiatr Scand Suppl 1990; **360**:94–97.
37. Timmings P et al. Intrahepatic cholestasis associated with moclobemide leading to death. Lancet 1996; **347**:762–763.
38. Benbow SJ et al. Paroxetine and hepatotoxicity. BMJ 1997; **314**:1387.

39. Odeh M et al. Severe hepatotoxicity with jaundice associated with paroxetine. Am J Gastroenterol 2001; **96:**2494–2496.

40. Dunbar GC. An interim overview of the safety and tolerability of paroxetine. Acta Psychiatr Scand Suppl 1989; **350:**135–137.

41. Kuhs H et al. A double-blind study of the comparative antidepressant effect of paroxetine and amitriptyline. Acta Psychiatr Scand Suppl 1989; **350:**145–146.

42. De Bree H et al. Fluvoxamine maleate: disposition in men. Eur J Drug Metab Pharmacokinet 1983; **8:**175–179.

43. Green BH. Fluvoxamine and hepatic function. Br J Psychiatry 1988; **153:**130–131.

44. Milne RJ et al. Citalopram. A review of its pharmacodynamic and pharmacokinetic properties, and therapeutic potential in depressive illness. Drugs 1991; **41:**450–477.

45. Lopez-Torres E et al. Hepatotoxicity related to citalopram (Letter). Am J Psychiatry 2004; **161:**923–924.

46. Colakoglu O et al. Toxic hepatitis associated with paroxetine. Int J Clin Pract 2005; **59:**861–862.

47. Rao N. The clinical pharmacokinetics of escitalopram. Clin Pharmacokinet 2007; **46:**281–290.

48. Suen CF et al. Acute liver injury secondary to sertraline. BMJ Case Rep 2013; **2013.**

49. Mayo MJ et al. Sertraline as a first-line treatment for cholestatic pruritus. Hepatology 2007; **45:**666–674.

50. Tran A et al. Pharmacokinetics of reboxetine in volunteers with hepatic impairment. Clin Drug Invest 2000; **19:**473–477.

51. Committee on Safety in Medicines. Lofepramine (Gamanil) and abnormal blood tests of liver function. Current Problems 1988; **23:**2.

52. Stadlmann S et al. Venlafaxine-induced cholestatic hepatitis: case report and review of literature. Am J Surg Pathol 2012; **36:**1724–1728.

53. Archer DF et al. Cardiovascular, cerebrovascular, and hepatic safety of desvenlafaxine for 1 year in women with vasomotor symptoms associated with menopause. Menopause 2013; **20:**47–56.

54. Baird-Bellaire S et al. An open-label, single-dose, parallel-group study of the effects of chronic hepatic impairment on the safety and pharmacokinetics of desvenlafaxine. Clin Ther 2013; **35:**782–794.

55. Bjornsson E. Hepatotoxicity associated with antiepileptic drugs. Acta Neurol Scand 2008; **118:**281–290.

56. Cohen LS et al. Lithium-induced hyperbilirubinemia in an adolescent. J Clin Psychopharmacol 1991; **11:**274–275.

57. Hazelwood RE. Ascites: a side effect of lithium? Am J Psychiatry 1981; **138:**257.

58. Krahenbuhl S et al. Mitochondrial diseases represent a risk factor for valproate-induced fulminant liver failure. Liver 2000; **20:**346–348.

59. Panei P et al. Safety of psychotropic drug prescribed for attention-deficit/hyperactivity disorder in Italy. Adverse Drug Reaction Bulletin 2010;999–1002.

60. Grattagliano I et al. Biochemical mechanisms in drug-induced liver injury: certainties and doubts. World J Gastroenterol 2009; **15:**4865–4876.

61. Rosalki SB et al. Liver function profiles and their interpretation. Br J Hosp Med 1994; **51:**181–186.

62. Rettenbacher MA et al. Association between antipsychotic-induced elevation of liver enzymes and weight gain: a prospective study. J Clin Psychopharmacol 2006; **26:**500–503.

CHAPTER 7

HIV infection

General principles of prescribing in HIV

Individuals with HIV/AIDs may experience symptoms of mental illness either as a direct consequence of (organic origin), a reaction to, or in addition to their underlying infection. In the first scenario, the focus of treatment should be the underlying infection. Where this is not feasible, or the presentation is not of organic origin, psychotropic medication will be the primary treatment.

When prescribing psychotropics, the following principles should be adhered to:

- Start with a low dose and titrate according to tolerability and response.
- Select the simplest dosing regime possible. (Remember that the patient's drug regime is likely to be complex already.)
- Select an agent with the fewest side-effects/interactions. Medical co-morbidity and potential drug interactions must be considered.
- Ensure that management is conducted in close cooperation with the HIV physicians and the rest of the multi-disciplinary team.

Although most psychotropic agents are thought to be safe in HIV-infected individuals, definitive data are lacking in many cases, and it has been suggested that this group may be more sensitive to higher doses, adverse side-effects and interactions.[1] Patients with low CD4 counts and high viral loads are more likely to have exaggerated adverse reactions to psychotropic medications.

Psychosis

Atypicals are usually used as a first-line. Risperidone is the most widely studied[2] and generally appears to be safe, although idiosyncratic interactions with ritonavir have been reported.[3,4] Quetiapine, aripiprazole and olanzapine may also be used.[5-7] The use of clozapine is not routinely recommended, although it may be useful in low doses in patients with higher CD4 counts who are otherwise medically stable. Clozapine may also be helpful in the treatment of individuals with HIV-associated psychosis with drug-induced parkinsonism.[8] Although it is not known whether patients with HIV have a greater risk of agranulocytosis, extremely close monitoring of the white cell count is recommended. Patients with HIV may be more susceptible to extrapyramidal side-effects,[9] neuroleptic malignant syndrome[10] and tardive dyskinesia.[11]

Delirium

Organic causes should be identified and treated. Short-term symptomatic treatment may include low-dose atypicals such as risperidone,[12] olanzapine,[13] quetiapine[14] or ziprasidone.[15] The concomitant use of short courses of low dose, short-acting benzodiazepines such as lorazepam may also be helpful, although use as a sole agent may worsen delirium.[6] Chlorpromazine and haloperidol have been successfully used.[16]

Depression

Depression is common in individuals with HIV, and a recent study estimated the prevalence in this population to be as high as 84%.[17] Of note, depression may be a risk factor for HIV,[18] and it has been further suggested that much of this depression is either unrecognised or insufficiently managed.[19] First-line agents include SSRIs, especially escitalopram/citalopram[5,20] (because it does not inhibit CYP2D6 or CYP3A4), with further treatment as per standard protocols. Oddly, the most recent study of escitalopram found no difference from placebo.[21] There is limited evidence that SSRIs enhance HIV-related immunity.[22] The risk of serotonin syndrome may be increased.[23] The use of TCAs may be appropriate in some cases, although side-effects may limit efficacy and compliance.[24] MAOIs are not recommended in this population. Other agents (bupropion,[25] mirtazapine,[26] reboxetine[27] and trazodone[28]) have been investigated, and although these agents were shown to reduce depressive symptoms, the high prevalence of side-effects limited their utility. Their routine use is therefore not recommended. Testosterone and stimulants have also been successfully used.[29]

Bipolar affective disorder

Mania is a recognised presentation in HIV[30] and individuals with HIV may be more sensitive to the side-effects of mood stabilisers such as lithium,[31] especially if they have neurocognitive dysfunction.[30] Conventional agents such as valproate, lamotrigine and gabapentin may be used cautiously, but carbamazepine should be avoided because of important interactions with antiretroviral agents such as ritonavir,[32] as well as the risk of neutropenia. In one case series lithium was shown to be poorly tolerated[33] and it may be advisable to limit its use to asymptomatic individuals with higher CD4 counts and to monitor closely these individuals. The use of antimanic antipsychotics such as risperidone, quetiapine and olanzapine is also an option.[5]

Anxiety disorders

Benzodiazepines may have some utility in the acute treatment of anxiety in individuals with HIV, but caution should be exercised because of the potential for both misuse and multiple, and in rare cases, potentially serious interactions. Some authorities suggest benzodiazepines are drugs of choice for anxiety in HIV.[5] SSRIs (remember interactions) and other antidepressants may be efficacious, and there is evidence that buspirone may be especially useful.[34]

HIV neurocognitive disorders

Individuals with HIV may present with cognitive impairment at any time in the course of their illness; this may range from mild forgetfulness ('minor cognitive and motor disorder') to severe and debilitating dementia. The mainstay of treatment is combination antiretroviral therapy,[35] with judicious, short-term use of an antipsychotic such as risperidone[36] if necessary. Treatment of these individuals is carried out primarily by HIV physicians, with liaison psychiatric input as required.

References

1. Ayuso JL. Use of psychotropic drugs in patients with HIV infection. Drugs 1994; 47:599–610.
2. Singh AN et al. Risperidone in HIV-related manic psychosis. Lancet 1994; 344:1029–1030.
3. Jover F et al. Reversible coma caused by risperidone-ritonavir interaction. Clin Neuropharmacol 2002; 25:251–253.
4. Kelly DV et al. Extrapyramidal symptoms with ritonavir/indinavir plus risperidone. Ann Pharmacother 2002; 36:827–830.
5. Freudenreich O et al. Psychiatric treatment of persons with HIV/AIDS: an HIV-Psychiatry Consensus Survey of Current Practices. Psychosomatics 2010; 51:480–488.
6. Brogan K et al. Management of common psychiatric conditions in the HIV-positive population. Curr HIV/AIDS Rep 2009; 6:108–115.
7. Singh D et al. Choice of antipsychotic in HIV-infected patients. J Clin Psychiatry 2007; 68:479–480.
8. Lera G et al. Pilot study with clozapine in patients with HIV-associated psychosis and drug-induced parkinsonism. Mov Disord 1999; 14:128–131.
9. Hriso E et al. Extrapyramidal symptoms due to dopamine-blocking agents in patients with AIDS encephalopathy. Am J Psychiatry 1991; 148:1558–1561.
10. Horwath E et al. NMS and HIV. Psychiatr Serv 1999; 50:564.
11. Shedlack KJ et al. Rapidly progressive tardive dyskinesia in AIDS. Biol Psychiatry 1994; 35:147–148.
12. Sipahimalani A et al. Treatment of delirium with risperidone. Int J Geriatr Psychopharmacol 1997; 1:24–26.
13. Sipahimalani A et al. Olanzapine in the treatment of delirium. Psychosomatics 1998; 39:422–430.
14. Schwartz TL et al. Treatment of delirium with quetiapine. Prim Care Companion J Clin Psychiatry 2000; 2:10–12.
15. Leso L et al. Ziprasidone treatment of delirium. Psychosomatics 2002; 43:61–62.
16. Breitbart W et al. A double-blind trial of haloperidol, chlorpromazine, and lorazepam in the treatment of delirium in hospitalized AIDS patients. Am J Psychiatry 1996; 153:231–237.
17. Anon. Depression is common among AIDS patients. Psych consult often is necessary. AIDS Alert 2002; 17:153–154.
18. McDermott BE et al. Diagnosis, health beliefs, and risk of HIV infection in psychiatric patients. Hosp Community Psychiatry 1994; 45:580–585.
19. Katz MH et al. Depression and use of mental health services among HIV-infected men. AIDS Care 1996; 8:433–442.
20. Currier MB et al. Citalopram treatment of major depressive disorder in Hispanic HIV and AIDS patients: a prospective study. Psychosomatics 2004; 45:210–216.
21. Hoare J et al. Escitalopram treatment of depression in human immunodeficiency virus/acquired immunodeficiency syndrome: a randomized, double-blind, placebo-controlled study. J Nerv Ment Dis 2014; 202:133–137.
22. Benton T et al. Selective serotonin reuptake inhibitor suppression of HIV infectivity and replication. Psychosom Med 2010; 72:925–932.
23. DeSilva KE et al. Serotonin syndrome in HIV-infected individuals receiving antiretroviral therapy and fluoxetine. AIDS 2001; 15:1281–1285.
24. Elliott AJ et al. Randomized, placebo-controlled trial of paroxetine versus imipramine in depressed HIV-positive outpatients. Am J Psychiatry 1998; 155:367–372.
25. Currier MB et al. A prospective trial of sustained-release bupropion for depression in HIV-seropositive and AIDS patients. Psychosomatics 2003; 44:120–125.
26. Elliott AJ et al. Mirtazapine for depression in patients with human immunodeficiency virus. J Clin Psychopharmacol 2000; 20:265–267.
27. Carvalhal AS et al. An open trial of reboxetine in HIV-seropositive outpatients with major depressive disorder. J Clin Psychiatry 2003; 64:421–424.
28. De WS et al. Efficacy and safety of trazodone versus clorazepate in the treatment of HIV-positive subjects with adjustment disorders: a pilot study. J Int Med Res 1999; 27:223–232.
29. Hill L et al. Pharmacotherapy considerations in patients with HIV and psychiatric disorders: focus on antidepressants and antipsychotics. Ann Pharmacother 2013; 47:75–89.
30. El-Mallakh RS. Mania in AIDS: clinical significance and theoretical considerations. Int J Psychiatry Med 1991; 21:383–391.
31. Tanquary J. Lithium neurotoxicity at therapeutic levels in an AIDS patient. J Nerv Ment Dis 1993; 181:518–519.
32. Berbel GA et al. Protease inhibitor-induced carbamazepine toxicity. Clin Neuropharmacol 2000; 23:216–218.
33. Parenti DM et al. Effect of lithium carbonate in HIV-infected patients with immune dysfunction. J Acquir Immune Defic Syndr 1988; 1:119–124.
34. Batki SL. Buspirone in drug users with AIDS or AIDS-related complex. J Clin Psychopharmacol 1990; 10:111S–115S.
35. Portegies P et al. Guidelines for the diagnosis and management of neurological complications of HIV infection. Eur J Neurol 2004; 11:297–304.
36. Belzie LR. Risperidone for AIDS-associated dementia: a case series. AIDS Patient Care STDS 1996; 10:246–249.

Drugs for HIV

Interactions

Table 7.26 lists drug–drug interactions that are included in the summary of product characteristics (SPCs: accessed May 2014) for antiretroviral agents. The concomitant prescribing of drugs that are highlighted in **bold** is **contraindicated**.

Table 7.26 Pharmacokinetic interaction with HIV drugs

Antiretroviral drug	Effect on CYP enzyme(s)	Anticipated clinical effect on psychotropic drug(s)	Anticipated clinical effect of psychotropic drug(s) on antiretroviral drug
Protease inhibitors – (mostly potent 3A4 inhibition)			
Atazanavir plus ritonavir (*as pharmacokinetic booster*) CYP3A4 substrates	Potent CYP3A4 inhibition Modest CYP3A4 induction Modest CYP2D6 inhibition	Psychotropic drug levels *increased*: **pimozide, oral midazolam, quetiapine**, buprenorphine, carbamazepine, parenteral midazolam, lurasidone Psychotropic drug levels *decreased*: Phenobarbital, phenytoin, lamotrigine	**St John's wort** (SJW, *Hypericum perforatum*), carbamazepine, phenytoin, phenobarbital: decreased atazanavir and ritonavir levels
Darunavir plus ritonavir (*as pharmacokinetic booster*) CYP3A4 substrates	Potent CYP3A4 inhibition Modest CYP3A4 induction Modest CYP2D6 inhibition CYP2C19 induction CYP2C9 induction	Psychotropic drug levels *increased*: **pimozide, oral midazolam, sertindole, quetiapine**, buprenorphine, carbamazepine, parenteral midazolam, lurasidone Psychotropic drug levels *decreased*: methadone, paroxetine, sertraline	**SJW, phenytoin, phenobarbital**: decreased darunavir and ritonavir levels
Fosamprenavir (active metabolite = amprenavir) **plus ritonavir** (*as pharmacokinetic booster*) CYP3A4 substrates	Potent CYP3A4 inhibition Modest CYP3A4 induction Modest CYP2D6 inhibition CYP2C9 induction CYP1A2 induction	Psychotropic drug levels *increased*: **pimozide, oral midazolam, quetiapine**, parenteral midazolam, tricyclic antidepressants (TCAs), lurasidone Psychotropic drug levels *decreased*: methadone and paroxetine, phenytoin	**SJW**, carbamazepine, phenobarbital: decreased fosamprenavir and ritonavir levels
Indinavir plus ritonavir (*as pharmacokinetic booster*) CYP3A4 substrates	Potent CYP3A4 inhibition Modest CYP3A4 induction Modest CYP2D6 inhibition CYP2C9 induction	Psychotropic drug levels *increased*: **alprazolam**, buspirone, **diazepam, oral midazolam, quetiapine**, carbamazepine, **flurazepam, pimozide**, parenteral midazolam, trazodone, phenytoin, phenobarbital, **clozapine**, lurasidone Psychotropic drug levels *decreased*: lamotrigine, valproic acid, methadone	**SJW**, carbamazepine, phenobarbital, phenytoin: decreased indinavir and ritonavir levels

(Continued)

Table 7.26 (*Continued*)

Antiretroviral drug	Effect on CYP enzyme(s)	Anticipated clinical effect on psychotropic drug(s)	Anticipated clinical effect of psychotropic drug(s) on antiretroviral drug
Lopinavir plus ritonavir (*as pharmacokinetic booster*) CYP3A4 substrates	Potent CYP3A4 inhibition Modest CYP3A4 induction Modest CYP2D6 inhibition CYP2B6 induction CYP2C9 induction CYP2C19 induction	Psychotropic drug levels *increased*: carbamazepine, phenobarbital, **pimozide**, **oral midazolam**, **quetiapine**, parenteral midazolam, trazodone, lurasidone Psychotropic drug levels *decreased*: bupropion, lamotrigine, valproate, methadone, phenytoin	**SJW**, carbamazepine, phenobarbital, phenytoin: decreased lopinavir and ritonavir levels
Ritonavir CYP3A4 substrate	Potent CYP3A4 inhibitor Modest CYP3A4 inducer Modest CYP2D6 inhibitor CYP2C9 inhibitor CYP2C9 inducer CYP2C19 inhibitor CYP2B6 inhibitor	Psychotropic drug levels *increased*: alprazolam, buprenorphine, buspirone, **diazepam, oral midazolam, quetiapine,** carbamazepine, **flurazepam, pimozide,** parenteral midazolam, trazodone, zolpidem, amitriptyline, amfetamine, **clozapine**, fluoxetine, haloperidol, imipramine, nortriptyline, paroxetine, risperidone, sertraline, lurasidone Psychotropic drug levels *decreased*: lamotrigine, phenytoin, valproic acid, bupropion, methadone	**SJW**: decreased ritonavir levels
Saquinavir plus ritonavir (*as pharmacokinetic booster*) CYP3A4 substrates	Potent CYP3A4 inhibition Modest CYP3A4 induction Modest CYP2D6 inhibition	Psychotropic drug levels *increased*: alprazolam, **clozapine**, diazepam, flurazepam, **haloperidol**, parenteral midazolam, **phenothiazines**, **pimozide, oral midazolam, trazodone**, **TCAs**, lurasidone Psychotropic drug levels *decreased*: **methadone**	**SJW**, carbamazepine, phenobarbital, phenytoin: decreased saquinavir levels

Table 7.26 (*Continued*)

Antiretroviral drug	Effect on CYP enzyme(s)	Anticipated clinical effect on psychotropic drug(s)	Anticipated clinical effect of psychotropic drug(s) on antiretroviral drug
Tipranavir plus ritonavir (*as pharmacokinetic booster*) CYP3A4 substrates	Potent CYP3A4 inhibition Modest CYP3A4 induction Modest CYP2D6 inhibition CYP 1A2, CYP2C9 and CYP2C19, inhibition CYP1A2 and to a much lesser extent, CYP2C9 induction	Psychotropic drug levels *increased*: carbamazepine, **pimozide, oral midazolam, quetiapine, sertindole,** parenteral midazolam, trazodone, lurasidone Psychotropic drug levels *decreased*: methadone, buprenorphine, bupropion	**SJW**, carbamazepine, phenobarbital, phenytoin: decreased tipranavir and ritonavir levels
Non-nucleoside reverse transcriptase inhibitors			
Efavirenz CYP3A4 substrate	CYP3A4 inducer and to a much lesser extent, CYP3A4 inhibitor CYP2C19 inhibitor CYP2B6 inhibitor	Psychotropic drug levels *increased*: lorazepam**, midazolam, pimozide**, lurasidone Psychotropic drug levels *decreased*: buprenorphine, **carbamazepine,** methadone, bupropion, sertraline	**SJW**, carbamazepine: decreased efavirenz levels
Etravirine CYP3A4 substrate CYP2C9 substrate CYP2C19 substrate	Weak CYP3A4 inducer Weak CYP2C9 inhibitor Weak CYP2C19 inhibitor	Psychotropic drug levels *increased*: diazepam	Carbamazepine, phenobarbital, phenytoin, **SJW**: decreased etravirine levels
Nevirapine CYP3A4 substrate	CYP3A4 inducer ?CYP2B6 inducer	Psychotropic drug levels *decreased*: methadone	**SJW**: decreased nevirapine levels
Rilpivirine CYP3A4 substrate	Nil activity of clinical relevance	Psychotropic drug levels *decreased*: methadone	**SJW**, carbamazepine, oxcarbazepine, phenobarbital, phenytoin: decreased rilpivirine levels
Nucleoside and nucleotide reverse transcriptase inhibitors			
Abacavir	Nil activity of clinical relevance	Levels *decreased*: methadone	Phenobarbital, phenytoin: decreased abacavir levels
Zidovudine			Methadone, valproic acid: increased zidovudine levels.
Didanosine	Nil activity of clinical relevance		
Emtricitabine	Nil activity of clinical relevance		
Stavudine	Nil activity of clinical relevance		

(*Continued*)

Table 7.26 (*Continued*)

Antiretroviral drug	Effect on CYP enzyme(s)	Anticipated clinical effect on psychotropic drug(s)	Anticipated clinical effect of psychotropic drug(s) on antiretroviral drug
Tenofovir	Nil activity of clinical relevance		
Lamivudine	Nil activity of clinical relevance		
Fusion inhibitor			
Enfuvirtide	Nil activity of clinical relevance		
Entry/integrase inhibitors			
Maraviroc CYP3A4 substrate	?CYP2D6 inhibitor		**SJW**: decreased maraviroc levels
Raltegravir	Nil activity of clinical relevance		
Elvitegravir CYP3A4 substrate	Modest CYP2C9, CYP1A2, CYP2C19, CYP3A, CYP2B6 and CYP2C8 induction	Psychotropic drug levels *increased*: buprenorphine	**SJW, carbamazepine, phenobarbital, phenytoin:** decreased elvitegravir levels
Dolutegravir CYP3A4 substrate			SJW, carbamazepine, oxcarbazepine, phenobarbital, phenytoin: decreased dolutegravir levels

Refer to the section on 'Cytochrome P450 (CYP) substrates, inhibitors and/or inducers' in this chapter to determine other potential drug–drug interactions.

Table 7.27 summarises the adverse psychiatric effects of antiretroviral drugs. Notes:

- The enzyme-modulating effect of ritonavir is dose-dependent. Anticipated drug–drug interactions may be more significant when ritonavir is used as an antiretroviral agent. When ritonavir is used as a 'pharmacokinetic booster' the details of potential drug–drug interactions with both ritonavir and the relevant protease inhibitor need to be considered.
- In clinical practice, all protease inhibitors are co-prescribed with ritonavir (used as a pharmacokinetic booster).
- Potential pharmacodynamic interactions are shown in Table 7.28.
- Use http://www.hiv-druginteractions.org/Interactions.aspx for information about individual drug–drug interactions involving psychotropic drugs with antiretroviral drugs.

Table 7.27 Adverse psychiatric effects of antiretroviral drugs

Adverse psychiatric effect	Implicated antiretroviral drug(s)
Abnormal dreams	Atazanavir, efavirenz, emtricitabine, etravirine, lopinavir, raltegravir, ritonavir, stavudine, darunavir, rilpivirine, dolutegravir
Agitation	Efavirenz
Amnesia	Raltegravir
Anxiety	Atazanavir, efavirenz, enfurvirtide, etravirine, lopinavir, raltegravir, ritonavir, stavudine, zidovudine, darunavir
Delusions/'psychosis-like behaviour'	Efavirenz
Depression	Atazanavir, maraviroc, raltegravir, stavudine, zidovudine, darunavir, efavirenz, rilpivirine, elvitegravir
Disorientation	Atazanavir, darunavir, etravirine
Fatal suicide	Efavirenz
Hypersomnia	Etravirine, raltegravir
Insomnia	Atazanavir, efavirenz, emtricitabine, etravirine, indinavir, lamivudine, maraviroc, lopinavir, raltegravir, ritonavir, stavudine, tipranavir, zidovudine, darunavir, rilpivirine, dolutegravir, elvitegravir
Irritability	Enfurvirtide
Mania	Efavirenz
Nightmare	Enfurvirtide, etravirine, raltegravir, darunavir
Panic attack	Raltegravir
Reduced libido	Lopinavir, saquinavir, darunavir
Severe/major depression	Efavirenz, raltegravir
Somnolence	Efavirenz, etravirine, raltegravir, ritonavir, stavudine, zidovudine darunavir, saquinavir, tipranivir, rilpivirine, elvitegravir
Suicidal ideation	Efavirenz, raltegravir, elvitegravir[29]
Suicide attempt	Efavirenz, raltegravir, elvitegravir[29]
'Abnormal thinking'	Stavudine, efavirenz
'Cognitive disorder'	Raltegravir
'Confusional state'	Raltegravir, darunavir, etravirine
'Disturbance in concentration'/ 'disturbance in attention'	Enfurvirtide, etravirine, raltegravir, ritonavir
'Emotional lability'	Stavudine, efavirenz
'Impaired concentration'	Efavirenz
'Memory impairment'	Raltegravir
'Sleep disorder'	Atazanavir, etravirine, raltegravir, saquinavir, tipranavir, darunavir, rilpivirine

*In patients with a pre-existing history of psychiatric illness.
All data derived from SPCs, accessed May 2014.

CHAPTER 7

Table 7.28 Potential pharmacodynamic interactions with HIV drugs

Potential adverse effect	Implicated antiretroviral drug(s)	Implications for psychotropic prescribing
Seizure(s)	Efavirenz, etravirine, lopinavir, darunavir, maraviroc, ritonavir, zidovudine, saquinavir	May increase seizure risk associated with certain psychotropic drugs
Metabolic abnormalities such as hypertriglyceridaemia, hypercholesterolaemia, insulin resistance, hyperglycaemia and hyperlactataemia	All combination antiretroviral therapy	May compound risk of metabolic adverse effects associated with certain psychotropic drugs
ECG changes	Atazanavir, lopinavir, ritonavir, saquinavir, darunavir	May increase risk of arrhythmias associated with certain psychotropic drugs
Raised creatine kinase (CK)	Emtricitabine, raltegravir	May be important to acknowledge associated link if diagnosis of NMS is being considered

ECG, electrocardiogram; NMS, neuroleptic malignant syndrome.

Reference

http://www.medicines.org.uk/emc/

Eating disorders

Eating disorders are increasingly common, especially in children and adolescents. Lifetime prevalence is 0.6% for anorexia nervosa, 1% for bulimia and 3% for binge eating disorder (rates for women are about three times higher than men).[1] There are many similarities between the different types of eating disorders and patients often traverse diagnoses, which can complicate treatment.[2] Other psychiatric conditions (particularly anxiety, depression and obsessive compulsive disorder) often coexist with eating disorders and this may in part explain the benefit seen with medication.

Anorexia nervosa carries considerable risk of mortality or serious physical morbidity. Patients may present with multiple physical conditions including amenorrhoea, muscle wasting, electrolyte abnormalities, cardiovascular complications and osteoporosis. Patients who purge through vomiting are at high risk of loss of tooth enamel, gastro-oesophageal erosion and dehydration.[2] Other modes of purging include laxative and diuretic misuse.

Any medicine prescribed should be accompanied by close monitoring to check for possible adverse reactions.

Anorexia nervosa

General guidance

There are few controlled trials to guide treatment with medicines for anorexia nervosa. Prompt weight restoration to a safe weight, family therapy and structured psychotherapy are the main interventions.[3,4] The aim of (physical) treatment is to improve nutritional health through re-feeding, with very limited evidence for the use of any pharmacological interventions other than those prescribed to correct metabolic deficiencies. Medicines may be used to treat co-morbid conditions,[3] but have a very limited role in weight restoration.[5] Olanzapine is the only one shown conclusively to have any effect on weight restoration in anorexia nervosa,[6–8] while early data for quetiapine were encouraging[9] but were not replicated in a more recent RCT.[10]

Dronabinol, a synthetic cannabinoid agonist, may induce slight weight gain[11] but remains an experimental treatment. The use of medicines to restore weight in anorexia nervosa is controversial, Behavioural interventions which have been shown to have a more long lasting effect are preferred.

Healthcare professionals should be aware of the risk of medicines that prolong the QT interval. All patients with a diagnosis of anorexia nervosa should have an alert placed in their prescribing record noting that they are at increased risk of arrhythmias secondary to electrolyte disturbances and potential cardiac complications associated with inadequate nutrition. ECG monitoring should be undertaken if the prescription of any medicine that may compromise cardiac functioning is essential.[3]

Physical aspects

Vitamins and minerals

Treatment with a multivitamin/multimineral supplement in oral form is recommended during both inpatient and outpatient weight restoration[3] (in the UK, Forceval or Sanatogen Gold one capsule daily may be used).

CHAPTER 7

Electrolytes

Electrolyte disturbances (e.g. hypokalaemia) may develop slowly over time and may be asymptomatic and resolve with re-feeding. Hypophosphataemia may also be precipitated by re-feeding. Rapid correction may be hazardous. Oral supplementation is therefore used to prevent serious sequelae rather than simply to restore normal levels. If supplements are used, urea and electrolytes, HCO_3, Ca, P and Mg need to be monitored and an ECG needs to be performed.[12]

Osteoporosis

Bone loss is a serious complication of anorexia with serious consequences. Hormonal treatment using oestrogen or dehydroepiandrosterone (DHEA) does not have a positive impact on bone density and oestrogen is not recommended in children and adolescents due to the risk of premature fusion of the bones.[3] Antipsychotics that raise prolactin levels can further increase the risk of bone loss and osteoporosis. Bisphosphonates are not generally recommended for women with anorexia nervosa due to the lack of data about both the benefits and also safety; they are not licensed for use in pre-menopausal girls.

Psychiatric aspects

Acute illness: antidepressants

A Cochrane review found no evidence from four placebo-controlled trials that antidepressants improved weight gain, eating disorder or associated psychopathology.[13] It has been suggested that neurochemical abnormalities in starvation may partially explain this non-response.[13] Co-prescribing nutritional supplementation (including tryptophan) with fluoxetine has not been shown to increase efficacy.[14]

Other psychotropic medicines

Antipsychotics (e.g. olanzapine), minor tranquilisers or antihistamines (e.g. promethazine) are often used to reduce the high levels of anxiety associated with anorexia nervosa but they are not usually recommended for the promotion of weight gain.[3] Case reports and retrospective studies have suggested that olanzapine may reduce agitation (and possibly improve weight gain).[15,16] One RCT[7] showed that 87.5% of patients given olanzapine achieved weight restoration (55.6% placebo). Quetiapine may improve psychological symptoms but there are few data.[9] Only prolactin-sparing antipsychotics should be considered. Many other medications[5] have been investigated in small placebo-controlled trials of varying quality and success, these include zinc,[17] naltrexone[18] and cyproheptadine.[19]

Relapse prevention

There is evidence from one small trial that fluoxetine may be useful in improving outcome and preventing relapse of patients with anorexia nervosa after weight restoration.[20] Other studies have found no benefit.[13,21] SSRIs can, albeit very rarely, elevate prolactin, so caution is required.

Co-morbid disorders

Antidepressants are often used to treat co-morbid major depressive disorder and obsessive compulsive disorder. However, caution should be used as these conditions may resolve with weight gain alone.[3]

Bulimia nervosa and binge eating disorder

Psychological interventions should be considered first-line for bulimia.[22] Adults with bulimia nervosa and binge eating disorder (BED) may be offered a trial of an antidepressant. SSRIs (specifically fluoxetine[23-24]) are the antidepressant of first choice. The effective dose of fluoxetine is 60 mg daily.[26] Patients should be informed that this can reduce the frequency of binge eating and purging but long-term effects are unknown.[3] Early response (at 3 weeks) is a strong predictor of response overall.[27]

Antidepressants may be used for the treatment of bulimia nervosa in adolescents but they are not licensed for this age group and there is little evidence for this practice. They should not be considered as a first-line treatment in adolescent bulimia nervosa.[3]

There is some reasonable evidence that topiramate reduces frequency of binge-eating[28] and limited evidence for the usefulness of bupropion[29], duloxetine,[30] lamotrigine,[31] zonisamide,[32,33] acamprosate[34] and sodium oxybate.[35]

Other atypical eating disorders

There have been no studies of the use of medicines to treat atypical eating disorders other than anorexia nervosa, bulimia nervosa and BED.[3,36] In the absence of evidence to guide the management of other atypical eating disorders (also known as 'eating disorders not otherwise specified'), it is recommended that the clinician considers following the guidance of the eating disorder that mostly resembles the individual patient's eating disorder.[3] See Box 7.11.

Box 7.11 Summary of NICE guidance on eating disorders[3]

Anorexia nervosa
- Psychological interventions are the treatments of choice and should be accompanied by monitoring of the patient's physical state.
- No pharmacological intervention is recommended. A range of medicines may be used in the treatment of co-morbid conditions.

Bulimia nervosa
- An evidence-based self-help programme or cognitive behaviour therapy for bulimia nervosa should be the first choice of treatment.
- A trial of fluoxetine may be offered as an alternative or additional first step.

Binge eating disorder
- An evidence based self-help programme of cognitive behavioural therapy for binge eating disorder should be the first choice of treatment.
- A trial of an SSRI can be considered as an alternative or additional first step.

Although this guidance is 10 years old, updates of literature reviews have not yet given NICE cause to change its advice.[37]

References

1. Treasure J et al. Eating disorders. Lancet 2010; 375:583–593.
2. Steffen KJ et al. Emerging drugs for eating disorder treatment. Expert Opin Emerg Drugs 2006; 11:315–336.
3. National Institute for Health and Clinical Excellence. Eating disorders: Core interventions in the treatment and management of anorexia nervosa, bulimia nervosa and related eating disorders. Clinical Guideline 9, 2004. http://www.nice.org.uk
4. American Psychiatric Association. Treatment of patients with eating disorders, third edition. Am J Psychiatry 2006; 163:4–54.
5. Crow SJ et al. What potential role is there for medication treatment in anorexia nervosa? Int J Eat Disord 2009; 42:1–8.
6. Dunican KC et al. The role of olanzapine in the treatment of anorexia nervosa. Annal Pharmacother 2007; 41:111–115.
7. Bissada H et al. Olanzapine in the treatment of low body weight and obsessive thinking in women with anorexia nervosa: a randomized, double-blind, placebo-controlled trial. Am J Psychiatry 2008; 165:1281–1288.
8. Leggero C et al. Low-dose olanzapine monotherapy in girls with anorexia nervosa, restricting subtype: focus on hyperactivity. J Child Adolesc Psychopharmacol 2010; 20:127–133.
9. Court A et al. Investigating the effectiveness, safety and tolerability of quetiapine in the treatment of anorexia nervosa in young people: a pilot study. J Psychiatr Res 2010; 44:1027–1034.
10. Powers PS et al. Double-blind placebo-controlled trial of quetiapine in anorexia nervosa. Eur Eat Disord Rev 2012; 20:331–334.
11. Andries A et al. Dronabinol in severe, enduring anorexia nervosa: a randomized controlled trial. Int J Eat Disord 2014; 47:18–23.
12. Connan F et al. Biochemical and endocrine complications. Eur Eat Disord Rev 2007; 8:144–157.
13. Claudino AM et al. Antidepressants for anorexia nervosa. Cochrane Database Syst Rev 2006; CD004365.
14. Barbarich NC et al. Use of nutritional supplements to increase the efficacy of fluoxetine in the treatment of anorexia nervosa. Int J Eat Disord 2004; 35:10–15.
15. Malina A et al. Olanzapine treatment of anorexia nervosa: a retrospective study. Int J Eat Disord 2003; 33:234–237.
16. La Via MC et al. Case reports of olanzapine treatment of anorexia nervosa. Int J Eat Disord 2000; 27:363–366.
17. Su JC et al. Zinc supplementation in the treatment of anorexia nervosa. Eat Weight Disord 2002; 7:20–22.
18. Marrazzi MA et al. Naltrexone use in the treatment of anorexia nervosa and bulimia nervosa. Int Clin Psychopharmacol 1995; 10:163–172.
19. Halmi KA et al. Anorexia nervosa. Treatment efficacy of cyproheptadine and amitriptyline. Arch Gen Psychiatry 1986; 43:177–181.
20. Kaye WH et al. Double-blind placebo-controlled administration of fluoxetine in restricting- and restricting-purging-type anorexia nervosa. Biol Psychiatry 2001; 49:644–652.
21. Walsh BT et al. Fluoxetine after weight restoration in anorexia nervosa: a randomized controlled trial. JAMA 2006; 295:2605–2612.
22. Vocks S et al. Meta-analysis of the effectiveness of psychological and pharmacological treatments for binge eating disorder. Int J Eat Disord 2010; 43:205–217.
23. Fluoxetine Bulimia Nervosa Collaborative Study Group. Fluoxetine in the treatment of bulimia nervosa. A multicenter, placebo-controlled, double-blind trial. Arch Gen Psychiatry 1992; 49:139–147.
24. Goldstein DJ et al. Long-term fluoxetine treatment of bulimia nervosa. Fluoxetine Bulimia Nervosa Research Group. Br J Psychiatry 1995; 166:660–666.
25. Romano SJ et al. A placebo-controlled study of fluoxetine in continued treatment of bulimia nervosa after successful acute fluoxetine treatment. Am J Psychiatry 2002; 159:96–102.
26. Bacaltchuk J et al. Antidepressants versus placebo for people with bulimia nervosa. Cochrane Database Syst Rev 2003; CD003391.
27. Sysko R et al. Early response to antidepressant treatment in bulimia nervosa. Psychol Med 2010; 40:999–1005.
28. Arbaizar B et al. Efficacy of topiramate in bulimia nervosa and binge-eating disorder: a systematic review. Gen Hosp Psychiatry 2008; 30:471–475.
29. White MA et al. Bupropion for overweight women with binge-eating disorder: a randomized, double-blind, placebo-controlled trial. J Clin Psychiatry 2013; 74:400–406.
30. Leombruni P et al. Duloxetine in obese binge eater outpatients: preliminary results from a 12-week open trial. Hum Psychopharmacol 2009; 24:483–488.
31. Guerdjikova AI et al. Lamotrigine in the treatment of binge-eating disorder with obesity: a randomized, placebo-controlled monotherapy trial. Int Clin Psychopharmacol 2009; 24:150–158.
32. Ricca V et al. Zonisamide Combined with Cognitive Behavioral Therapy in Binge Eating Disorder: A One-year Follow-up Study. Psychiatry (Edgmont) 2009; 6:23–28.
33. Guerdjikova AI et al. Zonisamide in the treatment of bulimia nervosa: an open-label, pilot, prospective study. Int J Eat Disord 2013; 46:747–750.
34. McElroy SL et al. Acamprosate in the treatment of binge eating disorder: a placebo-controlled trial. Int J Eat Disord 2011; 44:81–90.
35. McElroy SL et al. Sodium oxybate in the treatment of binge eating disorder: An open-label, prospective study. Int J Eat Disord 2011; 44:262–268.
36. Leombruni P et al. A 12 to 24 weeks pilot study of sertraline treatment in obese women binge eaters. Hum Psychopharmacol 2006; 21:181–188.
37. National Institute for Health and Care Excellence. Eating disorders: surveillance review decision December 2013. 2013. http://www.nice.org.uk/nicemedia/live/10932/66224/66224.pdf.

Further reading

Jackson CW et al. Pharmacotherapy of eating disorders. Nutr Clin Pract 2010; 25:143–159.
Reas DL et al. Review and meta-analysis of pharmacotherapy for binge-eating disorder. Obesity (Silver Spring) 2008; 16:2024–2038.

Acutely disturbed or violent behaviour

Acute behavioural disturbance can occur in the context of psychiatric illness, physical illness, substance abuse or personality disorder. Psychotic symptoms are common and the patient may be aggressive towards others secondary to persecutory delusions or auditory, visual or tactile hallucinations.

The clinical practice of rapid tranquillisation (RT) is used when appropriate psychological and behavioural approaches have failed to de-escalate acutely disturbed behaviour. It is, essentially, a treatment of last resort. Patients who require RT are often too disturbed to give informed consent and therefore participate in RCTs, but, with the use of a number of creative methodologies, the evidence base with respect to the efficacy and tolerability of pharmacological strategies is growing. Recommendations, however, remain based partly on research data, partly on theoretical considerations and partly on clinical experience.

Several studies supporting the efficacy of oral SGAs have been published.[1-4] The level of behavioural disturbance exhibited by the patients in these studies was moderate at most, and all subjects accepted oral treatment (this degree of compliance would be unusual in clinical practice). Note too that patients recruited to these studies received the SGA as antipsychotic monotherapy. The efficacy and safety of adding a second antipsychotic as 'prn' has not been explicitly tested in formal RCTs.

The efficacy of inhaled loxapine (in behavioural disturbance that is moderate in severity) is also supported by RCTs;[5,6] note that use of this preparation requires the co-operation of the patient, and that bronchospasm is an established side-effect.

Larger, placebo-controlled RCTs support the efficacy of IM preparations of olanzapine, ziprasidone and aripiprazole. When considered together these trials suggested that IM olanzapine is more effective than IM haloperidol which in turn is more effective than IM aripiprazole.[7] Again, the level of behavioural disturbance in these studies was moderate at most.

Five large RCTs have investigated the effectiveness of parenteral medication in 'real-life' acutely disturbed patients.

- Compared with IV midazolam alone, a combination of IV olanzapine or IV droperidol with IV midazolam was more rapidly effective and resulted in fewer subsequent doses of medication being required.[8]
- IM midazolam 7.5–15 mg was more rapidly sedating than a combination of haloperidol 5–10 mg and promethazine 50 mg (TREC 1).[9]
- Olanzapine 10 mg was as effective as a combination of haloperidol 10 mg and promethazine 25–50 mg in the short term, but the effect did not last as long (TREC 4).[10]
- A combination of haloperidol 5–10 mg and promethazine 50 mg was more effective and better tolerated than haloperidol 5–10 mg alone (TREC 3).[11]
- A combination of haloperidol 10 mg and promethazine 25–50 mg was more effective than lorazepam 4 mg (TREC 2).[12]

Note that TREC 3[11] found IM haloperidol alone to be poorly tolerated; 6% of patients had an acute dystonic reaction. Cochrane concludes that haloperidol alone is effective in the management of acute behavioural disturbance but poorly tolerated, and that co-administration of promethazine but not lorazepam improves tolerability.[13] However

NICE considers the evidence relating to the use of promethazine for this purpose to be inconclusive.[14]

In a meta-analysis that examined the tolerability of IM antipsychotics when used for the treatment of agitation, the incidence of acute dystonia with haloperidol was reported to be 5%, with SGAs faring considerably better.[15] Acute extrapyramidal symptoms may adversely affect longer-term compliance.[16] In addition, the SPC for haloperidol requires a pre-treatment ECG[17,18] and recommends that concomitant antipsychotics are not prescribed. The mean increase in QTc after 10 mg IM haloperidol has been administered has been reported to be 15 ms but the range is wide.[19] Note that promethazine may inhibit the metabolism of haloperidol;[20] a pharmacokinetic interaction that is potentially clinically significant given the potential of haloperidol to prolong QTc. While this is unlikely to be problematic if a single dose is administered, repeat dosing may confer risk.

A large observational study supports the efficacy and tolerability of IM olanzapine in clinical emergencies (where disturbance was severe).[21]

In an acute psychiatric setting, high dose sedation (defined as a dose of more than 10 mg of haloperidol, droperidol or midazolam in routine clinical practice) was not more effective than lower doses but was associated with more adverse effects (hypotension and oxygen desaturation).[22] Consistent with this, a small RCT supports the efficacy of low dose haloperidol, although both efficacy and tolerability were superior when midazolam was co-prescribed.[23] These data support the use of standard doses in clinical emergencies.

A small observational study supports the effectiveness of buccal midazolam in a psychiatric intensive care unit (PICU) setting.[24] Parenteral administration of midazolam, particularly in higher doses, may cause over-sedation accompanied by respiratory depression.[25] Lorazepam IM is an established treatment and TREC 2[12] supports its efficacy, although combining all results from the TREC studies suggests midazolam 7.5–15 mg is probably more effective. Cochrane supports the efficacy of benzodiazepines when used alone and concludes that there is no advantage of benzodiazepine-antipsychotic combinations over benzodiazepines alone.[26]

With respect to those who are behaviourally disturbed secondary to acute intoxication with alcohol or illicit drugs, there are fewer data to guide practice. A large observational study of IV sedation in patients intoxicated with alcohol found that combination treatment (most commonly haloperidol 5 mg and lorazepam 2 mg) was more effective and reduced the need for subsequent sedation than either drug given alone.[27] A case series (n = 59) of patients who received modest doses of oral, IM or IV haloperidol to manage behavioural disturbance in the context of phencyclidine (PCP) consumption, reported that haloperidol was effective and well tolerated (one case each of mild hypotension and mild hypoxia).[28]

Plans for the management of individual patients should ideally be made in advance. The aim is to prevent disturbed behaviour and reduce risk of violence. Nursing interventions (de-escalation, time out, seclusion[29]), increased nursing levels, transfer of the patient to a PICU and pharmacological management are options that may be employed. Care should be taken to avoid combinations and high cumulative doses of antipsychotic drugs. The monitoring of routine physical observations after RT is essential. Note that RT is often viewed as punitive by patients. There is little research into the patient experience of RT.

The aims of RT are threefold.

- To reduce suffering for the patient: psychological or physical (through self-harm or accidents).
- To reduce risk of harm to others by maintaining a safe environment.
- To do no harm (by prescribing safe regimes and monitoring physical health).

Note: Despite the need for rapid and effective treatment, concomitant use of two or more antipsychotics (antipsychotic polypharmacy) should be avoided on the basis of risk associated with QT prolongation (common to almost all antipsychotics). This is a particularly important consideration in RT where the patient's physical state predisposes to cardiac arrhythmia.

Table 7.29 outlines the interventions to use in an emergency situation. Remedial measures are shown in Table 7.30. Box 7.12 describes physical monitoring requirements in RT; Box 7.13 the use of flumazenil; and Box 7.14 shows guidelines for the use of zuclopenthixol acetate.

Table 7.29 Recommended interventions for patients showing acutely disturbed or violent behaviour

Step	Intervention	Comment
1	De-escalation, time out, placement, etc., as appropriate	
2	Offer **oral** treatment	
	If the patient is prescribed a regular antipsychotic, lorazepam 1–2 mg alone avoids the risks associated with combining antipsychotics	An oral antipsychotic is an option in patients not already taking a regular oral or depot antipsychotic
	Repeat after 45–60 minutes	■ Quetiapine 50–100 mg or
	Monotherapy with **buccal midazolam, 10–20 mg may avoid the need for IM treatment**	■ Olanzapine 10 mg or ■ Risperidone 1–2 mg or ■ Haloperidol 5 mg (best with promethazine 25 mg)
	Note that this preparation is unlicensed	
	Go to step 3 if two doses fail or sooner if the patient is placing themselves or others at significant risk	Note that the SPC for **haloperidol** recommends: ■ **Avoid concomitant antipsychotics** ■ **A pre-treatment ECG**
3	Consider **IM** treatment	
	Lorazepam 2 mg[a,b]	Have flumazenil to hand in case of benzodiazepine-induced respiratory depression
	Promethazine 50 mg[c]	IM promethazine is a useful option in a benzodiazepine-tolerant patient
	Olanzapine 10 mg[d]	IM olanzapine should NOT be combined with an IM benzodiazepine, particularly if alcohol has been consumed[30]
	Aripiprazole 9.75 mg	Less hypotension than olanzapine, but possibly less effective[3,7,31]
	Haloperidol 5 mg	**Haloperidol should be the last drug considered** ■ The incidence of acute dystonia is high; combine with IM promethazine and ensure IM procyclidine is available
	Repeat after 30–60 minutes if insufficient effect	■ The SPC recommends a pre-treatment ECG

(Continued)

CHAPTER 7

Table 7.29 (*Continued*)

Step	Intervention	Comment
4	Consider **IV** treatment Diazepam 10 mg over at least 5 minutes[b,e] Repeat after 5–10 minutes if insufficient effect (up to 3 times) Have flumazenil to hand	
5	**Seek advice** from a senior psychiatrist or senior clinical pharmacist[f]	

[a] Carefully check administration instructions, which differ between manufacturers. With respect to Ativan (the most commonly used preparation), mix lorazepam 1:1 with water for injections before injecting. Some centres use 2–4 mg. An alternative is midazolam 7.5–15 mg. The risk of respiratory depression is dose-related with both but generally greater with midazolam.

[b] Caution in the very young and elderly and those with pre-existing brain damage or impulse control problems, as disinhibition reactions are more likely.[32]

[c] Promethazine has a slow onset of action but is often an effective sedative. Dilution is not required before IM injection. May be repeated up to a maximum of 100 mg/day. Wait 1–2 hours after injection to assess response. Note that promethazine alone has been reported, albeit very rarely, to cause NMS[33] although it is an extremely weak dopamine antagonist. Note the potential pharmacokinetic interaction between promethazine and haloperidol (reduced metabolism of haloperidol) which may confer risk if repeated doses of both are administered.

[d] Recommended by NICE only for moderate behavioural disturbance, but data from a large observational study also support efficacy in clinical emergencies.

[e] Use Diazemuls to avoid injection site reactions. IV therapy may be used instead of IM when a very rapid effect is required. IV therapy also ensures near immediate delivery of the drug to its site of action and effectively avoids the danger of inadvertent accumulation of slowly absorbed IM doses. Note also that IV doses can be repeated after only 5–10 minutes if no effect is observed.

[f] Options at this point are limited. IM amylobarbitone and paraldehyde have been used in the past but are used now only extremely rarely. ECT is probably a better option. Behavioural disturbance secondary to the use of illicit drugs can be very difficult to manage. Time and supportive care may be safer than administering more sedative medication.

Box 7.12 Rapid tranquillisation: physical monitoring

After any parenteral drug administration, monitor as follows:

- temperature
- pulse
- blood pressure
- respiratory rate

every 10 minutes for 1 hour, and then half-hourly until the patient is ambulatory. Patients who refuse to have their vital signs monitored, or who remain too behaviourally disturbed to be approached, should be observed for signs/symptoms of pyrexia, hypotension, over-sedation and general physical wellbeing.

If the patient is asleep or **unconscious**, the continuous use of pulse oximetry to measure oxygen saturation is desirable. A nurse should remain with the patient until ambulatory.

ECG and haematological monitoring are also strongly recommended when parenteral antipsychotics are given, especially when higher doses are used.[34,35] Hypokalaemia, stress and agitation place the patient at risk of cardiac arrhythmia[36] (see section on 'QT prolongation' in Chapter 2). ECG monitoring is formally recommended for all patients who receive haloperidol.

Table 7.30 Remedial measures in rapid tranquillisation

Problem	Remedial measures
Acute dystonia (including oculogyric crises)	Give **procyclidine** 5–10 mg IM or IV
Reduced respiratory rate (<10/min) or oxygen saturation (<90%)	Give oxygen, raise legs, ensure patient is not lying face down
	Give **flumazenil** if benzodiazepine-induced respiratory depression suspected
	If induced by any other sedative agent: **transfer to a medical bed and ventilate mechanically**
Irregular or slow (<50/min) **pulse**	**Refer** to specialist medical care immediately
Fall in blood pressure (>30 mmHg orthostatic drop or <50 mmHg diastolic)	**Have patient lie flat**, tilt bed towards head. Monitor closely
Increased temperature	**Withold antipsychotics** (risk of NMS and perhaps arrhythmia). Check creatinine kinase urgently

IM, intramuscular; IV, intravenous; NMS, neuroleptic malignant syndrome.

Box 7.13 Guidelines for the use of flumazenil

Indication for use	If, after the administration of lorazepam, midazolam or diazepam, respiratory rate falls below 10/minute.
Contraindications	Patients with epilepsy who have been receiving long-term benzodiazepines.
Caution	Dose should be carefully titrated in hepatic impairment.
Dose and route of administration	*Initial:* 200 μg *intravenously* over 15 seconds – if required level of consciousness not achieved after 60 seconds, then, *subsequent dose:* 100 μg over 10 seconds.
Time before dose can be repeated	60 seconds.
Maximum dose	1 mg in 24 hours (one initial dose and eight subsequent doses).
Side-effects	Patients may become agitated, anxious or fearful on awakening. Seizures may occur in regular benzodiazepine users.
Management	Side-effects usually subside.
Monitoring	
What to monitor?	Respiratory rate
How often?	Continuously until respiratory rate returns to baseline level. Flumazenil has a short half-life (much shorter than diazepam) and respiratory function may recover and then deteriorate again.
	Note: If respiratory rate does not return to normal or patient is not alert after initial doses given, assume that sedation is due to some other cause.

> **Box 7.14** Guidelines for the use of Clopixol Acuphase (zuclopenthixol acetate)
>
> Acuphase should be used only after an acutely psychotic patient has required *repeated* injections of short-acting antipsychotic drugs such as haloperidol or olanzapine, or sedative drugs such as lorazepam. It is perhaps best reserved for those few patients who have a prior history of good response to Acuphase.
>
> Acuphase should be given only when enough time has elapsed to assess the full response to previously injected drugs: allow 15 minutes after IV injections; 60 minutes after IM.
>
> Acuphase should **never** be administered:
> - in an attempt to 'hasten' the antipsychotic effect of other antipsychotic therapy
> - for rapid tranquillisation (onset of effect is too slow)
> - at the same time as other parenteral antipsychotics or benzodiazepines (may lead to over-sedation which is difficult to reverse)
> - as a 'test dose' for zuclopenthixol decanoate depot
> - to a patient who is physically resistant (risk of intravasation and oil embolus).
>
> Acuphase should **never** be used for, or in, the following:
> - patients who accept oral medication
> - patients who are neuroleptic-naïve
> - patients who are sensitive to EPS
> - patients who are unconscious
> - patients who are pregnant
> - those with hepatic or renal impairment
> - those with cardiac disease.
>
> **Onset and duration of action**
> Sedative effects usually begin to be seen 2 hours after injection and peak after 12 hours. The effects may last for up to 72 hours. Note: Acuphase has no place in rapid tranquillisation: *its action is not rapid*. Cochrane concludes that Acuphase has no advantages over other options in the immediate management of an episode of behavioural disturbance but that patients who receive this preparation may need fewer subsequent injections in the medium term (7 days).[37]
>
> **Dose**
> Acuphase should be given in a dose of 50–150 mg (note there is no evidence to support any advantage of higher over lower doses),[37] up to a maximum of 400 mg over a 2-week period. This maximum duration ensures that a treatment plan is put in place. It does not indicate that there are known harmful effects from more prolonged administration, although such use should be very exceptional. There is no such thing as a 'course of Acuphase'. The patient should be assessed before each administration.
>
> Injections should be spaced at least 24 hours apart.
>
> Note: zuclopenthixol acetate was formerly widely misused as a sort of 'chemical straitjacket'. In reality it is a potentially toxic preparation with very little published information to support its use.[37]

References

1. Currier GW et al. Acute treatment of psychotic agitation: a randomized comparison of oral treatment with risperidone and lorazepam versus intramuscular treatment with haloperidol and lorazepam. J Clin Psychiatry 2004; **65**:386–394.
2. Ganesan S et al. Effectiveness of quetiapine for the management of aggressive psychosis in the emergency psychiatric setting: a naturalistic uncontrolled trial. Int J Psychiatry Clin Pract 2005; **9**:199–203.
3. Simpson JR, Jr. et al. Impact of orally disintegrating olanzapine on use of intramuscular antipsychotics, seclusion, and restraint in an acute inpatient psychiatric setting. J Clin Psychopharmacol 2006; **26**:333–335.
4. Hsu WY et al. Comparison of intramuscular olanzapine, orally disintegrating olanzapine tablets, oral risperidone solution, and intramuscular haloperidol in the management of acute agitation in an acute care psychiatric ward in Taiwan. J Clin Psychopharmacol 2010; **30**:230–234.

5. Lesem MD et al. Rapid acute treatment of agitation in individuals with schizophrenia: multicentre, randomised, placebo-controlled study of inhaled loxapine. Br J Psychiatry 2011; **198**:51–58.

6. Kwentus J et al. Rapid acute treatment of agitation in patients with bipolar I disorder: a multicenter, randomized, placebo-controlled clinical trial with inhaled loxapine. Bipolar Disord 2012; **14**:31–40.

7. Citrome L. Comparison of intramuscular ziprasidone, olanzapine, or aripiprazole for agitation: a quantitative review of efficacy and safety. J Clin Psychiatry 2007; **68**:1876–1885.

8. Chan EW et al. Intravenous droperidol or olanzapine as an adjunct to midazolam for the acutely agitated patient: a multicenter, randomized, double-blind, placebo-controlled clinical trial. Ann Emerg Med 2013; **61**:72–81.

9. TREC Collaborative Group. Rapid tranquillisation for agitated patients in emergency psychiatric rooms: a randomised trial of midazolam versus haloperidol plus promethazine. BMJ 2003; **327**:708–713.

10. Raveendran NS et al. Rapid tranquillisation in psychiatric emergency settings in India: pragmatic randomised controlled trial of intramuscular olanzapine versus intramuscular haloperidol plus promethazine. BMJ 2007; **335**:865.

11. Huf G et al. Rapid tranquillisation in psychiatric emergency settings in Brazil: pragmatic randomised controlled trial of intramuscular haloperidol versus intramuscular haloperidol plus promethazine. BMJ 2007; **335**:869.

12. Alexander J et al. Rapid tranquillisation of violent or agitated patients in a psychiatric emergency setting. Pragmatic randomised trial of intramuscular lorazepam v. haloperidol plus promethazine. Br J Psychiatry 2004; **185**:63–69.

13. Powney MJ et al. Haloperidol for psychosis-induced aggression or agitation (rapid tranquillisation). Cochrane Database Syst Rev 2012; **11**: CD009377.

14. National Institute for Health and Care Excellence. Evidence Summaries: Unlicensed/Off-Label Medicines: Rapid tranquillisation in mental health settings: promethazine hydrochloride (ESUOM 28), 2014. http://www.nice.org.uk/

15. Satterthwaite TD et al. A meta-analysis of the risk of acute extrapyramidal symptoms with intramuscular antipsychotics for the treatment of agitation. J Clin Psychiatry 2008; **69**:1869–1879.

16. van Harten PN et al. Acute dystonia induced by drug treatment. Br Med J 1999; **319**:623–626.

17. Pharmacovigilance Working Party. Public Assessment Report on Neuroleptics and Cardiac safety, in particular QT prolongation, cardiac arrhythmias, ventricular tachycardia and torsades de pointes, 2006. http://www.mhra.gov.uk

18. Janssen-Cilag Ltd. *Summary of Product Characteristics*. Haldol Injection, 2014. https://www.medicines.org.uk/

19. Miceli JJ et al. Effects of high-dose ziprasidone and haloperidol on the QTc interval after intramuscular administration: a randomized, single-blind, parallel-group study in patients with schizophrenia or schizoaffective disorder. Clin Ther 2010; **32**:472–491.

20. Suzuki A et al. Histamine H1-receptor antagonists, promethazine and homochlorcyclizine, increase the steady-state plasma concentrations of haloperidol and reduced haloperidol. Ther Drug Monit 2003; **25**:192–196.

21. Perrin E et al. A prospective, observational study of the safety and effectiveness of intramuscular psychotropic treatment in acutely agitated patients with schizophrenia and bipolar mania. Eur Psychiatry 2012; **27**:234–239.

22. Calver L et al. A prospective study of high dose sedation for rapid tranquilisation of acute behavioural disturbance in an acute mental health unit. BMC Psychiatry 2013; **13**:225.

23. Mantovani C et al. Are low doses of antipsychotics effective in the management of psychomotor agitation? A randomized, rated-blind trial of 4 intramuscular interventions. J Clin Psychopharmacol 2013; **33**:306–312.

24. Taylor D et al. Buccal midazolam for rapid tranquillisation. Int J Psychiatry Clin Pract 2008; **12**:309–311.

25. Spain D et al. Safety and effectiveness of high-dose midazolam for severe behavioural disturbance in an emergency department with suspected psychostimulant-affected patients. Emerg Med Australas 2008; **20**:112–120.

26. Gillies D et al. Benzodiazepines for psychosis-induced aggression or agitation. Cochrane Database Syst Rev 2013; **9**: CD003079.

27. Li SF et al. Safety and efficacy of intravenous combination sedatives in the ED. Am J Emerg Med 2013; **31**:1402–1404.

28. MacNeal JJ et al. Use of haloperidol in PCP-intoxicated individuals. Clin Toxicol (Phila) 2012; **50**:851–853.

29. Huf G et al. Physical restraints versus seclusion room for management of people with acute aggression or agitation due to psychotic illness (TREC-SAVE): a randomized trial. Psychol Med 2012; **42**:2265–2273.

30. Wilson MP et al. Potential complications of combining intramuscular olanzapine with benzodiazepines in emergency department patients. J Emerg Med 2012; **43**:889–896.

31. Villari V et al. Oral risperidone, olanzapine and quetiapine versus haloperidol in psychotic agitation. Prog Neuropsychopharmacol Biol Psychiatry 2008; **32**:405–413.

32. Paton C. Benzodiazepines and disinhibition: a review. Psychiatr Bull 2002; **26**:460–462.

33. Chan-Tack KM. Neuroleptic malignant syndrome due to promethazine. South Med J 1999; **92**:1017–1018.

34. Appleby L et al. Sudden unexplained death in psychiatric in-patients. Br J Psychiatry 2000; **176**:405–406.

35. Yap YG et al. Risk of torsades de pointes with non-cardiac drugs. Doctors need to be aware that many drugs can cause QT prolongation. BMJ 2000; **320**:1158–1159.

36. Taylor DM. Antipsychotics and QT prolongation. Acta Psychiatr Scand 2003; **107**:85–95.

37. Jayakody K et al. Zuclopenthixol acetate for acute schizophrenia and similar serious mental illnesses. Cochrane Database Syst Rev 2012; **4**: CD000525.

Further reading

National Institute for Health and Clinical Excellence. Violence – The short-term management of disturbed/violent behaviour in in-patient psychiatric settings and emergency departments. Clinical Guideline 25, 2005. www.nice.org.uk

Borderline personality disorder

Borderline personality disorder (BPD) is common in psychiatric settings with a reported prevalence of up to 20%.[2] In BPD, co-morbid depression, anxiety spectrum disorders and bipolar illness occur more frequently than would be expected by chance association alone, and the lifetime risk of having at least one co-morbid mental disorder approaches 100%.[3] The suicide rate in BPD is similar to that seen in affective disorders and schizophrenia.[4,5]

Although it is classified as a personality disorder, several 'symptoms' of BPD may intuitively be expected to respond to drug treatment. These include affective instability, transient stress-related psychotic symptoms, suicidal and self-harming behaviours, and impulsivity.[5] A high proportion of people with BPD are prescribed psychotropic drugs.[3,6,7] The prevalence of prescribing of antipsychotics, antidepressants and mood stabilisers in those with borderline personality disorder as a sole psychiatric diagnosis is not notably different than in those with borderline personality disorder and a co-morbid diagnosis of schizophrenia, depression or bipolar disorder respectively[7]. No drug is specifically licensed for the treatment of BPD.

NICE[1] recommend that:

- drug treatment should not be used routinely for borderline personality disorder or for the individual symptoms or behaviour associated with the disorder (for example, repeated self-harm, marked emotional instability, risk-taking behaviour and transient psychotic symptoms
- drug treatment may be considered in the overall treatment of co-morbid conditions
- short-term use of sedative medication may be considered as part of the overall treatment plan for people with borderline personality disorder in a crisis. The duration of treatment should be agreed with them but should be no longer than one week.

Since the publication of the NICE guideline for BPD, two further independent systematic reviews have been published.[8,9] Essentially the same studies were considered in all three reviews and where numerical data were combined in meta-analyses the results of these analyses were similar across all three systematic reviews. In addition, all noted that the majority of studies of drug treatment in BPD last for only 6 weeks and that the large number of different outcome measures that were used made it difficult to evaluate and compare studies.

NICE considered that the data were not robust enough to be the basis for recommendations to the NHS while the other two reviews concluded that some of the analyses showed promising results and that these were sufficiently cogent to inform clinical practice.

Antipsychotics

Open studies have found benefit for a number of first and second-generation antipsychotics over a wide range of symptoms. In contrast, placebo-controlled RCTs generally show more modest benefits for active drug over placebo. The symptoms/symptom clusters that may respond are affect dysregulation, impulsivity and cognitive-perceptual symptoms.[8-10] Open studies report reductions in aggression and self-harming behaviour with clozapine[11–13] and clozapine has been shown to have an anti-aggressive effect in people with schizophrenia.[14] A recent RCT showed clinically significant efficacy for quetiapine 150 mg/day.[15] Antipsychotic medications are associated with a wide range of adverse effects (see Chapter 2).

Antidepressants

Several open studies have found that SSRIs reduce impulsivity and aggression in BPD, but these findings have not been replicated in RCTs. It can be concluded with reasonable certainty that there is no robust evidence to support the use of antidepressants in treating depressed mood or impulsivity in people with BPD.[8,9]

Mood stabilisers

Up to a half of people with BPD may also have a bipolar spectrum disorder[16] and mood stabilisers are commonly prescribed.[3] There is some evidence that mood stabilisers reduce impulsivity, anger, and affect dysregulation in people with BPD.[8,9] Lithium is licensed for the control of aggressive behaviour or intentional self-harm.[17] A large RCT of lamotrigine is currently recruiting in the UK.[18]

Management of crisis

Drug treatments are often used during periods of crisis when 'symptoms' can be severe, distressing and potentially life-threatening. By their very nature, these symptoms can be expected to wax and wane.[4] Drug therapy may then be required intermittently. It is generally easy to see when treatment is required, but much more difficult to decide when modest gains are worthwhile and whether or not continuation is likely to be necessary.

NICE[1] recommend that during periods of crisis, time-limited treatment with a sedative drug may be helpful. Anticipated side-effect profile and potential toxicity in overdose should guide choice. For example, benzodiazepines (particularly short-acting drugs) can cause disinhibition in this group of patients,[19] potentially compounding problems; sedative antipsychotics can cause EPS and/or considerable weight gain (see section on 'Antipsychotics and weight gain' in Chapter 2), and tricyclic antidepressants are particularly toxic in overdose (see section on 'Psychotropics in overdose' in Chapter 8). A sedative antihistamine such as promethazine is quite well tolerated and may be a helpful short-term treatment when used as part of a co-ordinated care plan. Its adverse effects (dry mouth, constipation) and lack of clear anxiolytic effects may militate against longer term use.

References

1. National Institute for Health and Clinical Excellence. Borderline personality disorder: treatment and management. Clinical Guideline 78, 2009. http://www.nice.org.uk
2. Kernberg OF et al. Borderline personality disorder. Am J Psychiatry 2009; **166**:505–508.
3. Pascual JC et al. A naturalistic study of changes in pharmacological prescription for borderline personality disorder in clinical practice: from APA to NICE guidelines. Int Clin Psychopharmacol 2010; **25**:349–355.

4. Links PS et al. Prospective follow-up study of borderline personality disorder: prognosis, prediction of outcome, and Axis II comorbidity. Can J Psychiatry 1998; **43**:265–270.

5. Oldham JM. Guideline watch: practice guideline for the treatment of patients with borderline personality disorder. Focus 2005; **3**:396–400.

6. Baker-Glenn E et al. Use of psychotropic medication among psychiatric out-patients with personality disorder. Psychiatrist 2010; **34**:83–86.

7. Paton C. Prescribing for people with emotionally unstable personality disorder under the care of UK mental health services. J Clin Psychiatry 2014; submitted.

8. Lieb K et al. Pharmacotherapy for borderline personality disorder: Cochrane systematic review of randomised trials. Br J Psychiatry 2010; **196**:4–12.

9. Ingenhoven T et al. Effectiveness of pharmacotherapy for severe personality disorders: meta-analyses of randomized controlled trials. J Clin Psychiatry 2010; **71**:14–25.

10. Zanarini MC et al. A dose comparison of olanzapine for the treatment of borderline personality disorder: a 12-week randomized, double-blind, placebo-controlled study. J Clin Psychiatry 2011; **72**:1353–1362.

11. Benedetti F et al. Low-dose clozapine in acute and continuation treatment of severe borderline personality disorder. J Clin Psychiatry 1998; **59**:103–107.

12. Frogley C et al. A case series of clozapine for borderline personality disorder. Ann Clin Psychiatry 2013; **25**:125–134.

13. Chengappa KN et al. Clozapine reduces severe self-mutilation and aggression in psychotic patients with borderline personality disorder. J Clin Psychiatry 1999; **60**:477–484.

14. Volavka J et al. Heterogeneity of violence in schizophrenia and implications for long-term treatment. Int J Clin Pract 2008; **62**:1237–1245.

15. Black DW et al. Comparison of low and moderate doses of extended-release quetiapine in borderline personality disorder: a randomized, double-blind, placebo-controlled trial. Am J Psych 2014; **171**:1174–1182.

16. Deltito J et al. Do patients with borderline personality disorder belong to the bipolar spectrum? J Affect Disord 2001; **67**:221–228.

17. Sanofi. Summary of product characteristics. Priadel 400 mg prolonged release tablets, 2014. https://www.medicines.org.uk/

18. NHS National Institute for Health Research, Imperial College London. LABILE Clinical Trial - Lamotrigine and borderline personality disorder: investigating long-term effectiveness, 2013. http://www.labile.org/

19. Gardner DL et al. Alprazolam-induced dyscontrol in borderline personality disorder. Am J Psychiatry 1985; **142**:98–100.

Further reading

National Health and Medical Research Council. Clinical practice guideline for the management of borderline personality disorder. MH25, 2012. https://www.nhmrc.gov.au/guidelines/publications/mh25

Ripoll LH et al. Evidence-based pharmacotherapy for personality disorders. Int J Neuropsychopharmacol 2011; **14**:1257–1288.

Learning disabilities

General considerations[1]

Prescribing psychotropic medications for people with learning disabilities (LD) is a challenging and controversial area of psychiatric practice.[2,3] There are concerns that psychotropic drugs of all kinds (antipsychotics, antidepressants, benzodiazepines, both regular and as required, and anticonvulsants as mood stabilisers) are overprescribed with poor review and assessment of their benefit.

Although prescribing for individuals with mild or borderline intellectual impairment may be undertaken by mainstream mental health services, the assessment and treatment of behavioural and emotional disorders in people with more marked (or, as in the case of autism, atypical patterns of significant cognitive impairment) should be undertaken in the first instance by, or at least in consultation with, specialist clinicians.

The term 'dual diagnosis' in this context refers to the co-occurrence of an identifiable psychiatric disorder (mental illness, personality disorder) and LD. 'Diagnostic overshadowing' is the misattribution of emotional or behavioural problems to LD itself rather than a co-morbid condition. LD is an important risk factor for all psychiatric disorders (including dementia, particularly for individuals with Down's syndrome).[4] Where it is possible to diagnose a mental illness using conventional or modified criteria then drug treatment in the first instance should, in general, be similar to that in the population at large. Most treatment guidelines are increasingly stating their intended applicability to people with LD in this regard.

Mental illness may initially present in unusual ways, e.g. depression as self-injurious behaviour, persecutory ideation as complaints of being 'picked on'. Conversely, behaviours such as self-talk may be normal in some individuals but mistakenly identified as psychosis. In general, diagnosis becomes increasingly complex with severity of disability and associated communication impairment.

Co-morbid autistic spectrum disorder has special assessment considerations and in its own right is an important risk factor for psychiatric disorder, in particular anxiety and depression, bipolar spectrum disorder, severe obsessional behaviour, anger disorders and psychosis-like episodes that may not meet criteria for schizophrenia but nonetheless require treatment. Autistic traits are common amongst patients using LD services.

Key practice areas

Capacity and consent: it is uncommon for patients in LD services (who often represent a sub-population of those identified with special educational needs in childhood) to have sufficient understanding of their treatment in order to be able to make truly informed decisions, and there is inevitably an increased onus on the clinician to bear the weight of decision-making. Decision-making capacity, depending on the severity of intellectual impairment, may be improved through appropriate verbal and written communication. The involvement of carers in this process is generally essential.

Physical co-morbidity, especially epilepsy: epilepsy is over-represented in LD populations, becoming more prevalent as severity increases with approximately one third of

Table 7.31 Current and historically-used medications for behaviour disorder

Drug class	Clinical applications	Notes
Antipsychotics[5]	Used across a broad range of behavioural disturbances. Most consistently useful for aggression and irritability	The most widely used yet most controversial medication for behavioural problems.[6,7] Although a recent RCT[8] cast doubt on their efficacy the study was not without its problems and there is a significant body of other evidence supporting their use including a number of small RCTs in children with LD Discontinuation studies in long-term treatment commonly show re-emergence of problem behaviours Before the advent of atypicals the best evidence was for **haloperidol**[9] in the context of autism and for zuclopenthixol for behavioural disturbance[10] The best evidence is for **risperidone**[11,12] at low dose (0.5–2 mg) for aggression and mood instability **(now licensed for short-term use)**, particularly with associated autism though in non-autistic cases also. **Aripiprazole** has a FDA licence for behavioural disturbance in young people with autism[13,14] Some evidence to support **olanzapine**[15] and case reports of **clozapine**[16] for very severe cases of aggression though not widely used and unlikely to emerge outside highly specialist (inpatient) settings Results for **quetiapine** are modest at best[17]
SSRIs	Helpful for severe anxiety and obsessionality in autistic spectrum disorder. Use here is off-licence unless an additional diagnosis of anxiety disorder or OCD is made. Also used as a first-line alternative to antipsychotics for aggression and impulsivity	Commonly used in combination with antipsychotics though limited evidence base for combination treatment. Effectiveness in absence of mood or anxiety-spectrum disorder is unclear, however, and recent Cochrane Review pessimistic[18] about the evidence for their effectiveness for behaviour disorder in autistic children (who may be at heightened risk of adverse effects), though a little more encouraging in adults. Note quality of trials poor and effects may be exaggerated by use in less severe cases.[19] Caution needed because of the risk of precipitation of hypomania in this population.[20] Also major concerns about overprescribing
Anticonvulsants[21]	Aggression and self-injury	Some uncontrolled studies supporting **sodium valproate**[22] in LD populations though evidence not strong and research findings contradictory in this population. However, remains best supported of the anticonvulsants for mood lability and aggression partly because of positive studies in the non-LD groups[23] Limited studies of **lamotrigine**, mostly in children, suggest no effect, at least in autism and in the absence of affective instability[17] Data for **carbamazepine** also unconvincing, but it is still widely used[24]

Table 7.31 (Continued)

Drug class	Clinical applications	Notes
Lithium[25]	Licensed for the treatment of self-injurious behaviour and aggression	Some RCT evidence[26] for LD but no studies in this population for many years, although there has been one more recent positive RCT for aggression in adolescents without developmental impairment.[27] Experience suggests lithium can be very helpful in individual cases where other treatments have failed and is possibly underused though side-effects can be problematic. Perhaps best considered where there is a sub-syndromal or nonspecific 'affective component'. Some authorities suggest that, on close examination, challenging behaviour may occur in the context of very rapid cycling bipolar disorder in some individuals with severe and profound learning disability and that the diagnosis is easily missed
Naltrexone[28]	Has been used for severe self-injurious behaviour[29]	Evidence not strong and results are inconsistent. Use may still be an option in severe and intractable cases

FDA, Food and Drug Administration; LD, learning disability; OCD, obsessive compulsive disorder; RCT, randomised controlled trial; SSRI, selective serotonin reuptake inhibitor.

affected individuals developing a seizure disorder by early adulthood. Special consideration is needed when considering the use of medications that may lower seizure threshold.

Assessment of care environments: behavioural and emotional disturbance may sometimes be a reflection of problems or failings in the care environment. Different staff in a care home may have different thresholds of tolerance (or make different attributions) for these difficulties which can lead to varied reports of their significance and impact. Allowing for a period of prospective assessment and using simple assessment tools, (for example, simple ABC or sleep charts) can be very helpful to the clinician in making judgements about recommending medication. If medication is used in a care home, staff may need special education in its use and anticipated side-effects and, for 'as required' medications, clear guidelines for its use. This may make it difficult to initiate certain treatments in the community.

Side-effect sensitivity: it is widely thought that people with LD are especially sensitive to side-effects of psychotropics and more at risk of long-term effects such as the metabolic syndrome, however this is not supported by study evidence. It is good practice to start at lower doses and increase more slowly than might be usual in general psychiatric practice. Notable side effects include worsening of seizures, sedation, extrapyramidal reactions (including with risperidone at normal doses, especially in individuals who already have mobility problems), problems with swallowing (with clozapine and other antipsychotics) and worsening of cognitive function with anticholinergic medications (see section on 'Prescribing in dementia' in this chapter).

Psychological interventions: in the absence of an identifiable mental illness (including atypical presentations) with clear treatment implications, psychological interventions such as functional behavioural analysis should be considered as first-line intervention for all but the most serious or intractable presentations of behavioural disturbance. In studies where it has been possible to infer severity of challenging behaviour treatment, response is generally associated with more severe problems at baseline.

Table 7.31 shows current and historically-used medications for behaviour disorder in people with learning disabilities.

References

1. Deb S. The use of medications for the management of problem behaviours in adults who has Intellectual [Learning] Disabilities, 2012. http://www.intellectualdisability.info/mental-health/the-use-of-drugs-for-the-treatment-of-behaviour-disorders-in-adults-who-have-learning-intellectual-disabilities
2. Tyrer P et al. Drug treatments in people with intellectual disability and challenging behaviour. BMJ 2014; 349:g4323.
3. Glover G et al. Use of medication for challenging behaviour in people with intellectual disability. Br J Psychiatry 2014; 205:6–7.
4. Cooper SA et al. Mental ill-health in adults with intellectual disabilities: prevalence and associated factors. Br J Psychiatry 2007; 190:27–35.
5. Antochi R et al. Psychopharmacological treatments in persons with dual diagnosis of psychiatric disorders and developmental disabilities. Postgrad Med J 2003; 79:139–146.
6. Deb S et al. The effectiveness of antipsychotic medication in the management of behaviour problems in adults with intellectual disabilities. J Intellect Disabil Res 2007; 51:766–777.
7. Roy D et al. Pharmacologic Management of Aggression in Adults with Intellectual Disability. J Intellect Disabil Res 2013; 1:28–43.
8. Tyrer P et al. Risperidone, haloperidol, and placebo in the treatment of aggressive challenging behaviour in patients with intellectual disability: a randomised controlled trial. Lancet 2008; 371:57–63.
9. Malone RP et al. The role of antipsychotics in the management of behavioural symptoms in children and adolescents with autism. Drugs 2009; 69:535–548.
10. Malt UF et al. Effectiveness of zuclopenthixol compared with haloperidol in the treatment of behavioural disturbances in learning disabled patients. Br J Psychiatry 1995; 166:374–377.
11. Nagaraj R et al. Risperidone in children with autism: randomized, placebo-controlled, double-blind study. J Child Neurol 2006; 21:450–455.
12. Pandina GJ et al. Risperidone improves behavioral symptoms in children with autism in a randomized, double-blind, placebo-controlled trial. J Autism Dev Disord 2007; 37:367–373.
13. Owen R et al. Aripiprazole in the treatment of irritability in children and adolescents with autistic disorder. Pediatrics 2009; 124:1533–1540.
14. Marcus RN et al. A placebo-controlled, fixed-dose study of aripiprazole in children and adolescents with irritability associated with autistic disorder. J Am Acad Child Adolesc Psychiatry 2009; 48:1110–1119.
15. Fido A et al. Olanzapine in the treatment of behavioral problems associated with autism: an open-label trial in Kuwait. Med Princ Pract 2008; 17:415–418.
16. Zuddas A et al. Clinical effects of clozapine on autistic disorder. Am J Psychiatry 1996; 153:738.
17. Stigler KA et al. Pharmacotherapy of irritability in pervasive developmental disorders. Child Adolesc Psychiatr Clin N Am 2008; 17:739–752.
18. Williams K et al. Selective serotonin reuptake inhibitors (SSRIs) for autism spectrum disorders (ASD). Cochrane Database Syst Rev 2013; 8: CD004677.
19. Myers SM. Citalopram not effective for repetitive behaviour in autistic spectrum disorders. Evid Based Ment Health 2010; 13:22.
20. Cook EH, Jr. et al. Fluoxetine treatment of children and adults with autistic disorder and mental retardation. J Am Acad Child Adolesc Psychiatry 1992; 31:739–745.
21. Deb S et al. The effectiveness of mood stabilizers and antiepileptic medication for the management of behaviour problems in adults with intellectual disability: a systematic review. J Intellect Disabil Res 2008; 52:107–113.
22. Ruedrich S et al. Effect of divalproex sodium on aggression and self-injurious behaviour in adults with intellectual disability: a retrospective review. J Intellect Disabil Res 1999; 43 (Pt 2):105–111.
23. Donovan SJ et al. Divalproex treatment for youth with explosive temper and mood lability: a double-blind, placebo-controlled crossover design. Am J Psychiatry 2000; 157:818–820.
24. Unwin GL et al. Use of medication for the management of behavior problems among adults with intellectual disabilities: a clinicians' consensus survey. Am J Ment Retard 2008; 113:19–31.
25. Pary RJ. Towards defining adequate lithium trials for individuals with mental retardation and mental illness. Am J Ment Retard 1991; 95:681–691.
26. Craft M et al. Lithium in the treatment of aggression in mentally handicapped patients. A double-blind trial. Br J Psychiatry 1987; 150:685–689.
27. Malone RP et al. A double-blind placebo-controlled study of lithium in hospitalized aggressive children and adolescents with conduct disorder. Arch Gen Psychiatry 2000; 57:649–654.
28. Campbell M et al. Naltrexone in autistic children: an acute open dose range tolerance trial. J Am Acad Child Adolesc Psychiatry 1989; 28:200–206.
29. Barrett RP et al. Effects of naloxone and naltrexone on self-injury: a double-blind, placebo-controlled analysis. Am J Ment Retard 1989; 93:644–651.

Delirium

Delirium is a common neuropsychiatric condition that presents in medical and surgical settings and is known by various names including organic brain syndrome, intensive care psychosis and acute confusional state.[1]

Diagnostic criteria for delirium[2]

- Disturbance of *consciousness* (reduced clarity of awareness of the environment) with reduced ability to focus, sustain or shift attention.
- A change in *cognition* (such as memory deficit, disorientation, language disturbance or perceptual disturbance) not better explained by a pre-existing or evolving dementia.
- The disturbance develops over a *short period of time* (usually hours to days) and tends to fluctuate over the course of the day.
- There is often evidence from the history, physical examination or laboratory findings that the disturbance is due to concomitant medications, a medical condition, substance intoxication or substance withdrawal.

Tools for evaluation[3]

A brief cognitive assessment should be included in the examination of patients at risk of delirium. A standardised tool, the Confusion Assessment Method (CAM) is a brief, validated algorithm currently used to diagnose delirium. CAM relies on the presence of acute onset of symptoms, fluctuating course, inattention and either disorganised thinking or an altered level of consciousness.

Clinical subtypes of delirium[4-6]

- **Hyperactive delirium:** characterised by increased motor activity with agitation, hallucinations and inappropriate behaviour.
- **Hypoactive delirium:** characterised by reduced motor activity and lethargy (has a poorer prognosis).
- **Mixed delirium:** features of both increased and reduced motor activity.

Prevalence

Delirium is present in 10% of hospitalised medical patients and a further 10–30% develop delirium after admission.[4] Postoperative delirium occurs in 15–53% of patients and in 70–87% of those in intensive care.[7]

Risk factors

Delirium is almost invariably multifactorial and it is often inappropriate to isolate a single precipitant as the cause.[4] The most important risk factors have consistently emerged as:[4,5,8,9]

- prior cognitive impairment or dementia
- older age (>65 years)

- multiple comorbidities
- previous history of delirium, stroke, neurological disease, falls or gait disorder
- psychoactive drug use
- polypharmacy (>4 medications)
- anticholinergic drug use.

Outcome

Patients with delirium have an increased length of hospital stay, increased mortality and increased risk of long-term institutional placement.[1,5] Hospital mortality rates of patients with delirium range from 6% to 18% and are twice that of matched controls.[5] The one-year mortality rate associated with cases of delirium is 35–40%.[7] Up to 60% of individuals suffer persistent cognitive impairment following delirium and these patients are also three times more likely to develop dementia.[1,5]

Management

Preventing delirium is the most effective strategy for reducing its frequency and complications.[7] Delirium is a medical emergency and the identification and treatment of the underlying cause should be the first aim of management.[10]

Non-pharmacological or environmental support strategies should be instituted wherever possible. These include, co-ordinating nursing care, preventing sensory deprivation and disorientation, and maintaining competence.[5,11] Pharmacological treatment should be directed first at the underlying cause (if known) and then at the relief of specific symptoms of delirium.

The common errors in the pharmacological management of delirium are to use antipsychotic medications in excessive doses, give them too late or to overuse benzodiazepines.[4]

General principles[4,5,12–14]

- Keep the use of sedatives and antipsychotics to a minimum.
- Use one drug at a time.
- Tailor doses according to age, body size and degree of agitation.
- Titrate doses to effect.
- Use small doses regularly, rather than large doses less frequently.
- Review at least every 24 hours.
- Increase scheduled doses if regular 'as needed' doses are required after the initial 24-hour period.
- Maintain at an effective dose and discontinue 7–10 days after symptoms resolve.
- Ensure that the diagnosis of delirium is documented both in the patients hospital notes and in their primary health record (include in discharge letter or summary).

Pharmacological prophylaxis[15,16]

Data are sparse and conflicting around the use of medication to prevent delirium. Most studies use low dose haloperidol in patients deemed at high risk of developing delirium (elderly, post-surgical or ICU patients). Prophylactic low dose haloperidol (around

Table 7.32 Drugs used to treat delirium

Drug	Dose	Adverse effects	Notes
First-generation antipsychotics			
Haloperidol[1,5,7,11,18–20]	Oral 0.5–1 mg bd with additional doses every 4 hourly as needed (peak effect: 4–6 hours) IM 0.5–1 mg, observe for 30–60 minutes and repeat if necessary (peak effect: 20–40 minutes)	EPS can occur especially at doses above 3 mg Prolonged QT interval Increased risk of stroke in patients with dementia	Considered first-line agent. No trial data have demonstrated superiority of other antipsychotics over haloperidol, however care must be taken to monitor for EPS and cardiac side-effects Baseline ECG is recommended for all patients, and especially for the elderly or those with a family or personal history of cardiac disease Regular monitoring of the ECG and potassium levels should be carried out if there are other conditions present that may prolong the QT interval Avoid in Lewy body dementia and Parkinson's disease Avoid IV use where possible. However, in the medical ICU setting, IV is often used with close continuous ECG monitoring
Second-generation antipsychotics			
Amisulpride[11,12,21,22]	Oral 50–300 mg od, up to a maximum of 800 mg od Doses higher than 300 mg should be given in two divided doses	Prolonged QT interval Increased risk of stroke in patients with dementia	Very limited evidence As amisulpride is almost entirely excreted via the kidneys it is imperative to monitor renal function when used in medically ill or elderly patients
Aripiprazole[11,12,21–23]	Oral 5–15 mg/day, up to a maximum of 30 mg/day	Akathisia or worsening sleep cycle may be problematic Increased risk of stroke in patients with dementia	Very limited evidence The rapid-acting intramuscular preparation has not been assessed for the treatment of delirium
Olanzapine[1191–1195]	Oral 2.5–5 mg od, up to a maximum of 20 mg/day	EPS less likely than with haloperidol Sedation is the most commonly reported side effect Increased risk of stroke in patients with dementia	A trial comparing olanzapine, risperidone, haloperidol and quetiapine showed that all were equally efficacious and safe in the treatment of delirium, but the response rate to olanzapine was poorer in the older age group (>75 years)[29] The rapid-acting intramuscular preparations has not been assessed for the treatment of delirium

(Continued)

CHAPTER 7

Table 7.32 (Continued)

Drug	Dose	Adverse effects	Notes
Risperidone[26,27,30-35]	Oral 0.5 mg bd with additional doses every 4 hourly as needed. Usual maximum 4 mg/day	The most common reported side effects are hypotension and EPS Increased risk of stroke in patients with dementia	A trial comparing risperidone with olanzapine showed that both were equally effective in reducing delirium symptoms but the response to risperidone was poorer in the older age group (>70 years)[27]
Quetiapine[36-40]	Oral 12.5–50 mg bd This may be increased every 12 hours to 200 mg daily if it is well tolerated	Sedation and postural hypotension are the most common reported side effects Increased risk of stroke in patients with dementia	There is an increasing number of trials demonstrating safety and efficacy of low dose quetiapine compared with haloperidol both in and outside the medical ICU
Ziprasidone[41]	IM 10 mg every 2 hourly Usual maximum 40 mg/day	QT prolongation Increased risk of stroke in patients with dementia	Very limited evidence Not available in the UK
Benzodiazepines			
Lorazepam[1,5,7]	Oral/IM 0.25–1 mg every 2 to 4 hourly as needed Usual maximum 3 mg in 24 hours IV use is usually reserved for emergencies	More likely than antipsychotics to cause respiratory depression, over sedation and paradoxical excitement Associated with prolongation and worsening of delirium symptoms	Used in alcohol or sedative hypnotic withdrawal, Parkinson's disease and NMS Otherwise – avoid
Diazepam[42]	Starting oral dose of 5–10 mg In the elderly a starting dose of 2 mg is recommended	Much longer half life in comparison with lorazepam Associated with prolongation and worsening of delirium symptoms	Used in alcohol or sedative hypnotic withdrawal, Parkinson's disease and NMS Otherwise – avoid
Cholinesterase inhibitors			
Donepezil[43,44]	Oral 5 mg od	Reasonably well tolerated compared with placebo. Nausea, vomiting and diarrhoea are the most common adverse effects reported	Very limited evidence. In the small studies where it has been used, clinical benefits have not been convincing. Not recommended

Rivastigmine[45,44]	Oral 1.5–6 mg bd	A study which added rivastigmine to usual care (haloperidol), showed that rivastigmine did not decrease the duration of delirium but in fact was associated with a more severe type of delirium, a longer stay in intensive care and higher mortality compared with placebo	Use of rivastigmine to treat delirium in critically ill patients is not recommended
Other drugs		
Melatonin[47,48]	Oral 2 mg od		Very limited experience, used mainly to correct altered sleep-wake cycle. Not recommended
Trazodone[4,7]	25–150 mg nocte	Sedation is the most commonly reported adverse effect	Limited experience – used only in uncontrolled studies. Not recommended
Sodium valproate[49]	Oral/IM/IV 250 mg bd increased to plasma level of 50–100 mg/L	Over sedation is problematic	Some case reports of its use where antipsychotics and/or benzodiazepines are ineffective, otherwise not recommended
		Contraindicated in active liver disease	

bd, *bis die* (twice a day); ECG, electrocardiogram; EPS, extrapyramidal side-effects; ICU, intensive care unit; IM, intramuscular; IV, intravenous; NMS, neuroleptic malignant syndrome; nocte, at night; od, *omne in die* (once a day).

3 mg/day) may reduce the severity and duration of delirium episodes and shorten the length of hospital stay in patients at high risk of developing the condition, but further research is needed before routinely recommending this strategy. Some evidence exists to support non-drug measures to minimise the risk of delirium.[17] Even low dose antipsychotics have serious adverse effects in elderly patients.

Table 7.32 gives a summary of the drugs used to treat delirium.

References

1. van Zyl LT et al. Delirium concisely: condition is associated with increased morbidity, mortality, and length of hospitalization. Geriatrics 2006; **61**:18–21.
2. American Psychiatric Association. *Diagnostic and Statistical Manual of Mental Disorders, Fifth Edition (DSM-5)*. Arlington, VA: American Psychiatric Association; 2013.
3. Inouye SK et al. Clarifying confusion: the confusion assessment method. A new method for detection of delirium. Ann Intern Med 1990; **113**:941–948.
4. Nayeem K et al. Delirium. Clin Med 2003; **3**:412–415.
5. Potter J et al. The prevention, diagnosis and management of delirium in older people: concise guidelines. Clin Med 2006; **6**:303–308.
6. Fong TG et al. Delirium in elderly adults: diagnosis, prevention and treatment. Nat Rev Neurol 2009; **5**:210–220.
7. Inouye SK. Delirium in older persons. N Engl J Med 2006; **354**:1157–1165.
8. Saxena S et al. Delirium in the elderly: a clinical review. Postgrad Med J 2009; **85**:405–413.
9. Naja M et al. Delirium in geriatric medicine is related to anticholinergic burden. Eur Geriatr Med 2013; **4 Suppl** 1:S208.
10. Burns A et al. Delirium. J Neurol Neurosurg Psychiatry 2004; **75**:362–367.
11. Schwartz TL et al. The role of atypical antipsychotics in the treatment of delirium. Psychosomatics 2002; **43**:171–174.
12. Seitz DP et al. Antipsychotics in the treatment of delirium: a systematic review. J Clin Psychiatry 2007; **68**:11–21.
13. National Institute for Health and Clinical Excellence. Delirium: diagnosis, prevention and management. Clinical Guideline 103, 2010. http://www.nice.org.uk/
14. Donders E et al. Effect of haloperidol dosing frequencies on the duration and severity of delirium in elderly hip fracture patients. A prospective randomized trial. Eur Geriatr Med 2012; **3 Suppl** 1:S118–S119.
15. Siddiqi N et al. Interventions for preventing delirium in hospitalised patients. Cochrane Database Syst Rev 2007; CD005563.
16. van den Boogaard M et al. Haloperidol prophylaxis in critically ill patients with a high risk for delirium. Crit Care 2013; **17**:R9.
17. Clegg A et al. Interventions for preventing delirium in older people in institutional long-term care. Cochrane Database Syst Rev 2014; **1**: CD009537.
18. Fricchione GL et al. Postoperative delirium. Am J Psychiatry 2008; **165**:803–812.
19. Lonergan E et al. Antipsychotics for delirium (review). Cochrane Database Syst Rev 2007; CD005594.
20. Page VJ et al. Effect of intravenous haloperidol on the duration of delirium and coma in critically ill patients (Hope-ICU): a randomised, double-blind, placebo-controlled trial. Lancet Respir Med 2013; **1**:515–523.
21. Boettger S et al. Atypical antipsychotics in the management of delirium: a review of the empirical literature. Palliat Support Care 2005; **3**:227–237.
22. Leentjens AF et al. Delirium in elderly people: an update. Curr Opin Psychiatry 2005; **18**:325–330.
23. Boettger S et al. Aripiprazole and haloperidol in the treatment of delirium. Aust N Z J Psychiatry 2011; **45**:477–482.
24. Skrobik YK et al. Olanzapine vs haloperidol: treating delirium in a critical care setting. Intensive Care Med 2004; **30**:444–449.
25. Sipahimalani A et al. Olanzapine in the treatment of delirium. Psychosomatics 1998; **39**:422–430.
26. Duff G. Atypical antipsychotic drugs and stroke, 2004. http://www.mhra.gov.uk
27. Kim SW et al. Risperidone versus olanzapine for the treatment of delirium. Hum Psychopharmacol 2010; **25**:298–302.
28. Grover S et al. Comparative efficacy study of haloperidol, olanzapine and risperidone in delirium. J Psychosom Res 2011; **71**:277–281.
29. Yoon HJ et al. Efficacy and safety of haloperidol versus atypical antipsychotic medications in the treatment of delirium. BMC Psychiatry 2013; **13**:240.
30. Bourgeois JA et al. Prolonged delirium managed with risperidone. Psychosomatics 2005; **46**:90–91.
31. Gupta N et al. Effectiveness of risperidone in delirium. Can J Psychiatry 2005; **50**:75.
32. Liu CY et al. Efficacy of risperidone in treating the hyperactive symptoms of delirium. Int Clin Psychopharmacol 2004; **19**:165–168.
33. Horikawa N et al. Treatment for delirium with risperidone: results of a prospective open trial with 10 patients. Gen Hosp Psychiatry 2003; **25**:289–292.
34. Han CS et al. A double-blind trial of risperidone and haloperidol for the treatment of delirium. Psychosomatics 2004; **45**:297–301.
35. Hakim SM et al. Early treatment with risperidone for subsyndromal delirium after on-pump cardiac surgery in the elderly: a randomized trial. Anesthesiology 2012; **116**:987–997.
36. Torres R et al. Use of quetiapine in delirium: case reports. Psychosomatics 2001; **42**:347–349.
37. Sasaki Y et al. A prospective, open-label, flexible-dose study of quetiapine in the treatment of delirium. J Clin Psychiatry 2003; **64**:1316–1321.

38. Devlin JW et al. Efficacy and safety of quetiapine in critically ill patients with delirium: a prospective, multicenter, randomized, double-blind, placebo-controlled pilot study. Crit Care Med 2010; **38**:419–427.

39. Hawkins SB et al. Quetiapine for the treatment of delirium. J Hosp Med 2013; **8**:215–220.

40. Tahir TA et al. A randomized controlled trial of quetiapine versus placebo in the treatment of delirium. J Psychosom Res 2010; **69**:485–490.

41. Young CC et al. Intravenous ziprasidone for treatment of delirium in the intensive care unit. Anesthesiology 2004; **101**:794–795.

42. Chan D et al. Delirium: making the diagnosis, improving the prognosis. Geriatrics 1999; **54**:28–42.

43. Overshott R et al. Cholinesterase inhibitors for delirium. Cochrane Database Syst Rev 2008; CD005317.

44. Sampson EL et al. A randomized, double-blind, placebo-controlled trial of donepezil hydrochloride (Aricept) for reducing the incidence of postoperative delirium after elective total hip replacement. Int J Geriatr Psychiatry 2007; **22**:343–349.

45. Dautzenberg PL et al. Adding rivastigmine to antipsychotics in the treatment of a chronic delirium. Age Ageing 2004; **33**:516–517.

46. van Eijk MM et al. Effect of rivastigmine as an adjunct to usual care with haloperidol on duration of delirium and mortality in critically ill patients: a multicentre, double-blind, placebo-controlled randomised trial. Lancet 2010; **376**:1829–1837.

47. Hanania M et al. Melatonin for treatment and prevention of postoperative delirium. Anesth Analg 2002; **94**:338–9, table.

48. Cronin AJ et al. Melatonin secretion after surgery. Lancet 2000; **356**:1244–1245.

49. Bourgeois JA et al. Adjunctive valproic acid for delirium and/or agitation on a consultation-liaison service: a report of six cases. J Neuropsychiatry Clin Neurosci 2005; **17**:232–238.

Further reading

Donders E et al. Effect of haloperidol dosing frequencies on the duration and severity of delirium in elderly hip fracture patients. Eur Geriatr Med 2012; **3**(S118-119), 1878–7649.

Boettger S et al. Aripiprazole and haloperidol in the treatment of delirium. Aust NZ J Psychiat 2011; **45**(6):477–482.

Yoon H-J et al. Efficacy and safety of typical and atypical antipsychotic medications in the treatment of delirium. Int Psychogeriatrics 2013; **25**(S133):1041–6102.

Hakim SM, Othman AI, Naoum DO. Early treatment with risperidone for subsyndromal delirium after on-pump cardiac surgery in the elderly: a randomized trial. Anaesthesiology 2012; **116**(5):987–997

Hawkins SB et al. Quetiapine for the treatment of delirium. J Hosp Med 2013; **8**(4):215–220.

Page VJ et al. Effect of intravenous haloperidol on the duration of delirium and coma in critically ill patients (Hope-ICU): a randomised, double-blind, placebo-controlled trial. Lancet Resp Med 2013; **1**(7):515–523.

Tahir TA et al. A randomised controlled trial of quetiapine versus placebo in the treatment of delirium. J Psychosom Res 2010; **69**(5):485–490.

Naja M et al. Delirium in geriatric medicine is related to anticholinergic burden. Eur Geriatr Med 2013; **4**(S208).

Van Den Boogaard M et al. Haloperidol prophylaxis in critically ill patients with a high risk for delirium. Crit Care 2013; **17**:1–11.

Siddiqi H et al. Interventions for preventing delirium in hospitalised patients. Cochrane Database Syst Rev 2007; CD005563.

CHAPTER 7

Epilepsy

Depression and psychosis in epilepsy

The prevalence of depression in people with epilepsy is reported to range from 9% to 22%,[1,2] with higher rates in those with poor seizure control.[3] Depressive symptoms may occur in up to 60% of people with intractable epilepsy.[4] This association may be explained in part by serotonin; depletion of serotonin increases the risk of both depression and epilepsy.[5] Suicide rates in epilepsy have been estimated to be 4–5 times that of the general population.[1,2,6] The prevalence of psychotic illness in people with epilepsy is at least 4%.[4] A diagnosis of temporal lobe epilepsy does not seem to confer additional risk.[7]

Peri-ictal depression or psychosis (that is, symptoms temporally related to seizure activity) should initially be treated by optimising anticonvulsant therapy.[8] Interictal depression or psychosis (symptoms occurring independently of seizures) are likely to require treatment with antidepressants or antipsychotics.[2,8]

Use of antidepressants and antipsychotics in epilepsy

The prevalence of active epilepsy in adults under the age of 65 is 0.6% and the annual incidence 0.03%.[9] It is notable that the incidence of unprovoked seizures in the placebo arms of randomised controlled trials of antidepressants and antipsychotics is approximately 15-fold higher, suggesting that both depression and psychosis are risk factors for seizures.[10] Reports of seizures associated with drug treatment should be interpreted in the context of this background risk and single case reports treated with caution. Note also that almost all antidepressants and antipsychotics have been associated with hyponatraemia (see section on 'Hyponatraemia' in Chapter 4) and seizures may occur if this is severe.[11] Some antipsychotics and antidepressants can reduce the seizure threshold[1,2,12,13] and the risk is dose-related (see Table 7.33).

There are few systematic studies of antipsychotics or antidepressants in people with epilepsy. Data are mainly derived from animal studies, clinical trials, case reports and spontaneous reporting to regulatory bodies. Table 7.33 gives some general guidance. Treatment should be commenced at the lowest dose and this should be gradually increased until a therapeutic dose is achieved.[2,13,14] As a very general rule, the more sedating a drug is, the more likely it is to induce seizures,[13] although mirtazapine is a notable exception.[15]

Electroconvulsive therapy (ECT) has anticonvulsive properties and is worth considering in the treatment of depression in patients with unstable epilepsy.[1,2] ECT does not appear to cause epilepsy.[16]

Depression and psychosis associated with anticonvulsant drugs

Anticonvulsant drugs have been associated with new-onset depression and psychosis.[1] If anticonvulsants have recently been changed, this should always be considered as a potential cause of a new/worsening depressive or psychotic illness (for example a newly started or discontinued drug may have antidepressant effects, may worsen depression

Table 7.33 Psychotropics in epilepsy

	Safety in epilepsy	Special considerations
Antidepressant		
Moclobemide[30]	Good choice	Not known to be pro-convulsive
SSRIs[31] (not citalopram) Mirtazapine[15,32]	Good choice	SSRIs may be anticonvulsant at therapeutic doses[10,33] and protect against hypoxic damage;[34] no clear difference between drugs,[9] except citalopram[35]
Citalopram[35,36]/venlafaxine[37,38]	Care required	Venlafaxine and citalopram pro-convulsive in overdose Use with care
Duloxetine,[11,17] vortioxetine, agomelatine, reboxetine	Care required	Very limited data and clinical experience
Amoxapine[39] (not available in the UK) Amitriptyline Dosulepin (dothiepin)[40] Clomipramine[41] Bupropion[10]	Avoid	Most TCAs are epileptogenic,[42] particularly at higher doses, as is bupropion (amfebutamone) Ideally, should be avoided completely
Lithium[2]	Care required	Low pro-convulsive effect at therapeutic doses Marked pro-convulsive activity in overdose
Antipsychotic		
Trifluoperazine/haloperidol[2,13,43]	Good choice	Low pro-convulsive effect Carbamazepine increases the metabolism of some antipsychotics and larger doses of an antipsychotic may be required
Sulpiride[44]/amisulpride[45,46]	Good choice	Low pro-convulsive effect, very few reports of suspected drug-related seizures[47] No known interactions with anticonvulsants
Risperidone[10] Olanzapine[10] Quetiapine[10]	Care required	Doubts about safety in epilepsy Olanzapine may affect EEG[48] and myoclonic seizures have been reported[49,50] Seizures rarely reported with quetiapine[51] but also shown to have anticonvulsant activity in ECT[44] Both olanzapine and quetiapine may increase the seizure threshold up to two-fold[10] and are linked to higher rates of drug-related seizure[47]
Aripiprazole	Care required	Very limited data and clinical experience Seizures have been reported rarely[52,53]
Clozapine[8,12,54]	Avoid if possible	Very epileptogenic Approximately 5% who receive more than 600 mg/day develop seizures Sodium valproate or lamotrigine are the anticonvulsant of choice as they have a lower incidence of leucopenia than carbamazepine
Lurasidone, asenapine	Avoid if possible	Not thought to affect seizure threshold but experience is limited

(Continued)

CHAPTER 7

Table 7.33 (*Continued*)

	Safety in epilepsy	Special considerations
Chlorpromazine[8] Loxapine (not available in the UK)	Avoid	Most epileptogenic of the older drugs Ideally best avoided completely
Zotepine (now withdrawn in the UK)	Avoid	Has established dose-related pro-convulsive effect Best avoided completely
Depot antipsychotics	Avoid	None of the depot preparations currently available are thought to be epileptogenic, however: ■ the kinetics of depots are complex (seizures may be delayed) ■ if seizures do occur, the offending drug may not be easily withdrawn. Depots should be used with extreme care

This table contains information about the pro-convulsive effects of antidepressants and antipsychotics when used in therapeutic doses. See section on 'Psychotropics in overdose' in Chapter 8 for information about supra-therapeutic doses.

ECT, electroconvulsive therapy; EEG, electroencephalogram; SSRI, selective serotonin reuptake inhibitor; TCA, tricyclic antidepressant.

or may induce or inhibit hepatic CYP enzymes thus interfering with existing treatments for depression). Lowering of folate levels by some anticonvulsants may also influence the expression of depression.[1] Folate levels should be checked and remedied where necessary.

Psychosis[17]

Summary of product characteristics and/or case reports associate the following anti-convulsants with the onset of psychotic symptoms: carbamazepine, ethosuximide, gabapentin, lamotrigine,[18] levetiracetam,[19,20] piracetam, pregabalin,[21] primidone, tiagabine, topiramate,[22] valproate, vigabatrin and zonisamide.[23] Some of these reports may relate to the process of 'forced normalisation' in which a diminished frequency of seizures allows psychotic symptoms to emerge (a kind of 'reverse ECT').

Depression[17,24,25]

Summary of product characteristics and case reports associate the following anticon-vulsants with the onset of depressive symptoms: acetazolamide, barbiturates, carba-mazepine, ethosuximide, felbamate, gabapentin, levitiracetam*, phenytoin, piracetam, tiagabine*, topiramate*, vigabatrin* and zonisamide. Iatrogenic depression is more likely in patients with a history of depression. Risk may be increased by more rapid dosage titration; this has been shown for topiramate.[26] There is limited evidence that these anti-epileptic drugs that are associated with a higher incidence of depression in clinical trials (marked*) may increase the risk of self-harm and suicidal behaviour.[27] Lamotrigine has also been implicated.[28] Note also that carbamazepine and lamotrigine have antidepressant properties and gabapentin is anxiolytic.

Interactions

Pharmacokinetic interactions between anticonvulsants and antidepressants/antipsychotics are common. These interactions are primarily mediated through cytochrome P450 enzymes.[1,2] Fluoxetine and paroxetine are potent inhibitors of several hepatic CYP enzyme systems (CYP2D6, CYP3A4). Sertraline is a less potent inhibitor, but this effect is dose-related and higher doses of sertraline are commonly used. Citalopram is a weak inhibitor. Carbamazepine and phenytoin have a narrow therapeutic index and plasma levels can be increased by enzyme inhibitors. This is particularly important with phenytoin. Plasma levels should be monitored and dosage adjustment may be required.

Carbamazepine is an enzyme inducer (mainly CYP3A4) and can lower plasma levels of some antipsychotic drugs.[29] Many other medicines can cause problems in people with epilepsy by raising or reducing the seizure threshold or interacting with anticonvulsant drugs.

Epilepsy and driving

In the UK, people with epilepsy may not drive a car if they have had a seizure while awake in the previous year or, if seizures occur only during sleep, this has been an established nocturnal pattern for at least 3 years. The consequences of inducing seizure with antidepressants or antipsychotics can therefore be significant. For further information see www.dvla.gov.uk.

References

1. Harden CL et al. Mood disorders in patients with epilepsy: epidemiology and management. CNS Drugs 2002; **16**:291–302.
2. Curran S et al. Selecting an antidepressant for use in a patient with epilepsy. Safety considerations. Drug Saf 1998; **18**:125–133.
3. Dias R et al. Depression in epilepsy is associated with lack of seizure control. Epilepsy Behav 2010; **19**:445–447.
4. Lambert MV et al. Depression in epilepsy: etiology, phenomenology, and treatment. Epilepsia 1999; **40 Suppl** 10:S21–S47.
5. Bagdy G et al. Serotonin and epilepsy. J Neurochem 2007; **100**:857–873.
6. Mula M et al. Suicidality in epilepsy and possible effects of antiepileptic drugs. Curr Neurol Neurosci Rep 2010; **10**:327–332.
7. Adams SJ et al. Neuropsychiatric morbidity in focal epilepsy. Br J Psychiatry 2008; **192**:464–469.
8. Blumer D et al. Treatment of the interictal psychoses. J Clin Psychiatry 2000; **61**:110–122.
9. Montgomery SA. Antidepressants and seizures: emphasis on newer agents and clinical implications. Int J Clin Pract 2005; **59**:1435–1440.
10. Alper K et al. Seizure incidence in psychopharmacological clinical trials: an analysis of Food and Drug Administration (FDA) summary basis of approval reports. Biol Psychiatry 2007; **62**:345–354.
11. Maramattom BV. Duloxetine-induced syndrome of inappropriate antidiuretic hormone secretion and seizures. Neurology 2006; **66**:773–774.
12. Pisani F et al. Effects of psychotropic drugs on seizure threshold. Drug Saf 2002; **25**:91–110.
13. Marks RC et al. Antipsychotic medications and seizures. Psychiatr Med 1991; **9**:37–52.
14. Rosenstein DL et al. Seizures associated with antidepressants: a review. J Clin Psychiatry 1993; **54**:289–299.
15. Berling I et al. Mirtazapine overdose is unlikely to cause major toxicity. Clin Toxicol (Phila) 2014; **52**:20–24.
16. Ray AK. Does electroconvulsive therapy cause epilepsy? J ECT 2013; **29**:201–205.
17. Datapharm Communications Ltd. Electronic Medicines Compendium. 2014. https://www.medicines.org.uk/emc/
18. Brandt C et al. Development of psychosis in patients with epilepsy treated with lamotrigine: report of six cases and review of the literature. Epilepsy Behav 2007; **11**:133–139.
19. Youroukos S et al. Acute psychosis associated with levetiracetam. Epileptic Disord 2003; **5**:117–119.
20. Bhardwaj R et al. Levetiracetam-induced psychosis. Epilepsy Behav 2010; **17**:614.
21. Olaizola I et al. Pregabalin-associated acute psychosis and epileptiform EEG-changes. Seizure 2006; **15**:208–210.
22. Karslioaylu EH et al. Topiramate-induced psychotic exacerbation: case report and review of literature. Int J Psychiatry Clin Pract 2007; **11**:285–290.
23. Michael CT et al. Psychosis following initiation of zonisamide. Am J Psychiatry 2007; **164**:682.
24. Besag FM. Behavioural effects of the newer antiepileptic drugs: an update. Expert Opin Drug Saf 2004; **3**:1–8.
25. Barry JJ et al. Consensus statement: the evaluation and treatment of people with epilepsy and affective disorders. Epilepsy Behav 2008; **13 Suppl** 1:S1–29.

26. Mula M et al. The role of titration schedule of topiramate for the development of depression in patients with epilepsy. Epilepsia 2009; 50:1072–1076.
27. Andersohn F et al. Use of antiepileptic drugs in epilepsy and the risk of self-harm or suicidal behavior. Neurology 2010; 75:335–340.
28. Patorno E et al. Anticonvulsant medications and the risk of suicide, attempted suicide, or violent death. JAMA 2010; 303:1401–1409.
29. Tiihonen J et al. Carbamazepine-induced changes in plasma levels of neuroleptics. Pharmacopsychiatry 1995; 28:26–28.
30. Schiwy W et al. Therapeutic and side-effect profile of a selective and reversible MAO-A inhibitor, brofaromine. Results of dose-finding trials in depressed patients. J Neural Transm Suppl 1989; 28:33–44.
31. Wedin GP et al. Relative toxicity of cyclic antidepressants. Ann Emerg Med 1986; 15:797–804.
32. Zia Ul HM et al. Mirtazapine precipitated seizures: a case report. Prog Neuropsychopharmacol Biol Psychiatry 2008; 32:1076–1078.
33. Hamid H et al. Should antidepressant drugs of the selective serotonin reuptake inhibitor family be tested as antiepileptic drugs? Epilepsy Behav 2013; 26:261–265.
34. Bateman LM et al. Serotonin reuptake inhibitors are associated with reduced severity of ictal hypoxemia in medically refractory partial epilepsy. Epilepsia 2010; 51:2211–2214.
35. Judge BS et al. Antidepressant overdose-induced seizures. Psychiatr Clin North Am 2013; 36:245–260.
36. Reichert C et al. Seizures after single-agent overdose with pharmaceutical drugs: Analysis of cases reported to a poison center. Clin Toxicol (Phila) 2014; 52:629–634.
37. Juckel G et al. Epileptiform EEG patterns induced by mirtazapine in both psychiatric patients and healthy volunteers. J Clin Psychopharmacol 2003; 23:421–422.
38. Alldredge BK. Seizure risk associated with psychotropic drugs: clinical and pharmacokinetic considerations. Neurology 1999; 53:S68–S75.
39. Barry JJ et al. Consensus statement: the evaluation and treatment of people with epilepsy and affective disorders. Epilepsy Behav 2008; 13 Suppl 1:S1–29.
40. Buckley NA et al. Greater toxicity in overdose of dothiepin than of other tricyclic antidepressants. Lancet 1994; 343:159–162.
41. Stimmel GL et al. Psychotrophic drug-induced reductions in seizure threshold: incidence and consequences. CNS Drugs 1996; 5:3750.
42. Koster M et al. Seizures during antidepressant treatment in psychiatric inpatients--results from the transnational pharmacovigilance project"Arzneimittelsicherheit in der Psychiatrie" (AMSP) 1993-2008. Psychopharmacology (Berl) 2013; 230:191–201.
43. Darby JK et al. Haloperidol dose and blood level variability: toxicity and interindividual and intraindividual variability in the nonresponder patient in the clinical practice setting. J Clin Psychopharmacol 1995; 15:334–340.
44. Gazdag G et al. The impact of neuroleptic medication on seizure threshold and duration in electroconvulsive therapy. Ideggyogy Sz 2004; 57:385–390.
45. Patat A et al. Effects of 50 mg amisulpride on EEG, psychomotor and cognitive functions in healthy sleep-deprived subjects. Fundam Clin Pharmacol 1999; 13:582–594.
46. Tracqui A et al. Amisulpride poisoning: a report on two cases. Hum Exp Toxicol 1995; 14:294–298.
47. Lertxundi U et al. Antipsychotics and seizures: higher risk with atypicals? Seizure 2013; 22:141–143.
48. Amann BL et al. EEG abnormalities associated with antipsychotics: a comparison of quetiapine, olanzapine, haloperidol and healthy subjects. Hum Psychopharmacol 2003; 18:641–646.
49. Camacho A et al. Olanzapine-induced myoclonic status. Clin Neuropharmacol 2005; 28:145–147.
50. Rosen JB et al. Olanzapine-associated myoclonus. Epilepsy Res 2012; 98:247–250.
51. Dogu O et al. Seizures associated with quetiapine treatment. Ann Pharmacother 2003; 37:1224–1227.
52. Tsai JF. Aripiprazole-associated seizure. J Clin Psychiatry 2006; 67:995–996.
53. Thabet FI et al. Aripiprazole-induced seizure in a 3-year-old child: a case report and literature review. Clin Neuropharmacol 2013; 36:29–30.
54. Toth P et al. Clozapine and seizures: a review. Can J Psychiatry 1994; 39:236–238.

Further reading

Arana A et al. Suicide-related events in patients treated with antiepileptic drugs. N Engl J Med 2010; 363:542–551.
Farooq S et al. Interventions for psychotic symptoms concomitant with epilepsy. Cochrane Database Syst Rev 2008; CD006118.
Trimble M et al. Postictal psychosis. Epilepsy Behav 2010; 19:159–161.

Surgery

There are few worthwhile studies of the effects of non-anaesthetic drugs on surgery and the anaesthetic process.[1,2] Practice is therefore largely based on theoretical considerations, case reports, clinical experience and personal opinion. Any guidance given in this area is therefore somewhat speculative.

The decision as to whether or not to continue a drug during surgery and the perioperative period should take into account a number of interacting factors. Some general considerations include:

- Patients are at risk of aspirating their stomach contents during general anaesthesia. For this reason they are usually prevented from eating for at least 6 hours before surgery. However, clear fluids leave the stomach within 2 hours of ingestion and so fluids that enable a patient to take routine medication may be allowed up to 2 hours before surgery. A clear fluid is defined as one through which newspaper print can be read.[3]
- There are some drug interactions between drugs used during surgery and routine medication that require the drugs not to be administered concurrently. This is usually managed by the anaesthetist through their choice of anaesthetic technique. Significant drug interactions between medicines used during surgery and psychotropics include:
  - enflurane may precipitate seizures in patients taking tricyclic antidepressants[4-6]
  - pethidine and other serotonergic opioids may precipitate fatal 'excitatory' reactions in patients taking MAOIs and may cause serotonin syndrome in patients taking SSRIs.[4-7]

- Major procedures induce profound physiological changes, which include electrolyte disturbances and the release of cortisol and catecholamines.
- Postoperatively, surgical stress and some agents used in anaesthesia often lead to gastric or gastrointestinal stasis. Oral absorption is therefore likely to be compromised.

For the most part, psychotropic drugs should be continued during the perioperative period, assuming agreement of the anaesthetist concerned. Table 7.34 provides some discussion of the merits or otherwise of continuing individual psychotropics during surgery. Note, however, that psychotropic and other drugs are frequently (accidentally and/or unthinkingly) withheld from preoperative patients simply because they are 'nil by mouth'.[1] Patients may be labelled 'nil by mouth' for several reasons, including unconsciousness, to rest the gut postoperatively or as a result of the surgery itself. Patients may also develop an intolerance of oral medicines at any time during a stay in hospital, often because of nausea and vomiting. When it is decided to continue a psychotropic, this needs to be explicitly outlined to appropriate medical and nursing staff.

For many patients undergoing surgery and recovery in a hospital there will be little or no opportunity to smoke. Abrupt cessation is likely to affect mental state and may also result in drug toxicity if psychotropics are continued (see section on 'Psychotropics and smoking' in Chapter 8).

Alternative routes and formulations may be sought. When changing the route or formulation, care should be taken to ensure the appropriate dose and frequency is prescribed as these may not be the same as for the oral route or previous formulation. Oral preparations may sometimes be administered via a nasogastric (NG), percutaneous endoscopic gastrostomy (PEG) or jejunostomy tube.

Table 7.34 Psychotropic drugs and surgery

Drug or drug group	Considerations	Safe in surgery?	Alternative formulations
Anticonvulsants[4,15]	■ CNS depressant activity may reduce anaesthetic requirements ■ Drug level monitoring may be required	Probably, usually continued for people with epilepsy	Carbamazepine liquid or suppositories are available: 100 mg tablet = 125 mg suppository. Maximum by rectum 1 g daily in four divided doses Phenytoin is available IV or liquid: IV dose = oral dose Sodium valproate is available IV or liquid: IV dose = oral dose Before crushing tablets and mixing with water, confirm with either local guidelines or the drug company for stability information
Antidepressants – MAOIs[3,4,16–20]	■ Dangerous, potentially fatal interaction with pethidine and dextromethorphan (serotonin syndrome or coma/respiratory depression may occur) ■ Action of inhaled anaesthetics and neuromuscular blockers is reduced ■ Sympathomimetic agents may result in hypertensive crisis ■ Phenylephrine only agent safe for hypotension ■ MAO inhibition lasts for up to 2 weeks: early withdrawal is required ■ Switching to moclobemide 2 weeks before surgery allows continued treatment up until day of surgery (do not give moclobemide on the day of surgery)	Probably not, but careful selection of anaesthetic agents may reduce risks if continuation is essential	None
Antidepressants – SSRIs[4,6,7,19,21–24]	■ Danger of serotonin syndrome if administered with pethidine, fentanyl, pentazocine or tramadol ■ Occasional seizures reported ■ Cessation may result in withdrawal syndrome ■ Various interactions with drugs used in surgery ■ Venlafaxine may provoke opioid-induced rigidity ■ Increases risk of perioperative bleeding	Probably, but avoid other serotonergic agents	Liquid escitalopram, fluoxetine and paroxetine are available Oral disintegrating tablets of mirtazapine have been used perioperatively (for nausea)[25]

Antidepressants – TCAs[4,6,14,19,21,22,24]	■ α_1 blockade may lead to hypotension and interfere with effects of epinephrine/norepinephrine ■ Danger of serotonin syndrome (clomipramine; amitriptyline) if administered with pethidine, pentazocine or tramadol ■ Many drugs prolong QT interval so arrhythmia more likely ■ Most drugs lower seizure threshold ■ May decrease core hypothermia ■ Sympathomimetic agents may give exaggerated response ■ Effects persist for several days after cessation so will need to be stopped some time before surgery ■ Clomipramine, amitriptyline may increase bleeding risk	Unclear, but anaesthetic agents need to be carefully chosen Some authorities recommend slow discontinuation before surgery	Liquid amitriptyline is available. It is acidic and may interact with enteral feeds Dosulepin (dothiepin) capsules can be opened and mixed with water before flushing well. This is preferred over crushing tablets Most tricyclics have potent local anaesthetic effects – oral delivery in liquid form is likely to cause local anaesthesia
Antipsychotics[4,13,19,26-29]	■ Some antipsychotics widely used in anaesthetic practice ■ Increased risk of arrhythmia with most drugs ■ α_1 blockade may lead to hypotension and interfere with effects of epinephrine/norepinephrine ■ Most drugs lower seizure threshold ■ May enhance interoperative core hypothermia ■ Clozapine may delay recovery from anaesthesia ■ Gaseous anaesthetics may affect dopamine metabolism ■ Preoperative olanzapine reduces risk of delirium[30]	Probably, usually continued to avoid relapse	Liquid preparations of some antipsychotics are available Some 'specials' liquids can be made for nasogastric delivery Before crushing tablets and mixing with water, confirm with either local guidelines or the drug company for stability information
Benzodiazepines[4,15]	■ Reduced requirements for induction and maintenance anaesthetics ■ Many have prolonged action (days or weeks), so early withdrawal is necessary ■ Withdrawal symptoms possible	Probably; usually continued	Liquid, IM, IV and rectal diazepam are available (do not use IM route) Buccal liquid available for midazolam Sublingual (use normal tablets), IM, IV and lorazepam are available

(Continued)

Table 7.34 (Continued)

Drug or drug group	Considerations	Safe in surgery?	Alternative formulations
Lithium[3,4,19,31]	■ Prolongs the action of both depolarising and non-depolarising muscle relaxants ■ Surgery-related electrolyte disturbance and reduced renal function may precipitate lithium toxicity. Avoid dehydration and NSAIDs ■ Possible increased risk of arrhythmia	Probably safe in minor surgery but usually discontinued before major procedures and re-started once electrolytes normalise Slow discontinuation is essential – anaesthetists may not appreciate this[32]	The bioavailability of lithium varies between brands. Care is needed with equivalent doses of salts: lithium carbonate 200 mg = lithium citrate 509 mg. Liquid lithium citrate is available and is usually administered twice daily
Methadone[3,15]	■ May reduce opiate requirements ■ Naloxone may induce withdrawal ■ Methadone prolongs QT interval ■ When using opiates, use only full agonists (avoid buprenorphine)	Probably, usually continued	IM dose = oral dose
Modafinil[33,34]	■ Limited data suggest no interference with anaesthesia ■ Improves recovery after anaesthesia	Probably, data limited	None

CNS, central nervous system; IM, intramuscular; IV, intravenous; MAOI, monoamine oxidase inhibitor; NSAID, non-steroidal anti-inflammatory drug; SSRI, selective serotonin reuptake inhibitor; TCA, tricyclic antidepressant.

Risks associated with discontinuing psychotropics

- Relapse (especially if treatment ceased for more than a few days).[8]
- Worsening of condition. For example, abrupt cessation of lithium worsens outcome in bipolar affective disorder.[9]
- Suicide. Cessation of antidepressants may increase risk of suicide.[10]
- Discontinuation symptoms. These may complicate diagnosis in the perioperative period.
- Delirium. May be more common in those discontinuing antipsychotics[11] or antidepressants.[6]

Risks associated with continuing psychotropics

- Potential for interactions, both pharmacokinetic and pharmacodynamic.
- Increased likelihood of bleeding (e.g. with SSRIs).[12]
- Hypo/hypertension (depending on psychotropic).[13,14]
- Effects on core body temperature (e.g. with phenothiazines).

References

1. Noble DW et al. Interrupting drug therapy in the perioperative period. Drug Saf 2002; **25**:489–495.
2. Noble DW et al. Risks of interrupting drug treatment before surgery. BMJ 2000; **321**:719–720.
3. Anon. Drugs in the peri-operative period: 1--Stopping or continuing drugs around surgery. Drug Ther Bull 1999; **37**:62–64.
4. Smith MS et al. Perioperative management of drug therapy, clinical considerations. Drugs 1996; **51**:238–259.
5. Chui PT et al. Medications to withhold or continue in the preoperative consultation. Curr Anaesth Crit Care 1998; **9**:302–306.
6. Kudoh A et al. Antidepressant treatment for chronic depressed patients should not be discontinued prior to anesthesia. Can J Anaesth 2002; **49**:132–136.
7. Spivey KM et al. Perioperative seizures and fluvoxamine. Br J Anaesth 1993; **71**:321.
8. De Baerdemaeker L et al. Anaesthesia for patients with mood disorders. Curr Opin Anaesthesiol 2005; **18**:333–338.
9. Faedda GL et al. Outcome after rapid vs gradual discontinuation of lithium treatment in bipolar disorders. Arch Gen Psychiatry 1993; **50**:448–455.
10. Yerevanian BI et al. Antidepressants and suicidal behaviour in unipolar depression. Acta Psychiatr Scand 2004; **110**:452–458.
11. Copeland LA et al. Postoperative complications in the seriously mentally ill: a systematic review of the literature. Ann Surg 2008; **248**:31–38.
12. Paton C et al. SSRIs and gastrointestinal bleeding. BMJ 2005; **331**:529–530.
13. Kudoh A et al. Chronic treatment with antipsychotics enhances intraoperative core hypothermia. Anesth Analg 2004; **98**:111–115.
14. Kudoh A et al. Chronic treatment with antidepressants decreases intraoperative core hypothermia. Anesth Analg 2003; **97**:275–279.
15. Morrow JI et al. Essential drugs in the perioperative period. Curr Pract Surg 1990; **90**:106–109.
16. Rahman MH et al. Medication in the peri-operative period. Pharm J 2004; **272**:287–289.
17. Blom-Peters L et al. Monoamine oxidase inhibitors and anesthesia: an updated literature review. Acta Anaesthesiol Belg 1993; **44**:57–60.
18. Hill S et al. MAOIs to RIMAs in anaesthesia: a literature review. Psychopharmacology 1992; **106 Suppl**:S43–S45.
19. Huyse FJ et al. Psychotropic drugs and the perioperative period: a proposal for a guideline in elective surgery. Psychosomatics 2006; **47**:8–22.
20. Bajwa SJ et al. Psychiatric diseases: need for an increased awareness among the anesthesiologists. J Anaesthesiol Clin Pharmacol 2011; **27**:440–446.
21. Chui PT et al. Medications to withhold or continue in the preoperative consultation. Curr Anaesth Crit Care 1998; **9**:302–306.
22. Takakura K et al. Refractory hypotension during combined general and epidural anaesthesia in a patient on tricyclic antidepressants. Anaesth Intensive Care 2008; **34**:111–114.
23. Roy S et al. Fentanyl-induced rigidity during emergence from general anesthesia potentiated by venlafaxine. Can J Anaesth 2003; **50**:32–35.
24. Mahdanian AA et al. Serotonergic antidepressants and perioperative bleeding risk: a systematic review. Expert Opin Drug Saf 2014; **13**:695–704.
25. Chang FL et al. Efficacy of mirtazapine in preventing intrathecal morphine-induced nausea and vomiting after orthopaedic surgery. Anaesthesia 2010; **65**:1206–1211.
26. Doherty J et al. Implications for anaesthesia in a patient established on clozapine treatment. Int J Obstet Anesth 2006; **15**:59–62.
27. Geeraerts T et al. Delayed recovery after short-duration, general anesthesia in a patient chronically treated with clozapine. Anesth Analg 2006; **103**:1618.

28. Adachi YU et al. Isoflurane anesthesia inhibits clozapine- and risperidone-induced dopamine release and anesthesia-induced changes in dopamine metabolism was modified by fluoxetine in the rat striatum: an in vivo microdialysis study. Neurochem Internat 2008; 52:384–391.

29. Parlow JL et al. Single-dose haloperidol for the prophylaxis of postoperative nausea and vomiting after intrathecal morphine. Anesth Analg 2004; 98:1072–6.

30. Larsen KA et al. Administration of olanzapine to prevent postoperative delirium in elderly joint-replacement patients: a randomized, controlled trial. Psychosomatics 2010; 51:409–418.

31. Rahman MH et al. Medication in the peri-operative period. Pharm J 2004; 272:287–289.

32. Attri JP et al. Psychiatric patient and anaesthesia. Indian J Anaesth 2012; 56:8–13.

33. Larijani GE et al. Modafinil improves recovery after general anesthesia. Anesth Analg 2004; 98:976–81.

34. Doyle A et al. Day case general anaesthesia in a patient with narcolepsy. Anaesthesia 2008; 63:880–882.

CHAPTER 7

Velo-cardio-facial syndrome

Description

Velo-cardio-facial syndrome (VCFS), also known as DiGeorge or Shprintzen syndrome, and 22q11.2 syndrome, is a congenital disorder caused by a microdeletion of chromosome 22 at band q11.2. It has an estimated incidence of 1 in 5000 births.[1] Although considerable phenotypic variability occurs, with over 180 clinical features described, it is characterized by:

- Cardiac defects
- Abnormal facies
- Thymic hypoplasia
- Cleft palate
- Hypocalcaemia

These abnormalities have been collectively named **CATCH 22** (22 refers to chromosome 22),[2] a somewhat inappropriate name for a syndrome that can often be treated very effectively.[3] The typical facial features of patients with VCFS include a long face, prominent nose with bulbous tip and narrow orbital features.[4] Cardiac defects usually involve major structural abnormalities (tetralogy of Fallot). Hypocalcaemia is caused by parathyroid dysfunction.

Mental retardation and learning disabilities (including impairment in the development of language, reading, spelling and numeracy skills) are common. A high rate of psychiatric morbidity has also been identified in VCFS patients, with schizophrenia and bipolar disorder being most commonly reported.[4] This is probably related to partial deletion of the gene coding for catechol-o-methyltransferase (COMT) which effectively results in increased concentrations of dopamine and noradrenaline.[3]

There are currently limited data on the treatment of psychiatric disorders in VCFS, with most of the evidence coming from a small number of anecdotal reports. The majority of patients do not require medication to treat the behavioural symptoms associated with the syndrome.[3] However, the range of psychiatric disorders seen in VCFS has been observed to respond to standard treatment protocols in both children and adults.[1]

Adults

Neuropsychiatric symptoms

A large study evaluating rates of psychiatric disorders in adult patients with VCFS reported that about 30% had a psychotic disorder; with 24% fulfilling DSM-IV criteria for schizophrenia and 12% had major depression without psychotic features.[5] The most recent study found that 41% of VCFS patients over the age of 25 years had a diagnosable psychotic disorder.[6] Individuals with schizophrenia associated with VCFS often have fewer negative symptoms and a relatively later age of onset (mean = 26 years) compared with control patients who did not have VCFS.[7] Psychotic symptoms are transient in some.[8] Results from genetic studies have estimated the prevalence of schizophrenia in

VCFS patients as 22%, a much higher figure than the 0.5% prevalence of schizophrenia in the general population.[9,10] In fact, VCFS has been found to be the highest known risk factor for the development of schizophrenia.[11]

Management of psychiatric symptoms

It has been suggested that neuropsychiatric symptoms of VCFS only partially respond to typical antipsychotics.[4] While the early introduction of clozapine is favoured,[4] experience suggests newer atypical antipsychotics are also effective in the treatment of VCFS-related schizophrenia.[1] Quetiapine[12] and aripiprazole[13] have been successfully used. Caution is required with most antipsychotics in VCFS because of the potential for cardiac toxicity (see section on 'QT changes' in Chapter 2).

Drugs which act directly against catecholamine excess may also be effective. There are case studies of successful use of methyldopa[14] and the catecholamine depleter, metyrosine.[15]

The use of atypical antipsychotics in VCFS patients with general developmental disabilities has been investigated and studies have found them to be broadly effective against challenging behaviours such as self-injury and aggression.[16,17] In addition, they have been found to be better tolerated than typical antipsychotics in this population.[18] Most evidence supports the use of risperidone.[16] The frequency of use of clozapine in learning disabilities still lags behind its use in the general population, despite the higher prevalence of psychiatric disorders in these patients. Clozapine has been associated with marked improvements in psychosis and aggressive behaviours in learning disabled patients. However, although it showed no worsening of seizure control or provocation of seizures in one study, a reduction in seizure threshold is a well-established and potentially serious adverse effect of clozapine. Unlike the other antipsychotics that do not precipitate seizures in patients with intellectual disability who have no history of seizures, this is not the case with clozapine. Therefore special caution should be observed in this population.[19]

Depression and anxiety symptoms are also common in VCFS.[1328,1338] Studies of treatment are few and far between but S-adenosyl-L-methionine has been shown to be effective.[21] SSRIs are commonly used.[20]

Children

Neuropsychiatric symptoms

Children with VCFS have been reported to have high rates of bipolar II disorder (47%), attention deficit hyperactivity disorder (ADHD) (27%) and attention deficit disorder without hyperactivity (ADD) (13%). The most recent (and largest) study suggest ADHD, with a prevalence of 37%, is the most common psychiatric disorder in VCFS children.[6] Data suggests that the inattentive subtype is the most common subtype of ADHD in children with VCFS. These children are less likely to be hyperactive or impulsive than children with idiopathic ADHD.[22] Some studies have also shown high rates of autism spectrum disorder, anxiety disorders and emotional instability in children with VCFS.[1]

Management of psychiatric symptoms

Concern has been raised over the theoretical risk of inducing psychosis in children with VCFS and co-morbid ADHD by using the psychostimulant methylphenidate. This is of particular concern in older adolescents or young adults. However, standard treatment for ADHD is recommended following experience suggesting psychosis is not a significant clinical risk.[1] Low doses of methylphenidate (0.3 mg/kg) have been shown to be effective in controlling VCFS-related ADHD and were generally well tolerated.[23] Note that there is also evidence that ADHD is under treated in VCFS.[20]

References

1. Murphy KC. Annotation: velo-cardio-facial syndrome. J Child Psychol Psychiatry 2005; **46**:563–571.
2. Buchanan LM et al. Velocardiofacial syndrome or DiGeorge's anomaly. Lancet 2001; **358**:420.
3. Shprintzen RJ. Velo-cardio-facial syndrome: 30 years of study. Dev Disabil Res Rev 2008; **14**:3–10.
4. Gothelf D et al. Clinical characteristics of schizophrenia associated with velo-cardio-facial syndrome. Schizophr Res 1999; **35**:105–112.
5. Murphy KC et al. High rates of schizophrenia in adults with velo-cardio-facial syndrome. Arch Gen Psychiatry 1999; **56**:940–945.
6. Schneider M et al. Psychiatric disorders from childhood to adulthood in 22q11.2 deletion syndrome: results from the International Consortium on Brain and Behavior in 22q11.2 Deletion Syndrome. Am J Psychiatry 2014.
7. Murphy KC et al. Velo-cardio-facial syndrome: a model for understanding the genetics and pathogenesis of schizophrenia. Br J Psychiatry 2001; **179**:397–402.
8. Schneider M et al. Clinical and cognitive risk factors for psychotic symptoms in 22q11.2 deletion syndrome: a transversal and longitudinal approach. Eur Child Adolesc Psychiatry 2014; **23**:425–436.
9. Karayiorgou M et al. Schizophrenia susceptibility associated with interstitial deletions of chromosome 22q11. Proc Natl Acad Sci U S A 1995; **92**:7612–7616.
10. Monks S et al. Further evidence for high rates of schizophrenia in 22q11.2 deletion syndrome. Schizophr Res 2014; **153**:231–236.
11. Eliez S et al. Parental origin of the deletion 22q11.2 and brain development in velocardiofacial syndrome: a preliminary study. Arch Gen Psychiatry 2001; **58**:64–68.
12. Muller UJ et al. Successful treatment of long-lasting psychosis in a case of 22q11.2 deletion syndrome. Pharmacopsychiatry 2008; **41**:158–159.
13. Lin CE et al. Treatment of schizophreniform disorder by aripiprazole in a female adolescent with 22q11.2 deletion syndrome. Prog Neuropsychopharmacol Biol Psychiatry 2010; **34**:1141–1143.
14. O'Hanlon JF et al. Replacement of antipsychotic and antiepileptic medication by L-alpha-methyldopa in a woman with velocardiofacial syndrome. Int Clin Psychopharmacol 2003; **18**:117–119.
15. Carandang CG et al. Metyrosine in psychosis associated with 22q11.2 deletion syndrome: case report. J Child Adolesc Psychopharmacol 2007; **17**:115–120.
16. Aman MG et al. Atypical antipsychotics in persons with developmental disabilities. Ment Retard Dev Disabil Res Rev 1999; **5**:253–263.
17. Williams H et al. Use of the atypical antipsychotics olanzapine and risperidone in adults with intellectual disability. J Intellect Disabil Res 2000; **44** (Pt 2):164–169.
18. Connor DF et al. A brief review of atypical antipsychotics in individuals with developmental disability. Ment Health Aspects Dev Disabil 1998; **1**:93–101.
19. Gladston S et al. Clozapine treatment of psychosis associated with velo-cardio-facial syndrome: benefits and risks. J Intellect Disabil Res 2005; **49**:567–570.
20. Tang SX et al. Psychiatric disorders in 22q11.2 deletion syndrome are prevalent but undertreated. Psychol Med 2014; **44**:1267–1277.
21. Green T et al. The feasibility and safety of S-adenosyl-L-methionine (SAMe) for the treatment of neuropsychiatric symptoms in 22q11.2 deletion syndrome: a double-blind placebo-controlled trial. J Neural Transm 2012; **119**:1417–1423.
22. Antshel KM et al. Comparing ADHD in velocardiofacial syndrome to idiopathic ADHD: a preliminary study. J Atten Disord 2007; **11**:64–73.
23. Gothelf D et al. Methylphenidate treatment for attention-deficit/hyperactivity disorder in children and adolescents with velocardiofacial syndrome: an open-label study. J Clin Psychiatry 2003; **64**:1163–1169.

CHAPTER 7

Cytochrome (CYP) function

Information on the effect of drugs on cytochrome function helps predict or confirm suspected interactions which may not have been uncovered in regulatory trials or in clinical use (sometimes called prediction from 'first principles'). Using 'first principles' essentially means understanding and interpreting pharmacokinetic information and anticipating the net effect of combining two or more drugs *in vivo*.

Apart from the effect of co-administered drugs on CYP function, genetic polymorphism associated with some enzyme pathways (e.g. 2D6, 2C9, 2C19 enzymes) may also account for inter-individual variations in metabolism of certain drugs.

The effects of polymorphism and pharmacokinetic interaction are difficult to predict because some drugs are metabolised by more than one enzyme and an alternative pathway(s) may compensate if other enzyme pathways are inhibited.

Also note that the function of CYPs is not the only consideration. P-glycoprotein (P-gp) is a drug transporter protein found in the gut wall. P-gp can eject (active process) drugs that diffuse (passive process) across the gut wall. P-gp is also found in testes and in the blood–brain barrier. Drugs that inhibit P-gp are anticipated to increase the uptake of other drugs (that are substrates for P-gp) and drugs that induce P-gp are anticipated to reduce the uptake of drugs (that are substrates for P-gp). Many drugs that are substrates for CYP3A4 have also been found to be substrates for P-gp.

UDP-glucuronosyl transferase (UGT) has been identified as an enzyme that is responsible for phase II (conjugation) reactions. The increasing importance of drug–drug interactions associated with UGT is emerging.

Table 7.35 summarises the interactions of psychotropic drugs with cytochromes. It does not include details of the effects of non-psychotropics on CYP function.

Table 7.35 Interactions of psychotropic drugs with cytochromes

Substrates	Inhibitors	Inducers
CPY1A2		
Agomelatine	**Fluvoxamine**	**'Barbiturates'**
Amitriptyline*	Moclobemide	Carbamazepine
Asenapine	Perphenazine	Modafinil*
Bupropion*		**Phenobarbital**
Chlorpromazine		Phenytoin
Clomipramine*		Smoking
Clozapine		
Duloxetine		
Fluphenazine		
Fluvoxamine		
Imipramine*		
Melatonin		
Mirtazapine*		
Olanzapine		
Perphenazine		
?Pimozide*		
Zolpidem*		
CYP2A6		
Bupropion*	**Tranylcypromine**	Phenobarbital
Nicotine		
CPY2B6		
Bupropion	Fluoxetine*	Carbamazepine*
Methadone*	Fluvoxamine	Modafinil*
Nicotine	Memantine	Phenobarbital
Sertraline*	Paroxetine*	Phenytoin
	Sertraline*	
CYP2B7		
Buprenorphine*	Not known	Not known
CPY2C8		
Zopiclone*	Not known	Not known
CPY2C9		
Agomelatine*	Fluoxetine*	Carbamazepine
Amitriptyline	Fluvoxamine	SJW
Bupropion*	Modafinil	
Fluoxetine*	Valproic acid	
Lamotrigine		
Phenobarbital		
Phenytoin		
Sertraline*		
Valproic acid		

(Continued)

Table 7.35 (*Continued*)

Substrates	Inhibitors	Inducers

CPY2C19

Substrates	Inhibitors	Inducers
Agomelatine*	Escitalopram*	Carbamazepine
Amitriptyline	Fluvoxamine	SJW
Carbamazepine*	Moclobemide	
Citalopram	Modafinil	
Clomipramine*	Topiramate	
Diazepam		
Escitalopram		
Fluoxetine*		
Imipramine*		
?Melatonin		
?Methadone		
Moclobemide		
Phenytoin		
Sertraline*		
Trimipramine*		

CPY2D6

Substrates	Inhibitors	Inducers
Amitriptyline	**Amitriptyline**	Not known
'Amfetamines'	**Asenapine**	
Atomoxetine	**Bupropion**	
Aripiprazole	Chlorpromazine	
Chlorpromazine	Citalopram*	
Citalopram	Clomipramine	
Clomipramine	Clozapine	
Clozapine*	**Duloxetine**	
Donepezil*	Escitalopram	
Duloxetine	**Fluoxetine**	
Escitalopram	Fluphenazine	
Fluoxetine	Fluvoxamine*	
Fluvoxamine	Haloperidol	
Fluphenazine	Levomepromazine	
Galantamine	Methadone*	
Haloperidol	Moclobemide	
Iloperidone	**Paroxetine**	
Imipramine	Perphenazine	
Methadone*	Reboxetine*	
Mianserin	Risperidone	
Mirtazapine*	Sertraline	
Moclobemide	Venlafaxine*	
Nortriptyline		
Olanzapine		
Paroxetine		
Perphenazine		
Pimozide*		
Quetiapine*		
Risperidone		
Sertraline		
Trazodone*		
Trimipramine		
Venlafaxine		
Vortioxetine		
Zuclopenthixol		

CYP2E1

Substrates	Inhibitors	Inducers
Bupropion	**Disulfiram**	Ethanol
Ethanol	Paracetamol	

Substrates	Inhibitors	Inducers
CYP3A4		
Alfentanyl	**Fluoxetine**	**Asenapine?**
Alprazolam	Fluvoxamine	**Carbamazepine**
Amitriptyline	**Paroxetine**	**Modafinil**
Aripiprazole	Perphenazine	**Phenobarbital**
Buprenorphine	Reboxetine*	'and probably
Bupropion*		other
Buspirone		barbiturates'
Carbamazepine		**Phenytoin**
Chlorpromazine		**SJW**
Citalopram		Topiramate
Clomipramine*		
Clonazepam		
Clozapine*		
Diazepam		
Donepezil		
Dosulepin		
Escitalopram*		
Fentanyl		
Fluoxetine*		
?Flurazepam		
Galantamine		
Haloperidol		
Imipramine		
Lurasidone		
Methadone		
Midazolam		
Mirtazapine		
Modafinil		
Nitrazepam		
Perphenazine		
Pimozide		
Quetiapine		
Reboxetine		
Risperidone*		
Sertindole		
Sertraline*		
Trazodone		
Trimipramine*		
Venlafaxine		
Zaleplon		
Ziprasidone		
Zolpidem		
Zopiclone		

Drugs highlighted in **bold** indicate:
- predominant metabolic enzyme pathway or
- predominant enzyme activity (inhibition or induction).

Drugs annotated with * indicate:
- known to be a minor metabolic enzyme pathway or activity
  (i.e. not demonstrated to be clinically significant).

Drugs in normal font (not bold and without *) indicate:
- metabolic enzyme pathway(s) or activity where significance is unclear
  or unknown.

Information on CYP function derived from individual SPCs and US
Labelling (accessed June 2014).
SJW, St John's wort.

Psychiatric side-effects of non-psychotropic drugs

It is increasingly recognised that non-psychotropic medications can induce a wide range of psychiatric symptoms, with one report estimating that up to two thirds of all available medications may be implicated.[1] Additionally, individuals with psychiatric problems in general have increased rates of physical illness,[2] especially those with schizophrenia[3,4] which will necessitate additional medication treatment. These patients are thus more likely to be exposed to polypharmacy, both of psychotropics[5] as well as non-psychotropics.[6,7]

Table 7.36 summarises the main behavioural, cognitive and psychiatric, side-effects of commonly prescribed non-psychotropics, with information compiled from various sources.[8–15] The information presented below is inevitably incomplete, and is intended as a general guide only. For details of agents not listed below, additional sources of information should be consulted (especially references 14 and 15). In the majority of cases the evidence for these various psychiatric and behavioural side-effects is limited, with details obtained mainly from case reports and manufacturers' information sheets. Although cessation of the implicated agent in question may be indicated, such decisions should always be made with caution as many of these presentations are idiosyncratic and many may be unrelated to the suspected causative agent. It should be further noted that medical co-morbidity, psychiatric and non-psychiatric polypharmacy, and the effects of non-prescribed agents may all influence the clinical presentation and outcome. Note that neuropsychiatric effects of anti-HIV medications and psychiatric side-effects of psychotropics are summarised elsewhere in the *Guidelines*.

Table 7.36 Summary of psychiatric side-effects of commonly prescribed non-psychotropic drugs

Event	Implicated agent
Agitation	Amantadine, aminophylline, apomorphine, aspirin, atropine, baclofen, benazapril, benzhexol, captopril, cimetidine, clonidine, corticosteroids, co-trimoxazole, cyclizine, cyproheptadine, dantrolene, doxazosin, enalapril, ethionamide, ethotoin, famotidine, fentanyl, flumazenil, fosinopril, fosphenytoin, gabapentin, ganciclovir, glucocorticoids, hydralazine, ibuprofen, indomethacin, isoniazid, isosorbide dinitrate, isosorbide mononitrate, L-dopa, levothyroxine, mefenamic acid, mefloquine, methoxamine, mephenytoin, methyltestosterone, misoprostol, morphine, naltrexone, naproxen, neostigmine, nitroglycerin, octreotide, omeprazole, orphenadrine, pentazocine, phenobarbital, piperazine, piroxicam, prednisone, procyclidine, promethazine, pseudoephedrine, ranitidine, salbutamol, selegiline, sibutramine, streptokinase, theophylline, tizanidine, trimeprazine, vigabatrin, yohimbine
Abnormal dreams	Atenolol, baclofen, chloroquine, dantrolene, L-dopa, mefloquine, metoprolol, oxprenolol, propranolol, sotalol, stanozolol, tizanidine
Aggression	Amantadine, apomorphine, bromocriptine, carbamazepine, corticosteroids, dapsone, diazepam, flunitrazepam, lamotrigine, lisuride, odafinil, naloxone, nandrolone, omeprazole, oxandrolone, pergolide, selegeline, stanozolol, testosterone, vigabatrin
Anxiety	Acetazolamide, amantadine, apomorphine, aspirin, atropine, baclofen, bendroflumethiazide, benzhexol, benzthiazide, benzatropine, biperiden, bromocriptine, cabergoline, chloroquine, chlorthalidone, cimetidine, clonidine, corticosteroids, co-trimoxazole, ciclosporin, dantrolene, dichlorphenamide, doxazosin, famotidine, fentanyl, flumazenil, ganciclovir, glucocorticoids, hydralazine, ibuprofen, indomethacin, isoniazid, isosorbide dinitrate, isosorbide mononitrate, L-dopa, levothyroxine, lisuride, mefenamic acid, mefloquine, methoxamine, methyltestosterone, misoprostol, morphine, naltrexone, nandrolone, naproxen, neostigmine, nitroglycerin, octreotide, omeprazole, orphenadrine, penicillins, pentazocine, pergolide, phentolamine, piperazine, piroxicam, pramipexole, prazosin, prednisone, procyclidine, pseudoephedrine, quinidine, quinine, ranitidine, ropinirole, salbutamol, sibutramine, stanozolol, streptokinase, tacrolimus, terazosin, testosterone, theophylline, tizanidine, yohimbine
Asthenia/ lethargy	Aciclovir, corticosteroids, digitoxin, digoxin, lidocaine, magnesium, mexilitine, moricizine, procainamide, vigabatrin
Change of behaviour	Anabolic steroids, barbiturates, benzodiazepines, clonazepam, L-dopa
Cognitive impairment	Acebutolol, apomorphine, atenolol, bromocriptine, clonidine, ciclosporin, ethotoin, foscarnet sodium, fosphenytoin, interferons, isoniazid, L-dopa, lidocaine, lisuride, mephenytoin, mexilitine, moricizine, nadolol, pergolide, phenobarbital, pindolol, procainamide, propranolol, quinidine, selegiline, topiramate, vigabatrin
Decreased concentration	Amantadine, tetracyclines, topiramate
Delirium	Acetazolamide, acebutolol, aciclovir, adrenocorticotrophin, amantadine, α-methyldopa, α-methyl-p-tyrosine, amiloride, aminophylline, amiodarone, amphotericin B, anaesthetics, apomorphine, aspirin, atenolol, atropine, baclofen, barbiturates, benazapril, benzhexol, benzatropine, biperiden, bromocriptine, cabergoline, captopril, carbamazepine, cephalosporins, chloramphenicol, chloroquine, ciclosporin A, cimetidine, ciprofloxacin, clarithromycin, clonidine, corticosteroids, cycloserine, dantrolene, dichlorphenamide, digitoxin, digoxin, disopyramide, doxapram, doxazosin, enalapril, entacapone, ethosuximide, ethotoin, famotidine, fenoprofen, fosinopril, fosphenytoin, ganciclovir,

(Continued)

Table 7.36 (*Continued*)

Event	Implicated agent
	hydralazine, hydroxychloroquine, hypoglycaemics, ibuprofen, indomethacin, interferons, isoniazid, isosorbide dinitrate, isosorbide mononitrate, L-dopa, lidocaine, lisuride, magnesium, mefenamic acid, mefloquine, mentholatum, mephenytoin, methotrexate, methylprednisolone, metoprolol, methixene, methyldopa, mexilitine, misoprostol, moricizine, nabilone, nadolol, naproxen, nitroglycerin, oxprenolol, papaveretum, penicillin, pergolide, phenobarbital, phentolamine, phenytoin, pindolol, piperazine, piroxicam, pramipexole, prazosin, primidone, procainamide, propranolol, quinidine, quinine, ranitidine, rifampicin, ropinirole, scopolamine, selegiline, sotalol, spironolactone, streptomycin, sulfasalazine, sulindac, sulphadiazine, sulphonamides, tacrolimus, terazosin, theophylline, tramadol, triamcinolone
Depression	Acetazolamide, acebutolol, alimenazine, allopurinol, amantadine, α-methyldopa, α-methyl-p-tyrosine, amiodarone, aminophylline, anaesthetics, atenolol, baclofen, benazapril, calcium-channel blockers, captopril, cephradine, chloramphenicol, chloroquine, cimetidine, cinnarizine, clofazimine, clomifene, clonidine, clotrimazole, codeine, corticosteroids, co-trimoxazole, cycloserine, ciclosporin, danazol, dapsone, dexamethasone, dichlorphenamide, digitoxin, digoxin, diltiazem, diphenoxylate, enalapril, ephedrine, ethionamide, ethotoin, etretinate, felodipine, fentanyl, finasteride, lunisolide, flurbiprofen, fosinopril, fosphenytoin, ganciclovir, griseofulvin, guanethidine, hydralazine, hydroxyzine, imidapril, indomethacin, inositol, interferons, ketoconazole, L-dopa, lignocaine, mefloquine, mephenytoin, mesna, metoclopramide, methyldopa, metoprolol, metronidazole, mexilitine, mitramycin, nabilone, nadolol, nandrolone, nicardipine, nifedipine, oestrogens, omega 3 fatty acids, ondansetron, opioids, oral contraceptives, organophosphates, oxprenolol, pentazocine, phenobarbital, phenylpropanolamine, picamycin, pindolol, piperazine, pravastatin, prednisolone, prednisone, primaquine, procainamide, progestogens, propranolol, quinapril, quinidine, ramipril, ranitidine, reserpine, ribavirin, isotretinoin, simvastatin, sotalol, stanozolol, streptokinase, sulphazalazine, sulindac, sulphonamides, tacrolimus, tamoxifen, testosterone, theophylline, tiagabine, timolol, topiramate, tramadol, triamcinolone, trimeprazine, trimethoprim, vigabatrin, xylometazoline
Disorientation/ confusion	Amiloride, baclofen, dantrolene, enalapril, imidapril, quinapril, quinine, ramipril, spironolactone, tizanidine
Fatigue/ lethargy	Acebutolol, α-methyldopa, α-methyl-p-tyrosine, amlodipine, amantadine, amiloride, anticholinergics, aspirin, atenolol, benazapril, bepridil, captopril, chlorphenamine, cimetidine, clemastine, cyproheptadine, diphenhydramine, doxazosin, enalapril, famotidine, felodipine, flunarizine, foscarnet sodium, fosinopril, gabapentin, hydroxyzine, ibuprofen, indomethacin, L-dopa, lignocaine, mefenamic acid, mexilitine, nadolol, naproxen, nicardipine, phentolamine, pindolol, piroxicam, prazosin, procainamide, propranolol, ranitidine, spironolactone, terazosin, verapamil
Hallucinations	Acebutolol, amantadine, amoxicillin, anticholinergics, apomorphine, aspirin, atenolol, baclofen, benazapril, beta-blockers, bromocriptine, buprenorphine, cabergoline, captopril, celecoxib, cephalosporins, chloroquine, cimetidine, ciprofloxacin, clonidine, corticosteroids, dantrolene, dextromethorphan, digoxin, diltiazem, disopyramide, enalapril, entacapone, erythropoetin, famotidine, fenbufen, flucytosine, fosinopril, gentamicin, hydroxyurea, ibuprofen, indomethacin, itraconazole, L-dopa, lisuride, mefenamic acid, mefloquine, nadolol, naproxen, penicillins, pentazocine, pergolide, phenylephrine, phenylpropanolamine, pindolol, piroxicam, procainamide, promethazine, propranolol, pseudoephedrine, ranitidine, ropinirole, pramipexole, salbutamol, salicylates, selegeline, streptokinase, sulphasalazine, timolol, tizanidine, tolterodine, tramadol

Table 7.36 (Continued)

Event	Implicated agent
Insomnia	Baclofen, benzhexol, dantrolene, doxazosin, orphenadrine, phentolamine, prazosin, procyclidine, terazosin, tizanidine
Irritability	Amantadine, cycloserine, ethionamide, ethosuximide, levetiracetam, methotrexate, penicillins, vigabatrin
Mood changes/ lability	Amiodarone, amlodipine, aspirin, baclofen, bepridil, bromocriptine, dantrolene, diltiazem, disopyramide, ethosuximide, felopidine, flunarizine, foscarnet sodium, ganciclovir, ibuprofen, indomethacin, isoniazid, ketoconazole, L-dopa, lidocaine, mefenamic acid, mexilitine, moricizine, naproxen, nicardipine, opioids, piroxicam, primidone, procainamide, procyclidine, quinolones, tetracyclines, topiramate, verapamil
Mania, euphoria, hypomania	ACTH, aminophylline, amlodipine, amantadine, baclofen, beclomethasone, benazapril, bepridil, bromocriptine, buprenorphine, captopril, chloroquine, ciclosporin, cimetidine, clarithromycin, clonidine, corticosteroids, cortisone, cyclizine, cyproheptadine, dantrolene, dapsone, dexamethasone, dextromethorphan, digoxin, dihydroepiandrosterone, diltiazem, enalapril, felodipine, flunarizine, fosinopril, frovatriptan, hydralazine, hydrocortisone, indomethacin, interferon alpha, isoniazid, isosorbide dinitrate, isosorbide mononitrate, L-dopa, mepacrine, metoclopramide, nandrolone, nefopam, nicardipine, nitrofurans, nitroglycerin, omega 3 fatty acids, pentazocine, procainamide, procarbazine, procyclidine, propranolol, ranitidine, salbutamol, sildenafil, stanozolol, steroids, testosterone, tizanidine, tramadol, triptorelin, triamcinolone, tri-iodothyronine, verapamil
Misuse potential	Anabolic steroids, benzhexol, benzatropine, corticosteroids, orphenadrine, oxymetazoline, procyclidine
Nervousness	Amantadine, atropine, baclofen, co-trimoxazole, doxazosin, enalapril, fentanyl, flumazenil, ganciclovir, glucocorticoids, hydralazine, imidapril, isoniazid, L-dopa, levothyroxine, mefloquine, methoxamine, methyltestosterone, misoprostol, morphine, naltrexone, neostigmine, octreotide, omeprazole, pentazocine, piperazine, prednisone, pseudoephedrine, quinapril, ramipril, salbutamol, sibutramine, streptokinase, theophylline
Obsessive-compulsive symptoms	Cabergoline, colchicine, topiramate
Panic attacks/ disorder	Calcium lactate, carvedilol, chloroquine, co-trimoxazole, mefloquine, oxymetazoline, phenylephrine, sibutramine, steroids, sumatriptan, yohimbine
Personality change	Corticosteroids, methotrexate
Psychomotor restlessness	Apomorphine, bromocriptine, cabergoline, lisuride, pergolide, ropinirole, pramipexole
Psychosis	Acebutolol, aciclovir, adrenocorticotrophin, amantadine, α-methyldopa, α-methyl-p-tyrosine, amiloride, amiodarone, amlodipine, amphotericin B, amyl nitrate, apomorphine, aspirin, atenolol, atropine, baclofen, benzhexol, benzatropine, bepridil, beta-blockers, biperiden, bromocriptine, cabergoline, calcium lactate, carbaryl, carbimazole, cefuroxime, cephalexin, cephalothin, chloroquine, chlorphenamine, cimetidine, ciprofloxacin, clarithromycin, clomifene, clonidine, colistin, corticosteroids, cortisone, cycloserine, cyclizine, ciclosporin, cyproheptadine, dapsone, desmopressin, dextromethorphan, dicyclomine, digitoxin, digoxin, diphenhydramine, diltiazem, disopyramide, disulfiram, doxazosin, enalapril, erythromycin, ethosuximide, ethionamide, ethotoin, felodipine, flunarizine, foscarnet sodium, fosphenytoin, ganciclovir, griseofulvin, hydralazine, hyoscine, ibuprofen, indomethacin, interferon alpha,

(Continued)

CHAPTER 7

Table 7.36 (*Continued*)

Event	Implicated agent
	isoniazid, isosorbide dinitrate, isosorbide mononitrate, isotretoin, ketoconazole, L-dopa, levetiracetam, levofloxacin, lidocaine, lisuride, melatonin, mefenamic acid, mefloquine, mephenytoin, methixene, methyldopa, methylprednisolone, methyltestosterone, metronidazole, mexilitine, moricizine, nabilone, nadolol, nalidixic acid, nandrolone, naproxen, nicardipine, nifedipine, nitrofurans, nitroglycerin, opioids, orphenadrine, oxymetazoline, penicillin G, pentazocine, pergolide, phenobarbital, phenylephrine, phenylpropanolamine, pindolol, piroxicam, prednisone, procainamide, procaine, procyclidine, promethazine, propranolol, quinolones, ropinirole, pramipexole, primaquine, primidone, procaine, pyridostigmine, quinine, quinidine, reserpine, salbutamol, scopolamine, selegiline, sibutramine, stanozolol, sulindac, sulphonamides, tacrolimus, testosterone, tiagabine, tobramycin, tocainide, topiramate, tramadol, trimeprazine, trimethoprim, verapamil, vigabatrin
Sedation	Acetazolamide, acebutolol, amiodarone, apomorphine, atenolol, bendroflumethiazide, benzthiazide, benzatropine, biperiden, bromocriptine, cabergoline, chlorphenamine, chlorthalidone, clemastine, cyclizine, cyproheptadine, dichlorphenamide, digitoxin, digoxin, diphenhydramine, disopyramide, doxazosin, ethionamide, ethotoin, flucytosine, fosphenytoin, gabapentin, guanethidine, hydroxyzine, levetiracetam, lisuride, mephenytoin, nadolol, penicillins, pergolide, phenobarbital, phentolamine, pindolol, pramipexole, prazosin, primidone, promethazine, propranolol, reserpine, rifampicin, ropinirole, terazosin, tiagabine, trimeprazine
Sleep disturbance	Acebutolol, amantadine, α-methyldopa, α-methyl-p-tyrosine, aminophylline, amiodarone, apomorphine, aspirin, atenolol, baclofen, bendroflumethiazide, benzthiazide, bromocriptine, brompheniramine, cabergoline, carvedilol, cephalosporins, chlorthalidone, cinoxacin, ciprofloxacin, clomifene, clonidine, corticosteroids, dantrolene, dexamethasone, diclofenac, diflunisal, digoxin, diltiazem, entacapone, ethosuximide, ethotoin, fenoprofen, fosphenytoin, ganciclovir, griseofulvin, ibuprofen, indomethacin, interferons, isradipine, L-dopa, lisuride, lovastatin, mefenamic acid, mephenytoin, methyldopa, nadolol, naproxen, nitrofurans, pergolide, phenobarbital, pindolol, piroxicam, pramipexole, propranolol, propantheline, pseudoephedrine, quinolones, ranitidine, ropinirole, selegiline, sibutramine, simvastatin, sulfasalazine, sulindac, tetracyclines, theophylline, tolzamide, triamcinolone
Suicidal ideation	Chloroquine, clofazimine, interferons, mefloquine, reserpine
Visual hallucinations	Amantadine, benzhexol, benzatropine, biperiden, L-dopa, orphenadrine, procyclidine

References

1. Smith DA. Psychiatric side effects of non-psychiatric drugs. S D J Med 1991; **44**:291–292.
2. Goldman LS. Comorbid medical illness in psychiatric patients. Curr Psychiatry Rep 2000; **2**:256–263.
3. Jones DR et al. Prevalence, severity, and co-occurrence of chronic physical health problems of persons with serious mental illness. Psychiatr Serv 2004; **55**:1250–1257.
4. Leucht S et al. Physical illness and schizophrenia: a review of the literature. Acta Psychiatr Scand 2007; **116**:317–333.
5. Taylor D. Antipsychotic polypharmacy - confusion reigns. Psychiatrist 2010; **34**:41–43.
6. Davies SJ et al. PRN prescribing in psychiatric inpatients: potential for pharmacokinetic drug interactions. J Psychopharmacol 2007; **21**:153–160.
7. Bingefors K et al. Antidepressant-treated patients in ambulatory care long-term use of non-psychotropic and psychotropic drugs. Br J Psychiatry 1996; **168**:292–298.

8. Datapharm Communications Ltd. Electronic Medicines Compendium. 2014. https://www.medicines.org.uk/emc/

9. Joint Formulary Committee. *BNF* 67 March-September 2014 (online). London: Pharmaceutical Press; 2014. http://www.medicinescomplete.com/mc/bnf/current/

10. Sidhu KS et al. Watch for nonpsychotropics causing psychiatric side effects. Curr Psychiatry 2008; 7:61–74.

11. Turjanski N et al. Psychiatric side-effects of medications: recent developments. Adv Psychiatr Treat 2005; **11**:58–70.

12. Ashton HC. Psychiatric effects of drugs for other disorders. Medicine 2008; **36**:501–504.

13. Bazire S. *Psychotropic Drug Directory*. UK: Lloyd-Reinhold Communcations LLP; 2014.

14. American Pharmacists Association. *Drug Information Handbook 2014-2015*, 23rd edn. United States: Lexi-Comp; 2014.

15. Brown TM et al. *Psychiatric side-effects of prescription and over the counter medications: recognition and management*. Washington, DC: American Psychiatric Press; 1998.

Atrial fibrillation

Atrial fibrillation (AF) is the most common cardiac arrhythmia. It particularly affects older people but may occur in an important proportion of people under the age of 40. Risk factors include anxiety, obesity, diabetes, hypertension, long-standing aerobic exercise and high alcohol consumption.[1–3] AF itself is not usually life-threatening, but stasis of blood in the atria during fibrillation predisposes to clot formation and substantially increases the risk of stroke.[4] The use of warfarin or novel oral anticoagulants is therefore essential.[3]

AF can be defined as 'lone' or paroxysmal (occurring infrequently and spontaneously reverting to sinus rhythm), persistent (repeated and prolonged [> one week] episodes, which are usually, if temporarily, responsive to treatment) or permanent (unresponsive). Risk of stroke is increased in all three conditions.[3]

Treatment may involve DC conversion, rhythm control (usually flecainide, propafenone or amiodarone) or rate control (with diltiazem, verapamil or sotalol). With rhythm control the aim is to maintain sinus rhythm, although this is not always achieved. With rate control, atrial fibrillation is allowed to continue but ventricular response is controlled and ventricles are filled passively. Many people with paroxysmal or persistent AF can now be effectively cured of the condition by catheter or cryo-ablation of aberrant electrical pathways.[5,6]

Atrial fibrillation is commonly encountered in psychiatry not least because of the high rates of obesity, diabetes and alcohol misuse seen in mental health patients. When considering the use of psychotropics several factors need to be taken into account.

- Interactions between psychotropics and anticoagulant therapy (see section on 'SSRIs and bleeding' in Chapter 4).
- Arrhythmogenicity of psychotropics prescribed (AF usually results from cardiovascular disease; drugs affecting cardiac ion channels may increase mortality in these patients, especially those with ischaemic disease).[7,8]
- Effect on ventricular rate (some drugs induce reflex tachycardia via postural hypotension, others [clozapine, quetiapine] directly increase heart rate).
- Reported association between individual psychotropics and AF.
- Risk of interaction with co-prescribed antiarrhythmics or rate-controlling drugs.
- Whether AF is paroxysmal (aim to avoid precipitating AF), persistent (aim to avoid prolonging AF) or permanent (aim to avoid increasing ventricular rate).

Recommendations for using psychotropic drugs in AF are shown in Table 7.37.

Table 7.37 Recommendations for using psychotropic drugs in AF

Condition	Suggested drugs	Drugs to avoid
Schizophrenia/schizoaffective disorder (The condition itself may be associated with an increased risk of AF)[9]	In paroxysmal or persistent AF, **aripiprazole** or **lurasidone** may be appropriate choices. In permanent AF with rate control, drug choice is less crucial but probably best to avoid drugs with potent effects on the ECG (ziprasidone, pimozide, sertindole, etc.) and those which increase heart rate.	AF reported with clozapine,[10] olanzapine[11,12] and paliperidone.[13] Causation not established but avoid use in paroxysmal or persistent AF. Avoid QT-prolonging drugs in ischaemic heart disease (see section on QT prolongation in Chapter 2).
Bipolar disorder	**Valproate** **Lithium**	Mood stabilisers appear not to affect risk of AF.
Depression (note – untreated depression predicts recurrence of AF)[14]	SSRIs (may be beneficial in paroxysmal AF)[15] but beware interaction with warfarin and other anticoagulants.[16] Animal studies suggest an antiarrhythmic effect for SSRIs.[17,18] Venlafaxine does not directly affect atrial conduction[19] and may cardiovert paroxysmal AF.[20] No evidence that **agomelatine** affects cardiac conduction or clotting.	Avoid tricyclics in coronary disease.[21] Tricyclics may also provoke AF[22,23] but do not increase risk of haemorrhage when combined with warfarin.[16]
Anxiety disorders (anxiety symptoms increase risk of AF)[24]	**Benzodiazepines** **SSRIs** (see above)	Tricyclics (see above).
Alzheimer's disease	**Acetylcholinesterase inhibitors** (but beware bradycardic effects in patients with paroxysmal 'vagal' AF [paroxysmal AF provoked by low heart rate]) **Rivastigmine** has least interaction potential. **Memantine**	Avoid cholinesterase inhibitors in paroxysmal 'vagal' AF.

AF, atrial fibrillation; ECG, electrocardiogram; SSRI, selective serotonin reuptake inhibitor.

References

1. Chen LY et al. Epidemiology of atrial fibrillation: a current perspective. Heart Rhythm 2007; **4**:S1–S6.
2. Tully PJ et al. Anxiety, depression, and stress as risk factors for atrial fibrillation after cardiac surgery. Heart Lung 2011; **40**:4–11.
3. National Institute for Health and Care Excellence. Atrial fibrillation: the management of atrial fibrillation. Clinical Guideline 180, 2014. http://www.nice.org.uk/guidance/cg180
4. Lakshminarayan K et al. Clinical epidemiology of atrial fibrillation and related cerebrovascular events in the United States. Neurologist 2008; **14**:143–150.
5. Rodgers M et al. Curative catheter ablation in atrial fibrillation and typical atrial flutter: systematic review and economic evaluation. Health Technol Assess 2008; **12**:iii–xiii, 1.
6. Latchamsetty R et al. Catheter ablation of atrial fibrillation. Cardiol Clin 2014; **32**:551–561.

CHAPTER 7

7. Investigators, TCASTI. Effect of the antiarrhythmic agent moricizine on survival after myocardial infarction. N Engl J Med 1992; **327**:227–233.

8. Epstein AE et al. Mortality following ventricular arrhythmia suppression by encainide, flecainide, and moricizine after myocardial infarction. The original design concept of the Cardiac Arrhythmia Suppression Trial (CAST). JAMA 1993; **270**:2451–2455.

9. Emul M et al. P wave and QT changes among inpatients with schizophrenia after parenteral ziprasidone administration. Pharmacol Res 2009; **60**:369–372.

10. Low RA Jr. et al. Clozapine induced atrial fibrillation. J Clin Psychopharmacol 1998; **18**:170.

11. Waters BM et al. Olanzapine-associated new-onset atrial fibrillation. J Clin Psychopharmacol 2008; **28**:354–355.

12. Yaylaci S et al. Atrial fibrillation due to olanzapine overdose. Clin Toxicol (Phila) 2011; **49**:440.

13. Schneider RA et al. Apparent seizure and atrial fibrillation associated with paliperidone. Am J Health Syst Pharm 2008; **65**:2122–2125.

14. Lange HW et al. Depressive symptoms predict recurrence of atrial fibrillation after cardioversion. J Psychosom Res 2007; **63**:509–513.

15. Shirayama T et al. Usefulness of paroxetine in depressed men with paroxysmal atrial fibrillation. Am J Cardiol 2006; **97**:1749–1751.

16. Quinn GR et al. Effect of selective serotonin reuptake inhibitors on bleeding risk in patients with atrial fibrillation taking warfarin. Am J Cardiol 2014; **114**:583–586.

17. Pousti A et al. Effect of sertraline on ouabain-induced arrhythmia in isolated guinea-pig atria. Depress Anxiety 2009; **26**:E106–E110.

18. Pousti A et al. Effect of citalopram on ouabain-induced arrhythmia in isolated guinea-pig atria. Human Psychopharmacol 2003; **18**:121–124.

19. Emul M et al. The influences of depression and venlafaxine use at therapeutic doses on atrial conduction. J Psychopharmacol (Oxford, England) 2009; **23**:163–167.

20. Finch SJ et al. Cardioversion of persistent atrial arrhythmia after treatment with venlafaxine in successful management of major depression and posttraumatic stress disorder. Psychosomatics 2006; **47**:533–536.

21. Taylor D. Antidepressant drugs and cardiovascular pathology: a clinical overview of effectiveness and safety. Acta Psychiatr Scand 2008; **118**:434–442.

22. Moorhead CN et al. Imipramine-induced auricular fibrillation. Am J Psychiatry 1965; **122**:216–217.

23. Rosen BH. Case report of auricular fibrillation following the use of imipramine (Tofranil). J Mt Sinai Hosp NY 1960; **27**:609–611.

24. Eaker ED et al. Tension and anxiety and the prediction of the 10-year incidence of coronary heart disease, atrial fibrillation, and total mortality: the Framingham Offspring Study. Psychosom Med 2005; **67**:692–696.

Chapter 8

Miscellaneous conditions and substances

Psychotropic drugs in overdose

Suicide attempts and suicidal gestures are frequently encountered in psychiatric and general practice, and psychotropic drugs are often taken in overdose. This section gives brief details of the toxicity in overdose of commonly used psychotropics (Table 8.1). It is intended to help guide drug choice in those thought to be at risk of suicide and to help identify symptoms of overdose. This section gives no information on the treatment of psychotropic overdose and readers are directed to specialist poisons units. In all cases of suspected overdose, urgent referral to acute medical facilities is, of course, strongly advised.

Table 8.1 Psychotropic drugs in overdose

Drug or drug group	Toxicity in overdose	Smallest dose likely to cause death	Signs and symptoms of overdose
Antidepressants			
Agomelatine[1]	Probably low	No deaths reported. In early trials, 800 mg was maximum tolerated dose	Sedation
Bupropion[2–5]	Moderate	Around 4.5 g	Tachycardia, seizures, QRS prolongation, QT prolongation, arrhythmia
Duloxetine[6–8]	Low	Unclear – no deaths from single overdose reported	Drowsiness, bradycardia, hypotension. May be asymptomatic
Lofepramine[9–11]	Low	Unclear. Fatality unlikely if lofepramine taken alone	Sedation, coma, tachycardia, hypotension
MAOIs (not moclobemide)[9,12–14]	High	Phenelzine – 400 mg Tranylcypromine – 200 mg	Tremor, weakness, confusion, sweating, tachycardia, hypertension

(*Continued*)

The Maudsley Prescribing Guidelines in Psychiatry, Twelfth Edition. David Taylor, Carol Paton and Shitij Kapur.
© 2015 David Taylor, Carol Paton and Shitij Kapur. Published 2015 by John Wiley & Sons, Ltd.

Table 8.1 (*Continued*)

Drug or drug group	Toxicity in overdose	Smallest dose likely to cause death	Signs and symptoms of overdose
Mianserin[15–17]	Low	Unclear but probably more than 1 g. Fatality unlikely if mianserin taken alone	Sedation, coma, hypotension, hypertension, tachycardia, possible QT prolongation
Mirtazapine[2,18–21]	Low	Unclear but probably more than 2.25 g. Fatality unlikely in overdose of mirtazapine alone	Sedation; even large overdose may be asymptomatic. Tachycardia/hypertension sometimes seen
Moclobemide[22,23]	Low	Unclear, but probably more than 8 g. Fatality unlikely if moclobemide taken alone	Vomiting, sedation, disorientation
Reboxetine[2,24]	Low	Not known. Fatality unlikely in overdose of reboxetine alone	Sweating, tachycardia, changes in blood pressure
SSRIs[10,11,25–27]	Low	Unclear. Probably above 1–2 g. Fatality unlikely if SSRI taken alone	Vomiting, tremor, drowsiness, tachycardia, ST depression. Seizures and QT prolongation possible. Citalopram most toxic of SSRIs in overdose (coma, seizures, arrhythmia); escitalopram is less toxic[28,29]
Trazodone[7,30–33]	Low	Unclear but probably more than 10 g. Fatality unlikely in overdose of trazodone alone	Drowsiness, nausea, hypotension, dizziness. Rarely QT prolongation, arrhythmia
TCAs[9,12,13,34,35] (not lofepramine)	High	Around 500 mg. Doses over 50 mg/kg usually fatal	Sedation, coma, tachycardia, arrhythmia (QRS, QT prolongation), hypotension, seizures
Venlafaxine[2,36–41] (assume same for desvenlafaxine)	Moderate	Probably above 5 g, but seizures may occur after ingestion of 1 g	Vomiting, sedation, tachycardia, hypertension, seizures. Rarely QT prolongation, arrhythmia, rhabdomyolysis. Very rarely cardiac arrest/MI, heart failure
Vortioxetine[42]	Low	Unclear	Nausea, somnolence, diarrhoea, pruritis
Antipsychotics			
Amisulpride[43,43–45]	Moderate	Around 16 g	QT prolongation, arrhythmia, cardiac arrest
Aripiprazole[46–49]	Low	Unclear. Fatality unlikely when taken alone	Sedation, lethargy, gastrointestinal disturbance, drooling
Asenapine[50]	Probably low	Unclear. No deaths from overdose reported	Sedation, confusion, facial dystonia, benign ECG changes
Butyrophenones[51–53]	Moderate	Haloperidol – probably above 500 mg. Arrhythmia may occur at 300 mg	Sedation, coma, dystonia, NMS, QT prolongation, arrhythmia
Clozapine[54,55]	Moderate	Around 2 g, much less in non-tolerant individuals	Lethargy, coma, tachycardia, hypotension, hypersalivation, pneumonia, seizures

Table 8.1 (*Continued*)

Drug or drug group	Toxicity in overdose	Smallest dose likely to cause death	Signs and symptoms of overdose
Iloperidone[56,57]	Probably moderate	Unclear but probably more than 500 mg	Potent effect on QT interval. Sedation, tachycardia, hypotension likely
Lurasidone[58]	Probably low	Unclear	Very limited information. Minimal effect on QT interval
Olanzapine[54,59–61]	Moderate	Unclear. Probably substantially more than 200 mg	Lethargy, confusion, myoclonus, myopathy, hypotension, tachycardia, delirium. Possibly QT prolongation
Phenothiazines[51,62–64]	Moderate	Chlorpromazine 5–10 g	Sedation, coma, tachycardia, arrhythmia, pulmonary oedema, hypotension, QT prolongation, seizures, dystonia, NMS
Quetiapine[54,65–70]	Low	Unclear. Probably more than 5 g. Fatalities rare	Lethargy, delirium, tachycardia, QT prolongation, respiratory depression, hypotension, rhabdomyolysis, NMS
Risperidone[54,71,72] (assume same for paliperidone)	Low	Unclear. Fatality rare in those taking risperidone alone	Lethargy, dystonia, tachycardia, changes in blood pressure, QT prolongation. Renal failure with paliperidone
Ziprasidone[73–78]	Low	Around 10 g. Fatality unlikely when taken alone	Drowsiness, lethargy. QT prolongation, Torsades
Mood stabilisers			
Carbamazepine[79,80]	Moderate	Around 20 g, but seizures may occur at around 5 g	Somnolence, coma, respiratory depression, ataxia, seizures, tachycardia, arrhythmia, electrolyte disturbance
Lamotrigine[81–83]	Low	Unclear. No deaths from overdose reported	Drowsiness, vomiting, ataxia, tachycardia, dyskinesia
Lithium[84–87]	Low (acute overdose)	Acute overdose does not normally result in fatality. Insidious, chronic toxicity is more dangerous	Nausea, diarrhoea, tremor, confusion, weakness, lethargy, seizures, coma, cardiovascular collapse, bradycardia, arrhythmia, heart block
Valproate[88–92]	Moderate	Unclear but probably more than 20 g. Doses over 400 mg/kg cause severe toxicity	Somnolence, coma, cerebral oedema, respiratory depression, blood dyscrasia, hypotension, hypothermia, seizures, electrolyte disturbance (hyper ammonaemia)
Others			
Benzodiazepines[93,94]	Low	Probably more than 100 mg diazepam equivalents. Fatality unusual if taken alone. Alprazolam is most toxic	Drowsiness, ataxia, nystagmus, respiratory dysarthria, depression, coma

(*Continued*)

CHAPTER 8

Table 8.1 (*Continued*)

Drug or drug group	Toxicity in overdose	Smallest dose likely to cause death	Signs and symptoms of overdose
Methadone[95,96]	High	20–50 mg may be fatal in non-users. Co-ingestion of benzodiazepines increases toxicity	Drowsiness, nausea, hypotension, respiratory depression, coma, rhabdomyolysis
Modafinil[97,98]	Low	Unclear. Overdoses of >6 g have not caused death	Tachycardia, insomnia, agitation, anxiety, nausea, hypertension, dystonia
Zolpidem[99,100]	Low	Unclear. Probably >200 mg. Fatality rare in those taking zolpidem alone	Drowsiness, agitation, respiratory depression, tachycardia, coma
Zopiclone[93,101,102]	Low	Unclear. Probably >100 mg. Fatality rare in those taking zopiclone alone	Ataxia, nausea, diplopia, drowsiness, coma

ECG, electrocardiogram; MAOI, monoamine oxidase inhibitor; MI, myocardial infarction; NMS, neuroleptic malignant syndrome; SSRI, selective serotonin reuptake inhibitor; TCA, tricyclic antidepressant.

High = Less than 1 week's supply likely to cause serious toxicity or death
Moderate = 1–4 weeks' supply likely to cause serious toxicity or death
Low = Death or serious toxicity unlikely even if more than 1 month's supply taken

References

1. Howland RH. Critical appraisal and update on the clinical utility of agomelatine, a melatonergic agonist, for the treatment of major depressive disease in adults. Neuropsychiatr Dis Treat 2009; 5:563–576.
2. Buckley NA et al. 'Atypical' antidepressants in overdose: clinical considerations with respect to safety. Drug Saf 2003; 26:539–551.
3. Paris PA et al. ECG conduction delays associated with massive bupropion overdose. J Toxicol Clin Toxicol 1998; 36:595–598.
4. Curry SC et al. Intraventricular conduction delay after bupropion overdose. J Emerg Med 2005; 29:299–305.
5. Mercerolle M et al. A fatal case of bupropion (Zyban) overdose. J Anal Toxicol 2008; 32:192–196.
6. Menchetti M et al. Non-fatal overdose of duloxetine in combination with other antidepressants and benzodiazepines. World J Biol Psychiatry 2008;1-5.
7. White N et al. Suicidal antidepressant overdoses: a comparative analysis by antidepressant type. J Med Toxicol 2008; 4:238–250.
8. Darracq MA et al. A retrospective review of isolated duloxetine-exposure cases. Clin Toxicol (Phila) 2013; 51:106–110.
9. Cassidy S et al. Fatal toxicity of antidepressant drugs in overdose. Br Med J 1987; 295:1021–1024.
10. Henry JA et al. Relative mortality from overdose of antidepressants. BMJ 1995; 310:221–224.
11. Cheeta S et al. Antidepressant-related deaths and antidepressant prescriptions in England and Wales, 1998-2000. Br J Psychiatry 2004; 184:41–47.
12. Crome P. Antidepressant overdosage. Drugs 1982; 23:431–461.
13. Henry JA. Epidemiology and relative toxicity of antidepressant drugs in overdose. Drug Saf 1997; 16:374–390.
14. Waring WS et al. Acute myocarditis after massive phenelzine overdose. Eur J Clin Pharmacol 2007; 63:1007–1009.
15. Chand S et al. One hundred cases of acute intoxication with minaserin hydrochloride. Pharmacopsychiatry 1981; 14:15–17.
16. Scherer D et al. Inhibition of cardiac hERG potassium channels by tetracyclic antidepressant mianserin. Naunyn Schmiedebergs Arch Pharmacol 2008; 378:73–83.
17. Koseoglu Z et al. Bradycardia and hypotension in mianserin intoxication. Hum Exp Toxicol 2010; 29:887–888.
18. Bremner JD et al. Safety of mirtazapine in overdose. J Clin Psychiatry 1998; 59:233–235.
19. LoVecchio F et al. Outcomes after isolated mirtazapine (Remeron) supratherapeutic ingestions. J Emerg Med 2008; 34:77–78.
20. Hawton K et al. Toxicity of antidepressants: rates of suicide relative to prescribing and non-fatal overdose. Br J Psychiatry 2010; 196:354–358.
21. Berling I et al. Mirtazapine overdose is unlikely to cause major toxicity. Clin Toxicol (Phila) 2014; 52:20–24.
22. Hetzel W. Safety of moclobemide taken in overdose for attempted suicide. Psychopharmacology 1992; 106 Suppl:S127–S129.
23. Myrenfors PG et al. Moclobemide overdose. J Intern Med 1993; 233:113–115.
24. Baldwin DS et al. Tolerability and safety of reboxetine. Rev Contemp Pharmacother 2000; 11:321–330.
25. Barbey JT et al. SSRI safety in overdose. J Clin Psychiatry 1998; 59 Suppl 15:42–48.
26. Jimmink A et al. Clinical toxicology of citalopram after acute intoxication with the sole drug or in combination with other drugs: overview of 26 cases. Ther Drug Monit 2008; 30:365–371.

27. Tarabar AF et al. Citalopram overdose: late presentation of torsades de pointes (TdP) with cardiac arrest. J Med Toxicol 2008; 4:101–105.

28. Yilmaz Z et al. Escitalopram causes fewer seizures in human overdose than citalopram. Clin Toxicol (Phila) 2010; 48:207–212.

29. van GF et al. Clinical and ECG effects of escitalopram overdose. Ann Emerg Med 2009; 54:404–408.

30. Gamble DE et al. Trazodone overdose: four years of experience from voluntary reports. J Clin Psychiatry 1986; 47:544–546.

31. Martinez MA et al. Investigation of a fatality due to trazodone poisoning: case report and literature review. J Anal Toxicol 2005; 29:262–268.

32. Dattilo PB et al. Prolonged QT associated with an overdose of trazodone. J Clin Psychiatry 2007; 68:1309–1310.

33. Service JA et al. QT Prolongation and delayed atrioventricular conduction caused by acute ingestion of trazodone. Clin Toxicol (Phila) 2008; 46:71–73.

34. Power BM et al. Antidepressant toxicity and the need for identification and concentration monitoring in overdose. Clin Pharmacokinet 1995; 29:154–171.

35. Caksen H et al. Acute amitriptyline intoxication: an analysis of 44 children. Hum Exp Toxicol 2006; 25:107–110.

36. Huang SS et al. Low-dose venlafaxine-induced severe rhabdomyolysis: a case report. Gen Hosp Psychiatry 2012; 34:436–437.

37. Batista M et al. The spectrum of acute heart failure after venlafaxine overdose. Clin Toxicol (Phila) 2013; 51:92–95.

38. Whyte IM et al. Relative toxicity of venlafaxine and selective serotonin reuptake inhibitors in overdose compared to tricyclic antidepressants. QJM 2003; 96:369–374.

39. Howell C et al. Cardiovascular toxicity due to venlafaxine poisoning in adults: a review of 235 consecutive cases. Br J Clin Pharmacol 2007; 64:192–197.

40. Hojer J et al. Fatal cardiotoxicity induced by venlafaxine overdosage. Clin Toxicol (Phila) 2008; 46:336–337.

41. Taylor D. Venlafaxine and cardiovascular toxicity. BMJ 2010; 340:327.

42. Takeda Pharmaceuticals America Inc. Highlights of Prescribing Information: BRINTELLIX (vortioxetine) tablets. 2013. http://www.accessdata.fda.gov/drugsatfda_docs/label/2013/204447s000lbl.pdf

43. Isbister GK et al. Amisulpride deliberate self-poisoning causing severe cardiac toxicity including QT prolongation and torsades de pointes. Med J Aust 2006; 184:354–356.

44. Ward DI. Two cases of amisulpride overdose: A cause for prolonged QT syndrome. Emerg Med Australas 2005; 17:274–276.

45. Isbister GK et al. Amisulpride overdose is frequently associated with QT prolongation and torsades de pointes. J Clin Psychopharmacol 2010; 30:391–395.

46. Lofton AL et al. Atypical experience: a case series of pediatric aripiprazole exposures. Clin Toxicol (Phila) 2005; 43:151–153.

47. Seifert SA et al. Aripiprazole (abilify) overdose in a child. Clin Toxicol (Phila) 2005; 43:193–195.

48. Carstairs SD et al. Overdose of aripiprazole, a new type of antipsychotic. J Emerg Med 2005; 28:311–313.

49. Forrester MB. Aripiprazole exposures reported to Texas poison control centers during 2002-2004. J Toxicol Environ Health A 2006; 69:1719–1726.

50. Taylor JE et al. A case of intentional asenapine overdose. Prim Care Companion CNS Disord 2013; 15.

51. Haddad PM et al. Antipsychotic-related QTc prolongation, torsade de pointes and sudden death. Drugs 2002; 62:1649–1671.

52. Levine BS et al. Two fatalities involving haloperidol. J Anal Toxicol 1991; 15:282–284.

53. Henderson RA et al. Life-threatening ventricular arrhythmia (torsades de pointes) after haloperidol overdose. Hum Exp Toxicol 1991; 10:59–62.

54. Trenton A et al. Fatalities associated with therapeutic use and overdose of atypical antipsychotics. CNS Drugs 2003; 17:307–324.

55. Flanagan RJ et al. Suspected clozapine poisoning in the UK/Eire, 1992-2003. Forensic Sci Int 2005; 155:91–99.

56. Vigneault P et al. Iloperidone (Fanapt(R)), a novel atypical antipsychotic, is a potent HERG blocker and delays cardiac ventricular repolarization at clinically relevant concentration. Pharmacol Res 2012; 66:60–65.

57. Novartis Pharmaceuticals Corporation. Highlights of Prescribing Information. FANAPT® (iloperidone) tablets. 2014. http://www.pharma.us.novartis.com/product/pi/pdf/fanapt.pdf

58. Sunovion Pharmaceuticals Inc. Highlights of Prescribing Information: LATUDA (lurasidone hydrochloride) tablets. 2013. http://www.latuda.com/LatudaPrescribingInformation.pdf

59. Chue P et al. A review of olanzapine-associated toxicity and fatality in overdose. J Psychiatry Neurosci 2003; 28:253–261.

60. Waring WS et al. Olanzapine overdose is associated with acute muscle toxicity. Hum Exp Toxicol 2006; 25:735–740.

61. Morissette P et al. Olanzapine prolongs cardiac repolarization by blocking the rapid component of the delayed rectifier potassium current. J Psychopharmacol 2007; 21:735–741.

62. Buckley NA et al. Cardiotoxicity more common in thioridazine overdose than with other neuroleptics. J Toxicol Clin Toxicol 1995; 33:199–204.

63. Li C et al. Acute pulmonary edema induced by overdosage of phenothiazines. Chest 1992; 101:102–104.

64. Flanagan RJ. Fatal toxicity of drugs used in psychiatry. Hum Psychopharmacol 2008; 23 Suppl 1:43–51.

65. Langman LJ et al. Fatal overdoses associated with quetiapine. J Anal Toxicol 2004; 28:520–525.

66. Hunfeld NG et al. Quetiapine in overdosage: a clinical and pharmacokinetic analysis of 14 cases. Ther Drug Monit 2006; 28:185–189.

67. Strachan PM et al. Mental status change, myoclonus, electrocardiographic changes, and acute respiratory distress syndrome induced by quetiapine overdose. Pharmacotherapy 2006; 26:578–582.

68. Ngo A et al. Acute quetiapine overdose in adults: a 5-Year retrospective case series. Ann Emerg Med 2008; 52: 541–547.

69. Khan KH et al. Neuroleptic malignant syndrome induced by quetiapine overdose. Br J Hosp Med 2008; 69:171.

70. Alexander J. Delirium as a symptom of quetiapine poisoning. Aust N Z J Psychiatry 2009; 43:781.

71. Liang CS et al. Acute renal failure after paliperidone overdose: a case report. J Clin Psychopharmacol 2012; 32:128.

72. Lapid MI et al. Acute dystonia associated with paliperidone overdose. Psychosomatics 2011; 52:291–294.

CHAPTER 8

73. Gomez-Criado MS et al. Ziprasidone overdose: cases recorded in the database of Pfizer-Spain and literature review. Pharmacotherapy 2005; 25:1660–1665.

74. Arbuck DM. 12,800-mg ziprasidone overdose without significant ECG changes. Gen Hosp Psychiatry 2005; 27:222–223.

75. Insa Gomez FJ et al. Ziprasidone overdose: cardiac safety. Actas Esp Psiquiatr 2005; 33:398–400.

76. Klein-Schwartz W et al. Prospective observational multi-poison center study of ziprasidone exposures. Clin Toxicol (Phila) 2007; 45:782–786.

77. Tan HH et al. A systematic review of cardiovascular effects after atypical antipsychotic medication overdose. Am J Emerg Med 2009; 27:607–616.

78. Alipour A et al. Torsade de pointes after ziprasidone overdose with coingestants. J Clin Psychopharmacol 2010; 30:76–77.

79. Spiller HA. Management of carbamazepine overdose. Pediatr Emerg Care 2001; 17:452–456.

80. Schmidt S et al. Signs and symptoms of carbamazepine overdose. J Neurol 1995; 242:169–173.

81. Miller MA et al. Choreiform dyskinesia following isolated lamotrigine overdose. J Child Neurol 2008; 23:243.

82. Reimers A et al. Acute lamotrigine overdose in an adolescent. Ther Drug Monit 2007; 29:669–670.

83. Lofton AL et al. Evaluation of lamotrigine toxicity reported to poison centers. Ann Pharmacother 2004; 38:1811–1815.

84. Tuohy K et al. Acute lithium intoxication. Dial Transplant 2003; 32:478–481.

85. Chen KP et al. Implication of serum concentration monitoring in patients with lithium intoxication. Psychiatry Clin Neurosci 2004; 58:25–29.

86. Serinken M et al. Rarely seen cardiotoxicity of lithium overdose: complete heart block. Int J Cardiol 2009; 132:276–278.

87. Offerman SR et al. Hospitalized lithium overdose cases reported to the California Poison Control System. Clin Toxicol (Phila) 2010; 48:443–448.

88. Isbister GK et al. Valproate overdose: a comparative cohort study of self poisonings. Br J Clin Pharmacol 2003; 55:398–404.

89. Spiller HA et al. Multicenter case series of valproic acid ingestion: serum concentrations and toxicity. J Toxicol Clin Toxicol 2000; 38:755–760.

90. Sztajnkrycer MD. Valproic acid toxicity: overview and management. J Toxicol Clin Toxicol 2002; 40:789–801.

91. Eyer F et al. Acute valproate poisoning: pharmacokinetics, alteration in fatty acid metabolism, and changes during therapy. J Clin Psychopharmacol 2005; 25:376–380.

92. Robinson P et al. Severe hypothermia in association with sodium valproate overdose. N Z Med J 2005; 118:U1681.

93. Reith DM et al. Comparison of the fatal toxicity index of zopiclone with benzodiazepines. J Toxicol Clin Toxicol 2003; 41:975–980.

94. Isbister GK et al. Alprazolam is relatively more toxic than other benzodiazepines in overdose. Br J Clin Pharmacol 2004; 58:88–95.

95. Gable RS. Comparison of acute lethal toxicity of commonly abused psychoactive substances. Addiction 2004; 99:686–696.

96. Caplehorn JR et al. Fatal methadone toxicity: signs and circumstances, and the role of benzodiazepines. Aust N Z J Public Health 2002; 26:358–362.

97. Spiller HA et al. Toxicity from modafinil ingestion. Clin Toxicol (Phila) 2008;1-4.

98. Carstairs SD et al. A retrospective review of supratherapeutic modafinil exposures. J Med Toxicol 2010; 6:307–310.

99. Gock SB et al. Acute zolpidem overdose: report of two cases. J Anal Toxicol 1999; 23:559–562.

100. Garnier R et al. Acute zolpidem poisoning: analysis of 344 cases. J Toxicol Clin Toxicol 1994; 32:391–404.

101. Pounder D et al. Zopiclone poisoning. J Anal Toxicol 1996; 20:273–274.

102. Bramness JG et al. Fatal overdose of zopiclone in an elderly woman with bronchogenic carcinoma. J Forensic Sci 2001; 46:1247–1249.

Biochemical and haematological effects of psychotropics

Almost all psychotropics currently used in clinical practice have haematology or biochemistry-related adverse effects that may be detected using routine blood tests. While many of these changes are idiosyncratic and not clinically significant, others, such as the agranulocytosis associated with agents such as clozapine, will require regular monitoring of the full blood count. In general, where an agent has a high incidence of biochemical/haematological side-effects or a rare but potentially fatal effect, regular monitoring is required as discussed in other sections.

For other agents, laboratory-related side-effects are comparatively rare (prevalence usually less than 1%), are often reversible upon cessation of the putative offending agent and not always clinically significant although expert advice should be sought. It should further be noted that medical co-morbidity, polypharmacy and the effects of non-prescribed agents, including substances of abuse and alcohol, may also influence biochemical and haematological parameters. In some cases, where a clear temporal association between starting the agent and the onset of laboratory changes is unclear, then withdrawal and re-challenge with the agent in question may be considered. Where there is doubt as to the aetiology and significance of the effect, the appropriate source of expert advice should always be consulted.

Tables 8.2 and 8.3 summarise those agents with identified biochemical and haematological effects, with information compiled from various sources.[1-11] In many cases the evidence for these various effects is limited, with information obtained mostly from case reports, case series and information supplied by manufacturers. For further details about each individual agent, the reader is encouraged to consult the appropriate section of the *Guidelines* as well as other, specialist sources, particularly product literature relating to individual drugs.

CHAPTER 8

Table 8.2 Summary of biochemical changes associated with psychotropic drugs

Parameter	Reference range	Agents reported to raise levels	Agents reported to lower levels
Alanine transferase	0–45 IU/L (may be higher in males and obese subjects)	**Antipsychotics:** asenapine, benperidol, chlorpromazine, clozapine, haloperidol, olanzapine, quetiapine **Antidepressants:** agomelatine, duloxetine, mianserin, mirtazapine, moclobemide, monoamine oxidase inhibitors, SSRIs (especially paroxetine and sertraline); TCAs, trazodone, venlafaxine **Anxiolytics/hypnotics:** barbiturates, benzodiazepines, chloral hydrate, chlormethiazole, promethazine **Miscellaneous agents:** caffeine, dexamfetamine, disulfiram, opioids **Mood stabilisers:** carbamazepine, lamotrigine, valproate	Vigabatrin
Albumin	3.5–4.8 g/dL (gradually decreases after age 40)	Microalbuminuria may be a feature of metabolic syndrome secondary to psychotropic use (especially phenothiazines, clozapine, olanzapine and possibly quetiapine)	Chronic use of amfetamine or cocaine
Alkaline phosphatase	50–120 IU/L	Caffeine (excess/chronic use), carbamazepine, clozapine, disulfiram, duloxetine, galantamine, haloperidol, memantine, modafinil, nortriptyline, olanzapine, phenytoin, sertraline; also associated agents that induce neuroleptic malignant syndrome	None known
Amylase	<300 IU/L	Clozapine, donepezil, methadone, olanzapine, opiates, pregabalin, rivastigmine, SSRIs (rarely), valproate	None known
Aspartate aminotransferase	10–50 IU/L (values slightly higher in males)	As for alanine transferase	Trifluoperazine
Bicarbonate	22–30 mmol/L	None known	Agents associated with SIADH: all antidepressants, antipsychotics (clozapine, haloperidol, olanzapine, phenothiazines, pimozide, risperidone/paliperidone, quetiapine), carbamazepine
Bilirubin	3–20 μmol/L (total bilirubin)	Amitriptyline, benzodiazepines, carbamazepine, chlordiazepoxide, chlorpromazine, clomethiazole, disulfiram, imipramine, fluphenazine, meprobamate, phenothiazines, phenytoin, promethazine, trifluoperazine, valproate	None known

Table 8.2 (*Continued*)

Parameter	Reference range	Agents reported to raise levels	Agents reported to lower levels
C-reactive protein	<10 µg/mL	Buprenorphine (rare)	None known
Calcium (corrected)	2.2–2.6 mmol/L	Lithium (rare)	Barbiturates, haloperidol
Carbohydrate-deficient transferrin	1.9–3.4 g/L	None known	None known
Chloride	98–107 mmol/L	None known	Medications associated with SIADH: all antidepressants, antipsychotics (clozapine, haloperidol, olanzapine, phenothiazines, pimozide, risperidone/paliperidone, quetiapine), carbamazepine
Cholesterol (total)	<5.2 mmol/L	Antipsychotic treatment, especially those implicated in the metabolic syndrome (phenothiazines, clozapine, olanzapine and quetiapine). Rarely: aripiprazole, beta-blockers, disulfiram, memantine, mirtazapine, modafinil, phenytoin, rivastigmine, and venlafaxine	Ziprasidone
Creatine Kinase	<90 IU/L	Clozapine (when associated with seizures), donepezil, olanzapine; also associated with agents causing neuroleptic malignant syndrome and SIADH; cocaine, dexamfetamine	None known
Creatinine	60– 110 µmol/L	Clozapine, lithium,lurasidone, thioridazine, valproate, medications associated with rhabdomyolysis (benzodiazepines, dexamfetamine, pregabalin, thioridazine); may also be also associated with agents causing neuroleptic malignant syndrome and SIADH	None known
Ferritin	Males: 40–340 µg/L; Females: 14–150 µg/L	None known	None known
Gamma-glutamyl transferase	<60 IU/L (higher levels may be found in males)	**Antidepressants:** mirtazapine, SSRIs (paroxetine and sertraline implicated); TCAs, trazodone, venlafaxine **Anticonvulsants/mood stabilisers:** carbamazepine, lamotrigine, phenytoin, phenobarbitone, valproate **Antipsychotics:** benperidol, chlorpromazine, clozapine, fluphenazine, haloperidol, olanzapine, quetiapine, **Miscellaneous:** barbiturates, clomethiazole, dexamfetamine, modafinil	None known

(*Continued*)

Table 8.2 (*Continued*)

Parameter	Reference range	Agents reported to raise levels	Agents reported to lower levels
Glucose	Fasting: 2.8–6.0 mmol/L Random: <11.1 mmol/L	**Antidepressants:** MAOI*, SSRI, TCAs* **Antipsychotics:** chlorpromazine, clozapine, olanzapine*, quetiapine, and others **Substances of abuse:** methadone, opioids **Other:** beta-blockers*, bupropion, donepezil, galantamine, lithium All antipsychotics associated with hyperglycaemia (excluding amisulpride, lurasidone, aripiprazole and ziprasidone), glantamine, methadone, morphine, TCAs	Rarely with duloxetine, haloperidol, pregabalin, TCAs Medications associated with metabolic syndrome may result in raised or decreased glucose levels
Glycated haemoglobin	3.5–5.5% (4–6% in diabetics)	As above	Lithium, MAOIs, SSRIs
Lactate dehydrogenase	90–200 U/L (levels rise gradually with age)	TCAs (especially Imipramine), valproate, methadone, agents associated with neuroleptic malignant syndrome	None known
Lipoproteins: HDL	>1.2 mmol/L	Carbamazepine, phenobarbitone, phenytoin	Olanzapine, phenothiazines, valproate
Lipoproteins: LDL	<3.5 mmol/L	Beta-blockers, caffeine (controversial), chlorpromazine, clozapine, memantine, mirtazapine, modafinil, olanzapine, phenothiazines, quetiapine, risperidone/paliperidone, rivastigmine, venlafaxine	None known
Phosphate	0.8–1.4 mmol/L	Acamprosate, carbamazepine, dexamfetamine, agents associated with neuroleptic malignant syndrome	None known
Potassium	3.5–5.0 mmol/L	Pregabalin	Haloperidol, lithium, mianserin, reboxetine, rivastigmine, alcohol, caffeine, cocaine
Prolactin	Normal <350 mU/L; Abnormal >600 mU/L;	**Antidepressants:** especially MAOIs and TCAs, venlafaxine also implicated **Antipsychotics:** amisulpride, haloperidol, pimozide, risperidone/paliperidone, sulpiride (aripiprazole, asenapine, clozapine, lurasidone, olanzapine, quetiapine and ziprasidone have minimal effects on prolactin levels)	None known

Table 8.2 (Continued)

Parameter	Reference range	Agents reported to raise levels	Agents reported to lower levels
Protein (total)	60–80 g/L	None known	None known
Sodium	135–145 mmol/L	None known	Benzodiazepines, carbamazepine, chlorpromazine, donepezil, duloxetine, haloperidol, lithium, memantine, mianserin, phenothiazines, reboxetine, rivastigmine, SSRIs (especially fluoxetine), tricyclic antidepressants (especially amitriptyline) Hyponatraemia should be considered in any patient on an antidepressant who develops confusion, convulsions or drowsiness
Thyroid-stimulating hormone	0.3–4.0 mU/L	Aripiprazole, carbamazepine, lithium, rivastigmine	Moclobemide
Thyroxine	Free: 9–26 pmol/L; Total: 60–150 nmol/L	Dexamfetamine, moclobemide (rare)	Lithium (causes decreased T4 secretion), heroin, methadone (increase serum thyroxine-binding globulin), carbamazepine, phenytoin treatment. Rarely implicated: aripiprazole, quetiapine and rivastigmine
Triglycerides	0.4–1.8 mmol/L	Beta-blockers, chlorpromazine, clozapine, memantine, mirtazapine, modafinil, olanzapine, quetiapine, phenothiazines, rivastigmine, valproate, venlafaxine,	Ziprasidone (controversial)
Tri-iodothyronine	Free 3.0–8.8 pmol/L; Total: 1.2–2.9 nmol/L	Heroin, methadone, moclobemide	Free T3: valproate Total T3: carbamazepine, lithium
Urate (uric acid)	0.1–0.4 mmol/L	Rarely: rivastigmine	None known
Urea	1.8–7.1 mmol/L (levels increase slightly after age 40)	Rarely with agents associated with anticonvulsant hypersensitivity syndrome and rhabdomyolysis	None known

*may also be associated with hypoglycaemia.
HDL, high-density lipoprotein; LDL, low-density lipoprotein; MAOI, monoamine oxidase inhibitor; SIADH, syndrome of inappropriate antidiuretic hormone; SSRI, selective serotonin reuptake inhibitor; TCA, tricyclic antidepressant.

Table 8.3 Summary of haematological changes associated with psychotropic drugs

Parameter	Reference range	Agents reported to raise levels	Agents reported to lower levels
Activated partial thromboplastin time	25–39 seconds	Bupropion*, phenothiazines (especially chlorpromazine)	Modafinil (rare)
Basophils	0.0–0.10 × 10⁹/L	TCAs (especially desipramine)	None known
Eosinophils	0.04–0.45 × 10⁹/L	Amitriptyline, beta-blockers, carbamazepine, chloral hydrate, chlorpromazine, clonazepam, clozapine, donepezil, fluphenazine, haloperidol, imipramine, meprobamate, modafinil, nortriptyline, olanzapine, promethazine, quetiapine, SSRIs, tryptophan, valproate	None known
Erythrocytes	Males: 4.5–6.0 × 10¹²/L Females: 3.8–5.2 × 10¹²/L	None known	Carbamazepine, chlordiazepoxide, chlorpromazine, donepezil, meprobamate, phenytoin, trifluoperazine
Erythrocyte sedimentation rate	<20 mm/hour; Note: levels increase with age and are slightly higher in females	Buprenorphine, clozapine, dexamfetamine, levomepromazine, maprotiline, SSRIs	None known
Haemoglobin	Males: 14–18 g/dL Females: 12–16 g/dL	None known	Aripiprazole, barbiturates, bupropion, carbamazepine, chlordiazepoxide, chlorpromazine, donepezil, duloxetine, galantamine, MAOIs, memantine, meprobamate, mianserin, phenytoin, promethazine, rivastigmine, trifluoperazine
Lymphocytes	1.0–4.8 × 10⁹/L	Opioids, valproate	Chloral hydrate, lithium
Mean cell haemoglobin	27–37 pg Note: Levels are slightly higher in males and may be raised in the elderly	Medications associated with megaloblastic anaemia, e.g. all anticonvulsants	None known
Mean cell haemoglobin concentration	300–350 g/L		
Mean cell volume	80–100 fL		
Monocytes	0.21–0.92 × 10⁹/L	Haloperidol	None known
Neutrophils	2–9 × 10⁹/L Note: may be lower in people of African descent due to benign ethnic neutropenia	Bupropion, carbamazepine†, citalopram, chlorpromazine, clozapine†, duloxetine, fluphenazine, haloperidol, lithium, olanzapine, quetiapine, risperidone/paliperidone, rivastigmine, trazodone, venlafaxine	**Agents associated with agranulocytosis:** amitriptyline, amoxapine, aripiprazole, barbiturates, carbamazepine, chlordiazepoxide, chlorpromazine, clomipramine, clozapine‡, diazepam, fluphenazine, haloperidol, imipramine, meprobamate, mianserin, mirtazapine, nortriptyline, olanzapine, promethazine, tranylcypromine, valproate

Table 8.3 (*Continued*)

Parameter	Reference range	Agents reported to raise levels	Agents reported to lower levels
			Agents associated with leucopoenia: amitriptyline, amoxapine, bupropion, carbamazepine, chlorpromazine, citalopram, clomipramine, clonazepam, clozapine, duloxetine, fluphenazine, galantamine, haloperidol, lamotrigine, lorazepam, MAOIs, memantine, meprobamate, mianserin, mirtazapine, modafinil, olanzapine, oxazepam, pregabalin, promethazine, quetiapine, risperidone/paliperidone, tranylcypromine, valproate, venlafaxine **Agents associated with neutropenia:** trazodone, valproate
Packed cell volume	Adult males: 42–52% Adult females: 35–47% (levels slightly lower in pregnant versus non-pregnant women)	None known	None known
Platelets	150–400 × 10⁹/L	Lithium	Amitriptyline, barbiturates, bupropion, carbamazepine, clomipramine, chlordiazepoxide, chlorpromazine, clonazepam, clozapine, diazepam, donepezil, duloxetine, fluphenazine, imipramine, lamotrigine, MAOIs, meprobamate, mirtazapine, olanzapine, promethazine, risperidone/paliperidone, rivastigmine, sertraline, tranylcypromine, trazodone, trifluoperazine, valproate, cocaine, methadone **Agents associated with impaired platelet aggregation:** chlordiazepoxide, citalopram, diazepam, fluoxetine, fluvoxamine, paroxetine, sertraline
Prothrombin time/ International Normalised Ratio	10–13 seconds	Fluoxetine, fluvoxamine, disulfiram; bupropion, mirtazapine	Barbiturates, carbamazepine, phenytoin

(*Continued*)

Table 8.3 (*Continued*)

Parameter	Reference range	Agents reported to raise levels	Agents reported to lower levels
Red cell distribution width	11.5–14.5%	**Agents associated with anaemia:** carbamazepine, chlordiazepoxide, citalopram, clonazepam, diazepam, lamotrigine, mirtazapine, sertraline, tranylcypromine, trazodone, valproate, venlafaxine	None known
Reticulocyte count	0.5–1.5%	None known	Carbamazepine, chlordiazepoxide, chlorpromazine, meprobamate, phenytoin, trifluoperazine

*may raise or lower levels
†Rare, usually associated with leucopoenia.
‡Note that in rare cases clozapine has been associated with a 'morning pseudo-neutropenia' with lower levels of circulating neutrophil levels. As neutrophil counts may show circadian rhythms, repeating the FBC at a later time of day may be instructive.
FBC, full blood count; MAOI, monoamine oxidase inhibitor; SSRI, selective serotonin reuptake inhibitor; TCA, tricyclic antidepressant.

References

1. Balon R et al. Hematologic side effects of psychotropic drugs. Psychosomatics 1986; 27:119–127.
2. Bazire S. *Psychotropic Drug Directory*. UK: Lloyd-Reinhold Communcations LLP; 2014.
3. Joint Formulary Committee. *BNF 67* March-September 2014 (online). London: Pharmaceutical Press; 2014. http://www.medicinescomplete.com/mc/bnf/current/
4. Aronson JK. *Meyler's Side Effects of Drugs: The International Encyclopedia of Adverse Drug Reactions and Interactions*, 15th edn. Amsterdam: Elsevier Science; 2006.
5. Foster R. *Clinical Laboratory Investigation and Psychiatry. A Practical Handbook*. New York: Informa; 2008.
6. Jacobs DS et al. *Laboratory Test Handbook*, 5th edn. Hudson, Cleveland: Lexi-Comp Inc; 2001.
7. Livingstone C et al. The role of clinical biochemistry in psychiatry. Clin Biochem 2004; 6:59–65.
8. Oyesanmi O et al. Hematologic side effects of psychotropics. Psychosomatics 1999; 40:414–421.
9. Stubner S et al. Blood dyscrasias induced by psychotropic drugs. Pharmacopsychiatry 2004; 37 Suppl 1:S70–S78.
10. Martindale: The Complete Drug Reference. London: Pharmaceutical Press; 2014. http://www.medicinescomplete.com
11. Wu AHB. *Tietz Clinical Guide to Laboratory Tests*, 4th edn. Philadelphia, Pennsylvania: WB Saunders and Company; 2006.

Prescribing drugs outside their licensed indications ('off-label' prescribing)

A Product Licence (PL) is granted when regulatory authorities are satisfied that the drug in question has proven efficacy in the treatment of a specified disorder, along with an acceptable side-effect profile, relative to the severity of the disorder being treated and other available treatments. Licensed indications are preparation specific, outlined in the Summary of Product Characteristics (SPC), and may be different for branded and generic formulations of the same drug.[1] In the US product 'labelling' has a similar legal status to EU licensing.

The decision of a manufacturer to seek a PL for a given indication is essentially a commercial one; potential sales are balanced against the cost of conducting the necessary clinical trials. It therefore follows that drugs may be effective outside their licensed indications for different disease states, age ranges, doses and durations. The absence of a formal PL or labelling may simply reflect the absence of controlled trials supporting the drug's efficacy in these areas. In other cases (e.g. sertraline or quetiapine in generalised anxiety disorder) there is sufficient evidence but a licence has not been sought by the manufacturer. Importantly, however, it is possible that trials have been conducted but given negative results. Clinicians often assume that drugs with a similar mode of action will be similarly effective for a given indication, and in many cases this may be true. For example, the efficacy of aripiprazole, olanzapine, quetiapine and risperidone in reducing behavioural and psychological symptoms (BPSD) in people with dementia, is similar[2] yet only risperidone is licensed for this indication.

Prescribing a drug within its licence or labelling does not guarantee that the patient will come to no harm. Likewise, prescribing outside a licence does not mean that the risk–benefit ratio is automatically adverse. In the BPSD example given above, risperidone is not clearly better tolerated than other antipsychotics.[2] In the UK, prescribing outside a licence, usually called 'off-label', does confer extra responsibilities on prescribers, who will be expected to be able to show that they acted in accordance with a respected body of medical opinion (the Bolam test)[3] and that their action was capable of withstanding logical analysis (the Bolitho test).[4]

It has been suggested that off-label prescribing in psychiatry is less likely to be supported by a strong evidence base than off-label prescribing in other areas of medicine.[5] In psychiatry, small (underpowered) studies (with wide confidence intervals) often influence practice, particularly with respect to treatment resistant illness. When these small studies are combined in the form of a meta-analysis, considerable heterogeneity is often found suggesting publication bias (that is, that negative studies are not published). Treatments may therefore become incorporated into 'routine custom and practice' in the absence of any evidence supporting efficacy and/or tolerability, and these treatments may sometimes continue to be used despite the findings of later, larger, and more definitive negative studies.

The psychopharmacology special interest group at the Royal College of Psychiatrists has published a consensus statement on the use of licensed medicines for unlicensed uses.[6] They note that unlicensed use is common in general adult psychiatry with

CHAPTER 8

Box 8.1 Summary of the consensus statement on the use of licensed medicines for unlicensed uses

---

Before prescribing 'off-label':
1. Exclude licensed alternatives (e.g. they have proved ineffective or poorly tolerated).
2. Ensure familiarity with the evidence base for the intended unlicensed use. If unsure, seek advice.
3. Consider and document the potential risks and benefits of the proposed treatment. Share this risk assessment with the patient, and carers if applicable. Document the discussion and the patient's consent or lack of capacity to consent.
4. If prescribing responsibility is to be shared with primary care, ensure that the risk assessment and consent issues are shared with the GP.
5. Monitor for efficacy and side-effects.
6. Consider publishing the case to add to the body of knowledge.
The more experimental the unlicensed use is, the more important it is to adhere to the above guidance.

---

cross-sectional studies showing that up to 50% of patients are prescribed at least one drug outside the terms of its licence. They also note that the prevalence of this type of prescribing is likely to be higher in patients under the age of 18 or over 65, in those with a learning disability, in women who are pregnant or lactating and in those patients who are cared for in forensic psychiatry settings. The main recommendations in the consensus statement are summarised in Box 8.1.

Examples of acceptable use of drugs outside their Product Licences/Labels

Table 8.4 gives examples of common unlicensed uses of drugs in psychiatric practice. These examples would all fulfil the Bolam and Bolitho criteria in principle. An exhaustive list of unlicensed uses is impossible to prepare as:

- the evidence base is constantly changing
- the expertise and experience of prescribers varies. A strategy may be justified in the hands of a specialist in psychopharmacology based in a tertiary referral centre but be much more difficult to justify if initiated by someone with a special interest in psychotherapy who rarely prescribes.

Note that some drugs do not have a UK licence for any indication. Two commonly prescribed examples in psychiatric practice are immediate release formulations of melatonin (used to treat insomnia in children and adolescents) and pirenzepine (used to treat clozapine-induced hypersalivation). Awareness of the evidence base and documentation of potential benefits, side-effects and patient consent are especially important here.

Table 8.4 Common unlicensed uses of drugs in psychiatric practice

Drug/drug group	Unlicensed use(s)	Further information
Second-generation antipsychotics	Psychotic illness other than schizophrenia	Licensed indications vary markedly, and in most cases are unlikely to reflect real differences in efficacy between drugs
Clozapine	Rapid cycling bipolar disorder	Some evidence to support efficacy when standard treatments have failed to control symptoms
Cyproheptadine	Akathisia	Some evidence to support efficacy in this distressing and difficult to treat side-effect of antipsychotics
Fluoxetine	Maintenance treatment of depression	Few prescribers are likely to be aware that this is not a licensed indication in the UK
Melatonin (Circadin)	Insomnia in children	Licence covers adults > 55 years only. Probably preferable to unlicensed formulations of melatonin
Methylphenidate	ADHD in children under 6 years	Established clinical practice
	ADHD in people over 18 years	Supported by evidence base
Naltrexone	Self-injurious behaviour in people with learning disabilities	Limited evidence base. Acceptable in specialist hands
Sodium valproate	Treatment and prophylaxis of bipolar disorder	Established clinical practice

ADHD, attention deficit hyperactivity disorder.

References

1. Datapharm Communications Ltd. Summary of Product Characteristics. Electronic Medicines Compendium. 2014. http://www.medicines.org.uk/emc/
2. Maher AR et al. Efficacy and comparative effectiveness of atypical antipsychotic medications for off-label uses in adults: a systematic review and meta-analysis. JAMA 2011; **306**:1359–1369.
3. Bolam v Friern Barnet Hospital Management Committee. WLR 1957; **1**:582.
4. Bolitho v City and Hackney Health Authority. WLR 1997; **3**:1151.
5. Epstein RS et al. The many sides of off-label prescribing. Clin Pharmacol Ther 2012; **91**:755–758.
6. Royal College of Psychiatrists. College Report 142. Use of licensed medicines for unlicensed applications in psychiatric practice. 2007. http://www.rcpsych.ac.uk/publications/collegereports/cr/cr142.aspx

Further reading

Frank B et al. Psychotropic medications and informed consent: a review. Ann Clin Psychiatry 2008; **20**:87–95.
General Medical Council. Good practice in prescribing and managing medicines and devices. 2013. http://www.gmc-uk.org/guidance/ethical_guidance/14316.asp.

Observations on the placebo effect in mental illness

Target symptoms improve to varying degrees in approximately one-third of patients given a placebo.[1,2] Adverse effects also occur; the so-called nocebo effect.[2] Although pharmacologically inert, placebo can cause direct physiological effects, at least in the short term, that are consistent with the effects of active drugs. This has been demonstrated in neuroimaging studies.[3,4] The exact neurobiological response varies with the target illness.[2,5] In many psychiatric conditions the effect size of placebo is substantial;[6] often greater than the effect size of drugs used in general medicine.[7] Proving the efficacy of psychotropic drugs is thus challenging; much more challenging than in general medicine where placebo effects are often absent (e.g. type I diabetes).

The following considerations apply when interpreting the results of placebo-controlled studies. Although the references for each point are drawn from the depression literature, the same principles apply to the treatment of other disorders. The relative importance of each point will vary depending on the disorder that is being treated.

- Placebo is not the same as no care: patients who maintain contact with services have a better outcome than those who receive no care.[8]
- The placebo response is greater in mild illness.[9,10]
- Placebo tablets and controls for the non-specific effects of psychological interventions such as CBT may not be equitable,[11] leading to an overestimation of the benefits of psychological relative to pharmacological interventions.
- The higher the placebo response rate, the more difficult it is to power studies to show treatment effects. Where the placebo response rate exceeds 40%, studies have to recruit very large numbers of patients to be adequately powered to show differences between treatments.[12] For example, it has been demonstrated in a novel analysis that 39% of participants in placebo-controlled RCTs of escitalopram respond irrespective of treatment allocation, with just 19% of the total benefit attributable to active treatment.[10] The large placebo response rate results in a small overall absolute difference between the active and placebo arms but within this small 'effect size' a proportion of patients improve markedly with active treatment.
- It is difficult to separate placebo effects from spontaneous remission. The higher the spontaneous remission rate, the more difficult it is to power studies to show treatment effects.[8]
- Patients who enter RCTs generally do so when acutely unwell. Symptoms are likely to improve in the majority, irrespective of the intervention. This is so-called 'regression to the mean'.[11,13]
- The placebo response rate in published studies is increasing over time.[14] This may be because of increasing numbers of mildly ill patients being recruited into trials perhaps because of clinicians' reluctance to risk severely ill patients being randomised into placebo arms.
- 'Breaking the blind' may influence outcome. The resultant 'expectancy effect' may explain why active placebos are more effective than inert placebos.[15,16] That is, if patients or observers note adverse effects, the placebo effect is enhanced.
- Overt administration of placebo is more effective than covert administration.[2]
- Not all placebos are the same. Patients perceive two brightly coloured tablets to be more effective than one small white one. Capsules, injections and branding also

increase expectations of efficacy.[1] This may partly explain different placebo response rates in studies of similar design.

- Placebo effects may be cumulative, with two different placebo interventions used simultaneously giving a greater effect than one.[2]
- Most psychotropic drugs have side-effects such as sedation that may improve scores on rating scales without actually treating the target illness.
- Placebo response may be short-lived: studies are usually too short to pick up placebo relapsers.[17]
- Statistical significance and clinical significance are not the same thing: a study may report on a highly statistically significant difference in efficacy between active drug and placebo, but the magnitude of the difference may be too small to be clinically meaningful.
- Publication bias remains a problem.[18-20] Many negative studies are never published.[21,22] Underpowered positive studies often are. Reboxetine is a good example here – considering unpublished studies reveal the drug to have limited, if any, efficacy.[22]
- Placebo response increases according to expectancy. For example, placebo response is greater in studies randomising 2:1 active: placebo than in those randomising 1:1 (chance of receiving active is greater).[22]
- Placebo and nocebo mechanisms can be additive to those of drug treatment as treatment is given in a therapeutic context that has the potential to activate and modulate placebo mechanisms.[2,23]
- Note that other effects may operate: 'wish bias' probably exaggerates the efficacy of new drugs compared with established agents.[24]
- Placebo shows a dose-related effect. The more visits (assessments) in a trial, the better the effect of placebo.[25]

References

1. Rajagopal S. The placebo effect. Psychiatr Bull 2006; **30**:185–188.
2. Finniss DG et al. Biological, clinical, and ethical advances of placebo effects. Lancet 2010; **375**:686–695.
3. Scott DJ et al. Placebo and nocebo effects are defined by opposite opioid and dopaminergic responses. Arch Gen Psychiatry 2008; **65**:220–231.
4. Lidstone SC et al. Effects of expectation on placebo-induced dopamine release in Parkinson disease. Arch Gen Psychiatry 2010; **67**:857–865.
5. Brody H et al. Lessons from recent research about the placebo effect: from art to science. JAMA 2011; **306**:2612–2613.
6. Kirsch I et al. Initial severity and antidepressant benefits: a meta-analysis of data submitted to the Food and Drug Administration. PLoS Med 2008; **5**:e45.
7. Leucht S et al. Putting the efficacy of psychiatric and general medicine medication into perspective: review of meta-analyses. Br J Psychiatry 2012; **200**:97–106.
8. Andrews G. Placebo response in depression: bane of research, boon to therapy. Br J Psychiatry 2001; **178**:192–194.
9. Khan A et al. Severity of depression and response to antidepressants and placebo: an analysis of the Food and Drug Administration database. J Clin Psychopharmacol 2002; **22**:40–45.
10. Thase ME et al. Assessing the 'true' effect of active antidepressant therapy v. placebo in major depressive disorder: use of a mixture model. Br J Psychiatry 2011; **199**:501–507.
11. Jauhar S et al. Cognitive-behavioural therapy for the symptoms of schizophrenia: systematic review and meta-analysis with examination of potential bias. Br J Psychiatry 2014; **204**:20–29.
12. Thase ME. Studying new antidepressants: if there were a light at the end of the tunnel, could we see it? J Clin Psychiatry 2002; **63 Suppl** **2**:24–28.
13. McDonald CJ et al. How much of the placebo 'effect' is really statistical regression? Stat Med 1983; **2**:417–427.
14. Walsh BT et al. Placebo response in studies of major depression: variable, substantial, and growing. JAMA 2002; **287**:1840–1847.

15. Kirsch I et al. The Emperor's new drugs: An analysis of antidepressant medication data submitted to the US Food and Drug Administration. Prevention Treatment 2002; **5**:10–23.

16. Moncrieff J et al. Active placebos versus antidepressants for depression. Cochrane Database Syst Rev 2004; CD003012.

17. Ross DC et al. A typological model for estimation of drug and placebo effects in depression. J Clin Psychopharmacol 2002; **22**:414–418.

18. Lexchin J et al. Pharmaceutical industry sponsorship and research outcome and quality: systematic review. BMJ 2003; **326**:1167–1170.

19. Melander H et al. Evidence b(i)ased medicine–selective reporting from studies sponsored by pharmaceutical industry: review of studies in new drug applications. BMJ 2003; **326**:1171–1173.

20. Werneke U et al. How effective is St John's wort? The evidence revisited. J Clin Psychiatry 2004; **65**:611–617.

21. Turner EH et al. Selective publication of antidepressant trials and its influence on apparent efficacy. N Engl J Med 2008; **358**:252–260.

22. Eyding D et al. Reboxetine for acute treatment of major depression: systematic review and meta-analysis of published and unpublished placebo and selective serotonin reuptake inhibitor controlled trials. BMJ 2010; **341**:c4737.

23. Grelotti DJ et al. Placebo by proxy. BMJ 2011; **343**:d4345.

24. Barbui C et al. "Wish bias" in antidepressant drug trials? J Clin Psychopharmacol 2004; **24**:126–130.

25. Posternak MA et al. Therapeutic effect of follow-up assessments on antidepressant and placebo response rates in antidepressant efficacy trials: meta-analysis. Br J Psychiatry 2007; **190**:287–292.

Drug interactions with alcohol

Drug interactions with alcohol are complex. Many patient-related and drug-related factors need to be considered. It can be difficult to predict accurately outcomes because a number of processes may occur simultaneously or consequently.

Pharmacokinetic interactions[1–4]

Alcohol (ethanol) is absorbed from the gastrointestinal tract and distributed in body water. The volume of distribution is smaller in women and the elderly where plasma levels of alcohol will be higher for a given 'dose' of alcohol than in males. Approximately 10% of ingested alcohol is subjected to first pass metabolism by alcohol dehydrogenase (ADH). A small proportion of alcohol is metabolised by ADH in the stomach. The remainder is metabolised in the liver by ADH and CYP2E1; women have less capacity to metabolise via ADH than men. CYP2E1 plays a minor role in occasional drinkers but is an important and inducible metabolic route in chronic, heavy drinkers. CYP1A2, CYP3A4 and many other CYP enzymes also play a minor role.[5,6]

CYP2E1 and ADH convert alcohol to acetaldehyde which is both the toxic substance responsible for the unpleasant symptoms of the 'antabuse reaction' (e.g. flushing, headache, nausea, malaise), and the compound implicated in hepatic damage. Acetaldehyde is further metabolised by aldehyde dehydrogenase to acetic acid and then to carbon dioxide and water.

All of the enzymes involved in the metabolism of alcohol exhibit genetic polymorphism. For example, 40% of people of Asian origin are poor metabolisers via ADH. Chronic consumption of alcohol induces CYP2E1 and CYP3A4. The effects of alcohol on other hepatic metabolising enzymes have been poorly studied.

The metabolism of alcohol is summarised in Figure 8.1.

Interactions are difficult to predict in alcohol misusers because two opposing processes may be at work: competition for enzymatic sites during periods of intoxication (increasing drug plasma levels) and enzyme induction prevailing during periods of

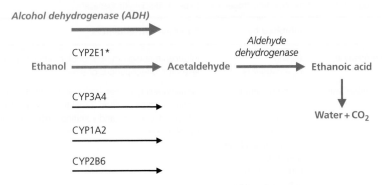

Figure 8.1 Metabolism of alcohol. *Minor route in occasional drinkers; major route in misusers and at higher blood alcohol concentration.

sobriety (reducing plasma levels). See Tables 8.5 and 8.6. In chronic drinkers, particularly those who binge drink, serum levels of prescribed drugs may reach toxic levels during periods of intoxication with alcohol and then be sub-therapeutic when the patient is sober. This makes it very difficult to optimise treatment of physical or mental illness.

Interactions of uncertain aetiology include increased blood alcohol concentrations in people who take verapamil and decreased metabolism of methylphenidate in people who consume alcohol.

Table 8.5 Co-administration of alcohol and substrates for CYP2E1 and CYP3A4

	Substrates for enzyme Note: this is not an exhaustive list	Effects in an intoxicated patient	Effects in a chronic, sober drinker
CYP2E1	Paracetamol Isoniazid Phenobarbitone Warfarin	Competition between alcohol and drug leading to reduced rates of metabolism of both compounds. Increased plasma levels may lead to toxicity	Activity of CYP2E1 is increased up 10-fold. Increased metabolism of drugs potentially leading to therapeutic failure
CYP3A4	Benzodiazepines Carbamazepine Clozapine Donepezil Galantamine Mirtazapine Risperidone Sildenafil Tricyclics Valproate Venlafaxine 'Z' hypnotics	Competition between alcohol and drug leading to reduced rates of metabolism of both compounds. Increased plasma levels may lead to toxicity	Increased rate of drug metabolism potentially leading to therapeutic failure. Enzyme induction can last for several weeks after alcohol consumption ceases.

Table 8.6 Drugs that inhibit alcohol dehydrogenase and aldehyde dehydrogenase

Enzyme	Inhibited by	Potential consequences
Alcohol dehydrogenase	Aspirin H$_2$ antagonists	Reduced metabolism of alcohol resulting in higher plasma levels for longer periods of time
Aldehyde dehydrogenase	Chlorpropamide Disulfiram Griseofulvin Isoniazid Isosorbide dinitrate Metronidazole Nitrofurantoin Sulphamethoxazole Tolbutamide	Reduced ability to metabolise acetaldehyde leading to 'antabuse' type reaction: facial flushing, headache, tachycardia, nausea and vomiting, arrhythmias and hypotension

Pharmacodynamic interactions[2–4,7]

Alcohol enhances inhibitory neurotransmission at gamma-aminobutyric acid (GABA) receptors and reduces excitatory neurotransmission at glutamate N-methyl-D-aspartate (NMDA) receptors. It also increases dopamine release in the mesolimbic pathway and may have some effects on serotonin and opiate pathways. Given these actions, alcohol alone would therefore be expected to cause sedation, amnesia, ataxia and give rise to feelings of pleasure (and/or worsen psychotic symptoms in vulnerable individuals). See Table 8.7.

Alcohol can cause or worsen psychotic symptoms by increasing dopamine release in mesolimbic pathways. The effect of antipsychotic drugs may be competitively antagonised, rendering them less effective.

Electrolyte disturbances secondary to alcohol-related dehydration can be exacerbated by other drugs that cause electrolyte disturbances such as diuretics.

Note that heavy alcohol consumption can lead to hypoglycaemia in people with diabetes who take insulin or oral hypoglycaemics. Theoretically there is an increased risk of lactic acidosis in patients who take metformin with alcohol. Alcohol can also increase blood pressure.

Chronic drinkers are particularly susceptible to the gastrointestinal irritant effects of aspirin and NSAIDs.

Table 8.7 Pharmacodynamic interactions with alcohol

Effect of alcohol	Effect exacerbated by	Potential consequences
Sedation	Other sedative drugs, e.g. Antihistamines Antipsychotics Baclofen Benzodiazepines Lofexidine Opiates Tizanidine Tricyclics Z-hypnotics	Increased CNS depression ranging from increased propensity to be involved in accidents through to respiratory depression and death
Amnesia	Other amnesic drugs, e.g. Barbiturates Benzodiazepines Z-hypnotics	Increased amnesic effects ranging from mild memory loss to total amnesia
Ataxia	ACE inhibitors Beta-blockers Calcium channel blockers Nitrates Adrenergic a-receptor antagonists, e.g. Clozapine Risperidone Tricyclics	Increased unsteadiness and falls

ACE, angiotensin-converting enzyme; CNS, central nervous system.

CHAPTER 8

Table 8.8 Psychotropic drugs: choice in patients who continue to drink

	Safest choice	Best avoided
Antipsychotics	**Sulpiride** and **amisulpride** **Paliperidone,** if depot required Non-sedative and renally excreted	**Very sedative antipsychotics** such as chlorpromazine and clozapine
Antidepressants	**SSRI – citalopram, sertraline** Potent inhibitors of CYP3A4 (fluoxetine, paroxetine) may decrease alcohol metabolism in chronic drinkers	**TCAs**, because impairment of metabolism by alcohol (while intoxicated) can lead to increased plasma levels and consequent signs and symptoms of overdose (profound hypotension, seizures, arrhythmias and coma) Cardiac effects can be exacerbated by electrolyte disturbances Combinations of TCAs and alcohol profoundly impair psychomotor skills **MAOIs** as can cause profound hypotension. Also potential interaction with tyramine- containing drinks which can lead to hypertensive crisis
Mood stabilisers	**Valproate** **Carbamazepine** Note: higher plasma levels achieved during periods of alcohol intoxication may be poorly tolerated	**Lithium**, because it has a narrow therapeutic index and alcohol-related dehydration and electrolyte disturbance can precipitate lithium toxicity

MAOI, monoamine oxidase inhibitor; SSRI, selective serotonin reuptake inhibitor; TCA, tricyclic antidepressant.

Note: in the presence of pharmacokinetic interactions, pharmacodynamic interactions will be more marked. For example, in a chronic heavy drinker who is sober, enzyme induction will increase the metabolism of diazepam which may lead to increased levels of anxiety (treatment failure). If the same patient becomes intoxicated with alcohol, the metabolism of diazepam will be greatly reduced as it will have to compete with alcohol for the metabolic capacity of CYP3A4. Plasma levels of alcohol and diazepam will rise (toxicity). As both alcohol and diazepam are sedative (via GABA affinity), loss of consciousness and respiratory depression may occur.

Note: be aware of the possibility of hepatic failure or reduced hepatic function in chronic alcohol misusers. See section on 'Hepatic impairment' in Chapter 7. Also note risk of hepatic toxicity with some recommended drugs (e.g. valproate). Psychotropic drugs of choice are given in Table 8.8.

References

1. Zakhari S. Overview: how is alcohol metabolized by the body? Alcohol Res Health 2006; **29**:245–254.
2. Tanaka E. Toxicological interactions involving psychiatric drugs and alcohol: an update. J Clin Pharm Ther 2003; **28**:81–95.
3. Wan Chih T. Alcohol-related drug interactions. Pharmacist's Letter/Prescriber's Letter 2008; **24**:240106.
4. Smith RG. An appraisal of potential drug interactions in cigarette smokers and alcohol drinkers. J Am Podiatr Med Assoc 2009; **99**:81–88.
5. Salmela KS et al. Respective roles of human cytochrome P-4502E1, 1A2, and 3A4 in the hepatic microsomal ethanol oxidizing system. Alcohol Clin Exp Res 1998; **22**:2125–2132.

CHAPTER 8

6. Hamitouche S et al. Ethanol oxidation into acetaldehyde by 16 recombinant human cytochrome P450 isoforms: role of CYP2C isoforms in human liver microsomes. Toxicol Lett 2006; **167**:221–230.
7. Stahl SM et al. *Essential Psychopharmacology: Neuroscientific Basis and Practical Applications*, 3rd edn. Cambridge: Cambridge University Press; 2008.

Further reading

Joint Formulary Committee. *BNF* 67 March-September 2014 (online). London: Pharmaceutical Press; 2014. http://www.medicinescomplete.com/mc/bnf/current/
Stockley's Drug Interactions. London: Pharamceutical Press; 2014. https://www.medicinescomplete.com/

Nicotine

The most common method of consuming nicotine is by smoking cigarettes. One-quarter of the general population, 40–50% of those with depression[1] and 70–80% of those with schizophrenia smoke.[2] Nicotine causes peripheral vasoconstriction, tachycardia and increased blood pressure.[3] Smokers are at increased risk of developing cardiovascular disease. People with schizophrenia who smoke are more likely to develop the metabolic syndrome, compared with those who do not smoke.[4] As well as nicotine, cigarettes also contain tar (a complex mixture of organic molecules, many carcinogenic), a cause of cancers of the respiratory tract, chronic bronchitis and emphysema.[5] Electronic cigarettes, it is claimed, contain only nicotine, which has very limited toxicity and is not thought to be carcinogenic. E-cigarettes are thus preferred for all smokers, albeit with some reservations in regard to quality control of content and the so-called re-normalisation of smoking.

Nicotine is highly addictive; an effect which may be at least partially genetically determined.[6] People with mental illness are 2–3 times more likely than the general population to develop and maintain a nicotine addiction.[1] Chronic smoking contributes to the increased morbidity and mortality from respiratory and cardiovascular disease that is seen in this patient group. Nicotine also has psychotropic effects. Smoking can affect the metabolism (and therefore the efficacy and toxicity) of drugs prescribed to treat psychiatric illness.[7] See section on 'Smoking and psychotropic drugs' in this chapter. Nicotine use may be a gateway to experimenting with other psychoactive substances.

Psychotropic effects

Nicotine is highly lipid-soluble and rapidly enters the brain after inhalation. Nicotine receptors are found on dopaminergic cell bodies and stimulation of these receptors leads to dopamine release.[1] Dopamine release in the limbic system is associated with pleasure: dopamine is the brain's 'reward' neurotransmitter. Nicotine may be used by people with mental health problems as a form of 'self-medication' (e.g. to alleviate the negative symptoms of schizophrenia or antipsychotic-induced extrapyramidal side-effects [EPS] or for its anxiolytic effect[8]). Drugs that increase the release of dopamine reduce the craving for nicotine. They may also worsen psychotic illness (see the section on 'Nicotine and smoking cessation' in Chapter 6).

Nicotine improves concentration and vigilance.[1] It also enhances the effects of glutamate, acetylcholine and serotonin.[8]

Schizophrenia

Seventy to eighty per cent of people with schizophrenia regularly smoke cigarettes[2] and this increased tendency to smoke predates the onset of psychiatric symptoms.[9] Possible explanations are as follows: smoking causes dopamine release, leading to feelings of well-being and a reduction in negative symptoms;[8] to alleviate some of the side-effects of antipsychotics such as drowsiness and EPS[1] and cognitive slowing;[10] as a means of structuring the day (a behavioural filler); a familial vulnerability[11] or as a means of alleviating the deficit in auditory gaiting that is found in schizophrenia.[12]

Nicotine may also improve working memory and attentional deficits.[13-15] Nicotinic receptor agonists may have beneficial effects on neurocognition,[16,17] although none is yet licensed for this purpose. Note though that cholinergic drugs may exacerbate nicotine dependence.[18] A single photon emission computed tomography (SPECT) study has shown that the greater the occupancy of striatal D_2 receptors by antipsychotic drugs, the more likely the patient is to smoke.[19] This may partly explain the clinical observation that smoking cessation may be more achievable when clozapine (a weak dopamine antagonist) is prescribed in place of a conventional antipsychotic. It has been suggested that people with schizophrenia find it particularly difficult to tolerate nicotine withdrawal symptoms.[7] Switching to nicotine replacement therapy (NRT) or e-cigarettes may thus be a preferred option.[20]

Depression and anxiety

In 'normal' individuals a moderate consumption of nicotine is associated with pleasure and a decrease in anxiety and feelings of anger.[21] The mechanism of this anxiolytic effect is not understood. People who suffer from anxiety and/or depression are more likely to smoke[22,23] and find it more difficult to stop.[21,24] This is compounded by the observation that nicotine withdrawal can precipitate or exacerbate depression in those with a history of the illness,[21] and cigarette smoking may directly increase the risk of symptoms of depression.[25] In marked contrast, a recent analysis suggests that stopping smoking actually improves depression and anxiety.[26] These contradictory findings are explained by the fact that early withdrawal worsens depression whereas successful cessation improves depression in the longer term.

Patients with depression are at increased risk of cardiovascular disease. By directly causing tachycardia and hypertension,[3] nicotine may, in theory, exacerbate this problem. More importantly, smoking is a well known independent risk factor for cardiovascular disease, probably because it hastens athlerosclerosis. A Cochrane review[27] suggests smoking cessation is achievable in depressed smokers.

Movement disorders and Parkinson's disease

By increasing dopaminergic neurotransmission, nicotine provides a protective effect against both drug-induced EPS and idiopathic Parkinson's disease. Smokers are less likely to suffer from antipsychotic-induced movement disorders than non-smokers[1] and use anticholinergics less often.[7] Parkinson's disease occurs less frequently in smokers than in non-smokers and the onset of clinical symptoms is delayed.[1,28] This may reflect the inverse association between Parkinson's disease and sensation seeking behavioural traits, rather than a direct effect of nicotine.[29]

Drug interactions

Polycyclic hydrocarbons in cigarette smoke are known to stimulate the hepatic microsomal enzyme system, particularly P4501A2,[8] the enzyme responsible for the metabolism of many psychotropic drugs. Smoking can lower the blood levels of some drugs by up to 50%.[8] This can affect both efficacy and side-effects and needs to be taken into account when making clinical decisions. The drugs most likely to be affected are: clozapine,[30] fluphenazine, haloperidol, chlorpromazine, olanzapine, many tricyclic antidepressants, mirtazapine, fluvoxamine and propranolol. See section on 'Smoking and psychotropic drugs' in this chapter.

Withdrawal symptoms[7]

Withdrawal symptoms occur within 6–12 hours of stopping smoking and include intense craving, depressed mood, insomnia, anxiety, restlessness, irritability, difficulty in concentrating and increased appetite. Nicotine withdrawal can be confused with depression, anxiety, sleep disorders and mania. Withdrawal can also exacerbate the symptoms of schizophrenia.

Smoking cessation

See section on 'Nicotine and smoking cessation' in Chapter 6.

References

1. Goff DC et al. Cigarette smoking in schizophrenia: relationship to psychopathology and medication side effects. Am J Psychiatry 1992; **149**:1189–1194.
2. Winterer G. Why do patients with schizophrenia smoke? Curr Opin Psychiatry 2010; **23**:112–119.
3. Benowitz NL et al. Cardiovascular effects of nasal and transdermal nicotine and cigarette smoking. Hypertension 2002; **39**:1107–1112.
4. Yevtushenko OO et al. Influence of 5-HT2C receptor and leptin gene polymorphisms, smoking and drug treatment on metabolic disturbances in patients with schizophrenia. Br J Psychiatry 2008; **192**:424–428.
5. Anderson JE et al. Treating tobacco use and dependence: an evidence-based clinical practice guideline for tobacco cessation. Chest 2002; **121**:932–941.
6. Berrettini W. Nicotine addiction. Am J Psychiatry 2008; **165**:1089–1092.
7. Ziedonis DM et al. Schizophrenia and nicotine use: report of a pilot smoking cessation program and review of neurobiological and clinical issues. Schizophr Bull 1997; **23**:247–254.
8. Lyon ER. A review of the effects of nicotine on schizophrenia and antipsychotic medications. Psychiatr Serv 1999; **50**:1346–1350.
9. Weiser M et al. Higher rates of cigarette smoking in male adolescents before the onset of schizophrenia: a historical-prospective cohort study. Am J Psychiatry 2004; **161**:1219–1223.
10. Harris JG et al. Effects of nicotine on cognitive deficits in schizophrenia. Neuropsychopharmacology 2004; **29**:1378–1385.
11. Ferchiou A et al. Exploring the relationships between tobacco smoking and schizophrenia in first-degree relatives. Psychiatry Res 2012; **200**:674–678.
12. McEvoy JP et al. Smoking and therapeutic response to clozapine in patients with schizophrenia. Biol Psychiatry 1999; **46**:125–129.
13. Jacobsen LK et al. Nicotine effects on brain function and functional connectivity in schizophrenia. Biol Psychiatry 2004; **55**:850–858.
14. Sacco KA et al. Effects of cigarette smoking on spatial working memory and attentional deficits in schizophrenia: involvement of nicotinic receptor mechanisms. Arch Gen Psychiatry 2005; **62**:649–659.
15. Smith RC et al. Effects of nicotine nasal spray on cognitive function in schizophrenia. Neuropsychopharmacology 2006; **31**:637–643.
16. Olincy A et al. Proof-of-concept trial of an alpha7 nicotinic agonist in schizophrenia. Arch Gen Psychiatry 2006; **63**:630–638.
17. Lieberman JA et al. Cholinergic agonists as novel treatments for schizophrenia: the promise of rational drug development for psychiatry. Am J Psychiatry 2008; **165**:931–936.
18. Kelly DL et al. Lack of beneficial galantamine effect for smoking behavior: a double-blind randomized trial in people with schizophrenia. Schizophr Res 2008; **103**:161–168.
19. de Haan L et al. Occupancy of dopamine D2 receptors by antipsychotic drugs is related to nicotine addiction in young patients with schizophrenia. Psychopharmacology 2006; **183**:500–505.
20. Caponnetto P et al. Impact of an electronic cigarette on smoking reduction and cessation in schizophrenic smokers: a prospective 12-month pilot study. Int J Environ Res Public Health 2013; **10**:446–461.
21. Glassman AH. Cigarette smoking: implications for psychiatric illness. Am J Psychiatry 1993; **150**:546–553.
22. Nunes SO et al. The shared role of oxidative stress and inflammation in major depressive disorder and nicotine dependence. Neurosci Biobehav Rev 2013; **37**:1336–1345.
23. Tsuang MT et al. Genetics of smoking and depression. Hum Genet 2012; **131**:905–915.
24. Wilhelm K et al. Clinical aspects of nicotine dependence and depression. Med Today 2004; **5**:40–47.

25. Boden JM et al. Cigarette smoking and depression: tests of causal linkages using a longitudinal birth cohort. Br J Psychiatry 2010; **196**:440–446.

26. Taylor G et al. Change in mental health after smoking cessation: systematic review and meta-analysis. BMJ 2014; **348**:g1151.

27. van der Meer RM et al. Smoking cessation interventions for smokers with current or past depression. Cochrane Database Syst Rev 2013; **8**: CD006102.

28. Scott WK et al. Family-based case-control study of cigarette smoking and Parkinson disease. Neurology 2005; **64**:442–447.

29. Evans AH et al. Relationship between impulsive sensation seeking traits, smoking, alcohol and caffeine intake, and Parkinson's disease. J Neurol Neurosurg Psychiatry 2006; **77**:317–321.

30. Derenne JL et al. Clozapine toxicity associated with smoking cessation: case report. Am J Ther 2005; **12**:469–471.

Further reading

Aguilar MC et al. Nicotine dependence and symptoms in schizophrenia: naturalistic study of complex interactions. Br J Psychiatry 2005;**186**:215–21.

Ziedonis D et al. Tobacco use and cessation in psychiatric disorders: National Institute of Mental Health report. Nicotine Tob Res 2008; **10**:1691–1715.

Smoking and psychotropic drugs

Tobacco smoke contains polycyclic aromatic hydrocarbons that induce (increase the activity of) certain hepatic enzymes (CYP1A2 in particular).[1] For some drugs used in psychiatry, smoking significantly reduces drug plasma levels and higher doses are required than in non-smokers.

When people stop smoking, enzyme activity reduces over a week or so. (Nicotine replacement or use of electronic cigarettes has no effect on this process.) Plasma levels of affected drugs will then rise, sometimes substantially. Dose reduction will usually be necessary. If smoking is re-started, enzyme activity increases, plasma levels fall and dose increases are then required. The process is complicated and effects are difficult to predict. Of course, few people manage to give up smoking completely, so additional complexity is introduced by intermittent smoking and repeated attempts at stopping completely. Close monitoring of plasma levels (where useful), clinical progress and adverse effect severity are essential.

Table 8.9 gives details of psychotropic drugs known to be affected by smoking status.

Table 8.9 Psychotropic drugs affected by smoking status

Drug	Effect of smoking	Action to be taken on stopping smoking	Action to be taken on re-starting
Agomelatine[2]	Plasma levels reduced	Monitor closely. Dose may need to be reduced	Consider re-introducing previous smoking dose
Benzodiazapines[3,4]	Plasma levels reduced by 0–50% (depends on drug and smoking status)	Monitor closely. Consider reducing dose by up to 25% over one week	Monitor closely. Consider re-starting 'normal' smoking dose
Carbamazepine[3]	Unclear, but smoking may reduce carbamazepine plasma levels to a small extent	Monitor for changes in severity of adverse effects	Monitor plasma levels
Chlorpromazine[3–5]	Plasma levels reduced. Varied estimates of exact effect	Monitor closely. Consider dose reduction	Monitor closely. Consider re-starting previous smoking dose
Clozapine[6–10]	Reduces plasma levels by up to 50%. Plasma level reduction may be greater in those receiving valproate	Take plasma level before stopping. On stopping, reduce dose gradually (over a week) until around 75% of original dose reached (i.e. reduce by 25%). Repeat plasma level one week after stopping. Anticipate further dose reductions	Take plasma level before re-starting. Increase dose to previous smoking dose over one week. Repeat plasma level
Duloxetine[11]	Plasma levels may be reduced by up to 50%	Monitor closely. Dose may need to be reduced	Consider re-introducing previous smoking dose
Fluphenazine[12]	Reduces plasma levels by up to 50%	On stopping, reduce dose by 25%. Monitor carefully over following 4-8 weeks. Consider further dose reductions	On re-starting, increase dose to previous smoking dose
Fluvoxamine[13]	Plasma levels decreased by around one-third	Monitor closely. Dose may need to be reduced	Dose may need to be increased to previous level

Table 8.9 (Continued)

Drug	Effect of smoking	Action to be taken on stopping smoking	Action to be taken on re-starting
Haloperidol[14,15]	Reduces plasma levels by around 20%	Reduce dose by around 10%. Monitor carefully. Consider further dose reductions	On re-starting, increase dose to previous smoking dose
Mirtazapine[16]	Unclear, but effect probably minimal	Monitor	Monitor
Olanzapine[17–20]	Reduces plasma levels by up to 50%	Take plasma level before stopping. On stopping, reduce dose by 25%. After one week, repeat plasma level. Consider further dose reductions	Take plasma level before restarting. Increase dose to previous smoking dose over one week. Repeat plasma level
Tricyclic antidepressants[3,4]	Plasma levels reduced by 25–50%	Monitor closely. Consider reducing dose by 10–25% over one week. Consider further dose reductions	Monitor closely. Consider re-starting previous smoking dose
Zuclopentixol[21,22]	Unclear, but effect probably minimal	Monitor	Monitor

Note: Only cigarette smoking induces hepatic enzymes in the manner described above – nicotine replacement and electronic cigarettes (which do not contain polycyclic aromatic compounds) have no effect on enzyme activity.

References

1. Kroon LA. Drug interactions with smoking. Am J Health Syst Pharm 2007; **64**:1917–1921.
2. Servier Laboratories Limited. Summary of Product Characteristics. Valdoxan. 2013. http://www.medicines.org.uk/emc/medicine/21830/SPC/Valdoxan/
3. Desai HD et al. Smoking in patients receiving psychotropic medications: a pharmacokinetic perspective. CNS Drugs 2001; **15**:469–494.
4. Miller LG. Recent developments in the study of the effects of cigarette smoking on clinical pharmacokinetics and clinical pharmacodynamics. Clin Pharmacokinet 1989; **17**:90–108.
5. Goff DC et al. Cigarette smoking in schizophrenia: relationship to psychopathology and medication side effects. Am J Psychiatry 1992; **149**:1189–1194.
6. Haring C et al. Influence of patient-related variables on clozapine plasma levels. Am J Psychiatry 1990; **147**:1471–1475.
7. Haring C et al. Dose-related plasma levels of clozapine: influence of smoking behaviour, sex and age. Psychopharmacology 1989; **99** Suppl:S38–S40.
8. Diaz FJ et al. Estimating the size of the effects of co-medications on plasma clozapine concentrations using a model that controls for clozapine doses and confounding variables. Pharmacopsychiatry 2008; **41**:81–91.
9. Murayama-Sung L et al. The impact of hospital smoking ban on clozapine and norclozapine levels. J Clin Psychopharmacol 2011; **31**:124–126.
10. Cormac I et al. A retrospective evaluation of the impact of total smoking cessation on psychiatric inpatients taking clozapine. Acta Psychiatr Scand 2010; **121**:393–397.
11. Fric M et al. The influence of smoking on the serum level of duloxetine. Pharmacopsychiatry 2008; **41**:151–155.
12. Ereshefsky L et al. Effects of smoking on fluphenazine clearance in psychiatric inpatients. Biol Psychiatry 1985; **20**:329–332.
13. Spigset O et al. Effect of cigarette smoking on fluvoxamine pharmacokinetics in humans. Clin Pharmacol Ther 1995; **58**:399–403.
14. Jann MW et al. Effects of smoking on haloperidol and reduced haloperidol plasma concentrations and haloperidol clearance. Psychopharmacology 1986; **90**:468–470.
15. Shimoda K et al. Lower plasma levels of haloperidol in smoking than in nonsmoking schizophrenic patients. Ther Drug Monit 1999; **21**:293–296.
16. Grasmader K et al. Population pharmacokinetic analysis of mirtazapine. Eur J Clin Pharmacol 2004; **60**:473–480.
17. Carrillo JA et al. Role of the smoking-induced cytochrome P450 (CYP)1A2 and polymorphic CYP2D6 in steady-state concentration of olanzapine. J Clin Psychopharmacol 2003; **23**:119–127.
18. Gex-Fabry M et al. Therapeutic drug monitoring of olanzapine: the combined effect of age, gender, smoking, and comedication. Ther Drug Monit 2003; **25**:46–53.
19. Bigos KL et al. Sex, race, and smoking impact olanzapine exposure. J Clin Pharmacol 2008; **48**:157–165.
20. Lowe EJ et al. Impact of tobacco smoking cessation on stable clozapine or olanzapine treatment. Ann Pharmacother 2010; **44**:727–732.
21. Jann MW et al. Clinical pharmacokinetics of the depot antipsychotics. Clin Pharmacokinet 1985; **10**:315–333.
22. Jorgensen A et al. Zuclopenthixol decanoate in schizophrenia: serum levels and clinical state. Psychopharmacology 1985; **87**:364–367.

Caffeine

Caffeine is probably the most popular psychoactive substance in the world. Mean daily consumption in the UK is 350–620 mg.[1] A quarter of the general population and half of those with psychiatric illness regularly consume over 500 mg caffeine/day.[2] Consumption of caffeine should be routinely discussed with an individual to assess its effect on their symptoms and presentation.[3] In particular, caffeine withdrawal can have a marked effect on mental and physical health. See Table 8.10 for the caffeine content of various drinks.

Chocolate also contains caffeine. Martindale lists over 600 medicines that contain caffeine.[4] Most are available without prescription and are marketed as analgesics or appetite suppressants.

General effects of caffeine

- Acute use can increase systolic and diastolic BP by up to 10 mmHg; for up to 4 hours.[3] Chronic moderate use probably has little effect on BP.[5]
- May enhance reinforcing effects of nicotine and possibly other drugs of abuse.[4,6]
- Caffeine has *de novo* psychotropic effects (Table 8.11), may worsen existing psychiatric illness, and interact with psychotropic drugs.
- Caffeine is an antagonist at adenosine A_1 and A_{2A} receptors, thus stimulating dopamine pathways.

Pharmacokinetics

- **Absorption**
  - rapid after oral administration, especially in liquid form
  - half-life of 2.5–4.5 hours.
- **Metabolism**
  - metabolised by CYP1A2, a hepatic cytochrome enzyme that exhibits genetic polymorphism, which may partially account for the large inter-individual differences that are seen in the ability to tolerate caffeine.[10] Note that CYP1A2 is induced by smoking and inhibited by a number of drugs such as fluvoxamine
  - metabolic pathways also become saturated at higher doses.[11]

Table 8.10 Caffeine content of drinks

Drink	Caffeine content
Brewed coffee	100 mg/cup
Red Bull	80 mg/can (other energy drinks may contain substantially more)
Instant coffee	60 mg/cup
BlackTea	45 mg/cup
Green Tea	20–30 mg/cup
Soft drinks	25–50 mg/can

Table 8.11 Psychotropic effects of caffeine

Dose	Psychotropic effect
Generally	CNS stimulation Increase catecholamine release, particularly dopamine[7]
Low to moderate dose	Elation[2] Peacefulness[2]
Large doses >600 mg/day (Sensitive individuals may experience affects at lower doses)	Anxiety[8] Insomnia[8] Psychomotor agitation[8] Excitement[8] Rambling speech[8] Sometimes delirium and psychosis[8] May inhibit benzodiazepine-receptor binding[8] Tolerance may develop to the affects Established withdrawal syndrome exists, symptoms include: headache, depressed mood, anxiety, fatigue, irritability, nausea, dysphoria and craving[9]

- **Interactions**
  - the potential effects of caffeine on the metabolism of other drugs, as well as the potential to induce a caffeine-withdrawal syndrome, should always be considered before substituting caffeine-free drinks (Table 8.12)
  - caffeine competitively inhibits CYP1A2. Plasma levels of some drugs may be reduced if caffeine is withdrawn.

Caffeine intoxication

The *Diagnostic and Statistical Manual of Mental Disorders* DSM-V[16] defines caffeine intoxication as the recent consumption of caffeine, usually in excess of 250 mg accompanied by five or more of the symptoms shown in Box 8.2.

In caffeine intoxication, these symptoms cause significant distress or impairment in social, occupational or other important areas of functioning and are not due to a general medical condition or better accounted for by another mental disorder (e.g. an anxiety disorder).

Caffeine abuse or dependence as a clinical syndrome has been reported[3] and Caffeine Use Disorder and Caffeine Withdrawal are both DSM-V diagnoses.

Energy drinks

So called energy drinks contain large amounts of caffeine along with sugar, vitamins and a number of other ingredients such as guarana. There is some evidence that these drinks can improve attention and short-term memory.[17] Marketing is targeted at adolescents and young adults, some of whom consume large volumes of these drinks, and seem to be particularly vulnerable to developing signs and symptoms of caffeine intoxication. Symptoms of anxiety and depression, frank suicidal behaviour and seizures have been associated with use of these products by young people.[18–20]

CHAPTER 8

Table 8.12 Interactions of caffeine

Interacting substance	Effect	Comment
CYP1A2 inhibitors: Oestrogens Cimetidine Fluvoxamine (may decrease caffeine clearance by 80%)[12] Disulfiram	Reduce caffeine clearance	Effects of caffeine may be prolonged or increased Adverse effects may be increased May precipitate caffeine toxicity
Cigarette smoke	CYP1A2 inducer – increasing caffeine metabolism[7]	Smokers may require higher doses to gain desired effects[7]
Lithium	High doses may reduce lithium levels	Caffeine withdrawal may cause a lithium level rise[13]
MAOIs	May enhance stimulant CNS effects	
Clozapine	Caffeine may increase plasma levels by up to 60%[14]	Thought to be through competitive inhibition of CYP1A2. Other drugs affected by the enzyme include olanzapine, imipramine and clomipramine
SSRIs	Large doses may increase risk of serotonin syndrome[15]	
Benzodiazepines	Caffeine may receptor binding, acting as an antagonist	Reduce the efficacy[8]

CNS, central nervous system; MAOI, monoamine oxidase inhibitor; SSRI, selective serotonin reuptake inhibitor.

Box 8.2 Symptoms of caffeine intoxication

- Restlessness
- Nervousness
- Excitement
- Insomnia
- Flushed face
- Diuresis
- Gastrointestinal disturbance
- Muscle twitching
- Rambling flow of thought and speech
- Tachycardia or cardiac arrhythmia
- Periods of inexhaustibility
- Psychomotor agitation

Schizophrenia

- Patients with schizophrenia often consume large amounts of caffeine-containing drinks[1] and they are twice as likely as controls to consume >200 mg caffeine/day.[7]
- This may be to relieve dry mouth (as a side-effect of antipsychotic drugs), for the stimulant effects of caffeine (to relieve dysphoria/sedation/negative symptoms)[7] or simply because coffee/tea drinking structures the day or relieves boredom.
- Schizophrenia may increase sensitivity to drug related cues.[7]
- Large doses of caffeine can worsen psychotic symptoms[7] (in particular elation and conceptual disorganisation) and result in the prescription of larger doses of antipsychotic drugs.

- The removal of caffeine from the diets of chronically disturbed (challenging behaviour) patients, may lead to decreased levels of hostility, irritability and suspiciousness[21] and may be of benefit in clozapine resistant schizophrenia,[22] although this may not hold true in less disturbed populations.[23]

Mood disorders

- Caffeine may elevate mood through increasing noradrenaline release[24] and modest caffeine consumption may protect against depression in those who do not have a pre-existing mood disorder.[25]
- People with mood disorders are more likely to consume caffeine, particularly when depressed.[13,26]
- Depressed patients may be more sensitive to the anxiogenic effects of caffeine.[27,28]
- Excessive consumption of caffeine may precipitate mania.[28–30]
- Caffeine can increase cortisol secretion (gives a false positive in the dexamethasone-suppression test),[31] increase seizure length during ECT[32] and increase the clearance of lithium by promoting dieresis.[33]

Anxiety disorders

- Increases vigilance, decreases reaction times, increases sleep latency and worsens subjective estimates of sleep quality, effects that may be more marked in poor metabolisers.
- May precipitate or worsen generalised anxiety and panic attacks;[34] vulnerability to these effects may be genetically determined.[6]
- Effects are so marked that caffeine intoxication should always be considered when patients complain of anxiety symptoms or insomnia.
- Symptoms may diminish considerably or even abate completely if caffeine is avoided.[35]

In summary, caffeine:

- is present in high quantities in coffee and some soft drinks, particularly energy drinks
- may worsen psychosis and anxiety; young people may be particularly vulnerable
- can increase plasma clozapine levels
- may induce intoxication which is characterised by psychomotor agitation and rambling speech
- may be associated with toxicity when co-administered with CYP1A2 inhibitors such as fluvoxamine
- can enhance the reinforcing effects of nicotine and possibly other drugs of abuse.

References

1. Rihs M et al. Caffeine consumption in hospitalized psychiatric patients. Eur Arch Psychiatry Clin Neurosci 1996; 246:83–92.
2. Clementz GL et al. Psychotropic effects of caffeine. Am Fam Physician 1988; 37:167–172.
3. Ogawa N et al. Clinical importance of caffeine dependence and abuse. Psychiatry Clin Neurosci 2007; 61:263–268.
4. Martindale: The Complete Drug Reference. London: Pharmaceutical Press; 2014. https://www.medicinescomplete.com/
5. O'Keefe JH et al. Effects of habitual coffee consumption on cardiometabolic disease, cardiovascular health, and all-cause mortality. J Am Coll Cardiol 2013; 62:1043–1051.
6. Bergin JE et al. Common psychiatric disorders and caffeine use, tolerance, and withdrawal: an examination of shared genetic and environmental effects. Twin Res Hum Genet 2012; 15:473–482.

7. Adolfo AB et al. Effects of smoking cues on caffeine urges in heavy smokers and caffeine consumers with and without schizophrenia. Schizophr Res 2009; **107**:192–197.

8. Sawynok J. Pharmacological rationale for the clinical use of caffeine. Drugs 1995; **49**:37–50.

9. Silverman K et al. Withdrawal syndrome after the double-blind cessation of caffeine consumption. N Engl J Med 1992; **327**:1109–1114.

10. Butler MA et al. Determination of CYP1A2 and NAT2 phenotypes in human populations by analysis of caffeine urinary metabolites. Pharmacogenetics 1992; **2**:116–127.

11. Kaplan GB et al. Dose-dependent pharmacokinetics and psychomotor effects of caffeine in humans. J Clin Pharmacol 1997; **37**:693–703.

12. Stockley's Drug Interactions. London: Pharamceutical Press; 2014. https://www.medicinescomplete.com/

13. Baethge C et al. Coffee and cigarette use: association with suicidal acts in 352 Sardinian bipolar disorder patients. Bipolar Disord 2009; **11**:494–503.

14. Carrillo JA et al. Effects of caffeine withdrawal from the diet on the metabolism of clozapine in schizophrenic patients. J Clin Psychopharmacol 1998; **18**:311–316.

15. Shioda K et al. Possible serotonin syndrome arising from an interaction between caffeine and serotonergic antidepressants. Hum Psychopharmacol 2004; **19**:353–354.

16. American Psychiatric Association. *Diagnostic and Statistical Manual of Mental Disorders*, 5th edn (DSM-5). Arlington, VA: American Psychiatric Association; 2013.

17. Wesnes KA et al. An evaluation of the cognitive and mood effects of an energy shot over a 6 h period in volunteers: a randomized, double-blind, placebo controlled, cross-over study. Appetite 2013; **67**:105–113.

18. Szpak A et al. A case of acute suicidality following excessive caffeine intake. J Psychopharmacol 2012; **26**:1502–1510.

19. Trapp GS et al. Energy drink consumption among young Australian adults: associations with alcohol and illicit drug use. Drug Alcohol Depend 2014; **134**:30–37.

20. Pennington N et al. Energy drinks: a new health hazard for adolescents. J Sch Nurs 2010; **26**:352–359.

21. De Freitas B et al. Effects of caffeine in chronic psychiatric patients. Am J Psychiatry 1979; **136**:1337–1338.

22. Dratcu L et al. Clozapine-resistant psychosis, smoking, and caffeine: managing the neglected effects of substances that our patients consume every day. Am J Ther 2007; **14**:314–318.

23. Koczapski A et al. Effects of caffeine on behavior of schizophrenic inpatients. Schizophr Bull 1989; **15**:339–344.

24. Achor MB et al. Diet aids, mania, and affective illness. Am J Psychiatry 1981; **138**:392.

25. Lucas M et al. Coffee, caffeine, and risk of depression among women. Arch Intern Med 2011; **171**:1571–1578.

26. Maremmani I et al. Are "social drugs" (tobacco, coffee and chocolate) related to the bipolar spectrum? J Affect Disord 2011; **133**:227–233.

27. Lee MA et al. Anxiogenic effects of caffeine on panic and depressed patients. Am J Psychiatry 1988; **145**:632–635.

28. Rizkallah E et al. Could the use of energy drinks induce manic or depressive relapse among abstinent substance use disorder patients with comorbid bipolar spectrum disorder? Bipolar Disord 2011; **13**:578–580.

29. Machado-Vieira R et al. Mania associated with an energy drink: the possible role of caffeine, taurine, and inositol. Can J Psychiatry 2001; **46**:454–455.

30. Ogawa N et al. Secondary mania caused by caffeine. Gen Hosp Psychiatry 2003; **25**:138–139.

31. Uhde TW et al. Caffeine-induced escape from dexamethasone suppression. Arch Gen Psychiatry 1985; **42**:737–738.

32. Cantu TG et al. Caffeine in electroconvulsive therapy. Ann Pharmacother 1991; **25**:1079–1080.

33. Mester R et al. Caffeine withdrawal increases lithium blood levels. Biol Psychiatry 1995; **37**:348–350.

34. Bruce MS. The anxiogenic effects of caffeine. Postgrad Med J 1990; **66 Suppl** 2:S18–S24.

35. Bruce MS et al. Caffeine abstention in the management of anxiety disorders. Psychol Med 1989; **19**:211–214.

Further reading

Caffeine: In AHFS Drug Information. American Society of Health Care Pharmacists. http://www.medicinescomplete.com

Paton C, Beer D. Caffeine: the forgotten variable. Int J Psychiatry Clin Pract 2002; **5**: 231–236.

Complementary therapies

Complementary therapies are those used alongside orthodox treatments with the aim of providing psychological and emotional support through the relief of symptoms. A wide range of treatments are available, most with limited or no scientific support. These therapies do not change or develop over time, there being almost no research aimed at determining best practice. Whenever an alternative treatment is shown to be active, it usually becomes part of mainstream practice.

A large proportion of the population currently use or have recently used complementary therapies (CTs).[1] Most users suffer from psychiatric conditions.[2,3] As health professionals are rarely consulted before purchase, a diagnosis is often not made and efficacy and side-effects are not monitored. The majority of those who use CTs are also taking conventional medicines and many people use more than one CT simultaneously.[4] Many do not tell their doctor.[5] The public associate natural products with safety and may be unwilling to report possible side-effects.[6] Herbal medicines, in particular, can be toxic as they contain pharmacologically active substances.[7] Many conventional drugs prescribed today were originally derived from plants. These include medicines as diverse as aspirin, digoxin and the vinca alkaloids used in cancer chemotherapy. Herbal medicines such as St John's wort, *Ginkgo biloba*, Yokukansan and Valerian are increasingly used as self-medication for psychiatric and neurodegenerative illnesses.[3,8–13]

Few CTs have been subject to randomised controlled trials, so efficacy is largely unproven. For some, Cochrane Reviews exist, but none support their use. These include the use of Chinese herbal medicine as an adjunct to antipsychotics in schizophrenia (promising, more evidence required)[14] aromatherapy for behavioural problems in dementia (insufficient evidence, but worth further study)[15,16] and hypnosis for schizophrenia (insufficient evidence, but worth further study).[17] Several complementary therapies are thought to be worthy of further study in the adjunctive management of substance misuse.[18] There is some preliminary, limited support for aromatherapy as an adjunct to conventional treatments in a range of psychiatric conditions.[19] Folic Acid[20] and Vitamin D[21] have been used in depression.

There is little systematic monitoring of side-effects caused by CTs, so safety is unknown. There are an increasing number of published case reports of significant drug–herb interactions;[22] these include ginkgo and aspirin or warfarin leading to increased bleeding, ginkgo and trazodone leading to coma, and ginseng and phenelzine leading to mania.[23,24] The wide range of drug interactions with St John's wort are outlined in the section 'Drug interactions with antidepressants' in Chapter 4.

Some herbs are known to be very toxic.[25,26] During consultation with patients or in the process of medicine reconciliation, the use of any specific complementary therapies should be explored and reviewed.

Whatever the perceived 'evidence base' for the use of complementary therapies, the feelings of autonomy engendered by (apparently) taking control of one's own illness and treatment can result in important psychological benefits irrespective of any direct therapeutic benefits of the CT; the placebo effect is likely to be important here. (See section on 'Observations on the placebo effect in mental illness' in this chapter.) There are many different complementary therapies, the most popular being homeopathy and herbal medicine with its branches of Bach's flower remedies, and Chinese and Ayurvedic

Table 8.13 An introduction to complementary therapies

	Health beliefs	Used for	Not suitable for	Side-effects and other information
Homeopathy[15,17,31,32]	■ Treatment is selected according to the individual characteristics of the patient (hair colour and personality are as important as symptoms) ■ Treatment stimulates the body to restore health (there is no scientifically plausible theory to support this claim) ■ Like is treated with like (e.g. substances that cause a fever, treat a fever) ■ The more diluted the preparation, the more potent it is thought to be ■ Very potent preparations are unlikely to contain even one molecule of active substance	■ A wide range of indications (except those outlined below) ■ May be taken with conventional treatments ■ Over 2000 remedies and many dilutions are available	■ Infection ■ Organ failure ■ Vitamin/mineral/ hormone deficiency	■ None known or anticipated ■ Said to be inactivated by aromatherapy and strong smells (e.g. coffee, peppermint, toothpaste) ■ Said to be inactivated by handling ■ Healing follows the law of cure: symptoms disappear down the body in the reverse order to which they appeared, move from vital to less vital organs and ultimately appear as a rash (which is a sign of cure)
Herbal medicine (phytotherapy)[25,26]	■ Treatment is selected according to the individual characteristics of the patient (as with homeopathy) ■ Herbs are believed to stimulate the body's natural defences and enhance the elimination of toxins by increasing diuresis, defecation, bile flow and sweating ■ Attention to diet is important ■ The whole plant is used, not the specific active ingredient (this is believed to reduce side-effects) ■ Active ingredients vary with the source of the herb (standardisation is contrary to the philosophy of herbal medicine) ■ Herbalists believe that if the correct treatment is chosen, treatment will be completely free of side-effects	■ Everything except as outlined below ■ May be taken with conventional treatments but many significant interactions are possible (some have been reported) ■ Advertised in the lay press for a wide range of indications	■ Use in pregnancy and lactation (many herbs are abortifacient) ■ Evening primrose oil should not be used in epilepsy	■ Herbal remedies are occasionally adulterated (with conventional medicines such as steroids or toxic substances such as lead) ■ Many side-effects can be anticipated (e.g. kelp and thyrotoxicosis, St John's wort and serotonin syndrome) ■ Overuse, adulteration, variation in plant constituents and misidentification of plants are common causes of toxicity. Some Chinese herbs are toxic

	Health beliefs	Used for	Not suitable for	Side-effects and other information
Aromatherapy[16,33]	<ul><li>Treatment is selected according to the individual characteristics of the patient (as with homeopathy and herbal medicine)</li><li>Illness is believed to be the result of imbalance in mental, emotional and physical processes, and aromatherapy is believed to promote balance</li><li>Purified oils are not used (the many natural constituents and believed to protect against adverse effects: similar to the beliefs held by herbalists)</li><li>There is no standard dose</li><li>Individual oils may be used for several unrelated indications</li></ul>	<ul><li>Everything except as outlined below</li><li>May be used as an adjunct to conventional treatments</li><li>Usually administered by massage onto the skin, which is known to relieve pain and tension, increase circulation and aid relaxation</li></ul>	<ul><li>Use in pregnancy (jasmine, peppermint, rose and rosemary may stimulate uterine contractions)</li><li>Rosemary should be avoided in epilepsy and hypertension</li></ul>	<ul><li>Skin sensitivity</li><li>**Significant systemic absorption** can occur during massage</li><li>Ingestion can cause liver/kidney toxicity</li><li>All aromatherapy products should be stored in dark containers away from heat to avoid oxidation</li></ul>

medicine. Non-drug therapies such as acupuncture and osteopathy are also popular. Aromatherapy is usually considered to be a non-pharmacological treatment but this may not be the case.[27] Physical exercise[28] and spirituality[29] have also been suggested.

To master one CT can sometimes take years of study. Therefore, to ensure safe and effective treatment, any referrals should be to a qualified practitioner with the Complementary and Natural Healthcare Council.[30]

Be aware, nonetheless, that scientific support for most complementary medicine is minimal and 'qualification' to practise may entail little in the way of examination or regulation. Moreover, much of what is taught and learned is palpable nonsense. The majority of doctors and pharmacists have no qualifications or specific training in CTs. Table 8.13 gives a brief introduction. Further reading is strongly recommended.

References

1. Posadzki P et al. Prevalence of use of complementary and alternative medicine (CAM) by patients/consumers in the UK: systematic review of surveys. Clin Med 2013; **13**:126–131.
2. Barnes J et al. *Herbal Medicines*, 3rd edn. London: Pharmaceutical Press; 2007.
3. Werneke U. Complementary medicines in mental health. Evid Based Ment Health 2009; **12**:1–4.
4. Fischer FH et al. High prevalence but limited evidence in complementary and alternative medicine: guidelines for future research. BMC Complementary and Alternative Medicine 2014; **14**:46.
5. Robinson A et al. Disclosure of CAM use to medical practitioners: a review of qualitative and quantitative studies. Complement Ther Med 2004; **12**:90–98.
6. Barnes J et al. Different standards for reporting ADRs to herbal remedies and conventional OTC medicines: face-to-face interviews with 515 users of herbal remedies. Br J Clin Pharmacol 1998; **45**:496–500.
7. Medicines and Healthcare Products Regulatory Agency. Public health risk with herbal medicines: an overview. London: MHRA; 2008. http://www.mhra.gov.uk/home/groups/es-herbal/documents/websiteresources/con023163.pdf
8. van der Watt G et al. Complementary and alternative medicine in the treatment of anxiety and depression. Curr Opin Psychiatry 2008; **21**:37–42.
9. Andreescu C et al. Complementary and alternative medicine in the treatment of bipolar disorder: a review of the evidence. J Affect Disord 2008; **110**:16–26.
10. Singh V et al. Review and meta-analysis of usage of ginkgo as an adjunct therapy in chronic schizophrenia. Int J Neuropsychopharmacol 2010; **13**:257–271.
11. Birks J et al. Ginkgo biloba for cognitive impairment and dementia. Cochrane Database Syst Rev 2009; CD003120.
12. Miyaoka T et al. Efficacy and safety of yokukansan (TJ-54) for treatment-resistant schizophrenia: a randomised placebo-controlled trial. Eur Neuropsychopharmacol 2013; **23 Suppl 2**:S476.
13. Matsuda Y et al. Yokukansan in the treatment of behavioral and psychological symptoms of dementia: a systematic review and meta-analysis of randomized controlled trials. Hum Psychopharmacol 2013; **28**:80–86.
14. Rathbone J et al. Chinese herbal medicine for schizophrenia: Cochrane systematic review of randomised trials. Br J Psychiatry 2007; **190**:379–384.
15. Thorgrimsen L et al. Aroma therapy for dementia. Cochrane Database Syst Rev 2003; CD003150.
16. Fung JK et al. A systematic review of the use of aromatherapy in treatment of behavioral problems in dementia. Geriatr Gerontol Int 2012; **12**:372–382.
17. Izquierdo de SA et al. Hypnosis for schizophrenia. Cochrane Database Syst Rev 2007; CD004160.
18. Dean AJ. Natural and complementary therapies for substance use disorders. Curr Opin Psychiatry 2005; **18**:271–276.
19. Perry N et al. Aromatherapy in the management of psychiatric disorders: clinical and neuropharmacological perspectives. CNS Drugs 2006; **20**:257–280.
20. Lazarou C et al. The role of folic acid in prevention and treatment of depression: an overview of existing evidence and implications for practice. Complement Ther Clin Pract 2010; **16**:161–166.
21. Li G et al. Efficacy of vitamin D supplementation in depression in adults: a systematic review. J Clin Endocrinol Metab 2013;jc20133450.
22. Hu Z et al. Herb-drug interactions: a literature review. Drugs 2005; **65**:1239–1282.
23. Chen XW et al. Clinical herbal interactions with conventional drugs: from molecules to maladies. Curr Med Chem 2011; **18**:4836–4850.
24. Izzo AA et al. Interactions between herbal medicines and prescribed drugs: a systematic review. Drugs 2001; **61**:2163–2175.
25. Ernst E. Serious psychiatric and neurological adverse effects of herbal medicines: a systematic review. Acta Psychiatr Scand 2003; **108**:83–91.
26. De Smet PA. Health risks of herbal remedies: an update. Clin Pharmacol Ther 2004; **76**:1–17.
27. Nguyen QA et al. The use of aromatherapy to treat behavioural problems in dementia. Int J Geriatr Psychiatry 2008; **23**:337–346.

28. Cooney GM et al. Exercise for depression. Cochrane Database Syst Rev 2013; **9**: CD004366.

29. Royal College of Psychiatrists' Spirituality and Psychiatry Special Interest Group Executive Committee. Spirituality and mental health. 2013. http://www.rcpsych.ac.uk/healthadvice/treatmentswellbeing/spirituality.aspx

30. Complementary and Natural Healthcare Council. What should I look for when choosing a complementary therapist? 2014. http://www.cnhc.org.uk

31. NHS Centre for Reviews and Dissemination. Homeopathy. Effect Health Care Bull 2002; **7**:1–12.

32. Davidson JR et al. Homeopathic treatments in psychiatry: a systematic review of randomized placebo-controlled studies. J Clin Psychiatry 2011; **72**:795–805.

33. Ernst E et al. *Oxford Handbook of Complementary Medicine*. Oxford: Oxford University Press; 2008.

Further reading

Rethink Mental Illness. Complementary Therapies. 2012. http://www.rethink.org/

Ernst E. Assessments of complementary and alternative medicine: the clinical guidelines from NICE. Int J Clin Pract 2010; **64**:1350–1358.

Enhancing medication adherence

Recommendations made in clinical guidelines regarding the use of medicines are based on evidence from clinical trials supplemented by clinicians' opinions of the balance between the potential benefits and potential risks of treatment. In clinical practice, however, a range of patient-related factors such as insight, health beliefs and the perceived efficacy and tolerability of treatment, influence whether medication is taken, and if so, for how long.

The patient and prescriber should agree jointly on the goals of treatment and how these can be reached. Sticking to this mutually agreed plan is termed concordance or adherence; non-adherence indicates that the treatment plan should be renegotiated, and not that the patient is at fault.

How common is non-adherence?

Reviews of adherence generally conclude that approximately 50% of people do not take their medication as prescribed, and that this proportion is similar across chronic physical and mental disorders.[1] This, however, may be an over-simplification in that it is probable that only a very small proportion of patients are fully adherent, the majority are partially adherent to varying degrees, and a few never take any medication at all of their own volition.[2]

There is some **variation in adherence** rates both **over time** and **across settings**. For example, ten days after discharge from hospital, up to 25% of patients with schizophrenia are partially or completely non-adherent and this figure rises to 50% at one year and 75% by 2 years.[3] In some mental healthcare settings the rate of non-adherence may be up to 90%.[4]

Poor adherence to medication is a major risk factor for poor outcomes including relapse in people with schizophrenia,[5–7] bipolar disorder[8] and depression.[9,10] Wider health benefits are also lost. For example, compared with depressed patients who take an antidepressant, those who do not have a 20% increased risk of an incident myocardial infarction.[10] As a rule of thumb, the lower the amount of prescribed medication that is taken, the poorer the outcome. There is no evidence that newer (presumed better tolerated) medicines are consistently associated with increased adherence.[2]

According to the World Health Organisation 'increasing the effectiveness of adherence interventions may have far greater impact on the health of the population than any improvements in specific medical treatments'; it has therefore been suggested that non-adherence should be a diagnosable condition for which active interventions are provided.[11] Indeed, analyses of data collected as part of the national confidential inquiry into suicide and homicide by people with mental illness, revealed that healthcare providers that had a policy in place regarding how to manage patients who are not taking their medication as prescribed, had 20% fewer suicides than providers that did not have such a policy.[12]

Not surprisingly, non-adherence is known to be more common when the patient disagrees with the need for treatment, the medication regimen is complex, or the patient perceives the side-effects of treatment to be unacceptable.[9] Adherence may also therefore be **medication specific**, where some medicines are taken regularly, others intermittently and others not at all. Notably, half of those who stop treatment don't tell their doctor. Psychiatrists generally prefer to use direct questioning over the use of more intrusive/objective methods of assessing adherence,[13] and so partial or non-adherence may go undetected.

Why don't people take medication?

Non-adherence can be intentional (sometimes termed 'intelligent' non-adherence) or unintentional or a mixture of both. Most non-adherence is intentional. Individual influences (which can change in any given patient over time) include the following factors.

- **Illness-related factors** such as denial of illness, specific symptoms such as grandiose or persecutory thoughts or delusions, or the impact of illness on lifestyle (e.g. cognitive deficits, disorganisation).
- **Treatment-related factors** such as the drug being perceived not to be effective or the side-effects intolerable; akathisia, weight gain and sexual dysfunction feature prominently here.
- **Clinician-related factors** such as not feeling listened to or consulted, perceiving the clinician as authoritative or dismissive, being given a poor explanation of treatment or having infrequent contact.
- **Patient-related factors** such as personal beliefs about illness, denial of illness/or lack of insight, perception of illness severity, being young and male, having co-morbid personality disorder(s) and/or substance misuse, personal beliefs about treatment such as concerns about dependency, concerns about long-term side-effects, a lack of knowledge about treatment, misunderstanding instructions or simply forgetting. Also, up to 25% of people with schizophrenia report missing their psychotic experiences,[14] when effectively treated.
- **Environmental and cultural factors** such as the family's beliefs about illness and treatment, religious beliefs and peer pressure.

NICE (2009)[15] recommend that, as long as the patient has capacity to consent, their right not to take medication should be respected. If the prescriber considers that this decision may have an adverse effect, the reasons for the patient's decision and the prescriber's concerns should be recorded.

Assessing attitudes to medication

A number of rating scales and checklists are available that help to guide and structure discussion around attitudes to medication. The most widely used is the Drug Attitude Inventory (DAI)[16] which consists of a mix of positive and negative statements about medication; 30 statements in its full form and 10 in its abbreviated form. It is designed to be completed by the patient who simply agrees or disagrees with each statement. The total score is an indicator of the patients overall perception of the balance between the benefits and harms associated with taking medication, and therefore likely adherence. Attitudes to medication as measured using the DAI have been shown to be a useful predictor of compliance over time.[17] Other available checklists include the Rating of Medication Influences Scale (ROMI),[18] the Beliefs about Medicines Questionnaire[19] and the Medication Adherence rating Scale (MARS).[7]

How can you assess adherence?

It is very difficult to be certain about whether or not a patient is taking prescribed medicines; partial and non-adherence are almost always covert until the patient relapses. Clinicians are known to overestimate adherence rates and patients may not openly acknowledge that they are not taking all or any of their medication. NICE recommend that the patient should be asked in a non-judgemental way if they have missed any doses over a specific time period such as the previous week.[15]

It is also important to ask the patient about perceived effectiveness and side-effects. More intrusive methods include checks that prescriptions have been collected, asking to see the patient's medication (pill counts) and asking family or carers. For some antipsychotics such as clozapine, olanzapine and risperidone, blood tests can be useful to directly assess plasma levels. It is important to note that plasma levels of these drugs achieved with a fixed dose vary somewhat and it is not possible to accurately determine partial non-adherence (i.e. total non-adherence will be readily revealed but partial and full adherence may be difficult to tell apart). See section on 'Plasma level monitoring' in Chapter 1.

Strategies for improving adherence

Note that few studies specifically recruit non-adherent patients (the refusal rate in such patients is likely to be high) and the specific barriers to adherence are rarely identified. The small effect size seen in many studies may simply be a consequence of this unfocused approach. Where barriers to adherence are identified and targeted interventions delivered, adherence is more likely to improve.[20]

NICE has reviewed the evidence for adherence over a range of health conditions.[15] They conclude that no specific intervention can be recommended for all patients but, in general, **adherence is maximised if:**

- the patient is **offered information about medicines** before the decision is taken to prescribe
- this information is actively **discussed,** taking into account the patient's understanding and beliefs about diagnosis and treatment
- the information includes the **name** of the medicine, how it works, the likely benefits and side-effects, and how long it should be continued
- the patient is given the opportunity to be **involved in making decisions** about prescribed medicines[21]
- at each contact, the patient is asked if they have any concerns about their medicines, and any identified **concerns are addressed**
- specific to schizophrenia, **good social and family support** has been shown to have a positive impact on adherence.[21]

NICE further recommend that any intervention that is used to increase adherence should be tailored to overcome the specific difficulties experienced or reported by a patient.

It is essential that the **patient's perspective is understood and respected and a treatment plan agreed jointly.** The following strategies may help to achieve this:

- explore aspirations for the future and **how medication could help,** e.g. staying out of hospital or not getting into trouble with the police

- help the patient and carer **understand** their experiences in a culturally sensitive way that recognises the place of medication in recovery
- work with the patient to elicit and explore the **positive and negative** things about taking/ not taking medication
- talk through past experiences of medication and exploring which medicines were helpful and less helpful **from the patient's perspective**
- **listen** to and **acknowledge** the **concerns** of patients and their carers about the use of medication and address any false beliefs
- **work collaboratively** with the patient to find a medication that the patient perceives to be helpful
- **systematically monitor the effectiveness and adverse effects** of medication so that the patient feels listened to and respected
- **manage adverse effects when they occur.** Consider dosage reduction, change of medication, alteration of the timing of doses, or additional medication for side-effects.

Overcoming **practical difficulties** can also help. Potentially useful strategies include:

- ensuring the patient knows how to **obtain medication** and is able to do this[22]
- keeping **medication regimes** as **simple** as possible
- using **reminders and prompts,** including electronic pill dispensers,[23] telephone follow-up or mobile phone text messaging[24,25]
- **maximising engagement** with services by introducing patients to their community team before discharge from hospital
- providing support, encouragement and **regular planned follow up.**

The need to consider multiple strategies tailored to the needs of individual patients is also the conclusion of a Cochrane review that examined medication adherence over a wide range of medical conditions.[1] Almost all of the interventions that were effective in improving adherence in long-term care were complex, and even the most effective interventions did not lead to large improvements in adherence and treatment outcomes. Haynes et al[1] emphasized that there is no evidence that low adherence can be 'cured'; efforts to improve adherence must be maintained for as long as treatment is needed.

'Compliance therapy' for schizophrenia

After early promise in improving insight, adherence, attitudes towards medication and rehospitalisation rates in an inpatient sample,[26] further studies of Compliance therapy have failed to replicate this finding. Compliance therapy has been shown to have no advantage over non-specific counselling in either inpatients[17] or outpatients,[27] or those who have been clinically unstable in the last year.[28]

Compliance aids

Compliance aids that contain compartments accommodating up to four doses of multiple medicines each day may be helpful in patients who are clearly motivated to take medication but find this difficult because of disorganisation or cognitive deficits. It should be noted that only 10% of non-compliant patients say that they forgot to take medication[29] and that compliance aids are not a substitute for lack of insight or lack of motivation to take medication. Some medicines are unstable when removed from blister packaging and placed in a compliance aid. These include oro-dispersible formulations which are often prescribed for non-adherent patients. In addition, compliance aids are labour intensive (expensive) to fill, it can be difficult to change prescriptions at short notice and the filling of these devices is particularly error-prone.[30]

Depot antipsychotics

Meta-analyses of clinical trials have shown that the relative and absolute risks of relapse with depot maintenance treatment were 30% and 10% lower respectively, than with oral treatment[31,32] when depots are used. In clinical practice, covert non-adherence is avoided; if the patient defaults from treatment, it will be immediately apparent. NICE recommends that depots are an option in patients who are known to be non-adherent to oral treatment and/or those who prefer this method of administration.[33] Depots are likely to be underused, for example a recent US study found that depot preparations were prescribed for fewer than one in five patients with a recent episode of non-adherence.[34] The introduction of so-called atypical depots may allow wider use of these formulations. Wider choice may lead to improved acceptability.

Paying patients to take their medication

There is evidence from controlled trials across a number of disease areas supporting the potential of financial incentives to enhance medication adherence. Paying people to take their medication is extremely controversial, though some clinicians have found this strategy to be successful in high risk patients with psychotic illness.[35] An RCT has demonstrated that modest payments improve adherence in patients with psychotic illness.[36]

References

1. Haynes RB et al. Interventions for enhancing medication adherence. Cochrane Database Syst Rev 2008; CD000011.
2. Masand PS et al. Partial adherence to antipsychotic medication impacts the course of illness in patients with schizophrenia: a review. Prim Care Companion J Clin Psychiatry 2009; 11:147–154.
3. Leucht S et al. Epidemiology, clinical consequences, and psychosocial treatment of nonadherence in schizophrenia. J Clin Psychiatry 2006; 67 Suppl 5:3–8.
4. Cramer JA et al. Compliance with medication regimens for mental and physical disorders. Psychiatr Serv 1998; 49:196–201.
5. Morken G et al. Non-adherence to antipsychotic medication, relapse and rehospitalisation in recent-onset schizophrenia. BMC Psych 2008; 8:32.
6. Knapp M et al. Non-adherence to antipsychotic medication regimens: associations with resource use and costs. Br J Psychiatry 2004; 184:509–516.
7. Jaeger S et al. Adherence styles of schizophrenia patients identified by a latent class analysis of the Medication Adherence Rating Scale (MARS): a six-month follow-up study. Psychiatry Res 2012; 200:83–88.
8. Lang K et al. Predictors of medication nonadherence and hospitalization in Medicaid patients with bipolar I disorder given long-acting or oral antipsychotics. J Med Econ 2011; 14:217–226.
9. Mitchell AJ et al. Why don't patients take their medicine? reasons and solutions in psychiatry. Adv Psychiatr Treat 2007; 13:336–346.
10. Scherrer JF et al. Antidepressant drug compliance: reduced risk of MI and mortality in depressed patients. Am J Med 2011; 124:318–324.
11. Marcum ZA et al. Medication nonadherence: a diagnosable and treatable medical condition. JAMA 2013; 309:2105–2106.
12. Appleby L, Kapur N, Shaw J, Hunt IM, While D, Flynn S et al. National Confidential Inquiry into Suicide and Homicide by People with Mental Illness. 2013. http://www.bbmh.manchester.ac.uk/cmhr/research/centreforsuicideprevention/nci/
13. Vieta E et al. Psychiatrists' perceptions of potential reasons for non- and partial adherence to medication: results of a survey in bipolar disorder from eight European countries. J Affect Disord 2012; 143:125–130.

14. Moritz S et al. Beyond the usual suspects: positive attitudes towards positive symptoms is associated with medication noncompliance in psychosis. Schizophr Bull 2013; 39:917–922.

15. National Institute for Health and Clinical Excellence. Medicines adherence: involving patients in decisions about prescribed medicines and supporting adherence. Clinical Guideline CG76, 2009. http://www.nice.org.uk/

16. Hogan TP et al. A self-report scale predictive of drug compliance in schizophrenics: reliability and discriminative validity. Psychol Med 1983; 13:177–183.

17. O'Donnell C et al. Compliance therapy: a randomised controlled trial in schizophrenia. BMJ 2003; 327:834.

18. Weiden P et al. Rating of medication influences (ROMI) scale in schizophrenia. Schizophr Bull 1994; 20:297–310.

19. Horne R et al. The beliefs about medicines questionnaire: The development and evaluation of a new method for assessing the cognitive representation of medication. Psychol Health 1999; 14:1–24.

20. Staring AB et al. Treatment adherence therapy in people with psychotic disorders: randomised controlled trial. Br J Psychiatry 2010; 197:448–455.

21. Wilder CM et al. Medication preferences and adherence among individuals with severe mental illness and psychiatric advance directives. Psychiatr Serv 2010; 61:380–385.

22. Valenstein M et al. Using a pharmacy-based intervention to improve antipsychotic adherence among patients with serious mental illness. Schizophr Bull 2011; 37:727–736.

23. Velligan D et al. A randomized trial comparing in person and electronic interventions for improving adherence to oral medications in schizophrenia. Schizophr Bull 2013; 39:999–1007.

24. Granholm E et al. Mobile Assessment and Treatment for Schizophrenia (MATS): a pilot trial of an interactive text-messaging intervention for medication adherence, socialization, and auditory hallucinations. Schizophr Bull 2012; 38:414–425.

25. Montes JM et al. A short message service (SMS)-based strategy for enhancing adherence to antipsychotic medication in schizophrenia. Psychiatry Res 2012; 200:89–95.

26. Kemp R et al. Randomised controlled trial of compliance therapy. 18-month follow-up. Br J Psychiatry 1998; 172:413–419.

27. Byerly MJ et al. A trial of compliance therapy in outpatients with schizophrenia or schizoaffective disorder. J Clin Psychiatry 2005; 66:997–1001.

28. Gray R et al. Adherence therapy for people with schizophrenia. European multicentre randomised controlled trial. Br J Psychiatry 2006; 189:508–514.

29. Perkins DO. Predictors of noncompliance in patients with schizophrenia. J Clin Psychiatry 2002; 63:1121–1128.

30. Barber ND et al. Care homes' use of medicines study: prevalence, causes and potential harm of medication errors in care homes for older people. Qual Safety Health Care 2009; 18:341–346.

31. Leucht C et al. Oral versus depot antipsychotic drugs for schizophrenia--a critical systematic review and meta-analysis of randomised long-term trials. Schizophr Res 2011; 127:83–92.

32. Leucht S et al. Antipsychotic drugs versus placebo for relapse prevention in schizophrenia: a systematic review and meta-analysis. Lancet 2012; 379:2063–2071.

33. National Institute for Health and Clinical Excellence. Schizophrenia: core interventions in the treatment and management of schizophrenia in adults in primary and secondary care (update). 2009. http://www.nice.org.uk/

34. West JC et al. Use of depot antipsychotic medications for medication nonadherence in schizophrenia. Schizophr Bull 2008; 34:995–1001.

35. Claassen D et al. Money for medication: financial incentives to improve medication adherence in assertive outreach. Psychiatr Bull 2007; 31:4–7.

36. Priebe S et al. Effectiveness of financial incentives to improve adherence to maintenance treatment with antipsychotics: cluster randomised controlled trial. BMJ 2013; 347:f5847.

Further reading

Barnes TR. Evidence-based guidelines for the pharmacological treatment of schizophrenia: recommendations from the British Association for Psychopharmacology. J Psychopharmacol 2011; 25:567–620.

CHAPTER 8

Driving and psychotropic medicines

Driving a car is important in maintaining independence and freedom. However, no one should drive if their performance is compromised. Everyone has a duty to drive reasonably and all drivers are legally responsible for accidents they cause.[1]

Many factors have been shown to affect driving performance. These include age, gender, personality, physical and mental state and being under the influence of alcohol, prescribed medicines, street drugs or over-the-counter medicines.[2,3] Studying the effects of any of these factors in isolation is extremely difficult. Some studies have attempted to categorize medicinal drugs according to how they affect driving performance.[4] Some studies have assessed the effect of medication on tests such as response-time and attention,[5] but these tests do not directly measure ability or inability to drive.

It has been estimated that up to 10% of people killed or injured in road traffic accidents (RTAs) are taking psychotropic medication.[5] See Table 8.14. Patients with personality disorders and alcoholism have the highest rates of motoring offences and are more likely to be involved in accidents.[5] People whose driving ability may be impaired through their illness or prescribed medication should inform their insurance company. Failure to do so is considered to be 'withholding a material fact' and may render the insurance policy void.

Effects of mental illness

Severe mental disorder is a prescribed disability for the purposes of the Road Traffic Act 1988.[19] Regulations define mental disorder as including mental illness, arrested or incomplete development of the mind, psychopathic disorder or severe impairment of intelligence or social functioning. The licence restrictions that apply to each disorder can be found in Table 8.15. Note that licence restrictions may also apply to people with diabetes, particularly if treated with insulin or if there are established micro or macro-vascular complications.

Many people with early dementia are capable of driving safely.[20] All drivers with new diagnoses of Alzheimer's disease and other dementias must notify the Drivers and Vehicle Licensing Agency (DVLA).[21,22] The doctor may need to make an immediate decision on safety to drive and ensure that the licensing agency is notified[23] There are no data to support ongoing driving assessments as a way of maintaining driving ability or improving road safety of drivers with dementia.[24]

Effects of psychiatric medicines

The Road Traffic Act does not differentiate between illicit drugs and prescribed medicines. In the UK, a new liability offence came into effect in the summer of 2014 for drivers who are impaired after recreational use of drugs.[25] Therefore, any person who drives in a public place while unfit due to any drug, is liable to prosecution. The DVLA list of 'recreational drugs' includes some that can be prescribed such as morphine, amfetamines and benzodiazepines (the full list can be found on the MHRA website). A comprehensive report[26] describing the evidence behind the new laws and legal limits for driving is available.

Table 8.14 Psychotropic drugs and driving

Drug	Effect
Alcohol	Alcohol causes sedation and impaired coordination, vision, attention and information-processing. Alcohol-dependent drivers are twice as likely to be involved in traffic accidents and offences than licensed drivers as a whole,[5] and a third of all fatal RTAs involve alcohol-dependent drivers.[5] Young drivers who use alcohol in combination with illicit drugs are particularly high risk[6,7]
Anticonvulsants	Initial, dose-related side-effects may affect driving ability (e.g. blurred vision, ataxia and sedation). There are strict rules regarding epilepsy and driving
Antidepressants	People who are prescribed an antidepressant have an increased risk of being involved in a RTA particularly at treatment initiation. SSRIs may have some advantages over TCAs but driving ability is still diminished compared with healthy individuals,[8] suggesting that depression itself may make a major contribution[9,10] Initiation effects caused by mirtazapine diminish to an extent when it is given as a single dose at night but many people experience substantial hangover. There is currently no available data on the effects of agomelatine and duloxetine on driving ability.[8]
Antipsychotics	Sedation and EPS can impair coordination and response time.[2] A high proportion of patients treated with antipsychotics may have an impaired ability to drive.[11,12] One study found patients with schizophrenia taking atypical antipsychotics or clozapine performed better in tests of skills related to car-driving ability than patients with schizophrenia taking typical antipsychotics.[13] Clinical assessment is required
Hypnotics and anxiolytics	Benzodiazepines cause sedation and impaired attention, information processing, memory and motor coordination, and along with opiates are the medicines most frequently implicated in RTAs.[14] When used as anxiolytics and hypnotics, benzodiazepines, zopiclone and zolpidem are associated with an increased risk of RTAs.[14] There is some gender variation in the pharmacokinetics of zolpidem with females having higher drug plasma concentrations than males for any given dose; the driving ability of females may therefore be particularly impaired.[3] Zaleplon and the newer hypnotics acting at melatonin or serotonin receptors have not been found to have any negative residual effects on driving ability[15]
Lithium	Lithium may impair visual adaptation to the dark[2] but the implications for driving safety are unknown. Elderly people who take lithium may be at increased risk of being involved in an injurious motor vehicle crash[16]
Methylphenidate	Some studies have demonstrated that reaction time is longer in patients with ADHD which may in turn be associated with increased driving risks.[17] Other studies have found that methylphenidate improved driving performance in adults with ADHD,[18] again suggesting that illness may make a bigger contribution to fitness to drive than the specific pharmacology of the treatment[18]

ADHD, attention deficit hyperactivity disorder; EPS, extrapyramidal side-effects; RTA, road traffic accident; SSRI, selective serotonin reuptake inhibitor; TCA, tricyclic antidepressant.

Many psychotropics can impair alertness, concentration and driving performance. Medicines that block H_1, α_1-adrenergic or cholinergic receptors may be particularly problematic. Effects are particularly marked at the start of treatment and after increasing the dose. Drivers must be made aware of any potential for impairment and advised to evaluate their driving performance at these times. They must stop driving if adversely affected.[27] The use of alcohol will further increase any impairment. Many antipsychotics and antidepressants lower the seizure threshold. The DVLA advises this

Table 8.15 Summary of DVLA regulations for psychiatric disorders (November 2013)[20]

To be read in conjunction with the section on 'Driving and psychotropic medicines'. It is the illness rather than the medication which is of prime importance. For cases which involve more than one condition, please consider all relevant regulations. Any psychiatric condition which does not fit neatly into the classifications below should be reported to the DVLA if it is felt that it could affect safe driving. DVLA notification by licence holder or applicant is required except where indicated.

Diagnosis	Group 1 Entitlement (cars and motorcycles)		Group 2 Entitlement (heavy goods or public service vehicles)	
	Notify DVLA?	Notes	Notify DVLA?	Notes
Uncomplicated anxiety or depression (without significant memory or concentration problems, agitation, behaviouraldisturbance or suicidal thoughts)	No	Consider effects of medication (see Table 8.14)	No	Very minor short-lived illnesses need not be notified to DVLA. Consider effects of medication (see Table 8.11)
Severe anxiety states or depressive illnesses (with significant memory or concentration problems, agitation, behavioural disturbance or suicidal thoughts)	Yes	Driving should cease pending the outcome of medical enquiry. A period of stability will be required before driving can be resumed	Yes	Driving may be permitted when person is well and stable for 6 months or if the illness is longstanding but maintained symptom free on medication which does not impair driving. DVLA may require psychiatric reports
Acute psychotic disorders of any type	Yes	Driving must cease during the acute illness. Relicensing can be considered when all of the following conditions can be satisfied: ■ has remained well and stable for at least 3 months ■ is compliant with treatment ■ has regained insight (hypomania/mania only) ■ is free from adverse effects of medication which would impair driving ■ subject to a favourable specialist report Drivers with a history of instability and/or poor compliance will require a longer period off driving	Yes	**DRIVING MUST CEASE** pending the outcome of medical enquiry by the DVLA panel. The normal requirement is that the person be well and stable for 3 years before driving can be resumed, on minimum effective antipsychotic dose, optimal tolerability achieved with no associated deficits that might impair driving ability. The risk if relapsed, treated or untreated should be appraised as low. DVLA will require a consultant report specifically addressing these issues before the licence can be considered

Table 8.15 (*Continued*)

| Diagnosis | Group 1 Entitlement (cars and motorcycles) | | Group 2 Entitlement (heavy goods or public service vehicles) | |
	Notify DVLA?	Notes	Notify DVLA?	Notes
Hypomania/mania	Yes	See 'Acute psychotic disorders of any type' **Repeated changes of mood**: when there have been four or more episodes of mood swing in the last 12 months, at least 6 months' stability is required under condition(a) above	Yes	As above
Chronic schizophrenia and other chronic psychoses	Yes	See 'Acute psychotic disorders of any type' **Continuing symptoms,** even with limited insight do not necessarily preclude driving. Symptoms should be unlikely to cause significant concentration problems, memory impairment or distraction whilst driving. Particularly dangerous are those drivers whose psychotic symptoms relate to other road users	Yes	As above
Dementia or any organic brain syndrome	Yes	Patient should inform DVLA (see Table 8.14). Decision regarding fitness to drive subject reports. In early dementia, licence may be issued based on medical reports subject to annual review. A formal driving assessment may be necessary	Yes	Refuse or revoke licence
Learning disability	Yes	Severe learning disability – licence application will be refused. Mild learning disability – possible if no relevant problems. Necessary to demonstrate adequate functional ability at the wheel: liaise with DVLA	Yes	Refusal or revocation if severe. Only persons with minor degrees of learning disability will be considered for a licence. When the condition is stable and there are no medical or psychiatric complications, licence may be restored
Developmental disorders including Asperger's syndrome, autism, severe communication disorders and ADHD	Yes	Diagnosis not in itself a bar to licensing. Factors such as impulsivity, lack of awareness of the impact of own behaviour on self or others need to be considered	Yes	Continuing minor symptomatology may be compatible with licensing. Cases considered individually

(Continued)

CHAPTER 8

Table 8.15 (*Continued*)

Diagnosis	Group 1 Entitlement (cars and motorcycles)		Group 2 Entitlement (heavy goods or public service vehicles)	
	Notify DVLA?	Notes	Notify DVLA?	Notes
Behaviour disorders (e.g. violent behaviour)	Yes	Licence revoked if behaviour is seriously disturbed. Licence reissued only after behaviour has been satisfactorily controlled. Medical report required	Yes	If behaviour is seriously disturbed, licence refused/revoked. Restoration of licence possible if psychiatric reports confirm stability
Personality disorders	Yes	If likely to be a source of danger at the wheel, licence would be revoked or refused. Can be permitted subject to medical report	Yes	Refusal/revocation if behaviour is likely to be a source of danger at the wheel. Restoration possible after psychiatrist's report confirms stability
Alcohol misuse 'persistent misuse of alcohol confirmed by medical enquiry'	Yes	Licence refused/revoked for confirmed, persistent alcohol misuse until minimum of 6 months' controlled drinking or abstinence attained. Patient to seek advice from medical or other sources during period off the road	Yes	Same as Group 1 except 1 year's controlled drinking or abstinence required. Patient to seek advice from medical or other sources during period off the road
Alcohol dependency (may include history of withdrawal symptoms, tolerance, detoxification(s) and/or alcohol-related fits)	Yes	Licence refused/revoked until a 1-year period free from alcohol problems attained. Abstinence usually required. Medical reports required. Restoration will require medical reports and may require independent medical examination and blood tests by DVLA. Consultant support/referral may be necessary	Yes	Licence not granted if there is a history of alcohol dependency in the past 3 years. Additional restrictions if seizures occur. Medical reports required. Restoration will require medical reports and may require independent medical examination and blood tests by DVLA. Consultant support/referral may be necessary
Alcohol-related seizures	Yes	Following an isolated seizure, licence is revoked for a minimum 6 months. If relevant, refer to alcohol dependency above. If more than one seizure, then epilepsy regulations will apply. Medical enquiry will be required before restoration. Independent medical assessment by DVLA normally necessary	Yes	Following an isolated seizure, licence is revoked/refused for a minimum of 5 years. Restoration subject to: ■ no structural cerebral abnormality ■ off anticonvulsant medication for at least 5 years ■ maintained abstinence from alcohol if previously dependent ■ review by addiction specialist and neurologist If more than one seizure or underlying structural abnormality, vocational epilepsy regulations apply

Table 8.15 (Continued)

Diagnosis	Group 1 Entitlement (cars and motorcycles)		Group 2 Entitlement (heavy goods or public service vehicles)	
	Notify DVLA?	Notes	Notify DVLA?	Notes
Alcohol-related disorders (e.g. hepatic cirrhosis with neuropsychiatric impairment or psychosis)	Yes	Licence refused/revoked until satisfactory recovery and medical standards are satisfied	Yes	Licence refused/revoked
Drug misuse and dependency: cannabis, amfetamines, ecstasy, ketamine and other psychoactive substances	Yes	If persistent use or dependency confirmed, licence is refused or revoked until a minimum 6 months drug-free period. For ketamine misuse, 6 months off driving, drug free and 12 months if dependent. Assessment and urine screen arranged by DVLA may be required	Yes	If persistent use or dependency, refusal or revocation for a minimum of 1 year drug free. Assessment and urine screen arranged by DVLA will be required
Heroin, morphine, methadone, cocaine methamfetamine	Yes	As above but for minimum of 1 year. Medical report may also be required on reapplication. (there are exceptions for those on a supervised maintenance programme)	Yes	As above but for a minimum of 3 years Medical report will also be required before relicensing (there are exceptions for those on a supervised maintenance programme)

Full information can be found at: https://www.gov.uk/government/publications/at-a-glance

is taken into consideration when prescribing for a driver. Further information about the effects of psychotropics on driving can be found in Table 8.14.

Medication-induced sedation

Many psychotropics are sedating. The more sedating a medicine is, the more likely it is to impair driving ability. Other medicines, either prescribed or bought over the counter, may also be sedative and/or affect driving ability (e.g. antihistamines[5]). One study found that 89% of patients taking other psychotropics in addition to antidepressants failed a battery of 'fitness to drive' tests.[28] Since the degree of sedation any individual will experience is very difficult to predict, patients prescribed sedating medicines should be advised not to drive if they feel sedated.

DVLA: duty of the driver

It is the legal responsibility of the licence holder or applicant to notify the DVLA of any medical condition which may affect safe driving. A list of relevant medical conditions can be found in the DVLA 'At a glance' guide.[20] Drivers must recognize signs of impaired driving performance due to medication or illness.

CHAPTER 8

DVLA: duty of the prescriber

Make sure the patient understands that their condition may impair their ability to drive. If the patient is incapable of understanding, notify the DVLA immediately. Explain to the patient that they have a legal duty to inform the DVLA.

Note: the DVLA guidance specifies that patients under S17 of the Mental Health Act must be able to satisfy the standards of fitness for their respective conditions and be free from any effects of medication which would affect driving adversely, before resuming driving. Very few patients will fulfil these criteria.

General Medical Council guidelines for prescribers[29]

- Patients who disagree with the diagnosis or the effect of the condition on their ability to drive should seek a second opinion and refrain from driving until this has been obtained.
- If the patient continues to drive while unfit, you should make every reasonable effect to persuade them to stop. This may include telling their next of kin if they agree you may do so.
- If they continue to drive, inform the DVLA. Tell the patient you are going to do this and write to the patient to confirm you have done so. Document the advice given clearly in the patient's notes.

References

1. Annas GJ. Doctors, drugs, and driving--tort liability for patient-caused accidents. N Engl J Med 2008; 359:521–525.
2. Metzner JL et al. Impairment in driving and psychiatric illness. J Neuropsychiatry Clin Neurosci 1993; 5:211–220.
3. Farkas RH et al. Zolpidem and driving impairment--identifying persons at risk. N Engl J Med 2013; 369:689–691.
4. Alvarez J, de Gier H, Mercier-Guyon C, Verstraete A. ICADTS Working Group: Catergorization system for medicinal drugs affecting driving performance. 2007. http://www.icadts.nl/medicinal.html
5. Noyes R, Jr. Motor vehicle accidents related to psychiatric impairment. Psychosomatics 1985; 26:569–580.
6. Biecheler MB et al. SAM survey on "drugs and fatal accidents": search of substances consumed and comparison between drivers involved under the influence of alcohol or cannabis. Traffic Inj Prev 2008; 9:11–21.
7. Oyefeso A et al. Fatal injuries while under the influence of psychoactive drugs: a cross-sectional exploratory study in England. BMC Public Health 2006; 6:148.
8. Brunnauer A et al. The effects of most commonly prescribed second generation antidepressants on driving ability: a systematic review: 70th Birthday Prof. Riederer. J Neural Transm 2013; 120:225–232.
9. Bramness JG et al. Minor increase in risk of road traffic accidents after prescriptions of antidepressants: a study of population registry data in Norway. J Clin Psychiatry 2008; 69:1099–1103.
10. Verster JC et al. Psychoactive medication and traffic safety. Int J Environ Res Public Health 2009; 6:1041–1054.
11. Grabe HJ et al. The influence of clozapine and typical neuroleptics on information processing of the central nervous system under clinical conditions in schizophrenic disorders: implications for fitness to drive. Neuropsychobiology 1999; 40:196–201.
12. Wylie KR et al. Effects of depot neuroleptics on driving performance in chronic schizophrenic patients. J Neurol Neurosurg Psychiatry 1993; 56:910–913.
13. Brunnauer A et al. The impact of antipsychotics on psychomotor performance with regards to car driving skills. J Clin Psychopharmacol 2004; 24:155–160.
14. Dassanayake T et al. Effects of benzodiazepines, antidepressants and opioids on driving: a systematic review and meta-analysis of epidemiological and experimental evidence. Drug Saf 2011; 34:125–156.
15. Verster JC et al. Hypnotics and driving safety: meta-analyses of randomized controlled trials applying the on-the-road driving test. Curr Drug Saf 2006; 1:63–71.
16. Etminan M et al. Use of lithium and the risk of injurious motor vehicle crash in elderly adults: case-control study nested within a cohort. BMJ 2004; 328:558–559.
17. Hashemian F et al. A comparison of the effects of reboxetine and placebo on reaction time in adults with Attention Deficit-Hyperactivity Disorder (ADHD). Daru 2011; 19:231–235.

18. Classen S et al. Evidence-based review on interventions and determinants of driving performance in teens with attention deficit hyperactivity disorder or autism spectrum disorder. Traffic Inj Prev 2013; **14**:188–193.

19. The National Archives. Road Traffic Act 1991. 1991. http://www.legislation.gov.uk/ukpga/1991/40/contents

20. Driver and Vehicle Licensing Agency. At a glance guide to the current medical standards of fitness to drive. 2013. https://www.gov.uk/government/publications/at-a-glance

21. DirectGov. Alzheimer's disease and driving. 2013. https://www.gov.uk/alzheimers-disease-and-driving

22. DirectGov. Dementia and driving. 2013. https://www.gov.uk/dementia-and-driving

23. Breen DA et al. Driving and dementia. BMJ 2007; **334**:1365–1369.

24. Martin AJ et al. Driving assessment for maintaining mobility and safety in drivers with dementia. Cochrane Database Syst Rev 2013; **8**: CD006222.

25. Medicines and Healthcare Products Regulatory Agency. New drug driving offence – implications for medicines packaging. London: MHRA; 2013. http://www.mhra.gov.uk/Howweregulate/Medicines/Medicinesregulatorynews/CON350699

26. Wolff K et al. UK Department of Transport - Driving under the Influence of Drugs. Report from the Expert Panel on Drug Driving. 2013. https://www.gov.uk/government/uploads/system/uploads/attachment_data/file/167971/drug-driving-expert-panel-report.pdf

27. Department of Transport. Medication and Road Safety: A Scoping Study. Road Safety Research Report No. 116. 2010. http://www.dft.gov.uk/

28. Grabe HJ et al. The influence of polypharmacological antidepressive treatment on central nervous information processing of depressed patients: implications for fitness to drive. Neuropsychobiology 1998; **37**:200–204.

29. General Medical Council. Good practice in prescribing and managing medicines and devices. 2013. http://www.gmc-uk.org/guidance/ethical_guidance/14316.asp

Covert administration of medicines within food and drink

In mental health settings, it is common for patients to refuse medication. Some patients with cognitive disorders may lack capacity to make an informed choice about whether medication will be beneficial to them or not. In these cases, the clinical team may consider whether it would be in the patient's best interests to conceal medication in food or drink. This practice is known as covert administration of medicines. Guidance from the Nursing and Midwifery Council[1–3] and the Royal College of Psychiatrists[4] exists in order to protect patients from the unlawful and inappropriate administration of medication in this way. The legal framework for such interventions would be either the Mental Capacity Act (MCA)[5] or, more rarely, the Mental Health Act (MHA).[6]

Assessment of mental capacity[5,7]

When it applies to the covert administration of medicines, the assessment of capacity regarding treatment is primarily a matter for doctors treating the patient.[5,7] Nurses will also have to be mindful of their own codes of professional practice and should be satisfied that the doctor's assessment is reasonable. In assessing capacity it is important to make the assessment in relation to the particular treatment proposed. Capacity can vary over time and the assessment should be made at the time of the proposed treatment. The assessment should be documented in the patient's notes and recorded in the care plan.

A patient is presumed to have the capacity to make treatment decisions unless he/she is unable to:

- understand the information relevant to the decision
- retain that information
- use or weigh that information as part of the process of making the decision, or
- communicate his/her decision (whether by talking, using sign language or any other means).

Guidance on covert administration

If a patient has the capacity to give a valid refusal to medication and is not detainable under the Mental Health Act, their refusal should be respected.

If a patient has the capacity to give a valid refusal and is either being treated under the Mental Health Act or is legally detainable under the Act, the provisions of the Mental Health Act with regard to treatment will apply, which are outside the scope of this chapter. In general, the Mental Health Act will only be used if the person is actively resisting admission and treatment. Someone who passively assents to admission and treatment can be admitted and treated without the Mental Health Act being used. If such a patient lacks capacity, the legal framework under which the patient is being treated is the Mental Capacity Act.

The administration of medicines to patients who lack the capacity to consent and who are unable to appreciate that they are taking medication (e.g. unconscious patients) should not need to be carried out covertly.

However, some patients who lack the capacity to consent would be aware, if they were not deceived into thinking otherwise.[8] For example a patient with moderate dementia who has no insight and does not believe he needs to take medication, but will take liquid medication if this is mixed with his tea without him being aware of this. It is this group to whom the rest of this guidance will apply.

Treatment may be given to people who lack capacity if it has been concluded that that treatment is in the patient's best interests (Section 5, MCA[5]) and proportionate to the harm to be avoided (Chapter 6.41, MCA Code of Practice.[8]) So, there should be a clear expectation that the patient will benefit from covert administration, and that this will avoid significant harm (either mental or physical) to the patient or others. The treatment must be necessary to save the patient's life, to prevent deterioration in health or to ensure an improvement in physical or mental health.[8]

The decision to administer medication covertly should not be made by a single individual but should involve discussion with the multidisciplinary team caring for the patient and the patient's relatives or informal carers. It is good practice to hold a 'best interests meeting'[9] (see below). Decisions should be carefully documented and each instance of covert administration recorded on the prescription chart.[10] The decision should be subject to regular review,[8] and the reviews also documented.

Summary of process

The process for covert administration of medicines should include the following safeguards.

- Assessment of capacity of the patient to make a decision regarding their treatment with medication. If the patient has capacity their wishes should be respected and covert medication not administered.
- A record of the examination of the patient's capacity must be made in the clinical notes, and evidence for incapacity documented.
- If the patient lacks capacity there should be a 'best interests meeting' which should be attended by relevant health professionals and a person who can communicate the views and interests of the patient (family member, friend or independent mental capacity advocate [IMCA]). If the patient has an attorney appointed under the Mental Capacity Act for health and welfare decisions, then this person should be present at the meeting.
- Those attending the meeting should ascertain whether the patient has made an Advanced Decision refusing a particular medication or treatment which can be used to guide decision-making.
- The 'best interests meeting' should consider whether a formal legal procedure such as the Mental Health Act or Deprivation of Liberty Safeguards (DoLs) is appropriate. Discussion of the indications and use of this legislation in the context of covert medication is outside the scope of this guidance, but specialist psychiatric and/or legal opinion should be sought in individual circumstances if necessary.
- Medication should not be administered covertly until a 'best interests meeting' has been held. If the situation is urgent it is acceptable for a less formal discussion to occur between carer/ nursing staff, prescriber and family/advocate in order to make an urgent decision, but a formal meeting should be arranged as soon as possible.
- After the meeting, there should be clear documentation of the outcome of the meeting. If the decision is to use covert administration of medication, a check should be made with the pharmacy to determine whether the properties of the medications are

likely to be affected by crushing and/or being mixed with food or drink. The prescription card should be amended to describe how the medication is to be administered.

- When the medication is administered in foodstuff, it is the responsibility of the dispensing nurse to ensure that the medication is taken. This can be facilitated by direct observation or by nominating another member of the clinical team to observe the patient taking the medication.
- A plan to review on a regular basis the need for continued covert administration of medicines should be made.

References

1. Nursing and Midwifery Council. *The Code: Standards of conduct, performance and ethics for nurses and midwives*. London: NMC; 2008. http://www.nmc-uk.org/Publications/Standards/The-code/Introduction/
2. Nursing and Midwifery Council. *Standards for medicines management*. London: NMC; 2007. http://www.nmc-uk.org/Documents/NMC-Publications/238747_NMC_Standards_for_medicines_management.pdf
3. Nursing and Midwifery Council. *Covert administration of medicines*. London: NMC; 2013. http://www.nmc-uk.org/Nurses-and-midwives/Regulation-in-practice/Medicines-management-and-prescribing/Covert-administration-of-medicines/
4. Royal College of Psychiatrists. College Statement on Covert Administration of Medicines. Psychiatr Bull 2004; 28:385–386.
5. Office of Public Sector Information. Mental Capacity Act 2005, Chapter 9. 2005. http://www.opsi.gov.uk/
6. The National Archives. Mental Health Act 2007. 2007. http://www.legislation.gov.uk/ukpga/2007/12/contents
7. British Medical Association et al. *Assessment of Mental Capacity*, 3rd edn. London: The Law Society; 2009.
8. Department for Constitutional Affairs. Mental Capacity Act 2005 - Code of Practice. 2005. http://www.justice.gov.uk/.
9. Joyce T. Best interests: guidance on determining the best interests of adults who lack the capacity to make a decision (or decisions) for themselves. England and Wales. A report published by the Professional Practice Board of the British Psychological Society. 2007. http://www.bps.org.uk/
10. Treloar A et al. Concealing medication in patients' food. Lancet 2001; 357:62–64.

Further reading

Haw C et al. Covert administration of medication to older adults: a review of the literature and published studies. J Psychiatr Ment Health Nurs 2010; 17:761–768.

Haw C et al. Administration of medicines in food and drink: a study of older inpatients with severe mental illness. Int Psychogeriatr 2010; 22:409–416.

For Scotland

Mental Welfare Commission for Scotland. Good Practice Guide: Covert administration. 2013. http://www.mwcscot.org.uk/media/140485/covert_medication_finalnov_13.pdf

Index

Note: page numbers in *italics* refer to figures; those in **bold** to tables or boxes.